ASSESSMENT OF DISORDERS IN CHILDHOOD AND ADOLESCENCE

Selected Works by the Editors

Assessment of Disorders in Childhood and Adolescence

FIFTH EDITION

Edited by
Eric A. Youngstrom
Mitchell J. Prinstein
Eric J. Mash
Russell A. Barkley

THE GUILFORD PRESS
New York   London

The authors have checked with sources believed to be reliable in their efforts to
provide information that is complete and generally in accord with the standards
of practice that are accepted at the time of publication. However, in view of the
possibility of human error or changes in behavioral, mental health, or medical
sciences, neither the authors, nor the editor and publisher, nor any other party
who has been involved in the preparation or publication of this work warrants
that the information contained herein is in every respect accurate or complete,
and they are not responsible for any errors or omissions or the results obtained
from the use of such information. Readers are encouraged to confirm the
information contained in this book with other sources.

Library of Congress Cataloging-in-Publication Data
Names: Youngstrom, Eric Arden, editor. | Prinstein, Mitchell J., 1970– editor. |
    Mash, Eric J., editor. | Barkley, Russell A., 1949– editor.
Title: Assessment of disorders in childhood and adolescence / edited by
    Eric A. Youngstrom, Mitchell J. Prinstein, Eric J. Mash, Russell A. Barkley.
Other titles: Treatment of disorders in childhood and adolescence.
Description: Fifth edition. | New York : The Guilford Press, [2020] |
Identifiers: LCCN 2019055651 | ISBN9781462543632 (hardcover)
Subjects: LCSH: Behavior disorders in children—Treatment. | Behavior
    therapy for children. | Affective disorders in children—Treatment. |
    Child psychopathology. | Child psychotherapy. | Behavioral assessment of
    children.
Classification: LCC RJ506.B44 T73 2020 | DDC 618.92/89—dc23
LC record available at *https://lccn.loc.gov/2019055651*

About the Editors

Eric A. Youngstrom, PhD, is Professor of Psychology and Neuroscience and Professor of Psychiatry at the University of North Carolina at Chapel Hill, where he is also Acting Director of the Center for Excellence in Research and Treatment of Bipolar Disorder. He was the inaugural recipient of the Early Career Award from the Society of Clinical Child and Adolescent Psychology of the American Psychological Association (APA), and is an elected full member of the American College of Neuropsychopharmacology. Dr. Youngstrom has consulted on DSM-5 and ICD-11. He is past president of the Society for Clinical Child and Adolescent Psychology and currently chairs the Work Group on Child Diagnosis for the International Society for Bipolar Disorders and serves as President (2020) of APA Division 5, Quantitative and Qualitative Methods.

Mitchell J. Prinstein, PhD, ABPP, is the John Van Seters Distinguished Professor of Psychology and Neuroscience at the University of North Carolina at Chapel Hill. His research examines interpersonal models of internalizing symptoms and health-risk behaviors among adolescents, with a focus on the unique role of peer relationships in the developmental psychopathology of depression, self-injury, and suicidality. An Associate Editor of the *Journal of Consulting and Clinical Psychology* and a member of the National Institutes of Health's Study Section on Psychosocial Development, Risk, and Prevention, Dr. Prinstein is a recipient of the Theodore Blau Early Career Award from the Society of Clinical Psychology of the APA, among other honors. He is a Fellow of the APA Society of Clinical Child and Adolescent Psychology.

Eric J. Mash, PhD, is Professor Emeritus of Psychology at the University of Calgary and Affiliate Professor in the Department of Psychiatry at Oregon Health and Science University. He is a Fellow of the Canadian Psychological Association and of the Society of Clinical Psychology, the Society for Child and Family Policy and Practice, the Society of Clinical Child and Adolescent Psychology, and the Society of Pediatric Psychology of the

APA. Dr. Mash is also a Fellow and Charter Member of the Association for Psychological Science. He has served as an editor, editorial board member, and editorial consultant for numerous journals and has published widely on child and adolescent psychopathology, assessment, and treatment.

Russell A. Barkley, PhD, ABPP, ABCN, is Clinical Professor of Psychiatry at the Virginia Commonwealth University School of Medicine. He has worked with children, adolescents, and families since the 1970s and is the author of numerous bestselling books for both professionals and the public, including *Taking Charge of ADHD* and *Your Defiant Child*. He has also published six assessment scales and more than 280 scientific articles and book chapters on ADHD, executive functioning, and childhood defiance, and is editor of the newsletter *The ADHD Report*. A frequent conference presenter and speaker who is widely cited in the national media, Dr. Barkley is past president of the Section on Clinical Child Psychology (the former Division 12) of the APA, and of the International Society for Research in Child and Adolescent Psychopathology. He is a recipient of awards from the American Academy of Pediatrics and the APA, among other honors.

Contributors

Jonathan S. Abramowitz, PhD, Department of Psychology and Neuroscience, University of North Carolina at Chapel Hill, Chapel Hill, North Carolina

Emma Adam, PhD, School of Education and Social Policy, Northwestern University, Evanston, Illinois

Anna M. Bardone-Cone, PhD, Department of Psychology and Neuroscience, University of North Carolina at Chapel Hill, Chapel Hill, North Carolina

Jennifer L. Buchholz, MA, Department of Psychology and Neuroscience, University of North Carolina at Chapel Hill, Chapel Hill, North Carolina

Jocelyn Smith Carter, PhD, Department of Psychology, DePaul University, Chicago, Illinois

Elizabeth Casline, MS, Department of Psychology, University of Miami, Coral Gables, Florida

Tammy A. Chung, PhD, Department of Psychiatry, Rutgers, The State University of New Jersey, New Brunswick, New Jersey

Joseph R. Cohen, PhD, Department of Psychology, University of Illinois at Urbana–Champaign, Champaign, Illinois

Margaret E. Crane, BA, Department of Psychology, Temple University, Philadelphia, Pennsylvania

BreAnne A. Danzi, PhD, Department of Psychology, University of South Dakota, Vermillion, South Dakota

Stefan C. Dombrowski, PhD, School Psychology Program, Rider University, Lawrenceville, New Jersey

Steven W. Evans, PhD, Center for Intervention Research in Schools, Ohio University, Athens, Ohio

Madison C. Feil, BS, Department of Psychology, University of Washington, Seattle, Washington

Nicole Fleischer, PsyD, Department of Psychology, Philadelphia College of Osteopathic Medicine, Philadelphia, Pennsylvania

Andrew J. Freeman, PhD, Department of Psychology, University of Nevada, Las Vegas, Las Vegas, Nevada

Paul J. Frick, PhD, Department of Psychology, Louisiana State University, Baton Rouge, Louisiana; Institute for Learning Science and Teacher Education, Australian Catholic University, Brisbane, Australia

Kathryn Grant, PhD, Department of Psychology, DePaul University, Chicago, Illinois

Max A. Halvorson, MA, Department of Psychology, University of Washington, Seattle, Washington

Benjamin L. Hankin, PhD, Department of Psychology, University of Illinois at Urbana–Champaign, Champaign, Illinois

Yo Jackson, PhD, ABPP, Department of Psychology, Penn State University, University Park, Pennsylvania

Amanda Jensen-Doss, PhD, Department of Psychology, University of Miami, Coral Gables, Florida

Randy W. Kamphaus, PhD, College of Education, University of Oregon, Eugene, Oregon

Julie B. Kaplow, PhD, ABPP, Trauma and Grief Center, Texas Children's Hospital/Baylor College of Medicine, Houston, Texas

Philip C. Kendall, PhD, ABPP, Department of Psychology, Temple University, Philadelphia, Pennsylvania

Kevin M. King, PhD, Department of Psychology, University of Washington, Seattle, Washington

Kevin S. Kuehn, MS, Department of Psychology, University of Washington, Seattle, Washington

Annette M. La Greca, PhD, ABPP, Department of Psychology, University of Miami, Coral Gables, Florida

Ilana E. Ladis, BA, Department of Psychology, Wesleyan University, Middletown, Connecticut; Department of Psychiatry, Massachusetts General Hospital, Boston, Massachusetts

Christopher M. Layne, PhD, National Center for Child Traumatic Stress and Department of Psychiatry and Biobehavioral Sciences, David Geffen School of Medicine, University of California, Los Angeles, Los Angeles, California

Catherine Lord, PhD, Department of Psychiatry and Biobehavioral Sciences, David Geffen School of Medicine, University of California, Los Angeles, Los Angeles, California

Samantha M. Margherio, MA, Department of Psychology, Ohio University, Athens, Ohio

Jon M. McClellan, MD, Division of Child and Adolescent Psychiatry, Department of Psychiatry and Behavioral Sciences, University of Washington, Seattle, Washington

Ryan J. McGill, PhD, Department of School Psychology and Counselor Education, William & Mary School of Education, College of William & Mary, Williamsburg, Virginia

Bryce D. McLeod, PhD, Department of Psychology, Virginia Commonwealth University, Richmond, Virginia

Robert J. McMahon, PhD, Department of Psychology, Simon Fraser University, Burnaby, British Columbia, Canada; Brain, Behaviour, & Development, BC Children's Hospital Research Institute, Vancouver, British Columbia, Canada

Lisa J. Meltzer, PhD, Department of Pediatrics, National Jewish Health, Denver, Colorado

Alexander J. Millner, PhD, Department of Psychology, Harvard University, Cambridge, Massachusetts

Helen M. Milojevich, PhD, Department of Psychology and Neuroscience, University of North Carolina at Chapel Hill, Chapel Hill, North Carolina

Emma E. Morton, PhD, Department of Psychiatry, Faculty of Medicine, University of British Columbia, Vancouver, British Columbia, Canada

Greg Murray, PhD, Centre for Mental Health, Swinburne University of Technology, Hawthorne, Victoria, Australia

Matthew K. Nock, PhD, Department of Psychology, Harvard University, Cambridge, Massachusetts

Julie Sarno Owens, PhD, Center for Intervention Research in Schools, Ohio University, Athens, Ohio

Zabin Patel, MPH, MS, Department of Psychology, University of Miami, Coral Gables, Florida

Mitchell J. Prinstein, PhD, Department of Psychology and Neuroscience, University of North Carolina at Chapel Hill, Chapel Hill, North Carolina

Katherine Seldin, BA, Department of Psychology, University of Washington, Seattle, Washington

Aditi Sharma, MD, Division of Child and Adolescent Psychiatry, Department of Psychiatry and Behavioral Sciences, University of Washington, Seattle, Washington

Elisabeth Sheridan, PhD, Department
of Psychiatry, Weill Cornell Medicine,
White Plains, New York

Michele R. Smith, EdM, Department of Psychology,
University of Washington, Seattle, Washington

Kara M. Styck, PhD, Department of Psychology,
Northern Illinois University, DeKalb, Illinois

Berta J. Summers, PhD, Department
of Psychiatry, Massachusetts General Hospital,
Boston, Massachusetts

Anna Van Meter, PhD, Institute
of Behavioral Science, The Feinstein Institutes
for Medical Research, Northwell Health,
Manhasset, New York; Donald and Barbara
Zucker School of Medicine at Hofstra/Northwell,
Hempstead, New York

Kristin M. von Ranson, PhD, Department
of Psychology, University of Calgary,
Calgary, Alberta, Canada

Emily Walden, MA, College of Education,
University of Oregon, Eugene, Oregon

Toni M. Walker, MS, Department of Psychology,
Louisiana State University, Baton Rouge, Louisiana

Frances L. Wang, PhD, Department of Psychiatry,
University of Pittsburgh, Pittsburgh, Pennsylvania

Hilary Weingarden, PhD, OCD and Related
Disorders Program, Massachusetts General Hospital,
Boston, Massachusetts; Department of Psychology,
Harvard University, Cambridge, Massachusetts

Sabine Wilhelm, PhD, OCD and Related
Disorders Program, Massachusetts General Hospital,
Boston, Massachusetts; Department of Psychology,
Harvard University, Cambridge, Massachusetts

Vicky Veitch Wolfe, PhD, IWK Health Centre,
Halifax, Nova Scotia, Canada

John Young, PhD, Department of Psychology,
University of Mississippi, University, Mississippi

Eric A. Youngstrom, PhD, Department
of Psychology, University of North Carolina
at Chapel Hill, Chapel Hill, North Carolina

Contents

VII. Problems of Adolescence and Emerging Adulthood

VIII. Health-Related Issues

Selected tools and resources discussed throughout the book
can be obtained online at the open-access Wikiversity page on
Evidence-Based Assessment, developed by Youngstrom, Prinstein,
Ong, and Helping Give Away Psychological Science (HGAPS.org):
https://en.wikiversity.org/wiki/Evidence-based_assessment.

PART I

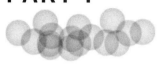

General Principles and Skills

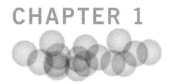

CHAPTER 1

Introduction to Evidence-Based Assessment
A Recipe for Success

Eric A. Youngstrom and Mitchell J. Prinstein

We all eat. Sometimes we do it thoughtlessly, stuffing whatever is fast and convenient into our mouths. Other times we do it more mindfully. For special events, we may make a particularly elaborate meal to celebrate or go to a restaurant that has a reputation for great food. Some people hire dietary coaches or trainers to help them achieve specific goals, and others take classes to learn how to cook better themselves.

Psychology as a discipline has a broad and flexible set of skills and job opportunities. We can offer therapy, conduct and interpret psychological assessments, do research, consult with other professionals, engage with policymakers, and fill many other roles that connect with a variety of different stakeholders. But psychological assessment is our special forte. Depending on state regulations, therapy can be done by social workers, nurses, counselors, psychiatrists (and in some countries, philosophers!). Any discipline with a doctorate does some form of research. "Psychological assessment"—that has our name baked into the title. We are the discipline that invented the methods, refined them, and honed the skills needed for advancing the science and also delivering the goods to consumers. We have classes, books, and journals devoted to the basics and the finer points of the topic, and we have supervision and training crafted to initiate you into the methods.

The term "cookbook" is often used in a pejorative way, insinuating that the skills are being reduced to a formulaic recipe that requires neither skill nor creativity, and that does not take thought (and may even turn off thinking). The implication is that cookbooks are beneath professionals. We would be surprised to go to a fancy restaurant with an open kitchen, and see the staff thumbing through a recipe book after we placed our order.

A good class teaches the principles, not just the recipes, though. Understanding the principles not only gives us the "why" behind the recipe's steps but it also empowers us to improvise, to make substitutions when we are missing an ingredient, and to innovate when we understand something unique about the needs or goals of the particular situation. No eggs? Using applesauce instead will work for making muffins. No parent available because the youth is incarcerated or in foster care? Interviewing the case manager or adding some performance measures might be a workaround.

In both cooking and assessment, the sequencing of steps matters. Planning the order makes it possible to get more done in the same amount of time, letting the professional work smarter, and not harder. We can chop vegetables while bringing the broth to a boil, start the marinade the night before—versus discovering at Step 5 that things are supposed to soak in the marinade for at least 3 hours, forcing us to order takeout or reschedule dinner. Similarly, we can organize and batch assessment methods, so that some can be done before the first session, others during the main intake or evaluation appointment, and still others rolled out in the feedback session or over the course of treatment. Having a plan for the sequence lets us gather more data (at least three courses instead of one), and it also adds the special ingredient of time, allowing us a better sense of how things are developing and changing. We can make adjustments to the recipe as we learn more about the person, individualizing the menu and meal of intervention.

The first four chapters of this book (including this one) go through the principles. They cover the "why" and the "how" of assessment methods. Their order follows the arc of the clinical encounter. They go from even before the first appointment is scheduled (preparation phase), to assessments that can be mailed ahead, done online, or completed in the waiting room (prediction phase), then to things done during the intake or evaluation session (prescription and case formulation phase), and finally to the feedback session or through the course of therapy to successful termination and monitoring (process, progress, and outcome phase). These chapters walk through the principles, using a case (Ty Lee) to show how these would work in practice with a person. Note, all of the case material included in this book is fictional/composite or thoroughly disguised.

The rest of the book goes in depth on particular problems or issues you are likely to encounter when working with clients. There are some key features. The topics focus on the "vital few": Whereas the fifth edition of the *Diagnostic and Statistical Manual of Mental Disorders* (DSM-5; American Psychiatric Association, 2013) has more diagnoses than there are days of the year, we focus on the most frequent referral issues. If you have the tools and principles to work with externalizing, anxiety, mood, attention problems, and trauma, then you have what you need to make good headway with four out of five clients at most clinics (Rettew, Lynch, Achenbach, Dumenci, & Ivanova, 2009; Youngstrom & Van Meter, 2016). Add some crosscutting issues, such as sleep problems and cognitive functioning, and we have an excellent foundation. Having the basics covered frees us to use our supervision and "research and development" time to learn how to address the exceptions and build expertise in specialized areas.

Another feature of the later chapters is that they are modular and self-sufficient, yet they have a shared layout. They typically start with the clinical picture and any relevant diagnostic criteria, then proceed through checklists and scales to interview strategies and progress and outcome tracking. The structure makes it easy to find what we need, in the order that we are likely to use it. Most use case examples. Content chapters use new cases to keep the person-centered focus, while adding more variations that show how things change in the real world. Algorithms can break. The better chef knows when and how to change the recipe—the principles are the power to improvise and create, achieving the goals despite the constraints, challenges, and needs of a particular individual.

The chapters also recommend a "starter kit" of checklists, rating scales, interviews, and progress measures. The kits make a point of including the best of the free available options. Often there are free measures with strong psychometrics and a good or excellent research base. "Free" eliminates a cost barrier, but it has the unintended consequence of making them harder to find. There is no advertising budget, and commercial publishers are not including them in their websites or glossy catalogs. Having the content experts identify them for us is a big step toward better dissemination. We have gathered copies of the measures and put them online at a free website where you can get them and more details about the supporting evidence and how to score and use them. This is a second big step towards implementation support. Think of it as a shared pantry that is already stocked with many of the best free ingredients, organized in a way that follows the principles and organization of the book. Even better than a physical pantry, the ingredients never run out—clicking a link or downloading a PDF does not "use up" the resource. The pantry is built in a way that makes it easy to update, so as new resources and updated versions become available, we all have one place to go and find the newest tools and evidence. This will be much faster than waiting for the next edition of the book to come out!

Preparation: Organizing the Assessment Materials to Address Common Issues

This first chapter covers the preparation phase. These are things that can be done before the client even schedules an appointment. When you move to a new apartment, you know that you are going to need to eat, and you have a sense of the basics that you want to stock to get through the week. With a clinic, the same principles apply: Knowing what the common needs are lets us stock the testing cabinet effectively. The professors and teaching fellows running the class have already made sure that there are enough copies of the assessment booklets on hand and ordered anything that was low. Practicing clinicians can scan their caseload and referral pattern, and compare it with materials in their cabinet. Any gaps help add to the shopping list the next time they order out for supplies.

Diagnostic Criteria/Presenting Features

A Pragmatic View of Diagnosis

Mental health diagnoses are strange things. They look different when viewed through the eyes of a scientist, a clinician, a client, and the general public. They serve multiple functions, too. In a philosophical sense, they may or may not be "real," and many of the ones that we work with in this book are unlikely to be clear categories with well-defined edges (Haslam, Holland, & Kuppens, 2012). For those of us interested in philosophy of science or in research, these phenomenological and epistemological questions can be not only fascinating but also rich enough to sustain a research program in its own right. For the rest of us, diagnoses play important practical roles even if they are fuzzy constructs. We use them as a shorthand to query the research literature, to organize our resources, to match a recipe for assessment and treatment with a particular individual. Another currently inescapable value of diagnosis is that it unlocks reimbursement for our services in many parts of the health care system. We need a diagnosis to bill Medicaid or insurance companies.

For the diagnosis to have any chance of being valid, we need to use consistent definitions. If the same label means different things to different people, then one person's experience and research on "depression" will not transfer to another clinician who has something different in mind. When we borrow each other's recipes for clinical work, we will not get the same results because we are not working on the same issue.

The chapter authors are amazing researchers and have written chapters designed to be clinically practical. We do not spend a lot of ink on the scientific validity of the diagnoses (that is coming in the third book in the series!). Instead, we concentrate on practical aspects of diagnosis. When a research study says that it used DSM-5 definitions of depression based on a semistructured diagnostic interview, that shorthand tells us that everyone in the study had a change in mood and energy that affected at least five symptoms out of a list of nine (and they asked about all nine), and it was a clear change in functioning that lasted at least 2 weeks, caused impairment in at least one important aspect of their lives, and was not due to a general medical condition. Like the term "a meatball," "DSM depression" compresses a lot of information into shorthand. A formal diagnosis provides a consistent list of symptom ingredients and steps for assembling the diagnosis, much like a standardized list for making a meatball. Is the "standard meatball" the only scientifically valid definition? When does something change from meatball to a mini-hamburger, köfte, or sausage? These are great research topics, and also things that a good clinical chef could think about as they apply to an individual case. As we are learning to cook, having a standard recipe lets us transfer the knowledge from books and articles into our work, helps us match the client's needs and goals with our plan, and makes it easier to get paid for our services.

Classification Systems

There are two major official classification systems in the world of mental health. The *Diagnostic and Statistical Manual of Mental Disorders* of the American Psychiatric Association has been the most commonly used system in the United States, and it has guided most U.S. research until recently. It is the system used in most textbooks about psychopathology. DSM-5 was published in 2013, whereas the previous edition of this handbook was published in 2007. Thus, the official recipes for diagnoses changed roughly halfway in between editions of the assessment handbook. Given how long it takes to do research and get it published, most of the studies cited in the chapters will still have used the older (DSM-IV) definitions, but you are probably using the newer definitions in your classes and billing. The chapter authors do a good job of alerting us to changes in the recipe. For many conditions (depression, oppositional defiant disorder) there were few or only small tweaks. For others (autism, posttraumatic stress disorder), the changes are much more substantial (for synopses, see Sheridan & Lord, Chapter 12, and La Greca & Danzi, Chapter 15, this volume).

The World Health Organization (WHO) organizes the *International Classification of Diseases* (ICD), which just released its 11th edition. There are several key differences versus the DSM. The ICD is managed by an international organization, not a U.S. one, and it covers all areas of medicine, not just psychiatry. It is also freely available (*https://icd.who.int/browse11/l-m/en*, and then expand section 06 to see the list of "Mental, behavioural or neurodevelopmental disorders"), whereas the DSM costs a sizable amount per copy. The ICD is translated into multiple languages, too. It is less well known in the United States. A little-known fact is that all of our insurance billing codes are mapped to ICD diagnoses—every country that is a member of the United Nations is treaty-bound to report mental health statistics to the WHO using ICD definitions. Anyone who is a fan of open-source things, and people who want to promote international cooperation, cultural representation, and sharing, will be fans of the ICD.

Until ICD-11, the mental health part of ICD used to follow the DSM closely. With ICD-11, there are some significant departures from DSM-5. For those of us working with kids, a big difference is how to conceptualize kids who get extremely moody and aggressive, yet do not meet criteria for bipolar disorder (see Deshawn on Wikiversity for a case example). DSM-5 added a new diagnosis of disruptive mood dysregulation disorder (DMDD) and put it in the depression chapter, to signal that it was not something bipolar, and not ordinary oppositional defiant disorder (ODD). In contrast, the ICD reviewed two sets of literature—everything it could find about the relevant diagnoses, and also the developmental psychopathology work about longitudinal trajectories of externalizing problems (Evans et al., 2017), and decided

(1) not to include the new DMDD diagnosis; (2) to conceptualize cases fitting this clinical picture as having externalizing problems, not depression; and (3) to add a specifier to ODD, so that the clinician can tag the case to alert that there are significant mood issues that should also be a part of the treatment plan.

The distinction matters. Confronted with a case (see Deshawn on Wikiversity), we have to decide whether to evaluate for depression or externalizing problems, or both. In the context of this book, we want a plan that uses what we know about the person to decide whether to go more in depth around depression (see Hankin & Cohen, Chapter 7, this volume), bipolar disorder (Youngstrom, Morton, & Murray, Chapter 8, this volume), or conduct problems (Walker, Frick, & McMahon, Chapter 6, this volume), while also not missing important comorbidities or other contributing factors. The difference in conceptualization matters at least as much in terms of treatment plans, too. Using a broadband measure, such as the Achenbach System of Empirically Based Assessment (ASEBA), the Behavior Assessment System for Children (BASC), or the Child and Adolescent Symptom Inventory (CASI), or a starter kit designed for broad coverage (see Table 1.2 for some sample menus and Wikiversity for free options for each) will help to gather a lot of information quickly to compare different hypotheses.

There are other classification systems, too, that we do not discuss in as much depth in this book. The Research Domain Criteria (RDoC) approach is a major re-visioning of basic research, moving away from diagnosis to focus on basic dimensions of functioning (Cuthbert & Insel, 2010, 2013). The RDoC system has led to changes in grant proposals and active studies, but it will be several more years before there are clear clinical applications. RDoC is analogous to a research and development investment in fundamental changes to food processing and preparation—it will take time to find its way to the table, but it has the potential for big improvements when it arrives.

At the other extreme is the educational classification system, which guides placement for special education, giftedness, and other educational resources and tracking. We need to be aware of the system and have a sense of how it works in order to help youth get services they need. Surprisingly, schools do not use DSM or ICD criteria directly. Diagnoses are not exactly irrelevant, either. Instead, diagnoses are one factor in a multifactored educational evaluation, and they are helpful inasmuch as they are linked to behaviors and emotional disturbance that make it difficult for the youth to learn. The chapters on intellectual disability (Kamphaus & Walden, Chapter 13, this volume) and learning disability (McGill, Styck, & Dombrowski, Chapter 14, this volume) go into detail about the evaluation aspects, and companion chapters in the treatment book (Matson et al., 2019; McGill & Ndip, 2019) provide more context and ideas for resources and recommendations. Other chapters provide specific methods for getting teacher perspectives, perhaps using formal rating scales, daily report cards, or other methods to be able to assess functioning and progress (see, e.g., Owens, Evans, & Margherio, Chapter 5, this volume).

Clinical Presentation

Experienced clinicians and chefs, like any expert performer, use sophisticated pattern recognition to evaluate what is going on. Experts focus on a different set of details rather than the general background knowledge, and chunk facts and information together (Epstein, 2019). Newer clinicians or cooks need to have more of the general background information, as well as a prototype to give a mental picture of how all of the facts might fit together (Straus, Glasziou, Richardson, & Haynes, 2011). The clinical snapshot in many abnormal psychology texts describes the "classic" presentation, providing a clear illustration of the concept. Much like the retouched professional pictures in recipe books and cooking shows, these are best-case scenarios of clarity that we might occasionally see in our own work. It is still worth having the picture in mind but better to also remember that the reality is usually more complicated. Mental health challenges usually have many facets and contributing factors. Every family is different, though they often struggle with some archetypal issues. The teaching cases that we use, particularly the online ones, all have a realistic degree of complexity and "plot twists" as the assessment process unfolds.

Prevalence and Clinical Benchmarks

Some clinical issues are common, others are less so, and most of the ones listed in the ICD or DSM are rare. What we see depends on where we are working. There may be regional differences. Suicide rates vary across countries (much higher in Korea and Japan than the global average), within

countries (higher in the Mountain Time Zone than the rest of the United States), and even within states (higher in western North Carolina than in the rest of the state). What families seek services for, and how they describe the problem, also may vary by region.

Epidemiological studies help give us a scouting report of how common different issues are. This is a valuable starting point: It helps identify the most common problems and public health priorities. Anyone working with young children should be prepared to evaluate potential anxiety disorders (Fleischer, Crane, & Kendall, Chapter 10, this volume) and attention-deficit/hyperactivity disorder (ADHD), which likely affect between 8 and 20% of the general population of children and teens (Table 1.1).

Other problems come and go with age. Separation anxiety tends to decrease, whereas depression, bipolar disorder, conduct problems, eating disorders, and psychosis all increase in adolescence. Knowing the age group with which we are working lets us stock the ingredients to be able to work with the most common problems. The principle is the law of the "Vital Few": There is a subset of clinical issues that will apply to the bulk of our cases. Pareto was the economist who popularized the "80:20 Rule": 80% of the cases will be linked with 20% of the diagnoses or issues. Getting prepared for the vital few ahead of time lets us set a menu of assessments that cover the needs of most of our cases (Youngstrom & Van Meter, 2016). This makes our work more efficient, and it frees us to use our precious discretionary time to explore the exceptions and to individualize our evaluations. Rather than making every pasta sauce from scratch, we are stocking a good basic sauce, then seasoning and garnishing for the client.

Clinical Benchmarks

Most epidemiological studies focus on the general population, which means that the rates include people who are not seeking treatment. Sometimes this is because the problems are mild (Berkson, 1946), leading to debate about whether epidemiological studies are identifying "true" cases (Bird et al., 1990). More often, it is because there are barriers to getting services: There are not enough psychologists or psychiatrists in most parts of the world to meet the mental health needs of the population. There also is a lot of stigma related to mental health, which makes people reluctant to admit that they have a problem and shy or

TABLE 1.1. Prevalence Benchmarks for Clinical Issues Discussed in This Volume

Condition	Chapter	CDC	Outpatient (Rettew et al., 2009)		General population[c]
			DAU	SDI	
ADHD	5	11% or 6.8%[a]	23%		
Conduct problems	6	3.5%[a]	17% CD, 37% ODD	25% CD, 38% ODD	1.5–3.2% antisocial[b]
Mood disorders			17% MDD, 10% dysthymia	26% MDD, 8% dysthymia	
Depression	7	2.1%[a]	—	—	
Bipolar	8	—	—	—	2.9%[NCS-A], 1% bipolar I, 2–4% spectrum (Chapter 8, this volume)
Self-injurious thought and behavior					
Nonsuicidal self-injury	9				
Ideation					
Attempt					
Anxiety		3.0%[a]			
Child and adolescent	10		8%	18%	
Specific and social phobia		—	6% (social)	20% (social)	9% social and 19% specific[NCS-A]
Panic and agoraphobia		—	12% (panic)	11% (panic)	2.4% agoraphobia, 2.3% panic[NCS-A]
Generalized anxiety disorder		—	5%	10%	2.2%[NCS-A]
Obsessive–compulsive disorder	11	—	9%	12%	1–2%
Posttraumatic stress disorder	15	—	3%	9%	5%[NCS-A], 3.6%[NCS18-54]
Substance use disorders	19	4.7%[a]	14%	17%	
Alcohol use disorder		4.2%[a]	10%	13%	
Schizophrenia	20	—	—	—	0.014% child
Personality disorders		—	—	—	
Cluster A					3–6% life[b]
Cluster B (antisocial separate)					1–5% life[b]
Cluster C					2–4% life[b]
Couple distress		—	—	—	~50% divorce rate
Eating disorders	21	—	—	—	
Sleep–wake disorders	23	—	—	—	

Note. Adapted from Youngstrom and Van Meter (2016); *https://en.wikiversity.org/wiki/Evidence-based_assessment*; CC-BY-SA 4.0. CDC, Centers for Disease Control and Prevention; DAU, diagnosis as usual; SDI, standardized diagnostic interview; CD, conduct disorder; ODD, oppositional defiant disorder; MDD, major depressive disorder; NCS-A, National Comorbidity Survey—Adolescent Supplement; NCS18-54 is the age 18–54 cohort of the National Comorbidity Survey.
[a]Perou et al. (2013).
[b]Roth and Fonagy (2005).
[c]Epidemiological rates refer to general population, not treatment-seeking samples, and so often represent a lower bound of what might be expected at a clinic.

ashamed about seeking services (Corrigan, Druss, & Perlick, 2014; Hinshaw & Cicchetti, 2000). Language and cultural differences can create further barriers to access. All of these factors mean that what the epidemiologist reports will not look like the mix of issues we see at our clinic.

What would be more helpful in our own work would be to know the common issues and needs at our own clinic. If we have an electronic medical record, or if we have sufficient time and motivation, we could do a chart review and come up with a summary ourselves. It is a fair amount of work: It would be like a restaurant combing through a year's worth of receipts and trying to find the patterns to tune the offerings on the menu. To give a sense of ballpark figures, the content chapters include benchmarks from different clinical settings. These show how the chances of working with different disorders or problems change across levels of care. Bipolar or suicidal behaviors are rare in the general population, for example, but become a larger slice of referrals in outpatient settings, and an even bigger portion in partial hospital, forensic, or residential treatment; and they are among the most common problems in inpatient and emergency room settings (e.g., Blader & Carlson, 2007). Over the course of my training and licensure, one of us (E. A. Youngstrom) has worked in each of those settings (during internship, across six different settings in 1 year), and the amount of bipolar disorder changed with each rotation.

The content chapters give a sense of how the prevalence benchmarks change across levels of care. Table 1.1 organizes the information a different way. Rather than going deep across many settings for one disorder, Table 1.1 casts wide across many disorders for just two settings: the general population and outpatient clinics. Outpatient clinics are the best approximation of the setting in which students usually see their first clients, and where the bulk of private practitioners continue to work. The Centers for Disease Control and Prevention (CDC) tracks rates of some diagnoses (but there are surprising omissions—e.g., it does not report figures for conduct disorder), and the Substance Abuse and Mental Health Services Administration (SAMHSA) publishes rates from a subset of states (but the diagnoses include throwbacks from DSM-III). Perhaps more helpfully, Rettew and colleagues (2009) performed a meta-analysis examining diagnostic agreement between clinical diagnoses as usual (an unstructured interview) versus diagnoses using a more structured interview with the same people. The meta-analysis gives an extremely helpful snapshot of the mix at clinics.

We can use these numbers to make a good list of the most common referrals we see. Based on the meta-analysis, our "vital few" should include ADHD, conduct problems, anxiety, depression, substance misuse, obsessive–compulsive disorder, and trauma and posttraumatic stress disorder (PTSD). This list maps to eight chapters in the book. We could round out the menu by adding some things that are rare but clinically crucial (Morrison, 2014), such as self-harm. We also can think beyond traditional diagnoses and apply developmental science to consider issues related to sleep, which changes markedly from childhood to adolescence and adulthood and plays a major role in starting or worsening a lot of cognitive and emotional problems when sleep is disrupted (Meltzer, Chapter 23, this volume). If we work with a narrower age group, or if we have a specialty clinic, then we can probably tweak the menu even further. Working with mostly adolescents, for example, we would expect to see more eating disorders (Bardone-Cone & von Ranson, Chapter 21, this volume), body dysmorphia (Summers, Ladis, Weingarden, & Wilhelm, Chapter 22, this volume), mood disorders (Hankin & Cohen, Chapter 7, this volume), psychosis (Sharma & McClellan, Chapter 20, this volume), or obsessive–compulsive disorder (Abramowitz & Buchholz, Chapter 11, this volume).

It is reassuring when the numbers from the meta-analysis or the CDC align with what we see at our clinic. When we see differences, this should make us stop and think—is there something unusual about our referral pattern? Or is there an opportunity to tune our practice to better meet the needs of our clients? There can be gaps in our training or tradition—many training curricula historically have not had much information about assessing substance problems, for example. There also can be changes in what are common problems. The rate of nonsuicidal self-injury has jumped from rare to common in the space of a few decades (Millner & Nock, Chapter 9, this volume), and there are shifts in rates of depression (Twenge et al., 2010; Twenge & Nolen-Hoeksema, 2002). Social media and screen time may be contributing to rapid changes in anxiety and risk-taking behavior (Nesi, Miller, & Prinstein, 2017; Nesi & Prinstein, 2019) as well as sleep problems (Burkhart & Phelps, 2009; Meltzer, Chapter 23, this volume). All of these can be opportunities to customize our assessment toolkit to better match the needs of the people seeking our help.

Prediction: Gathering Data to Guide the Evaluation

There are two different common scenarios for clinical assessment. One is the "psychological evaluation," in which the assessment itself is the main goal of the referral. Evaluations for educational placement—giftedness, special education, learning disability, early enrollment in kindergarten—are frequent examples. Neuropsychological evaluations after an injury or illness would be another, as would diagnostic workups at medical centers or forensic evaluations. Each of these would involve a written report, including the assessment results, interpretation, and recommendations about what to do next. A second scenario occurs when we are seeing the client for therapy ourselves. In this case, there usually is no written report about the assessment, and we work from our session notes and treatment plan. The differences are as pronounced as those between a multipage, detailed review of a restaurant versus grabbing lunch at one of our regular haunts, sometimes ordering on autopilot. We believe that with a little bit of planning, it is possible to improve the impact our work in either scenario. One of the strategies is to gather information before the first session. Questionnaires, rating scales, and checklists about risk factors are things that we can send ahead of time or have clients fill out in the waiting room before we meet. If they do these electronically, we can have all of the information scored and in front of us as we meet.

We offer some assessment starter menus, which are samples of what a "core battery" might look like (see Table 1.2). These could be sets of scales and questions that get done ahead of the first session, either sent ahead of time or filled out in the waiting room. There are several options that cover a range of topics by design, often referred to as "broadband" measures because of the broad range of content. The ASEBA (Achenbach & Rescorla, 2001) and the BASC (Reynolds & Kamphaus, 2015) are two of the most widely used examples. The CASI (Gadow & Sprafkin, 1994, 1997) is an alternative system that hews closely to DSM symptoms and definitions. These contenders have moderate to huge amounts of research with them, and each has versions that may be completed by parents, teachers, and the youth themselves (age and reading ability permitting). The ASEBA and the BASC also have normative data that are fantastic for helping get a sense of what is typical behavior for boys and girls at different ages. Note that the CASI does not have the same kind of detailed norms, instead concentrating on mapping to diagnoses.

These all also cost money. The cost is low considering the amount of information that is gathered, and one of the most expensive ingredients in building the instrument is developing an accurate set of norms. Still, the cost creates a barrier to use in many settings (Jensen-Doss & Hawley, 2010, 2011). There also are gaps in coverage due to changes in the science and shifts in the issues that families need assessed. The original items for the ASEBA were written in the late 1970s and published in the early 1980s, for example. These predate DSM-III. When the items were written, there was little research on autism and even less on bipolar disorder in youth, and both were considered too rare to be worth including in a broad measure. Eating disorders, nonsuicidal self-injury (NSSI), and Internet addiction also were not included. The first version of the ASEBA is older than the Internet, and much older than the iPhone! See Figure 1.1 for a timeline with changes in assessment and in technology more broadly.

TABLE 1.2. Examples of Starter Menus for Topics to get Initial Information about "Vital Few" Topics

Parent about youth	Youth about self	Adult about self
ADHD	(ADHD)[a]	ADHD
Depression	Depression	Depression
Anxiety	Anxiety	Anxiety
Abuse/PTSD	Abuse/PTSD	Abuse/PTSD
Bipolar disorder	Bipolar disorder	Bipolar disorder
Substance use	Substance use	Substance use
ODD and CD	ODD and CD	

[a]Many experts do not recommend self-report as a way of evaluating ADHD. See Owens et al. (Chapter 5, this volume) for details.

1999 — SurveyMonkey founded

— Youth Outcome Questionnaire developed

2000 — Outcome Questionnaire published

2001 — Current norms for the ASEBA ages 6–18 years

2002 — ChronoRecord Web-based life charting introduced

STARD Guidelines published — 2003 — Wechsler Intelligence Scale for Children, Fourth Edition
(Bossuyt et al., 2003)   (WISC-IV) published

Lambert (2003) Meta-analysis —

2004 — PROMIS launched

EBA Special Issues: 2005

Psychological Assessment —

Journal of Clinical Child —
and Adolescent Psychology

2006

Annual Review of Clinical Psychology EBA — **2007** — iPhone released June 29; Fitbit founded
(1.0) published (Hunsley & Mash, 2007)

Assessment of Childhood Disorders (ACD) —

Guide to Assessment That Works (GATW) — 2008 — Wechsler Adult Intelligence Scales–IV published
(Hunsley & Mash, 2008)

STROBE Guidelines (von Elm et al., 2008) —

2009 — REDCap general release

2010

HONEES Guidelines — 2011 — IBM Watson beat human champion at Jeopardy
(Youngstrom et al., 2011)

Rebooting Psychotherapy —   — MATRICS neurocognitive consensus battery
(Kazdin & Blase, 2011)   commercialized

— Fitbit sells 0.2 million units

2012 — PROMIS rollout of paper and CAT versions for
pediatrics, primary care

— Fitbit sells 1.3 million units

— 8.7 billion devices connected to the Internet of Things

Future Directions in Assessment — 2013 — SurveyMonkey reaches 15 million users
(Youngstrom, 2013)

— IBM Watson applied to decision support in health care

— IDC: Internet of Things global market of $1.3 trillion

Ready to ROC Primer (Youngstrom, 2014) — 2014 — WISC-V published with tablet administration, online
scoring

— Woodcock–Johnson-IV published with only online
scoring (no manual)

— Fitbit sells 10.9 million units

(continued)

FIGURE 1.1. Timeline of major reviews of evidence-based assessment and parallel developments in psychological assessment and related technological changes. Copyright © 2019 E. Youngstrom: CC-BY 4.0.

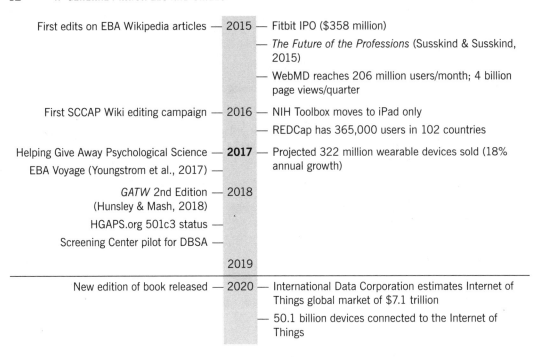

FIGURE 1.1. *(continued)*

Thus, our starter menus supplement the broad measures with some newer, focused scales to round out the offerings and try to avoid missing any of the vital few. As you change where you work, or learn more about your practice, you can adapt the menu to fit your needs. If you are working in a setting where costs are a major concern, then we also have sample menus that are built around the best of the free options. Here "best" means that they are supported by published data showing good reliability and validity in samples that are likely to look similar to what clinicians would see at an outpatient clinic (Beidas et al., 2015). None of these are official endorsements, saying "use this and nothing else." They are ideas to get you started, and they are examples of "good-enough" options rather than anointing any of them as best in class.

Screening Tools and Diagnostic Aids

When we have the client or family fill out scales and forms, we should look at them. This sounds obvious, but in many settings, we slip into a habit of filling out paperwork for its own sake, and not thinking about it as information. Clients do not mind filling out forms if they help improve their care (Suppiger et al., 2009), but they hate doing useless paperwork at least as much as we do.

At a minimum, we should scan the results to make sure that they are complete and to see what the major themes are. Some, such as the ASEBA, have write-in boxes where the person can give an example. We are supposed to read these and use clinical judgment to decide whether they are clinically concerning, discuss with the client as needed, then rescore the item as necessary. Busy practitioners and research assistants often forget (Drotar, Stein, & Perrin, 1995).

Some scales also include items asking about sensitive content, such as suicidal ideation or substance use. These are topics about which people are often more likely to volunteer information when asked on paper or by a computer rather than an unfamiliar person (Lucas, Gratch, King, & Morency, 2014; Shaffer, Fisher, Lucas, Dulcan, & Schwab-Stone, 2000). Reviewing the scales with clients helps show them that they are connected to the evaluation, and it provides a great basis for conversations that solicit their input and perspectives.

A more powerful way of using the information is as a scouting report or a tasting menu to guide where to focus attention during the interview. The simple strategy is to see which scores are elevated. A more advanced approach is to think in terms of probability, much as we are used to doing with weather forecasts, elections, and sporting events now (Silver, 2015). We can actually estimate the client's probability of different issues by taking the starting probability—our clinic's base rate of the problem—then personalizing the probability on the basis of the assessment results (Straus et al., 2011). The idea has been around for a few centuries (Bayes & Price, 1763), and both Meehl (1954) and evidence-based medicine have been advocating it for a couple decades (Jaeschke, Guyatt, & Sackett, 1994). The technique is taking off now with Web and smartphone apps, and IBM Watson putting it on tablets and other devices (cf. Epstein, 2019). The chapter on prediction (Van Meter, Chapter 2, this volume) walks us through the process in detail. The content chapters and Wikiversity pages gather the effect size that we would use to apply the result to the individual client, a "diagnostic likelihood ratio" (DLR), so that they are easy to find. Van Meter also talks about the older concepts of sensitivity, specificity, and predictive powers; but you may decide to skip using those older methods when you get the hang of thinking in terms of probability.

The probability estimates are not intended to replace case formulation, but rather to serve up a lot of information quickly. They are the microwave oven of assessment—not preparing a gourmet meal, but using technology to speed up parts of the process. Like a microwave oven, they also provide much more consistency in the processing than working freestyle over different burners would do. Clinicians using these probability methods with the same inputs are much more likely to agree about next steps than when they eyeball the same facts and use their intuition and experience to decide what to do next (Jenkins, Youngstrom, Washburn, & Youngstrom, 2011; Jenkins, Youngstrom, Youngstrom, Feeny, & Findling, 2012).

Cross-Informant Assessment

One of the biggest differences about working with youth versus adults is that the evaluation almost always involves at least one adult as well. We get information from one or more parents or teachers, as well as working directly with the youth. It often will be the grown-up who sought services, made the appointment, and brought the youth. We want to consider both the adult and the youth perspective in developmentally appropriate ways,

similar to how a restaurant would have different things on a kids' section of the menu. Youth age and cognitive development change the sources of information available for the assessment process, and also perhaps the weight that we assign to different perspectives. Younger children cannot read, so they are not able to fill out self-report questionnaires, and older youth may still have difficulty with complicated reading. At the same time, we also need to consider what the adult wants out of the evaluation. In addition to the information value, at a pragmatic level, it is usually the adult who is paying the bill and deciding whether the family will come back—yet another way that the restaurant analogy holds. If the person paying the check does not like the service, the family probably is not coming back.

With adolescents, the parent report still remains valuable, but the self-report becomes more viable and informative. We want to think through the processes that might underlie apparent disagreements. Teens may have low insight into how their behavior is seen by others (egocentrism is part of typical adolescent development). If the teen did not schedule the appointment, he or she is likely to be less motivated to be at the clinic, and that also can lead to underreporting symptoms, because he or she does not want to be there. Conversely, parents' stress levels can lead to overreporting, although not so much that we should ignore their views (Youngstrom, Ackerman, & Izard, 1999).

One of the most shocking things when we start doing assessment is how low the agreement between different people is when we are asking about the same youth. The correlation between parent, teacher, and youth reports is statistically significant, but it hovers in the small to medium range of correlation ($r \sim .28$ in two huge meta-analyses; Achenbach, McConaughy, & Howell, 1987; De Los Reyes et al., 2015). In the research context, the correlations are statistically significant, and each informant is contributing different reliable information about varying situations and facets of behavior. But when we are trying to figure out what is going on with one client or one family, it feels more like a detective story than a scientific study. Do not panic when one person's responses are clinically worrying (usually the person who made the appointment) and the other perspectives all seem more typical. If two or three people agree about a problem, it is usually more serious (Carlson & Youngstrom, 2003; Youngstrom, Findling, & Calabrese, 2003); when only one is clearly worried, then it takes some sleuthing to decide what is the best formulation, and some creative cooking to have something that each person likes in in the feedback to get them to come back for future sessions. Both the chapters on prediction (Van Meter, Chapter 2, this volume) and prescription and case formulation (Jensen-Doss, Casline, Patel, & McLeod, Chapter 3, this volume) present ideas about how to make sense of the different informant perspectives—the prediction phase generates hypotheses that we will be able to quickly test and revise during the interview.

Norms and Standardization

Norms help us compare our client's situation to what is typical (Achenbach, 2001). They are built with a defined reference group, such as "youth ages 6–18 years, living in the United States." Similar to doing a political poll, the goal is to include a representative mix of people that matches the population of interest. To be useful, the sample needs to be large. Size makes it likely that the results fall close to the "true" values. Very large samples also make it possible to see whether results differ by age, sex, or other features. For tests of cognitive ability, age is the variable of primary importance—older youth tend to know more facts, have bigger working memory capacity, and faster processing speed. The improvements with age can be so rapid that most measures of cognitive ability stratify their samples in 3-month segments. When we give a case a Weschler, we are comparing the client's score to a group of more than 200 youth within a 3-month age window (Wechsler, 2014).

Emotional and behavior problems also change with age. Younger children tend to be more active and have more difficulty staying focused, whereas adolescents are more likely to have moodiness and some depressive symptoms. These changes are much slower than the cognitive changes, though. Most measures of mood and behavior problems split the standardization sample into bands defined by 5 or more years (e.g., Achenbach & Rescorla, 2001; Reynolds & Kamphaus, 2015) instead of the 3-month chunks with cognitive measures. Another difference is that many have separate norms for males and females. Whereas sex differences in cognitive performance tend to be small, differences in behavior may be more substantial. Norms help to tease apart what is typical for young boys or adolescent women, and provide a statistical definition of what is abnormal.

With norms, the standard deviation is also a powerful piece of information, conveying how much youth tend to differ from each other on that feature. Combining the mean and the standard deviation lets us construct percentiles and standard scores. Percentiles seem easy to understand, but they have quirks that can make them misleading (see Sattler, 2002). We tend to rely on standardized scores instead. Three common ways of scaling them are standard scores with $M = 100$, $SD = 15$—used for most composite scores on ability and achievement tests, T scores with $M = 50$, $SD = 10$—typical of most behavior scales such as the ASEBA and the BASC, and also used with several personality measures, and z scores with $M = 0$ and $SD = 1$, used in most statistics classes. When we do a comprehensive evaluation, different tests often use different scales, similar to putting together a banquet in which some of the recipes are in metric grams and liters, and others are in imperial tablespoons and ounces. Using the z-score lets us convert the units. An IQ of 130 is two standard deviations above average, so $z = 2.0$, which would be a value of 70 in T-score units. Any of those would indicate that the person scored in the 97.5% percentile compared to his or her normative group. Whenever we use norms, we should ask ourselves whether our client looks similar to the standardization sample on the variables that are important for the construct. If there are differences, the follow-up question is whether the difference is likely to affect the scores. Many variations may not matter, but we do not want to miss ones that make the normative comparison inappropriate.

Risk and Protective Factors and Moderators

Another set of ingredients that is great to gather before the main interview includes risk and protective factors, as well as things that might alter the types of treatment we might recommend. *Risk factors* include things that are bad in their own right, as well as things that increase the risk of other diagnoses or bad outcomes. Three things we want to ask about routinely are threats to self (suicidal ideation and behavior; Millner & Nock, Chapter 9, this volume), threats to others (homicidal ideation or plans, as well as impulsive aggression with access to a weapon; Walker, Frick, & McMahon, Chapter 6, this volume), or abuse (physical, sexual, or neglect; Milojevich & Wolfe, Chapter 18, this volume). Any of these three needs to be addressed in the case formulation and treatment plan, and each has its own obligations in terms of safety plan and reporting. Like other sensitive topics, it is worth asking more than once, and in different ways—people may be more willing to disclose on paper than in person. Make sure that you know what the clinic policies are for managing these before you ask—these are hot potatoes that you want to be able to handle quickly and safely, and they are crucial opportunities to help the person.

Examples of risk factors that could change the probability of other diagnoses or outcomes include exposure to drugs during pregnancy, head injury, or exposure to a natural disaster (La Greca & Danzi, Chapter 15, this volume). Family history is often the single most useful risk factor to check: Whether there is a genetic or multigenerational environmental component, many problems run in families (Smoller & Finn, 2003; Weissman et al., 2000). Leaving aside causality, knowing the common themes and issues in a family can help narrow the list of suspects and improve the formulation. Often, drawing the parallel between the youth's situation and that of other family members helps us understand and communicate, and if other relatives have had success addressing issues, then this can provide an excellent recipe for treatment. Personalized medicine is rediscovering that treatment response, not just the problem, runs in families, too.

Moderators are things that would change the choice of treatment or the likely outcome. Diagnosis itself can be a moderator, inasmuch as it guides a different treatment selection or predicts a different response. ODD, parent–child conflict, and PTSD all lead to a lot of irritable mood and stress, but they would not all respond equally well to family therapy (see the online Wikiversity case example of Tamika). Comorbidity is another moderator: Cases with more diagnoses and problems are likely to be more difficult to treat, and often show smaller improvements. Personality disorders and substance misuse (Chung & Wang, Chapter 19, this volume) also complicate treatment. When more than one thing is an issue, we can often add modules of treatment, pairing an intervention strategy with a facet of a problem (Weisz et al., 2012). Discrepancies in informant perspective also are likely to be moderators. An excessively worried parent might benefit from psychoeducation to normalize his or her expectations, or from getting support him- or herself, whereas a disengaged youth in denial might suggest the addition of motivational interviewing, rapport building, or other tactics to

get him or her engaged and unstuck. Cognitive ability and age are two more moderators—the older and more verbal the person is, the more he or she will benefit from cognitive elements of treatment, whereas younger, less verbal, or more functionally impaired clients often benefit more from behavioral interventions (Jensen-Doss et al., Chapter 3, this volume).

Challenges in Obtaining Family History

In spite of its proven clinical value, it may not always be possible to gather a good family history. Fathers often do not participate directly in the clinical evaluation process. In many families, the biological father may have been absent from the child's life for years, or even since conception. When a parent is not directly evaluated, the clinician has to rely on information provided by the other available adult. Parents are often unfamiliar with the details of the other adult's mental health history, especially in childhood. Indirect interviews are also prone to reporter bias. If the parents had an abusive relationship or an ugly divorce, then these circumstances could easily color the report about mental health history. If the child is placed in foster care, or adopted, then there may be little or no information available about the biological parents. In school-based or forensic clinics, parents may not routinely be involved in clinical evaluations, and it may be difficult to include them (Milojevich & Wolfe, Chapter 18, this volume).

Another thing to keep in mind is that historical diagnoses themselves may not have been accurate. A family history diagnosis is almost always based on a prior clinical, not research, evaluation. Thus a historical diagnosis is prone to all of the limitations of clinical diagnoses in general (Garb, 1998). Yet more fog gets added by imperfect awareness of other family members' diagnoses, as well as imperfect memory. Even worse are the factors related to race and ethnicity that can increase the chances of things going undetected or misdiagnosed. "Schizophrenia," "psychotic disorder," "antisocial personality," "drug and alcohol problems," or "conduct disorder" are all labels that could signify an undiagnosed bipolar illness, particularly in minority families (Youngstrom et al., Chapter 8, this volume). Finally, family members typically do not have formal clinical training themselves, so their labels are more likely to be filtered through their own cultural lenses. A relative with bipolar disorder might be described as having "bad nerves," a "hot temper," or "anxiety attacks," for example (Carpenter-Song, 2009). As we work longer in a given setting, we learn more about members of the community we serve and become more comfortable using their language to develop a shared formulation.

Cognitive Debiasing

Our brains evolved to process huge amounts of information quickly, using cognitive shortcuts called *heuristics*. These often work well, which is why evolution favored them (Gigerenzer, 2001). When they fail, they fail in predictable ways, too (Kahneman, 2011). We are learning to harness them and debug them. This lets us learn a powerful set of principles that can become good habits.

Croskerry (2002, 2003) has made a career out of studying the thought processes of emergency room doctors, and others have applied the lessons to psychiatry and psychology (Galanter & Patel, 2005). Van Meter (Chapter 2, this volume) describes several of the most common mental shortcuts that can go awry, along with some fast and free techniques that debug them. Always having more than one hypothesis about what might explain the symptoms, forcing the hypotheses to compete with each other, and remembering that people often have more than one issue (comorbidity being the rule instead of the exception) are examples of debugging methods that produce big improvements in the accuracy of our case formulations and agreement about what actions to take next with clients (Jenkins et al., 2011). Van Meter introduces the debugging techniques at the beginning of Chapter 2, this volume, but they can also be very useful when skimming the results of the scales and getting ready for the face-to-face interview.

Prescription and Case Formulation

The next phase of assessment concentrates on what we do with the client during the first appointment. If therapy is a journey, then the evaluation session, and resulting case formulation, is the GPS that takes into account where the client is stuck, sets the desired destination, and suggests an optimal route to get there (Youngstrom et al., 2017). If psychological services are a multicourse meal, then the evaluation session is the main course: It is the centerpiece that provides the bulk of the sustenance, and it builds off the earlier assessment appetizers and guides the subsequent

courses of treatment and outcome. If we are seeing the case for therapy, then the first session is when we get to know the person, understand his or her problem and goals, and pull it all together in a "case formulation" that guides our work. If we are doing a psychological assessment that leads to a written report and recommendations, then we may use more than one session to gather data because it can take several hours to get through the interview and tests involved. Either way, we focus on how the assessment improves our understanding of what is going on, and how it informs next actions for the client. We may add some more narrow and specific rating scales to gather data about specific hypotheses; then we definitely are going to do an interview in which we talk about the scores and responses, and start comparing the findings to different diagnoses or other ways of formulating our conceptualization. We explore the history of how the person and the problems developed, and learn about the person's personal preferences, so that the recommendations are individualized and more appetizing.

Focused, Incremental Assessments

Sometimes it makes sense to add additional assessment instruments to go deeper into particular topics. These are not things that we do with all clients, but they make sense to add on a case-by-case basis. Each addition should add incremental value and help predict some key target, prescribe a change in the treatment approach, or inform the process of working together (Youngstrom, 2013).

Many of these more focused assessments may be more narrow checklists and questionnaires. If the client has high levels of internalizing problems, then following up with more detailed questionnaires about anxiety and depression may help tease apart which aspects of internalizing problems are most important for this person (Fleischer et al., Chapter 10, and Hankin & Cohen, Chapter 7, this volume). Similarly, when there are concerns about depression, adding some mania scales helps to ascertain "which type of mood disorder" (Youngstrom et al., Chapter 8, this volume). In many settings, bipolar disorder is not common enough to warrant including mania scales in the core battery used with all clients. Saving the mania scales for a second tier of evaluation saves time and reduces the burden by not administering them needlessly; it also provides motivation and context when we do use them. Similarly, autism scales (e.g., Sheridan & Lord, Chapter 12, this volume), neurocognitive evaluations of attention and processing speed, and teacher report about attention problems are all great additions to the menu when the referral question or initial hypotheses tag these as considerations, but they do not need to be on the default menu for the clinic.

If the concern is mentioned in the presenting problem, or the referral pattern of the clinic, then the supplemental tools can be picked ahead of time and included in the first package, potentially before the first interview. Some of these also may be done in the waiting room. Other parts—especially the cognitive and achievement measures (Kamphaus & Walden, Chapter 13, and 2020; McGill et al., Chapter 14, this volume)—may become the focus of a separate session in their own right. Some larger practices have psychometric technicians administer these, score them, then present summary data to the psychologist. On a recent visit to Shanghai, one of us (Youngstrom) saw a hospital that had a room with more than 50 computers set up in cubicles for waves of patients to complete questionnaires and neurocognitive tests. We are not recommending it, but it offers an extreme example of what is possible with cafeteria-style organization. Depending on the order in which the data are gathered, findings from these additional focal assessments may help to guide discussion and probing during the interview, or it may be compared and synthesized with the interview material later to make the case formulation, assessment summary, and recommendation.

The Interview

The assessment interview is the time to pull together a lot of information. We want to hear about the presenting problem in the person's own words, and translate it into hypotheses that we can evaluate to build a formulation that guides the person through choices of action to improve his or her situation. We want to have a sense of developmental history, contextual factors, diagnoses, and any cognitive or cultural factors that might change the problem or solution. It is a lot to try to accomplish. The task gets even more difficult inasmuch as we have additional paperwork we have to jam into the session—confidentiality, insurance and billing review, mandated reporting, the location of the bathroom, how to pay for parking—big issues and tiny details that all compete for time and attention.

The most common approach is to treat the interview as a question-and-answer session, follow-ing threads of conversation that seem interesting or important to the clinician. This gives the clinician a sense of control and reliance on his or her experience and training (Meehl, 1997). It also is prone to confirmation bias, missing a fair amount of comorbidity or complicating factors, as well as getting derailed by loquacious parents (Youngstrom et al., 2017). Jensen-Doss and colleagues (Chapter 3, this volume) do a great job reviewing the range of options from fully unstructured interviews through semistructured to fully structured interviews. A fully structured interview is completely scripted, with all the questions asked exactly the same way, and following the same logic. Fully computerized interviews are the obvious culmination of the fully structured approach, and they have been used in different platforms for more than 20 years (Shaffer et al., 2000).

Fully structured approaches often feel comfortable at early stages of our training. They provide clarity and scaffolding, literally telling us what to say and do. They are a detailed recipe for the interview. They rapidly come to feel confining, even boring, as we get more confident. We want the freedom to use our own words, to ask our own follow-up questions. We want to add our own seasoning, not be a line cook following a recipe to the letter. As practitioners, we often stop using them as soon as we are allowed to make our own independent choices. Our rationalizations for stopping—that they take too long, that clients do not like them, that they will hurt rapport—have all been disproven (see Jensen-Doss et al., Chapter 3, this volume, for review). Clients actually prefer more structured approaches, perceiving them as more thorough and leading to better understanding (Suppiger et al., 2009). The reliability is much higher, too.

A hybrid approach might keep the best features of both structured and clinician-directed approaches. One blend is the semistructured interview, with set content areas, but with latitude in how to ask the questions (e.g., Kaufman et al., 1997). Another option is to select modules or content based on the hypotheses and scouting report from the initial assessment (Youngstrom et al., 2017). Yet another option is to have a computer or technician do the structured interview, then have the clinician discuss and probe the diagnoses to decide what to confirm and what to adjust. Any of these can keep the advantages of more comprehensive coverage and enhanced consistency (i.e., better interrater reliability) while being less confining to the clinician. Done well, they put us in the role of the head chef making adjustments to the meal after the basics are prepared, but before it is served to the client. In our training clinic, we often start by teaching a structured interview first, then encouraging interviewers to use it in a semistructured way as they get more confident or see other factors to explore in a particular formulation. In the content chapters, experts recommend both structured and semistructured interview options that may be appropriate.

Younger children tend to be less psychologically minded and often have difficulty both sitting thorough formal interviews and providing meaningful responses. Because referrals in outpatient practice are usually driven by parental concerns, youth are frequently less motivated to cooperate with the interview. At a minimum, it seems like good practice to meet with the child to understand his or her concerns, to assess the motivation for treatment, and also to make behavioral observations that can (1) support or counter parent report; (2) provide a sense of whether cognitive ability, a pervasive developmental disorder, a speech or language problem, some other medical factor, a cultural consideration, or some mix of them, might be contributing to the problem; and (3) gather some initial information about how the child responds interpersonally.

With adolescents, more thorough assessment of substance use should be a prominent feature of case formulation (Chung & Wang, Chapter 19, this volume). ADHD, disruptive behavior, and mood disorders are all linked to great increases in risk of alcohol and drug use. Discussions about sexual activity may also be necessary, as the impulsivity and fluctuating self-esteem associated with adolescence get amplified by impulse control and affective disorders, increasing the risk of pregnancy, infection, and poorer choice of partners (e.g., Stewart et al., 2012). Impulsivity and risky behavior are such important aspects of adolescence that we have added a new chapter devoted to the topic in this edition (King et al., Chapter 24, this volume). These are easier conversations to have privately; just be sure before jumping in that everyone understands the rules about confidentiality and what the exceptions are.

Developmental History

Developmental history influences the assessment process in important ways. The details are important to gather, but it can be a challenge to sift out signal from noise. Does it matter if the umbilical cord was wrapped around the baby's neck and he or she was blue at delivery now that he or she is in gifted classes at high school? Does it matter that he or she had chickenpox at 7? At 17? There are some helpful big-picture questions to keep in mind while asking about developmental history:

• *Are the presenting problems old or new?* This simple question can expose a wealth of information. If the problems are a recent development, then we know that there is a change in functioning. Asking about how the client was doing before things fell apart gives a sense of baseline that will be helpful for setting treatment goals. Knowing that it is a change, versus a more chronic or insidious presentation, leads to a different set of hypotheses, and raises or demotes the probability of different diagnoses. Abrupt changes in functioning can be more suggestive of mood disorders, substance use, exposure to trauma, or new environmental stressors, whereas more chronic presentation of the same symptoms might be more indicative of anxiety disorders, ADHD, autistic spectrum or personality disorders, learning disability, and other conditions that have a long-standing neurocognitive or temperamental aspect (Morrison, 2014). Of course, it is not a perfect mapping: People with ADHD or a learning disability may appear to suddenly develop problems when the classwork exceeds their ability to keep up, and mood disorders may include cyclothymic disorder or persistent depressive disorder (previously called "dysthymia") with episodes that last for years. *Old versus new* is still a powerful question for learning and organizing a lot of data quickly.

• *Are the problems limited to one setting or evident across several?* If the problems occur mostly in one place or relationship, then the focus often shifts to the environment rather than to a more neurodevelopmental or biological explanation. A good behavioral analysis may help a lot (Shapiro & Skinner, 1990). What are the antecedents, and what are the consequences or reinforcers that happen around the problem behavior? What is different at home versus at school? Or with the younger brother versus the older sister? When similar problems are noted by multiple people and across a variety of settings, the problem is often more severe and associated with more impairment (Carlson & Youngstrom, 2003). Conversely, problems that are worse in a single context provide clues about how to change the environment and reinforcers to change the behavior (Vollmer & Northup, 1996).

When we gather input from more than one person, the similarities and differences in their views have important implications for treatment and their chances of sticking with it, as well as for our initial formulation (much more on this below!).

• *Are there other potential explanations for what is going on?* DSM-IV used a five-axis system for formulating diagnostic impressions; Axis III was devoted to considering "other medical conditions" that might be affecting mental health and interpersonal functioning. DSM-5 dropped the multiaxial formulation system but asserts that it still is crucial to do a holistic evaluation that considers social and biological factors. Unfortunately, taking away the axes is more likely make it harder to remember to do this, similar to decluttering the kitchen of sticky notes yet reminding staff that it is still important to do all the things that were jotted down. We still need to check for potential medical explanations. We just have fewer cues to remind us. As psychologists, following through on the principle most often means considering the point of view of pediatricians, who have the medical expertise and in the United States see almost every youth at least once a year. At a minimum, we can ask clients whether they have talked about the problems with the pediatrician. We can ask to see notes or results (with the appropriate release), and we can coach the family about specific questions to ask at their next visit. We are not going to become MDs, but there is plenty that we can do to facilitate communication. When we establish a practice, growing relationships with local pediatricians can be a major source of referrals, too.

In addition to potential medical explanations, the developmental history may also inform us about familial, social, and cultural factors that may be involved. Unfortunately, there is not yet a great crosscutting checklist or method to use. The good news is that many of the themes and risk factors are not specific to one problem. It turns out that physical or sexual abuse, or traumatic events, are examples of things that could contribute to anxiety, mood problems, substance misuse, or externalizing behaviors. The data are clear that these are worth asking about, then factoring into the formulation. Multiple chapters of this book include discussions of bereavement (Layne & Kaplow, Chapter 17) and other stressful events (Grant, Carter, Adam, & Jackson, Chapter 16), abuse (Milojevich & Wolfe, Chapter 18), and trauma (La Greca & Danzi, Chapter 15), making use of different options for information gathering

and assessment. Lots of material is available on the Wikiversity pages, including copies of many of the recommended tools.

• *How does a client's age and developmental stage change things?* The younger the individual, the less likely some diagnoses or mechanisms are for a set of problems. We might think of this as changes in the base rates of different problems at different ages. Separation anxiety is much more common in young children, and panic disorder occurs more frequently in late adolescence and adulthood, for example. Risky behaviors (King et al., Chapter 24, this volume), mood disorders (Hankin & Cohen, Chapter 7, and Youngstrom et al., Chapter 8, this volume), substance misuse (Chung & Wang, Chapter 19, this volume) all become more common after puberty. But puberty often starts younger than we expect. One practical ingredient to add to our assessments would be a quick assessment of pubertal status. The Petersen Pubertal Development Scale (Petersen, Crockett, Richards, & Boxer, 1988) is one of the most widely used in research and happens to have free versions that can be completed by the youth or the parent. Shockingly, perhaps 20% of 8-year-old girls are starting to enter puberty, so it is worth considering adding the Petersen to the assessment packet for youth ages 8 and up, then thinking through the implications in terms of peer functioning and risky behavior, as well as changes in probability of different diagnoses.

Normal development involves testing of limits, tantrums, and some aggression (Emery, 1992), and these all can interact powerfully with the family environment and parenting to produce coercive cycles of aggressive behavior (McMahon & Frick, 2005; Patterson, DeBaryshe, & Ramsey, 1989). If we detect them, then these patterns can be a powerful choice of target for therapy, especially parent training and family-based interventions. There are several free measures of parenting and family conflict that might be helpful to add (see Walker et al., Chapter 6, this volume, for some suggestions). Additionally, many childhood disorders, including anxiety disorders, pervasive developmental disorders, and unipolar depression, frequently have irritable mood and poor frustration tolerance as part of their presentation. In the behavioral genetics literature, these are sometimes described as potential "phenocopies," or processes that produce a similar-looking set of behaviors, but for different reasons (Youngstrom & Algorta, 2014).

• *Comorbidity* is another challenge in case formulation. It is not parsimonious to diagnose children showing both anxiety and explosive, irritable mood as having multiple disorders, unless it can be shown that the two appear at separate times in at least some of the person's life (American Psychiatric Association, 2013). Nor is it prudent from a risk management perspective to simultaneously start medications for both "comorbid" conditions—instead, the assessment process should clarify which problems are "primary"—in the sense of producing the biggest therapeutic gains and reductions in burden—and concentrate on alleviating them first. "Comorbidity" in the initial presentation might provide some useful distinctions about treatment selection in the future, but it often is more a marker of severity. From a case formulation perspective, "comorbidity" may also provide a shorthand for a list of topics to revisit later in treatment, to "mop up" whatever has not resolved along with treatment of the primary problems. With a good developmental history, understanding the sequencing may inform treatment selection, too (Cummings, Caporino, & Kendall, 2013).

Learning about Personal Preferences

The interview is an excellent opportunity to learn about personal preferences. The more that we learn about the client, the more we can adjust the flavor of the assessment and recommendations to taste. Providing clients with some psychoeducation about options, then having open discussion, are core ideas of shared decision making (Barratt, 2008; Harter & Simon, 2011). Helping clients understand the menu of options, as well as the rationale and the evidence behind them, empowers them and increases their engagement. It is also a great way to approach where the sidewalk ends in terms of research evidence: Clinical work inevitably involves situations in which there are no high-quality studies to guide our decision. There is a tension between rigor and relevance: Sometimes strong evidence is only available for a subset of cases, and what is relevant to the individual client may require improvisation (Schon, 1983). The combination of strong knowledge of principles plus ongoing conversations with the client and frequent check-ins is a recipe for better treatment.

Culture matters a lot, too. There are major differences in perspective on what childhood, adolescence, and adulthood should look like, on the appropriate roles and realms of authority for parents versus teens, expectations about schoolwork, and extracurricular activities, there are equally large variations in whether problems are con-

ceived as being behavioral, emotional, biological, or spiritual (Carpenter-Song, 2009). Think about our different cultural definitions of what counts as "food"—from cheesecake to crickets, from kale to kimchee, from pizza to pig's feet. The range of perspectives about parenting and about psychological treatment is at least as wide, and once we understand that, there will still be much to learn about how to tweak the seasoning, so that our formulation and recommendations are more palatable to the family. Hankin and Cohen (Chapter 7, this volume) do a beautiful job of showing how we can explore facets of racial, ethnic, and gender identity as they might connect with assessment and formulation. A balance of confidence that we have something to offer with curiosity and respect about clients and their beliefs not only helps with rapport, but it also increases our own cultural competence.

Ethical and Legal Issues

Assessment of youth raises multiple ethical and legal issues. Who is responsible for seeking and accepting treatment? And how do we proceed when the youth and the parent or teacher do not agree about what the problems are (or even whether there is a problem)?

The issue of responsibility for seeking and adhering to treatment can be complicated. Youth under age 18 years are in the legal custody of a parent or other caregiver (who ultimately is responsible for seeking and approving of treatment). We usually cannot provide services without custodial consent, so we need to understand and acknowledge their concerns. If treatment is going to be individual therapy, we may have a disconnect between what the parent wants and what the youth sees as important. Psychosis, substance use, and bipolar disorder are all examples of real problems that can reduce children's and teen's insight into their behavior. Furthermore, many of the symptoms of these problems are not distressing to the youth, whereas they are annoying or threatening to the people around him or her. Behavior that feels "spontaneous" and "alive" to youth can be perceived as obnoxious or threatening by others. The lack of insight may lessen their motivation for therapy, and it can raise ethical concerns about continuing to treat them even when they are actively opposed to therapy. It also challenges the conventional definitions of impairment that emphasize the symptoms causing distress (Wakefield, 1997).

Cross-informant agreement raises a second, related set of issues. Clinicians are often unimpressed by the level of agreement between parents and other informants. We should consider the possibility that parents' own stress might bias their description of child behavior. This needs to be balanced against youth's tendency toward lack of insight to undermine the validity of self-report. Because most often it is parents who initiate most outpatient referrals, parents, on average, are the most concerned party. Many legitimate cases are referred by parents who themselves experience epochs of stress and mood disturbance. Parent report appears to be one of the most valid indicators of many problems on average, even when the adult also is affected by mood disorder (Youngstrom et al., 2011).

Process, Progress, and Outcome Measurement

Planning about how to measure what should happen next for the client, and embedding these tools in our suggestions and recommendations sections, leads to better reports. Similarly, adding more ongoing progress and process measures in our therapy is likely to lead to better outcomes. Both are ways of thinking differently about assessment, making it an ongoing process rather than a single event. We can mix short and fast updates with more in-depth assessments to get a "big-picture" sense of progress. Doing therapy also may produce a lot of information about how the work is going, and a little creativity can turn the notes and appointment schedules into helpful data. If all goes well, then we can use assessment both to measure our successes with the client and to develop a monitoring system to help him or her stay well and continuing thriving after we are done.

Goal Measurement

Having a clearer definition of a goal helps us reach it. By writing it down we make sure that we are on the same page as our client. When we pick the goals, we can do it using benchmarks based on norms or clinical data (a nomothetic approach), or using personalized goal tracking (idiographic measurement). Freeman and Young (Chapter 4, this volume) go into detail about both process and outcome. The clinically significant change model developed by Jacobson, Roberts, Berns, and McGlinchey (1999) or the minimally important difference framework (Streiner, Norman, & Cairney,

2015) are similar to the *Consumer Reports* guide to restaurant reviews: They are frameworks for taking what we know about a particular measure and norms in clinical and nonclinical samples, then applying that to the individual case or meal. Freeman and Young go into detail about how to build the benchmarks, provide a starter set for several widely used scales, then walk through how to apply them to a case. Several clinical vignettes on Wikiversity also walk through the steps in detail.

Progress Measures

Progress measures track whether we are making headway toward our goals. Their key feature is sensitivity to treatment effects. If therapy helps, then the score should change. If the score changes for other reasons, then this is not so good: It actually makes it harder to tell whether the change is due to treatment versus other factors. In research, that sort of instability contributes to high placebo response and failed studies. On the other hand, measures of personality traits and things that change slowly, if at all, are not going to be good markers of short- and medium-term progress in treatment. Retest reliability and reproducibility (Bland & Altman, 1986) are two ways of measuring the stability of scores outside of treatment, and effect sizes from clinical trials with a comparison group provide the best evidence of treatment sensitivity for a measure. On Wikiversity, we indicate whether scales have shown treatment sensitivity, and the top-tier scales in this category are the ones that have detected effects in two or more independent studies.

Progress measures ideally are short, and fast to administer and to score. This is even more true if we want to do them every session, or on a daily or weekly schedule. Brevity is at cross-purposes with one of the most common ways people measure reliability: Cronbach's alpha and scores for internal consistency are higher for longer scales. When we pick short forms or one- or two-item "check-in" measures, the alpha looks like trash. For a progress measure, we should not worry, especially if the scale has shown treatment sensitivity, or if we are using it in a way that combines many data points—such as making a chart of progress across days or sessions. In fact, a scale having a very high alpha may be a clue that it is a poor choice for a progress measure—it is likely to be either obnoxiously long or narrowly focused and repetitive (Youngstrom, Salcedo, Frazier, & Algorta, 2019).

All of these statistics refer to how the measure does for a group of cases. What we and our clients want to know is how the individual client is doing. The standard error of the difference score, the reliable change index, and the minimally important difference (MID) are three different ways of quantifying how individual change compares to the stability of the measure, or to perceptions of whether the change is even noticeable (MID). Freeman and Young (Chapter 4, this volume) go into more detail. These more clinically helpful statistics are less likely to be included in journal articles. We include these for several common measures in the Chapter 4, as well as for content measures in their respective chapters and Wikiversity pages, making it easier to find the information we need to track change better with our clients.

Taken to a logical extreme, a single item is the shortest possible evaluation. It can be as simple as "So, how are you doing this week?" but with a number attached. In the Top Problems approach (Weisz et al., 2011), therapist and client pick one to three things to track together every session, then use a 0 (*no problem at all, no symptoms*) to 10 (*as bad as it can get*) scaling system, that is, defining a set of up to three scales of one item each. It is impossible to estimate an internal consistency for a single-item scale. In clinical mode, we do not much care, so long as the scale shows treatment sensitivity. The Top Problems approach does. Another powerful feature is that it is "idiographic"— the client gets to define what he or she personally wants to track. This is tremendous in terms of getting buy-in. Other examples of intensive progress measures that you will see include daily report cards (often used with ADHD; Owens et al., Chapter 5, this volume), mood charts (often used with mood disorders; Hankin & Cohen, Chapter 7, and Youngstrom et al., Chapter 8, this volume), and ecological momentary assessment (EMA; e.g., sending a few questions as text messages several times a day or week). EMA is rapidly moving out of the realm of research into the proof of concept phase, with many treatment grants and app developers. As discussed by Freeman and Young (Chapter 4, this volume), tracking progress over the course of therapy is likely to be one of the most "disruptive innovations" in psychological work. What you will be able to do with your clients is going to be worlds apart from what was possible when your instructors and supervisors were training. Peek at Figure 1.1 again and you will have a sense of the speed of the change.

Another approach would be to use longer measures but less often. We are familiar with such a framework in teaching: We might combine weekly quizzes with a longer midterm and final exam (Youngstrom et al., 2017). The longer measures we used in the preparation and prediction/formulation phases could be repeated as a "midterm" six sessions into treatment, then again when we think we are nearing planned termination. We could streamline things even more by having the client repeat only the scales that started with the highest scores, or pick one or two that are the main targets for treatment. An advantage of adding a midterm or outcome test is that we can pick a measure that has norms, which opens up a set of benchmarks to see whether treatment has moved the person's functioning out of the clinical range, back into the nonclinical range, or at least significantly closer to the nonclinical range. Jacobson and colleagues (1999) developed the model using external norms to define benchmarks for clinically significant change at the individual level. Freeman and Young (Chapter 4, this volume) go into detail about the model and provide benchmarks for several widely used instruments. Some of the chapters have benchmarks for disorder-specific instruments (e.g., mania and depression scales; Youngstrom et al., Chapter 8), and many of the Wikiversity pages have these for disorder-specific measures, too. As in teaching, it is possible to do both—have a quick quiz about how things are going each session, combined with longer midterm and outcome evaluations with target benchmarks.

Process Measures

Process measures focus on how the therapy work itself is going rather than whether the symptoms or functioning are changing. An old joke goes: "How many therapists does it take to change a lightbulb? Only one . . . but the lightbulb has to be ready to change." To that, we would add, the lightbulb has to actually do some work. Process measures are ways of tracking whether the work is getting done. They might be as simple as looking at whether the appointments are kept versus constantly getting rescheduled, or even worse, having "no-shows." This is a fundamental measure of whether the client is even showing up (and the client showing has important fiscal implications for our practice, too!). Did the client do the homework in between sessions? Did he or she "forget" to do the mood chart? All of these behaviors represent data about engagement. They become more helpful and informative when we track them.

Researchers also often measure process variables using scales or physiological measures to test whether their theory is right about the mechanism of change. Researchers often talk about "mediators" as a label for these sorts of process variables. How does cognitive-behavioral therapy reduce depression? The theory is that changing automatic thoughts changes the way that the person feels. Good therapy → [Fewer negative automatic thoughts] → Less depression. The client signed up for the "less depression" part. He or she may or may not care about the change in his or her automatic thoughts along the way to reaching that goal. In a similar way, people who are changing their diet with a particular goal in mind, such as weight loss or increased muscle mass, may or may not be fascinated by details about how the diet works. They definitely will care whether it works. Progress measures are the bottom line—did it work or not? Process measures help us understand why it works or is not working.

Our hunch is that clinicians will prefer process measures that (1) are easy and inexpensive, (2) incrementally improve outcomes, (3) quickly reveal when and why clients are "stuck," and (4) improve client retention and satisfaction. Some of the measures that researchers are using to test theories are going to add time and burden, and if they do not add value in terms of client satisfaction, retention, or outcome, then they may not have clinical rele-

vance in resource-constrained settings. Other process measures may be short and on point enough to be worth adding to routine care. Single-item measures of working alliance (e.g., McLaughlin, Keller, Feeny, Youngstrom, & Zoellner, 2014), rapport, or asking "How was the session for you?" might be examples. Tracking process is another place where technology is likely to transform the tools available to us swiftly and substantially (Chapter 4, this volume).

When our process measures show that the client is not doing the work, it is helpful to step back and ask why. Think about concordance and adherence as two separate parts of the puzzle. Adherence is what we are measuring with our process tools—is the client doing the work or not? Concordance is asking whether client and therapist are aligned in the goals. Put another way, is the client motivated? Does he or she understand the treatment rationale? When our process measures indicated trouble, thinking about concordance helps problem solve rapidly. Table 1.3 walks through four scenarios. High concordance + High adherence = Favorite client; the client loves our recommendations and put them into action. Good things usually follow. Such a client is a great customer—he or she keeps coming back, leaves us great reviews, and is fun to work with. High concordance + Low adherence is

TABLE 1.3. Adherence and concordance as Key Dimensions in Understanding How the Work Is Going with Our Clients

	Concordant	Not concordant
Adherent	*Process measures:* they are doing the work • Motivated client • Good understanding of the rationale for treatment elements • Aligned on goals *Example:* Our favorite clients!	*Process measures:* they are coming to session, may be doing the work • But they do now want to be there • Unmotivated clients (often the adult's idea for the youth to be in treatment) • Likely to quit as soon as no one is making them come • Less likely to maintain any gains after treatment *Example:* Youth dragged to appointment scheduled by parent.
Not adherent	*Process measures:* There is a problem, but . . . • Motivated client, and good alignment. • Problems are implementation challenges (forgetting; chaotic lives; or did not understand instructions). *Example:* Going on a diet. Excellent intentions, and the hard part is following through.	*Process measures:* Definite problem • Clients are not motivated • Alignment poor—clients do not share goal • Not sure how treatment will help them—may not get the rationale, may not be culturally or personally appropriate • Likely to drop out if we do not change something about treatment quickly *Example:* Many treatment dropouts.

many people's experience with going on a diet—they understand the goal and are on board with it, but sticking to the diet is hard. Our job in this scenario is to help them problem-solve: What is getting in the way? What are ways of working around the problem? Are the missed appointments simply a matter of forgetting? Helping clients set notifications on their calendar might be a solution, or setting an alarm when it is time to start the bedtime routine (not just using it to wake up).

The Low adherence + Low concordance quadrant is a challenging one. The client is not following the recommendations because he or she does not see how they would help. Revisiting the rationale, psychoeducation, and motivational interviewing all are tools that we could use to increase engagement. Alternatively, we could explore other treatment options and see whether there is something else on the menu that would be a better fit for the client personally. Having the process measures alert us to this creates an opportunity to avoid client dropout ("premature termination" in the treatment literature), which is the worst outcome for both client and therapist.

The High adherence + Low concordance scenario is an interesting one. The client is coming to session and may even be doing some work, but he or she does not want to. We often see this with kids who are getting dragged to us by their parents or sent to us by their teachers. We can bet this is coming when we see big differences in scores on similar measures from parent, teacher, and the youth. Having a plan about how to increase alignment and engagement not only helps make the therapy more fun but also is likely longer lasting. Knowing how to make it less aversive to eat the vegetables makes mealtime both less stressful and healthier in the long run.

Long-Term Monitoring

Congratulations! When we make it to the long-term monitoring phase, we have accomplished a lot with the client! We have done excellent work together, met our goals, and are ready to wrap up treatment. When we get to plan a good-bye together, that is bittersweet, but it also is an opportunity to celebrate the successes. It also is a window for us to help plan for hiccups and triggers that might lead to relapse. There are helpful articles about termination (e.g., Swift, Greenberg, Whipple, & Kominiak, 2012; Ward, 1984). In assessment mode, we would suggest a couple of specific additions.

Make a list of risk factors. Have you ever seen a horror movie? A cliché is the fake ending—the monster is vanquished! But the movie does not end yet. From the audience's perspective, where the monster is lurking is so predictable. From a therapist's perspective, where life is going to ambush the client and push for a relapse may be equally predictable. These are clinical issues where it is even more important to have a plan for not only prevention but also early detection and what to do when we see danger signs. Crises are obvious triggers to us; the proactive practitioner walks through the plan ahead of time: "If your parents do get divorced, remember that it is normal to be stressed. What are three things you could do that might help you get support?" Developmental transitions, such as going to middle school (especially if several elementary schools all feed into a much larger middle school) or moving out of the house, are milestones that often have a lot of stress and disruption associated with them, even though they are normal.

We can use termination sessions to build a care package for the client's future self. It might include a "message in a bottle" with coaching tips and personalized (idiographic!) assessment ideas. "Dear Future Me: Congratulations on kicking depression's butt! Remember that depression often tries to come back. That's not you being weak; that's just what depression does. Pay attention to how you are sleeping. When you can't sleep, or start sleeping through the whole weekend, those are early signs that things are going wrong. That would be a great time to make an appointment and get a boost." If the client is using a sleep tracking log or app, or a life chart, then he or she has a long-term monitoring plan that is already a habit. It is a small but powerful thing to have the client look at this as an early warning system. The client can also include notes about what worked best for him or her in therapy, what he or she tried and did not like (so that the client can skip it, if and when he or she returns to therapy), and what things worked well for self-care. These are personalized checklists and simple rules for maintaining the gains and nipping any new problems in the bud. Although not normally the realm of clinical or school psychology, nothing would stop us from stealing a page from the "life coaching" book and including ideas about performance enhancement and promoting positive functioning, either. In fact, thinking about how to best package and market our services is an important topic in its own right (see Appendix 1.1, the Fourth "P": Payment).

Conclusion

Now you have the overview of how assessment helps— from when we first meet the client through the course of our work together, to providing recommendations about how to keep doing well in the future. The assessment model advocated in this book is heavily influenced by the recommendations of evidence-based medicine (Guyatt & Rennie, 2002; Sackett, Straus, Richardson, Rosenberg, & Haynes, 2000). In the next chapters we walk through the "how-to" aspects, providing in-depth tutorials in the principles. The content-area-oriented chapters then provide the specific ingredients to apply the principles for each given topic. The book and the Wikiversity pages aim to make it easier than ever before to find the tools and the information you need to be able to put it all into practice.

Using the evidence-based methods described here will help you make the best use of the assessment tools available to make more accurate formulations, build better treatment plans, and improve treatment processes and outcomes. Evidence-based assessment (EBA) helps strike the balance between being open to the possibility of rare diagnoses and situations while also avoiding overdiagnosis of uncommon yet sometimes popularized conditions. By using a sequenced approach to assessment, it is possible to work smarter and not harder, getting better results without increasing the cost or burden to the clinician or the family. You are about to learn the principles and sequence to become an excellent cook, able to do great assessment of common problems quickly and well, and to know how to customize and improvise to meet people's needs in clinical practice. Assessment is the skill that sets psychology apart from the rest of the caring professions and social sciences. Be patient while you learn the hands-on skills, and enjoy the results as you give feedback and deliver improved outcomes.

REFERENCES

Achenbach, T. M. (2001). What are norms and why do we need valid ones? *Clinical Psychology: Science and Practice, 8,* 446–450.

Achenbach, T. M., McConaughy, S. H., & Howell, C. T. (1987). Child/adolescent behavioral and emotional problems: Implication of cross-informant correlations for situational specificity. *Psychological Bulletin, 101,* 213–232.

Achenbach, T. M., & Rescorla, L. A. (2001). *Manual for the ASEBA School-Age Forms and Profiles.* Burlington: University of Vermont.

American Psychiatric Association. (2013). *Diagnostic and statistical manual of mental disorders* (5th ed.). Arlington, VA: Author.

Barratt, A. (2008). Evidence based medicine and shared decision making: The challenge of getting both evidence and preferences into health care. *Patient Education and Counseling, 73,* 407–412.

Bayes, T., & Price, R. (1763). LII. An essay towards solving a problem in the doctrine of chance (by the late Rev. Mr. Bayes, communicated by Mr. Price, in a letter to John Canton, M. A. and F. R. S.). *Philosophical Transactions of the Royal Society of London, 53,* 370–418.

Beidas, R. S., Stewart, R. E., Walsh, L., Lucas, S., Downey, M. M., Jackson, K., . . . Mandell, D. S. (2015). Free, brief, and validated: Standardized instruments for low-resource mental health settings. *Cognitive and Behavioral Practice, 22,* 5–19.

Berkson, J. (1946). Limitations of the application of fourfold table analysis to hospital data. *Biometrics Bulletin, 2,* 47–53.

Bird, H. R., Yager, T. J., Staghezza, B., Gould, M. S., Canino, G., & Rubio-Stipec, M. (1990). Impairment in the epidemiological measurement of childhood psychopathology in the community. *Journal of the American Academy of Child and Adolescent Psychiatry, 29,* 796–803.

Blader, J. C., & Carlson, G. A. (2007). Increased rates of bipolar disorder diagnoses among U.S. child, adolescent, and adult inpatients, 1996–2004. *Biological Psychiatry, 62,* 107–114.

Bland, J. M., & Altman, D. G. (1986). Statistical methods for assessing agreement between two methods of clinical measurement. *Lancet, 1,* 307–310.

Bossuyt, P. M., Reitsma, J. B., Bruns, D. E., Gatsonis, C. A., Glasziou, P. P., Irwig, L. M., . . . de Vet, H. C. W. (2003). Towards complete and accurate reporting of studies of diagnostic accuracy: The STARD initiative. *British Medical Journal, 326,* 41–44.

Burkhart, K., & Phelps, J. R. (2009). Amber lenses to block blue light and improve sleep: A randomized trial. *Chronobiology International, 26,* 1602–1612.

Carlson, G. A., & Youngstrom, E. A. (2003). Clinical implications of pervasive manic symptoms in children. *Biological Psychiatry, 53,* 1050–1058.

Carpenter-Song, E. (2009). Caught in the psychiatric net: Meanings and experiences of ADHD, pediatric bipolar disorder and mental health treatment among a diverse group of families in the United States. *Culture, Medicine, and Psychiatry, 33,* 61–85.

Corrigan, P. W., Druss, B. G., & Perlick, D. A. (2014). The impact of mental illness stigma on seeking and participating in mental health care. *Psychological Science in the Public Interest, 15,* 37–70.

Croskerry, P. (2002). Achieving quality in clinical decision making: Cognitive strategies and detection of bias. *Academic Emergency Medicine, 9,* 1184–1204.

Croskerry, P. (2003). The importance of cognitive errors in diagnosis and strategies to minimize them. *Academic Medicine, 78*, 775–780.

Cummings, C. M., Caporino, N. E., & Kendall, P. C. (2013). Comorbidity of anxiety and depression in children and adolescents: 20 years after. *Psychological Bulletin, 140*, 816–845.

Cuthbert, B. N., & Insel, T. R. (2010). Toward new approaches to psychotic disorders: The NIMH Research Domain Criteria project. *Schizophrenia Bulletin, 36*, 1061–1062.

Cuthbert, B. N., & Insel, T. R. (2013). Toward the future of psychiatric diagnosis: The seven pillars of RDoC. *BMC Medicine, 11*, 126.

De Los Reyes, A., Augenstein, T. M., Wang, M., Thomas, S. A., Drabick, D. A., Burgers, D. E., & Rabinowitz, J. (2015). The validity of the multi-informant approach to assessing child and adolescent mental health. *Psychological Bulletin, 141*, 858–900.

Drotar, D., Stein, R. E. K., & Perrin, E. C. (1995). Methodological issues in using the Child Behavior Checklist and its related instruments in clinical child psychology research [Special issue]. *Journal of Clinical Child Psychology, 24*, 184–192.

Emery, R. (1992). Family conflicts and their developmental implications: A conceptual analysis of meanings for the structure of relationships. In W. Hartup & C. Shantz (Eds.), *Family conflicts* (pp. 270–298). New York: Cambridge University Press.

Epstein, D. (2019). *Range: How generalists triumph in a specialized world*. London: Macmillan.

Evans, S. C., Burke, J. D., Roberts, M. C., Fite, P. J., Lochman, J. E., de la Pena, F. R., & Reed, G. M. (2017). Irritability in child and adolescent psychopathology: An integrative review for ICD-11. *Clinical Psychology Review, 53*, 29–45.

Gadow, K. D., & Sprafkin, J. (1994). *Child Symptom Inventories manual*. Stony Brook, NY: Checkmate Plus.

Gadow, K. D., & Sprafkin, J. (1997). *Adolescent Symptom Inventory: Screening manual*. Stony Brook, NY: Checkmate Plus.

Galanter, C. A., & Patel, V. L. (2005). Medical decision making: A selective review for child psychiatrists and psychologists. *Journal of Child Psychology and Psychiatry, 46*, 675–689.

Garb, H. N. (1998). *Studying the clinician: Judgment research and psychological assessment*. Washington, DC: American Psychological Association.

Gigerenzer, G. (2001). The adaptive toolbox: Toward a darwinian rationality. *Nebraska Symposium on Motivation, 47*, 113–143.

Guyatt, G. H., & Rennie, D. (Eds.). (2002). *Users' guides to the medical literature*. Chicago: American Medical Association Press.

Harter, M., & Simon, D. (2011). Do patients want shared decision making and how is this measured? In G. Gigerenzer & J. A. Muir Gray (Eds.), *Better doctors, better patients, better decisions* (pp. 53–58). Cambridge, MA: MIT Press.

Haslam, N., Holland, E., & Kuppens, P. (2012). Categories versus dimensions in personality and psychopathology: A quantitative review of taxometric research. *Psychological Medicine, 42*, 903–920.

Hinshaw, S. P., & Cicchetti, D. (2000). Stigma and mental disorder: Conceptions of illness, public attitudes, personal disclosure, and social policy. *Development and Psychopathology, 12*, 555–598.

Hunsley, J., & Mash, E. J. (2007). Evidence-based assessment. *Annual Review of Clinical Psychology, 3*, 29–51.

Hunsley, J., & Mash, E. J. (Eds.). (2008). *A guide to assessments that work*. New York: Oxford University Press.

Hunsley, J., & Mash, E. J. (Eds.). (2018). *A guide to assessments that work* (2nd ed.). New York: Oxford University Press.

Jacobson, N. S., Roberts, L. J., Berns, S. B., & McGlinchey, J. B. (1999). Methods for defining and determining the clinical significance of treatment effects: Description, application, and alternatives. *Journal of Consulting and Clinical Psychology, 67*, 300–307.

Jaeschke, R., Guyatt, G. H., & Sackett, D. L. (1994). Users' guides to the medical literature: III. How to use an article about a diagnostic test. B: What are the results and will they help me in caring for my patients? *Journal of the American Medical Association, 271*, 703–707.

Jenkins, M. M., Youngstrom, E. A., Washburn, J. J., & Youngstrom, J. K. (2011). Evidence-based strategies improve assessment of pediatric bipolar disorder by community practitioners. *Professional Psychology: Research and Practice, 42*, 121–129.

Jenkins, M. M., Youngstrom, E. A., Youngstrom, J. K., Feeny, N. C., & Findling, R. L. (2012). Generalizability of evidence-based assessment recommendations for pediatric bipolar disorder. *Psychological Assessment, 24*, 269–281.

Jensen-Doss, A., & Hawley, K. M. (2010). Understanding barriers to evidence-based assessment: Clinician attitudes toward standardized assessment tools. *Journal of Clinical Child and Adolescent Psychology, 39*, 885–896.

Jensen-Doss, A., & Hawley, K. M. (2011). Understanding clinicians' diagnostic practices: Attitudes toward the utility of diagnosis and standardized diagnostic tools. *Administration and Policy in Mental Health, 38*, 476–485.

Kahneman, D. (2011). *Thinking, fast and slow*. New York: Farrar, Straus & Giroux.

Kaufman, J., Birmaher, B., Brent, D., Rao, U., Flynn, C., Moreci, P., . . . Ryan, N. (1997). Schedule for Affective Disorders and Schizophrenia for School-Age Children—Present and Lifetime version (K-SADS-PL): Initial reliability and validity data. *Journal of the American Academy of Child and Adolescent Psychiatry, 36*, 980–988.

Kazdin, A. E., & Blase, S. L. (2011). Rebooting psychotherapy research and practice to reduce the burden of mental illness. *Perspectives on Psychological Science*, 6, 21–37.

Lambert, M. J. (2003). Is it time for clinicians to routinely track patient outcome?: A meta-analysis. *Clinical Psychology: Science and Practice*, 10, 288–301.

Lucas, G. M., Gratch, J., King, A., & Morency, L.-P. (2014). It's only a computer: Virtual humans increase willingness to disclose. *Computers in Human Behavior*, 37, 94–100.

Matson, J. L., Matheis, M., Estabillo, J. A., Burns, C. O., Issarraras, A., Peters, W. J., & Jiang, X. (2019). Intellectual disability. In M. J. Prinstein, E. A. Youngstrom, E. J. Mash, & R. A. Barkley (Eds.), *Treatment of disorders in childhood and adolescence* (4th ed., pp. 416–447). New York: Guilford Press.

McGill, R. J., & Ndip, N. (2019). Learning disabilities. In M. J. Prinstein, E. A. Youngstrom, E. J. Mash, & R. A. Barkley (Eds.), *Treatment of disorders in childhood and adolescence* (4th ed., pp. 448–492). New York: Guilford Press.

McLaughlin, A. A., Keller, S. M., Feeny, N. C., Youngstrom, E. A., & Zoellner, L. A. (2014). Patterns of therapeutic alliance: Rupture–repair episodes in prolonged exposure for posttraumatic stress disorder. *Journal of Consulting and Clinical Psychology*, 82(1), 112–121.

McMahon, R. J., & Frick, P. J. (2005). Evidence-based assessment of conduct problems in children and adolescents. *Journal of Clinical Child and Adolescent Psychiatry*, 34, 477–505.

Meehl, P. E. (1954). *Clinical versus statistical prediction: A theoretical analysis and a review of the evidence.* Minneapolis: University of Minnesota Press.

Meehl, P. E. (1997). Credentialed persons, credentialed knowledge. *Clinical Psychology: Science and Practice*, 4, 91–98.

Morrison, J. (2014). *Diagnosis made easier: Principles and techniques for mental health clinicians* (2nd ed.). New York: Guilford Press.

Nesi, J., Miller, A. B., & Prinstein, M. J. (2017). Adolescents' depressive symptoms and subsequent technology-based interpersonal behaviors: A multi-wave study. *Journal of Applied Developmental Psychology*, 51, 12–19.

Nesi, J., & Prinstein, M. J. (2019). In search of likes: Longitudinal associations between adolescents' digital status seeking and health-risk behaviors. *Journal of Clinical Child and Adolescent Psychology*, 48, 740–748.

Patterson, G. R., DeBaryshe, B. D., & Ramsey, E. (1989). A developmental perspective on antisocial behavior: Children and their development: Knowledge base, research agenda, and social policy application [Special issue]. *American Psychologist*, 44, 329–335.

Perou, R., Bitsko, R. H., Blumberg, S. J., Pastor, P., Ghandour, R. M., Gfroerer, J. C., . . . Huang, L. N. (2013). Mental health surveillance among children—United States, 2005–2011. *Morbidity and Mortality Weekly Report*, 62, 1–35.

Petersen, A. C., Crockett, L., Richards, M., & Boxer, A. (1988). A self-report measure of pubertal status: Reliability, validity, and initial norms. *Journal of Youth and Adolescence*, 17, 117–133.

Rettew, D. C., Lynch, A. D., Achenbach, T. M., Dumenci, L., & Ivanova, M. Y. (2009). Meta-analyses of agreement between diagnoses made from clinical evaluations and standardized diagnostic interviews. *International Journal of Methods in Psychiatric Research*, 18, 169–184.

Reynolds, C. R., & Kamphaus, R. (2015). *Behavior Assessment System for Children (BASC)* (3rd ed.). Bloomington, MN: Pearson Clinical Assessment.

Roth, A., & Fonagy, P. (2005). *What works for whom?: A critical review of psychotherapy research* (2nd ed.). New York: Guilford Press.

Sackett, D. L., Straus, S. E., Richardson, W. S., Rosenberg, W., & Haynes, R. B. (2000). *Evidence-based medicine: How to practice and teach EBM* (2nd ed.). New York: Churchill Livingstone.

Sattler, J. M. (2002). *Assessment of children: Behavioral and clinical applications* (4th ed.). La Mesa, CA: Author.

Schon, D. A. (1983). *The reflective practitioner: How professionals think in action.* New York: Basic Books.

Shaffer, D., Fisher, P., Lucas, C. P., Dulcan, M. K., & Schwab-Stone, M. E. (2000). NIMH Diagnostic Interview Schedule for Children Version IV (NIMH DISC-IV): Description, differences from previous versions, and reliability of some common diagnoses. *Journal of the American Academy of Child and Adolescent Psychiatry*, 39, 28–38.

Shapiro, E. S., & Skinner, C. H. (1990). Principles of behavioral assessment. In C. R. Reynolds & R. W. Kamphaus (Eds.), *Handbook of psychological and educational assessment of children: Personality, behavior, and context* (Vol. 2, pp. 343–363). New York: Guilford Press.

Silver, N. (2015). *The signal and the noise: Why so many predictions fail—but some don't.* New York: Penguin.

Smoller, J. W., & Finn, C. T. (2003). Family, twin, and adoption studies of bipolar disorder. *American Journal of Medical Genetics C: Seminars in Medical Genetics*, 123, 48–58.

Stewart, A. J., Theodore-Oklota, C., Hadley, W., Brown, L. K., Donenberg, G., & DiClemente, R. (Project Style Study Group). (2012). Mania symptoms and HIV-risk behavior among adolescents in mental health treatment. *Journal of Clinical Child and Adolescent Psychology*, 41, 803–810.

Straus, S. E., Glasziou, P., Richardson, W. S., & Haynes, R. B. (2011). *Evidence-based medicine: How to practice and teach EBM* (4th ed.). New York: Churchill Livingstone.

Streiner, D. L., Norman, G. R., & Cairney, J. (2015). *Health Measurement Scales: A practical guide to their development and use* (5th ed.). New York: Oxford University Press.

Suppiger, A., In-Albon, T., Hendriksen, S., Hermann,

E., Margraf, J., & Schneider, S. (2009). Acceptance of structured diagnostic interviews for mental disorders in clinical practice and research settings. *Behavior Therapy, 40*, 272–279.

Susskind, R., & Susskind, D. (2015). *The future of the professions: How technology will transform the work of human experts.* New York: Oxford University Press.

Swift, J. K., Greenberg, R. P., Whipple, J. L., & Kominiak, N. (2012). Practice recommendations for reducing premature termination in therapy. *Professional Psychology: Research and Practice, 43*, 379–387.

Twenge, J. M., Gentile, B., DeWall, C. N., Ma, D., Lacefield, K., & Schurtz, D. R. (2010). Birth cohort increases in psychopathology among young Americans, 1938–2007: A cross-temporal meta-analysis of the MMPI. *Clinical Psychology Review, 30*, 145–154.

Twenge, J. M., & Nolen-Hoeksema, S. (2002). Age, gender, race, socioeconomic status, and birth cohort difference on the children's depression inventory: A meta-analysis. *Journal of Abnormal Psychology, 111*, 578–588.

Vollmer, T. R., & Northup, J. (1996). Some implications of functional analysis for school psychology. *School Psychology Quarterly, 11*, 76–92.

von Elm, E., Altman, D. G., Egger, M., Pocock, S. J., Gotzsche, P. C., & Vandenbroucke, J. P. (2008). The Strengthening the Reporting of Observational Studies in Epidemiology (STROBE) statement: Guidelines for reporting observational studies. *Journal of Clinical Epidemiology, 61*, 344–349.

Wakefield, J. C. (1997). When is development disordered?: Developmental psychopathology and the harmful dysfunction analysis of mental disorder. *Development and Psychopathology, 9*, 269–290.

Ward, D. E. (1984). Termination of individual counseling: Concepts and strategies. *Journal of Counseling and Development, 63*, 21–25.

Wechsler, D. (2014). *Wechsler Intelligence Scale for Children—5th edition.* San Antonio, TX: NCS Pearson.

Weissman, M. M., Wickramaratne, P., Adams, P., Wolk, S., Verdeli, H., & Olfson, M. (2000). Brief screening for family psychiatric history: The family history screen. *Archives of General Psychiatry, 57*, 675–682.

Weisz, J. R., Chorpita, B. F., Frye, A., Ng, M. Y., Lau, N., Bearman, S. K., . . . Hoagwood, K. E. (2011). Youth Top Problems: Using idiographic, consumer-guided assessment to identify treatment needs and to track change during psychotherapy. *Journal of Consulting and Clinical Psychology, 79*, 369–380.

Weisz, J. R., Chorpita, B. F., Palinkas, L. A., Schoenwald, S. K., Miranda, J., Bearman, S. K., . . . Research Network on Youth Mental Health. (2012). Testing standard and modular designs for psychotherapy treating depression, anxiety, and conduct problems in youth: A randomized effectiveness trial. *Archives of General Psychiatry, 69*, 274–282.

Youngstrom, E. A. (2013). Future directions in psychological assessment: Combining evidence-based

medicine innovations with psychology's historical strengths to enhance utility. *Journal of Clinical Child and Adolescent Psychology, 42*, 139–159.

Youngstrom, E. A. (2014). A primer on Receiver Operating Characteristic analysis and diagnostic efficiency statistics for pediatric psychology: We are ready to ROC. *Journal of Pediatric Psychology, 39*, 204–221.

Youngstrom, E. A., Ackerman, B. P., & Izard, C. E. (1999). Dysphoria-related bias in maternal ratings of children. *Journal of Consulting and Clinical Psychology, 67*, 905–916.

Youngstrom, E. A., & Algorta, G. P. (2014). Pediatric bipolar disorder. In E. J. Mash & R. A. Barkley (Eds.), *Child psychopathology* (3rd ed., pp. 264–316). New York: Guilford Press.

Youngstrom, E. A., Findling, R. L., & Calabrese, J. R. (2003). Who are the comorbid adolescents?: Agreement between psychiatric diagnosis, parent, teacher, and youth report. *Journal of Abnormal Child Psychology, 31*, 231–245.

Youngstrom, E. A., LaKind, J. S., Kenworthy, L., Lipkin, P. H., Goodman, M., Squibb, K., . . . Anthony, L. G. (2010). Advancing the selection of neurodevelopmental measures in epidemiological studies of environmental chemical exposure and health effects. *International Journal of Environmental Research and Public Health, 7*, 229–268.

Youngstrom, E. A., Salcedo, S., Frazier, T. W., & Algorta, G. P. (2019). Is the finding too good to be true?: Moving from "more is better" to thinking in terms of simple predictions and credibility. *Journal of Clinical Child and Adolescent Psychology, 48*(6), 811–824.

Youngstrom, E. A., & Van Meter, A. (2016). Empirically supported assessment of children and adolescents. *Clinical Psychology: Science and Practice, 23*, 327–347.

Youngstrom, E. A., Van Meter, A., Frazier, T. W., Hunsley, J., Prinstein, M. J., Ong, M.-L., & Youngstrom, J. K. (2017). Evidence-based assessment as an integrative model for applying psychological science to guide the voyage of treatment. *Clinical Psychology: Science and Practice, 24*, 331–363.

Youngstrom, E. A., Youngstrom, J. K., Freeman, A. J., De Los Reyes, A., Feeny, N. C., & Findling, R. L. (2011). Informants are not all equal: Predictors and correlates of clinician judgments about caregiver and youth credibility. *Journal of Child and Adolescent Psychopharmacology, 21*, 407–415.

APPENDIX 1.1. The Fourth "P": Payment

Whether we are students, practitioners, or applied researchers, there are economic considerations that affect our work. Being aware of the fiscal aspects is crucial for the sustainability and success of our practices. We need to think through how to support ourselves, while also making sure that our services are accessible. There is a tension between maximizing reach as opposed to revenue and prestige. Do we want to position ourselves like the neighborhood taco truck, known for tasty, filling, low-cost food that will serve the community regardless of resources? Or are we aiming to be a private-pay, concierge-level gourmet service? Both are viable models, and there is plenty of range in between the two. Because psychological assessment is a unique service in mental health, it adds great value, and our professional monopoly on it gives us a lot of latitude in terms of pricing and business models.

While we are students, it is common for our training clinics to use a sliding scale, or offer services at a discounted rate compared to local practices. We may even offer some services pro bono (at no charge). It is worth keeping in mind that the discount is not because we are offering lower quality services. With good supervision, research shows that the products and outcomes are as good or better than what is available in the free market (especially when considering the plethora of options that families will find when they search Google). The discount is more about ensuring that there is a stream of referrals to help students grow their skills on a schedule, and to give back to the local community. So feel good about the work you are doing when you are starting out, even if you do not feel confident at first.

There some things to keep in mind if you move into starting your own practice. When you take assessment classes, the cabinet is magically stocked with ingredients. They were selected by the professors and clinic directors, and paid for with training funds or revenue from the clinic. If you are starting an independent practice, you get to pick how to stock the cabinet, and you are also doing the buying. This book and the Wikiversity pages will be excellent resources yet again. Treat the book like a shopping list: What are the essentials you want to be sure to stock to be ready for the "vital few" common problems? What are the issues in which you would like to specialize? These chapters provide the supplemental ingredients to add to your stock. Remember how the experts made a point of including the best of the free options? That just provides a huge cost savings as you are starting your practice, and continued savings for as long as the tools are helpful. The weakest links in the chain connecting research to practice have often been awareness and access—the Wikiversity site is addressing both of those shortcomings. The same site that was helpful for students is built to stay helpful over the long haul.

When we think about costs, time is also money. The time that it takes us to find materials, to score them, and to find the interpretive information has an opportunity cost for us. Once again, Wikiversity is organized to help us keep cooking like a professional. There are limits to what clients will accept in terms of burden, so the emphasis on shorter versions is a helpful default. The more in-depth options are also there for when they clearly add value.

The economic landscape will change over the course of our careers. Part of that is the developmental arc of our professional growth. As students, a fellowship is not tied to clinical productivity, and we charge discounted fees at our training clinics. When we become professionals, we choose a setting and practice model. In medical settings and in private practice, there is a much tighter connection between our income and service provision. Assessment is an invaluable tool: It commands a higher rate than an hour of therapy; it unlocks access to more intensive services; and we are the specialists—no other profession has the skills or the mandate to fill that role in systems of care.

The landscape also is changing in terms of insurance and competition. Measurement based care and paying for quality are major shifts. Assessment is integral—we are the best positioned profession to work with that change in tastes. The most disruptive threat comes from technology: Companies such as Google, 23 and Me, Amazon, and Facebook are using machine learning to make diagnoses and dabble with offering services. If they succeed—and this is no certain thing—they will fill the fast-food franchise niche of mental health. They will excel at automation and scale, and they may do a workable job with routine problems and with psychoeducation. But psychology is one of the disciplines least likely to get automated away: Humans are complex, and their needs and tastes may be so individualized that it takes sophistication to understand, and a lot of soft skills to engage them and promote change (Susskind & Susskind, 2015). We will continue to have successful roles, including catering to those with more complex or rare issues, providing bespoke services in private pay settings, or mixing some ingredients from technology services into an individualized approach—such as using chicken tenders, some off-the-shelf ingredients, and creativity to make a delicious stir fry. Understanding the principles of assessment is the edge that ensures we will remain as the cooks and chefs delivering and designing quality and personalized care.

CHAPTER 2

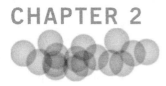

The Prediction Phase
of Evidence-Based Assessment

Anna Van Meter

The fifth edition of the *Diagnostic and Statistical Manual of Mental Disorders* (DSM-5) provides us with hundreds of diagnostic options—more when we take into account subtypes and qualifiers (American Psychiatric Association, 2013). Related, the publishing industry and independent authors have produced thousands of assessment tools for determining whether an individual meets criteria for one or more of these diagnoses (Carlson, Geisinger, & Jonson, 2017). Each new case presents nearly unlimited options—so many possible diagnoses, so many methods for determining which diagnosis best fits the presenting problems. For a clinician with unlimited time and a family with no urgency in reducing its distress, this could be an exciting opportunity, a chance to really delve into the youth's symptoms and history from multiple angles, to try on different diagnoses until finding the best fit. However, for clinicians

practicing under normal circumstances, in which time is one's most precious—and limited—resource, and for families who are often desperate for help, this approach is a nonstarter. Arriving at the right diagnosis, so that an appropriate treatment can be selected and the clinician can work with family members to effectively meet their needs, is important, but efficiency is also a key consideration: There are more families in need than we have hours in the day.

The first stage of assessment—*prediction*—offers a process by which clinicians can improve their efficiency by focusing their clinical questions without sacrificing accuracy or rapport (Youngstrom, 2008). At the end of the prediction phase of assessment, a clinician will have whittled down the list of probable diagnoses to a few contenders and will be aware of factors that might influence his or her work with the client and family. The goal of the prediction phase is to prepare for the *prescription* phase, in which diagnoses will be determined and treatment plans developed, and for the *process* phase, during which progress toward treatment goals and, ultimately, outcomes, will be assessed. Prediction helps set you and the client on track for a successful course of treatment, and although it requires some groundwork, it will quickly improve both the efficiency and effectiveness of the assessment process (Youngstrom, 2008,

2012; Youngstrom, Choukas-Bradley, Calhoun, & Jensen-Doss, 2014; Youngstrom & Van Meter, 2016; Youngstrom et al., 2017).

After a hectic Monday, you check your mailbox and retrieve three newly completed intake forms. On top of the stack is Ty Lee. According to Ty's form, he is 12 and lives with his mom and older sister. His mom reports "bad temper, lack of effort on homework, and slipping grades." This sounds like the majority of your middle school–age clients. You see that Ty and his mom are scheduled to meet with you for an intake appointment the following Monday at 3:00 P.M. Beyond the basics of the case, included on the screening form, what would help you get the most out of your 60-minute intake? What are your goals for the appointment? Ideally, you would like to be able to give the family members a diagnosis and start talking to them about potential treatment options, but a semistructured interview can take an hour or more, and you would like to talk with Ty and his mom separately, which could double that time. Plus, you need to go through the consent process, learn about Ty's development, and get a family history. It does not feel possible to do a comprehensive assessment in the time allotted. Luckily, you have a few strategies for learning more about Ty before he arrives, so that you can get the most out of the time you have with him and his mom.

Avoiding Decision-Making Biases

Ty's symptoms, listed on the screening form, are pretty nonspecific and do not give you much of a clue about what the most likely diagnosis/es are. You might be tempted to start thinking about other 12-year-old boys you have seen and mentally match what you know about Ty with the presenting problems of these other boys. Is he more like the boy who ended up having oppositional defiant disorder (ODD) and responded well to a behavioral intervention? Or like the guy who was so anxious about his grades that he avoided his homework and nearly failed out of school? Our brains are well trained to look for patterns and, in most situations, this skill helps us be more efficient (Tversky & Kahneman, 1974). However, when it comes to clinical decision making, relying on patterns—often referred to as "heuristics"—or other mental shortcuts can seriously derail the accuracy of our evaluation before we even get started (Lilienfeld & Lynn, 2014; Patel, Kaufman, & Arocha, 2002).

Being aware of this tendency to rely on heuristics is the first step in trying to ensure the accuracy of your clinical decision-making process. Although it is natural to think back to estimate the prevalence of different disorders and to consider how well your new case matches past "prototypical" cases, this sort of back-of-the-envelope estimate is likely to be inaccurate. Large discrepancies between our estimate of the rates of diagnoses at our clinic (what we see most often) and the true rates could have serious consequences (Meehl, 1954). If you work on an inpatient unit, you probably see cases of serious mood disorders and psychosis most often, so if you are a betting person, you might wager that the next person admitted to the unit would have a mood or psychotic disorder and be reasonably confident about your odds of being right. On the other hand, if you work at a specialty anxiety clinic, you probably see relatively few severe mood or psychotic disorder cases. If you were to bet, you might be smarter going for generalized anxiety disorder or separation anxiety—disorders that are less likely to be seen by your colleague on the inpatient unit. This might seem obvious, but clinicians often engage in *base rate neglect*—an error that, unfortunately, is common enough that it has its own name (Croskerry, 2003). There are multiple factors that contribute to base rate neglect, some of which are described below, but the best way to combat making this error is by knowing the base rates of the most common diagnoses in your setting (more on this later). Knowing the base rates can help you to avoid diagnosing a lower prevalence disorder when a more common disorder could account for the presenting problems—we are tempted to see zebras, but more often than not, we are actually faced with a horses (Fiedler, Brinkmann, Betsch, & Wild, 2000). What other decision-making errors might we make in the prediction phase?

Availability Heuristic

Clinicians often overestimate the probability of easily recalled events and underestimate events that are harder to recall (Elstein & Schwarz, 2002; Galanter & Patel, 2005). For example, although schizophrenia is very rare among children, these cases are memorable, which can make the phenotype more "available" in a clinician's mind and could lead to overdiagnosis if new cases seem to match a prominent prototype in one's mind. However, for most clinicians, who will not have seen many—if any—cases of childhood schizophrenia, this phenotype would be relatively "unavailable" and, as a result, may not be diagnosed even when it would be the appropriate diagnosis. Inexperienced clinicians tend to rely more on prototypes than do those with more experience, who may be more aware of the probability of specific diagnoses (Croskerry, 2002). The availability heuristic is also more likely to result in misdiagnosis of disorders with heterogeneous presentations because they are, by nature, less "prototypical" and may not fit with what the clinician expects or has previously seen in cases with the same diagnosis.

Confirmation Bias

Confirmation bias occurs when a clinician forms a hypothesis about a patient, then seeks evidence to confirm the hypothesis, rather than inquiring more broadly about the symptoms the patient is experiencing. Additionally, confirmation bias can lead clinicians to ignore or reject evidence that is not consistent with his or her hypothesis (Elstein, 1999; Galanter & Patel, 2005). Confirmation bias is especially likely when a client has an existing diagnosis or comes in with a hypothesis about his or her own (or his or her child's) diagnosis—"Based on what I read online, I'm almost certain my child has generalized anxiety!" (Lighthall & Vazquez-Guillamet, 2015). For example, upon hearing that your new client, Ty, has oppositional behavior and slipping grades, it would be natural to hypothesize about oppositional defiant disorder or perhaps attention-deficit/hyperactivity disorder (ADHD); these are common diagnoses, so the availability heuristic might also be at play here, easily populating your mind with past, similar cases. This could lead to a series of questions during the intake about behavioral problems and impulse control to the exclusion of other inquiries about internalizing behavior. When Ty's mom confirms that, yes, he is impulsive, but no, he is not oppositional with other adults, you might be inclined to think that "impulsivity, poor school performance, irritability—sounds like ADHD" and then fail to continue your assessment because you have "confirmed" your initial hypothesis due to the confirmation bias (Lighthall & Vazquez-Guillamet, 2015). This can feel like a very efficient way to get to the diagnostic answer, but if you "confirm" the wrong diagnosis or fail to recognize comorbid conditions, treatment is unlikely to proceed effectively and you may need to reassess Ty's diagnosis when his symptoms do not improve, ultimately leading to more suffering and a longer course of treatment than necessary.

Satisficing

Clinicians may also engage in a shortcut known as *search satisficing*. Satisficing occurs when a clinician completes the evaluation when he or she has arrived at a diagnosis that is compatible with the child's presentation. In doing so, the clinician satisfies the clinical question, but without probing further to ensure that a different diagnosis is not a better fit and to assess for comorbid conditions. The results of this evaluation are not valid, and this approach is not in the best interests of the client and his or her family (Jenkins & Youngstrom, 2016).

Representativeness Heuristic Bias

The *representativeness heuristic bias* is similar to the availability heuristic in that it occurs when a clinician attempts to match a new client to prototypical clients with particular diagnoses. However, whereas the availability heuristic leads to errors related to how memorable (or not) past cases have been, the representative heuristic is related more to a failure to take into account the base rate of a certain diagnosis. This can lead to over- or underestimating the likelihood that a new client has a certain diagnosis (Bruchmüller & Meyer, 2009; Elstein, 1999; Galanter & Patel, 2005). Interestingly, this heuristic is more likely to be used when there is perceived familiarity with a diagnostic group—thus, more experienced clinicians implement this heuristic more frequently. For example, an expert in pediatric bipolar disorder might hear about Ty's symptoms of irritability and decline in functioning and determine that he is likely to have bipolar disorder because he or she has seen other clients who also experience these problems, even though other, more common diagnoses (e.g., ADHD) would also account for these symptoms (Lighthall & Vazquez-Guillamet, 2015).

Irrelevant Information Bias

Clinicians may also fail to take a systematic approach to assessment when the patient (or caregiver) provides an alternative reason that may explain the presenting symptoms (Bruchmüller & Meyer, 2009). For example, if Ty's mother mentions that his new teacher is very strict and has high standards, the clinician might attribute Ty's academic problems to a changing environment rather than an inability to focus in class (or some other explanation; Galanter & Patel, 2005). Thus, even though a teacher's standards have little clinical relevance, clinicians tend to weigh such information heavily in their diagnostic process (Bruchmüller & Meyer, 2009; Wolkenstein, Bruchmüller, Schmid, & Meyer, 2011).

Under other circumstances in our lives, using heuristics enables us to make decisions quickly and to function efficiently in our environments, but relying on these cognitive shortcuts can impede clinical assessment. Being aware of our propensity to use heuristics is important to limiting their influence on our clinical decision making. It is also worth noting that these heuristics are not mutually exclusive; a clinician may employ multiple shortcuts in a given case. Relying on heuristics can feel like being guided by carefully honed clinical instinct, but our clients are best served by a more systematic approach to assessment. Additionally, although the biases described above are related to decision-making errors, diagnosis is also negatively impacted by biases related to client demographics or other characteristics (Garb, 1998) that contribute to disparities in care based on sex and race (Ely, Graber, & Croskerry, 2011). These biases may be more difficult to notice in ourselves, which further emphasizes the importance of taking an approach designed to reduce the influence of biases, regardless of source.

Using Screening Tools to Focus the Clinical Question

At this point, you have only very basic information about Ty, but it is standard operating procedure at your clinic to have each family complete a few assessments online before the initial intake. On the Thursday before Ty's Monday intake session, you log on to your clinic's secure server and see that Ty's mom has completed her assessments and Ty has completed one of the questionnaires he is supposed to do. Mom filled out the Child Behavior Checklist (CBCL; Achenbach, 1991a) and a developmental and family history form, and Ty completed the Youth Self-Report (YSR; Achenbach, 1991a). As you suspected, based on the intake form, Ty has elevated Externalizing scores on his mom's CBCL (77) but not his YSR (42). Additionally, Ty's mom rates him as having elevated Internalizing T-scores on the CBCL (72), though his YSR score is again much lower (44). You are a little surprised by this, but you also know that youth are more likely to be brought for treatment due to externalizing symptoms. Externalizing symptoms

bother people around the youth—like his or her parents—and are more likely to motivate treatment seeking than internalizing symptoms, which tend to bother the client most (Freeman, Youngstrom, Freeman, Youngstrom, & Findling, 2011).

It is also worth thinking about how the referral question might affect the way Ty and his mom completed the assessments. Based on the intake form, you know that Ty's mom is especially concerned about his "bad temper, lack of effort on homework, and slipping grades." These problems are her main reason for seeking treatment now, and when she completed the CBCL, she probably focused on these problems and on communicating to you that they need help. This does not mean that there are not other issues affecting Ty and his family, and the fact that Ty's Internalizing scores are also elevated gives you a clue that his temper and school performance may not be the whole story.

Reading through the developmental and family history form that Ty's mom completed, you notice that she reported that Ty's father suffers from depression. You know that a family history can often increase the probability for a specific diagnosis, so you make a note to find out more about this at the appointment, so that you can incorporate this information into your clinical decision making. Otherwise, Ty's history is not noteworthy for any developmental delays, traumatic events, or history of other mental health problems. It does say that Ty's parents are separated, which would almost certainly affect Ty, so you also make a note of this. It is helpful to have even this basic information before the first appointment, so that you know ahead of time that you want to inquire about the circumstances of the separation and that you need to set up a phone call or meeting with Ty's dad to ask about his history with depression and to get his impressions of Ty.

You are now aware of the clinical decision-making traps that have been set, but how do you avoid them? Without relying first on patterns, how do you integrate and make sense of all the information you will collect as you get to know a new client? You know what Ty's presenting problem is, you have both his and his mom's reports about his general symptoms, and you are aware that he may have a first-degree relative with depression, and that he has gone through a likely upsetting event with his parents' separation. Are you any closer to making a diagnosis or to understanding how to best help Ty and his family? Yes, and what you do next will be really important to help ensure the accuracy of your clinical decisions. You could easily rely on heuristics here—what other clients have had similar scores? What did their diagnoses turn out to be? But, as we learned, this could result in an inaccurate and/or incomplete diagnosis. A better approach is to use the information you have to statistically determine what is the most probable diagnosis/es affecting Ty. You may be wondering how statistics can help you make sense of the information you have collected—in fact, there are a few different statistical approaches that might be helpful.

Bayes' Theorem

First, do not forget that you also know (or can determine) the base rate for the most common diagnoses at your clinic. Without any other information, the average prevalence of different disorders gives you a rough starting point for the probability of different diagnoses. This is helpful, but an even more informative approach is to use Bayes' theorem to combine the base prevalence with other pieces of information to arrive at a revised "posterior probability" of having a specific diagnosis. Bayes' theorem can be summarized as the probability of an event given the occurrence of other events. In psychology, we often try to determine the probability that a child has a certain diagnosis, or that he or she will develop a particular outcome, given a certain set of symptoms, genetic/biological risk factors, and developmental results. Bayes' theorem gives us a way to integrate the known pieces of information in order to solve for the unknown diagnosis or outcome and to plan our next clinical steps accordingly. The IBM medical decision-making tool run by Watson uses a Bayesian approach to revise the probabilities of different conditions based on information as it is collected, providing information on the current leading hypotheses, and a recommendation about whether more assessment or treatment is indicated (Youngstrom et al., 2017). So, if you use Bayes' theorem, you will be in good company!

Diagnostic Likelihood Ratios

In order to incorporate different pieces of information using Bayes' theorem, we first need to transform our risk information into a form that can be combined. The most common way of doing this is by calculating the likelihood ratio associated with a certain piece of information. A *diagnostic likelihood ratio (DLR)* is the technical name for a

change in risk, and it is estimated by comparing the rate at which individuals who have a certain characteristic (e.g., an above-threshold score, a risky family history) and meet criteria for the diagnosis of interest (true positives) with the rate at which people who have the diagnosis, but do not have the characteristic (false negative; American Educational Research Association, 2014; Sackett, Straus, Richardson, Rosenberg, & Haynes, 2000). A DLR is an effect size and can take on any value from almost zero to infinity; DLRs greater than one increase the probability of a certain diagnosis or outcome, DLRs between zero and one decrease the probability. A DLR of one means that the characteristic or risk factor is equally likely in people who have the diagnosis and those who do not—it will not be helpful in making your diagnostic decisions. The further away from one you get, the more influential the DLR is; values >10 (or smaller than .10) can be diagnostic (i.e., the characteristic is *almost only* present or absent in the population that has the diagnosis). DLRs around 5 (or .2) are helpful and can change the probability of a diagnosis in a meaningful way, and DLRs between .5 and 2 are generally not very informative (Youngstrom et al., 2017). In some cases, papers about the association between a characteristic/risk factor and a diagnosis report the likelihood ratio, but more often, it is something that you need to calculate. Fortunately, this is a simple math problem once you know the sensitivity and specificity associated with the characteristic/risk factor (see Figure 2.1). Whenever authors of chapters in this book report sensitivity and specificity, they include the DLRs for you.

Sensitivity and Specificity

The DLR is derived from the *sensitivity* and *specificity* associated with a characteristic or risk factor. These terms tell us how good the assessment finding (usually this refers to an above-threshold score on a self-report or other scale) is at discriminating between people who have the disorder (or other outcome) of interest and those who do not. Sensitivity is the proportion of people who have the outcome (or diagnosis) of interest and the characteristic (true positive)—this is how good the tool is at picking up *all* the true cases. People with the outcome of interest will always score above threshold on a tool with 100% sensitivity. However, this high sensitivity usually comes at a price; if I set the threshold for my measure low enough that every single true case is guaranteed to score positive, chances are that a lot of people who *do not* have

For scores that are above the threshold or the presence of a risk factor:

$$\text{Likelihood ratio} + = \frac{\text{sensitivity}}{1 - \text{specificity}} = \frac{\text{probability of a person with the condition testing positive}}{\text{probability of a person \textbf{without} the condition testing positive}}$$

For scores that are below the threshold or the absence of a risk factor:

$$\text{Likelihood ratio} - = \frac{1 - \text{sensitivity}}{\text{specificity}} = \frac{\text{probability of a person with the condition testing negative}}{\text{probability of a person \textbf{without} the condition testing negative}}$$

FIGURE 2.1. Diagnostic likelihood ratio formulas.

the outcome of interest will also score positive. For example, if I create a measure for anxiety disorders and ask three questions—(1) "Do you ever feel anxious?"; (2) "Do you ever feel nervous?"; (3) "Do you ever worry about things?"—and say that anyone who answers "yes" to one or more questions has a score that is positive for anxiety, it is likely that almost all people with anxiety disorders will score positive, but because worry/anxiety (just like many symptoms of psychopathology) are also experienced, to a lesser degree, by people without a clinical diagnosis, my measure would also identify a lot of people who do not have impairing anxiety.

Although we want people who have the outcome of interest to score positive, we also want people who do not have the outcome to score negative. The proportion of people who do not have the disorder and score negative is known as *specificity*. If I wanted to be sure my anxiety measure had very high specificity, I might set the cutoff score to 3. This would reduce the number of false positives by a lot, but many people with anxiety disorders might not endorse all three questions, so I would also increase the number of false negatives.

You can see that the sensitivity and specificity associated with a questionnaire varies depending on the score threshold(s) meant to distinguish between "positive" and "negative" scores or between various levels of risk. Typically, cutoff scores for a given measure are determined by the optimal balance between sensitivity and specificity, making a trade-off between identifying as many "true positives" as possible, while minimizing "false positives." Dichotomizing results in this way can be problematic (does a 1-point difference really mean someone goes from being at risk to not being at risk?), so it may be prudent for researchers to calculate multiple thresholds, allowing different levels of risk to be represented. For example, in a study of the utility of the Achenbach System of Empirically

Based Assessment (ASEBA; Achenbach, 1991a, 1991b, 1991c; Achenbach & Rescorla, 2001) for identifying childhood anxiety disorders, scores were split into five ranges—scores in the highest range doubled the probability of an anxiety disorder, while scores in the lowest range effectively ruled out anxiety (Van Meter et al., 2014). There are also some situations in which a balance between sensitivity and specificity will not best meet your clinical needs. For example, when assessing for suicide risk, it may make sense to maximize sensitivity because you do not want to miss any at-risk cases, even if it means having to follow-up with a higher number of false positives (Van Meter et al., 2018).

In addition to being used to calculate a likelihood ratio, knowing the sensitivity and specificity associated with a scale score or characteristic can be informative in a couple of other ways. When the cutoff score of a certain measure is associated with very high sensitivity, it can help us rule out a diagnosis (Straus, Tetroe, & Graham, 2011). Going back to the example of the three-question anxiety measure, we note that a score of 1 (endorsing any one of the anxiety-related questions) would likely identify nearly all cases of anxiety (plus a large number of people without clinically significant anxiety). Because a score of 1 on this measure is associated with high sensitivity, someone who scores a 0 is very *unlikely* to have an anxiety disorder. There is a mnemonic to help us remember this: SnNOut—on a highly Sensitive test, a Negative result rules the diagnosis Out (Straus, Glasziou, Richardson, & Haynes 2011). Related, if we have a cutoff score that is associated with high specificity, we can be confident that positive score means the person has the diagnosis of interest. The mnemonic associated with this is SpPIn—on a test with high Specificity, a Positive test rules the diagnosis In.

The sensitivity and specificity of each possible score (or result) from a given tool are calculated using receiver operating characteristic (ROC) analysis (see Youngstrom, 2014, if you want details about how to do ROC analysis yourself). A ROC analysis plots the sensitivity and specificity (technically, 1-specificity) for each possible result. The graph this produces gives us an area under the curve (AUC; see Figure 2.2). This effect size is helpful in summarizing the overall performance of a tool; it tells us the probability that a person with the disorder will be *more likely* to have a positive test result than someone without the disorder (when comparing two people in a randomly selected pair). AUCs close to .5 correspond roughly with chance—you are just as likely to accurately identify someone with your outcome of interest with a coin flip as you are with this tool (go for the coin flip, it's probably quicker!). An AUC of 1 would mean that every person is correctly classified using this measure. So, you should look for tools with AUCs close to 1, right? Not exactly.

The sensitivity and specificity of a tool are affected by the population in which the tool is tested because the AUC reflects how much the score distributions of the "positive" and "negative" groups overlap. In the earlier anxiety questionnaire example, if I decide to validate my measure in a sample of youth from a specialty mood and anxiety disorders clinic, the measure is likely to have a smaller AUC (perform more poorly) than if I validate it by comparing scores between a group of youth with anxiety disorders and a group of psychologically

healthy youth. Because many symptoms of psychopathology overlap, youth with mood disorders are likely to endorse some of the anxiety-related questions; as a result, the score distributions (the bell curves of all scores) for the youth with mood disorders and for the youth with anxiety disorders are likely to overlap significantly. This makes it harder to tell the two groups apart, based on their scores. On the other hand, youth with no psychopathology are likely to have an average close to 0, making it relatively easy to distinguish them from the youth with anxiety disorders based on their scores (see Figure 2.3). This type of situation, in which the score distributions barely overlap, will yield AUCs close to 1. Although this might seem like a sign of a really great measure, more likely, it is a problem. It is not often that you administer a questionnaire because you are wondering whether a child has a mental health disorder or *no disorder at all*. When measures are validated by comparing a clinical group to a typically developing group, this is the question being addressed. For clinical applications, what you want to find is a measure that does a good job distinguishing between treatment-seeking youth at a setting similar to yours. Studies conducted in clinical samples typical of what we see in practice will yield smaller AUCs, but the results are much more relevant and likely to replicate when you use the measure with your clients (Youngstrom, Genzlinger, Egerton, & Van Meter, 2015; Youngstrom, Meyers, Youngstrom, Calabrese, & Findling, 2006a). When you are reading about potential measures to use, it is worth paying attention to the composition of the validation sample—if you cannot find a study in a similar population, it does not mean you should avoid the measure, but you do need to be aware of how the population in which the measure was validated will influence your interpretation.

Positive and Negative Predictive Value

Another helpful clinical term is "positive predictive value" (PPV; Kraemer, 1992). The PPV is the percentage of individuals scoring positive on a test (or endorsing a family history, etc.) who also have the condition of interest. It is a measure of how often the result from a particular test would correctly indicate that the individual did have the diagnosis of interest. Although the PPV provides potentially helpful information, it comes with a large caveat: Because the PPV is based on the proportion of "test positive" people who have the diagnosis (vs. those who test positive but do not have

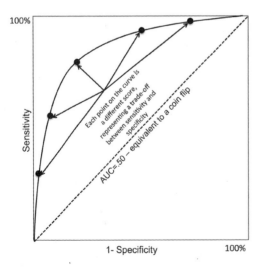

FIGURE 2.2. Receiver operating characteristic curve.

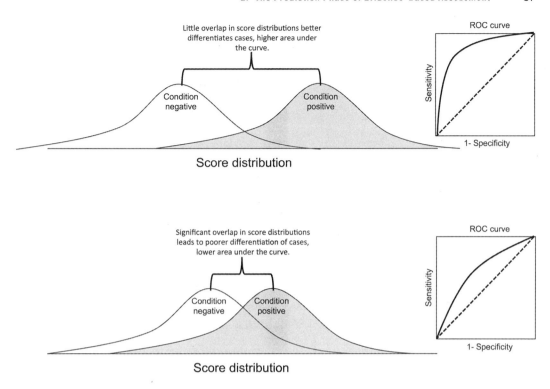

FIGURE 2.3. Illustration of the association among score distribution, area under the curve, and diagnostic efficiency: (1) representation of nonoverlapping distributions and (2) representation of overlapping distributions.

the diagnosis), it is strongly affected by the base rate of the diagnosis in the sample from which it was calculated. Consequently, it would be incorrect to apply a published PPV to your client unless the base rate of the disorder of interest is very similar in your clinic and the published sample. It is also possible to calculate a "negative predictive value" (NPV); this would tell you how accurate a negative test score is, but it is subject to the same bias as the PPV and should only be applied across very similar populations. To understand the associations between PPV, NPV, sensitivity, and specificity, see Figure 2.4.

The Nomogram

Unlike the PPV and NPV, likelihood ratios are not significantly biased by sample base rates, so you can use a likelihood ratio across populations more confidently. Once you have a likelihood ratio, either because it was reported or you calculated it from the sensitivity and specificity, what do you do with it? Here is where Bayes' theorem comes in handy. Using Bayes' theorem, you can combine

your base rate and the likelihood ratio(s) you have. Fortunately, although applying a theorem sounds like it requires advanced math, a couple of simple tools can help you do this easily. The first is the probability nomogram (Figure 2.5). A *nomogram* is a tool that uses a graphical interface to calculate a mathematical function. Rather than using algebra or other, more complicated approaches to solve for an unknown value, a nomogram enables you to do so literally by connecting dots because the corresponding values have been built into the graphical scales. There are different nomograms for use with different types of information. For our purposes, we use a probability nomogram, which allows us to graphically plot the relationships between our initial risk (most likely the base rate), the likelihood ratio associated with a self-report scale, risk factor, or other characteristic, and the revised probability of a particular outcome. In Figure 2.5, the left column is the starting point, where you would indicate the starting probability. In the middle column, you find the number associated with your likelihood ratio, then draw a line through these two points, connecting to the

	Condition		
	(A) *Meets criteria* diagnosis or outcome of interest	(B) *Does not meet criteria* for diagnosis or outcome of interest	
Test or risk factor — (C) *Above threshold* score or *Positive* for risk factor	(D) True Positive	(E) False Positive	Positive Predictive Value = $\dfrac{\text{True Positive (D)}}{\textit{Above threshold} \text{ score (C)}}$
(F) *Below threshold* score or *Negative* for risk factor	(G) False Negative	(H) True Negative	Negative Predictive Value = $\dfrac{\text{True Negative (H)}}{\textit{Below threshold} \text{ score (F)}}$
	Sensitivity = $\dfrac{\text{True Positive (D)}}{\textit{Meets criteria} \text{ (A)}}$	Specificity = $\dfrac{\text{True Negative (H)}}{\textit{Does not meet criteria} \text{ (B)}}$	

FIGURE 2.4. Associations among sensitivity, specificity, positive predictive value, and negative predictive value.

third line on the right side. The point where the line intersects the right-hand line is the posterior probability—the probability that a case will meet criteria for a diagnosis given the base rate at your setting and the likelihood ratio associated with a certain characteristic/risk factor.

In spite of the intimidation factor that comes from mentioning a theorem and the nomogram, this process is simple once you have the necessary pieces (the base rate and the likelihood ratio). Even better, this approach is precise and unlikely to be influenced by biases, the way your thought process might be if you tried to weigh and integrate these pieces of information on your own—plus there is evidence that using the nomogram makes big differences in the accuracy and consistency of diagnostic decisions of practicing clinicians (Jenkins, Youngstrom, Washburn, & Youngstrom, 2011). If the process of marking down the prior probability and likelihood ratio and drawing a line seems clunky, you may instead want to utilize an online calculator (e.g., *http://araw.mede.uic.edu/cgi-bin/testcalc.pl* or *https://appadvice.com/app/docnomo/901279945*) or program the formula (see Figure 2.6) into a spreadsheet and save it on your computer. Even if the nomogram is new to you, this type of approach probably is not; as detailed data about individuals are increasingly available (think genetics, family history, blood pressure, cholesterol levels), medicine is becoming more sophisticated in its ability to forecast the likelihood of different health events (e.g., heart attack

or stroke). Psychology and psychiatry are working to catch up by quantifying the associations we have long observed between risk or protective factors and outcomes, and by developing our own risk calculators to predict individual risk (Cannon et al., 2016; Fusar-Poli et al., 2017; Hafeman et al., 2017). The nomogram enables you to do this on a small scale and to personalize it to your individual client.

Multiple-Informant Reports

One of the best attributes of the nomogram is that allows you to integrate multiple sources of information to arrive at a posterior probability. As a child mental health professional, you have the benefit, in many cases, of having information from the child, one or more caregivers, and—sometimes—you also have access to input from a teacher or other third party. This gives you a much fuller picture of what is going on, but it can also introduce challenges—rare are the cases in which youth and caregiver agree completely, and sometimes their accounts do not seem to overlap at all (Jensen-Doss, Youngstrom, Youngstrom, Feeny, & Findling, 2014; Youngstrom, Findling, & Calabrese, 2003). What do you do in these situations? There are rules of thumb—caregivers are more accurate when reporting about externalizing symptoms, youth are better able to report on their internal states—but the process of integrating reports from multiple informants is more complicated

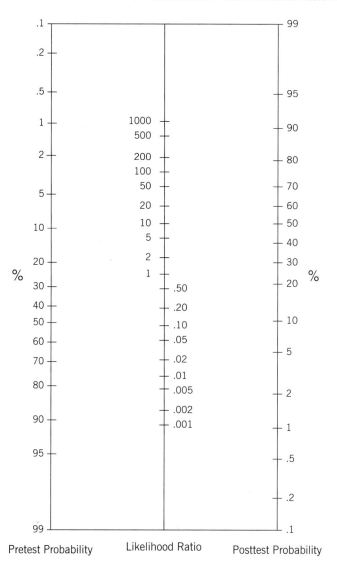

FIGURE 2.5. Probability nomogram.

$$\frac{\dfrac{\text{prior probability}}{(1-\text{prior probability})} * DLR}{1+\dfrac{\text{prior probability}}{(1-\text{prior probability})} * DLR}$$

FIGURE 2.6. Posterior probability formula.

than that (Carlson & Youngstrom, 2011; De Los Reyes & Kazdin, 2005; Ferdinand, van der Ende, & Verhulst, 2004; Youngstrom et al., 2011). Informants bring their own perspective, and biases, to the situation; a caregiver who calls for treatment because she is fed-up with her son's oppositional behavior may unconsciously elevate her report of the boy's symptoms because she is frustrated and she feels the need to justify her call for help. Related, a child who can think of many ways he would rather spend Thursday afternoons than in therapy, might be motivated to downplay problems he has been experiencing (Carlson & Youngstrom, 2011). In general, agreement between informants (whether caregiver–child, teacher–child, or other dyad) tends to be low (De Los Reyes et al., 2015); when one person in the dyad rates clinically significant problems, the other is likely to rate the same symptom/behavior as being within normal limits (Youngstrom et al., 2006b). It is also important to consider factors such as the developmental stage of the child (Does he or she have the ability to articulate internal states?), the relationship between the caregiver and child (Is there conflict that could be influencing the degree of disagreement?), and other psychosocial variables that might impact how symptoms are reported (Is the family under financial or other stressors? Are there other children or elderly relatives who also require care? Does the parent have his or her own psychopathology?) (Ringoot et al., 2015; Youngstrom et al., 2011). This does not mean that one person is wrong and the other is right—it just reflects differences in each person's primary focus and perspective of the problem(s).

When you start thinking about the motivations of patients and their family members, and how that should impact how you weigh their reports, the likelihood of falling back on cognitive biases or heuristics increases—you are asking your brain to process a lot of potentially disparate information, which is tough to do in an objective way without help. Here is where the nomogram can come to the rescue. Earlier you read a description of the process for integrating the base rate and a likelihood ratio associated with a risk factor. The likelihood ratios for other sources of information—self reports, caregiver-completed checklists—can be incorporated in the same way. With each new piece of information, you simply replace the starting probability (left-hand line) with the posterior probability indicated by the previous data (right-hand line). If you start with your clinic base rate and add a DLR for family history to arrive

at a posterior probability of 60%, this number can then be moved to the left side of the nomogram, and your DLR for youth self-report (or caregiver report) added to the middle line. Just connect these new dots and you have your revised posterior probability, which can then be moved to the left side to add another DLR. In addition to clinic base rates, historical data, and checklist scores, you could also include the DLR associated with a neuropsychological test or a behavioral task (e.g., the continuous performance task; Jarrett, Van Meter, Youngstrom, Hilton, & Ollendick, 2018).

An important caveat to this approach is that *you can only include one piece of information from each source.* This is because Bayes' theorem assumes independence of each piece of information, and responses from the same source are likely to be highly correlated, which—if integrated—will bias your result (Youngstrom et al., 2014). For example, you know both Ty's Internalizing and Externalizing *T*-scores for both the CBCL and YSR, but because Ty and his mom each contributed two of these scores, you have to choose whether you want to include the YSR—Internalizing or YSR—Externalizing and the CBCL—Internalizing or the CBCL—Externalizing. Luckily, there is a strategy to the selection process. Remember that the size of a likelihood ratio is related to its influence, with very small (<.10) and very large (10+) likelihood ratios being nearly diagnostic, whereas likelihood ratios close to 1 do not really change the probability of a diagnosis. Consequently, it often makes sense to use the pieces of information you have that are most influential (this could mean a large or small likelihood ratio). If you have given a battery of measures, or one measure with multiple scales, articulate your clinical question (e.g., "What is the probability that Ty has ODD?") and use the likelihood ratio most likely to influence the posterior probability. At this stage in your assessment, you may only have a broad symptoms measure, such as the YSR and CBCL, but in the next stage of your evidence-based assessment, you will begin to incorporate more targeted assessment tools, intended to evaluate symptoms specific to the most probable diagnoses. These assessments are likely to be associated with more clinically meaningful DLRs.

Okay, so now you know to avoid using heuristics and falling into other clinical decision-making traps, and you have learned how to use the nomogram to incorporate different pieces of information that you might learn about Ty. What should that information be? As I stated at the beginning of this chapter, there are literally thousands of measures that you could administer, each of which would yield a separate DLR. Plus, there are a lot of facts about Ty that might be important to consider: Did he meet his developmental milestones on time? Do his age or sex put him at higher risk for some disorders? Was there a traumatic event that precipitated his symptoms? Given all the questions you might ask, how do you prioritize?

Assembling Your Assessment Toolkit

It is not practical (or a good use of time) to prepare for all imaginable clinical situations. You want to be well prepared for the clients who constitute the bulk of your practice and prepared enough to identify an unusual case as such when it arrives. Pareto's 80/20 rule can come in handy here—80% of cases are likely to have 20% of possible diagnoses (Burr, 1990). Put another way, it is worth spending the time to know the base rates for the disorders that make up 80% of your practice, to know the psychometric properties for measures (both youth and caregiver) that are effective at identifying—and distinguishing between—these disorders, and you want to be well versed in the treatment protocols that address these concerns. You also want to have a couple of broad measures that can do a decent job alerting you when you might be facing someone from the 20% (e.g., in outpatient clinics, a tool that inquires about psychotic symptoms in addition to anxiety and behavioral problems). As you encounter these more unusual cases, you can take the time to investigate the best assessment tools and treatments—this way you keep growing your "assessment toolkit," without having to commit a huge amount of time upfront.

A well-equipped toolkit should include the following:

- Base rates for the most common diagnoses or problems at your clinic (or a close approximation) (see Youngstrom & Prinstein, Chapter 1, this volume)
- Information about how common risk factors affect the probability of common diagnoses (e.g., sex differences, family history)
- At least one broad measure that assesses for symptoms across the spectrum of psychopathology and offers scale scores to guide the administration of more specialized scales, plus the scoring instructions and corresponding DLRs for these scales (many of the chapters include

information for the ASEBA, and the Wikiversity pages include information for other alternatives)
- Specialized scales or behavioral tasks designed to assess for specific domains of symptoms (youth and caregiver report, if possible); scoring instructions and corresponding DLRs (the DLRs for positive scores on these are above 2 ideally—otherwise they may not add much beyond the general scales to your decision-making process)
- A modular semi-structured interview to inquire more comprehensively about the diagnostic criteria for the common diagnoses (see Jensen-Doss, Patel, Casline, & McLeod, Chapter 3, this volume)
- Manuals for evidence-based treatments appropriate to the population and disorders you see most often (think about whether family or individual treatment is most appropriate, along with the developmental stage of the client; see Jensen-Doss et al., Chapter 3, this volume, for more on this)
- Scales sensitive to assessing change over time (see Freeman & Young, Chapter 4, this volume, for more on this)

Time to start building your toolkit! Knowing the *base rate* for the most commonly seen disorders/problems in your setting will give you some sense for what you are likely to encounter when your next client walks through the door. For example, at an outpatient clinic, like the one where you are seeing Ty, a typical patient population might comprise youth with behavior disorders (ADHD, ODD), anxiety, and mood disorders. Even without the information from the screening form, you know—based on the rates of diagnoses at your clinic—that there is a 38% chance that Ty has ADHD, a 38% chance that he has ODD, a 40% chance that he has an anxiety disorder, and a 26% chance that he has depression (rates add up to more than 100% because comorbidity is also common at your clinic). This is not diagnostic, but combined with other information you will learn about Ty, it can help to further narrow the diagnoses under consideration.

Determining the most commonly diagnosed disorders at your setting can require a little work, but it will pay off. In some settings, it may be possible to query an electronic medical record to determine the prevalence of each diagnosis over the past year. In settings without this technological advantage, you might need to enlist help to pull a random sample of charts and record the diagnoses, or to see what the most common *International Classification of Diseases* (ICD) codes are in the billing records. As you compile these data, it is a good idea to think about whether you can institute a system for tracking diagnoses moving forward; this will enable you to update the prevalence rates more easily in the future.

At this stage—remember, you have not even met Ty yet!—your main goal should be to create a list of the diagnoses you want to evaluate more closely when you do meet with Ty and his mom. If you go into your intake appointment with a focused list of two or three high-probability diagnoses, you can get a fuller picture about the important details without sacrificing time collecting broad information necessary to focus your intake. Collecting data most likely to influence the posterior probability *before* your first session is a good way to whittle down the list of probable diagnoses ahead of the appointment, making better use of the precious time when you meet with the family.

Finding Effective Clinical Tools

How do you know which questionnaires or other tools are most informative? There are a number of psychometric characteristics you should consider. For example, the internal consistency of a measure tells you whether patient responses are related across items, suggesting that the measure (or scale within a measure) is assessing a single construct. High internal consistency provides some assurance that your measure is assessing the symptom domain on which you are focused and not psychopathology more broadly. When considering which assessment tools to use in your practice—in most cases—you will also want to prioritize those that demonstrate a good balance of sensitivity and specificity, which gives you the best chance at limiting the number of false positives or false negatives. Remember that when you are evaluating which tools to use in your practice, it is important to be aware of the potential for an AUC to be "too good." It is best to seek out validation studies conducted in samples relevant to your practice—if you work in an outpatient clinic, look for psychometric data from an outpatient sample of a similar age; likewise for inpatient, school, or specialty clinics. If you cannot find a study conducted in a similar sample, you can use the data you do find, but keep in mind how differences might influence the results. For example, a typically developing comparison group inflates effect sizes, whereas a more

seriously ill group might lead to an unnecessarily high cutoff score.

Seeking psychometric data about the measures of interest can be challenging. When you search, use terms that are likely to yield useful information, such as "diagnostic likelihood ratio," "predictive power," "sensitivity," "specificity," "receiver operating characteristic curve," "ROC," "area under the curve." Most studies report the means for the target group and the comparison group, along with the reliability of a measure, but, unfortunately, these statistics do not directly inform an evidence-based approach to assessment. When searching for articles about assessment tools (or therapeutic interventions or psychosocial risk factors) it can be helpful to organize your search in a specific way; think about the *patient* group in which you are interested, the *intervention* (or assessment) of interest, the *comparison* intervention (or assessment), and the *outcome*. This approach is known as PICO (Straus et al., 2011). Not every clinical question fits neatly into this framework, but it is good for organizing your search before diving into the library databases. For example, if you were interested in finding a good measure to screen for ADHD, you might start with a background search to get a sense of some common measures (e.g., attention-deficit/hyperactivity disorder AND screen AND youth AND sensitivity). Once you have a couple of contenders, you can refine your search into a PICO framework—Patient: youth with ADHD; Assessment: Vanderbilt ADHD Diagnostic Rating Scale; Comparison: Conners' Parent Rating Scale; Outcome: Diagnosis (you might also include some of the terms suggested earlier; e.g., sensitivity/specificity or likelihood ratio to increase the chances of finding an article that has the information you need).

The TRIP database (*www.tripdatabase.com/#pico*) is a great resource for PICO questions, as it builds the framework right into its interface. Like TRIP, other databases that you might use (e.g., PsycINFO, PubMED) have their own interface and method for indexing terms. It is worth spending some time to learn how each works, so that you can tailor your searches accordingly. Searching for "anxiety" "youth" "measure" will yield thousands of hits, the majority of which will not be relevant. Using some of the assessment-specific terms listed earlier and capitalizing on database features (e.g., you can filter to get just results with youth samples, rather than including all papers that have "youth" in the text) will work to your advantage. You will also want to look for meta-analyses and systematic reviews. These are great because (as long as they are relatively recent) someone else has gone to the trouble of reviewing all the existing options for you, and you can quickly surmise what will be the best option, based on its psychometric properties, length/reading level, and cost. Although we all learned how to do an online search ages ago, it is also worthwhile to make an appointment with a reference librarian to get his or her guidance about how to best conduct these clinical searches. Reference librarians are search ninjas and always have some nifty insider tricks—these can help you find what you need much more quickly, and without scrolling through endless abstracts.

Of course, measures are not the only source of information to inform the assessment process; you may also be interested in finding the sensitivity/specificity or DLR for other factors that are likely to change the probability of a certain outcome, such as family history or sex. It is worth searching for the necessary statistics associated with these factors, too, but you may be more likely to find that risk related to individual characteristics is reported as odds ratios (ORs). The nomogram included with this chapter works using Bayes' theorem and cannot directly incorporate ORs. However, if you know the number of people who have the risk factor and the diagnosis (or outcome), and the number who do not, you can calculate both the OR and the DLR (Page & Attia, 2003; see Figure 2.7).

Back to those thousands of questionnaires: Should you figure out the DLRs for all of them? How long would that take? Too long is the answer. Remember the 80/20 rule we applied to figuring out the diagnostic base rates at your setting? It can help here, too. If your setting does not often serve youth with neurodevelopmental disorders, you

$$\text{Diagnostic likelihood ratio} + = \frac{\dfrac{\text{True Positive}}{\text{Condition Positive}}}{1 - \dfrac{\text{True Negative}}{\text{Condition Negative}}}$$

$$\text{Diagnostic likelihood ratio} - = \frac{1 - \dfrac{\text{True Positive}}{\text{Condition Positive}}}{\dfrac{\text{True Negative}}{\text{Condition Negative}}}$$

$$\text{Odds ratio} = \frac{\text{True Positive} * \text{True Negative}}{\text{False Positive} * \text{False Negative}}$$

FIGURE 2.7. Calculating odds ratios and diagnostic likelihood ratios.

probably do not need to figure out the DLRs for the Ages and Stages Questionnaire. Prioritize your time to figure out the best measures for the disorders you are most likely to see and calculate the DLRs for those. Many of the most common scenarios and most studied assessment tools have the details listed on Wikiversity (*https://en.wikiversity.org/wiki/Evidence-based_assessment/Which_Questionnaire_Should_I_Use%3f*). As unique cases come along, you will have reason to research measures and risk factors related to the disorders that fall outside the 80%, but you do not need to plan for everything as you are creating your assessment toolbox.

Applying What You Have Learned

Now you have determined the base rates for the diagnoses/outcomes that affect 80% of your clients, you have researched the tools that are most efficient at identifying these diagnoses/outcomes, you have calculated the DLRs that correspond to the recommended cutoff score(s), and you have your ruler ready for the nomogram. How is this preparation going to help you with Ty? As a reminder, Ty's mother is bringing him in due to "bad temper, lack of effort on homework, and slipping grades." Based on this information, you could probably justify hypothesizing about most childhood disorders—it could be ADHD that was not noticed earlier due to low academic expectations, it could be an internalizing disorder leading to irritable mood and lack of goal-directed activity, or it could be a behavior disorder like ODD. These diagnoses are even more probable given that they are all common in the outpatient clinic where you work. Although there are occasionally youth who present with more serious psychopathology, such as bipolar disorder or psychosis, you are not going to focus on those for now.

Because your clinic has all families complete the Achenbach measures before their intake appointment, you have found or calculated the DLRs for the most common diagnoses as part of your assessment toolkit. For example, the literature suggests that scores above 70 on the Externalizing subscale of the CBCL are associated with a DLR around 2 for ADHD (Raiker et al., 2017). At your clinic, the base rate for ADHD is 38% (if you want to go further, you could calculate rates for males and females separately, since boys are more likely to have ADHD). Pulling out your nomogram, you can put a dot on the mark for .38 on the left side, and a mark for your DLR of 2 in the middle. Drawing a line from .38 through 2, you arrive at a posterior probability of 55% (see Figure 2.8).

In contrast, Ty is reporting fewer externalizing problems than would be typical for a 12-year-old male. Taken at face value, that would be a strike against a diagnosis of ADHD. We can be more precise. Using the DLR for Ty's YSR Externalizing score takes you from 55% through 0.83 (the DLR for ADHD associated with his score of 44, based on Table 3 in Raiker et al., 2017) to ~50% (see Figure 2.8). On the one hand, Ty and his mom have contradictory perspectives. On the other hand, they do not exactly cancel out. The DLRs tell us that we should give more weight to the mom's report on this particular issue (2.0 vs. .83), and the net result is to move the probability of ADHD up from 38 to 50%.

Repeating this process for the other common diagnoses gives you a sense for what you need to investigate further and what you probably do not need to spend time on during the intake. For example, the posterior probability for any anxiety disorder is 37% given the base rate of 40%, a DLR of 1.51 associated with the CBCL score of 72, and

a DLR of 0.57 for Ty's YSR score of 44 (Figure 2.9; Van Meter et al., 2014). Here, the two perspectives come closer to canceling out. There is nothing that makes you more worried about anxiety, but neither is there anything too reassuring that anxiety is not an issue. Given how common anxiety problems are, it still would be worth exploring when you meet the family.

Similarly, you can also calculate the probability of a depression diagnosis; given a depression base rate of 26% and a DLR of 1.74 associated with his CBCL score and a DLR of 0.92 for his YSR score of 44, Ty's probability of depression is 36%. Finally, given the 38% base rate of ODD, a DLR of 1.72 for a CBCL score of 75, and a DLR of .80 for a YSR Externalizing score of 42, Ty's posterior probability of ODD is 46%.

Wait–Test–Treat

It can be helpful to think about three zones of action following each step of the assessment process (Straus, Glasziou, Richardson, & Haynes, 2011; Youngstrom et al., 2017). The Wait zone encom-

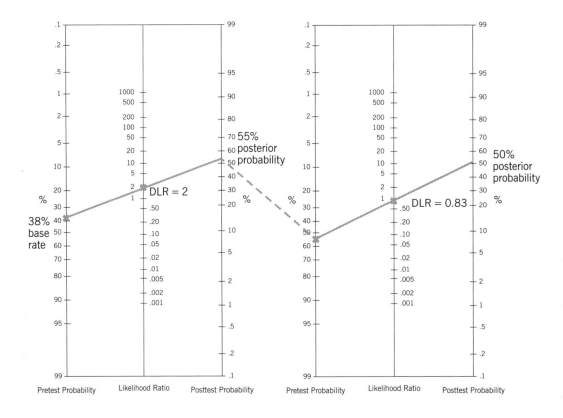

FIGURE 2.8. Using the nomogram to calculate the probability of ADHD.

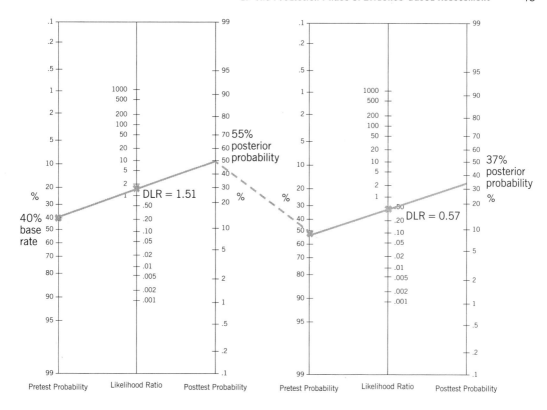

FIGURE 2.9. Using the nomogram to calculate the probability of an anxiety disorder.

passes probabilities low enough that the diagnosis is effectively ruled out unless new information later changes the probability. Probabilities in the Test zone require further assessment to determine whether treatment is warranted. The Treat zone is relevant when the probability is high enough that it makes sense to initiate an intervention. The thresholds between the Wait, Test, and Treat zones are not set at a specific probability. The reason for this is that the risks and benefits associated with different diagnoses vary, and this approach gives you flexibility to decide, with the family's input, when you might want to initiate treatment at a lower probability (e.g., for a low-burden intervention like mindfulness) or to hold off until you have more information and can be more confident about pursuing a more targeted treatment (e.g., referring the client to a psychiatrist for treatment with an antipsychotic medication). It can be helpful to associate the Wait, Test, and Treat zones with the colors of a stoplight: In the green Wait zone, there is no concern; in the yellow Test zone, you should slow down and carefully consider the situation; and in the red Treat zone, you should

stop and develop a plan to address the clinical problem.

Based on the presenting problem, the common disorders at your clinic, and the scores from the CBCL and YSR, you may not be able to rule anything out yet, but you can plan your intake appointment. Rather than knowing only that Ty's mom is worried about "bad temper, lack of effort on homework, and slipping grades," you know that you should be prepared to further assess for ADHD and also need to be prepared to assess for internalizing symptoms given the relatively high posterior probabilities for anxiety and depression. You also know to ask about known risk factors, such as family history, that may affect the probability of mood and anxiety disorders, in particular (Lieb, Isensee, Hofler, Pfister, & Wittchen, 2002; Moffitt et al., 2007). Additionally, because youth and their caregivers are likely to have different perspectives about internalizing and externalizing symptoms (De Los Reyes & Kazdin, 2005; Freeman et al., 2011), it is important that you talk to both Ty and his mom, and have each complete the measures that will offer specific information about the probable diagnoses. Before Ty and his mom arrive on Monday, you can collect the disorder-specific measures you want to use, take a few notes to guide your clinical interview, and print out a few nomograms to update probabilities as you go.

Conclusion

The focus of this chapter has been the Prediction phase of evidence-based assessment. The Prediction phase is crucial for focusing your clinical questions and preparing to conduct an evaluation that is efficient and that effectively minimizes the influence of bias, enabling you to make an accurate diagnosis/es and appropriately inform treatment (Youngstrom, 2008). You have learned how to narrow the list of probable diagnoses by administering screening measures early in the process, and how to avoid letting cognitive heuristics and other biases (often masquerading as clinical instinct!) derail your assessment. You know the importance of an assessment toolkit—comprised of the base rates of common disorders in your setting, both broad and disorder-specific measures (plus their DLRs), knowledge of how individual factors influence diagnostic risk, and other assessment tools to be described by Jensen-Doss and colleagues (Chapter 3) and Freeman and Young (Chapter 4) in the this volume—and should feel confident about your ability to assemble your toolkit, relying on EMR queries or chart reviews and well-designed database searches. Implementing the Prediction phase requires you to do a little work before your intake—you need to invest the time to assemble your toolkit. It can be challenging to find the extra hours, but this is a task that can be split among coworkers or approached in an incremental way, prioritizing the most common disorders. Like other investments, once you have your toolkit, it will pay off in both time and clinical performance. You also need to spend some time before the intake to distribute and score broad measures and to calculate the posterior probabilities based on the referral question. However, the evidence is overwhelming that using screening tools and a Bayesian approach to diagnostic decision making will improve both the accuracy and the overall efficiency of your diagnostic process (Croskerry, 2009; Elstein, 1999; Ely et al., 2011; Youngstrom, 2012; Youngstrom & Duax, 2005), and set your client up for the greatest odds of a successful treatment. Following the process outlined here will prepare you for the Prescription phase, when diagnoses are determined and treatment plans developed, and for the Process phase, during which progress toward treatment goals and, ultimately, outcomes, will be assessed. The Prediction phase is the foundation of your clinical work and will set you on track to bring your clients swift relief from their distress and positive treatment outcomes.

REFERENCES

Achenbach, T. (1991a). *Manual for the Child Behavior Checklist.* Burlington: Department of Psychiatry, University of Vermont.

Achenbach, T. (1991b). *Manual for the Youth Self-Report and 1991 profile.* Burlington: Department of Psychiatry, University of Vermont.

Achenbach, T. (1991c). *Teacher Report Form.* Burlington: Department of Psychiatry, University of Vermont.

Achenbach, T. M., & Rescorla, L. A. (2001). *Manual for the ASEBA School-Age Forms and Profiles.* Burlington: Department of Psychiatry, University of Vermont.

American Educational Research Association. (2014). *The standards for educational and psychological testing.* Washington, DC: American Psychological Association.

American Psychiatric Association. (2013). *Diagnostic and statistical manual of mental disorders* (5th ed.). Arlington, VA: Author.

Bruchmüller, K., & Meyer, T. D. (2009). Diagnostically irrelevant information can affect the likelihood of a diagnosis of bipolar disorder. *Journal of Affective Disorders, 116,* 148–151.

Burr, J. T. (1990). The tools of quality: Part VI. Pareto charts. *Quality Progress, 23,* 59–61.

Cannon, T. D., Yu, C., Addington, J., Bearden, C. E., Cadenhead, K. S., Cornblatt, B. A., . . . Kattan, M. W. (2016). An individualized risk calculator for research in prodromal psychosis. *American Journal of Psychiatry, 173,* 980–988.

Carlson, G. A., & Youngstrom, E. A. (2011). Two opinions about one child—What's the clinician to do? *Journal of Child and Adolescent Psychopharmacology, 21,* 385–387.

Carlson, J. F., Geisinger, K. F., & Jonson, J. L. (2017). *The twentieth mental measurements yearbook.* Lincoln, NE: Buros Center for Testing.

Croskerry, P. (2002). Achieving quality in clinical decision making: Cognitive strategies and detection of bias. *Academic Emergency Medicine, 9,* 1184–1204.

Croskerry, P. (2003). The importance of cognitive errors in diagnosis and strategies to minimize them. *Academic Medicine, 78,* 775–780.

Croskerry, P. (2009). Clinical cognition and diagnostic error: Applications of a dual process model of reasoning. *Advances in Health Sciences Education, 14,* 27–35.

De Los Reyes, A., Augenstein, T. M., Wang, M., Thomas, S. A., Drabick, D. A., Burgers, D. E., & Rabinowitz, J. (2015). The validity of the multi-informant approach to assessing child and adolescent mental health. *Psychological Bulletin, 141*, 858–900.

De Los Reyes, A., & Kazdin, A. E. (2005). Informant discrepancies in the assessment of childhood psychopathology: A critical review, theoretical framework, and recommendations for further study. *Psychological Bulletin, 131*, 483–509.

Elstein, A. S. (1999). Heuristics and biases: Selected errors in clinical reasoning. *Academic Medicine, 74*, 791–794.

Elstein, A. S., & Schwarz, A. (2002). Evidence base of clinical diagnosis: Clinical problem solving and diagnostic decision making: Selective review of the cognitive literature. *British Medical Journal, 324*, 729–732.

Ely, J. W., Graber, M. L., & Croskerry, P. (2011). Checklists to reduce diagnostic errors. *Academic Medicine, 86*, 307–313.

Ferdinand, R. F., van der Ende, J., & Verhulst, F. C. (2004). Parent–adolescent disagreement regarding psychopathology in adolescents from the general population as a risk factor for adverse outcome. *Journal of Abnormal Psychology, 113*, 198–206.

Fiedler, K., Brinkmann, B., Betsch, T., & Wild, B. (2000). A sampling approach to biases in conditional probability judgments: Beyond base rate neglect and statistical format. *Journal of Experimental Psychology: General, 129*, 399–418.

Freeman, A., Youngstrom, E., Freeman, M., Youngstrom, J., & Findling, R. (2011). Is caregiver–adolescent disagreement due to differences in thresholds for reporting manic symptoms? *Journal of Child and Adolescent Psychopharmacology, 21*, 425–432.

Fusar-Poli, P., Rutigliano, G., Stahl, D., Davies, C., Bonoldi, I., Reilly, T., & McGuire, P. (2017). Development and validation of a clinically based risk calculator for the transdiagnostic prediction of psychosis. *JAMA Psychiatry, 74*, 493–500.

Galanter, C. A., & Patel, V. L. (2005). Medical decision making: A selective review for child psychiatrists and psychologists. *Journal of Child Psychology and Psychiatry, 46*, 675–689.

Garb, H. N. (1998). *Studying the clinician: Judgment research and psychological assessment.* Washington, DC: American Psychological Association.

Hafeman, D. M., Merranko, J., Goldstein, T. R., Axelson, D., Goldstein, B. I., Monk, K., . . . Birmaher, B. (2017). Assessment of a person-level risk calculator to predict new-onset bipolar spectrum disorder in youth at familial risk. *JAMA Psychiatry, 74*, 841–847.

Jarrett, M. A., Meter, A. V., Youngstrom, E. A., Hilton, D. C., & Ollendick, T. H. (2018). Evidence-based assessment of ADHD in youth using a receiver operating characteristic approach. *Journal of Clinical Child and Adolescent Psychology*, 1–13.

Jenkins, M. M., & Youngstrom, E. A. (2016). A randomized controlled trial of cognitive debiasing improves assessment and treatment selection for pediatric bipolar disorder. *Journal of Consulting and Clinical Psychology, 84*(4), 323–333.

Jenkins, M., Youngstrom, E., Washburn, J., & Youngstrom, J. (2011). Evidence-based strategies improve assessment of pediatric bipolar disorder by community practitioners. *Professional Psychology: Research and Practice, 42*, 121–129.

Jensen-Doss, A., Youngstrom, E. A., Youngstrom, J. K., Feeny, N. C., & Findling, R. L. (2014). Predictors and moderators of agreement between clinical and research diagnoses for children and adolescents. *Journal of Consulting and Clinical Psychology, 82*, 1151–1162.

Kraemer, H. C. (1992). *Evaluating medical tests: Objective and quantitative guidelines.* Newbury Park, CA: SAGE.

Lieb, R., Isensee, B., Hofler, M., Pfister, H., & Wittchen, H.-U. (2002). Parental major depression and the risk of depression and other mental disorders in offspring: A prospective-longitudinal community study. *Archives of General Psychiatry, 59*, 365–374.

Lighthall, G. K., & Vazquez-Guillamet, C. (2015). Understanding decision making in critical care. *Clinical Medicine and Research, 13*, 156–168.

Lilienfeld, S. O., & Lynn, S. J. (2015). Errors/biases in clinical decision making. In R. L. Cautin & S. O. Lilienfeld (Eds.), *The encyclopedia of clinical psychology* (Vol. 2). New York: Wiley-Blackwell.

Meehl, P. E. (1954). *Clinical versus statistical prediction: A theoretical analysis and a review of the evidence.* Minneapolis: University of Minnesota Press.

Moffitt, T. E., Caspi, A., Harrington, H., Milne, B. J., Melchior, M., Goldberg, D., & Poulton, R. (2007). Generalized anxiety disorder and depression: Childhood risk factors in a birth cohort followed to age 32. *Psychological Medicine, 37*, 441–452.

Page, J. H., & Attia, J. (2003). Using Bayes' nomogram to help interpret odds ratios. *ACP Journal Club, 139*, A11–A12.

Patel, V. L., Kaufman, D. R., & Arocha, J. F. (2002). Emerging paradigms of cognition in medical decision-making. *Journal of Biomedical Informatics, 35*, 52–75.

Raiker, J. S., Freeman, A. J., Perez-Algorta, G., Frazier, T. W., Findling, R. L., & Youngstrom, E. A. (2017). Accuracy of Achenbach scales in the screening of attention-deficit/hyperactivity disorder in a community mental health clinic. *Journal of the American Academy of Child and Adolescent Psychiatry, 56*, 401–409.

Ringoot, A. P., van der Ende, J., Jansen, P. W., Measelle, J. R., Basten, M., So, P., . . . Tiemeier, H. (2015). Why mothers and young children agree or disagree in their reports of the child's problem behavior. *Child Psychiatry and Human Development, 46*, 913–927.

Sackett, D. L., Straus, S. E., Richardson, W. S., Rosenberg, W., & Haynes, R. B. (2000). *Evidence-based medicine: How to practice and teach EBM* (2nd ed.). New York: Churchill Livingstone.

Straus, S. E., Glasziou, P., Richardson, W. S., & Haynes, R. B. (2011). *Evidence-based medicine: How to practice and teach EBM* (4th ed.). New York: Churchill Livingstone.

Straus, S., Tetroe, J., & Graham, I. D. (2011). *Knowledge translation in health care: Moving from evidence to practice.* London: BMJ Books.

Tversky, A., & Kahneman, D. (1974). Judgment under uncertainty: Heuristics and biases. *Science, 185,* 1124–1131.

Van Meter, A. R., Algorta, G. P., Youngstrom, E. A., Lechtman, Y., Youngstrom, J. K., Feeny, N. C., & Findling, R. L. (2018). Assessing for suicidal behavior in youth using the Achenbach system of empirically based assessment. *European Child and Adolescent Psychiatry, 27,* 159–169.

Van Meter, A., Youngstrom, E., Youngstrom, J. K., Ollendick, T., Demeter, C., & Findling, R. L. (2014). Clinical decision making about child and adolescent anxiety disorders using the Achenbach system of empirically based assessment. *Journal of Clinical Child and Adolescent Psychology, 43,* 552–565.

Wolkenstein, L., Bruchmüller, K., Schmid, P., & Meyer, T. D. (2011). Misdiagnosing bipolar disorder: Do clinicians show heuristic biases? *Journal of Affective Disorders, 130,* 405–412.

Youngstrom, E. (2008). Evidence-based strategies for the assessment of developmental psychopathology: Measuring prediction, prescription, and process. In W. Craighead, D. Miklowitz, & L. Craighead (Eds.), *Developmental psychopathology* (pp. 34–77). New York: Wiley.

Youngstrom, E. A. (2012). Future directions in psychological assessment: Combining evidence-based medicine innovations with psychology's historical strengths to enhance utility. *Journal of Clinical Child and Adolescent Psychology, 42,* 139–159.

Youngstrom, E. A. (2014). A primer on receiver operating characteristic analysis and diagnostic efficiency statistics for pediatric psychology: We are ready to ROC. *Journal of Pediatric Psychology, 39,* 204–221.

Youngstrom, E. A., Choukas-Bradley, S., Calhoun, C. D., & Jensen-Doss, A. (2014). Clinical guide to the evidence-based assessment approach to diagnosis and treatment. *Cognitive and Behavioral Practice, 22,* 20–35.

Youngstrom, E., & Duax, J. (2005). Evidence-based assessment of pediatric bipolar disorder: Part I. Base rate and family history. *Journal of the American Academy of Child and Adolescent Psychiatry, 44,* 712–717.

Youngstrom, E., Findling, R., & Calabrese, J. (2003). Who are the comorbid adolescents?: Agreement between psychiatric diagnosis, youth, parent, and teacher report. *Journal of Abnormal Child Psychology, 31,* 231–245.

Youngstrom, E. A., Genzlinger, J. E., Egerton, G. A., & Van Meter, A. R. (2015). Multivariate meta-analysis of the discriminative validity of caregiver, youth, and teacher rating scales for pediatric bipolar disorder: Mother knows best about mania. *Archives of Scientific Psychology, 3,* 112–137.

Youngstrom, E. A., Meyers, O. I., Youngstrom, J. K., Calabrese, J. R., & Findling, R. L. (2006a). Comparing the effects of sampling designs on the diagnostic accuracy of eight promising screening algorithms for pediatric bipolar disorder. *Biological Psychiatry, 60,* 1013–1019.

Youngstrom, E., Meyers, O., Youngstrom, J. K., Calabrese, J. R., & Findling, R. L. (2006b). Diagnostic and measurement issues in the assessment of pediatric bipolar disorder: Implications for understanding mood disorder across the life cycle. *Development and Psychopathology, 18,* 989–1021.

Youngstrom, E. A., & Van Meter, A. (2016). Empirically supported assessment of children and adolescents. *Clinical Psychology: Science and Practice, 23,* 327–347.

Youngstrom, E. A., Van Meter, A., Frazier, T. W., Hunsley, J., Prinstein, M. J., Ong, M.-L., & Youngstrom, J. K. (2017). Evidence-based assessment as an integrative model for applying psychological science to guide the voyage of treatment. *Clinical Psychology: Science and Practice, 24,* 331–363.

Youngstrom, E. A., Youngstrom, J. K., Freeman, A. J., De Los Reyes, A., Feeny, N. C., & Findling, R. L. (2011). Informants are not all equal: Predictors and correlates of clinician judgments about caregiver and youth credibility. *Journal of Child and Adolescent Psychopharmacology, 21,* 407–415.

CHAPTER 3

The Prescription Phase
of Evidence-Based Assessment

Amanda Jensen-Doss, Zabin Patel, Elizabeth Casline,
and Bryce D. McLeod

The prescription phase of assessment sets the stage for subsequent treatment. This phase begins at the intake assessment, building off of the more general information on symptoms and risk factors gathered during the prediction phase. The data collected during the previous phase are used to identify areas in need of more in-depth assessment. Given that the tools associated with the prescription phase are often more time and cost intensive, data from the prediction phase and the youth psychopathology and treatment literature may be used to focus the assessment on issues most relevant to the client. The prescription phase ends when the initial case conceptualization is generated and treatment begins, leading directly into the process/progress/outcome phase.

According to Youngstrom and colleagues' (2017) evidence-based assessment (EBA) model, the prescription phase includes (1) use of focused, incremental assessments (e.g., problem-specific rating scales) to narrow the diagnostic possibilities (Step 6); (2) application of intensive methods to finalize the diagnoses (Step 7); and (3) gathering relevant data to develop a case conceptualization for treatment planning (Step 8). Throughout the prescription phase, client and caregiver preferences (Step 9) are incorporated into decisions such as who should be involved in the assessment and in treatment, what problems should be prioritized in treatment, and what treatment components should be selected.

In this chapter, we discuss the assessment tools and strategies associated with the prescription phase. Given the focus of the prescription phase on case conceptualization, we have organized the chapter around the stages of generating a case conceptualization, drawn from the science-informed case conceptualization model (Christon, McLeod, & Jensen-Doss, 2015; McLeod, Jensen-Doss, &

Ollendick, 2013a). As we discuss in detail below, the stages from this model map nicely onto EBA model (Youngstrom et al., 2017) steps for the prescription phase. To orient the reader, we present a general discussion of case conceptualization (i.e., the process of pulling assessment data together into a "map" of the client's problems that can be used to guide treatment). Next, we go through each stage of the process. Within each stage, we detail the applicable *assessment tools*, including psychometric and other considerations involved in choosing which tools to apply to specific clients. We also describe salient *assessment strategies*, or procedures for interpreting, integrating, or utilizing assessment data to make clinical decisions for each stage. To set the stage for this discussion, however, we first provide a brief introduction to psychometric considerations relevant to the prescription phase.

Psychometric Considerations of the Prescription Phase

In their 2017 article outlining the EBA model, Youngstrom and colleagues provide a rubric for evaluating the score reliability, validity, and utility of assessment tools and strategies. They also organize psychometric parameters based on the assessment objective, or the three P's of the treatment processes, to underscore that selection of assessment strategies depends on the goal. For example, a 60-minute structured diagnostic interview may help determine whether a client meets diagnostic criteria, and thus be useful for the prescription phase; however, the same interview may not capture client symptom changes over treatment and may thus be less useful (and less practical!) for the process phase. In addition to the clinical objective, the selection of an assessment tool depends on who is being assessed. Thus, an instrument's quality should be evaluated in consideration of client demographics (Newman, Rugh, & Ciarlo, 2004). For example, a 30-item depression rating scale may be reliable when used with an adolescent but be less developmentally appropriate for a young child.

The key psychometric properties relevant to the prescription phase include interrater reliability, content validity, construct validity, prescriptive validity, and validity generalization. As we discuss below, these psychometric characteristics must also be balanced with the clinical utility of instruments, or whether they are practical for use in a specific clinical setting.

Interrater Reliability

Broadly, *reliability* refers to the degree to which results from an instrument are consistent over multiple measurements (Anastasi, 1988). For example, a weighing scale is considered reliable if it indicates the same weight of an object each time. Although reliability is assessed in multiple ways (e.g., internal consistency, test–retest, parallel forms), interrater reliability (IRR) is the measure of reliability most relevant to the prescription phase. IRR refers to the extent that two clinicians assign the same diagnosis using the same diagnostic tool, or two observers generate the same ratings when using observational methods. Thus, it is a method of quantifying the degree of agreement between two clinicians who make independent ratings about a client's symptoms or behavior (Hallgren, 2012).

Traditionally, IRR has been reported as percentage of "agreement among clinicians" across diagnoses (McHugh, 2012). For example, if agreement between diagnoses is 80%, this is directly interpreted as the percentage of diagnoses that are correct, while 20% of the diagnoses are considered incorrect due to disagreement. However, as an indicator of IRR, percentage agreement is problematic, as it does not account for chance agreement between two clinicians, which would lead percentage agreement to be higher for rare diagnoses (McHugh, 2012).

Cohen's (1960) kappa is therefore preferred to percentage agreement, as this method accounts for the level of agreement between clinicians when they do not know the correct diagnoses but are merely guessing. Kappa is a standardized value that ranges from –1 to +1, where 0 represents the *amount of agreement that can be expected from random chance*, and 1 represents *perfect agreement*. Since kappa is standardized, it can be used to compare IRR across studies and diagnoses. Kappa is traditionally interpreted using the following values: ≤ 0 indicates no agreement between clinicians; .01–.2 indicates slight agreement; .21–.4 indicates fair agreement; .41–.60 indicates moderate agreement; .61–.8 indicates substantial agreement; and .81–1.0 indicates almost perfect agreement (Cohen, 1960; Landis & Koch, 1977). However, some consider this standard too high for a complex activity such as diagnostic assessment and have argued for lower cutoffs (Kraemer, Kupfer, Clarke, Narrow, & Regier, 2012).

IRR is also used for observational assessment methods, such as the Autism Diagnostic Observation Schedule (e.g., Lord et al., 2012), in which clinicians observe and code client behavior using a standard coding system. Whereas kappa is useful for assessing the IRR of categorical codes, such as whether a client meets criteria for an autism spectrum disorder diagnosis, the IRR of continuous codes (e.g., severity rating of symptoms) is typically assessed using the intraclass correlation coefficient (ICC; Hallgren, 2012). The ICC is preferred over other correlation coefficients because it captures both consistency between raters (i.e., whether they are correlated) and their level of absolute agreement (i.e., whether they agree on the values); without accounting for both, it is possible that one rater could be consistently rating 2 points lower than the other rater. ICC values range from –1 to 1, with an ICC estimate of 1 indicating *perfect agreement* and 0 indicating *random agreement* (Hallgren, 2012). IRR using ICC values can be interpreted using the following criteria: <.40 indicates *poor agreement*, .40–.59 indicates *fair agreement*, .60–.74 indicates *good agreement*, and .75–1.00 indicates *excellent* (Cicchetti, 1994).

Other indices of reliability that are relevant to the prescription phase are internal consistency (i.e., whether all items of a scale "hang together" and assess the same construct) and test–retest reliability (i.e., whether a scale provides the same score over multiple administrations). These reliability indicators are especially relevant when rating scales are incorporated into the assessment and, in the case of retest reliability, when a clinician anticipates that a particular characteristic is relatively stable (e.g., intellectual ability). These issues are discussed in more depth in Van Meter (Chapter 2, this volume) and Freeman and Young (Chapter 4, this volume), so interested readers are referred to these chapters for more information about these concepts.

Validity

Although the results of an assessment may be reliable, this does not demonstrate that the results are valid, or accurate (Anastasi, 1988). For example, a weighing scale is considered valid if it provides the true weight of an object. In discussing validity, it important to emphasize that validity does not refer to the instrument itself (e.g., an assessment tool is not valid or invalid). Rather, assessment data have more or less validity to support interpretation of scores for a specific purpose, at a given time, with a particular client (Downing, 2003; Furr & Bacharach, 2008). To support score validity, the interpretation of assessment data must be grounded

in psychological theory and research, bridging together data collection and testing, critical evaluation, and logical inference (Downing, 2003). Thus, determining score validity may be viewed as an evidence-based argument to demonstrate a relation between scores on an assessment tool and what it claims to assess (Furr & Bacharach, 2008). This evidence can be used to support, or not support, the use of an assessment tool, but it is a requirement of the assessment process (Downing, 2003). Without evidence of score validity, data collected from psychological assessment have little or no intrinsic meaning (Downing, 2003).

Content Validity

Content validity refers to the degree that an instrument's content represents all aspects of the domain of interest (e.g., a specific disorder). For example, a tool used to assess a depressive episode would demonstrate content validity if it included items about the range of symptoms and behaviors found in the fifth edition of the *Diagnostic and Statistical Manual of Mental Disorders* (DSM-5; American Psychiatric Association, 2013), such as change in sleep and appetite, low energy, and mood shifts, instead of narrowly focusing on sadness. Content validity is not established via statistical procedures, but through expert review. A common approach used to establish content validity is to first define the target domain, develop items to represent that domain, then ask experts to rate whether the items reflect important aspects of the disorder being measured (Jensen et al., 2007; McLeod, Jensen-Doss, & Ollendick, 2013b).

Construct Validity

Psychological disorders are abstract, theoretical models that explain patterns in functioning (Kendell & Jablensky, 2003). Broadly, *construct validity* is a dimensional term that refers to the degree that an individual's assessment data (e.g., depressive symptom count) correlate with the theoretical disorder the test was designed to assess (e.g., depression). In the prescription phase, construct validity can be applied to both the diagnostic construct being assessed and the data collected from an assessment instrument. In the case of diagnosis, construct validity refers to the extent that a diagnosis has evidentiary support (e.g., major depression represents a distinct syndrome; Aboraya, France, Young, Curci, & Lepage, 2005). Regarding assessment tools, construct validity is reflected in the structure of the item scores and the extent to which those scores capture a client's symptoms and behaviors associated with a disorder (Aboraya et al., 2005). Construct validity can be evaluated in several ways and is considered an overarching term under which evidence is gathered from multiple sources to build a case to support the score validity of an instrument. In the prescription phase of assessment, two key sources of validity are considered: concurrent validity and predictive validity.

Concurrent validity refers to whether scores on the tool are related to scores on other instruments at the same point in time. For instance, if a clinician diagnosed a client with depression based on the results of a diagnostic interview and the client scored in the clinical range on a symptom checklist for depression, this would be evidence of concurrent validity. Concurrent validity can be *convergent, discriminant,* or *discriminative. Convergent validity* helps establish what an instrument actually assesses and is demonstrated through an association with other instruments of the same construct (e.g., Do scores on an instrument designed to assess depression converge with scores produced by other depression instruments?). Discriminant validity helps establish what an instrument does not assess and is demonstrated by low correlations with instruments of unrelated constructs (e.g., Do scores on an instrument designed to assess depression evidence low correlations with scores on a disruptive behavior disorder instrument?). *Discriminative validity* refers to whether the instrument can differentiate between distinct groups of individuals. For example, DSM-5 (American Psychiatric Association, 2013), differentiates between dysthymia and major depression, even though their respective symptoms overlap. Scores on an instrument would demonstrate discriminative validity if they distinguish between those disorders. Indicators of discriminative validity are the area under the curve from a receiver operator characteristic (ROC) analysis, and the diagnostic sensitivity and specificity attached to a score threshold or range, which are discussed in detail by Van Meter (Chapter 2, this volume). Finally, predictive validity is another indicator of construct validity, which indicates whether assessment data accurately predict a criterion. "Prognostic validity" narrowly refers to prediction of a criterion that will occur in the future, whereas "predictive validity" is a more general term that could include regression models predicting a criterion measured at the same time as other predictors.

Prescriptive Validity

Prescriptive validity, also referred to as "treatment validity" or "treatment utility," refers to the extent to which an instrument has evidentiary support to guide treatment selection, especially as distinct from predicting a diagnosis (Mash & Hunsley, 2005; Youngstrom et al., 2017). It is considered crucial for the prescription phase due to its role in treatment selection (Chambless & Hollon, 2012; Cone, 1997; Nelson-Gray, 2003).

Whereas treatment–outcome studies ask "How effective is treatment?", research that evaluates prescriptive validity asks "Does having these pieces of assessment data contribute to successful treatment outcome?" (Nelson-Gray, 2003). Although little research has examined prescriptive validity, in recent years it has become easier for clinicians to identify treatments that are associated with the remission of a particular diagnosis or a cluster of diagnoses. For example, Division 53, the Society of Clinical Child and Adolescent Psychology, of the American Psychological Association created the Effective Child Therapy website (*www.effectivechildtherapy.org*) that publishes a list of treatments that are "well established" or "probably efficacious" in treating children with specific diagnoses. Because knowing a client's diagnosis or target problem is required to use these lists to match clients to treatments, the assumption underlying these lists is that diagnostic data have prescriptive validity. However, this assumption has rarely been evaluated empirically.

When selecting a treatment to address a client's presenting problem, it is important to consider treatment moderators (Chambless & Hollon, 2012; Youngstrom et al., 2017). Certain client characteristics may predict better outcomes when using one treatment compared to another. For example, the Multimodal Treatment Study of Children with ADHD Cooperative group (1999) found that behavior treatment was more effective than community care, but only for youth with comorbid anxiety; in this case, anxiety comorbidity may be a moderator with prescriptive validity.

Validity Generalization

In research studies, the score reliability and validity of an assessment tool are evaluated among those enrolled in the study, or the study sample (Dekkers, von Elm, Algra, Romijn, & Vandenbroucke, 2010). Thoughtful study design, careful data collection, and appropriate statistical analysis are at the core of "internal validity," or the application of results to the study population (Kukull & Ganguli, 2012). Although internal validity has been widely investigated, validity generalization has received less attention (Sutton & Higgins, 2008). Instead of focusing on threats to causal inferences, validity generalization is concerned with the application of study findings to populations different than the study sample, such as using an instrument with research support in a community clinic setting.

The local context may differ in important ways from a controlled research setting, which can serve as an obstacle to using research evidence to guide selection of an assessment tool. Primary factors that impact validity generalization include client demographics (e.g., sex, age, racial and cultural background, language) and the setting in which clients are being assessed (e.g., clinic, school, home; Dekkers et al., 2010; Hunsley & Mash, 2018). It is important to understand the characteristics of the samples used to establish the score reliability and validity of each instrument, and whether findings have been consistent across groups with different characteristics. Ideally, the normative sample used to develop an instrument should be large and diverse, inclusive of clinical and nonclinical populations, and representative of the population of interest (Anastasi, 1988; Hunsley & Mash, 2018). If a given client is different from members of the sample used to develop and test the instrument, then scores on the instrument may not yield valid data. For example, individuals from a different population may have trouble understanding interview questions, or the scoring algorithms might not accurately capture their psychopathology. Guidelines that have been published for the process of translation and cross-cultural validation of instruments (Beaton, Bombardier, Guillemin, & Ferraz, 2000; Guillemin, Bombardier, & Beaton, 1993) typically involve item analysis, field testing, and psychometric validation.

Clinical Utility

Finally, practicality is important to consider when selecting an assessment instrument. Factors that influence administration decisions include cost, time spent scoring, ease of interpretation, and level of required training. A clinician must consider the acceptability of an instrument to clients and its potential negative impact on the therapeutic relationship (Mash & Hunsley, 2005). Furthermore, clinicians must take into consideration

whether an instrument is available in the client's native language (Doss, Cook, & McLeod, 2008). There are now pages on Wikipedia and Wikiversity that emphasize the best freely available tools (Beidas et al., 2015) for assessing different constructs and clinical issues (*https://en.wikiversity.org/wiki/Evidence-based_assessment/Which_Questionnaire_Should_I_Use%3f*), and many translated versions are available on these pages as well.

The Goal of the Prescription Phase: The Case Conceptualization

The ultimate goal of the prescription phase is to generate a case conceptualization to guide treatment. A *case conceptualization* is broadly defined as a set of hypotheses about the causes, antecedents, and maintaining factors of a client's treatment targets (Eells, 2007; Haynes, O'Brien, & Kaholokula, 2011; Nezu, Nezu, & Lombardo, 2004). Generated from the initial assessment data and guided by empirical and theoretical literature, a case conceptualization provides a road map for selecting the best treatment approach for a given client. Once developed, the case conceptualization guides ongoing assessment and treatment by identifying treatment targets and candidate mechanisms of change (Eells & Lombart, 2004).

Case conceptualization is best thought of as an ongoing process, wherein hypotheses are generated and then tested using ongoing assessment during treatment. Consistent with the probabilistic approach to assessment, the initial case conceptualization can be considered a "best guess" of how to proceed in treatment, and the treatment plan should include an assessment plan that will support the ongoing testing and possible revision of the conceptualization. It is important that the conceptualization be grounded in empirically supported developmental and psychopathology theories regarding the development and maintenance of target behaviors observed in a particular client (Haynes et al., 2011; Hunsley & Mash, 2007). A well-designed case conceptualization directly informs (1) treatment planning (e.g., selection of treatment targets), (2) treatment selection (i.e., the interventions designed to alter the causal and maintaining factors most relevant to the client), and (3) treatment monitoring.

Case conceptualization is considered a core competency for mental health professionals (e.g., American Psychological Association, 2011; British Psychological Society, 2017) and a central activity in the evidence-based practice of psychology (EBPP; APA Presidential Task Force on Evidence-Based Practice, 2006). Approaches to case conceptualization can be broadly classified into two groups. *Theory-specific* approaches to case conceptualization typically start from a specific theoretical perspective (e.g., cognitive theory, behavioral theory), and subsequently organize assessment data within that framework (e.g., Haynes et al., 2011; Persons, 2008). *General* approaches organize information into hypotheses grounded in whatever theories best fit a client's causal and maintaining factors (e.g., Eells, 2015; McLeod et al., 2013a).

Despite the centrality of case conceptualization to clinical practice, little research evaluates what type of case conceptualization approach is best, or even what an "empirically supported" approach to case conceptualization should look like. While some research shows that clinicians can demonstrate reliable case conceptualizations guided by particular theories, findings are mixed, and the methodological rigor of these studies is variable (Flinn, Braham, & das Nair, 2015). Limited research has focused on understanding the validity of case conceptualizations (Mumma, 2011). As such, it is important to remember that the collection of ongoing treatment progress and process data creates a feedback loop that can be used to assess the validity of any client's case conceptualization (Mumma & Fluck, 2016).

Given that multiple theoretical approaches may be empirically supported for the same target problem (e.g., cognitive-behavioral treatment and interpersonal treatment for adolescent depression; Weersing, Jeffreys, Do, Schwartz, & Bolano, 2017), our position is that taking a more general approach to case conceptualization helps avoid taking a "one size fits all" approach to treatment selection, while acknowledging that this position is in need of future research. One general model developed specifically from a developmental psychopathology perspective is the science-informed case conceptualization model (Christon et al., 2015; McLeod et al., 2013a), which emphasizes utilizing the developmental psychopathology and treatment literatures to generate hypotheses that can subsequently be tested over the course of treatment through the assessment process. Throughout the rest of this chapter, we detail the stages of this model and describe the assessment tools and strategies relevant to each stage (see Table 3.1). As noted throughout the discussion, some tools and strategies are relevant to multiple stages of the process. It is also important to note that case conceptualization is an iterative rather than a linear process. We use the Ty case example to illustrate each stage.

Conceptualization Stage 1: Identify and Quantify Presenting Problems and Causal/Maintaining Factors

The goals of the first stage are to generate a list of target problems, characterize them in order to determine their relative importance, and identify factors that might be causing or maintaining

TABLE 3.1. The Science-Informed Case Conceptualization Model

Stage	Relevant tools	Relevant strategies
Stage 1: Identify and quantify presenting problems and causal/maintaining factors.	• Rating scales • Idiographic tools • Interviews	• Functional analysis
Stage 2: Assign diagnoses.	• Interviews • Observational methods • Cognitive tests	• Bayesian approaches • LEAD procedures • DSM model for differential diagnosis
Stage 3: Develop initial case conceptualization.	• Data gathered in Stages 1 and 2	• Addressing informant discrepancies
Stage 4: Proceed with treatment plan and selection.	• Data gathered in Stages 1 and 2 • Evidence-based treatments literature	• Shared decision-making strategies
Stage 5: Monitor and evaluate treatment outcomes and revise case conceptualization as necessary.	• Rating scales • Idiographic tools • Monitor relevant process variables (e.g., therapy alliance, mastery of treatment strategies)	• Functional analysis

them. Something can be important because it is likely to occur, or because it is serious (Morrison, 2014). Suicide is a rare event, but it is so serious that it deserves assessment consideration, for example. It is a good strategy to always have multiple hypotheses early in the assessment process and have them compete. Building a list helps avoid the well-documented traps of confirmation bias and calling off the search when the first idea is confirmed (Galanter & Patel, 2005).

Once the target problems have been identified, additional variables are identified that can form the basis of the conceptualization. *Historical events* are nonmalleable factors that set the stage for the current problems (e.g., a genetic history of anxiety, or a head injury in a car accident). Whereas historical events cannot be addressed in treatment, these events often result in specific *causal factors* (e.g., avoidant coping style, negative cognitive styles) that can be targeted. It is also important to determine the *antecedent factors* that surround each target problem, including where and when the problem occurs. Identifying antecedent conditions for each target problem can help guide both diagnosis and treatment planning. Finally, *maintaining factors* are either internal or external conditions that reinforce or punish target problems.

Assessment Tools Relevant to Conceptualization Stage 1

The first three steps of the EBA model are relevant to this first stage of case conceptualization. Information from the incremental, focused assessment in Step 6 and from the more intensive methods in Step 7 can be used to identify potential target problems, while the assessments for treatment planning and goal setting (Step 8) can be used to identify the historical, causal, antecedent, and maintaining factors. Potential target problems can be identified using idiographic assessment tools, elevations on rating scales, or symptoms endorsed through interviews. Historical, causal, antecedent, and maintaining factors can also be identified through interviews or rating scales.

Rating Scales

As noted by Van Meter (Chapter 2), broad rating scales quickly provide the clinician with information about a client's problem areas. In the prediction phase, problem-focused rating scales can help gather more nuanced and specific information to help narrow down diagnostic possibilities before utilizing more intensive assessment strategies. As

noted by Youngstrom and colleagues (2017), more specific rating scales have greater diagnostic accuracy than broad instruments, but they can still have high rates of false positives, so using broad instruments to narrow the diagnostic possibilities in the prediction phase before moving to more specific rating scales can be a good balance between assessment efficiency and accuracy. The diagnostic likelihood ratio process outlined by Van Meter (Chapter 2, this volume) can utilize results from these narrow rating scales to refine the probabilities generated by the broad instruments.

In addition to assessing psychopathology, rating scales can aid in assessing other variables relevant to the case conceptualization. For example, rating scales can be used to assess causal factors such as emotional avoidance (e.g., the Emotional Avoidance Strategy Inventory for Adolescents [EASI-A]; Kennedy & Ehrenreich-May, 2017), cognitive style (e.g., the Adolescent Coping Style Questionnaire [ACSQ]; Hankin & Abramson, 2002), or parental psychopathology. Some rating scales also examine the function of target problems, such as the School Refusal Assessment Scale, which examines whether school refusal is a function of avoidance of negative affect, avoidance of social situations, pursuit of attention from others, or pursuit of some other tangible reinforcement (Kearney, 2002).

Because rating scales were covered in depth by Van Meter (Chapter 2, this volume), we refer readers to that chapter for a discussion of relevant psychometric considerations when choosing a rating scale.

Idiographic Tools

Idiographic, or individualized, instruments stem from the behavioral assessment tradition (Cone, 1986) and are traditionally used to track within-individual change on specific, tailored assessment targets, such as tantrums or incidents of self-harm. Although these instruments are most relevant to the process phase and are discussed in more detail by Freeman and Young (Chapter 4, this volume), the process of setting up idiographic assessment can help identify the treatment targets most important to clients and caregivers via a collaborative process. For example, Weisz and colleagues' (2011) Top Problems assessment tool asks clients and caregivers to identify up to three problems that are most important to focus on in treatment and to rate how big a problem it is for the client on a scale from 0 (*not at all*) to 10 (*very, very much*). The problems listed and the relative rankings of each can be helpful in identifying target problems. While the problems identified through instruments such as the Top Problems tool typically correspond to items from rating scales, they often provide more specific information tailored to the unique problems experienced by individual clients (e.g., Weisz et al. provide the example of a Top Problem item of "Sad because she doesn't have a dad anymore" versus a rating scale item of "Sad, unhappy, depressed"). Eliciting information about individualized treatment goals also helps emphasize client goals and priorities and may promote client and caregiver engagement in treatment (McGuire et al., 2014; Sales & Alves, 2012).

Interviews

Information relevant to Stage 1 can also be generated through a variety of interview strategies, including both unstandardized (i.e., interviews with open-ended questions, tailored to the client, often used at the beginning of the assessment to gather general information about the client) and standardized interviews (i.e., interviews with set questions and scoring algorithms designed to gather assessment data for a specific purpose). Because interviews are most closely aligned with assigning diagnoses, we discussed them in depth under Stage 2. However, we wish to note here that diagnostic interviews can help identify target problems and contextual factors (e.g., that a client's anxiety is related to separating from caregivers) as well as specific historical, casual, antecedent, or maintaining factors (e.g., Structured Developmental History Interview for the Behavioral Assessment System for Children [BASC-3]; Reynolds & Kamphaus, 2015).

Assessment Strategies Relevant to Conceptualization Stage 1

Once a list of target problems has been generated, their relative importance can be determined through a variety of strategies that include examining severity ratings on rating scales and asking clients or caregivers to rate the frequency, intensity, or functional impact of each problem through idiographic tools, or through a shared decision-making process with the client and caregiver (see "Assessment Strategies Relevant to Stage 4").

One strategy that is particularly relevant to fleshing out the variables in this stage is functional assessment. Cone (1997) describes the functional approach as a strategy for "identifying controlling variables for problem behavior" (p. 260), and

breaks it down into two component parts. *Functional assessment* involves collection of data regarding the target problem and generating hypotheses regarding variables that may be related to that problem via either operant (i.e., serve as punishers or reinforcers) or classical (i.e., are linked with the target problem via temporal relationships) conditioning principles. *Functional analysis* refers to testing these hypotheses via systematically manipulating hypotheses causal and maintaining factors, often via treatment. The functional assessment process is essentially what is happening in Stage 1 of the science-informed case conceptualization model, although that model does not limit itself to treatment approaches that are grounded in operant or classical conditioning, which was the original purpose of functional approaches.

In a very helpful primer, in which he uses the term "functional analysis" to refer to both the assessment and analysis phase, Yoman (2008) outlines the steps of functional analysis. In the first step, clients are asked about the "ultimate outcomes" they desire from treatment, or their long-term hopes, such as increased life satisfaction. Identification of these ultimate outcomes then informs the second step of the process, which is identifying target problems. During this step, target problems are described in detail and can be prioritized, based on the likelihood that they will contribute to the desired ultimate outcome. In the third step, data are collected on the behavior of interest and its antecedents and consequences. Consistent with the behavioral assessment tradition that views observational strategies as more objective, Yoman advocates using self-monitoring or direct observation to gather these data, but, as we discussed earlier, interviews or other strategies can also be applied during the treatment intake to begin the assessment process. The later steps of Yoman's model map onto later stages of the science-informed conceptualization model, which includes formulating provisional hypotheses regarding the target problem (see Stage 3, below) and incorporating additional assessment as needed to strengthen them, selecting an intervention to test the hypotheses (see Stage 4, below), then testing the hypotheses via ongoing assessment during treatment (see Stage 5, below).

Application of Conceptualization Stage 1 to Ty

As discussed by Van Meter (Chapter 2, this volume), according to his mother, Ty's initial presenting problems were his "bad temper, lack of effort on homework, and slipping grades." In the prein-take assessment, we learned that although mild levels of externalizing symptoms were present, Ty also had clinically significant levels of internalizing symptoms.

At the intake assessment, we separately gathered assessment data from Ty and his mother, using a combination of unstandardized interviews, rating scales, and structured interviews. During the unstandardized interview with Ty's mother, she reported struggles coping with Ty's attitude and behavior since she and her husband had separated about a year earlier and Ty only sees his father on weekends. According to the mother, Ty's older sister is a "straight-A student" and has "never had any problems" like Ty's. Ty's mother feels frustrated by his behavior and is very worried that he is putting his future in jeopardy due to his slipping academic performance. She described experiencing a lot of stress over her new role as a primarily single parent and has had to work more hours to increase her income.

We first talked with Ty in an unstandardized way to begin establishing rapport and defining treatment goals. During this time, he reported experiencing a lot of academic pressure, especially because he has to take high school placement tests this year. He also expressed worries about being the "man of the house" now that his father is not in the home. He described his mother as "on him" and critical all of the time. He said she does not notice the good things he does. He reported having "a few friends," but he does not spend time with them outside of school. In the past, he played soccer but had to quit because his mother is not able to pick him up after practice. Ty said he spends a lot of time home alone after school, primarily playing video games. When his mother does come home, the two of them fight about his not doing homework.

Based on the preintake rating scale results and the additional information received during the unstandardized interview, we decided to administer the Mood and Feelings Questionnaire (MFQ; Angold, Costello, Messer, & Pickles, 1995) and the Screen for Child Anxiety Related Emotional Disorders (SCARED; Birmaher et al., 1999) to both Ty and his mother to get more specific symptom information. We also had his mother complete the Vanderbilt Assessment Scales to get more information about his inattention, impulsivity, and disruptive behavior (Wolraich et al., 2003). All of these instruments are free, and copies are available on Wikiversity. We also worked with Ty and his

mother to identify "top problems," following Weisz and colleagues (2011). As discussed in more detail under Stage 2, we administered sections of the Mini-International Neuropsychiatric Interview for Children and Adolescents (MINI-KID; Sheehan et al., 2010). The results of these assessments suggested three potential target problems for treatment: (1) Ty's refusal to do his schoolwork, (2) Ty's irritable mood, and (3) Ty's worries about his academic future and his family.

The unstandardized part of our interview also yielded information about other variables important to fleshing out the case conceptualization. Important *historical factors* included the parents' separation and Ty's subsequent withdrawal from soccer. Moreover, Ty's parents had immigrated to the United States from Korea, so it was important for us to consider the possible impact of cultural factors. We used questions from the DSM-5 Cultural Formulation Interview (American Psychiatric Association, 2013) to explore this possibility with Ty and his mother. When answering these questions, Ty's mother reported that academic success was very important in her family, and that her children needed to work hard to succeed in the United States. Ty indicated that he was aware that his mother felt this way, but he felt like her views were old-fashioned. He reported that he was tired from the pressure to do well in school and to be a "model Korean kid," and that he felt like he would never be as "perfect" as his sister. These cultural differences between Ty and his mother were seen by both as contributing to their ongoing conflicts over schoolwork.

Our initial interview and the general psychopathology literature related to anxiety and depression also pointed to potential *causal factors* that could be a focus of treatment. Given Ty's mother's description of her stress level following separation from her husband, we asked her to complete the Caregiver Strain Questionnaire—Short Form 7 (Brannan, Athay, & de Andrade, 2012), which indicated that she was experiencing high levels of stress related to Ty's difficulties. Additionally, given the role that cognitive vulnerabilities can play in both depression and anxiety (e.g., Hankin et al., 2016), we administered the ACSQ (Hankin & Abramson, 2002) to Ty; results indicated Ty tended to make negative inferences about the causes of events, the consequences of those events, and the implications of those events for himself. Finally, we noted that Ty continued not doing his homework, although he recognized his life would be easier in many ways if he just did it. This raised the possibility that Ty was engaged in avoidance. We explored this possibility by administering the EASI-A (Kennedy & Ehrenreich-May, 2017); from the EASI-A, we learned that Ty engaged in high levels of avoidance of thoughts and feelings, and used distraction as a form of coping.

As a final step, we conducted a functional interview focused on identifying *antecedents* and *maintaining factors* (Ollendick, McLeod, & Jensen-Doss, 2013). This part of the interview indicated that two antecedent situations appeared to trigger Ty's problems. Requests from his mother that he do his homework were associated with an irritable mood, worry that he would not do well on his work, and refusal to do the work. Ty also indicated that spending long afternoons home alone increased his negative mood and gave him time to worry more about both academics and his family situation. We also identified several potential maintaining factors. Ty's difficulties with irritable mood were maintained by his poor grades, his conflicts with his mother, and his social withdrawal. His poor grades and social withdrawal also helped maintain his worries. Finally, we identified a loop wherein Ty's refusal to do his homework resulted in poor grades, which increased his conflict with his mother. This conflict increased his irritable mood, which in turn made it more likely that he would refuse to do his homework the next time his mother asked.

Conceptualization Stage 2: Generate a Diagnosis

Under the science-informed case conceptualization model, a diagnosis is considered an important step in the case conceptualization, but primarily as an entrée into the relevant psychopathology and treatment literature, as simply knowing that a diagnosis does not necessarily point to the correct treatment for a given client. Linking a client's diagnoses to the developmental psychopathology literature can help identify candidate causal and maintaining factors to flesh out the case conceptualization. Diagnoses are also a useful avenue for identifying potential evidence-based treatment options and relevant progress monitoring strategies.

Assessment Tools Relevant to Conceptualization Stage 2

Stage 2 maps most closely onto Youngstrom and colleagues' (2017) assessment Step 7, applying

more intensive assessment methods to finalize diagnoses. It often helps to combine the results of these more intensive tools with the assessment results from the other assessment steps in order to yield a finalized set of diagnoses.

Interviews

Interviews are assessments that traditionally involve an assessor asking a client or caregiver questions, although computer-administered interviews also exist (e.g., Diagnostic Interview Schedule for Children; Shaffer, Fisher, Lucas, Dulcan, & Schwab-Stone, 2000). There are three main types of interviews that vary based on their level of standardization, or the degree to which the interview approach uses consistent administration and scoring procedure across clients and conditions (Barrios & Hartmann, 1986): (1) unstandardized interviews, (2) structured interviews, and (3) semistructured interviews.

The traditional method of diagnosis is the *unstandardized diagnostic interview (UDI)*, in which a clinician relies solely on clinical expertise in lieu of standardized questions and scoring algorithms. UDIs are conversational in nature, allowing the clinician to focus on the client's experience, tailor questions to the client, and apply clinical expertise to probe for additional information. They can take many forms, such as being used as just one tool within a broader diagnostic assessment battery, or as a stand-alone diagnostic method. Surveys indicate that the unstandardized clinical interview is the assessment method used most often by clinicians (e.g., Cashel, 2002; Connors, Arora, Curtis, & Stephan, 2015; Cook, Hausman, Jensen-Doss, & Hawley, 2017).

During *structured interviews*, the clinician administers a set of standardized questions guided by strict rules for administration and scoring, without the use of clinical judgment. These standardized questions are organized into diagnostic "modules" that cover DSM or ICD criteria for specific diagnoses. These interviews typically have contingency rules to guide the questioning. For example, if a parent answers "yes" to the question "Has your child felt depressed in the past year?", the interviewer then asks a standard set of questions about the frequency, duration, and impairment associated with the symptoms of depression. If the parent answered "no" to this question, then the interviewer would move on and ask about a symptom from a different module. Structured interviews also follow standardized scoring procedures, wherein the yes–no responses are entered into scoring algorithms that yield diagnoses. Structured interviews are also referred to as *respondent-based interviews (RBIs)*, in that they follow a set script whose scoring is based solely on the respondent's responses (Angold & Fisher, 1999).

Semistructured interviews fall somewhere in between unstandardized and structured approaches, relying on standardized questions and scoring algorithms but allowing some clinical judgment in both administration and scoring. Like structured interviews, semistructured interviews have standard questions or topics that are covered and standard scoring algorithms, and these two types of interviews are sometimes collectively referred to as *standardized diagnostic interviews (SDIs)*. However, in semistructured interviews, clinicians can add follow-up questions, clarify meaning, or adjust the wording of the standardized questions to match the child's developmental level or the family's conceptualization of symptoms (e.g., substituting "frustrated" for "irritable" or "stressed" for "worried"). Semistructured interviews also typically incorporate some clinical judgment into determining whether symptoms are present or not, rather than just recording yes/no answers, and in deciding how to weigh symptoms when assigning diagnoses. Because the interviewer determines what questions are asked and how responses are scored, semistructured interviews are also referred to as *interviewer-based interviews (IBIs)* (Angold & Fisher, 1999).

Psychometric Considerations in Choosing an Interview

The decision to use an unstandardized or standardized approach to diagnostic assessment has important implications for the reliability and validity of generated diagnoses, the clinical practicality of the assessment process, and the quality of the case conceptualization. While SDIs have become nearly ubiquitous in research settings, the majority of practicing clinicians rely solely on a UDI approach (Anderson & Paulosky, 2004; Bruchmüller, Margraf, Suppiger, & Schneider, 2011; Cook et al., 2017; Jensen-Doss & Hawley, 2011). This discrepancy is significant because the clinical judgment used to guide UDIs is prone to a number of information gathering and interpretation biases that impact diagnostic rates and accuracy (Angold & Fisher, 1999; Garb, 1998, 2005). As discussed in the prediction phase (Van Meter, Chapter 2, this volume), these biases can negatively influence the accuracy of the information-gathering and decision-making processes.

Perhaps not surprising given the potential for the introduction of bias into the assessment process without standardized procedures, studies have generally indicated that unstandardized interviews have poor content validity. For example, a review of inpatient UDIs found that almost half of the key diagnostic criteria necessary to rule in and rule out disorders were unassessed, and that many diagnoses were assigned without sufficient evidence (Miller, 2002; Miller, Dasher, Collins, Griffiths, & Brown, 2001). This finding is consistent with studies that indicate clinicians seek information to confirm a diagnosis, while ignoring information that is inconsistent with it and often base diagnostic decisions on whether a client conforms to a predetermine cognitive schema of the prototypical client with the diagnosis (Garb, 2005). Clinical decisions guided by invalid or incomplete assessments can have a negative downstream impact on the validity and interrater reliability of assigned diagnoses (Cook et al., 2017). In contrast, reviews of SDIs have found strong psychometric support for many interviews, covering a range of childhood disorders (Leffler, Riebel, & Hughes, 2015).

Studies comparing UDIs to SDIs have found that, in general, UDIs result in fewer diagnoses and a greater assignment of not otherwise specified or unspecified diagnoses (e.g., Hughes et al., 2005; Jensen & Weisz, 2002; Matuschek et al., 2016). UDIs also underidentify subclinical conditions and miss the presence of significant comorbidities, including substance use and suicidal thoughts and behaviors (Aronen, Noam, & Weinstein, 1993; Bongiovi-Garcia et al., 2009; Jensen-Doss, Youngstrom, Youngstrom, Feeny, & Findling, 2014; Kramer, Robbins, Phillips, Miller, & Burns, 2003). A meta-analysis of this literature found that the average agreement for youth diagnoses between these two approaches is kappa = .39 (Rettew, Lynch, Achenbach, Dumenci, & Ivanova, 2009), suggesting that overall agreement is considered "poor" (Landis & Koch, 1977).

While the lack of agreement between the two approaches does not directly equate to the SDIs being correct and UDIs being incorrect, youth whose diagnoses match SDIs have been found to have better treatment engagement and outcomes (Jensen-Doss & Weisz, 2008; Kramer et al., 2003; Pogge et al., 2001). Other studies have also indicated that SDIs typically demonstrate more favorable validity than UDIs. SDIs have been found to have higher concordance than unstandardized interviews with "gold standard diagnoses" generated by experts who reviewed all available information

(Basco et al., 2000; Miller et al., 2001). Additional research has indicated higher predictive validity for SDIs when diagnoses for both types of interviews were compared to external validity indicators such as daily behavior reports (Jewell, Handwerk, Almquist, & Lucas, 2004) and impaired functioning (Tenney, Schotte, Denys, van Megen, & Westenberg, 2003). Taken together, these data suggest that current research does not support the psychometric quality of unstandardized interviews alone as a method of diagnosis (Miller et al., 2001).

Despite possessing stronger psychometric properties, SDIs do have limitations related to clinical utility. SDIs require considerable time to administer, usually up to two hours per informant (although some exceptions do exist, e.g., the MINI-KID [Sheehan et al., 2010]). Moreover, there is no single interview that adequately covers all diagnoses, and the currently available SDIs may not be as useful for diagnosing disorders such as attention-deficit/hyperactivity disorder (ADHD) (Pelham, Fabiano, & Massetti, 2005) and pediatric bipolar disorder (Youngstrom, Findling, Youngstrom, & Calabrese, 2005). Surveys of community-based clinicians indicate that lack of training and cost of use of standardized assessment are the primary clinician-reported barrier to their use (Bruchmüller et al., 2011; Cook et al., 2017; Whiteside, Sattler, Hathaway, & Douglas, 2016). In addition to these practical concerns, many clinicians report believing that SDIs are unacceptable to clients and have the potential to damage the therapeutic relationship (Bruchmüller et al., 2011). Data gathered from clients, however, do not support this concern (Suppiger et al., 2009).

A final concern is that SDIs are limited in their coverage of historical events and casual, antecedent, and maintaining factors that are important for case conceptualization. They also provide limited guidance in making differential diagnoses or interpreting discrepancies in interinformant reports (for an exception, see the description of the K-SADS-PL below).

Semistructured approaches do provide more opportunities to ground diagnostic questions in context (e.g., "Does your child experience more fear of embarrassment around peers or with adults?") than do structured interviews. This ability to make adjustments may be particularly beneficial when an interview has not demonstrated cross-cultural validity for a given client's background, and alternative language may improve the client's understanding of interview questions. However, to employ this flexibility in a reliable manner requires a high level of training, whereas training is more straightforward for fully structured interviews. Therefore, the selection of an interview depends on the goals of the assessment and available personnel and time resources. A long-term goal for one's practice might be to use more structured approaches early in training, then streamline to semistructured approaches, perhaps using checklists to make sure that the more unstandardized interview still is covering key elements, and that there is enough information to confirm a diagnosis or formulation.

A hybrid approach can use the prediction phase to integrate screening, risk factors, and checklists to inform the selection of which SDI to use, or which specific issues to drill down during the interview (e.g., selecting modules from the Kiddie Schedule for Affective Disorders and Schizophrenia [K-SADS]). This shortens the battery, allaying clinical concerns about burden, and empowers clinicians to add their judgment and refine hypotheses on the basis of new information. The sequencing also demonstrates "medical necessity" for the interview and subsequent assessment components, changing the potential level of reimbursement by third-party payers.

Structured Interview Example: The MINI-KID

The MINI-KID is a structured diagnostic interview for children ages 6–17 (Sheehan et al., 2010). It assesses suicidality and 24 psychiatric disorders using DSM-5 and ICD-10 criteria. The interview can be administered to the child and parent together or separately, and there is also a parent-only version (MINI-KID-P). It takes about 30 minutes to administer. The MINI-KID is organized into diagnostic modules, and all questions are in a yes–no format. The instrument uses branching tree logic, in that two to four screening questions are asked for each disorder and, if endorsed, additional symptom questions are administered. For example, if a child responds "yes" to the screening question "Have you felt sad or depressed, down or empty, or grouchy or annoyed most of the day, nearly every day for the past 2 weeks?", the clinician would administer the corresponding depression module. For internalizing disorders, the MINI-KID assesses all anxiety disorders, common mood disorders, and associated mood disorders. The externalizing disorders modules assess all disruptive behaviors, substance abuse, and substance dependence. Several studies have demonstrated good reliability, ranging from .41 to 1, and internal consistency, alpha = .41 to .87 (Duncan et al., 2019; Sheehan et al., 2010).

There are several advantages to using the MINI-KID. Given that it only focuses on establishing current diagnoses, administration is brief. Sheehan and colleagues (2010) compared administration times between the MINI-KID and a semistructured interview, the Kiddie Schedule for Affective Disorders and Schizophrenia—Present and Lifetime Version (K-SADS-PL; Kaufman et al., 2016; see below). Administration of the MINI-KID for children with any internalizing or externalizing disorder took 35–40 minutes, compared to 95–120 minutes for the K-SADS P/L. Moreover, the MINI-KID is available in multiple languages, can be administered by a trained layperson, and has been tested in both clinical and nonclinical samples (Duncan et al., 2018). However, criticisms have been directed at the MINI-KID's screening questions (Leffler et al., 2015), as the same screening questions are used for multiple diagnoses, and a single screening question may cover a range of symptoms. The MINI-KID also has a fee for each administration, which may be prohibitive in some settings.

Semistructured Interview Example: The K-SADS-PL

The K-SADS-PL (Kaufman et al., 1997, 2016) is a semistructured interview designed to evaluate current and past psychiatric conditions in children and adolescents ages 6–18. The K-SADS-PL-5 assesses 23 DSM-5 disorders, including internalizing disorders, externalizing disorders, neurodevelopmental disorders, elimination disorders, and psychosis. The interview is conducted with the parent and child separately, with each interview taking approximately 1.5 hours (Ambrosini, 2000). In addition to the categorical (i.e., diagnosis) approach used in prior versions of the K-SADS-PL, the DSM-5 version takes a dimensional (e.g., severity) approach to assessment. Specifically, prior to administering the diagnostic screening portion of the interview, the parent and child each complete a self-report DSM-5 crosscutting symptoms measure. The interviewer also conducts a brief, guided unstandardized interview with each informant to help establish rapport, obtain psychiatric history, and assess current functioning. The screening interview portion of the K-SADS-PL is modularized and uses a series of skip-out rules to assess for the presence of diagnostic criteria and symptom severity. The majority of the interview modules provide multiple illustrative examples of questions that could be used to assess different diagnostic criteria. For example, Criterion A for separation anxiety disorder ("excessive anxiety concerning separation from home or from those to whom the individual is attached") is assessed through variations on the question "Did you ever worry that something bad might happen to you where you would never see your parents again? Like getting lost, kidnapped, killed, or getting into an accident?" Supplemental modules are also administered as necessary to aid the clinician in making differential diagnoses. The K-SADS has been translated into 16 different languages including Spanish (Ulloa et al., 2006), Mandarin (Chen, Shen, & Gau, 2017), Korean (Kim et al., 2004), and Farsi (Ghanizadeh, Mohammadi, & Yazdanshenas, 2006). Psychometric studies of the K-SADS-PL for DSM-IV have shown strong interrater (kappa by diagnosis = .80–.90) and test–retest reliability (kappa by diagnosis = .38–.87) and construct validity (Birmaher et al., 2009; Kaufman et al., 1997; Shahrivar, Kousha, Moallemi, Tehrani-Doost, & Alaghband-Rad, 2010). A recent study of the Spanish version of the K-SADS-PL-5 found good construct validity and good interrater reliability (kappa > .70) for the majority of diagnostic categories (de la Pena et al., 2018).

Observational Methods

Although observational methods are more traditionally used in behaviorally oriented research (e.g., in multiple baseline studies of classroom interventions), there is also evidentiary support for standardized observational methods in diagnostic assessment. Observational methods involve either observing a child in his or her naturalistic environment or placing a child into standard situations and coding his or her behavior (Reitman, McGregor, & Resnick, 2013). In the case of diagnostic behavioral assessment, the demonstrated behaviors can then be compared to the norming sample to assess the typical behavior elicited by the situation.

The Autism Diagnostic Observational Schedule (ADOS-2; Lord et al., 2012) is a semistructured observational tool used to diagnose autism spectrum disorders using DSM-5 criteria. During administration of the ADOS-2, a child engages in a series of standardized communication, social, and play activities to elicit behaviors associated with autism spectrum disorder. These behaviors are then coded by trained observers to determine whether they are developmentally typical. There is evidentiary support for the ADOS-2 among both clinical and research samples (Hus & Lord, 2014; Langman et al., 2017; Pugliese et al., 2015).

While observational tools do not currently have strong support as diagnostic tools for other disorders, they are potentially useful to generate information to use during Stage 1 of the case conceptualization process. For example, the Dyadic Parent–Child Interaction Coding System (Eyberg & Robinson, 1981), which assesses the quality of parent–child social interaction, and the Disruptive Behavior Diagnostic Observation System (Wakschlag et al., 2008), which that assesses disruptive behavior in preschool children, are two observational instruments that can be used for this purpose. Data from these instruments can give good insight into the quality of behavior, its age appropriateness, and the context in which it occurs. These provide a rubric for coding behaviors, without going so far as to have formal norms. There is value in incorporating information from behavioral observations into the case conceptualization process because it can help with differential diagnoses. However, the time and training requirements for standardized observational tools often make them prohibitive for use by practicing clinicians.

Cognitive Tests

Cognitive ability tests are a widely used for psychoeducational evaluations (McGill & Ndip, 2019) and play a role in evaluating potential cognitive disability (Matson et al., 2019). For these referral issues, they are a core part of a comprehensive evaluation. When the referral focuses more on emotional or behavioral problems, and formulation is oriented toward potential treatment, then the value of cognitive testing is more circumscribed. Youth with higher verbal ability are more likely to be able to use words, metacognition, and metaemotion to engage in treatment. Put another way, being older and more cognitively developed may help with using the more cognitive aspects of cognitive-behavioral and interpersonal interventions, whereas behavioral treatment elements may be more likely to get traction with less verbal clients.

The potential value added by cognitive tests for treatment planning may not require the addition of a lengthy test to the intake assessment. Often a review of school records, group-based standardized tests, and other records is sufficient. If additional testing seems indicated, a well-designed two- or four-subtest battery usually offers valid and precise enough information to inform next steps with regard to treatment. Although there is a large literature and considerable clinical lore about using factor score or subtest discrepancies to form hypotheses or evaluate neurobehavioral disorders, there are much less expensive, faster, and more accurate ways of assessing these constructs (Canivez, 2013). For example, rather than using an apparent weakness on the Arithmetic subtest on a Wechsler to infer that the child might have ADHD, parent and teacher checklists are not only less costly and burdensome but their validity coefficients for association with ADHD are also substantially higher (cf. Raiker et al., 2017; Watkins, Kush, & Glutting, 1997).

Assessment Strategies Relevant to Conceptualization Stage 2

Although diagnostic interviews are designed to yield diagnostic recommendations, there are many reasons why they cannot be treated as a "gold standard" method of diagnosis (Spitzer, 1983). In youth clients, for example, youth- and parent-report interviews often generate different sets of diagnoses for the same client, so additional work is needed to determine what the "true" diagnosis is. Several strategies have been proposed in the literature for integrating assessment data to generate a final diagnosis.

Bayesian Approaches

One approach to integrating assessment data to generate a diagnosis is a Bayesian approach that stems from the evidence-based medicine tradition (Straus, Glasziou, Richardson, & Haynes, 2011). Within this framework, diagnosis is conceptualized as a process of moving from a pretest probability (i.e., the clinician's initial "best guess" about how likely a client is to meet criteria for a particular disorder) to a series of posttest probabilities (i.e., the likelihood that a client meets criteria for that disorder after additional assessment data have been gathered). Under the EBA model, probabilities are refined during the prediction phase by incorporating data on risk factors and scores on broad-band instruments. During the prediction phase, these probabilities are further refined through more focused assessments (e.g., problem-specific rating scales) before conducting more intensive assessments for disorders that continue to seem likely. In this way, the assessment can focus more on problems that seem likely, and clinicians can even choose to administer only sections of interviews that seem relevant to a given client and skip others that seem unlikely based on other stages of data collection. Other authors have noted that Bayesian principles can also be applied within diagnostic interviews, creating algorithms to make the interviews themselves more efficient (Chorpita & Nakamura, 2008). The Bayesian approach is covered in depth by Van Meter (Chapter 2, this volume).

LEAD Procedures

Spitzer (1983) proposed the LEAD (i.e., Longitudinal, Expert, and All Data) standard for incorporating diagnostic data; this approach has been used in dozens of research studies to generate final diagnoses.

Consistent with the iterative nature of case conceptualization, the LEAD standard first states that a diagnostic assessment should not be limited to a single evaluation, but should be considered an ongoing Longitudinal process by which diagnoses are revised as new information becomes available (Spitzer, 1983). Diagnoses should be generated by a team of Expert clinicians who have been trained to generate reliable diagnoses using All Data available to the team. Utilizing information available in clinical records and gathered through all of the assessment steps rather than just the diagnostic interview, Spitzer recommends that team members make independent diagnoses, then come together to discuss any discrepancies before coming to a final consensus diagnosis.

DSM Model for Differential Diagnosis

Given that similar symptoms may present across conditions and that different diagnostic categories exist for certain causal factors (e.g., stress, substance use, medical conditions), the process of differential diagnosis, or choosing between different diagnoses that share common symptoms, can be complicated (Morrison, 2014). Knowing what are competing hypotheses for similar clinical presentations can prevent jumping to a premature diagnosis or formulation. To assist clinicians in this process, the American Psychiatric Association has published the *DSM-5 Handbook of Differential Diagnosis* (First, 2014). Similar to other books that outline a step-by-step process for diagnosis (e.g., Morrison, 2014), the manual describes a six-step framework using decision trees to facilitate the diagnostic process.

First, to avoid malingering or reports of a fictitious disorder, First (2014) recommends assessing whether reported symptoms are real. Although few formal tests of malingering have been validated for youth samples, clinicians should consider whether clients or parents might be motivated to report symptoms for external incentives (e.g., to qualify for financial support, to influence custody decisions, or for forensic evaluations in criminal cases). Rating scales also often have built-in validity scales that can also be used to assess whether respondents show inconsistent or overly negative responding patterns. For example, the BASC-3 F Index (Reynolds & Kamphaus, 2015) flags responding patterns that may be excessively negative. In cases where this index is elevated, the clinician can reinterview the respondent and seek additional information about possible drivers of that score, which includes asking about how the respondent interpreted the items or his or her Likert anchors, asking for specific examples of symptoms that sound overly severe, and assessing any motivations they might have to "fake bad" (e.g., a desire to qualify for services).

Second, clinicians should evaluate whether a symptom may be the result of a substance (e.g., drug use, toxin exposure). First (2014) provides a decision tree for determining the relation between substance use and the client's symptoms to help the clinicians decide whether to assign a substance-induced disorder diagnosis (e.g., if there is a temporal relationship between use and the disorder, if substance use is the result of a disorder rather than the cause). If substances have been ruled out as a cause for the symptoms, then in Step 3, the manual also provides a decision tree to rule out any medical causes for the symptoms.

Once substance-related and medical causes have been ruled out, the clinician can move on to assigning the client's diagnosis. To support differential diagnosis, First (2014) presents a series of decision trees grouped by presenting symptoms (e.g., a decision tree to guide clinicians through the diagnostic possibilities for a child with behavior problems). At this stage, the clinician may have determined a diagnosis. However, if the client is experiencing symptoms that do not clearly fit a diagnostic category, the clinician moves on to consider whether the symptoms may be better captured by a diagnosis of adjustment disorder or one of the residual, "Other Specified" or "Unspecified" categories.

An adjustment disorder diagnosis would indicate that symptoms are attributable to a specific event the client has experienced (e.g., divorce, grief from losing a loved one). Selection of an "Other Specified" or "Unspecified" label would indicate that symptoms do not meet criteria for the more specific variant of the diagnosis, with "Other Specified" being used to denote a presentation that does not meet criteria for another diagnostic category (e.g., a period of depression without enough symptoms to meet criteria for a depressive episode) and "Unspecified" being used when distress or impairment is present but the clinician either does not wish to specify the reason or does not have enough information to assign a diagnosis. It is worth noting that these "Other Specified" diagnoses are meant to be used after considering the other options, not used first as a broad umbrella—which appears often to be the case with billing diagnoses in practice (Jensen-Doss et al., 2014).

In the final step, the clinician must evaluate whether the client's symptoms cause clinically significant distress and impairment, and thus lead to a diagnosis. Given that many symptoms are common and DSM-5 does not define "clinically significant," the clinician should gather from the client and his or her parents how symptoms may impact functioning. Once assessment data point to a potential diagnosis or diagnoses, a clinician can use this information to guide treatment planning. Although First (2014) developed his framework using DSM-5, the principles certainly apply to diagnoses using the ICD-11 classification, too.

Application of Conceptualization Stage 2 to Ty

Adding the MFQ, the SCARED, and the Vanderbilt provided more information about some of the contending hypotheses. Ty's scores on the SCARED were relatively low, according to both Ty and his mother. In contrast, his depression scores were high compared to published cutoffs, and his self-report was much higher than his mother's ratings on the same items. Apparently, the conversation and rapport building got him to open up.

When administering a questionnaire or checklist, we want to make sure to skim the responses to look for skipped items, comments about content, and anything else that might get lost in a simple number. Some instruments have "write-in" boxes for examples. Sometimes this factors into the scoring—the Achenbach manual explicitly tells us to read the written details, probe if needed, then change the scoring depending on our clinical judgment. Another crucial thing is to make sure to read any "critical" items, such as those asked about self-harm,

suicidal ideation or behavior, threats to others, or physical or sexual abuse. These provide key knowledge from a risk-management perspective, and they also may have mandatory reporting requirements or other legal obligations. People often are more likely to volunteer information on a questionnaire or a computer than they are in a conversation, especially when they are first meeting a clinician, so these are valuable ways of scouting for additional things to address in the case formulation. The MFQ has several items asking about suicidal ideation (numbers 15–19, with 19 being "I thought about killing myself"). His mother did not report any concerns, but Ty checked "sometimes" to three of the hopeless and passive ideation items. We checked with him to make sure he wasn't experiencing suicidal ideation, and documented it in our notes.

We can also do better than just eyeballing the scores and thinking, "That looks high . . . and that one looks low." Diagnostic likelihood ratios are available for the MFQ for depression, the SCARED for anxiety disorders, and the Vanderbilt for ADHD. When the same person fills out multiple instruments, they are highly correlated with each other—they share the same source, and factors such as demoralization or social desirability tend to raise or lower all scores. When two scales are trying to assess the same construct, they will be redundant. If we are going to estimate the probabilities using a nomogram or a calculator, we should pick the best score from each informant for each construct. "Best" means "most valid," not necessarily the highest score. The MFQ would be a better choice for assessing depression than the Internalizing, Anxious/Depressed, or even DSM-oriented mood scales from the ASEBA—it has more coverage of depression.

Swapping in the diagnostic likelihood ratios for the SCARED demoted the probability of anxiety, and the MFQ scores raised the probability of depression (see Ty's page on Wikiversity for details). The plot twist was the Vanderbilt score. Ty's mother endorsed a lot of inattention items but not the hyperactive or impulsive items. ADHD is a common problem in Ty's age group, and the Vanderbilt score pushed the probability up enough that we made a point of covering it in our interview as well.

Based on these probabilities, we administered the MINI-KID (Sheehan et al., 2010) Anxiety, Mood Disorders, and ADHD sections to both Ty and his mother. Given the mother's view that the presenting problem was oppositional behavior and the mild elevations in externalizing symptoms in the preintake instruments, we also administered the Oppositional Defiant Disorder section of the MINI-KID to help rule out externalizing problems. The results of the MINI-KID indicated that Ty met criteria for major depressive disorder but not any anxiety disorders. The mood episode was sufficient to explain the internalizing symptoms, and they were a change for Ty, whereas anxiety would be more likely to be long-standing or chronic. Taken together with other information gathered through the interview and the results of the rating scales, we assigned Ty with a diagnosis of major depressive disorder, single episode, moderate, with anxious distress. He also met criteria for ADHD, inattentive type, but we consider this a provisional diagnosis because many of the symptoms also may be due to depression, and it was difficult to tease apart whether some of the inattention predated the depression. Another possibility is that his mother's expectations are high, and she may be concerned about behaviors that might not be unusual for a young male. We decided to have Ty's teachers fill out the Vanderbilt to get more information about his history of inattention and how it compares to those of his peers.

Conceptualization Stage 3: Develop the Initial Case Conceptualization

The goal of this stage is to pull data from the previous two stages into a set of working hypotheses about factors that contribute to and maintain the client's problems. In these hypotheses, each presenting problem is thought of as a dependent variable that the clinician will work to change during treatment. The causal and maintaining factors identified during Stage 1 become the independent variables through which treatment will work to change the presenting problems. We recommend first writing out these hypotheses, then mapping them into a figural drawing of the conceptualization, incorporating relevant historical and antecedent factors.

Strategies Related to Conceptualization Stage 3

At this stage of the case conceptualization process, the focus moves from assessment to integrating assessment data into a case conceptualization. This does not use new tools. However, a major focus at this phase is reconciling data from multiple informants.

A central challenge of the multi-informant approach to child assessment is that rates of agreement across informants are low to moderate (De Los Reyes et al., 2015). Traditionally, informant discrepancies have been attributed to measurement error, including differences in validity and scale interpretations across reporters (De Los Reyes et al., 2011; Dirks, De Los Reyes, Briggs-Gowan, Cella, & Wakschlag, 2012). The belief that discrepancies are a product of error has resulted in many clinicians dismissing incongruent reports as biased or invalid. Recent studies, however, indicate that discrepant reports can be reliable, valid, and uniquely predictive of the child's psychopathology and functioning (De Los Reyes et al., 2011; Dirks, Boyle, & Georgiades, 2011; van Dulmen & Egeland, 2011). Therefore, an important aspect of finalizing the case conceptualization is to effectively integrate interinformant discrepancies.

Over the past decade, evidence has been growing in support of the attribution bias context (ABC) model (De Los Reyes & Kazdin, 2005), a framework that provides guidance for making sense of interinformant discrepancies. This model posits that discrepancies in child assessment result from meaningful differences in informant perspectives and variability in child symptom presentation across contexts (De Los Reyes & Kazdin, 2005; Dirks et al., 2012).

First, informant discrepancies may result from differences in informant attributions about the cause of the child's problems (De Los Reyes & Kazdin, 2005). Specifically, observers of the child, including parents and teachers, are more likely to attribute problems to the child's characteristics (e.g., "The child is a troublemaker"), whereas children more often attribute them to the environment (e.g., "My teacher is too strict").

Attribution differences between reporters also influence informant perspectives regarding the nature of the problem and need for treatment. Similar to ways in which clinician judgment can be influenced by mental shortcuts, an observer's predetermined attributions about a child's traits may impact his or her report (De Los Reyes & Kazdin, 2005). For example, parents who perceive a child to be oppositional may more easily access information about the child's defiance. Observers may also be prone to generalizing problems to contexts in which they do not observe the child (e.g., a teacher assuming that a child who is disruptive in class also misbehaves at home). This would subsequently strengthen the view that treatment is warranted. In contrast, children who perceive their problem as resulting from a specific situation may be less likely to identify a need for treatment.

Importantly, these perspectives also vary in their relation to the goal of the clinical process, which is to assess whether treatment is warranted by collecting negative information about the child. For children, this likely contributes to discrepancies, as they are less likely than other informants to want to provide this type of information.

The ABC model also states that informant discrepancies arise from observable differences in a child's behavior across contexts. Contexts may vary both in their expectation or demand for particular behaviors and their tolerance or threshold of them. For example, a classroom may demand higher levels of attention from a child and have lower tolerance for hyperactivity than the child's home environment. As such, teacher and parent reports may differ in both the number of ADHD symptoms endorsed and in how problematic the symptoms are viewed to be. Expectations and tolerance for child behavior can also be culturally bound and influenced by the child's developmental stage (e.g., Weisz & Weiss, 1991).

Although the ABC model provides a framework for understanding data gathered from multiple informants, there is limited empirical evidence to guide data integration. Moreover, there is little consensus that patterns of agreement map onto differences in need for treatment, disorder severity, or prognosis (Dirks et al., 2012). Thus, without an evidence-based approach to integrate discrepant reports, there is potential for clinical judgment to negatively bias the assessment process. It is thus crucial that clinicians integrate reports through an empirical, hypothesis-testing approach that identifies factors, such as context, culture, perceptual differences, or development, that might account for differences across informants (De Los Reyes, Thomas, Goodman, & Kundey, 2013; McLeod et al., 2013b), and also apply clinical judgment about which informants are providing credible reports (Youngstrom et al., 2011).

As such, the process of integrating informant reports is synonymous with a strong case conceptualization. Target problems hypothesized within the case conceptualization as having context-specific antecedents would be predicted to result in greater informant discrepancies among reporters observing the child within and outside this context. To test hypotheses about informant discrepancies, a behavioral assessment plan designed to inform case conceptualization should also be guided by the ABC model (McLeod et al., 2013b). For example, direct observation of a child's behavior in school and at home can help the clinician under-

stand whether teachers and parents are reporting on the same types of behaviors. Assessment could also reduce the impact of different informant perspectives by (1) identifying reporter attributions about the cause of the child's behavior and (2) asking general (e.g., "Does your child experience anxiety when separated from you?") and context-specific (e.g., "Does your child experience anxiety when separated from you to attend playdates with peers?") questions (McLeod et al., 2013b). In addition, informant discrepancies should not be perceived as a problematic component of the child assessment process, but rather as a meaningful source of information for refining the case conceptualization and understanding how the various respondents are "on the same page" regarding the client's problems and functioning.

Application of Conceptualization Stage 3 to Ty

Figure 3.1 presents the figural drawing that we generated for Ty's case conceptualization. We based this drawing on the following clinical hypotheses:

1. The stress of marital separation, combined with the mismatch between her cultural beliefs about academic success and Ty's behavior, is leading to significant caregiver strain for Ty's mother. This strain interferes with her own functioning, as well as her ability to effectively parent Ty. These historical factors also relate to Ty's irritable mood and worry.
2. Ty's avoidant coping style leads him to avoid doing his homework.
3. Ty's negative cognitive style contributes to his irritability and worries about his family and his academics.
4. Requests from Ty's mother to do his homework trigger Ty's academic worries and his irritability, which in turn lead him to refuse to do his homework.
5. Since Ty can no longer take part in soccer, he spends a lot of time alone. This time alone contributes to his irritable mood and worry.
6. Ty's avoidance of his schoolwork is reinforced by immediate reductions in anxiety, but the subsequent poor grades serve to increase his worry in the long term.
7. Ty's irritable mood is maintained by his conflicts with his mother, which stem from his refusal to do schoolwork and his irritability.
8. Ty's irritable mood and worry lead him to withdraw socially, which in turn increases his irritability and worry.

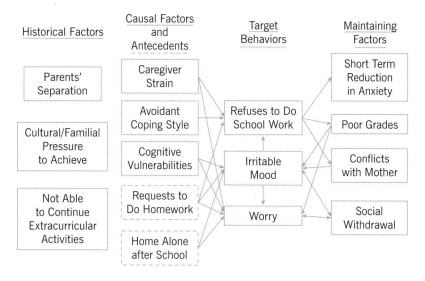

FIGURE 3.1. Case conceptualization figural drawing for Ty.

Conceptualization Stage 4: Proceed with Treatment Plan and Selection

In this stage, the conceptualization helps prioritize treatment goals and select appropriate treatment strategies to help the client meet those goals. In situations in which a client has multiple goals, clinician, client, and caregiver should work together to order treatment goals in terms of priority, which will guide selection of the initial treatment plan. The hypotheses generated in Stage 3 can be used to identify interventions that can target the independent variables (i.e., the causal and maintaining factors) in order to impact the dependent variable (i.e., the target problems). The treatment literature can then be consulted to select an appropriate evidence-based treatment that includes interventions that are of highest priority. As we discuss further below, this stage is another important time to engage in shared decision making with clients and their caregivers to generate a plan that fits the conceptualization, is acceptable to the family, and is feasible within the constraints of the practice setting.

Strategies for Conceptualization Stage 4

As with Stage 3, Stage 4 does not involve additional assessment tools, but rather involves using the case conceptualization to guide treatment selection. As such, the only new "tool" incorporated at this stage is the evidence-based treatment literature, which can be reviewed to pick treatments that match the client's diagnoses and include techniques that match the hypotheses present in the case conceptualization. In addition, to the extent that moderators of treatment effects are known (e.g., that the treatment works better for older than for younger children), this information can also be incorporated into treatment selection. Chorpita, Bernstein, and Daleiden (2011) have also proposed a process called "relevance mapping" that suggests comparing client characteristics (e.g., sex, diagnosis, race/ethnicity) to the composition of the studies used to support a given treatment, to determine whether a treatment has been tested with similar individuals.

Although client perspectives (Youngstrom et al., 2017, Step 9) should be incorporated into all stages of the model, this often becomes most salient at the treatment selection phase. *Shared decision making* (SDM) is a broad term that refers to providers and consumers of health care working together to make decisions about treatment (Cheng et al., 2017; Langer & Jensen-Doss, 2018). SDM is consistent with an EBA to practice, which should incorporate client preferences (APA Presidential Task Force on Evidence-Based Practice, 2006), and also facilitates individualized and culturally sensitive treatment (Langer & Jensen-Doss, 2018). Although widely studied within medicine, the application of SDM is relatively understudied in youth mental health. Cheng and colleagues (2017) recently did a systematic review of SDM interventions in youth mental health and found that most approaches target either caregivers or youth, but not both, and the quality of existing studies is quite variable. The sole focus on one set of decision-makers is a major limitation given that youth mental health treatment often involves reconciling disparate assessment results and treatment preferences across caregivers and clients.

Langer and Jensen-Doss (2018) recently proposed a sample SDM protocol for youth mental health involving the following steps. First, the clinician should initiate a discussion of whether and how caregivers and youth would like to be involved in treatment planning. Second, the individuals who wish to be involved in decision making should specify which decisions need to be made. These decisions might include issues such as the focus of treatment, who will be involved in sessions, how confidentiality will be managed, or what type of treatment will be utilized. Third, grounded in the case conceptualization, the few top choices for each decision should be presented. Fourth, discussion can focus on the pros and cons of each choice, facilitating perspectives from all individuals who are involved in the decision. The pros and cons can then be used to choose an initial treatment approach, then ongoing progress monitoring to determine whether this plan was the best one and to facilitate ongoing check-ins.

Application of Conceptualization Stage 4 to Ty

Our hypotheses from Stage 3 indicated that individual treatment with Ty might include *behavioral activation* (Hypotheses 2, 5, and 8), *exposures* (Hypotheses 2 and 6), *cognitive restructuring* (Hypothesis 3), or *work to help him navigate his new family situation and his acculturation differences with his mother* (Hypothesis 1). In addition, conjoint sessions might focus on *communication training* for Ty and his mother (Hypotheses 4 and 7), and *parent training* or *individual adult treatment* for Ty's mother might also be helpful (Hypothesis 1). We searched PubMed for "treatments for adolescent depression" and the first "best match" citation was for a treatment review by Weersing and colleagues (2017) that identified two well-established treatments for adolescent depression: cognitive-behavioral therapy (CBT) and interpersonal therapy (IPT). We thought CBT would be a good fit for Ty's conceptualization, as it often includes behavioral activation and cognitive restructuring. In addition, exposure therapy, found in CBT protocols for anxiety, is consistent with a CBT approach and is sometimes grouped together with behavioral activation under the umbrella of anti-avoidance strategies (e.g., Chu et al., 2016). However, we also thought IPT would be a good fit given its focus on framing and addressing adolescent depression within the context of significant interpersonal transitions, such as parental separation and interpersonal conflicts (Mufson, Dorta, Moreau, & Weissman, 2004). Finally, we also considered using a treatment considered "probably efficacious" by Weersing and colleagues, attachment-based family therapy (Diamond, Reis, Diamond, Siqueland, & Isaacs, 2002), given its focus on the parent–child relationship. However, we felt that decreasing Ty's irritability and worry through CBT would be the best first step and might lead to relationship improvements as Ty became less irritable and avoidant. Unless the teacher report raises more concerns about ADHD, inattentive type, we plan to see whether treatment focused on the mood issues is enough to address the problems with concentration and schoolwork.

We presented the case conceptualization to Ty and his mother, and our recommendation that treatment proceed with CBT focused on Ty's irritable mood and anxiety. Ty was amenable to this plan, but his mother expressed concern that treatment would not immediately focus on Ty's schoolwork. We helped Ty and his mother discuss the pros and cons of focusing on irritability and anxiety rather than schoolwork. After this discussion, Ty's mother continued to have concerns about the plan, but she agreed to try focusing on his mood while monitoring to see whether his schoolwork improved as a result.

Updating the Conceptualization: Revise as Needed While Monitoring Process and Outcome

As we discussed earlier, case conceptualization is a "living document" that should evolve as new data emerge. As such, the fifth stage of the science-informed case conceptualization model is development of a treatment monitoring plan that allows ongoing monitoring of both client progress and process variables to test the hypotheses in the case conceptualization. Although our initial plan for Ty seems sound and acceptable to the family, it is possible that IPT would have been a better choice, or that Ty's mother would be less engaged in a treatment that is not focused on schoolwork. A good plan monitors these possibilities and adjusts as new information emerges. This is discussed in greater detail by Freeman and Young (Chapter 4, this volume).

REFERENCES

Aboraya, A., France, C., Young, J., Curci, K., & Lepage, J. (2005). The validity of psychiatric diagnosis revisited: The clinician's guide to improve the validity of psychiatric diagnosis. *Psychiatry, 2*, 48–55.

Ambrosini, P. (2000). Historical development and present status of the Schedule for Affective Disorders and Schizophrenia for School-Age Children (K-SADS). *Journal of the American Academy of Child and Adolescent Psychiatry, 39*, 49–58.

American Psychiatric Association. (2013). *Diagnostic and statistical manual of mental disorders* (5th ed.). Arlington, VA: Author.

American Psychological Association. (2011). Competency benchmarks in professional psychology. Retrieved from *www.apa.org/ed/graduate/competency.aspx*.

Anastasi, A. (1988). *Psychological testing*. New York: MacMillan.

Anderson, D. A., & Paulosky, C. A. (2004). A survey of the use of assessment instruments by eating disorder professionals in clinical practice. *Eating and Weight Disorders, 9*, 238–241.

Angold, A., Costello, E. J., Messer, S. C., & Pickles, A. (1995). Development of a short questionnaire for use in epidemiological studies of depression in children and adolescents. *International Journal of Methods in Psychiatric Research, 5*, 237–249.

Angold, A., & Fisher, P. W. (1999). Interviewer-based interviews. In D. Shaffer, C. P. Lucas, & J. E. Richters (Eds.), *Diagnostic assessment in child and adolescent psychopathology* (pp. 34–64). New York: Guilford Press.

APA Presidential Task Force on Evidence-Based Practice. (2006). Evidence-based practice in psychology. *American Psychologist, 61*, 271–285.

Aronen, E. T., Noam, G. G., & Weinstein, S. R. (1993). Structured diagnostic interviews and clinicians' discharge diagnoses in hospitalized adolescents. *Journal of the American Academy of Child and Adolescent Psychiatry, 32*, 674–681.

Barrios, B., & Hartmann, D. P. (1986). The contributions of traditional assessment: Concepts, issues, and methodologies. In R. O. Nelson & S. C. Hayes (Eds.), *Conceptual foundations of behavioral assessment* (pp. 81–110). New York: Guilford Press.

Basco, M. R., Bostic, J. Q., Davies, D., Rush, A. J., Witte, B., Hendrickse, W., & Barnett, V. (2000). Methods to improve diagnostic accuracy in a community mental health setting. *American Journal of Psychiatry, 157*(10), 1599–1605.

Beaton, D. E., Bombardier, C., Guillemin, F., & Ferraz, M. B. (2000). Guidelines for the process of cross-cultural adaptation of self-report measures. *Spine, 25*(24), 3186–3191.

Beidas, R. S., Stewart, R. E., Walsh, L., Lucas, S., Downey, M. M., Jackson, K., . . . Mandell, D. S. (2015). Free, brief, and validated: Standardized instruments for low-resource mental health settings. *Cognitive and Behavioral Practice, 22*, 5–19.

Birmaher, B., Brent, D. A., Chiappetta, L., Bridge, J., Monga, S., & Baugher, M. (1999). Psychometric properties of the Screen for Child Anxiety Related Emotional Disorders (SCARED): A replication study. *Journal of the American Academy of Child and Adolescent Psychiatry, 38*, 1230–1236.

Birmaher, B., Ehmann, M., Axelson, D. A., Goldstein, B. I., Monk, K., Kalas, C., . . . Brent, D. A. (2009). Schedule for Affective Disorders and Schizophrenia for School-Age Children (K-SADS-PL) for the assessment of preschool children—a preliminary psychometric study. *Journal of Psychiatric Research, 43*, 680–686.

Bongiovi-Garcia, M. E., Merville, J., Almeida, M. G., Burke, A., Ellis, S., Stanley, B. H., . . . Oquendo, M. A. (2009). Comparison of clinical and research assessments of diagnosis, suicide attempt history and suicidal ideation in major depression. *Journal of Affective Disorders, 115*, 183–188.

Brannan, A. M., Athay, M. M., & de Andrade, A. R. V. (2012). Measurement quality of the Caregiver Strain Questionnaire—Short Form 7 (CGSQ-SF7). *Administration and Policy in Mental Health and Mental Health Services Research, 39*, 51–59.

British Psychological Society. (2017). BPS Practice Guidelines, Third edition. Retrieved from *www.bps.org.uk/news-and-policy/practice-guidelines*.

Bruchmüller, K., Margraf, J., Suppiger, A., & Schneider, S. (2011). Popular or unpopular?: Therapists' use of structured interviews and their estimation of patient acceptance. *Behavior Therapy, 42*, 634–643.

Canivez, G. L. (2013). Psychometric versus actuarial interpretation of intelligence and related aptitude batteries. In D. H. Saklofske, V. L. Schwean, & C. R. Reynolds (Eds.), *The Oxford handbook of child psychological assessments* (pp. 84–112). New York: Oxford University Press.

Cashel, M. L. (2002). Child and adolescent psychological assessment: Current clinical practices and the impact of managed care. *Professional Psychology: Research and Practice, 33*, 446–453.

Chambless, D. L., & Hollon, S. D. (2012). Treatment validity for intervention studies. In H. Cooper, P. M. Camic, D. L. Long, A. T. Panter, D. Rindskopf, & K. J. Sher (Eds.), *APA handbook of research methods in psychology: Vol. 2. Research designs: Quantitative, qualitative, neuropsychological, and biological* (p. 529–552). Washington, DC: American Psychological Association.

Chen, Y. L., Shen, L. J., & Gau, S. S. (2017). The Mandarin version of the Kiddie-Schedule for Affective Disorders and Schizophrenia—Epidemiological version for DSM-5—a psychometric study. *Journal of the Formosa Medical Association, 116,* 671–678.

Cheng, H., Hayes, D., Edbrooke-Childs, J., Martin, K., Chapman, L., & Wolpert, M. (2017). What approaches for promoting shared decision-making are used in child mental health?: A scoping review. *Clinical Psychology and Psychotherapy, 24*(6), 1495–1511.

Chorpita, B. F., Bernstein, A., & Daleiden, E. L. (2011). Empirically guided coordination of multiple evidence-based treatments: An illustration of relevance mapping in children's mental health services. *Journal of Consulting and Clinical Psychology, 79,* 470–480.

Chorpita, B. F., & Nakamura, B. J. (2008). Dynamic structure in diagnostic structured interviewing: A comparative test of accuracy and efficiency. *Journal of Psychopathology and Behavioral Assessment, 30,* 52–60.

Christon, L. M., McLeod, B. D., & Jensen-Doss, A. (2015). Evidence-based assessment meets evidence-based treatment: An approach to science-informed case conceptualization. *Cognitive and Behavioral Practice, 22,* 36–48.

Chu, B. C., Crocco, S. T., Esseling, P., Areizaga, M. J., Lindner, A. M., & Skriner, L. C. (2016). Transdiagnostic group behavioral activation and exposure therapy for youth anxiety and depression: Initial randomized controlled trial. *Behaviour Research and Therapy, 76,* 65–75.

Cicchetti, D. V. (1994). Guidelines, criteria, and rules of thumb for evaluating normed and standardized assessment instruments in psychology. *Psychological Assessment, 6,* 284–290.

Cohen, J. (1960). A coefficient of agreement for nominal scales. *Educational and Psychological Measurement, 20,* 37–46.

Cone, J. D. (1986). Idiographic, nomothetic, and related perspectives in behavioral assessment. In R. O. Nelson & S. C. Hayes (Eds.), *Conceptual foundations of behavioral assessment* (pp. 111–128). New York: Guilford Press.

Cone, J. D. (1997). Issues in functional analysis in behavioral assessment. *Behaviour Research and Therapy, 35,* 259–275.

Connors, E. H., Arora, P., Curtis, L., & Stephan, S. H. (2015). Evidence-based assessment in school mental health. *Cognitive and Behavioral Practice, 22,* 60–73.

Cook, J. R., Hausman, E. M., Jensen-Doss, A., & Hawley, K. M. (2017). Assessment practices of child clinicians. *Assessment, 24,* 210–221.

de la Pena, F. R., Villavicencio, L. R., Palacio, J. D., Felix, F. J., Larraguibel, M., Viola, L., . . . Ulloa, R. E. (2018). Validity and reliability of the Kiddie Schedule for Affective Disorders and Schizophrenia Present and Lifetime Version DSM-5 (K-SADS-PL-5) Spanish version. *BMC Psychiatry, 18,* 193.

De Los Reyes, A., Augenstein, T. M., Wang, M., Thomas, S. A., Drabick, D. A., Burgers, D. E., & Rabinowitz, J. (2015). The validity of the multi-informant approach to assessing child and adolescent mental health. *Psychological Bulletin, 141,* 858–900.

De Los Reyes, A., & Kazdin, A. E. (2005). Informant discrepancies in the assessment of childhood psychopathology: A critical review, theoretical framework, and recommendations for further study. *Psychological Bulletin, 131,* 483–509.

De Los Reyes, A., Thomas, S. A., Goodman, K. L., & Kundey, S. M. (2013). Principles underlying the use of multiple informants' reports. *Annual Review of Clinical Psychology, 9,* 123–149.

De Los Reyes, A., Youngstrom, E. A., Pabon, S. C., Youngstrom, J. K., Feeny, N. C., & Findling, R. L. (2011). Internal consistency and associated characteristics of informant discrepancies in clinic referred youths age 11 to 17 years. *Journal of Clinical Child and Adolescent Psychology, 40,* 36–53.

Dekkers, O. M., von Elm, E., Algra, A., Romijn, J. A., & Vandenbroucke, J. P. (2010). How to assess the external validity of therapeutic trials: A conceptual approach. *International Journal of Epidemiology, 39,* 89–94.

Diamond, G. S., Reis, B. F., Diamond, G. M., Siqueland, L., & Isaacs, L. (2002). Attachment-based family therapy for depressed adolescents: A treatment development study. *Journal of the American Academy of Child and Adolescent Psychiatry, 41,* 1190–1196.

Dirks, M. A., Boyle, M. H., & Georgiades, K. (2011). Psychological symptoms in youth and later socioeconomic functioning: Do associations vary by informant? *Journal of Clinical Child and Adolescent Psychology, 40,* 10–22.

Dirks, M. A., De Los Reyes, A., Briggs-Gowan, M., Cella, D., & Wakschlag, L. S. (2012). Annual research review: Embracing not erasing contextual variability in children's behavior—theory and utility in the selection and use of methods and informants in developmental psychopathology. *Journal of Child Psychology and Psychiatry, 53,* 558–574.

Doss, A. J., Cook, K. T., & McLeod, B. D. (2008). Diagnostic issues. In M. Hersen & D. Reitman (Eds.), *Handbook of psychological assessment, case conceptualization, and treatment: Vol 2. Children and adolescents* (pp. 25–52). Hoboken: Wiley.

Downing, S. M. (2003). Validity: On the meaningful interpretation of assessment data. *Medical Education, 37,* 830–837.

Duncan, L., Comeau, J., Wang, L., Vitoroulis, I., Boyle, M. H., & Bennett, K. (2019). Research Review: Test–retest reliability of standardized diagnostic interviews to assess child and adolescent psychiatric disorders: A systematic review and meta-analysis. *Journal of Child Psychology and Psychiatry, 60*(1), 16–29.

Duncan, L., Georgiades, K., Wang, L., Lieshout, R. J. V., Macmillan, H. L., Ferro, M. A., . . . Boyle, M. H. (2018). Psychometric evaluation of the Mini International Neuropsychiatric Interview for Children and Adolescents (MINI-KID). *Psychological Assessment, 30*(7), 916–928.

Eells, T. D. (2007). *Handbook of psychotherapy case formulation* (2nd ed.). New York: Guilford Press.

Eells, T. D. (2015). *Psychotherapy case formulation*. Washington, DC: American Psychological Association.

Eells, T. D., & Lombart, K. G. (2004). Case formulation: Determining the focus in brief dynamic psychotherapy. In D. P. Charman (Ed.), *Core processes in brief psychodynamic psychotherapy: Advancing effective practice* (pp. 119–144). Mahwah, NJ: Erlbaum.

Eyberg, S. M., & Robinson, E. A. (1981). *Dyadic parent–child interaction coding system: A manual*. Washington, DC: American Psychological Association.

First, M. B. (2014). *DSM-5™ handbook of differential diagnosis*. Arlington, VA: American Psychiatric Publishing.

Flinn, L., Braham, L., & das Nair, R. (2015). How reliable are case formulations?: A systematic literature review. *British Journal of Clinical Psychology, 54,* 266–290.

Furr, R. M., & Bacharach, V. R. (2008). *Psychometrics: An introduction*. Thousand Oaks, CA: SAGE.

Galanter, C. A., & Patel, V. L. (2005). Medical decision making: A selective review for child psychiatrists and psychologists. *Journal of Child Psychology and Psychiatry, 46*(7), 675–689.

Garb, H. N. (1998). *Studying the clinician: Judgment research and psychological assessment*. Washington, DC: American Psychological Association.

Garb, H. N. (2005). Clinical judgment and decision making. *Annual Review of Clinical Psychology, 1,* 67–89.

Ghanizadeh, A., Mohammadi, M. R., & Yazdanshenas, A. (2006). Psychometric properties of the Farsi translation of the Kiddie Schedule for Affective Disorders and Schizophrenia—Present and Lifetime Version. *BMC Psychiatry, 6,* 10.

Guillemin, F., Bombardier, C., & Beaton, D. (1993). Cross-cultural adaptation of health-related quality of life measures: Literature review and proposed guidelines. *Journal of Clinical Epidemiology, 46*(12), 1417–1432.

Hallgren, K. A. (2012). Computing inter-rater reliability for observational data: An overview and tutorial. *Tutorials in Quantitative Methods for Psychology, 8,* 23–34.

Hankin, B. L., & Abramson, L. Y. (2002). Measuring cognitive vulnerability to depression in adolescence: Reliability, validity and gender differences. *Journal of Clinical Child and Adolescent Psychology, 31,* 491–504.

Hankin, B. L., Snyder, H. R., Gulley, L. D., Schweizer, T. H., Bijttebier, P., Nelis, S., . . . Vasey, M. W. (2016). Understanding comorbidity among internalizing problems: Integrating latent structural models of psychopathology and risk mechanisms. *Development and Psychopathology, 28,* 987–1012.

Haynes, S. N., O'Brien, W. H., & Kaholokula, J. K. A. (2011). *Behavioral assessment and case formulation*. Hoboken, NJ: Wiley.

Hughes, C. W., Emslie, G. J., Wohlfahrt, H., Winslow, R., Kashner, T. M., & Rush, A. J. (2005). Effect of structured interviews on evaluation time in pediatric community mental health settings. *Psychiatric Services, 56,* 1098–1103.

Hunsley, J., & Mash, E. J. (2007). Evidence-based assessment. *Annual Review of Clinical Psychology, 3,* 29–51.

Hunsley, J., & Mash, E. J. (2018). *A guide to assessments that work* (2nd ed.). New York: Oxford University Press.

Hus, V., & Lord, C. (2014). The Autism Diagnostic Observation Schedule, Module 4: Revised algorithm and standardized severity scores. *Journal of Autism and Developmental Disorders, 44*(8), 1996–2012.

Jensen, A. L., & Weisz, J. R. (2002). Assessing match and mismatch between practitioner-generated and standardized interview-generated diagnoses for clinic-referred children and adolescents. *Journal of Consulting and Clinical Psychology, 70,* 158–168.

Jensen, P. S., Youngstrom, E. A., Steiner, H., Findling, R. L., Meyer, R. E., Malone, R. P., . . . Vitiello, B. (2007). Consensus report on impulsive aggression as a symptom across diagnostic categories in child psychiatry: Implications for medication studies. *Journal of the American Academy of Child and Adolescent Psychiatry, 46,* 309–322.

Jensen-Doss, A., & Hawley, K. M. (2011). Understanding clinicians' diagnostic practices: Attitudes toward the utility of diagnosis and standardized diagnostic tools. *Administration and Policy in Mental Health and Mental Health Services Research, 38,* 476–485.

Jensen-Doss, A., & Weisz, J. R. (2008). Diagnostic agreement predicts treatment process and outcomes in youth mental health clinics. *Journal of Consulting and Clinical Psychology, 76,* 711–722.

Jensen-Doss, A., Youngstrom, E. A., Youngstrom, J. K., Feeny, N. C., & Findling, R. L. (2014). Predictors and moderators of agreement between clinical and research diagnoses for children and adolescents. *Journal of Consulting and Clinical Psychology, 82,* 1151–1162.

Jewell, J., Handwerk, M., Almquist, J., & Lucas, C. (2004). Comparing the validity of clinician-generated diagnosis of conduct disorder to the Diagnostic Interview Schedule for Children. *Journal of Clinical Child and Adolescent Psychology, 33,* 536–546.

Kaufman, J., Birmaher, B., Axelson, D. A., Perepletchikova, F., Brent, D., & Ryan, N. (2016). Schedule for Affective Disorders and Schizophrenia for School-Age Children—Present and Lifetime Version for DSM-5 (K-SADS-PL DSM-5). Retrieved from *https://pediatricbipolar.pitt.edu/resources/instruments.*

Kaufman, J., Birmaher, B., Brent, D., Rao, U., Flynn, C., Moreci, P., . . . Ryan, N. (1997). Schedule for affective disorders and schizophrenia for school-age children-present and lifetime version (K-SADS-PL): Initial reliability and validity data. *Journal of the American Academy of Child and Adolescent Psychiatry, 36,* 980–988.

Kearney, C. A. (2002). Identifying the function of school refusal behavior: A revision of the School Refusal Assessment Scale. *Journal of Psychopathology and Behavioral Assessment, 24,* 235–245.

Kendell, R., & Jablensky, A. (2003). Distinguishing between the validity and utility of psychiatric diagnoses. *American Journal of Psychiatry, 160,* 4–12.

Kennedy, S. M., & Ehrenreich-May, J. (2017). Assessment of emotional avoidance in adolescents: Psychometric properties of a new multidimensional measure. *Journal of Psychopathology and Behavioral Assessment, 39,* 279–290.

Kim, Y. S., Cheon, K.-A., Kim, B.-N., Chang, S.-A., Yoo, H.-J., Kim, J., . . . Leventhal, B. (2004). The reliablity and validity of the Kiddie-Schedule for Affective Disorders and Schizophrenia—Present and Lifetime Version—Korean Version (K-SADS-PL-K). *Yonsei Medical Journal, 45,* 81–89.

Kraemer, H. C., Kupfer, D. J., Clarke, D. E., Narrow, W. E., & Regier, D. A. (2012). DSM-5: How reliable is reliable enough? *American Journal of Psychiatry, 169,* 13–15.

Kramer, T. L., Robbins, J. M., Phillips, S. D., Miller, T. L., & Burns, B. J. (2003). Detection and outcomes of substance use disorders in adolescents seeking mental health treatment. *Journal of the American Academy of Child and Adolescent Psychiatry, 42,* 1813–1826.

Kukull, W. A., & Ganguli, M. (2012). Generalizability: The trees, the forest, and the low-hanging fruit. *Neurology, 78,* 1886–1891.

Landis, J. R., & Koch, G. G. (1977). The measurement of observer agreement for categorical data. *Biometrics, 33,* 159–174.

Langer, D. A., & Jensen-Doss, A. (2018). Shared decision-making in youth mental health care: Using the evidence to plan treatments collaboratively. *Journal of Clinical Child and Adolescent Psychology, 47,* 821–831.

Leffler, J. M., Riebel, J., & Hughes, H. M. (2015). A review of child and adolescent diagnostic interviews for clinical practitioners. *Assessment, 22,* 690–703.

Lord, C., Rutter, M., DiLavore, P. C., Risi, S., Gotham, K., & Bishop, S. (2012). *Autism Diagnostic Observation Schedule* (2nd ed.). Torrance, CA: Western Psychological Services.

Mash, E. J., & Hunsley, J. (2005). Evidence-based assessment of child and adolescent disorders: Issues and challenges. *Journal of Clinical Child and Adolescent Psychology, 34,* 362–379.

Matson, J. L., Matheis, M., Estabillo, J. A., Burns, C. O., Issarraras, A., Peters, W. J., & Jiang, X. (2019). Intellectual disability. In M. J. Prinstein, E. A. Youngstrom, E. J. Mash, & R. A. Barkley (Eds.), *Treatment of disorders in childhood and adolescence* (4th ed., pp. 416–447). New York: Guilford Press.

Matuschek, T., Jaeger, S., Stadelmann, S., Dolling, K., Grunewald, M., Weis, S., . . . Dohnert, M. (2016). Implementing the K-SADS-PL as a standard diagnostic tool: Effects on clinical diagnoses. *Psychiatry Research, 236,* 119–124.

McGill, R. J., & Ndip, N. (2019). Learning disabilities. In M. J. Prinstein, E. A. Youngstrom, E. J. Mash, & R. A. Barkley (Eds.), *Treatment of disorders in childhood and adolescence* (4th ed., pp. 448–492). New York: Guilford Press.

McGuire, J. F., Sukhodolsky, D. G., Bearss, K., Grantz, H., Pachler, M., Lombroso, P. J., & Scahill, L. (2014). Individualized assessments in treatment research: An examination of parent-nominated target problems in the treatment of disruptive behaviors in youth with Tourette syndrome. *Child Psychiatry and Human Development, 45,* 686–694.

McHugh, M. L. (2012). Interrater reliability: The kappa statistic. *Biochemia Medica, 22,* 276–282.

McLeod, B. D., Jensen-Doss, A., & Ollendick, T. H. (2013a). Case conceptualization, treatment planning, and outcome monitoring. In B. D. McLeod, A. Jensen-Doss, & T. H. Ollendick (Eds.), *Diagnostic and behavioral assessment in children and adolescents: A clinical guide* (pp. 77–100). New York: Guilford Press.

McLeod, B. D., Jensen-Doss, A., & Ollendick, T. H. (2013b). Overview of diagnostic and behavioral assessment. In B. D. McLeod, A. Jensen-Doss, & T. H. Ollendick (Eds.), *Diagnostic and behavioral assessment in children and adolescents: A clinical guide* (pp. 3–33). New York: Guilford Press.

Miller, P. R. (2002). Inpatient diagnostic assessments: 3. Causes and effects of diagnostic imprecision. *Psychiatry Research, 111,* 191–197.

Miller, P. R., Dasher, R., Collins, R., Griffiths, P., & Brown, F. (2001). Inpatient diagnostic assessments: 1. Accuracy of structured vs. unstructured interviews. *Psychiatry Research, 105,* 255–264.

Morrison, J. (2014). *Diagnosis made easier: Principles and techniques for mental health clinicians* (2nd ed.). New York: Guilford Press.

Mufson, L. H., Dorta, K. P., Moreau, D., & Weissman, M. M. (2004). *Interpersonal psychotherapy for depressed adolescents* (2nd ed.). New York: Guilford Press.

Multimodal Treatment Study of Children with ADHD Cooperative Group. (1999). Moderators and mediators of treatment response for children with attention-deficit/hyperactivity disorder: The multimodal treatment study of children with attention-deficit/hyperactivity disorder. *Archives of General Psychiatry, 56,* 1088–1096.

Mumma, G. H. (2011). Validity issues in cognitive-behavioral case formulation. *European Journal of Psychological Assessment, 27,* 29–49.

Mumma, G. H., & Fluck, J. (2016). How valid is your case formulation?: Empirically testing your cognitive behavioural case formulation for tailored treatment. *The Cognitive Behaviour Therapist, 9,* e12.

Nelson-Gray, R. O. (2003). Treatment utility of psychological assessment. *Psychological Assessment, 15,* 521–531.

Newman, F. L., Rugh, D., & Ciarlo, J. A. (2004). Guidelines for selecting psychological instruments for treatment planning and outcomes assessment. In M. E. Maruish (Ed.), *The use of psychological testing for treatment planning and outcomes assessment: General considerations* (Vol. 1, 3rd ed., pp. 197–214). Mahwah, NJ: Erlbaum.

Nezu, A. M., Nezu, C. M., & Lombardo, E. (2004). *Cognitive-behavioral case formulation and treatment design: A problem-solving approach.* New York: Springer.

Ollendick, T. H., McLeod, B. D., & Jensen-Doss, A. (2013). Behavioral assessment. In B. D. McLeod, A. Jensen-Doss, & T. H. Ollendick (Eds.), *Diagnostic and behavioral assessment in children and adolescents: A clinical guide* (pp. 56–76). New York: Guilford Press.

Pelham, W. E., Jr., Fabiano, G. A., & Massetti, G. M. (2005). Evidence-based assessment of attention deficit hyperactivity disorder in children and adolescents. *Journal of Clinical Child and Adolescent Psychology, 34*(3), 449–476.

Persons, J. B. (2008). *The case formulation approach to cognitive-behavior therapy.* New York: Guilford Press.

Pogge, D. L., Wayland-Smith, D., Zaccario, M., Borgaro, S., Stokes, J., & Harvey, P. D. (2001). Diagnosis of manic episodes in adolescent inpatients: Structured diagnostic procedures compared to clinical chart diagnoses. *Psychiatry Research, 101,* 47–54.

Pugliese, C. E., Kenworthy, L., Bal, V. H., Wallace, G. L., Yerys, B. E., Maddox, B. B., . . . Herrington, J. D. (2015). Replication and comparison of the newly proposed ADOS-2, module 4 algorithm in ASD without ID: A multi-site study. *Journal of Autism and Developmental Disorders, 45*(12), 3919–3931.

Raiker, J. S., Freeman, A. J., Perez-Algorta, G., Frazier, T. W., Findling, R. L., & Youngstrom, E. A. (2017). Accuracy of Achenbach Scales in the screening of attention-deficit/hyperactivity disorder in a community mental health clinic. *Journal of American Academy of Child and Adolescent Psychiatry, 56,* 401–409.

Reitman, D., McGregor, S., & Resnick, A. (2013). Direct observation. In B. D. McLeod, A. Jensen-Doss, & T. H. Ollendick (Eds.), *Diagnostic and behavioral assessment in children and adolescents: A clinical guide* (pp. 164–195). New York: Guilford Press.

Rettew, D. C., Lynch, A. D., Achenbach, T. M., Dumenci, L., & Ivanova, M. Y. (2009). Meta-analyses of agreement between diagnoses made from clinical evaluations and standardized diagnostic interviews. *International Journal of Methods in Psychiatric Research, 18,* 169–184.

Reynolds, C. R., & Kamphaus, R. W. (2015). *Behavioral Assessment System for Children manual* (3rd ed.). Bloomington, MN: Pearson.

Sales, C., & Alves, P. C. (2012). Individualized patient-progress systems: Why we need to move towards a personalized evaluation of psychological treatments. *Canadian Psychology, 53,* 115–121.

Shaffer, D., Fisher, P., Lucas, C. P., Dulcan, M. K., &

Schwab-Stone, M. E. (2000). NIMH Diagnostic Interview Schedule for Children Version IV (NIMH DISC-IV): Description, differences from previous versions, and reliability of some commond diagnoses. *Journal of American Academy of Child and Adolescent Psychiatry, 39,* 28–38.

Shahrivar, Z., Kousha, M., Moallemi, S., Tehrani-Doost, M., & Alaghband-Rad, J. (2010). The reliability and validity of Kiddie-Schedule for Affective Disorders and Schizophrenia—Present and Life-time Version—Persian Version. *Child and Adolescent Mental Health, 15,* 97–102.

Sheehan, D. V., Sheehan, K. H., Shytle, R. D., Janavs, J., Bannon, Y., Rogers, J. E., . . . Wilkinson, B. (2010). Reliability and validity of the Mini International Neuropsychiatric Interview for Children and Adolescents (MINI-KID). *Journal of Clinical Psychiatry, 71,* 313–326.

Spitzer, R. L. (1983). Psychiatric diagnosis: Are clinicians still necessary? *Comprehensive Psychiatry, 24,* 399–411.

Straus, R. L., Glasziou, P., Richardson, W. S., & Haynes, R. B. (2011). *Evidence-based medicine: How to practice and teach EBM* (4th ed.). New York: Churchill Livingstone.

Suppiger, A., In-Albon, T., Hendriksen, S., Hermann, E., Margraf, J., & Schneider, S. (2009). Acceptance of structured diagnostic interviews for mental disorders in clinical practice and research settings. *Behavior Therapy, 40,* 272–279.

Sutton, A. J., & Higgins, J. P. T. (2008). Recent developments in meta-analysis. *Statistics in Medicine, 27,* 625–650.

Tenney, N. H., Schotte, C. K. W., Denys, D. A. J. P., van Megen, H. J. G. M., & Westenberg, H. G. M. (2003). Assessment of DSM-IV personality disorders in obsessive–compulsive disorder: Comparison of clinical diagnosis, self-report questionnaire, and semi-structured interview. *Journal of Personality Disorders, 17,* 550–561.

Ulloa, R. E., Ortiz, S., Higuera, F., Nogales, I., Fresán, A., Apiquian, R., . . . de la Peña, F. (2006). Interrater reliability of the Spanish version of Schedule for Affective Disorders and Schizophrenia for School-Age Children—Present and Lifetime version (K-SADS-PL). *Actas Espana Psiquiatrica, 35,* 36–40.

van Dulmen, M. H. M., & Egeland, B. (2011). Analyzing multiple informant data on child and adolescent behavior problems: Predictive validity and comparison to aggregation procedures. *International Journal of Behavioral Development, 35,* 84–92.

Wakschlag, L. S., Hill, C., Carter, A. S., Danis, B., Egger, H. L., Keenan, K., . . . Burns, J. (2008). Observational assessment of preschool disruptive behavior: Part I. Reliability of the Disruptive Behavior Diagnostic Observation Schedule (DB-DOS). *Journal of the American Academy of Child and Adolescent Psychiatry, 47,* 622–631.

Watkins, M. W., Kush, J. C., & Glutting, J. J. (1997). Discriminant and predictive validity of the WISC-III ACID profile among children with learning disabilities. *Psychology in the Schools, 34,* 309–319.

Weersing, V. R., Jeffreys, M., Do, M.-C. T., Schwartz, K. T. G., & Bolano, C. (2017). Evidence base update of psychosocial treatments for child and adolescent depression. *Journal of Clinical Child and Adolescent Psychology, 46,* 11–43.

Weisz, J. R., Chorpita, B. F., Frye, A., Ng, M. Y., Lau, N., Bearman, S. K., . . . Hoagwood, K. E. (2011). Youth top problems: Using idiographic, consumer-guided assessment to identify treatment needs and to track change during psychotherapy. *Journal of Consulting and Clinical Psychology, 79,* 369–380.

Weisz, J. R., & Weiss, B. (1991). Studying the "referability" of child clinical problems. *Journal of Consulting and Clinical Psychology, 59*(2), 266.

Whiteside, S. P. H., Sattler, A. F., Hathaway, J., & Douglas, K. V. (2016). Use of evidence-based assessment for childhood anxiety disorders in community practice. *Journal of Anxiety Disorders, 39,* 65–70.

Wolraich, M. L., Lambert, W., Doffing, M. A., Bickman, L., Simmons, T., & Worley, K. (2003). Psychometric properties of the Vanderbilt ADHD Diagnostic Parent Rating Scale in a referred population. *Journal of Pediatric Psychology, 28,* 559–567.

Yoman, J. (2008). A primer on functional analysis. *Cognitive and Behavioral Practice, 15,* 325–340.

Youngstrom, E. A., Findling, R. L., Youngstrom, J. K., & Calabrese, J. R. (2005). Toward an evidence-based assessment of pediatric bipolar disorder. *Journal of Clinical Child and Adolescent Psychology, 34*(3), 433–448.

Youngstrom, E. A., Van Meter, A., Frazier, T. W., Hunsley, J., Prinstein, M. J., Ong, M. L., & Youngstrom, J. K. (2017). Evidence-based assessment as an integrative model for applying psychological science to guide the voyage of treatment. *Clinical Psychology: Science and Practice, 24,* 331–363.

Youngstrom, E. A., Youngstrom, J. K., Freeman, A. J., De Los Reyes, A., Feeny, N. C., & Findling, R. L. (2011). Informants are not all equal: Predictors and correlates of clinician judgments about caregiver and youth credibility. *Journal of Child and Adolescent Psychopharmacology, 21,* 407–415.

CHAPTER 4

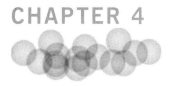

Assessing Process
Are We There Yet?

Andrew J. Freeman and John Young

Psychotherapy can be defined as the use of a thera-peutic relationship between a trained healer (e.g., therapist) and a sufferer (e.g., client, patient) by fo-cusing on changing attitudes, thoughts, affect, be-havior, social context, and/or development (Brent & Kolko, 1998). Psychotherapy is often described as a journey. Each of the three P's of assessment fit within this analogy. The *prediction* phase focuses on accurately and efficiently selecting a meaning-ful destination. The *prescription* phase provides an initial set of directions. The *process* phase an-swers the age-old question "Are we there yet?" The process phase of assessment helps us determine where in treatment we are. Are the roads clear, free of construction and accidents? If so, treatment should maintain its course and continue as is. Is there construction, an accident, traffic? If so, the course of treatment might need to be rerouted and revised. Have we reached our destination? If so,

then the termination phase of treatment can be started, and planning for the future should com-mence. The destination of treatment is the mean-ingful difference made in a person's everyday life as a result of treatment (Kazdin, 1999). Our purpose in this chapter is to provide a general conceptual framework for the process phase of assessment and to highlight the practical implementation of the process phase of assessment in the context of an individual case example—Ty.

What Is the *Process* Phase of Assessment?

Process in the context of psychotherapy has many definitions. Early reviews of psychotherapy re-search distinguished between psychotherapeutic process and outcome (Luborsky, 1959). Process often refers narrowly to the interpersonal context of psychotherapy (e.g., working alliance) or the mechanism of treatment (e.g., common vs. spe-cific factors) (Shirk & Karver, 2006). However, in the context of evidence-based assessment, the pro-cess phase of assessment refers to a broader set of information that includes psychotherapeutic pro-cess and outcomes. Outcomes are the meaningful, practical effects of treatment on an individual's everyday life. Process assessment could include measurement of many domains: (1) the interper-sonal context of treatment, (2) mechanisms of treatment, (3) treatment adherence, or (4) treatment outcomes. Therefore, the purpose of the process phase of assessment is to focus measurement on information that directly informs the clinician and the client about how the course of treatment is unfolding.

The process phase of assessment is based on the principles of measurement-based care. In surveys of clinicians, most report informally checking in with clients on how treatment is progressing but not engaging in routine outcome monitoring (Hatfield & Ogles, 2004; Ionita & Fitzpatrick, 2014; Overington, Fitzpatrick, Drapeau, & Hunsley, 2016). Most clinicians report that they have not been exposed to or trained in formal outcome monitoring during formal training experiences (Overington et al., 2016). When introduced to routine outcomes assessment, clinicians report concerns that it would take too much time, be too expensive, add too much client burden, and not have enough utility (Hatfield & Ogles, 2007; Jensen-Doss & Hawley, 2010). However, process monitoring can be brief, low or no cost, low burden, and has utility (Bickman, Kelley, Breda, de Andrade, & Riemer, 2011). Assessing the treatment process could be as simple as tracking a weekly verbal response to "How was your week?" or as complex as tracking multiple goals via formal measurement. Regardless of specific method, the process phase represents a systematic assessment focused on measuring what matters to the client. For the clinician, systematic assessment of what matters to the client provides the opportunity to collaboratively identify treatment goals/outcomes and a method for benchmarking progress in treatment (Meehl, 1973). For the client, the process phase asks the client to engage in shared decision making, with what matters to the client providing the benchmark for success. Therefore, the process phase of assessment provides an opportunity for the clinician and client to identify treatment goals/outcomes, determine how goals/outcomes are measured, then routinely monitor the goals/outcomes to inform how treatment is progressing.

Conceptual Framework

Many treatment sessions start with some version of "How are you doing?" Depending on therapeutic approach, a client's response to this question could result in a range of clinician responses, from an interpersonal nicety to meaningful information gathering that may not be integrated into the session, to the purpose of the session. The conceptual framework outlined below does not dictate a therapeutic response to this or any other potential assessment. Instead, the framework provides a foundation on which gathered information can be integrated into clinical practice. Therefore, the key step in the process phase of assessment is to record the assessment process for future use in either formal progress notes or informal psychotherapy notes.

Routine outcome monitoring forms the basis of a feedback loop about the performance of treatment. Feedback interventions are not new. Feedback interventions are routinely applied in many domains outside of clinical practice (Kluger & DeNisi, 1996). For example, Toyota relies on the Toyota Production System to improve quality and reduce cost (Holweg, 2007). A core principle of this lean approach to management is to routinely measure processes, so that any weaknesses in the production line can be identify and fixed quickly. Technology companies rely on management philosophies focused on improving measurable outcomes and purposefully building mechanisms to collect the data (e.g., Doerr & Page, 2018). In education, teachers trained using practice with performance feedback improve their teaching ability more than other versions of training, such as minicourses (Rose & Church, 1998). Despite a general focus on routine gathering and use of information in the broader culture, most clinicians report not engaging in routine outcome monitoring. In adult mental health, routine outcome monitoring with feedback has been consistently demonstrated to improve outcomes even for those adults who are initially worsening or not improving (Hawkins, Lambert, Vermeersch, Slade, & Tuttle, 2004). In child and adolescent mental health, routine outcome monitoring with feedback at each session is associated with greater improvement in youth outcomes than general outcome monitoring at longer intervals (Bickman et al., 2011). Youth in psychotherapy hold generally favorable views of routine outcome monitoring because it helps structure therapy sessions, increase self-awareness, and improve communication with the clinician (Duong, Lyon, Ludwig, Wasse, & McCauley, 2016). Therefore, the second key step to the process phase of assessment is to use systematically collected information as feedback.

In evidence-based assessment, the process phase consists of three formal steps and integrates a fourth step (Youngstrom, 2013; Youngstrom et al., 2017). The first step of the process phase of assessment is setting treatment goals/targets. The second step is to systematically measure the treatment goals. The third step is to plan for long-term self-monitoring. Across these steps, client preferences should be integrated via shared decision making. However, these steps do not occur only in a treatment room between a clinician and client. Process assessment scales throughout the system of care and specific measurements likely vary at different levels of care. Therefore, each section below outlines the framework for considering each step of the process phase across both clinician–client dyads and the context of care systems.

How Do I Set Goals?

The first step of process assessment is setting treatment goals. The discussion of *prescription* (Jensen-Doss, Patel, Casline, & McLeod, Chapter 3, this volume) provides a detailed review of how to build a scientifically based case conceptualization. One way to help jump-start the treatment goal process is to record the answer to the first question asked of a child and parent: "What brings you to the clinic?" This question brings out the top problems to focus on in treatment, which often are consistent with specific symptoms measured on questionnaires (Weisz et al., 2011). In building a case conceptualization, clinicians are also making explicit the treatment targets. Briefly, clinicians should (1) identify target behaviors and causal/maintaining factors, (2) arrive at a diagnosis, (3) form an initial case conceptualization, and (4) select and plan the initial course of treatment. Treatment goals often flow from the case conceptualization. For example, if the youth's top problem and target behavior is school refusal, then a treatment goal might be increased school attendance. The outcome to monitor is the treatment goal—school attendance. For treatment that is oriented toward active change, the relationship between treatment goal and treatment monitoring is strong. However, not all youth start treatment ready for change. For these youth, treatment goals should focus on remoralization or increasing motivation for change versus goals oriented toward remediation and/or rehabilitation (Lueger, 1998; Martinovich, 1998). Therefore, vital to treatment is the setting of appropriate treatment goals to inform not only the course of treatment but also what will be assessed, and how it will be assessed.

Good goals should be shared by the therapist, client, and family. The process of developing and sharing treatment goals improves the efficacy of treatment (Harkin et al., 2016; Marshall, Haywood, & Fitzpatrick, 2006; Tryon & Winograd, 2011). Clinicians should (1) develop case conceptualization-driven treatment goals, (2) set goals with youth, (3) set goals with parent, and (4) share clinician-, youth-, and parent-derived goals to create jointly shared treatment goals. When given the opportunity, youth and parents will independently create overlapping but unique treatment goals (Jacob, Edbrooke-Childs, Holley, Law, & Wolpert, 2016). Youth tend to create treatment goals that focus on how the youth copes with specific difficulties (e.g., "I will reduce the symptom/problem") and how he or she might achieve personal growth or independence (e.g., "I want to be more responsible for myself"). Parents tend to create treatment goals that focus on how the parent manages a specific difficulty (e.g., "I want to help my child reduce the symptom/problem") and how he or she can improve (e.g., "I want to be a better parent when my child engages in this behavior"). Notice that these are similar treatment goals, but the mechanism of change and the target of treatment vary. Sharing the clinician-, youth-, and parent-generated treatment goals with each other allows for the development of joint goals, which improves both the child's perception and the parent's engagement, which are associated with less dropout and better outcomes (Fisher, Bromberg, Tai, & Palermo, 2017; McPherson, Scribano, & Stevens, 2012; Ormhaug & Jensen, 2018). Jointly negotiated goals tend to focus on managing specific symptoms/problems (e.g., goals focused on behavior management or symptom reduction), parent-specific goals (e.g., goals focused on improving parental skills and understanding), self-confidence and understanding goals (e.g., goals related to family functioning), and hopes for the future (e.g., goals related to increasing child and parent independence).

The question remains: "What makes a good treatment goal?" Imagine a child who has frequently refused to attend school. What would be a good treatment goal for this child? Good goals have specific characteristics. First, good goals are approach-oriented, not avoidance-oriented. Approach-oriented goals focus on a positive end states, while avoidance-oriented goals focus on staying away from negative end states. For example, an avoidance-oriented goal is "I will avoid anxiously worrying about school," whereas an approach-oriented goal is "I will discuss my evening plans with my mom on the way to school." Approach-oriented goals are associated with greater symptom reduction than are avoidance-oriented goals (Wollburg & Braukhaus, 2010).

Second, good goals are also SMART goals. Goals should be Specific, not general. A general goal is "I will attend school," while a specific goal is "I will attend school 4 days per week." Goals should be Measurable. Most specific goals are also measurable (i.e., the number of days attended is our measurement). Goals should be Achievable. Goals that are one or two steps ahead of a youth or family's current functioning level are better than ideal outcome goals. For example, ideally, a child would attend school each school day for the entire school year. Most children miss at least one day of school and thus fail at this goal. For a child who is currently only attending one day of school a week, an initial realistic goal might be one step further: "I will attend school 2 days." Good goals have a time frame in which they will be established (e.g., "I will attend school 2 days next week"). SMART goals are also Relevant, which means that client and therapist agree that they are important, and Time based, so that there is a clear definition of when to measure and how fast to look for change.

Third, good goals are dynamic. Treatment goals should be updated frequently and not simply be "fixed," long-term goals (Fuchs, Fuchs, & Hamlett, 1989). Frequently resetting goals is associated with larger treatment gains (Benito et al., 2018). Putting this all together, clinicians should focus on building treatment goals that are approach-oriented SMART goals and revise these goals as they are accomplished or in need of change. In the context of the school refusal example, an approach-oriented SMART goal might be "I will attend school two times next week," and if the child achieves that goal, then it should be revised: "I will attend school three times next week."

What Are the General Principles of Measuring Change?

Once positive, approach-oriented goals have been established, the next step to consider is how to measure these goals. For some goals, the measurement is explicit in the goal. For example, a goal of "I will attend school two times next week" defines what and when to measure—frequency of school attendance in a 7-day period. However, for broader, longer-term goals, the measurement of outcomes may not be as explicit in the goal. For example, goals may focus on reduction of symptoms; functioning with families, peers, at school, and/or the work environment; or more broadly on improving health and well-being (Sederer, Dickey, & Eisen, 1997). Regardless of the specific treatment goal, measurements should target malleable characteristics. For example, consider intervention with a youth with intellectual disability. Measuring treatment progress via the repeated assessment of cognitive abilities (i.e., IQ) would likely be unhelpful, as it is unlikely to change even with intervention. In contrast, measuring a malleable skill such as self-care is likely to result in detectable change if the intervention works and the measurement is appropriate. An instrument's ability to detect change in a construct over time is called *responsiveness* (Mokkink et al., 2010).

Responsive scales are pivotal for the detection of change during treatment. Ideally, *process* phase measures have high responsiveness in that they are able to detect change when it is present (i.e., true positive) and indicate no change when change has not occurred (i.e., true negative). Measures that are low in responsiveness are less sensitive to change and are more likely to fail to detect change when change has occurred (i.e., false negative). Use of outcome measures that have low responsiveness has multiple risks. First, receiving feedback that the youth is not improving may result in demoralization or early termination of therapy. Second, clinicians might be engaged in a successful treatment plan that is then changed because the measure indicates no change. Third, when quality demonstration is part of the reimbursement system (e.g., program evaluation contexts), failure to demonstrate change that has occurred may result in the loss of resources to a successful program or clinician.

Sensitivity to change, or responsiveness, is the detection of an effect due to an intervention or general development (Ebesutani, Bernstein, Chorpita, & Weisz, 2012). Typically, construction of many of the measures used in psychological research such as symptom checklists is based on individual differences, with the goal of assessing a specific construct. Measures that are well suited for the prediction phase of assessment and have a strong ability to distinguish psychopathology may or may not be as well suited for measuring treatment change (Hays & Hadorn, 1992). There are four main reasons to consider why responsiveness might be limited in many of our traditional checklists. First, limited response options may result in too coarse of measurement to detect change, resulting in a false negative (Ebesutani et al., 2012; Guyatt, Deyo, Charlson, Levine, & Mitchell, 1989; Lipsey, 1990). Second, many traditional measures are built to cover defined constructs and include symptoms that define the disorder but are not relevant to the individual (Fitzpatrick, Ziebland, Jenkinson, Mowat, & Mowat, 1992). For any individual, the items on a general measure may be more or less sensitive to the individual's presentation. For example, imagine treating a child with mild oppositional behavior. Asking whether the child misbehaves in dangerous ways is unlikely to be elevated at baseline because only children with very high levels of disruptive behavior endorse this behavior with any frequency and, as a result, this item is unlikely to be responsive for a child with mild oppositional behavior (Wakschlag et al., 2014). Third, the instructions for a measure are not conducive to rapid, repeated assessment. For example, asking how a person's functioning is over the past 3 months when the assessment is occurring on a monthly basis will result in overlapping windows of measurement that make change difficult to assess (Vermeersch, Lambert, & Burlingame, 2000). Fourth, standardized measures of psychopathology may not cover the breadth of a construct adequately or consistently, resulting in relevant behaviors, emotions, or thoughts not being assessed. For example, a content review of the seven most common depression scales indicated that only 12% of the assessed depression symptoms appeared across all scales in some form and that 40% of symptoms asked about appeared on only one scale (Fried, 2017). In summary, traditional measures of psychopathology may not be adequately responsive to change due to design characteristics that improve their ability to discriminate among presentations but are flaws in the context of being sensitive to change.

A growing area of clinically meaningful research is identifying whether measures are responsive to change. Fundamentally, a measure is responsive to change if (1) the measurement of the construct changes when the construct changes and (2) the measurement indicates no change when no change in the construct occurs (de Vet, Terwee, Mokkink, & Knol, 2011). One design for assessing a scale's responsiveness is to measure it and a "gold standard" simultaneously. If the results are strongly correlated, then the scale can be considered responsive. For example, consider using exposures to treat a person with posttraumatic stress disorder (PTSD) or anxiety. Phasic changes in physiological activity (e.g., heart rate and skin conductance) are indicative of arousal and historically difficult to implement in everyday clinical practice. In contrast, subjective units of distress

(SUDs) are relevant, simple, uncomplicated, and comprehensive of the construct of arousal. If SUDs change in the predicted direction during an exposure in line with changes in physiological arousal, then one can conclude that SUDs are responsive to change. In fact, SUDs and physiological arousal typically change together (cf. Marx et al., 2012). An alternative approach to developing general responsive measures is to switch to idiographic approaches. For example, the repeated assessment of a youth's top presenting problem (Weisz et al., 2011) represents this approach. One shortcoming of idiographic assessment is that large-scale, systems-level evaluations of treatment typically require normative measures, so that all individuals can be compared to each other. In summary, the development of validated, responsive measures for everyday clinical practice is needed.

How Often Should I Assess a Client?

Over the course of treatment, clinically meaningful change can occur on three time scales: immediate, intermediate, and final changes (Greenberg, 1986). Immediate treatment progress outcomes can be measured within session. Immediate progress outcomes are typically observable and/or easily measurable in the moment. Changes in facial expressions, overt behavior, the content of a person's thought, or heart rate reflect potential observable immediate outcomes, while SUDs reflect a potential immediate outcome. In the context of treating anxiety with exposure therapy, immediate outcomes are typically measured via changes in SUDs or physiological measures such as heart rate or skin conductance. In the context of child directed play (i.e., free-play in which the parent attends to the child's behavior without directions or questions), clinicians assess the frequency and content of the parent's speech (e.g., positive praise, description of the child's behavior). In summary, assessing immediate outcomes within the context of therapy sessions requires simple, easy-to-use, uncomplicated, and targeted assessments that reflect the hypothesized therapy change process.

Repeated changes in immediate progress outcomes are hypothesized to lead to intermediate changes. Intermediate progress monitoring is changes that occur in everyday life. Intermediate changes that occur across sessions and assessment of intermediate outcomes are often referred to as "routine outcome monitoring." Like immediate change assessment, intermediate change assessment should be simple, teachable, easy to use, and uncomplicated. Intermediate progress assessment should also directly assess progress toward treatment goals; be systematic, compatible with practice, and have utility; and be relevant to the youth's treatment needs (Lambert, Huefner, & Nace, 1997). It is crucial that these measures be administered quickly, as clinicians report being unlikely to implement any approach that takes more than 5 minutes to complete, score, and interpret (Brown, Dreis, & Nace, 1999). Intermediate progress assessment has undergone tremendous growth since the 1990s. Developing measures that are highly repeatable over short periods of time (e.g., 7 days) and responsive to change is relatively new in children's mental health. The earliest formal approach to assessing intermediate change was to repeatedly assess symptoms with symptom checklists. However, recent developments based on effectiveness studies focus on either idiographic measures or general measures. In both idiographic and general measures, scores are plotted against time to visually identify treatment trends.

Idiographic measures of intermediate change such as the Youth Top Problems (YTP; Weisz et al., 2011) provide formal boundaries to good practice. The YTP can be used with multiple informants such as youth self-report and caregiver or teacher report. Early in treatment, the clinician asks the informant what his or her top problems are and lists them in order. Most youth- (98%) and caregiver-identified (96%) top problems match individual items on the Youth Self-Report (YSR) and the Child Behavior Checklist (CBCL), respectively (Weisz et al., 2011). Measuring the specific, identified top problem only measures the target of psychotherapy at each session to determine whether the treatment is creating change. At each session, the clinician assesses how each problem is using a scale of 1 (*not a problem*) to 10 (*very big problem*). Recent versions of the YTP use a scale of 1 (*not a problem*) to 3 (*very big problem*). While the 1- to 3-point scale matches the scaling of many standardized assessment measures, the 1- to 10-point scale is likely to be more responsive to changes in treatment. For a client, the top problems are tracked over time visually on a graph. Visual analysis of change or lack of change in scores indicates treatment utility.

In contrast to idiographic measures of intermediate change, two types of general measures have been developed. The first type of general measure is brief forms that assess the same set of symptoms for all clients. The Symptoms and Functioning

Severity Scale (SFSS) in the Peabody Treatment Progress Battery is an excellent example of this approach (Bickman et al., 2010). The 13-item short forms of the SFSS measure Internalizing symptoms (i.e., anxiety and depression) and Externalizing symptoms (i.e., hyperactivity, impulsivity, and disruptive behavior). The SFSS is designed to be measured one time every 2 weeks. In contrast to asking about specific symptoms, the second type of general measure is global measures of functioning or distress. The Child Outcome Rating Scale (CORS) is an example of a general measure of change (Duncan, 2012). Using a visual analog scale, the CORS assesses a youth's subjective beliefs about how he or she is doing, and how family, school, and everything in general is going. Specific symptoms are not assessed. Instead, the CORS assesses the youth's subjective well-being. Each approach has its strengths. Symptom measurement using the SFSS is based on modern test theory and mimics treatment trials. One downside of this approach is that while internalizing and externalizing problems are the dominant presentation in outpatient community mental health services, not all youth present with internalizing and externalizing problems. As a result, monitoring treatment change with the SFSS may not be possible with some youth, particularly in more specialized settings. In contrast, assessing subjective well-being focuses on the impairment for which a youth is seeking services. One downside of this is that the youth can report high levels of subjective well-being while being impaired. In summary, both symptom-specific and subjective well-being approaches offer a standardized, responsive method for assessing intermediate change.

Intermediate change is hypothesized to lead to treatment outcome, sometimes referred to as "final change" (Kiesler, 2004). Treatment trials report treatment outcomes. In everyday clinical practice, *successful treatment* is treatment that results in meaningful, practical changes in a person's life (Kazdin, 1999). Similar to both immediate and intermediate progress monitoring, outcome assessment should be driven by treatment goals. For example, clinicians working with youth in foster care settings may not have a primary treatment goal of symptom reduction. Instead, the primary treatment goal might be to increase placement stability because placement instability is associated with poor long-term outcomes (Pecora et al., 2006). In this context, outcome assessment would determine whether the youth maintained placement stability. However, many treatment providers base their outcome assessment on proxy measures of clinically meaningful change, such as symptom reduction. Assessing symptom reduction is easy to standardize across presenting problems and mimics treatment trials, and many measures are available. In the context of outcome assessment, longer comprehensive measures of psychopathology that are given infrequently over the course of treatment are good options for measuring treatment outcome. Broad measures of psychopathology allow for the assessment of specific presenting problems, while also attending to the potential for change in other domains. Broad measures of psychopathology include the CBCL or YSR from the Achenbach System of Empirically Based Assessment (Achenbach & Rescorla, 2001) and the BASC-3 (Reynolds & Kamphaus, 2015). Alternatives to measuring treatment change via symptom reduction include directly assessing treatment outcomes, quality of life, or general functioning, such as with the Child and Adolescent Needs and Strengths (CANS; Lyons & Fernando, 2016). A treatment provider should choose the relevant final change assessment that serves the individual client's needs, as well as the needs of the greater health care system.

Did My Client Get Better?

At the end of the day, assessing change in psychotherapy boils down to answering a simple question: "Did the intervention make a real, genuine, practical difference in my client's everyday life?" Measuring outcomes is one method for demonstrating genuine, practical change. Assessment can take many forms, and the principles described below apply to different methods. Developing positive, approach-oriented treatment goals provides the framework for assessing treatment outcomes. However, assessing individualized treatment goals can make it difficult to systematically assess the quality of treatment for a wide variety of youth. As a result, treatment outcomes are measured via proxy measures (e.g., quality of life, symptom reduction). Therefore, the following presentation provides a clinically useful framework for evaluating change in psychotherapy using commonly available, standardized assessment instruments.

Graphical Approaches to Assessing Change

The simplest method for assessing change in treatment is to graph scores on the outcome measure over time. Whether the outcome is immediate,

intermediate, or final, the systematic plotting of outcomes is a fast, low-cost, efficient method for evaluating change in everyday clinical practice (Cone, 2001). Graphical representation of treatment scores takes advantage of our human ability to recognize complex patterns (Kim, Helal, & Cook, 2010). In fact, clinicians readily identify deviations from expected treatment trajectories (Hooke, Sng, Cunningham, & Page, 2018) and potentially harmful trajectories (Kashyap, Hooke, & Page, 2015). Therefore, systematically graphing treatment progress provides clinicians with one easy method for identifying the course of treatment.

Figure 4.1 provides an example of change in symptoms over time for immediate change (panels A and B), intermediate change (panels C and D), and final outcomes (panels E and F). In each panel, the x-axis represents a metric of time, and the y-axis represents the score on a measure. At each time point, the clinician adds a dot representing the youth's current score and connects the current score to previous scores. The resulting lines present a visually appealing and easy-to-interpret representation of treatment progress.

Panels A and B (Figure 4.1) depict immediate change over time of SUDs during an exposure. An exposure session typically occurs over a relatively short period of time (40–90 minutes), and SUDs are used as the outcome. During an exposure, SUDs are hypothesized to decrease in line with habituation. Panel A represents a hypothetical course of a successful exposure. At the beginning of the exposure, the youth's SUDs are elevated, and over time they decrease. In contrast, panel B displays a more complicated pattern. In this hypothetical exposure session, the youth's SUDs started at an elevated level, declined, but then between 30 and 35 minutes increased. Plotting the SUDs in session as the youth reports them, the uptick between 30 and 35 minutes indicates a potential hot spot that may require additional exposures or processing. As a clinician, blending the graphical results with the content of the session may provide guidance on how to titrate treatment.

Panel C (Figure 4.1) depicts intermediate outcome assessment using the YTP scale. Inspecting the panel, notice that at baseline, Problem 1 is more impairing than Problem 2, which is more impairing than Problem 3. Over the course of sessions, Problem 1 changed more rapidly than Problem 2 or Problem 3, and Problems 2 and 3 remained relatively stable. A youth, caregiver, clinician, or clinical supervisor might look at this

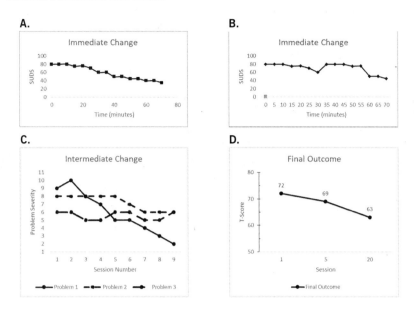

FIGURE 4.1. Graphs of Ty's immediate, intermediate, and outcome change.

figure and hypothesize that treatment has likely focused on Problem 1 and not Problems 2 and 3. Additionally, treatment of Problem 1 appears to be successful. Therefore, this graph indicates the youth's treatment is most likely ready for a change in treatment goals.

Panel D (Figure 4.1) tracks the youth's T-score on the Internalizing scale of the CBCL. At the beginning of treatment, the youth scored in the clinical range. Over the course of treatment, the youth's score declined to the normal range. Even though not all top problems have been resolved (see panel C), the overall internalizing score decreased. Visually, the youth's score appears to indicate treatment success. In summary, graphical approaches to assessing change provide easy, quick visual assessments of clinical change that can indicate how well the course of treatment is unfolding.

Statistical Methods for Determining Change

For many clinicians, sharing simple graphic displays with clients provides meaningful clinical information. In fact, regularly evaluating graphical displays of treatment progress and sharing the progression with clients is associated with better treatment outcomes in children and adolescents (Bickman et al., 2011). However, graphical displays of scores can be misleading and do not lend

themselves to evaluation of treatment progress across many clients. Three concepts regarding change are helpful in evaluating whether a youth has changed in treatment. First, did the youth's scores change to a meaningful degree? The minimally important difference (MID) is the smallest change in a treatment outcome that would indicate change as a result of treatment (Schünemann & Guyatt, 2005; Wright, Hannon, Hegedus, & Kavchak, 2012). Second, classical test theory dictates that observed scores are equal to true scores plus some amount of error (Lord & Novick, 1968). Reliable change is the amount of change necessary to be more change than random fluctuations in measurement error might predict (Jacobson & Truax, 1991). Third, scores can change reliably and more than the MID but not represent clinically significant change. Clinically significant change provides a set of goalposts that identify whether a youth's scores have changed reliably and meaningfully (Jacobson & Truax, 1991). Below are brief presentations of each concept.

The MID is the smallest change in a treatment outcome that an informed individual would identify as important and indicative of change in treatment for better or worse (Schünemann & Guyatt, 2005). In randomized controlled trials, p-values are often an indicator of whether treatment has an effect for a group of individuals relative to a control group. The MID is developed from a desire to have a consistent benchmark that would allow researchers, clinicians, and individual patients to see progress from subjective informant-report measures. The MID for a measure is usually set via one of two primary approaches.

First, distributional methods use the spread of scores on the measure (e.g., standard deviation, standard error of the measure) to build a definition based on typical variation. Each approach to setting the MID leads to slightly different MID estimates. However, the value of the MID in psychotherapy is that it can alert youth and their caregivers to meaningful change that occurs during treatment. Approximately 20–40% of youth display sudden changes in treatment (Dour, Chorpita, Lee, & Weisz, 2013). For youth demonstrating sudden changes, the MID is likely less important. For the 60–80% of youth whose change occurs gradually, MIDs provide a method for alerting youth and their caregivers to how treatment is unfolding.

Distributional methods for MID rely on the spread of the measure at baseline. The standard deviation (*SD*) is among the most commonly reported measures of spread and represents the average difference of individuals from the mean. An early systematic review of the MID indicated that across quality-of-life measures and diseases, 0.5 standard deviations was a remarkably consistent MID (Norman, Sloan, & Wyrwich, 2003). An alternative distribution-based method to using the standard deviation is to use the standard error of the measure (SE_m), which represents the variability in scores due to the unreliability of the measure. As a measure's reliability increases, the standard error of the measure decreases, indicating that the observed score is more likely due to an individual's true score and less likely due to measurement error. One recommendation is that a reasonable MID is at least one standard error of the measure because it is often equivalent to 0.5 standard deviations when the internal consistency is equal to .75 (Copay, Subach, Glassman, Polly, & Schuler, 2007).

However, distribution-based MIDs have been criticized as "meaning free." Distribution-based MIDs represent statistical change as it relates to measurement error and not necessarily whether the observed change is actually a meaningful MID for a patient (Crosby, Kolotkin, & Williams, 2003). Anchor-based methods, the second approach to defining MID, compare change in scores to an "anchor" or reference score. Distribution-based MIDs also tend to be substantially more conservative estimates of MID relative to anchor-based MID (Revicki, Hays, Cella, & Sloan, 2008). In summary, distributional approaches to setting MID rely on the measurement properties of the scale in question.

In contrast to distribution-based methods, anchor-based methods reflect shared decision making in which patients define the meaningful outcome (Revicki et al., 2008). An informed judge (e.g., youth, caregiver) is typically presented with an "anchor" case presentation or score profile that represents a typical presentation at the beginning of treatment. The judge compares the anchor presentation to a series of other presentations and rates whether they are different. This is performed across many judges, and the MID represents the average minimum change presentation. Unfortunately, very few studies apply anchor-based methods to determine MIDs in the context of psychopathology, let alone the treatment of children and adolescents. Of the studies that have, anchor-based methods typically result in MIDs that are equivalent to changes of approximately ~0.25 standard deviations (e.g., Button et al., 2015; Chatham et al., 2018; Cuijpers, Turner, Koole, van Dijke, & Smit, 2014; Thissen et al., 2016). In summary, anchor-based MIDs are typically less conservative than distributional-based MIDs and represent patient, not clinician-defined change.

The concept of MID has been most readily applied to patient-reported outcomes in physical health settings (e.g., oncology). As described earlier, this gives mental health professionals rules of thumb for what to use as an MID in the absence of published psychology studies. Conservatively, distribution-based methods suggest approximately 0.5 standard deviations. More liberally, patient-based estimates suggest that changes of only 0.25 standard deviations are typically considered important. However, each of these methods is fundamentally attempting to identify a common metric that patients would agree represents the minimal amount of meaningful change in their life that would be important. Similar to goal setting, discussed previously in this chapter, clinicians could consider using an idiographic qualitative approach to identifying MID. Asking the youth, caregiver, or teacher what is his or her minimally acceptable long-term outcome represents a practical qualitative approach to setting the MID for an individual youth (Carragee & Cheng, 2010). In this approach, each individual sets his or her minimally acceptable outcome. The disadvantage of this approach is that the MID is inconsistent across patients and difficult to use in the context of program evaluation. The advantage of this is approach is that the MID is formed as part of the treatment goal-setting process and is meaningful to each individual youth.

The *reliable change index* (RCI; Jacobson & Truax, 1991) developed as a method for accounting for change in a challenging measurement environment. First, the course of psychopathology is intrinsically variable, resulting in variability in observed scores. Second, observed scores include measurement error and naturally vary as a result. Third, change in psychopathology results in variability of observed scores. Therefore, the challenge of assessing change is to determine whether the observed change is greater than change that can be attributed to measurement error.

Unless the measurement instrument or process is faulty, measurement error can be assumed to distribute normally. This assumption means that the properties of the normal distribution apply to measurement errors. The distribution of the errors is symmetrical and has a mean of 0 and standard deviation of 1. The standard deviation of the measurement error distribution is $SE_m = s\sqrt{1 - r_{xx}}$, where s is the standard deviation of the measure and r_{xx} is the reliability of the measure. However, the RCI focuses on change, so the standard error of the measure must be converted to the standard error of the difference (SE_d). $SE_d = \sqrt{2(SE_m^2)}$ and represents the standard deviation of the difference scores. The conversion means that the standard error of the difference is always greater than the standard error of the measure. Having thus defined measurement error, we can now ask the question "Did the observed change in a youth's score from Time 1 to Time 2 occur due to measurement error?" Mathematically, the difference is $X_1 - X_2$, where X_1 is the youth's score at baseline and X_2 is the youth's score at a future measurement point. The null hypothesis is that no change occurred (i.e., $X_1 - X_2 = 0$). The alternative hypothesis is that change occurred. Applying the logic of a *T*-test, RCI = $x_2 - x_1/SE_d$. The resulting RCI is distributed as a z-score. Using alpha = .05, z-scores more extreme than ±1.96 are considered statistically significant. Using alpha = .05 for RCI reflects the general rule of thumb for null hypothesis testing in psychology that observations that occur less than 1 time in 20 by chance are worth investigating. In statistics, many commentators have critiqued the default use of alpha = .05 (e.g., Lakens et al., 2018). Clinicians should also consider whether using alpha = .05 (i.e., $|z| \geq 1.96$) is too stringent.

The RCI originated in a challenging measurement environment in which change is expected and answers the question of whether change is more than measurement error. For everyday clinical use, the process of using the RCI can be simplified. The RCI as calculated is a z-test. Instead of calculating the z-test for each client, a clinician could identify the critical z-value that represents reliable change for the measure of interest. This can be done using alpha * SE_d. As a clinician, one could keep a table (e.g., Table 4.1) that contains the RCI for the common outcome measures administered. Then, one only has to compare the observed change in scores to the table to determine whether the amount of change could be considered reliable change.

The RCI has some limitations. First, it is a special case of a distribution-based MID. As identified previously, the SE_m is one metric used to define a distribution-based MID. Given that the SE_d is always greater than the SE_m, the RCI is a very conservative metric of change relative to the MID. Individuals with chronic conditions tend to expect relatively little change (Wise, 2004), so the RCI might be particularly conservative for youth with more chronic presentations. Second, the RCI could experience floor or ceiling effects. For example, a youth with very severe symptoms could score near the maximum possible on a measure. If the youth's condition deteriorates, the measure would be unable to observe the deterioration, and as a result no reliable change would be observed. Third, multiple investigators have suggested corrections to the RCI formula to account for statistical issues such as regression to the mean, imperfect measurement at Time 1, imperfect measurement at Times 1 and 2, and practice effects. However, multiple different analyses of the RCI and its variations indicate that the RCI as proposed by Jacobson and Truax (1991) works extremely well (e.g., Bauer, Lambert, & Nielsen, 2004; McGlinchey, Atkins, & Jacobson, 2002). Despite its problems, the RCI represents a very conservative method for determining whether an outcome has changed over the course of therapy (Youngstrom et al., 2013).

Clinically significant change is an expansion of RCI. The RCI focuses on change that is reliably more than change one could expect due to measurement error. Imagine treating a youth with a very severe presentation. The youth earns a *T*-score of 82 (i.e., 2.2 standard deviations above the mean) on a measure of his or her symptoms and the reliable change score is 8 points. After intensive treatment, the youth's *T*-score is now 73. The youth has demonstrated reliable change;

TABLE 4.1. Benchmarks of Common Instruments for Minimally Important Differences and Clinical Significant Change

Measure	Cutoff scores[a]			Critical change (unstandardized scores)			Minimally important difference (MID)	
	A	B	C	95%	90%	$SE_{difference}$	$d \sim 0.5$	$d \sim 0.25$
Achenbach System of Empirically Based Assessment (ASEBA)								
CBCL T-scores (2001 norms)								
Externalizing	49	70	58	7	6	3.4	5	2.5
Internalizing	n/a	70	56	9	7	4.5	5	2.5
Attention Problems	n/a	66	58	8	7	4.2	5	2.5
TRF T-scores (2001 norms)								
Externalizing	n/a	70	56	6	5	3.0	5	2.5
Internalizing	n/a	70	55	9	7	4.4	5	2.5
Attention Problems	n/a	66	57	5	4	2.3	5	2.5
YSR T-scores (2001 norms)								
Externalizing	n/a	70	54	9	8	4.6	5	2.5
Internalizing	n/a	70	54	9	8	4.8	5	2.5
Behavior Assessment System for Children, Third Edition (BASC-3)								
Parent Rating Scales T-scores								
Externalizing	34	70	56	9	8	4.75	5	2.5
Internalizing	35	70	56	9	7	4.47	5	2.5
Hyperactivity	37	70	56	13	11	6.74	5	2.5
Self-Report of Personality T-scores								
School Problems	31	70	52	9	8	4.55	5	2.5
Internalizing	32	70	53	6	5	3.22	5	2.5
Inattention/Hyperactivity	33	70	52	9	7	4.41	5	2.5
Teacher Rating Scales T-scores								
Externalizing	29	70	54	7	6	3.49	5	2.5
Internalizing	34	70	56	10	8	4.93	5	2.5
School Problems	35	70	53	7	6	3.30	5	2.5
Hyperactivity	32	70	54	9	7	4.32	5	2.5

[a]A, away from the clinical range; B, back into the nonclinical range; C, closer to the nonclinical than to clinical mean.

however, most would agree that the youth is still impaired and still requires treatment. Clinically significant change is a statistically based method for identifying when reliable change has resulted in a meaningful amount of change (Jacobson & Truax, 1991).

Clinically significant change is based on two assumptions of what would be clinically significant. First, a person seeking treatment would prefer to not to be seeking treatment. An individual's score would fall outside of the treatment-seeking population's distribution of scores. Second, a person seeking treatment would prefer to be "typical" or "normal." An individual's score would fall within the distribution of healthy individuals' scores on the measure. Clinically significant change re-

quires reliable change that fulfills at least one two clinically significant criteria. When change is applied to these two criteria, three clinically significant thresholds result. First, a youth's score could move away from the treatment-seeking distribution. Practically, this would occur when a youth's score starts within the treatment-seeking distribution at Time 1 and at Time 2 is now more than two standard deviations away from the treatment-seeking distribution's mean. Second, a youth's score could move back into the healthy population's distribution. Practically, this would occur when a youth's score starts two standard deviations above the healthy population's mean at Time 1 and at Time 2 is now within two standard deviations of the healthy population's mean. Third, a youth's score could be crossing the threshold from the treatment-seeking population's distribution to the healthy population's distribution. Practically, this would occur when a youth's score crosses the threshold at which point scores could come from either distribution equally. Mathematically, the final threshold is defined as $([\overline{S}_h * \overline{ts}] + [\overline{S}_{tx} * \overline{h}])/(\overline{S}_h + \overline{S}_{ts})$, where S means standard deviation, h means healthy population, and ts means treatment-seeking population. In summary, outcomes could be monitored for whether an individual reliably changes and (A) moves away from the treatment-seeking distribution, (B) moves back into the healthy population's distribution, and (C) crosses over from the treatment-seeking distribution to the health population's distribution.

Clinically significant change provides an extremely high bar for demonstrating treatment effectiveness. Critics of clinically significant change have pointed out several potential flaws. First, the accurate defining of treatment-seeking and healthy (or non-treatment-seeking) populations is difficult (Tingey, Lambert, Burlingame, & Hansen, 1996). Many measures used in clinical populations may not have normative data from non-treatment-seeking or healthy youth. The lack of this data results in the loss of two thresholds—there is no nonclinical distribution to get "back" into for B, or numbers to pool and get the C threshold (Jacobson, Follette, & Revenstorf, 1984). Second, the cutoffs for clinically significant change (i.e., A, B, C) need a lot of separation between the clinical and nonclinical distributions to work well (i.e., large effect size differences between populations). Even measures with large differences between the treatment-seeking and non-treatment-seeking distributions can have substantial overlap. This can result in thresholds that are mathematically impossible (e.g., a negative threshold on a measure whose scores are only positive) or a treatment-seeking youth's starting scores already being too low to cross some of the thresholds. Third, youth who begin treatment with very severe presentations (e.g., T-score of 70) may meet RCI criteria without crossing thresholds A, B, or C. In this case, the youth is demonstrating reliable improvement, but the treatment effect has not been large enough to be considered clinically significant.

Despite these mathematical challenges, clinically significant change as a concept focuses the discussion of change onto meaningful change. The primary conceptual critique of clinically significant change is that clinically meaningful change does not require reliable change in symp-

toms (Kazdin, 1999). A youth can benefit from treatment despite the amount of change in symptoms demonstrated. This last critique serves as a reminder that while clinically significant change provides a framework for evaluating treatment progress, proper evaluation of outcomes should focus on more than symptom reduction.

Application of Process Stage to Ty

As discussed previously in Chapters 2 and 3, Ty's mother reported that Ty, an adolescent male, has a "bad temper, lack of effort on homework, slipping grades." At initial evaluation, Ty presented with clinically elevated internalizing symptoms and mildly elevated externalizing behavior. After completing a thorough differential diagnosis, Ty was conceptualized as experiencing a single major depressive episode of moderate severity with anxious distress. In the prescription phase of assessment, Ty and his mother identified three primary problem areas: (1) Ty's refusal to complete schoolwork, (2) Ty's irritable mood, and (3) Ty's worry about his academic future. We developed clinical hypotheses about what was maintaining each problem area (e.g., Ty's avoidance of homework is reinforced by immediate reductions in anxiety but exacerbated by his poor grades in the long term) that were used to inform treatment. Imagine that you are Ty's clinician and have chosen to implement a modular approach to treatment (e.g., Weisz et al., 2012), so that your course of treatment can flexibly address Ty's presenting problems.

The process phase of assessment focuses on determining how the course of Ty's treatment is unfolding. During your intake session, in which you developed Ty's case conceptualization, you had asked about Ty's top problems and collected the CBCL and YSR. These scores serve as your baseline for monitoring treatment progress. The process phase of assessment requires the systematic assessment of outcomes, so that as the first step you use a progress tracking spreadsheet to create a graph of Ty's treatment progress, as seen in Figure 4.1 (panels C and D).

The second step of process assessment is identifying approach-oriented treatment goals. According to his mother, Ty's top problem is his refusal to do schoolwork. This is an excellent treatment *target*, but it is a poor treatment *goal* because it is framed as avoidance. Working with Ty and his mother, you state the problem and ask what Ty should do. Both Ty and his mother state a longer-term outcome goal of "my/his homework." Early in treatment, it is key to make this approach-oriented goal SMART. To do this, you ask about the frequency with which Ty does homework, intensity (i.e., how much of any one assignment he completes), number of different class assignments he attempts, and duration of his attempts. Ty reports that he has not tried to do any homework for any classes in 3 months. You ask Ty, "What's the minimal amount of change that would be important to you?" Ty responds that trying at least two classes' homework would represent meaningful change to him. You ask Ty, "How could you tell that you tried two classes' homework?" Ty responds that he could tell that he tried if he did at least one page of his homework packet for each class. At this point, you can set a SMART intermediate goal by adding a time frame. After a brief discussion, Ty and his mother agree that a reasonable goal is that Ty will complete at least 1 page of homework for two different classes over the next week. The following week, you start your session by asking Ty how his top problems are going and graph them. As seen in Figure 4.1 (panel C), you see that Ty's score for homework problems has increased, which means that it was becoming a bigger problem for him. Clinically, this might prompt a discussion of what happened that week. Ty reports that his mother "nagged me every day about me failing to meet my goals." This leads you to a brief round of problem solving, after which Ty is able to plan out how he might accomplish his goal, and he contracts with his mother about how she should support him. Each session, you continue to check in with Ty about how his homework is going. As seen in Figure 4.1 (panel C), his homework completion problem is lessening each week. So each week, the goal is iteratively updated.

As seen in Figure 4.1 (panel C), Ty demonstrates rapid improvement in his top problem—homework completion, but his next two top problems have maintained a relatively stable course so far in treatment. This pattern suggests that it is time to focus treatment on his next problem and new treatment goal. To address his irritable mood in the context of depression, you choose to implement pleasant activity scheduling because of clinical hypotheses that his withdrawal was a maintaining factor. After showing Ty and his mother the graph of Ty's treatment progress, Ty agrees to give pleasant activity scheduling a try because he is hopeful that he can be less grumpy with others. Ty has a smartphone, and you encourage him to download a mood tracking app so that

he can easily track his mood multiple times a day. Mood tracking represents an immediate outcome. Ty tracks his mood multiple times a day and can see how it varies throughout the day. When he is engaged in his scheduled pleasant activities, his mood improves. When he is home alone, his mood worsens. Both he and his mother agree tell you that he should probably try scheduling an activity for after school, and before she gets home from work, as that seems to be the toughest time of his day. On Ty's intermediate change tracker (Figure 4.1, panel C), you see that Ty's irritability is starting to become less of a problem.

Treatment continues to progress. After four sessions, you have Ty complete the YSR, and his mother completes the CBCL to help track outcomes because four sessions is the average number of sessions youth receive in community mental health (Gopalan et al., 2010). Follow-up CBCLs and YSRs are administered every 3 months or when YTP indicates large enough reductions in Ty's top problems to indicate treatment is nearing readiness for termination. The YSR and CBCL are scored as T-scores with a mean of 50 and standard deviation of 10. As seen in Figure 4.1 (panel D), Ty's outcome scores appear to be improving. For outcomes, anchor-based MIDs for the YSR and CBCL are not available. Using the more liberal translation of anchor-based MID change, typically approximately 0.25 standard deviations, you consider any observed change of more than 2.5 points to indicate an MID has occurred. The RCI and clinically significant change thresholds for the YSR and CBCL are in Table 4.1. Between Session 1 and Session 5, Ty's score improves by 3 points. Ty's improvement at this point is not reliable change or clinically significant change; however, Ty has demonstrated an MID. Comparing Session 5 to Session 9, Ty has demonstrated another MID. However, the course of treatment is one of improvement since the beginning. Comparing Sessions 1 and 9, Ty's score has improved 9 points. This is right at the reliable change for the Internalizing scale, suggesting that Ty's improvement is reliable. Notice that Ty has crossed the B threshold but not the C threshold. Ty's Internalizing score has moved back into the healthy distribution but is still more likely to come from a youth seeking treatment than from a healthy youth. By using the principles of the process phase of assessment, you are able to show to Ty, his mother, and any other stakeholders that treatment is helping him, but he still has clinically meaningful room for more improvement.

REFERENCES

Achenbach, T. M., & Rescorla, L. A. (2001). *Manual for the ASEBA School-Age Forms and Profiles.* Burlington: Department of Psychiatry, University of Vermont.

Bauer, S., Lambert, M. J., & Nielsen, S. L. (2004). Clinical significance methods: A comparison of statistical techniques. *Journal of Personality Assessment, 82,* 60–70.

Benito, K. G., Machan, J., Freeman, J. B., Garcia, A. M., Walther, M., Frank, H., . . . Franklin, M. (2018). Measuring fear change within exposures: Functionally-defined habituation predicts outcome in three randomized controlled trials for pediatric OCD. *Journal of Consulting and Clinical Psychology, 86,* 615–630.

Bickman, L., Athay, M. M., Riemer, M., Lambert, M. J., Kelley, S. D., Breda, C., . . . Vides de Andrade, A. R. (2010). Manual of the Peabody Treatment Progress Battery PTPB 2010. Retrieved from *https://peabody. vanderbilt.edu/docs/pdf/cepi/ptpb_2nd_ed/ptpb_2010_ entire_manual_update_31212.pdf.*

Bickman, L., Kelley, S. D., Breda, C., de Andrade, A. R., & Riemer, M. (2011). Effects of routine feedback to clinicians on mental health outcomes of youths: Results of a randomized trial. *Psychiatric Services, 62,* 1423–1429.

Brent, D. A., & Kolko, D. J. (1998). Psychotherapy: Definitions, mechanisms of action, and relationship to etiological models. *Journal of Abnormal Child Psychology, 26,* 17–25.

Brown, J., Dreis, S., & Nace, D. K. (1999). What really makes a difference in psychotherapy outcome?: Why does managed care want to know? In M. A. Hubble, B. L. Duncan, & S. D. Miller (Eds.), *The heart and soul of change: What works in therapy* (pp. 389–406). Washington, DC: American Psychological Association.

Button, K. S., Kounali, D., Thomas, L., Wiles, N. J., Peters, T. J., Welton, N. J., . . . Lewis, G. (2015). Minimal clinically important difference on the Beck Depression Inventory–II according to the patient's perspective. *Psychological Medicine, 45,* 3269–3279.

Carragee, E. J., & Cheng, I. (2010). Minimum acceptable outcomes after lumbar spinal fusion. *The Spine Journal, 10,* 313–320.

Chatham, C. H., Taylor, K. I., Charman, T., Liogier D'ardhuy, X., Eule, E., Fedele, A., . . . Bolognani, F. (2018). Adaptive behavior in autism: Minimal clinically important differences on the Vineland-II. *Autism Research, 11,* 270–283.

Cone, J. D. (2001). *Evaluating outcomes: Empirical tools for effective practice.* Washington, DC: American Psychological Association.

Copay, A. G., Subach, B. R., Glassman, S. D., Polly, D. W., & Schuler, T. C. (2007). Understanding the minimum clinically important difference: A review of concepts and methods. *The Spine Journal, 7,* 541–546.

Crosby, R. D., Kolotkin, R. L., & Williams, G. R. (2003). Defining clinically meaningful change in health-related quality of life. *Journal of Clinical Epidemiology, 56,* 395–407.

Cuijpers, P., Turner, E. H., Koole, S. L., van Dijke, A., & Smit, F. (2014). What is the threshold for a clinically relevant effect?: The case of major depressive disorders. *Depression and Anxiety, 31,* 374–378.

de Vet, H. C. W., Terwee, C. B., Mokkink, L. B., & Knol, D. L. (2011). *Measurement in medicine: A practical guide.* New York: Cambridge University Press.

Doerr, J., & Page, L. (2018). *Measure what matters: How Google, Bono, and the Gates Foundation rock the world with OKRs.* New York: Portfolio.

Dour, H. J., Chorpita, B. F., Lee, S., & Weisz, J. R. (2013). Sudden gains as a long-term predictor of treatment improvement among children in community mental health organizations. *Behaviour Research and Therapy, 51,* 564–572.

Duncan, B. L. (2012). The Partners for Change Outcome Management System (PCOMS): The Heart and Soul of Change Project. *Canadian Psychology, 53,* 93–104.

Duong, M. T., Lyon, A. R., Ludwig, K., Wasse, J. K., & McCauley, E. (2016). Student perceptions of the acceptability and utility of standardized and idiographic assessment in school mental health. *International Journal of Mental Health Promotion, 18,* 49–63.

Ebesutani, C., Bernstein, A., Chorpita, B. F., & Weisz, J. R. (2012). A transportable assessment protocol for prescribing youth psychosocial treatments in real-world settings: Reducing assessment burden via self-report scales. *Psychological Assessment, 24,* 141–155.

Fisher, E., Bromberg, M. H., Tai, G., & Palermo, T. M. (2017). Adolescent and parent treatment goals in an Internet-delivered chronic pain self-management program: Does agreement of treatment goals matter? *Journal of Pediatric Psychology, 42,* 657–666.

Fitzpatrick, R., Ziebland, S., Jenkinson, C., Mowat, A., & Mowat, A. (1992). Importance of sensitivity to change as a criterion for selecting health status measures. *Quality in Health Care, 1,* 89–93.

Fried, E. I. (2017). The 52 symptoms of major depression: Lack of content overlap among seven common depression scales. *Journal of Affective Disorders, 208,* 191–197.

Fuchs, L. S., Fuchs, D., & Hamlett, C. L. (1989). Effects of alternative goal structures within curriculum-based measurement. *Exceptional Children, 55,* 429–438.

Gopalan, G., Goldstein, L., Klingenstein, K., Sicher, C., Blake, C., & McKay, M. M. (2010). Engaging families into child mental health treatment: Updates and special considerations. *Journal of the Canadian Academy of Child and Adolescent Psychiatry, 19,* 182–196.

Greenberg, L. S. (1986). Change process research. *Journal of Consulting and Clinical Psychology, 54,* 4–9.

Guyatt, G. H., Deyo, R. A., Charlson, M., Levine, M. N., & Mitchell, A. (1989). Responsiveness and validity in health status measurement: A clarification. *Journal of Clinical Epidemiology, 42,* 403–408.

Harkin, B., Webb, T. L., Chang, B. P. I., Prestwich, A.,

Conner, M., Kellar, I., . . . Sheeran, P. (2016). Does monitoring goal progress promote goal attainment?: A meta-analysis of the experimental evidence. *Psychological Bulletin, 142,* 198–229.

Hatfield, D. R., & Ogles, B. M. (2004). The use of outcome measures by psychologists in clinical practice. *Professional Psychology: Research and Practice, 35,* 485–491.

Hatfield, D. R., & Ogles, B. M. (2007). Why some clinicians use outcome measures and others do not. *Administration and Policy in Mental Health and Mental Health Services Research, 34,* 283–291.

Hawkins, E. J., Lambert, M. J., Vermeersch, D. A., Slade, K. L., & Tuttle, K. C. (2004). The therapeutic effects of providing patient progress information to therapists and patients. *Psychotherapy Research, 14,* 308–327.

Hays, R. D., & Hadorn, D. (1992). Responsiveness to change: An aspect of validity, not a separate dimension. *Quality of Life Research, 1,* 73–75.

Holweg, M. (2007). The genealogy of lean production. *Journal of Operations Management, 25,* 420–437.

Hooke, G. R., Sng, A. A. H., Cunningham, N. K., & Page, A. C. (2018). Methods of delivering progress feedback to optimise patient outcomes: The value of expected treatment trajectories. *Cognitive Therapy and Research, 42,* 204–211.

Ionita, G., & Fitzpatrick, M. (2014). Bringing science to clinical practice: A Canadian survey of psychological practice and usage of progress monitoring measures. *Canadian Psychology, 55,* 187–196.

Jacob, J., Edbrooke-Childs, J., Holley, S., Law, D., & Wolpert, M. (2016). Horses for courses?: A qualitative exploration of goals formulated in mental health settings by young people, parents, and clinicians. *Clinical Child Psychology and Psychiatry, 21,* 208–223.

Jacobson, N. S., Follette, W. C., & Revenstorf, D. (1984). Psychotherapy outcome research: Methods for reporting variability and evaluating clinical significance. *Behavior Therapy, 15,* 336–352.

Jacobson, N. S., & Truax, P. (1991). Clinical significance: A statistical approach to defining meaningful change in psychotherapy research. *Journal of Consulting and Clinical Psychology, 59,* 12–19.

Jensen-Doss, A., & Hawley, K. M. (2010). Understanding barriers to evidence-based assessment: Clinician attitudes toward standardized assessment tools. *Journal of Clinical Child and Adolescent Psychology, 39,* 885–896.

Kashyap, S., Hooke, G. R., & Page, A. C. (2015). Identifying risk of deliberate self-harm through longitudinal monitoring of psychological distress in an inpatient psychiatric population. *BMC Psychiatry, 15,* 81.

Kazdin, A. E. (1999). The meanings and measurement of clinical significance. *Journal of Consulting and Clinical Psychology, 67,* 332–339.

Kiesler, D. J. (2004). Intrepid pursuit of the essential ingredients of psychotherapy. *Clinical Psychology: Science and Practice, 11,* 391–395.

Kim, E., Helal, S., & Cook, D. (2010). Human activity recognition and pattern discovery. *IEEE Pervasive Computing, 9,* 48–53.

Kluger, A. N., & DeNisi, A. (1996). The effects of feedback interventions on performance: A historical review, a meta-analysis, and a preliminary feedback intervention theory. *Psychological Bulletin, 119,* 254–284.

Lakens, D., Adolfi, F. G., Albers, C. J., Anvari, F., Apps, M. A. J., Argamon, S. E., . . . Zwaan, R. A. (2018). Justify your alpha. *Nature Human Behaviour, 2,* 168–171.

Lambert, M. J., Huefner, J. C., & Nace, D. K. (1997). The promise and problems of psychotherapy research in a managed care setting. *Psychotherapy Research, 7,* 321–332.

Lipsey, M. W. (1990). *Design sensitivity: Statistical power for experimental research.* Thousand Oaks, CA: SAGE.

Lord, F. M., & Novick, M. R. (1968). *Statistical theories of mental test scores.* Oxford, UK: Addison-Wesley.

Luborsky, L. (1959). Psychotherapy. *Annual Review of Psychology, 10,* 317–344.

Lueger, R. J. (1998). Using feedback on patient progress to predict the outcome of psychotherapy. *Journal of Clinical Psychology, 54,* 383–393.

Lyons, J. S., & Fernando, A. D. (2016). *Child and Adolescent Needs and Strengths [Standard CANS Comprehensive]* (2nd ed.). Chicago: Praed Foundation.

Marshall, S., Haywood, K., & Fitzpatrick, R. (2006). Impact of patient-reported outcome measures on routine practice: A structured review. *Journal of Evaluation in Clinical Practice, 12,* 559–568.

Martinovich, Z. (1998). *Evaluating a phase model of psychotherapy outcome: An application of hierarchical logistic modeling.* Ann Arbor, MI: ProQuest Information & Learning.

Marx, B. P., Bovin, M. J., Suvak, M. K., Monson, C. M., Sloan, D. M., Fredman, S. J., . . . Keane, T. M. (2012). Concordance between physiological arousal and subjective distress among Vietnam combat veterans undergoing challenge testing for PTSD. *Journal of Traumatic Stress, 25,* 416–425.

McGlinchey, J. B., Atkins, D. C., & Jacobson, N. S. (2002). Clinical significance methods: Which one to use and how useful are they? *Behavior Therapy, 33,* 529–550.

McPherson, P., Scribano, P., & Stevens, J. (2012). Barriers to successful treatment completion in child sexual abuse survivors. *Journal of Interpersonal Violence, 27,* 23–39.

Meehl, P. E. (1973). Some methodological reflections on the difficulties of psychoanalytic research. *Psychological Issues, 8*(2, Mono. 30), 104–117.

Mokkink, L. B., Terwee, C. B., Patrick, D. L., Alonso, J., Stratford, P. W., Knol, D. L., . . . de Vet, H. C. W. (2010). The COSMIN checklist for assessing the methodological quality of studies on measurement properties of health status measurement instruments: An international Delphi study. *Quality of Life Research, 19,* 539–549.

Norman, G. R., Sloan, J. A., & Wyrwich, K. W. (2003). Interpretation of changes in health-related quality of life: The remarkable universality of half a standard deviation. *Medical Care, 41,* 582–592.

Ormhaug, S. M., & Jensen, T. K. (2018). Investigating treatment characteristics and first-session relationship variables as predictors of dropout in the treatment of traumatized youth. *Psychotherapy Research, 28,* 235–249.

Overington, L., Fitzpatrick, M., Drapeau, M., & Hunsley, J. (2016). Perspectives of internship training directors on the use of progress monitoring measures. *Canadian Psychology, 57,* 120–129.

Pecora, P. J., Kessler, R. C., O'Brien, K., White, C. R., Williams, J., Hiripi, E., . . . Herrick, M. A. (2006). Educational and employment outcomes of adults formerly placed in foster care: Results from the Northwest Foster Care Alumni Study. *Children and Youth Services Review, 28,* 1459–1481.

Revicki, D., Hays, R. D., Cella, D., & Sloan, J. (2008). Recommended methods for determining responsiveness and minimally important differences for patient-reported outcomes. *Journal of Clinical Epidemiology, 61,* 102–109.

Reynolds, C. R., & Kamphaus, R. W. (2015). *Behavior assessment system for children* (3rd ed.). Bloomington, MN: NCS Pearson.

Rose, D. J., & Church, R. J. (1998). Learning to teach: The acquisition and maintenance of teaching skills. *Journal of Behavioral Education, 8,* 5–35.

Schünemann, H. J., & Guyatt, G. H. (2005). Commentary—Goodbye M(C)ID! Hello MID, Where do you come from? *Health Services Research, 40,* 593–597.

Sederer, L. I., Dickey, B., & Eisen, S. V. (1997). Assessing outcomes in clinical practice. *Psychiatric Quarterly, 68,* 311–325.

Shirk, S., & Karver, M. (2006). Process issues in cognitive-behavioral therapy for youth. In P. C. Kendall (Ed.), *Child and adolescent therapy: Cognitive-behavioral procedures* (3rd ed., pp. 465–491). New York: Guilford Press.

Thissen, D., Liu, Y., Magnus, B., Quinn, H., Gipson, D. S., Dampier, C., . . . DeWalt, D. A. (2016). Estimating minimally important difference (MID) in PROMIS pediatric measures using the scale-judgment method. *Quality of Life Research, 25,* 13–23.

Tingey, R. C., Lambert, M. J., Burlingame, G. M., & Hansen, N. B. (1996). Clinically significant change: Practical indicators for evaluating psychotherapy outcome. *Psychotherapy Research, 6,* 144–153.

Tryon, G. S., & Winograd, G. (2011). Goal consensus and collaboration. *Psychotherapy, 48,* 50–57.

Vermeersch, D. A., Lambert, M. J., & Burlingame, G. M. (2000). Outcome Questionnaire: Item sensitivity to change. *Journal of Personality Assessment, 74,* 242–261.

Wakschlag, L. S., Briggs-Gowan, M. J., Choi, S. W., Nichols, S. R., Kestler, J., Burns, J. L., . . . Henry, D. (2014). Advancing a multidimensional, developmental spectrum approach to preschool disruptive behavior. *Journal of the American Academy of Child and Adolescent Psychiatry, 53,* 82–96.

Weisz, J. R., Chorpita, B. F., Frye, A., Ng, M. Y., Lau, N., Bearman, S. K., . . . Research Network on Youth Mental Health. (2011). Youth Top Problems: Using idiographic, consumer-guided assessment to identify treatment needs and to track change during psychotherapy. *Journal of Consulting and Clinical Psychology, 79,* 369–380.

Weisz, J. R., Chorpita, B. F., Palinkas, L. A., Schoenwald, S. K., Miranda, J., Bearman, S. K., . . . Gibbons, R. D. (2012). Testing standard and modular designs for psychotherapy treating depression, anxiety, and conduct problems in youth: A randomized effectiveness trial. *Archives of General Psychiatry, 69,* 274–282.

Wise, E. A. (2004). Methods for analyzing psychotherapy outcomes: A review of clinical significance, reliable change, and recommendations for future directions. *Journal of Personality Assessment, 82,* 50–59.

Wollburg, E., & Braukhaus, C. (2010). Goal setting in psychotherapy: The relevance of approach and avoidance goals for treatment outcome. *Psychotherapy Research, 20,* 488–494.

Wright, A., Hannon, J., Hegedus, E. J., & Kavchak, A. E. (2012). Clinimetrics corner: A closer look at the minimal clinically important difference (MCID). *Journal of Manual and Manipulative Therapy, 20,* 160–166.

Youngstrom, E. A. (2013). Future directions in psychological assessment: Combining evidence-based medicine innovations with psychology's historical strengths to enhance utility. *Journal of Clinical Child and Adolescent Psychology, 42,* 139–159.

Youngstrom, E. A., Van Meter, A., Frazier, T. W., Hunsley, J., Prinstein, M. J., Ong, M., & Youngstrom, J. K. (2017). Evidence-based assessment as an integrative model for applying psychological science to guide the voyage of treatment. *Clinical Psychology: Science and Practice, 24,* 331–363.

Youngstrom, E. A., Zhao, J., Mankoski, R., Forbes, R. A., Marcus, R. M., Carson, W., . . . Findling, R. L. (2013). Clinical significance of treatment effects with aripiprazole versus placebo in a study of manic or mixed episodes associated with pediatric bipolar I disorder. *Journal of Child and Adolescent Psychopharmacology, 23,* 72–79.

PART II

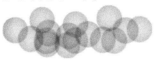

Behavior Disorders

CHAPTER 5

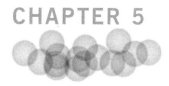

Attention-Deficit/Hyperactivity Disorder

Julie Sarno Owens, Steven W. Evans, and Samantha M. Margherio

Clinical assessment is critical to every aspect of mental health service delivery for children and adolescents with attention-deficit/hyperactivity disorder (ADHD), from the initial referral through the diagnostic evaluation and feedback process, as well as during treatment planning and when evaluating the client's response to treatment. Researchers and practitioners have developed a compendium of evidence-based assessment techniques that can be leveraged at each phase of service delivery to enhance the accuracy of the process and enhance positive outcome for youth, families, and society. With the fifth edition of this book, the editors challenge clinicians to think about assessment at every phase of service delivery and to utilize new resources to facilitate efficiency in our decision making and effectiveness of our services.

Readers are encouraged to conceptualize the assessment process as a funnel that starts with broad hypotheses and becomes narrowed and refined with additional information and data-driven hypothesis testing. This chapter is divided into four sections that mirror the funneling process. In the first section (on the preparation phase), readers learn important information about ADHD, prevalence rates, and common issues related to the diagnosis. This information lays the foundation for an assessment starter kit. In the second section (on the prediction phase), readers learn about psychometric properties of screening tools and diagnostic aids included in a starter kit, and about factors that may influence interpretation of data obtained from these tools (e.g., development, gender, race, informants). In the third section (on the prescription phase), readers learn about assessment tools and strategies for arriving at a comprehensive diagnostic picture, case conceptualization, and treatment plan. In this phase, clinicians should consider the client's profile of strengths, impairments, comorbidities, family preferences, and how each aligns with evidence-based treatment options. In the final section (on the progress, process, and outcome measurement phase), readers learn about how to assess treatment processes (e.g., integrity) and proximal and distal outcomes.

The Preparation Phase and Assessment Starter Kit

Diagnosis

ADHD is a chronic neurobehavioral disorder characterized by developmentally inappropriate symptoms of inattention and/or hyperactivity–impulsivity that create impairment in functioning (American Psychiatric Association, 2013). ADHD typically manifests in early childhood, and the symptoms and associated impairments persist into adulthood for most persons with the diagnosis (Barkley, Fischer, Smallish, & Fletcher, 2002; Klein et al., 2012). ADHD is a highly heritable disorder; the diagnostic likelihood increases four- to five-fold among children with a first-degree relative with ADHD (Frazier, Youngstrom, & Hamilton, 2006).

To meet current criteria for ADHD according to the fifth edition of the *Diagnostic and Statistical Manual of Mental Disorders* (DSM-5; American Psychiatric Association, 2013), the child (up to age 16) (1) must demonstrate at least six symptoms of inattention and/or hyperactivity–impulsivity that are excessive for the child's development; (2) some symptoms must manifest in at least two settings (e.g., home and school); (3) the symptoms must have been present prior to age 12; (4) the symptoms must cause impairment in social or academic/work-related functioning; and (5) the symptoms must not be better accounted for by another mental disorder. For persons age 17 and older, there must be at least five symptoms of either inattention and/or hyperactivity–impulsivity. Based on symptom profile, a child can be diagnosed with one of three ADHD presentations: predominantly inattentive presentation (DSM-5: 314.00; ICD-10: F90.0); predominantly hyperactive–impulsive presentation (DSM-5: 314.01; ICD-10: F90.1), or combined presentation (DSM-5: 314.01; ICD-10: F90.2) (American Psychiatric Association, 2013). Although ADHD is a chronic disorder for most individuals, there is limited stability in the specific presentation over time (Lahey, Pelham, Loney, Lee, & Willcutt, 2005), and limited evidence that the presentation has prescriptive utility (Pelham, 2001); that is, ADHD presentation has not been found to moderate treatment outcome (e.g., MTA Cooperative Group, 1999).

Although the same general criteria are used to assess for a diagnosis of ADHD in children of all genders and ages, clinicians must be aware of two considerations. First, symptoms must be ex-cessive for the child's development level. Thus, clinicians must have an understanding of typical development, and symptoms must be evaluated relative to same-age peers. For example, interrupting multiple times in 1 hour is not excessive for a kindergartner, but it would be consider excessive for a seventh grader. Second, the manifestations of symptoms and associated impairments are qualitatively different depending on the child's developmental level. For example, in childhood, excessive hyperactivity may manifest as running, climbing, and getting out of one's seat, whereas in adolescence and young adulthood, excessive hyperactivity may manifest as internal restlessness. Similarly, in childhood, excessive impulsivity manifests as taking someone's toy, difficulty waiting one's turn, and acting without thinking (e.g., darting across a street without looking). In adolescence, excessive impulsivity manifests as impulsive decision making in risky situations, for example, when driving, experimenting with substances, spending money, or engaging in intimate relationships (Barkley & Cox, 2007; Flory, Molina, Pelham, Gnagy, & Smith, 2006; Molina & Pelham, 2003). Furthermore, according to teacher ratings in normative datasets, rates of traditional hyperactive–impulsive symptoms decline with age, whereas rates of inattentive symptoms remain consistent across ages (DuPaul, Power, Anastopoulos, & Reid, 2016; Evans et al., 2013). Clinicians must be aware of these developmentally specific presentations.

Prevalence

According to DSM-5 (American Psychiatric Association, 2013), ADHD is prevalent in 5% of children. Similarly, according to a meta-analytic study summarizing over 130 articles reporting ADHD prevalence rates obtained from seven continents and global regions, the worldwide pooled prevalence of ADHD was 5.9%, with a range of 3–12% across geographic regions (Polanczyk, de Lima, Horta, Beiderman, & Rohde, 2007; Polanczyk, Willcutt, Salum, Kieling, & Rhode, 2014). In the United States, data from two national parent-based surveys indicate that the prevalence of ADHD in children ages 4–17 years has increased over the last two decades, from 6–7% to 10–11% in 2011 (Visser et al., 2014; Xu, Strathearn, Liu, Yang, & Bao, 2018).

Several factors are related to the rise in diagnostic rates across time, including our knowledge and societal awareness of the disorder, decreased mortality of low birth weight infants, and change in education policy (see Hinshaw, 2018, for review). However, the variability in diagnostic rates across studies is largely accounted for by variations in diagnostic criteria use (e.g., use of the impairment criterion, whether reports from both teachers and parents are included) (Martel, Schimmack, Nikolas, & Nigg, 2015; Polanczyk et al., 2014). Furthermore, it is important to note that basing a diagnosis on parent report alone is not consistent with DSM-5 criteria, previously defined evidence-based practices for the assessment for ADHD (Pelham, Fabiano, & Massetti, 2005), or current evidence (see the third section). When considering data derived from the assessment of symptoms and impairment from both parents and teachers, diagnostic base rates are closer to 5–7% (Polzanczyk et al., 2014). Because prevalence rates of ADHD vary across settings (e.g., schools, clinics serving children with a variety of problems, or an ADHD specialty clinic), clinicians are encouraged to keep records of the prevalence of ADHD within their setting so that such data can be incorporated into nomograms that inform diagnostic likelihood rates (see the second section).

Disorder-Associated Impairment

Most youth with ADHD experience academic impairment. Across development, inattentive symptoms are more predictive of academic impairment than are hyperactive–impulsive symptoms (Zoromski, Owens, Evans, & Brady, 2015). One meta-analysis reported a large effect size ($d = 0.71$) for the academic problems of children with ADHD relative to typically developing children (Frazier, Youngstrom, Glutting, & Watkins, 2007). In preschool and kindergarten, children with ADHD tend to lag behind typically developing peers in basic academic readiness skills and efficient acquisition of new skills (DuPaul, McGoey, Eckert, & VanBrakle, 2001). In elementary school, children with ADHD symptoms demonstrate poorer academic skills (low test scores, grades, and work accuracy and completion) and academic enablers (behaviors that enable academic success; e.g., motivation, cooperative learning skills, and engagement) (Loe & Feldman, 2007) than typically-developing peers (McConaughy, Volpe, Antshel, Gordon, & Eiraldi, 2011). ADHD symptoms incrementally predict low achievement test scores relative to what is expected based on intellectual ability (Barry, Lyman, & Klinger, 2002). As aca-

demic demands increase during the middle school years, adolescents with ADHD experience greater difficulty with homework completion (Langberg et al., 2011) and organization skills, and tend to experience declining grade point averages (GPAs) over the school year (Evans et al., 2016). High school students with ADHD are also more likely to fail courses, repeat a grade, and drop out of school than their peers (Kent et al., 2011). Thus, it is important for clinicians to assess for developmentally relevant indicators of academic impairment.

In addition, 40–60% of children with ADHD experience difficulties in peer relationships (Hoza, 2007) and family relationships (Johnston & Mash, 2001). In elementary school-age youth, hyperactive–impulsive symptoms are more predictive of social impairment than are inattentive symptoms (Zoromski, Owens, et al., 2015). However, in high school youth, inattentive symptoms are more predictive of social impairment than are hyperactive–impulsive symptoms (possibly because the current hyperactive–impulsive symptoms do not adequately capture this dimension in older youth with the disorder). Regardless of development level, however, as a group, children with ADHD tend to have fewer friends and experience greater peer rejection than their typically developing peers (Hoza, 2007). Some children with ADHD have difficulty accurately evaluating their own behavior (Owens, Goldfine, Evangelista, Hoza, & Kaiser, 2007), possibly making it more likely they will continue to engage in alienating behaviors. In adolescence, individuals with ADHD are more likely than typically developing peers to use illicit substances (Molina & Pelham, 2003), spend time with peers who engage in deviant behaviors (Marshal, Molina, & Pelham, 2003), and experience greater conflict with their parents (Johnston & Mash, 2001). Last, children younger than age 6 (particularly boys) and young adults (ages 18–36) with ADHD are significantly more likely to have accidents (e.g., head injuries, open wounds, poisoning, intoxication) that result in hospitalization than are same-age peers without ADHD (Lindemann, Langner, Banascheewski, Garbe, & Mikolajczyk, 2017).

When assessing impairment, it is important to consider both the level of child functioning and adults' expectations, as both contribute to the determination of impairment; that is, adults' expectations often adjust to a child's level of functioning, and these adjustments may influence the determination of impairment. For example, parents who find it difficult to get their child to do chores may stop expecting him or her to complete them. Thus, when clinicians ask about this domain of impairment, the parents may report that there are no problems related to household chores. In addition, adolescents with ADHD who persistently fail to complete homework assignments may have expectations modified to eliminate the requirement of homework. As a result, their grades may improve, and parents may report a lesser degree of impairment in the academic domain. These examples demonstrate how measuring function at home and school without measuring the extent to which the adults' expectations are age-appropriate can lead to inaccurate estimates of impairment. Assessment of such expectations most often can be completed in the context of interviews with parents and teachers (see the third section).

Purposes of Assessment

When families seek an assessment for behavior problems, the primary referral question is often to determine whether the child meets criteria for ADHD and/or any other mental health problem. However, beyond determining diagnostic status, clinicians in any setting (school, primary care office, clinic) must consider two other assessment goals and engage in activities that meet these goals. First, clinicians should assess impairment in multiple domains (e.g., academic, social, family, occupational). The impairment profile will (1) indicate whether the symptoms are causing impairment at a level that warrants treatment and (2) guide the treatment planning process (see the third section), as interventions that best address academic impairment are different from those that address impairment in social or family functioning (Evans, Owens, Wymbs, & Ray, 2018).

Second, clinicians should be aware of the systems involved in supporting the child's physical health, mental health, and educational success. Clinicians will likely need to educate parents about the implications of the assessment for possible pharmacological treatment and possible educational support services, and the sequencing and interaction of these services (Evans, Owens, Mautone, DuPaul, & Power, 2014; Fabiano & Pyle, 2019). With regard to educational services, it is important for parents to consider how they would like to communicate the findings to the child's school. Clinicians can help parents advocate for the highest quality services in the least restrictive environment. Clinicians can collaborate with teachers to facilitate the use of general classroom

management strategies (e.g., use of routines, rules, specific praise) and/or classroom interventions such as a daily report card (Vujnovic, Holdaway, Owens, & Fabiano, 2014), both of which can enhance student academic engagement and reduce disruptive behavior (Owens, Holdaway, et al., 2018) within the general education classroom.

Alternatively, parents also need to be aware that if their child meets criteria for ADHD, he or she may be eligible for protections and services under section 504 of the Americans with Disabilities Act (ADA) or the Individuals with Disabilities Education Improvement Act (IDEIA) (DuPaul, Power, Evans, Mautone, & Owens, 2016). Thus, it is important for clinicians to be aware of the eligibility requirements for these federal laws and to conduct assessments and write their reports in a manner that aligns with these requirements, so that school district personnel can use the diagnostician's assessment as they consider the student's eligibility. Helpful parent handouts about student educational rights can be found here within the ADHD Toolkit developed by National Institute for Children's Health Quality (NICHQ; *www.ihi.org/resources/pages/otherwebsites/nichq.aspx*).

Assessment Starter Kit

In this section, we have provided information about diagnostic criteria, prevalence rates and possible factors that impact these rates, developmental manifestations of the disorder, and the common goals of an assessment for ADHD. Having provided this foundational knowledge, we recommend that the following be included in an assessment starter kit:

- Broad-band rating scales from parent and teacher
- ADHD symptom rating scales from parent and teacher
- Impairment ratings from parent and teacher
- Checklist including family mental health history and birth information

Evidence of the utility of this starter kit has led the American Academy of Pediatrics (2011) and the American Academic of Child and Adolescent Psychiatry (Pliszka & AACAP Work Group on Quality Issues, 2007) to include the above in their recommended steps for assessing for ADHD. In the second section, we describe the empirical evidence that provides the rationale for this kit and highlight specific tools that may be used.

The Prediction Phase

Screening Tools and Diagnostic Aids

Broad-Band Rating Scales

Consistent with the metaphor of funneling, the initial assessment strategy should cover a wide variety of clinical diagnoses. Broad-band measures such as (1) the Child Behavior Checklist (CBCL) and Teacher's Report Form (TRF; Achenbach & Rescorla, 2001) within the Achenbach System of Empirically Based Assessment (ASEBA), (2) the Behavior Assessment System for Children, Third Edition (BASC-3; Reynolds, Kamphaus, & Vannest, 2015), and (3) the Strengths and Difficulties Questionnaire (SDQ; Goodman, 2001) may be particularly helpful in the development and refinement of hypotheses early in the assessment process. Each of these assessments have evidence of predictive utility in identifying children with ADHD and differentiating between referred and nonreferred children.

The parent- and teacher-reported Attention Problems subscales on the CBCL and TRF have demonstrated better clinical utility in identifying youth with ADHD than general scales such as the Externalizing Problems subscale (Hudziak, Copland, Stanger, & Wadsworth, 2004). Even among clinically-referred youth, the Attention Problems subscale discriminates between children with and without a diagnosis of ADHD, such that youth with scores in the clinical range on the TRF or CBCL Attention Problems subscale have a 15% increased likelihood of an ADHD diagnosis (Raiker et al., 2017). However, in another sample of referred youth, the Attention Problems subscale demonstrated clinical utility in identifying youth with ADHD, predominantly combined presentation, but not youth with ADHD, predominantly inattentive presentation (Jarrett, Van Meter, Youngstrom, Hilton, & Ollendick, 2018). Thus, the Attention Problems subscale is particularly useful for detecting youth with ADHD within clinical samples, although its utility in detecting youth with inattentive presentation remains questionable.

Similarly, the Attention Problems subscale of the BASC-3 parent and teacher report has demonstrated clinical utility in discriminating between nonclinical youth and referred youth with ADHD (Zhou, Reynolds, Zhu, Kamphaus, & Zhang, 2018). Youth with ADHD were also rated higher than the normative sample on the Hyperactivity scale (d_{par} = 1.18; d_{tch} = 0.43) and Attention Problems scale (d_{par} = 2.06; d_{tch} = 0.91). Furthermore, high scores on Executive Functioning and Learning Problems, coupled with low scores on Functional Communication and Resiliency also distinguished youth with ADHD, beyond the subscales of Attention Problems and Hyperactivity. Thus, by focusing on these four scales on the BASC-3 and utilizing diagnostic likelihood ratios (see discussion below), clinicians can significantly improve their diagnostic accuracy relative to focusing on just the Attention Problems and Hyperactivity subscales.

The SDQ parent- and teacher-report forms have demonstrated high sensitivity in detecting youth with ADHD within a community sample (Goodman, Ford, Simmons, Gatward, & Meltzer, 2003). The SDQ's computerized algorithm for detecting difficulties with hyperactivity–inattention has demonstrated moderate agreement with clinician ADHD diagnoses in referred adolescents (Kendall's tau-b = .44; Mathai, Anderson, & Bourne, 2004). Furthermore, in a longitudinal examination of the SDQ algorithms, this hyperactivity–inattention algorithm had a sensitivity of 45.6% and specificity of 97.2% in predicting later ADHD diagnoses in nonreferred preschool children (Rimvall et al., 2014).

This evidence, coupled with other indicators of reliability and validity (see Jensen-Doss, Patel, Casline, & McLeod, Chapter 3, this volume), suggests that these three broad-band rating scales are useful tools for this starter kit. When determining which tool to use, the relevant weaknesses of each should also be considered, including the cost of both the ASEBA and BASC systems, and the less-comprehensive nature of the SDQ. Given the wealth of research demonstrating the predictive validity of the Behavioral and Emotional Screening System (BESS) with important indicators of school success (Kamphaus, DiStefano, Dowdy, Eklund, & Dunn, 2010; Owens et al., 2016), the BESS may be an appropriate choice when a youth is referred within a school setting. Alternatively, given the well-documented clinical utility of the CBCL and the TRF in identifying youth with clinical diagnoses, the ASEBA system may be the appropriate broad-band rating scale for use in clinics. Although the SDQ is less comprehensive than the ASEBA or the BASC-2 and has slightly lower internal consistency, its accessibility (free and publicly available) may make it an attractive and acceptable option in settings with limited resources.

Broad-band screening measures tend to have high sensitivity and low specificity, resulting in an overinclusive pattern of identification. Thus, they should be reserved for screening and guiding the selection of other measures rather than valued as prescriptive. After administration of a broad-band measure, hypotheses should be reevaluated. If scores on scales associated with hyperactivity–impulsivity or inattention are elevated on these broad-band measures, it may be necessary to specifically assess ADHD symptoms with a narrow-band symptom rating scale.

Narrow-Band ADHD Symptom Rating Scales

The most commonly used and empirically supported narrow-band symptom rating scales for ADHD are the Conners Rating Scales (Conners-3; Conners, 2008), the Disruptive Behavior Disorder Rating Scale (DBD; Pelham, Gnagy, Greenslade, & Milich, 1992), the Vanderbilt ADHD Rating Scales (VADRS; Wolraich et al., 2003), the ADHD Rating Scale–5 Home and School Versions (ADHD-5; DuPaul, Reid, et al., 2016), and the Swanson, Nolan, and Pelham Rating Scale (SNAP; Swanson, 1992). One notable difference among these scales is that some are derived directly from 18 ADHD symptoms listed in the DSM (e.g., ADHD-5, DBD, SNAP), whereas others (e.g., Conners–3, Vanderbilt) include both items similar to DSM symptoms and related problems (i.e., executive functioning and learning problems). Table 5.1 reviews and rates the psychometric properties of each of these scales using the assessment grading rubric in Youngstrom and colleagues (2017). Given the importance of discriminative validity at the prediction phase (see Youngstrom et al., 2017), more research is needed using area under the receiver operating characteristic (ROC) curve calculations to determine the discriminative validity of each scale in the diagnosis of ADHD.

The efficiency of the measure (i.e., cost, number of items, ages and areas assessed) should also be considered when selecting a narrow-band symptom rating scale, and these tools vary across these indices (see Table 5.1). For example, given the high comorbidity of externalizing disorders, measures that also assess for symptoms of oppositional defiant disorder (ODD) and conduct disorder (CD) are desirable, particularly if a child exhibits elevated problems on externalizing dimensions on the broad-band rating scale. Additionally, because a diagnosis of ADHD requires impairment, the inclusion of indices of impairment further improves the efficiency of the assessment protocol. In summary, the most commonly used narrow-band

symptoms scales for ADHD are relatively similar in the strength of their psychometric properties; therefore, the decision of which scale to place in the assessment starter kit may rely on careful consideration of the efficiency of each measure. For example, although the SNAP and VADRS are both free, their lack of norms for older adolescents would make them an inappropriate choice for high school settings or clinics with several adolescent referrals. Similarly, the DBD is based on DSM-IV criteria; therefore, it does not include the DSM-5 updated behavior descriptors and examples for symptom presentation in adolescents, and this may limit the generalizability of the DBD for adolescents. Alternatively, the Conners–3, the only tool with a self-report version available, and the ADHD-5 may be the preferred options for settings with a large caseload of older adolescents.

Impairment Rating Scales

The presence of ADHD symptoms is not enough to confirm a diagnosis of ADHD. Impairment in functioning (e.g., academic, social, or occupational) related to the symptoms is also a requirement for the diagnosis (American Psychiatric Association, 2013). Furthermore, the experience of functional impairment, rather than symptoms, is typically the precipitant for youth being referred to services (Becker, Chorpita, & Daleiden, 2011). It is important to note that symptoms and impairment are related, yet distinct constructs, and some youth may experience an adequate number of ADHD symptoms without clinically significant impairment (Gathje, Lewandowski, & Gordon, 2008), and vice versa (Sibley et al., 2012; Waschbush & King, 2006). Furthermore, there is evidence that ADHD-related impairment, but not the number and type of ADHD symptoms, is predictive of a persistent course of ADHD (Biederman, Petty, Clarke, Lomedico, & Faraone, 2011). Thus, measuring impairment is a critical component of the assessment process, as it facilitates accurate diagnoses and quality treatment planning, and should serve as a focus of assessing progress in treatment.

Over the course of an evaluation, assessing for impairment may take place through the parent and teacher ratings, clinical interview, and/or review of records. However, the assessment starter kit should include parent and teacher rating scales of impairment. According to DSM-5, a diagnosis of ADHD requires impairment in social, academic, or occupational domains. Many rating scales measure domains of impairment other than these three, and

TABLE 5.1. Grading Rubric for Symptom Rating Scales

			Conners–3		
Rater	No. of items	Age	Comorbid disorders	Cost	Languages
Parent	ParFull: 110; ParShort: 45	Par: 6–18	CD; ODD; screening items for anxiety and depression; includes impairment items	$403 startup; $3–4.25 per form	English Spanish
Teacher	TchFull: 115; TchShort: 41	Tch: 6–18			
Self	SelfFull: 99; SelfShort: 41	Self: 8–18			

Criterion	Rating	Explanation
Norms	Excellent	Nationally representative samples including both clinical and nonclinical
Internal consistency	Par: Excellent Tch: Excellent Self: Good	
Interrater reliability	Less than adequate	Adequate among similar raters; intraclass correlations among different raters <.70
Test–retest reliability	Par: Good Tch: Excellent Self: Good	
Content validity	Adequate	Contains items typical of ADHD measures based on DSM-5 criteria, in addition to items relating to other behaviors and difficulties likely in children, such as learning problems and aggression
Construct validity	Adequate	Nonindependent examinations demonstrated moderate to high correlations with related ASEBA, BASC-2, and BRIEF scales; Some independent support for factor structure, with some debate regarding independence of Inattention and Learning Problems subscales
Discriminative validity	Adequate	Scores between clinical and nonclinical groups are significantly different, with moderate to large effect sizes
Validity generalization	Good	The Conners–3 has demonstrated adequate to good psychometric properties in clinical and nonclinical samples, in samples from diverse backgrounds
Treatment sensitivity	TBD	
Clinical utility	Adequate	

Citations: Conners (2008); Kao and Thomas (2010); Norfolk and Floyd, 2016; Schmidt et al. (2013)

			Vanderbilt ADHD Diagnostic Rating Scale (VADRS)		
Rater	No. of items	Age	Comorbid disorders	Cost	Language
Parent	ParFull: 55	Par: 6–12	CD; ODD; screening items for anxiety and depression; includes impairment items	Free	English
Teacher	TchFull: 43 F/U version: 26	Tch: 6–12			

Criterion	Rating	Explanation
Norms	Tch: TBD Par: TBD	Tch version norms have been collected from multiple, diverse, large samples of nonclinical elementary school children; Par version norms provided in one large, diverse community sample of elementary and middle school children
Internal consistency	Par: Excellent Tch: Excellent	
Interrater reliability	Less than adequate	Adequate among similar raters; low parent–teacher agreement

(continued)

TABLE 5.1. *(continued)*

Vanderbilt ADHD Diagnostic Rating Scale (VADRS) *(continued)*		
Criterion	Rating	Explanation
Test–retest reliability	Adequate	One examination of test–retest reliability demonstrated correlations of >.80 over approximately 2 weeks
Content validity	Adequate	Contains items typical of ADHD measures based on DSM-IV criteria, as well as items relating to relevant behaviors and difficulties in children
Construct validity	Adequate	Nonindependent examinations demonstrated moderate to high correlations with related SDQ and DISC subscales in clinical and nonclinical samples; factor structure is generally supported
Discriminative validity	TBD	
Validity generalization	Good	The VADRS psychometric properties have been supported in elementary and middle school clinical and nonclinical samples in the United States, as well as Spain and Germany
Treatment sensitivity	TBD	
Clinical utility	Adequate	

Citations: Bard et al. (2013); Becker et al. (2012); Wolraich et al. (2003, 2013)

ADHD Rating Scale–5					
Rater	No. of items	Age	Comorbid disorders	Cost	Languages
Parent	Par: 30	Child: 5–10	None; includes impairment items	$140.25 one-time fee	English Spanish
Teacher	Tch: 30	Adol.: 11–17			

Criterion	Rating	Explanation
Norms	Excellent	Nationally representative samples including both clinical and nonclinical
Internal consistency	Par: Excellent Tch: Excellent	
Interrater creliability	TBD	TBD for 5; ADHD Rating Scale–IV had low parent–teacher agreement
Test–retest reliability	Par: Adequate Tch: Adequate	.80–.93 over approximately 6 weeks
Content validity	Adequate	Contains items typical of ADHD measures based on DSM-5 criteria, in addition to items relating to other behaviors and difficulties likely in children such as learning problems, poor peer relations, and low self-esteem
Construct validity	Adequate	Nonindependent examinations demonstrate moderate to high correlations with relevant Conners–3 subscales, IRS, and observation data; factor structure supported in a nonindependent examination
Discriminative validity	Adequate	Statistically significant prediction of ADHD diagnostic status
Validity generalization	Good	Used in school and clinical settings with psychometric support in a representative sample; available in both English and Spanish versions
Treatment sensitivity	TBD	TBD for 5; ADHD Rating Scale–IV was sensitive to behavioral and pharmacological treatment in multiple studies
Clinical utility	Good	

Citations: DuPaul et al. (2016)

(continued)

TABLE 5.1. *(continued)*

Disruptive Behavior Disorder (DBD) Rating Scale

Rater	No. of items	Age	Comorbid disorders	Cost	Language
Parent	Par: 45	Par: 5–18	CD, ODD	Free	English
Teacher	Tch: 45	Tch: 5–18			

Criterion	Rating	Explanation
Norms	Adequate	Norms are provided from multiple moderate-size, predominantly European American clinical and nonclinical samples
Internal consistency	Par: Excellent Tch: Good	
Interrater reliability	Less than adequate	Adequate among similar raters; low parent–teacher agreement
Test–retest reliability	Adequate	
Content validity	Adequate	The DBD assesses all DSM-IV symptoms of ADHD, ODD, and CD; does not include information regarding impairment or other relevant difficulties
Construct validity	Adequate	Moderate to high correlations with relevant subscales of the DISC and SSQ (Speech, Spatial and Qualities of Hearing Scale); three-factor structure has been supported
Discriminative validity	TBD	
Validity generalization	Good	The DBD has been used in school and clinical settings from preschool to high school-age children; however, generalization to ethnically diverse samples, particularly African American youth, has been questioned
Treatment sensitivity	Good	Sensitive to behavioral and pharmacological treatment in multiple studies
Clinical utility	Adequate	

Citations: Antrop et al. (2002); DuPaul et al. (1998); Evans et al. (2011); Pelham et al. (1992)

SNAP Rating Scale

Rater	No. of items	Age	Comorbid disorders	Cost	Language
Parent	ParFull: 90; ParShort: 26	5–11	ODD; full version also screens for all other childhood disorders listed in DSM-IV	Free	English
Teacher	TchFull: 90; TchShort: 26				

Criterion	Rating	Explanation
Norms	Short: Adequate Long: Less than adequate	Norms for the short version are provided from one large sample of African American and European American elementary students, including both clinical and nonclinical students
Internal consistency	Par: Good Tch: Excellent	
Interrater reliability	Less than adequate	Adequate among similar raters; low parent–teacher agreement
Test–retest reliability	TBD	
Content validity	Adequate	Contains items typical of ADHD measures based on DSM-IV criteria, in addition to items relating to other behaviors and difficulties likely in children such as learning problems, poor peer relations, and low self-esteem

(continued)

TABLE 5.1. *(continued)*

		SNAP Rating Scale *(continued)*
Criterion	Rating	Explanation
Construct validity	Good	Independent and nonindependent studies demonstrate small to moderate associations with relevant measures of academics, observation measures, parent-reported concern of ADHD, and DISC subscales; factor structure supported in a nonindependent examination
Discriminative validity	Adequate	Statistically significant prediction of ADHD diagnostic status
Validity generalization	Good	Used in school and clinical settings, with psychometric support in representative samples
Treatment sensitivity	Good	Sensitive to behavioral and pharmacological treatment in multiple studies
Clinical utility	Good	

Citations: Bussing et al. (2008); MTA Cooperative Group (1999); Swanson (1992)

problems in those domains may not be relevant to a diagnosis (e.g., self-esteem). After hypotheses have been narrowed about relevant domains of impairment, elevated domains can be explored further via interviews with parents, teachers, and adolescents, and self-report ratings of impairment (with adolescents) before finalizing the diagnosis and treatment plan (see the third section).

Several rating scale approaches to assessing impairment have been utilized, including global assessments, multidimensional measures, and domain-specific measures. Global ratings that estimate an overall level of impairment tend to be efficient and sensitive to treatment effects (Jensen et al., 2007). However, global assessments of impairment fail to indicate whether impairment varies across settings, and they do not identify domains of impairment that may be targeted in further assessment and treatment.

Conversely, multidimensional measures of impairment provide information about specific domains in which the youth is experiencing impairment that may better inform diagnoses and treatment planning. Multidimensional measures of impairment include the SDQ's Supplemental Impact questions, the CBCL and TRF Competence and Adaptive subscales, and several BASC subscales, including Aggression and Learning Problems. Thus, if the SDQ, BASC, or CBCL/ TRF are given as screening measures, they may also offer a time-saving means for gauging the specific domains of impairment a youth experiences.

Some ADHD rating scales, such as the Conners-3, Vanderbilt, and ADHD-5, include items assessing ADHD-related impairment. However, to date, assessment of the psychometric properties of these items is limited (e.g., Becker, Langberg, Vaughn, & Epstein, 2012). In addition, some of these scales do not assess critical domains of functioning (e.g., Conners-3 does not include items about classroom behavior; the Vanderbilt does not include items about homework) nor symptom-specific impairment (a requirement of a DSM diagnosis).

The ADHD-5 impairment items assess several domains of impairment (e.g., familial relations, peer relations, academic functioning, behavioral functioning, homework functioning, self-esteem) as they relate to inattention symptoms and hyperactive–impulsive symptoms separately, potentially allowing for greater specificity within the impairment assessment. Power and colleagues (2017) provide normative data from a large, representative, nonclinical sample, in which they found that each of the six domains of impairment assessed in the ADHD-5 represented a distinct construct, and each domain of impairment was impacted by both inattention and hyperactivity–impulsivity symptoms. These findings speak to the need to assess each of these impairment domains as they relate to each dimension of ADHD symptoms. In summary, more assessment of the psychometric properties of impairment subscales on symptom rating scales is needed, yet extant data suggest that the ADHD-5 impairment ratings are promising.

Other multidimensional measures of impairment may be added to the assessment process, such as the Child and Adolescent Functional Assessment Scale (CAFAS; Hodges & Wong, 1996), the Impairment Rating Scale (IRS; Fabiano et al., 2006), the Weiss Functional Impairment Rating Scale (WFIRS; Weiss, 2000), and the Barkley Functional Impairment Scale—Children and Adolescents (BFIS-CA; Barkley, 2012). The CAFAS is associated with behavioral indices of impairment and is sensitive to treatment effects (Hodges, Doucette-Gates, & Liao, 1999). However, the CAFAS contains 164 items, costs approximately $3 per administration, and is clinician-administered, thus diminishing the clinical utility of the CAFAS as a screening tool. Alternatively, the IRS, WFIRS, and BFIS-CA are more appropriate screening measures given their relative brevity and low cost. Table 5.2 reviews and rates the psychometric properties of these scales using the assessment grading rubric in Youngstrom and colleagues (2017). Each of these scales was specifically designed to assess domains of impairment relevant for children and adolescents with ADHD. Each of these scales has demonstrated at least adequate psychometric properties, although it is worth noting the BFIS-CA has limited evaluation relative to the other two scales. Furthermore, although the WFIRS does not have normative data available, the WFIRS is the only multidimensional rating scale to include self-report and to assess risky behaviors, and it therefore may be the most appropriate tool for assessing impairment in older adolescents. The availability of a teacher-report version of the IRS and the evidence supporting its psychometric properties suggests it is an appropriate tool for children ages 3–18.

Clinicians can request that parents provide information from existing records, such as grade cards, school disciplinary records, and/or court involvement requests. Academic records that include information such as GPAs or disciplinary referrals may act as a proxy for teacher-rated impairment when the teacher report is either unavailable or conflicts with other reports. Although objective measures of impairment offer rich information, they can be difficult to obtain for clinicians outside of schools, and may only be available for some domains of functioning. Finally, objective measures are also influenced by contextual factors (e.g., peers in the classroom, student–teacher relationship), which limits comparisons over time and across clients. Because rating scale scores (e.g., the

IRS) correlate with objective measures of impairment (Fabiano et al., 2006), rating scales are likely an acceptable indicator of impairment during this phase; additional measures of impairment can be obtained later in the assessment process.

Developmental Considerations

Recent evidence suggests that our conceptualization of ADHD symptoms as a bifactor construct (i.e., inattention and hyperactivity–impulsiveness) is appropriate for preschool and elementary school children, and adolescents (Allan & Lonigan, 2019). However, the manifestations of ADHD symptoms are influenced by the youth's developmental stage, and to meet diagnostic criteria, must be excessive for his or her own developmental level. Thus, symptom severity should be considered relative to age-specific norms and context.

ADHD-related impairments are unique to developmental state. In preschool children, by carefully considering impairment of preschool youth *in addition to symptoms*, clinicians can substantially reduce the rate of false-positive diagnoses relative to relying on symptom criteria (Healey, Miller, Castelli, Marks, & Halperin, 2008). In preschool children, the primary area of impairment is likely to be within the mother–child relationship; however, injuries and hospitalization rates may serve as objective indicators of impairment (Lindemann et al., 2017). In addition, if the child is enrolled in a preschool or day care, impairment is also likely to be present with peers and other adults (DuPaul et al., 2001). Currently, the IRS is the only multidomain impairment rating scale that has been studied children as young as age 3 (Fabiano et al., 2006). Otherwise, clinicians will need to use domain-specific rating scales to assess parenting stress and/or family functioning.

Assessing ADHD symptoms and related impairment in adolescents can be challenging for two primary reasons. First, adolescents with a childhood history of ADHD may fail to meet the symptom threshold for diagnosis, despite continuing to experience clinically significant impairment (Sibley et al., 2012). This may occur as a function of the natural decline in hyperactivity over development (DuPaul et al., 2016; Evans et al., 2013) and/or because the symptoms of impulsivity in the DSM (e.g., blurts out, interrupts, difficulty waiting turn) do not adequately assess impulsivity in adolescents (Zoromoski, Owens, et al., 2015). At this stage, impulsivity may manifest as impulsive

TABLE 5.2. Grading Rubric for Impairment Rating Scales

Impairment Rating Scale (IRS)

Rater	No. of items	Age	Domains assessed	Cost	Language
Parent	Par: 7	3–18	Relations with peers, siblings, and parents; academic progress; self-esteem; family functioning; classroom functioning	Free	English
Teacher	Tch: 6				

Criterion	Rating	Explanation
Norms	Good	Normative data provided from multiple relevant samples including clinical and nonclinical; only the Tch IRS has normative data available for youth >12 years old
Internal consistency	N/A	
Interrater reliability	Less than adequate	Low parent–teacher agreement
Test–retest reliability	Good	Strong correlations over 6 months; ages 3–12 only
Content validity	Adequate	Contains items typical of impairment rating scales
Construct validity	Adequate	Weak to moderate correlations with relevant subscales on the DISC, CGAS, and DBD
Discriminative validity	Adequate	Statistically significant prediction of ADHD diagnostic status beyond ADHD symptoms; using the IRS in diagnosis predicted impairment 8 years later
Validity generalization	Adequate	Evidence supports its use in clinical and school settings; more research is needed to support its use in older youth
Treatment sensitivity	Good	Sensitive to psychosocial treatment in multiple studies
Clinical utility	Adequate	

Citations: Evans et al. (2011); Fabiano et al. (2006); Massetti et al. (2008)

Weiss Functional Impairment Rating Scale (WFIRS)

Rater	No. of items	Age	Domains assessed	Cost	Languages
Parent	Par: 50	5–19	Learning and school, life skills, self-concept, social activities, risky activities	Free	18 languages, including English, Spanish, French, Chinese, etc.
Self	Self: 69				

Criterion	Rating	Explanation
Norms	None	
Internal consistency	Excellent	
Interrater reliability	Adequate	Low to moderate self- and informant agreement
Test–retest reliability	Adequate	Strong correlations over 1–4 weeks
Content validity	Adequate	Contains items typical of impairment rating scales, including items specific to adolescent risky behavior
Construct validity	Adequate	Weak to moderate correlations with CGI, CGAS, and ADHD-Rating Scale; mixed evidence for factor structure across studies
Discriminative validity	Good	AUC was .91 for WFIRS-P in one sample
Validity generalization	Good	The psychometric properties of the WFIRS have been supported in numerous diverse populations, including 18 translated versions; its lack of teacher report inhibits its utility in schools
Treatment sensitivity	Good	Sensitive to psychosocial treatment in multiple studies
Clinical utility	Good	

Citations: Thompson et al. (2017); Weiss (2000); Weiss et al. (2018)

(continued)

TABLE 5.2. *(continued)*

Barkley Functional Impairment Scale: Children and Adolescents (BFIS-CA)					
Rater	No. of items	Age	Domains assessed	Cost	Language
Parent	15	6–17	Home, school, community, leisure	$140.25 one-time fee	English

Criterion	Rating	Explanation
Norms	Adequate	High test–retest reliability over a 3- to 5-week interval
Internal consistency	Excellent	
Interrater reliability	TBD	
Test–retest reliability	Adequate	High test–retest reliability over a 3- to 5-week interval
Content validity	Adequate	Contains items typical of impairment rating scales
Construct validity	Adequate	Nonindependent examinations demonstrate high correlations with relevant rating scales of executive functioning and ADHD symptoms; factor structure supported in a nonindependent examination
Discriminative validity	TBD	
Validity generalization	Good	The BFIS-CA has demonstrated adequate to good psychometric properties in clinical and nonclinical samples, in samples from diverse backgrounds
Treatment sensitivity	TBD	
Clinical utility	Adequate	

Citations: Barkley (2012)

decisions in the context of dating, driving, and experimentation with substances, and these behaviors are not captured by DSM-5 symptoms.

Second, impairment in adolescence is likely exhibited in different domains than in childhood. Adolescents with ADHD likely continue not only to experience difficulties in academic, social, and family functioning, but they also likely begin to experience functional impairments more characteristic of adulthood, including substance use, driving problems, justice involvement, and risky sexual behavior (Barkley & Cox, 2007; Flory et al., 2006; Molina et al., 2007). Currently, most impairment rating scales do not include assessment of these domains of impairment. One exception is the WFIRS (Weiss, 2000). Thus, clinicians may find this impairment scale to be particularly useful with older adolescents.

Thus, there is now evidence that (1) diagnoses based on developmentally appropriate norm-based symptom thresholds are associated with higher diagnostic persistence (meeting criteria at multiple time points) than are diagnoses based strictly on a six-symptom, DSM-based symptom count criterion (Sibley et al., 2012) and (2) the inclusion of impairment criterion can enhance diagnostic accuracy at multiple ages (Allan & Lonigan, 2019; Sibley et al., 2012). Including impairment ratings

for preschoolers may address false positives, and careful consideration of impairment in adolescents with ADHD may correct for false negatives. Although, additional research is still needed to replicate these findings and to guide further modification of DSM criteria (e.g., change in impulsivity symptoms and symptom count threshold for adolescents), these findings can guide the tools that clinicians use in their assessment starter kit based on the ages of clients they are assessing.

Gender Considerations

There is evidence that the factor structure of the symptoms underlying the disorder are invariant across gender (DuPaul et al., 2016). In addition, broadly speaking, the types of impairments experienced by children and adolescents with ADHD (i.e., difficulty with schoolwork and homework, difficulty getting along with peers and family members) are similar across genders (DuPaul et al., 2015; Evans et al., 2013). However, disorder prevalence rates are higher in males than in females (three to seven times higher in clinical populations; American Psychiatric Association, 2013), possibly related to the presence of gender differences in the parent and teacher symptom and impairment ratings (DuPaul et al., 2015; Evans et al.,

2013), and in observational studies of classroom behavior (Abikoff et al., 2002). For example, on average, in normative samples, parents and teachers rate boys higher than girls in symptoms and impairment at all ages, although this difference diminishes in parent ratings of teenagers, and teacher ratings of 11th and 12th graders (DuPaul et al., 2015; Evans et al., 2013). Last, one study indicated that some females experienced significant impairment but fell just short of the ADHD symptom count criteria (Waschbusch & King, 2006). This pattern was not found for males. Although this suggests that gender-specific thresholds could capture false negatives among girls, this only applied to a small subset of the sample, and the finding has not been replicated.

Given the current state of the science, there is insufficient evidence for the use of gender-specific norms for diagnosis. This aligns with current DSM and ICD recommendations, and current societal thresholds for impairment in functioning. For example, thresholds for competence are defined by the setting and context (e.g., grades, rules in sports games) and are typically not gender specific. Thus, to employ gender-specific norms for impairment would be equivalent to saying "She is functioning well in this domain *for a girl*," yet this is not how we consider thresholds for competence in society.

Conversely, we do recommend careful consideration of gender-specific data as they relate to interpreting symptom severity, engaging in case conceptualization, and treatment planning; that is, gender-specific norms can give clinicians some information about how the child is perceived by parents and teachers (i.e., her level of inattention is rated as more severe than 80% of girls her age). In addition, because there is evidence that some girls may be demonstrating impairment at a subthreshold level of symptoms, clinicians should consider making recommendations for intervention and use the child's impairment profile when designing the treatment plan.

Race and Ethnicity Considerations

Considerations related to the child's race and ethnicity are quite similar to those we mentioned for gender; that is, the factor structure of symptoms does not differ substantially across ethnic or racial groups (i.e., Hispanic and non-Hispanic; European American and African American) (DuPaul et al., 2015). Furthermore, there is evidence that average scores of symptoms and impairments are higher for African American high school students than for European American high school students (Evans et al., 2013), and for non-Hispanic African American students (K–12) than non-Hispanic European American and Hispanic children (DuPaul et al., 2015), with some evidence of an interaction between teacher race and ethnicity and student race and ethnicity. Thus, these nuances should be considered as clinicians are interpreting the severity of ratings for their client. Given that impairment is context-specific and driven by the expectations of adults in that setting, failing to meet the expectations (i.e., impairment) may be influenced by race or ethnicity to the extent that the expectations are influenced by race or ethnicity. Thus, although modifying impairment measures to better align with language used by parents and teachers of a given culture may assist in obtaining valid perceptions of impairment (Haack, Gerdes, Schneider, & Hurtado, 2011), in some cases, measuring expectations in the setting may be more helpful than adapting the measure.

Risk and Protective Factors

Knowledge about the risk and protective factors related to ADHD is necessary to understand the constellation of symptoms and impairment the child is experiencing. Risk and protective factors can help inform the likelihood of a diagnosis, the estimated prognosis, and the treatment plan. Several environmental and biological risk factors for ADHD have been investigated. A wealth of literature points to neurological underpinnings of ADHD, including evidence of dysfunction across neural systems involved in higher-level cognitive functions and sensorimotor processes (see Cortese et al., 2012), and neurotransmitter dysfunction, particularly in dopamine pathways (see Swanson, Baler, & Volkow, 2011). However, currently these neurological risk factors are unlikely to be diagnostic and they are not reviewed here.

Alternatively, a substantial risk factor for ADHD lies within genes, which can be indirectly assessed noninvasively and can contribute to diagnostic decision making. For example, the heritability coefficient of ADHD across many studies exceeds .80 (Boomsma, Cacioppo, Muthén, Asparouhov, & Clark, 2007; Larsson, Chang, D'Onofrio, & Lichtenstein, 2014). This large effect size is clinically informative, as the likelihood of an individual having ADHD increases four- to fivefold if he or she has a first-degree relative with ADHD (see Frazier, Youngstrom, & Hamilton, 2006). Thus, determining a family history of mental health difficulties is a crucial component of assessment for ADHD.

Through the process of epigenetics, a number of environmental risk factors may confer risk for ADHD during the critical vulnerability periods of pregnancy and early childhood (Schuch, Utsumi, Costa, Kulikowski, & Muszkat, 2015). Environmental risk factors for ADHD include low birth weight (less than 5.5 pounds; Nigg & Breslau, 2007), which may be specifically related to symptoms of inattention (Indredavik et al., 2004). Low birth weight may be confounded with other factors such as maternal smoking, maternal weight, low socioeconomic status (SES), stress, and pregnancy complications, which are also likely risk factors for the development of ADHD. However, evidence from a large within-twin pair design study suggests that low birth weight is independently related to ADHD, even after researchers control for all known environmental and genetic confounds (Pettersson et al., 2015). Despite the significance of this association, across studies, the effect sizes of birth weight on ADHD tend to be small; therefore, this risk factor is unlikely to be clinically informative for the average client. Similarly, effect sizes for risk factors such as maternal smoking during pregnancy and familial SES tend to be small to moderate (Larsson, Sariaslan, Långström, Donofrio, & Lichtenstein, 2014; Nigg & Breslau, 2007). Thus, these environmental risk factors are of questionable utility when determining a diagnosis. However, because environmental effects can influence the symptoms, course, and comorbidities of the disorder (Flouri, Midouhas, Ruddy, & Moulton, 2017), a thorough assessment of prenatal and perinatal factors can enhance the case conceptualization.

Social factors may exacerbate or attenuate ADHD symptoms and impairment, but they are unlikely to be causal of ADHD. For example, poor parental supervision and family conflict contribute to worsening symptoms, development of comorbidities (Flouri et al., 2017), and substance use (Molina et al., 2012), as does association with deviant peers (Marshal et al., 2003). Given the substantial contribution of genetic and neurobiological factors to ADHD, research has been limited in identifying protective factors for the development of ADHD. However, it is likely that malleable social factors may be protective against worsening ADHD symptoms and impairment. Thus, similar to most disorders of childhood, parental support, authoritative parenting, positive parent–child relationship, and social supports outside of the nu-

clear family are likely to play a protective role in ADHD, potentially protecting against worsening symptoms, further impaired functioning, and development of comorbidities.

One efficient method for obtaining information about risk and protective factors is to create a checklist covering the topics reviewed here (e.g., familial history of ADHD, prenatal and perinatal factors, family SES, family support, peer networks), and ask the family members to check mark items relevant for their child. The clinician can obtain additional information about endorsed items during a clinical interview with the parent(s) (see the third section).

Cross-Informant Assessment

The diagnosis of ADHD requires that the symptoms are present in two or more settings (e.g., at home and at school, American Psychiatric Association, 2013), calling for multi-informant assessments of ADHD. However, integrating these multi-informant assessments is challenging, as the low to moderate agreement among children, parents, and teachers in their ratings is well documented (for a review, see De Los Reyes et al., 2015). Although each source may provide unique information regarding the child's symptoms, comorbidities, and levels of functioning, few guidelines exist for how to best integrate these multi-informant reports. However, each information source also offers unique limitations that need to be considered when planning for and integrating multi-informant assessments.

Youth Self-Report

Children with ADHD tend to underreport ADHD symptoms and impairment (Aebi et al., 2017; Sibley et al., 2012); therefore, the incremental benefit of adding self-report rating scales has been questioned (Pelham et al., 2005). Indeed, consistent with literature investigating positive illusory bias (PIB; for a review, see Owens et al., 2007) relative to parents and teachers, youth with ADHD likely underreport impairment in academic and social domains. Thus, the addition of self-report rating scales adds little incremental validity to establishing a diagnosis of ADHD (Raiker et al., 2017; Sibley et al., 2012). However, children and adolescents are likely able to provide information regarding comorbidities and risk and protective factors not otherwise gleaned from parent or teacher report. For example, youth self-report has been discussed as a valid measure of internalizing symptoms (Aebi et al., 2017; Klein, Dougherty, & Olino, 2005; Silverman & Ollendick, 2005). Given the elevated rates of depression and anxiety in youth with ADHD relative to typically developing peers (Schatz & Rostain, 2006), screening for these symptoms within the assessment process is warranted. Additionally, adolescents may be able to provide additional information about risk and protective factors and impairment, such as describing their relationship with their parents or their risky behaviors (i.e., substance use, sexual behaviors). Collecting self-reports on broad-band rating scales may be useful for identifying areas of internalizing difficulties and impairments.

Parent Report

Current evidence-based recommendations prioritize gathering parent and teacher reports (Pelham et al., 2005), yet these reports offer limited agreement (Sibley et al., 2012), and parents may tend to report greater symptom severity than do teachers (Narad et al., 2015), particularly if parents have advanced education or psychopathology (Yeguez & Sibley, 2016). Given the high heritability estimates associated with ADHD, it is likely that parents are experiencing some ADHD symptomatology, which may inflate their ratings (Chronis-Tuscano et al., 2008), although findings regarding this hypothesis are mixed (Faraone, Monuteaux, Biederman, Cohan, & Mick, 2003). It may also be that parents with elevated psychopathology provide a more chaotic home life for the child, which in turn could contribute to elevated child symptoms at home, thus offering a context-specific hypothesis to explain these parents' elevated ratings. Interestingly, when examining both mother and father ratings of ADHD, the ratings demonstrated large shared variance, indicating that only one parent report may be necessary in diagnosing ADHD (Martel et al., 2015). Thus, if there are concerns regarding potentially inflated parent ratings and another parent is available, it may be appropriate to obtain the other parent's ratings, although this approach has not specifically been examined.

When selecting a parent to provide ratings, the gender of the parent may be an important factor to consider. Using the normative sample from the ADHD-5, Anastopoulos and colleagues (2018) found that males, but not females, were rated as having more inattentive symptoms and impairment if rated by their mothers than if rated by their fathers. Although the effect size of these di-

mensional differences were negligible (eta-squared = 0.002), mothers' ratings of male children resulted in 7.7% of males being identified as being at risk for ADHD compared to 4.2% when fathers completed the rating scale.

In addition to gender of the caregiver, clinicians should consider the potential influence of the caregiver's race. African American mothers provided significantly higher ratings of inattentive and hyperactive–impulsive symptoms than did European American mothers after watching a videotape of an African American or European American boy displaying similar levels of ADHD-related behaviors, regardless of child race (Barrett & DuPaul, 2018). This finding remained when maternal age and SES were held constant, indicating that caregiver race may uniquely influence ADHD symptom ratings. Thus, maternal race may be more important than child race when accounting for differences in ADHD symptom ratings between African American and European American boys.

In summary, although potential biases of parent report should be considered, the value of obtaining parent reports of symptoms, impairment, and risk and protective factors is vital to the ADHD assessment. If possible, obtaining ratings of ADHD symptoms and impairment from two caregivers may be preferred in order to balance variations in ratings due to rater psychopathology or gender. Teacher ratings may also help balance potential biases present within parent ratings.

Teacher Report

Teacher report may be ideal for capturing the constellation of symptoms and impairment present within the school setting. Some evidence suggests that teacher report may even outperform parent ratings in terms of sensitivity and specificity of identifying youth with ADHD (diagnosis based on rating scales and a structured interview with a parent; Tripp, Schaughency, & Clarke, 2006). However, teacher report has its own limitations. For example, Lawson, Nissley-Tsiopinis, Nahmias, McConaughy, and Eiraldi (2017) found that teachers, but not parents, rated children from low SES homes and African American children as having higher levels of symptoms than their peers. Yet observer ratings did not vary by SES, and observers actually rated African American youth as having lower levels of hyperactivity–impulsivity than their European American peers. Similarly, Evans and colleagues (2013) found that teachers rated

African American youth as having greater impairment than their peers, although parent report was not gathered in this study. Thus, it is possible that teachers report symptoms and impairment differentially by cultural factors, indicating the necessity of exploring cultural factors when integrating multi-informant reports.

Furthermore, the gender of the teacher and student may differentially influence teachers' ratings, such that male students, but not female students, are rated as having more hyperactive symptoms and impairment if rated by a female teacher compared to a male teacher (Anastopoulos et al., 2018). As a result, female teachers may identify twice as many male students as being at risk for ADHD compared to male teachers (12 vs. 5%). Because these findings are similar to those of parent ratings, clinicians may try to select raters of different genders when conducting assessments with male youth, if possible. In addition to selecting both male and female raters when possible, this pattern of findings also points to the need for using a multi-informant averaging approach to integrating multi-informant ratings rather than "and" or "or" rules, which tend to overemphasize a single informant's ratings (see below).

Another important consideration when gathering teacher reports is the grade level of the child. Specifically, as youth enter middle and high school settings, they begin to interact with several teachers, who may only observe the youth for a limited period of time throughout the week. Thus, choosing which teachers to ask about middle and high school students' symptoms and functioning is a challenging task. Although it may appear intuitive to choose a teacher who knows a child well, even this approach may not yield an accurate picture of the child's academic and behavioral difficulties. Middle school teachers tend to disagree with one another in their ratings of ADHD symptoms, specifically, such that general education teachers may report fewer symptoms than other teachers (Evans, Allen, Moore, & Strauss, 2005), and special education teachers may report more symptoms than other teachers (Yeguez & Sibley, 2016). Teacher ratings also tend to disagree with observer ratings (Evans et al., 2005). Importantly, observer ratings and teacher ratings significantly vary by classroom (Evans et al., 2005), indicating that teacher expectations, subject matter, and the social environment of each particular classroom are often unique, and it may be best to treat each classroom as a separate setting. Thus, relying on the report of a teacher who knows a child well may yield significantly different findings than if one relies on another teacher. However, there currently is no "best practice" method for choosing teachers to provide ratings, and variables such as availability of teachers, willingness to complete rating scales, and the family's preferences for school contact likely influence the decision of which teacher(s) to ask about the child's symptoms and functioning.

Integrating Multi-Informant Ratings

Although multi-informant methods are recommended for the assessment of ADHD, few guidelines exist for how best to integrate these ratings. In terms of symptom rating scales, a diagnosis of ADHD may be determined by use of the "or" or "and" rule. These commonly used rules state that a symptom should be counted if either informant endorses a specific symptom ("or" rule), or if both informants endorse a specific symptom ("and" rule). There is some evidence that the "or" rule has better predictive validity of future psychopathology and impairment among youth with ADHD than parent-only, teacher-only, and "and" rule approaches to symptom rating scales (Shemmassian & Lee, 2016). Both of these rules are easily implemented, easily standardized, and simple. However, in both approaches, a single rater could dominate the decision if the rater is particularly acquiescent or nay-saying. Furthermore, with the "or" rule, an individual could meet the symptom criterion (six symptoms) without having symptoms in two settings (which is required for diagnosis).

An alternative approach proposed by Martel and colleagues (2015) involves counting each rater's symptoms (either overall or within the symptom domains) and calculating the multi-informant average number of symptoms. Martel and colleagues found that multi-informants generally agreed on latent factors of inattention and hyperactivity–impulsivity, despite disagreeing at the individual symptom level. Thus, this approach reduces dominance by any one rater, allows for several raters, requires that the symptom threshold be reached by at least one rater, and is easy to implement. It is important to note that further investigation of this approach to diagnosis with rating scales is warranted, but calculating the average number of symptoms across raters is likely an improvement over the "and/or" approaches.

In addition to considering the "and/or" rule, clinicians can determine whether the child meets the thresholds for the presence of sufficient symptoms by a "count" method; that is, on a 4-point rating scale (ranging from 0 = *not at all present* to 3 = *very much present*), any symptom that is endorsed as a 2 (*pretty much*) or 3 (*very much*), is considered "present" and is counted toward the six-symptom threshold. This is a widely used practice in several federally funded randomized treatment trials (Evans et al., 2016; Langberg et al., 2018). However, it is important to recognize that a child could meet the "count" threshold with six items rated as *pretty much* but have an average score for a given symptom dimension that is well within one standard deviation of the normative mean for his or her age (and gender). Alternatively, the average rating per item (ARI) can be used to easily average across parent and teacher ratings, and can be compared to the scale's respective norms to determine a child's relative standing in relations to peers' symptom levels. Thus, if the clinician is using a count method, it is also prudent to ensure that the symptoms are excessive for the child's age. This requires careful consideration both counts and severity ratings, which can be achieved by calculating the ARI.

There is an underlying assumption that each informant carries a unique and valid perspective of the youth, and discrepancies arise in part due to contextual variations (De Los Reyes et al., 2015), as well as rater biases and informant mental health. Thus, cross-informant discrepancies are not merely "noise" but reveal important considerations regarding the child's presentation, prognosis, or response to treatment; De Los Reyes and colleagues (2015) recommend that individuals conducting assessments handle multi-informant ratings by first familiarizing themselves with the literature regarding multi-informant discrepancies, including awareness of multi-informant agreement and potential rater biases. Similarities and differences between home and school contexts in terms of management of the child's behavior and expectations should be probed. With this information, the clinician may be able to predict patterns of informant discrepancies. The clinician can then structure the assessment to identify factors that may explain informant discrepancies, such as including an observation of the child in different settings or gathering information about a parent's mental health. Another approach to handling informant discrepancies is to integrate each informant's report into a multi-tier diagnostic likelihood ratio (DLR) nomogram. This method would weight each informant's report equally to adjust the probability that the child or adolescent has ADHD.

Revising Probabilities Based on Screening Information

As described previously, rating scales tend to have a combination of high sensitivity and low specificity, which may be more helpful in ruling a condition out than ruling it in. This pattern of psychometric properties coupled with cognitive heuristics, such as confirmation bias, can place clinicians at risk for making false-positive judgments. Proposed methods for reducing the rate of false positives in assessments have included a greater reliance on actuarial methods, including DLRs, which can be determined for multiple levels of test results, including multi-informant reports, to provide an understandable and convenient measure for determining posttest probability of a disorder. Mathematically, the DLR represents the ratio of the diagnostic sensitivity to the false alarm rate, or the rate among those with the condition divided by the rate in those without the condition (e.g., 1-specificity). Interpreting the DLR involves considering base rates of the disorder in question, calculating a DLR based on assessment results, combining the DLR with the base rates using a form of Bayes's theorem, and determining the posttest probability. Probability nomograms are graphical approaches to easily incorporate these methods into the assessment by connecting the pretest probability to the posttest probability with a straight line. DLRs and nomograms also provide a straightforward method for integrating multi-informant, multimethod test results. The combination of DLRs with base rate probabilities offers several improvements over clinical judgment, including decreases in overdiagnosis and improvements in clinician consistency (Jenkins, Youngstrom, Washburn, & Youngstrom, 2011). Importantly, nomogram approaches can be implemented following brief (30-minute) training, require no cost to implement (beyond training), and, after receiving feedback about their improved performance, 89% of clinicians reported they would use nomogram approaches in their own practice (Jenkins et al., 2011). In summary, nomogram approaches offer a feasible, cost-effective solution for reducing bias in decision making.

The nomogram approach for assessment of ADHD has been investigated using parent, teacher, and self-reports from the ASEBA system (Raiker et al., 2017), and using parent and teacher reports from the BASC-3 (Zhou et al., 2018). On the ASEBA scales, the use of the nomogram resulted in diagnostic agreement between the costly, time-consuming interview and the relatively brief, low-cost screening measure, and demonstrated that little clinical utility was lost if teacher- and self-report forms were removed from the assessment (Raiker et al., 2017). Similarly, on the BASC-3, the DLR approach was an efficient approach to integrating multiple scales and informant ratings, and resulted in excellent agreement between parent and teacher ratings and diagnosis (Zhou et al., 2018).

We walk through an example using the DLR in an ADHD assessment. See Figure 5.1 for the nomogram visual to aid understanding of the example. If you worked in a clinic with an established local base rate of ADHD of 30%, every client who walks through the door has a pretest probability of 30%, which can be plotted on the left side of the nomogram. Within the screening procedures, it may be standard to administer the parent SDQ,

and the parent SDQ's Hyperactivity subscale has a sensitivity of 74% and a specificity of 92% for detecting ADHD (Goodman, 2001). The positive DLR is calculated by dividing the sensitivity by one minus the specificity, or .74/(1 − .92). The resulting positive DLR is 9.25. The negative DLR is calculated by dividing one minus the sensitivity by the specificity, or (1 − .74)/.92. The negative DLR is therefore .28. If a parent's Hyperactivity subscale report is above the preestablished cutoff, then the positive DLR (9.25) is plotted in the middle of the nomogram (see Figure 5.1). If the score is below the cutoff, then .28 is plotted. By using a straight line, a clinician can connect the two plotted points and extend the line to the edge of the nomogram to plot the posttest probability. If the parent reports elevated hyperactivity characteristics on the SDQ, the posttest probability that the youth has ADHD is 80%. This new probability can inform the clinician of the need for focused assessment of ADHD, and can be combined with other measures to complete a multilevel DLR that considers teacher ratings as well (see Raiker et al., 2017, for more examples). It is important to note that incorporating nomogram approaches does not equate questionnaire results with diagnoses, but posttest probabilities of the DLR approach can help clinicians prioritize diagnostic procedures and narrow their hypotheses.

The Prescription Phase

Finalizing Diagnoses

After gathering screening data and rating scales completed by parents and teachers, the clinician should have hypotheses about whether the child is likely to meet diagnostic criteria for ADHD. If the clinician has applied local base rates and sensitivity and specificity data about the rating scales within a nomogram, he or she can adjust the probability and confidence in a diagnosis of ADHD (Frazier et al., 2006). Hypotheses about potential comorbid conditions are also likely identifiable by these rating scale data. Regardless of the confidence the clinician has in the diagnosis at this point, there are limitations to relying exclusively on ratings in making a diagnosis that can mislead clinicians into making incorrect diagnoses. Given these limitations, we recommend that clinicians use a combination of the following tools in an assessment refinement kit to improve diagnostic accuracy and rule out disorders with insufficient evidence:

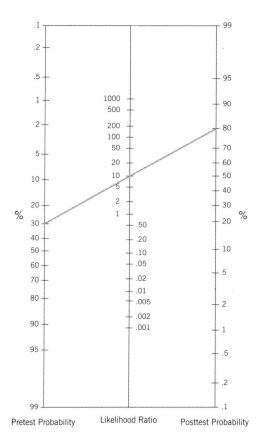

FIGURE 5.1. Nomogram for combining probability with diagnostic likelihood ratios. Copyright © 2019 E. Youngstrom: CC-BY 4.0.

- Semistructured diagnostic interview with parents
- Semistructured diagnostic interview with adolescents
- Interview with teacher(s)
- Observation of the child

Below, we describe the rationale and evidence for use of these tools. In addition, we discuss the evidence and the lack thereof for tools assessing executive functioning. Then, we describe how clinicians can use all information gathered to formulate a case conceptualization and treatment plan, with consideration of factors that may moderate treatment outcome and treatment selection.

Diagnostic Interviews with Parents

There are advantages and disadvantages to conducting diagnostic interviews with parents in an assessment for ADHD. With regard to benefits, a well-planned semistructured interview may be the mechanism through which clinicians can obtain information about the child's developmental history (e.g., exposure to toxins during pregnancy, birth weight), additional information about family history of ADHD and other mental health problems, and more details about symptom presentation (e.g., onset, intensity, duration, course) and related impairments. This information can facilitate an understanding of risk and protective factors for ADHD, the relative presence of comorbid conditions, and potentially influence the diagnostic likelihood of ADHD and other disorders. In addition, gaining an understanding of the expectations within various settings can help the clinician understand reports of impairment and eventually shape treatment recommendations. Last, the diagnostic interview presents an opportunity to build an alliance with the family members and understand their treatment preferences, which can facilitate subsequent treatment engagement (Hawley & Weisz, 2005). As a result, it is important to recognize that regardless of confidence in diagnoses indicated by rating scales, family history, and demographic information, the administration of a semistructured diagnostic interview can improve not only diagnostic accuracy but also the course of treatment.

There are also limitations to parent interviews; that is, there is limited research on the incremental utility of using a diagnostic interview, and the evidence that does exist does not show incremental benefit of structure diagnostic interviews in the identification of ADHD (e.g., Vaughn & Hoza, 2013) over rating scales. In addition, the administration of diagnostic interviews can take 1–2 hours. Thus, if there is limited incremental benefit, the cost outweighs the benefits.

However, it is important to recognize the limitations of the research on the incremental validity of diagnostic interviews. First, incremental validity studies tend to focus on a specific diagnosis of interest (e.g., ADHD) and fail to examine the incremental validity of identifying comorbid conditions. Even if the probability of an ADHD diagnosis is high following the screening phase, a semistructured interview could be useful in determining comorbid diagnosis, which may have important implications for treatment planning. Second, there is some evidence that unstructured interviews (Jensen-Doss et al., 2014) and computerized structured interviews (i.e., Diagnostic Interview Schedule for Children; Vaughn & Hoza, 2013) do not offer benefits in determining an ADHD diagnosis. Yet the incremental benefits of a *semistructured interview* in the identification of ADHD has not been tested. Semistructured interviews allow clinicians to gather additional information about each symptom (e.g., frequency and intensity relative to same-age children, degree to which the symptom causes problems), the age of onset of the symptoms and impairment, and to build alliance through conversation and understanding. They also allow clinicians to clarify the intended meaning of items on rating scales and discuss parent responses and interpretations.

Last, no study has tested the incremental validity of allowing the clinician to administer only the interview modules pertaining to the primary and likely comorbid diagnoses; this could create efficiency and accuracy. Thus, clinicians may wish to limit the interview to modules pertaining to the potential primary and comorbid diagnoses (as identified by the broad-band rating scales). This can reduce the time of administration, while maintaining the value of the interview; yet simultaneous empirical evaluation of this approach is warranted. In summary, although there are pros and cons to conducting an interview, a semistructured or structured interview has several benefits that go beyond diagnostic accuracy and may benefit the course of treatment. More research is needed to identify methods of streamlining these lengthy interviews.

Developmental Considerations

When conducting the interview, clinicians must consider the developmental history and context of the child. Although DSM-5 requires that symptoms be present prior to age 12, for a vast majority of youth with ADHD, symptoms and impairment begin much earlier. For children older than 12 years of age, identifying the onset of problems and history may not only confirm the diagnosis but also provide useful information to prescribe treatments (see below for discussion on informing prescribing). Asking parents about a history of school problems related to disruptive behavior, failure to complete tasks, and difficulties getting along with peers can often provide useful information. If the pattern reveals consistency over time and settings, rather than sudden onset in fourth grade or presenting in a singular setting, clinicians gain confirming evidence that the pattern is consistent with ADHD instead of another cause. However, occasionally, the onset may appear sudden when environmental factors were previously mitigating the impairment. For example, exceptional teachers can compensate for this impairment in young children. Parents can also minimize the impairment by communicating regularly with the teachers and managing the child's time at home to ensure the completion of any assignments. As children enter intermediate grades, the ability of parents and teachers to sufficiently compensate for the problems is reduced, and by middle school, it is often not possible. Thus, it can be helpful to ask about how much parents helped their child complete schoolwork or remember to take material back and forth to school to identify signs of excessive parent involvement. Parents are also good at reporting problems outside of school, including problems with community activities such as church groups, Scouts, and even playdates with peers. Parents of preschool children with ADHD often report having trouble finding a consistent babysitter, taking the child to a restaurant or church, and finding supportive day care. Furthermore, children with ADHD have often had multiple trips to the emergency room due to the consequences of impulsive behavior (Lindemann et al., 2017). Asking parents about these situations can help determine age of onset of the disorder and the extent to which patterns of symptoms and impairment are consistent with those commonly observed in children with ADHD.

Diagnostic Interview with Adolescents

The inclusion of the child in the interview will likely depend on the child's developmental stage. As we mentioned previously, children and adolescents tend to underreport the presence of externalizing symptoms (Aebi et al., 2017; Sibley et al., 2012). Thus, the amount of time it takes to conduct a structured diagnostic interview is not likely to produce benefits that outweigh the costs, as least with children and young adolescents, when the diagnostic focus is ADHD or ODD. However, if rating scales used in the assessment starter kit reveal the elevations on internalizing scales (anxiety, depression, withdrawn, somatic problems), then clinicians should consider administering a structured or semistructured diagnostic interview to further assess for comorbid internalizing problems and/or determine whether these problems are manifesting behaviors that resemble ADHD. Because there is low agreement between adolescent and parent report of symptoms and levels of functioning, each provides unique information (Sibley et al., 2012) that may help in determining the presence of comorbid anxiety and depressive disorders (Goodman et al., 2003; Klein et al., 2005).

Teacher Interview

We are unaware of any study that has examined the incremental utility of a teacher interview beyond teacher rating scales in the diagnosis of ADHD; indeed, such an interview may not enhance the diagnostic decision. However, with parent consent, a teacher interview (either by phone or in person) may offer clarifying information when parent and teacher ratings are highly discrepant and provide contextual information that helps the clinician determine impairment. In addition, this interview may lay an important foundation for engaging the teacher in a classroom intervention. First, teachers may be more willing to share contextual information (e.g., peer dynamics in the classroom, history of the home–school relationship) with a clinician verbally than in a written document (e.g., rating scale). Second, in an interview, clinicians can gain additional information about antecedent conditions that may trigger inappropriate behavior in the child, and possible consequences and reinforcement patterns that may be serving to maintain the disruptive behavior in the classroom. Such information can give clinicians information about the function of some behaviors, and this may serve to confirm and/or disconfirm hypotheses about ADHD and alternative explanations for the behavior. Third, this interpersonal interaction can set the stage for future collaboration in several ways. In some cases, the parent–teacher relationship is adversarial. By contacting the teacher, clinicians can initiate a relationship with the teacher and communicate directly (i.e., not filtered through the parent) about the purposes of the assessment and options for consultation with the school once recommendations are made. This allows the teacher to provide his or her perspective on the case, and once the teacher understands that this has been considered, he or she may be more willing to accept the outcomes of the assessment. Sample semistructured teacher interviews for the elementary level can be found on the websites (resources pages) of centers focused on assessment and treatment of ADHD (*http://oucirs.org/daily-report-card*; *https://ccf.fiu.edu/about/resources/index.html*).

Observations of the Child

Because rating scale data and interviews with parents and/or teachers are susceptible to bias, objective observations of classroom behavior and/or parent–child interactions may help clinicians make diagnostic decisions, particularly when there are large discrepancies between informants. Several systematic observation systems have been developed for observing ADHD-related behaviors in elementary school classrooms (see Volpe, DiPerna, Hintze, & Shapiro, 2005, for review). Most of these observation systems have acceptable cross-informant reliability, can differentiate elementary school students with and without classroom behavior problems, and can detect change in behavior as a function of interventions (Owens, Evans, et al., 2018). Examples include the Behavioral Observation of Students in Schools (BOSS; Shapiro, 2011) and the Student Behavior Teacher Response (SBTR; Pelham, Greiner, & Gnagy, 2008). One study also demonstrated incremental utility of the Direct Observation Form (DOF; McConaughy & Achenbach, 2009) of the ASEBA system. McConaughy and colleagues (2010) found that the DOF scales (obtained via three to four 10-minute observations) were significant predictors of the categorical diagnostic classifications of ADHD-C (combined presentation) versus non-ADHD and ADHD-C versus ADHD-IN (inattentive presentation), beyond the variance accounted for by the CBCL and TRF Attention Problem subscales. These observation systems are time consuming (most take 15–30 minutes and it may take four observations to obtain a dependable sample of student behavior; Volpe et al., 2005) and may not be feasible for clinical practice (i.e., not reimbursable). Nonetheless, they offer great value in school-based assessments, as these tools provide an objective assessment of student behavior (e.g., time on-task, rule violations) that are less vulnerable to subjective bias.

Executive Functioning

It has become common practice to consider measuring aspects of executive functioning (EF) to help with evaluation of an individual who may have ADHD. The rationale for measuring EF to help with a diagnosis is based on theory that suggests individuals with ADHD have deficits in EF that account for much of their impairment. However, there is not a clear definition of EF that operationally clarifies its measurement and, as a result, there are many nuanced approaches. Approaches to measurement have typically taken one of two forms: performance tasks (i.e., neuropsychological tests, continuous performance tasks) and rating scales.

Some professional guidelines for conducting evaluations address the use of EF-related neuropsychological measures to enhance evaluations. For example, the guidelines from the British Association for Psychopharmacology conclude that neuropsychological tests have good positive predictive power but poor negative predictive power, and as a result do not recommend their use (Nutt et al., 2007). Similarly, the guidelines for the American Academy of Child and Adolescent Psychiatry (AACAP) recommend that neuropsychological tests are not necessary to determine ADHD diagnoses (Pliszka & AACAP Work Group on Quality Issues, 2007). Indeed, even more recent work (e.g., Wodka et al., 2008) continues to support these conclusions as they relate to subscales of The Delis–Kaplan Executive Function System (D-KEFS; Delis, Kaplan, & Kramer, 2001) and the continuous performance task (CPT; Jarrett et al., 2018; Leth-Steensen, Elbaz, & Douglas, 2000).

The lack of supporting evidence for these tasks raises logistical questions. There is cost and time involved in administering a CPT or D-KEFS (20 minutes), and the value of the data appears limited to occasions when rating scale data are inconclusive. Instead, clinicians could use ADHD symptom and impairment rating scales, and consider administering an ADHD-specific diagnostic interview with the parents with the time saved not administering the CPT or D-KEFS. By administering these measures, one would have information similar to what is often considered the "gold standard" or criterion diagnosis in this type of research.

Finally, it is unclear to what extent reaction time variability data (e.g., from the CPT) are helpful in distinguishing a diagnosis of ADHD from another disorder. Results of a meta-analysis raise doubts about the utility of this variable, as reaction time variability was primarily associated with general psychopathology and not ADHD specifically (Kofler et al., 2013). This, combined with the conclusion by Nutt and colleagues (2007) that neuropsychological tests, broadly considered, lack specificity, the consensus of these findings appears to suggest that these tests are not useful in differentiating youth with ADHD from youth with any other clinical disorder.

An alternative approach to assessing EF via performance tasks is to use a rating scale that purportedly assesses EF. One concern about this approach is that many of the items on these measures are nearly synonymous with ADHD symptoms of inattention or academic impairment (vocational impairment for adults). As a result of asking similar questions across these measures, it is not surprising that EF rating scores are related to both symptoms and academic functioning (Langberg, Dvorsky, & Evans, 2013). Furthermore, there is evidence that scores from EF rating scales and EF performance measures are differentially related to functioning (Weyandt et al., 2013) and therefore assess different constructs (Toplak, West, & Stanovich, 2013).

Thus, although there is considerable theoretical support for deficits in EF accounting for much of the impairment in individuals with ADHD, there are serious limitations regarding its definition and measurement that limit the potential clinical utility of EF. It is worth noting that the evidence related to working memory (WM), one aspect of EF, suggests that performance measures of WM are associated with symptoms of ADHD and various areas of impairment (Kofler et al., 2018). The focus on a narrow aspect of EF with a better definition may be what leads to greater support for the role of WM than EF.

Assessments to Rule Out Alternatives and Inform Prescription

Up to this point, we have addressed assessment that can determine the extent to which a child meets diagnostic criteria for ADHD and comorbid conditions. Additional assessment can determine whether there are alternative reasons other than a diagnosis of ADHD that can account for the symptoms and impairment, and inform prescribing.

There are many common alternative explanations for inattention and problems with task completion. Children with low cognitive abilities and those with learning disabilities in reading, math, or language may have problems with attention and task completion. In addition, children who have vision or hearing problems, iron deficiencies, or thyroid problems may demonstrate symptoms consistent with ADHD. Furthermore, difficulties with attention is a symptom of many DSM-5 disorders (e.g., depression, anxiety). It is usually not feasible to evaluate all possible alternatives, but it is possible to screen for common alternatives. For example, cognitive abilities and academic achievement in the normal range for grade can reduce the likelihood that learning problems account for the inattention-related problems. It is often possible to obtain estimates of cognitive abilities and achievement from a child's school to make this decision. Similarly, clinicians can ask about the results of a child's most recent hearing and vision test and/or blood work, or recommend that parents seek out such testing. Furthermore, some common DSM-5 disorders that may account for inattention, such as internalizing difficulties, can be quickly screened. For example, a diagnosis of major depression requires that the child demonstrated either depressed mood/irritability or loss of interest or pleasure for at least 2 weeks. If neither were present, then there is no need to assess any further when considering a diagnosis of depression. As the base rate of children with ADHD is higher than that of children with other disorders in the community (Merikangas et al., 2010) and at clinics, a reasonable approach to the consideration of alternative diagnoses is to gather screening data that may rule them out.

The consideration of alternative explanations for presenting symptoms and impairment can be further informed by hypotheses specific to the child being evaluated. For example, information from an interview about history of the problems can provide rich data for consideration. If the onset of symptoms occurs in the context of a trauma or major life event, this can raise clinician concern for alternatives to ADHD. Many of these potential explanations may be unrelated to pathology if considered in a developmental context. For example, for a young child, experiencing a change in teachers in the middle of the year (e.g., maternity leave) or a stressful family event can negatively impact functioning. Other events can raise doubts about an ADHD diagnosis, such as a dramatic reduction in functioning without evidence of previous problems. ADHD is considered a chronic disorder, and impairment is usually evident over the course of a lifetime; thus, if a child's problems have a sudden onset, then additional data collection is warranted. It is possible that ADHD may be first expressed or exacerbated in reaction to a stressor or an increase in behavioral and/or academic expectations. However, clinicians should look for additional confirming evidence of ADHD, as many children who do not have ADHD can experience significant problems when expectations increase and/or stressors are present.

Using Assessment Data to Form a Case Conceptualization and Treatment Plan

At this point in the assessment process, the clinician likely has sufficient information about the diagnosis of ADHD and the presence of comorbid conditions. The clinician must integrate information about risk and protective factors, child history, family environment, and parent preferences to form a case conceptualization and treatment plan. Whereas a diagnosis can be considered a static piece of information, a case conceptualization is a multicomponent, theoretically driven individualized psychological portrait. It should explain symptoms and functional presentations; describe how past and present environment, interpersonal, and intrapersonal factors have shaped this presentation; and attempt to explain possible discrepancies between conflicting symptoms or presentations. In forming this conceptualization, a useful heuristic to consider is the 6 P's (Presenting Problems, Predisposing Factors, Precipitating Factors, Perpetuating Factors, Protective Factors, Prognosis; F. Wymbs, personal communication, January 21, 2019), as this rubric offers a means of communicating about the risk and protective factors, and moderators that may influence client response to treatment.

The case conceptualization can assist the clinician in formulating a treatment plan. The clinician should consider the evidence-based treatments for ADHD (Evans et al., 2018) and comorbid conditions (*www.effectivetherapy.org*). For ADHD, the evidence-based treatments (EBTs) include (1) behavioral management interventions implemented by parents (i.e., behavioral parent training programs), teachers (i.e., daily report cards and behavioral classroom interventions), and in therapeutic camp settings (e.g., the Summer Treatment Program for ADHD); (2) training interventions such as organization interventions, or interpersonal skills group for adolescents;

(3) pharmacological interventions (i.e., central nervous system stimulants or U.S. Food and Drug Administration [FDA]–approved nonstimulants); and (4) the combination of multiple psychosocial interventions or a psychosocial and pharmacological intervention.

Treatment Recommendations

Although symptoms are important for determining a diagnosis, clinicians should rely on impairment profiles, child age, and comorbid and contextual factors when recommending treatments (see Table 3 in Evans et al., 2018, for EBTs by age group). For example, if the child is in preschool or elementary school and the primary impairments are occurring within the context of the parent–child relationship, clinicians may recommend participation in a behavioral parenting program and consider adding pharmacological intervention if the parenting program is insufficient in producing desired change. It is important to note that one study found this sequence leads to significantly better parent engagement than if parents first use medication before being referred to a parenting program (Pelham et al., 2016). Furthermore, if the child is also experiencing significant impairment in school, clinicians may collaborate with teachers for a daily report card intervention (Volpe & Fabiano, 2013) and with parents on a homework program. However, if the child is in secondary school, school-based impairment may be best addressed via a training intervention for organization and planning and a homework management plan specific to the needs of teenagers (Evans et al., 2016; Langberg et al., 2011). Below, we discuss additional factors that may influence treatment recommendations and delivery as a function of data obtained in a comprehensive assessment.

Comorbid Diagnoses as Possible Treatment Moderators

The presence of comorbid ODD and CD should not significantly impact treatment selection for two reasons. First, most studies have not found strong differential responses to psychosocial or pharmacological treatment between those with and without comorbid ODD or CD (Langberg et al., 2016; MTA Cooperative Group, 1999). Second, particularly with ODD, the evidence-based psychosocial treatments for ADHD and ODD are similar for children, that is, behavioral parent training and/or modifications in environmental contingencies in the school (Evans et al., 2018). However, for comorbid CD, it is noteworthy that in addition to parenting-based interventions (like those provided for youth with ADHD and ODD), EBT for aggression and CD involves working directly with the child or adolescent (e.g., via an anger coping group) and/or taking a multisystemic family-based approach (see McCart & Sheidow, 2016).

In contrast, the presence of a comorbid learning disability (LD) does have important implications for treatment selection. First, when implementing daily report card or a home-based homework management plan, it is important to set the goals for performance at an academic level that is appropriate for the child's abilities and skills, considering his or her area of disability. Second, it is important that assessment and progress monitoring tools include both academic (e.g., grades, work completion and accuracy, progress in academic subskills) and behavioral (e.g., time on-task, rule following, academic enablers) outcomes. Third, children with ADHD and LD benefit from treatment targeting each specific disorder but do not experience crossover effects for either treatment (e.g., treatments for ADHD impacting reading outcomes) or an additive benefit of a combined treatment (Tannock et al., 2018). Fourth, a recent review indicated small, mixed results for medication alone on academic tasks (Froehlich et al., 2018). Thus, it is important to select interventions to address both the academic difficulties that are secondary to ADHD (i.e., deficits in sustained attention and attending to details), and the academic skills deficits associated with the LD (e.g., systematic reading instruction).

With regard to anxiety, there are few studies with samples large enough to look at treatment response in those with ADHD and comorbid anxiety. The one study suggests that the presence of anxiety in children with ADHD (with or without ODD/CD) actually confers some benefits in responsiveness to behavioral treatments for ADHD (Jensen et al., 2001), relative to pharmacological treatment. The results also suggest that the assessment of anxiety and ODD/CD in youth with ADHD is important, as combined psychosocial and pharmacological intervention may be needed to address the needs of those with both comorbidities, whereas behavioral intervention alone may be sufficient for those with ADHD + anxiety. We are not aware of any empirical study evaluating psychosocial treatment for ADHD and comorbid depression. Thus, until there are further data directly related to this population, it is recommended that clinicians apply the EBTs specific to each disorder.

Cultural Considerations as Possible Treatment Moderators

Family SES and racial and/or ethnic minority status warrant consideration when developing a treatment plan. With regard to SES, there is ample evidence that lower SES, single-parent status, and higher levels of parental stress are associated with lower rates of enrollment, lower rates of adherence, and higher rates of treatment attrition in behavioral parenting programs (Rieppi et al., 2002). Furthermore, children of parents who completed higher levels of education may make greater gains in treatment than children of parents with less education (Rieppi et al., 2002). In addition, lower rates of parent stress are predictive of better outcomes for secondary students participating in a school-based intervention (Langberg et al., 2016). These findings imply that clinicians should obtain information about client SES, assess its potential impact on parent initiation and engagement with treatment, and take active steps to help families overcome barriers to treatment completion (see Chacko, Wymbs, Chimiklis, Wymbs, & Pelham, 2012, for discussion).

We are not aware of any studies that have found moderating effects of race or ethnicity on treatment outcomes for youth with ADHD. Thus, although culturally contextualized treatments specific to race or ethnicity have intuitive appeal, until researchers identify (1) a specific cultural context that creates specific risk factors to be treated, (2) culturally specific protective factors to be leveraged in treatment, or (3) evidence that a minority group responds poorly to an evidence-based practice, clinicians should feel comfortable offering current EBTs to all families. Nonetheless, Eiraldi, Mazzuca, Clarke, and Power (2006) developed a reformulated model of help seeking that is specific to ADHD and accounts for the sociocultural factors likely producing disparities in health care for youth with ADHD. The model helps clinicians assess and consider the impact of culture on thresholds of problem recognition, willingness to seek services, and the importance of providing psychoeducation about a child's disorder and EBTs, so that parents can make more informed decisions about treatment.

Parent Psychopathology as a Possible Treatment Moderator

Unfortunately, parental psychopathology can have a substantial negative impact on child psychopathology (Chronis-Tuscano et al., 2008) and treatment outcomes (e.g., Jans et al., 2015). Thus, it is recommended that clinicians consider screening for parental depression and/or ADHD. If resources allow, this screening could occur universally for all referred clients. Alternatively, screening could occur more selectively, only if barriers to treatment engagement or progress are witnessed. Chronis-Tuscano and colleagues (2013) developed a program that integrates cognitive-behavioral treatment for depression into a traditional behavioral parent training program for depressed mothers of children with ADHD and found outcomes that surpassed those achieved via the traditional behavioral parenting training. In contrast, Jans and colleagues (2015) examined the effects of pharmacological treatments for maternal ADHD (followed by individual behavioral parent training) on child outcomes relative to a control group (which received 12 weeks of supportive counseling only). Although the mothers in the experimental condition experienced significant reduction of their own ADHD symptoms, there were no differences between the treatment groups on child outcomes. Thus, although there may be promise for the impact of treating maternal depression on child outcomes (Chronis-Tuscano et al., 2013), treating maternal ADHD to improve child ADHD outcomes may be more complicated (Chronis-Tuscano et al., 2008; Jans et al., 2015). Clinicians may need to consider simultaneous psychosocial treatment for maternal ADHD, titrating the presentation of information offered in individual parent training (e.g., to ensure mastery before moving onto a new parenting skill), and recommending the pursuit of medication for the child to potentially compensate for a lower or slower dose of the parent training intervention.

School District Resources as Possible Treatment Moderators

There are many effective school-based interventions for children with ADHD (Fabiano & Pyle, 2019) and their willingness to collaborate can substantially enhance or limit the potential benefits of treatment. By conducting an interview with the client's teacher, clinicians can assess the extent to which school staff members may collaborate to implement interventions and facilitate alliance building to enhance the likelihood of collaboration. Clinicians can facilitate collaboration with school personnel by expressing gratitude for what school staff members have done to date (e.g., completing rating scales in the assessment process), highlighting the common goals across all stakeholders (i.e.,

student success, reduction in classroom disruption by the student), and offering resources toward meeting that goal (e.g., guidance to parents for homework management, consultation with teachers regarding a daily report card or organizational intervention). It may also help to remind school personnel that problems related to ADHD are unlikely to improve without intervention (Evans et al., 2016; Owens, Murphy, Richerson, Girio, & Himawan, 2008), and that by addressing the child's problems proactively (i.e., via intervention), the student–teacher relationship is likely to improve and teacher stress is likely to decrease.

An additional step that clinicians can take to facilitate school-based services for the client is to educate families about the child's rights under section 504 of the ADA or IDEIA (see DuPaul, Power, Evans, et al., 2016). Clinicians can help parents understand how to advocate for their child's needs in order to garner school support rather than create an adversarial relationship. If possible, the clinician may consider accompanying the parents to a meeting with the school personnel to help with this communication (or conduct a conjoint meeting over the phone). The evaluation of the client can be a very valuable resource for the parents and school officials when determining the type of services to be provided and deciding whether the student meets criteria for services under the ADA or IDEIA. It is important for clinicians to recognize that the determination of that eligibility will occur within a process conducted by the school, and statements that a child is eligible for special education in the evaluation report should be carefully worded (i.e., requesting consideration for eligibility rather than recommending eligibility), as strong recommendations can increase the risk of an adversarial relationship (see Zoromski, Evans, Gahagan, Serrano, & Holdaway, 2015). Providing a careful explanation of why the student meets diagnostic criteria for ADHD and the nature of the associated school-related impairment can facilitate this process.

Client Preferences

In addition to considering these factors, it is important that clinicians assess parent treatment preferences in the context of the assessment, as this knowledge can shape the manner in which clinicians provide feedback and recommendations to parents. For example, Waschbusch and colleagues (2011) documented that a large portion of treatment-seeking parents (70%) prefer to avoid the use of medication. If clinicians are aware of this, they can offer parents information about the advantages and disadvantages of pharmacological treatment, but perhaps do so after offering recommendations for psychosocial treatment. In addition, Fiks, Mayne, DeBartolo, Power, and Guevara (2013) found that parents with different outcome goals (e.g., academic achievement vs. behavioral compliance) had differential patterns of treatment initiation (medication vs. behavior parent training, respectively). Thus, if clinicians obtain an understanding of parents' priorities and desired outcomes throughout the assessment process, they can educate parents on the relative match or mismatch between each treatments and each desired outcome domain. For example, if parents are hoping to improve their elementary school-age child's peer relationships but have a preference for medication, then it would be prudent for the clinician to inform the parents that medication is unlikely to substantially improve peer relations. Instead, they may need to take a more active role in the child's treatment, such as engaging in parental friendship coaching, home–school interventions, and strategies that target and reinforce the child's use of prosocial skills. Furthermore, in a sample of parents of children at risk for ADHD, Wymbs and colleagues (2016) found that 59% of parents reported a preference for individual behavioral parenting training over a group program, and that a sizable minority (20%) of parents (those with the most severe levels of parental depression and a symptomatic child) preferred minimal involvement in treatment. Because some parent preferences are not well aligned with EBT, clinicians may also need to engage in motivational interviewing strategies to enhance parent participation in the most effective treatment for their child's problems.

Progress, Process, and Outcome Measurement

Once the diagnoses, case conceptualization, and treatment plan have been shared with the family, the assessment tasks shift to the assessment of treatment process and treatment progress (short-term and long-term outcomes). We describe the following assessment procedures:

• Defining target behaviors
• Obtaining a baseline assessment of target behaviors
• Assessing proximal target behaviors and distal functioning over time

• Assessing treatment integrity and working alliance
• Assessing maintenance of treatment gains

Progress Monitoring: Assessment of Target Behaviors and Treatment Goals

It has long been recognized that treatment should focus on changing the child's impairments and functioning (peer relationships, academic achievement, family functioning) rather than changing the symptoms of inattention, impulsivity, and hyperactivity (e.g., Pelham et al., 2005), as impairment is typically the impetus for seeking treatment. Furthermore, reliable change in symptoms lacks correspondence with reliable change in impairment (Karpenko, Owens, Evangelista, & Dodd, 2009). Thus, target behaviors and treatment goals should be determined by the client's impairment profile, with consideration given to possible moderating factors, family strengths, and preferences (see the third section).

Broadly speaking, the goal of each EBT (e.g., behavioral parent training, daily report card in the classroom, homework management, organizational skills) is to move the child's behavior into the normative range. However, it is important to recognize two factors when setting treatment goals. First, several studies reveal that a substantial portion of children who receive EBTs do not achieve levels of symptoms or behavior that fall in the normative range (see Table 3 in Evans et al., 2018). Thus, although normalization may be the ultimate goal, achieving reliable improvement may be a more realistic goal and may still have a substantial impact on changing the trajectory of negative outcomes. Second, observing reliable improvement in child behavior can take time (e.g., 10–16 weeks of parent training, 2–4 months of a daily report cards, or 1 year of organizational training). Thus, it is important to give parents (and teachers) not only hope and optimism about treatment but also realistic expectations for the time and investment needed to obtain positive outcomes.

The first assessment task is to obtain a baseline measure of the behaviors to be targeted in treatment. Clinicians should help parents and teacher prioritize the behaviors that create the most impairment, operationally define the behaviors of concern, and encourage them to track the frequency of these behaviors (e.g., interrupting, aggression, noncompliance) for 1 week. These data should be used to set initial short-term goals that allow the child (and the parent and/or the teacher) to experience success early in treatment. For example, if, on average, the child is making 10 disrespectful comments to peers per day, teachers may initially reinforce the child for reducing this to eight comments per day (while engaging in other skills such as praising respectful behavior) and gradually change the criterion for reinforcement to shape the behavior into the normal range. The baseline data can also serve as points of comparison over time to determine whether the intervention is working. Similar principles apply to home-based target behaviors.

The second assessment task is to monitor change in the proximal target behaviors over time, and change in distal domain-specific impairment. To effectively assess a child's response to an intervention, it is necessary to use repeated assessments, often in a short cycle (e.g., at every session in a clinic, monthly at school), to determine whether the child's behavior is improving, maintaining, or worsening with the application of the selected intervention. It is important to recognize that assessment tools used for diagnostic purposes may or may not be the same tools needed for progress monitoring, as progress monitoring tools must have not only the psychometric properties of reliability and validity but also adequate treatment sensitivity (Gresham, 2005). "Treatment sensitivity" refers to the ability of an assessment tool to detect small changes in behavior. Considerably less attention has been paid to the development of progress monitoring tools relative to diagnostic assessment tools. In addition to those listed in Table 5.1, we review tools that have been tested for treatment sensitivity.

School-Based Target Behaviors

Because the field of education has focused on a movement toward response to intervention (RTI) in the last decade, most progress monitoring tools are those related to change in school-based behavior, primarily at the elementary school level. For example, the Academic Performance Rating Scale (APRS; DuPaul, Rapport, & Perriello, 1991) is a 19-item scale assessing teacher perception of children's academic functioning. The Academic Success (i.e., accuracy, quality) and Academic Productivity (i.e., attention to details, persistence) subscales have acceptable internal consistency (.72–.95), stability (.88–.95), and criterion-related validity, and have been shown to be sensitive to change in child behavior as a function of pharmacological (DuPaul & Rapport, 1993) and behav-

ioral interventions (Murray, Rabiner, Schulte, & Newitt, 2008). The structured classroom observations reviewed in Section 3 that assess classroom rule violations, disruptive behavior, and on/off task behaviors are also sensitive to intervention (Owens et al., 2018).

Another measure that has undergone significant empirical testing for treatment sensitivity for elementary and middle school children is a daily behavior rating (DBR), which is a short rating scale (one to six items) that assesses behavior that is observable, operationally defined, and closely tied to the teacher's primary concern (e.g., arguing, being out of one's seat, interrupting). This behavior is rated by the teacher as it naturally occurs (e.g., in a classroom or on the playground), and the ratings provide a means of quantifying the frequency or severity of the behavior in a period of time (e.g., class period, day, or week). The earliest work on DBRs focused on single-item scales (DBR-SIS). Over 25 published studies have helped to establish convincing evidence that the data obtained from DBR-SIS demonstrate adequate treatment sensitivity (Miller, Crovello, & Chafouleas, 2017), and are considered to be feasible and acceptable by teachers. It is important to recognize that when using a one-item scale, clinicians need to obtain seven to 10 ratings of a student's behavior to achieve an adequate level of dependability (Chafouleas, Riley-Tillman, & Christ, 2009). Additional information about this assessment tool may be found on the University of Connecticut's DBR website (*https://dbr.education.uconn.edu*).

Because DBR-SISs have focused on three behaviors (disruptive behavior, academic engagement, and disrespect), and may require up to 10 measurement occasions, additional studies have examined the benefits of multi-item DBRs (DBR-MIS; Daniels, Volpe, Briesch, Gadow, 2017), which can reduce the number of measurement occasions without substantially increasing the burden on teachers (e.g., use of five or six items). Volpe and colleagues have developed a set of five-item DBR-MISs that assess a wider range of target behaviors, including the domains Disruptive, Oppositional, Interpersonal Conflict, Conduct Problems, Socially Withdrawn, and Anxious-Depressed (Daniels, Volpe, Briesh, & Owens, 2019), with evidence of adequate treatment sensitivity for some scales (Hustus, Owens, Volpe, Briesch, & Daniels, 2018) and anticipation of further testing for others.

Last, the daily report card can serve as both an intervention and a progress monitoring tool; that is, once target behaviors are selected, teachers are asked to provide feedback to the child each day about the target behaviors (i.e., number of interruptions; percentage of work completed in math) and to document the rates of these behaviors on a daily basis. These data can reveal change in child behavior and be used to shape the child's behavior into the appropriate range; that is, as the child makes progress toward initial goals (e.g., raises his or her hand to speak, with eight or fewer violations), these goals can be gradually reduced (e.g., with six or fewer violations) over time. Owens and colleagues analyzed rates of behavior change that occur when using a daily report card (Holdaway et al., 2018; Owens et al., 2012) and provide benchmarks for the magnitude of change that can be expected with each month of intervention (for up to 4 months). The data reveal that changes of large magnitude can be achieved with 1 month of intervention, with small incremental benefits continuing each month thereafter.

For adolescents, the most well-studied school-based interventions focus on improving organization and planning behaviors (Evans et al., 2016; Langberg et al., 2018). The proximal indicators of treatment response are the student's organization checklist, which indicates the criteria for an organized planner, binder, bookbag, or locker (e.g., with a different-colored folder for each subject and separate locations for completed and uncompleted assignments). Each time the criteria and materials are reviewed with the student, the student receives a percent complete score, and these scores can be monitored over time to gauge progress in gaining competency in independently organizing belongings. Recent evidence documents that progress in this proximal indicator is a significant predictor of the distal outcome of GPA in the semester and year following participation in an organization intervention (Evans, Allan, Margherio, Xiang, & Owens, 2019). Like the daily report card, organization interventions have progress monitoring built into the intervention itself. Other school-based interventions do not, and with these interventions, DBRs or other progress monitoring data will be needed to measure progress monitoring.

Home-Based Target Behaviors

From a clinical standpoint, most home-based target behaviors are idiosyncratic and are monitored via parent tracking of the behavior frequency (e.g., number of temper tantrums, instances of noncompliance). Research decades ago by Arnold, Levine, and Patterson (1975) documented that such frequency counts in diagnosed children, and their siblings were sensitive to change as a function of parent and/or child participation in treatment. However, we are unaware of any recent studies focused on documenting the psychometric properties of such behaviors. Nevertheless, like the school-based progress monitoring measures described earlier, many of the behavioral home-based interventions include progress monitoring elements. For example, token economies are administered in a manner similar to the daily report card, but they operate in the home, and parents provide behavioral contingencies directly. Tracking target behaviors is required in order to consistently implement the token economy. Similarly, parent–adolescent behavioral contracts and homework management plans also require tracking behaviors to inform contingencies. These data can be used to assess change over time (Sibley et al., 2016). To facilitate high-quality tracking of target behaviors, clinicians can provide checklists to parents weekly at parenting sessions, and can graph the data, so that parents can observe the benefits of the data and the intervention.

Process Monitoring: Assessment of Treatment Integrity

There is now ample evidence that treatment process variables influence treatment outcome. One well studied process variable in the treatment of ADHD is that of treatment integrity. Integrity is a multidimensional construct and has most commonly been represented by either adherence scores (i.e., the extent to which an intervention is implemented as intended) or dosage (e.g., number of sessions received). Because home- and school-based interventions for ADHD require that parents and teachers implement the intervention, measurement of their adherence to procedures is critically important to interpreting outcomes. For example, if a child is not making adequate progress, it is important to know whether this is because the interventions are not being applied with high integrity or whether they are being applied with high quality and the child is not a responder to this type of intervention.

School-Based Treatments

With elementary school samples, there is evidence from both single-case design studies (Reinke, Lewis-Palmer, & Merrell, 2008; Sanetti, Collier-Meek, Long, Kim, & Kratochwill, 2014) and randomized controlled group designs (e.g., Conroy et al., 2015) that there is a functional relationship between teachers' intervention integrity and change in student behavior in the classroom. Owens and colleagues (2018) found that the relationship between teacher implementation behavior and negative student behavior increases in magnitude as teachers enhance their use of effective practices (e.g., r's < .35 at baseline; r's > .50 after 3–4 months of implementation), suggesting the importance of this process variable over time. Furthermore, this study revealed that although higher integrity is better, even helping teachers achieve a minimum benchmark of 51% adherence has an important impact on student outcomes (Owens et al., 2018); that is, teachers who achieved this benchmark witnessed about half the rule violations (among target students and other students) compared to teachers who did not achieve this benchmark (effect sizes were medium to large). Thus, as clinicians collaborate with teachers to implement a classroom intervention, it is important to attempt to periodically assess integrity. This may be achieved via periodic classroom observations, review of completed daily report cards or tracking sheets, and/or technology that facilitates the teacher's entry of implementation data that can serve as a close proxy for integrity (e.g., see *www.oucirs.org/daily-report-card-preview*).

With secondary school samples, we are aware of only one study that has examined the relationship between intervention dose and student outcomes. Evans, Schultz, and DeMars (2014) conducted a pilot study with 36 high school students, assessing the preliminary efficacy of a multicomponent intervention that included a 10-session parenting group (90 minutes each) with a focus on homework management planning, a 10-session adolescent interpersonal skills training group (90 minutes each), and brief (15–20 minutes) biweekly organizational skills training sessions throughout the school year. The authors used probit regression to examine the relationship between dose (i.e., total number of sessions) and reliable improvement in functioning. In both academic and family functioning domains, the regression model predicted that less than 15% of adolescents would achieve reliable improvement without coaching, whereas more than three times as many adolescents would achieve reliable improvement with 50 sessions or more over the school year. Although this demonstrates the importance of dose, there is a lack of research to provide guidance on best methods for measuring both dose and adherence. Furthermore,

we are unaware of any studies that evaluated the relationship between treatment adherence and outcomes in secondary schools. Nonetheless, clinicians are encourage to develop idiosyncratic methods to attempt to assess these important process variables.

Another important process variable is alliance. Within school-based organization training interventions, there is evidence that the therapeutic alliance, as perceived by the adolescent (but not the intervention coach) is predictive of treatment outcomes (Langberg et al., 2016). Thus, clinicians could assess adolescent perceptions of alliance using the short version of the Working Alliance Inventory (WAI-Short; Tracey & Kokotovic, 1989), which assesses agreement on tasks and goals, and the bond between the adolescent and the intervention coach.

Home-Based Treatments

For behavioral parent training interventions, the dose of treatment can be monitored by the number of sessions the parent attends. This is important to track for two reasons. First, of the parents who choose to attend behavioral parenting programs, 40–90% fail to complete the intended protocol (Pelham et al., 2016). Second, although attendance may not be sufficient to produce desired outcomes (Clarke et al., 2015), it is likely a necessary foundational condition for success. Factors including low SES, single-parent status, high levels of stress, and/or parent psychopathology are known barriers to participation (Chacko et al., 2012; Chronis-Tuscano et al., 2013). Thus, clinicians should consider these factors and help parents problem-solve possible barriers to participation.

However, some studies fail to reveal a significant relationship between attendance and treatment outcomes (e.g., Clarke et al., 2015), likely because parent adherence to recommended procedures is the more important mediator of desired outcomes. Indeed, Clarke and colleagues (2015) found that parent application of between session homework assignments was a significant predictor of multiple treatment outcomes for the parent (e.g., parenting self-efficacy) and the child (homework productivity), whereas attendance was not. Furthermore, using data from the Multimodal Treatment Study of ADHD (MTA), Hinshaw and colleagues (2000) demonstrated that reductions in negative and ineffective parent discipline mediated improvement in teacher-rated child social skills, indicating that parent adherence to parenting interventions was partially responsible for the desired change in child behavior. In group-based parent training, parent adherence can be assessed by having parents turn in homework assignments that document their use of a given strategy each week and via discussion. Clarke and colleagues rated completion using a 3-point scale (0 = *homework was not attempted or submitted*, 1 = *submitted homework was attempted but incomplete*, and 2 = *submitted homework was completed*). In the context of individual parent training or a research protocol, actual demonstration of parenting skills could be assessed by observations of behavior in the context of structured parent–child interactions such as a 5-minute free-play activity, a 10-minute homework task, or a clean-up task. Parent–child interactions during these tasks can be reliably coded using the Dyadic Parent–Child Interaction Coding System (DPICS; Eyberg, Nelson, Duke, & Boggs, 2004). Alternatively, a set of brief, carefully designed questions can be sent to the parents in a daily e-mail or asked on the telephone to assess adherence and changes in adherence over time (e.g., Evans, Vallano, & Pelham, 1994).

Last, clinicians are also encouraged to continuously assess the alliance between the parent and the intervention provider, as the parent–therapist alliance is a predictor of parent and child attendance and engagement in treatment (Hawley & Weiss, 2005). This can be assessed with the parent version of the Working Alliance Inventory (WAI; Tracey & Kokotovic, 1989).

Assessing Maintenance of Treatment Gains

Because ADHD is a chronic disorder, a chronic care model that includes ongoing assessment of child functioning at each developmental stage is warranted (Evans, Owens, et al., 2014). However, to date, only a minority of treatment–outcome studies have assessed long-term follow-up effects, and most studies find that the effects diminish from posttreatment to follow-up time periods (6 months to 3 years later; e.g., Jensen et al., 2007). In their most recent review of EBTs for ADHD, Evans and colleagues (2018) documented that only six of 30 studies conducted a follow-up assessment with adequate control conditions, and only one of these studies had maintained equivalent or increasing benefits from posttreatment to follow-up (Evans et al., 2016). As a result, most treatments are time-limited, and strategically implementing them at

the optimal times over development is only possible with good assessment.

The need for treatment across development can change due to age and situation. Thus, consistent assessment of functioning critical to each client is warranted. Even when there may be no active treatments, the continuation of assessment is consistent with care for a chronic condition and has the potential to identify the onset of problems before they are serious. Transition points are especially important times for assessment, as they include important changes in the environment (e.g., elementary to middle school, high school to adulthood, parent divorce) and changes in the child (e.g., puberty). Thus, clinicians should encourage parents to reconsider the need to re-engage with treatment in each developmental milestone and/or transition. Understanding patterns of assessment data over time can provide a great benefit to a child and family, and suggests that there may be benefits to coordinating care under one primary provider who has expertise in assessment and development across contexts (e.g., entry into middle school or high school).

Conclusion

High-quality assessment takes time. Thus, clinicians are continuously challenged to strike a balance between the demands of time and quality given the resources in their setting. In this chapter, we have reviewed the state of the science with regard to assessment at each of four stages in the service delivery process. We hope that by selecting as least some of the tools within this chapter, clinicians can find a balance between comprehensiveness and conducting a "good enough" assessment (Youngstrom et al., 2017, p. 336). Furthermore, we have attempted to describe throughout the chapter that best practice involves both assessment and treatment, and that these processes are inextricably intertwined. Although each can be completed alone, the lack of an integrated process will limit the potential benefit for a child with ADHD and his or her family. We hope that we have broadened readers' perspective on assessment, so that they consider the critical issues in preparation, prediction, planning, and progress monitoring, and that we have pointed out to them a variety of resources that can be combined to enhance quality and efficiency, and meet the needs of clinicians and clients in a diverse array of settings.

REFERENCES

Abikoff, H. B., Jensen, P. S., Arnold, L. E., Hoza, B., Hechtman, L., Pollack, S., . . . Vitiello, B. (2002). Observed classroom behavior of children with ADHD: Relationship to gender and comorbidity. *Journal of Abnormal Child Psychology, 30*(4), 349–359.

Achenbach, T. M., & Rescorla, L. A. (2001). *Manual for the ASEBA School-Age Forms and Profiles.* Burlington: University of Vermont, Research Center for Children, Youth, & Families.

Aebi, M., Kuhn, C., Banaschewski, T., Grimmer, Y., Poustka, L., Steinhausen, H. C., & Goodman, R. (2017). The contribution of parent and youth information to identify mental health disorders or problems in adolescents. *Child and Adolescent Psychiatry and Mental Health, 11*(1), 23.

Allan, D. M., & Lonigan, C. J. (2019). Examination of the structure and measurement of inattentive, hyperactive, and impulsive behaviors from preschool to grade 4. *Journal of Abnormal Child Psychology, 47*(6), 975–987.

American Academy of Pediatrics. (2011). ADHD: Clinical practice guideline for the diagnosis, evaluation, and treatment of ADHD in children and adolescents. *Pediatrics, 128*(5), 1–18.

American Psychiatric Association. (2013). *Diagnostic and statistical manual of mental disorders* (5th ed.). Arlington, VA: Author.

Anastopoulos, A. D., Beal, K. K., Reid, R. J., Reid, R., Power, T. J., & DuPaul, G. J. (2018). Impact of child and informant gender on parent and teacher ratings of attention-deficit/hyperactivity disorder. *Psychological Assessment, 30*(10), 1390–1394.

Antrop, I., Roeyers, H., Oosterlaan, J., & Van Oost, P. (2002). Agreement between parent and teacher ratings of disruptive behavior disorders in children with clinically diagnosed ADHD. *Journal of Psychopathology and Behavioral Assessment, 24*(1), 67–73.

Arnold, J. E., Levine, A. G., & Patterson, G. R. (1975). Changes in sibling behavior following family intervention. *Journal of Consulting and Clinical Psychology, 43*(5), 683–688.

Bard, D. E., Wolraich, M. L., Neas, B., Doffing, M., & Beck, L. (2013). The psychometric properties of the Vanderbilt Attention-Deficit Hyperactivity Disorder Diagnostic Parent Rating Scale in a community population. *Journal of Developmental and Behavioral Pediatrics, 34*(2), 72–82.

Barkley, R. A. (2012). *Barkley Functional Impairment Scale—Children and Adolescents (BFIS-CA).* New York: Guilford Press.

Barkley, R. A., & Cox, D. (2007). A review of driving risks and impairments associated with attention-deficit/hyperactivity disorder and the effects of stimulant medication on driving performance. *Journal of Safety Research, 38*(1), 113–128.

Barkley, R. A., Fischer, M., Smallish, L., & Fletcher, K. (2002). The persistence of attention-deficit/hyperactivity disorder into young adulthood as a function of reporting source and definition of disorder. *Journal of Abnormal Psychology, 111*(2), 279–289.

Barrett, C., & DuPaul, G. J. (2018). Impact of maternal and child race on maternal ratings of ADHD symptoms in black and white boys. *Journal of Attention Disorders, 22*(13), 1246–1254.

Barry, T. D., Lyman, R. D., & Klinger, L. G. (2002). Academic underachievement and attention-deficit/hyperactivity disorder: The negative impact of symptom severity on school performance. *Journal of School Psychology, 40*(3), 259–283.

Becker, K. D., Chorpita, B. F., & Daleiden, E. L. (2011). Improvement in symptoms versus functioning: How do our best treatments measure up? *Administration and Policy in Mental Health and Mental Health Services Research, 38*(6), 440–458.

Becker, S. P., Langberg, J. M., Vaughn, A. J., & Epstein, J. N. (2012). Clinical utility of the Vanderbilt ADHD diagnostic parent rating scale comorbidity screening scales. *Journal of Developmental and Behavioral Pediatrics, 33*(3), 221–228.

Biederman, J., Petty, C. R., Clarke, A., Lomedico, A., & Faraone, S. V. (2011). Predictors of persistent ADHD: An 11-year follow-up study. *Journal of Psychiatric Research, 45*(2), 150–155.

Boomsma, D. I., Cacioppo, J. T., Muthén, B., Asparouhov, T., & Clark, S. (2007). Longitudinal genetic analysis for loneliness in Dutch twins. *Twin Research and Human Genetics, 10*(2), 267–273.

Bussing, R., Fernandez, M., Harwood, M., Hou, W., Garvan, C. W., Eyberg, S. M., & Swanson, J. M. (2008). Parent and teacher SNAP-IV ratings of ADHD symptoms: Psychometric properties and normative ratings from a school district sample. *Assessment, 15*(3), 317–328.

Chacko, A., Wymbs, B. T., Chimiklis, A., Wymbs, F. A., & Pelham, W. E. (2012). Evaluating a comprehensive strategy to improve engagement to group-based behavioral parent training for high-risk families of children with ADHD. *Journal of Abnormal Child Psychology, 40,* 1351–1362.

Chafouleas, S. M., Riley-Tillman, T. C., & Christ, T. J. (2009). Direct Behavior Rating (DBR): An emerging method for assessing social behavior within a tiered intervention system. *Assessment for Effective Intervention, 34*(4), 195–200.

Chronis-Tuscano, A., Clarke, T. L., O'Brien, K. A., Raggi, V. L., Diaz, Y., Mintz, A. D., . . . Seeley, J. (2013). Development and preliminary evaluation of an integrated treatment targeting parenting and depressive symptoms in mothers of children with attention-deficit/hyperactivity disorder. *Journal of Consulting and Clinical Psychology, 81*(5), 918–925.

Chronis-Tuscano, A., Raggi, V. L., Clarke, T. L., Rooney, M. E., Diaz, Y., & Pian, J. (2008). Associations between maternal attention-deficit/hyperactivity disorder symptoms and parenting. *Journal of Abnormal Child Psychology, 36*(8), 1237–1250.

Clarke, A. T., Marshall, S. A., Mautone, J. A., Soffer, S. L., Jones, H. A., Costigan, T. E., . . . Power, T. J. (2015). Parent attendance and homework adherence predict response to a family–school intervention for children with ADHD. *Journal of Clinical Child and Adolescent Psychology, 44*(1), 58–67.

Conners, C. K. (2008). *Conners 3rd edition manual*. Toronto: Multi-Health Systems.

Conroy, M. A., Sutherland, K. S., Algina, J. J., Wilson, R. E., Martinez, J. R., & Whalon, K. J. (2015). Measuring teacher implementation of the BEST in CLASS intervention program and corollary child outcomes. *Journal of Emotional and Behavioral Disorders, 23*(3), 144–155.

Cortese, S., Kelly, C., Chabernaud, C., Proal, E., Di Martino, A., Milham, M. P., & Castellanos, F. X. (2012). Toward systems neuroscience of ADHD: A meta-analysis of 55 fMRI studies. *American Journal of Psychiatry, 169*(10), 1038–1055.

Daniels, B., Briesch, A. M., Volpe, R. J., & Owens, J. S. (2019). Content validation of direct behavior rating multi-item scales for assessing problem behaviors. *Journal of Emotional and Behavioral Disorders.* [Epub ahead of print]

Daniels, B., Volpe, R. J., Briesch, A. M., & Gadow, K. D. (2017). Dependability and treatment sensitivity of multi-item Direct Behavior Rating Scales for interpersonal peer conflict. *Assessment for Effective Intervention, 43*, 48–59.

De Los Reyes, A., Augenstein, T. M., Wang, M., Thomas, S. A., Drabick, D. A., Burgers, D. E., & Rabinowitz, J. (2015). The validity of the multi-informant approach to assessing child and adolescent mental health. *Psychological Bulletin, 141*(4), 858–900.

Delis, D. C., Kaplan, E., & Kramer, J. H. (2001). *Delis-Kaplan Executive Function System® (D-KEFS®): Examiner's manual: Flexibility of thinking, concept formation, problem solving, planning, creativity, impulse control, inhibition*. Bloomington, MN: Pearson.

DuPaul, G. J., McGoey, K. E., Eckert, T. L., & VanBrakle, J. (2001). Preschool children with ADHD: Impairments in behavioral, social, and school functioning. *Journal of the American Academy of Child and Adolescent Psychiatry, 40*(5), 508–515.

DuPaul, G. J., Power, T. J., Anastopoulos, A. D., & Reid, R. (1998). *ADHD Rating Scale—IV: Checklists, norms, and clinical interpretation*. New York: Guilford Press.

DuPaul, G. J., Power, T. J., Anastopoulos, A. D., & Reid, R. (2016). *ADHD Rating Scale–5 for children and adolescents: Checklists, norms, and clinical interpretation*. New York: Guilford Press.

DuPaul, G. J., Power, T. J., Evans, S. W., Mautone, J. A., & Owens, J. S. (2016). Students with ADHD and Section 504 Regulations: Challenges, obligations, and opportunities for school psychologists. *Communique, 45*(3), 1–26.

DuPaul, G. J., & Rapport, M. D. (1993). Does methylphenidate normalize the classroom performance of children with attention deficit disorder? *Journal of the American Academy of Child and Adolescent Psychiatry, 32*(1), 190–198.

DuPaul, G. J., Rapport, M. D., & Perriello, L. M. (1991). Teacher ratings of academic skills: The development of the Academic Performance Rating Scale. *School Psychology Review, 20*(2), 284–300.

DuPaul, G. J., Reid, R., Anastopoulos, A. D., Lambert, M. C., Watkins, M. W., & Power, T. J. (2016). Parent and teacher ratings of attention-deficit/hyperactivity disorder symptoms: Factor structure and normative data. *Psychological Assessment, 28*, 214–225.

Eiraldi, R. B., Mazzuca, L. B., Clarke, A. T., & Power, T. J. (2006). Service utilization among ethnic minority children with ADHD: A model of help-seeking behavior. *Administration and Policy in Mental Health and Mental Health Services Research, 33*(5), 607–622.

Evans, S. W., Allan, D., Margherio, S., Xiang, J., & Owens, J. S. (2019). *Organization interventions as a mechanism of change for grades in the challenging horizons program*. Manuscript under review.

Evans, S. W., Allen, J., Moore, S., & Strauss, V. (2005). Measuring symptoms and functioning of youth with ADHD in middle schools. *Journal of Abnormal Child Psychology, 33*(6), 695–706.

Evans, S. W., Brady, C. E., Harrison, J. R., Bunford, N., Kern, L., State, T., & Andrews, C. (2013). Measuring ADHD and ODD symptoms and impairment using high school teachers' ratings. *Journal of Clinical Child and Adolescent Psychology, 42*, 197–207.

Evans, S. W., Langberg, J. M., Schultz, B. K., Vaughn, A., Altaye, M., Marshall, S. A., & Zoromski, A. K. (2016). Evaluation of a school-based treatment program for young adolescents with ADHD. *Journal of Consulting and Clinical Psychology, 84*, 15–30.

Evans, S. W., Owens, J. S., Mautone, J. A., DuPaul, G. J., & Power, T. J. (2014). Toward a comprehensive life-course model of care for youth with attention-deficit/hyperactivity disorder. In M. D. Weist, N. A. Lever, C. P. Bradshaw, & J. S. Owens (Eds.), *Handbook of school mental health* (2nd ed., pp. 413–426). New York: Springer Science + Business Media.

Evans, S. W., Owens, J. S., Wymbs, B. T., & Ray, A. R. (2018). Evidence-based psychosocial treatments for children and adolescents with attention deficit/hyperactivity disorder. *Journal of Clinical Child and Adolescent Psychology, 47*(2), 157–198.

Evans, S. W., Schultz, B. K., & DeMars, C. E. (2014). High school-based treatment for adolescents with attention-deficit/hyperactivity disorder: Results from a pilot study examining outcomes and dosage. *School Psychology Review, 43*(2), 185–203.

Evans, S. W., Schultz, B. K., DeMars, C. E., & Davis, H. (2011). Effectiveness of the Challenging Horizons after-school program for young adolescents with ADHD. *Behavior Therapy, 42*(3), 462–474.

Evans, S. W., Vallano, G., & Pelham, W. (1994). Treatment of parenting behavior with a psychostimulant: A case study of an adult with attention-deficit hyperactivity disorder. *Journal of Child and Adolescent Psychopharmacology, 4*(1), 63–69.

Eyberg, S. M., Nelson, M. M., Duke, M., & Boggs, S. R. (2004). *Manual for the Dyadic Parent–Child Interaction Coding System, Third Edition.* Gainesville: University of Florida.

Fabiano, G. A., Pelham, W. E., Jr., Waschbusch, D. A., Gnagy, E. M., Lahey, B. B., Chronis, A. M., . . . Burrows-MacLean, L. (2006). A practical measure of impairment: Psychometric properties of the impairment rating scale in samples of children with ADHD and two school-based samples. *Journal of Clinical Child and Adolescent Psychology, 35*(3), 369–385.

Fabiano, G. A., & Pyle, K. (2019). Best practices in school mental health for attention-deficit/hyperactivity disorder: A framework for intervention. *School Mental Health, 11,* 72–91.

Faraone, S. V., Monuteaux, M. C., Biederman, J., Cohan, S. L., & Mick, E. (2003). Does parental ADHD bias maternal reports of ADHD symptoms in children? *Journal of Consulting and Clinical Psychology, 71*(1), 168–175.

Fiks, A. G., Mayne, S., DeBartolo, E., Power, T. J., & Guevara, J. P. (2013). Parental preferences and goals regarding ADHD treatment. *Pediatrics, 132*(4), 692–702.

Flory, K., Molina, B. S., Pelham, W. E., Jr., Gnagy, E., & Smith, B. (2006). Childhood ADHD predicts risky sexual behavior in young adulthood. *Journal of Clinical Child and Adolescent Psychology, 35*(4), 571–577.

Flouri, E., Midouhas, E., Ruddy, A., & Moulton, V. (2017). The role of socio-economic disadvantage in the development of comorbid emotional and conduct problems in children with ADHD. *European Child and Adolescent Psychiatry, 26*(6), 723–732.

Frazier, T. W., Youngstrom, E. A., Glutting, J. J., & Watkins, M. W. (2007). ADHD and achievement: Meta-analysis of the child, adolescent, and adult literatures and a concomitant study with college students. *Journal of Learning Disabilities, 40*(1), 49–65.

Frazier, T. W., Youngstrom, E. A., & Hamilton, J. D. (2006). Evidence-based assessment of attention-deficit/hyperactivity disorder: Using multiple sources of information. *Journal of the American Academy of Child and Adolescent Psychiatry, 45*(5), 614–620.

Froehlich, T. E., Fogler, J., Barbaresi, W. J., Elsayed, N. A., Evans, S. W., & Chan, E. (2018). Using ADHD medications to treat coexisting ADHD and reading disorders: A systematic review. *Clinical Pharmacology and Therapeutics, 104*(4), 619–637.

Gathje, R. A., Lewandowski, L. J., & Gordon, M. (2008). The role of impairment in the diagnosis of ADHD. *Journal of Attention Disorders, 11*(5), 529–537.

Goodman, R. (2001). Psychometric properties of the strengths and difficulties questionnaire. *Journal of the American Academy of Child and Adolescent Psychiatry, 40*(11), 1337–1345.

Goodman, R., Ford, T., Simmons, H., Gatward, R., &

Meltzer, H. (2003). Using the Strengths and Difficulties Questionnaire (SDQ) to screen for child psychiatric disorders in a community sample. *International Review of Psychiatry, 15*(1–2), 166–172.

Gresham, F. M. (2005). Response to intervention: An alternative means of identifying students as emotionally disturbed. *Education and Treatment of Children, 28*(4), 328–344.

Haack, L. M., Gerdes, A. C., Schneider, B. W., & Hurtado, G. D. (2011). Advancing our knowledge of ADHD in Latino children: Psychometric and cultural properties of Spanish-versions of parental/family functioning measures. *Journal of Abnormal Child Psychology, 39*(1), 33–43.

Hawley, K. M., & Weisz, J. R. (2005). Youth versus parent working alliance in usual clinical care: Distinctive associations with retention, satisfaction, and treatment outcome. *Journal of Clinical Child and Adolescent Psychology, 34*(1), 117–128.

Healey, D. M., Miller, C. J., Castelli, K. L., Marks, D. J., & Halperin, J. M. (2008). The impact of impairment criteria on rates of ADHD diagnoses in preschoolers. *Journal of Abnormal Child Psychology, 36*(5), 771–778.

Hinshaw, S. P. (2018). ADHD: Controversy, developmental mechanisms, and multiple levels of analysis. *Annual Review of Clinical Psychology, 14,* 291–316.

Hinshaw, S. P., Owens, E. B., Wells, K. C., Kraemer, H. C., Abikoff, H. B., Arnold, L. E., . . . Hoza, B. (2000). Family processes and treatment outcome in the MTA: Negative/ineffective parenting practices in relation to multimodal treatment. *Journal of Abnormal Child Psychology, 28*(6), 555–568.

Hodges, K., Doucette-Gates, A., & Liao, Q. (1999). The relationship between the Child and Adolescent Functional Assessment Scale (CAFAS) and indicators of functioning. *Journal of Child and Family Studies, 8*(1), 109–122.

Hodges, K., & Wong, M. M. (1996). Psychometric characteristics of a multidimensional measure to assess impairment: The Child and Adolescent Functional Assessment Scale. *Journal of Child and Family Studies, 5*(4), 445–467.

Holdaway, A. S., Owens, J. S., Evans, S. W., Coles, E. K., Egan, T. E., & Himawan, L. K. (2018, October). *Incremental benefits of a daily report card over time for youth with or at-risk for ADHD: Replication and extension.* Poster presented at the annual conference on Advancing School Mental Health, Las Vegas, NV.

Hoza, B. (2007). Peer functioning in children with ADHD. *Journal of Pediatric Psychology, 32*(6), 655–663.

Hudziak, J. J., Copeland, W., Stanger, C., & Wadsworth, M. (2004). Screening for DSM-IV externalizing disorders with the Child Behavior Checklist: A receiver-operating characteristic analysis. *Journal of Child Psychology and Psychiatry, 45*(7), 1299–1307.

Hustus, C. L., Owens, J. S., Volpe, R. J., Briesch, A. M., & Daniels, B. J. (2018). Treatment sensitivity of direct behavior rating–multi-item scales in the context of a daily report card intervention. *Journal of Emotional and Behavioral Disorders.* [Epub ahead of print]

Indredavik, M. S., Vik, T., Heyerdahl, S., Kulseng, S., Fayers, P., & Brubakk, A. M. (2004). Psychiatric symptoms and disorders in adolescents with low birth weight. *Archives of Disease in Childhood Fetal and Neonatal Edition, 89*(5), F445–F450.

Jans, T., Jacob, C., Warnke, A., Zwanzger, U., Groß-Lesch, S., Matthies, S., . . . Retz, W. (2015). Does intensive multimodal treatment for maternal ADHD improve the efficacy of parent training for children with ADHD?: A randomized controlled multicenter trial. *Journal of Child Psychology and Psychiatry, 56*(12), 1298–1313.

Jarrett, M. A., Van Meter, A., Youngstrom, E. A., Hilton, D. C., & Ollendick, T. H. (2018). Evidence-based assessment of ADHD in youth using a receiver operating characteristic approach. *Journal of Clinical Child and Adolescent Psychology, 47*(5), 808–820.

Jenkins, M. M., Youngstrom, E. A., Washburn, J. J., & Youngstrom, J. K. (2011). Evidence-based strategies improve assessment of pediatric bipolar disorder by community practitioners. *Professional Psychology: Research and Practice, 42*(2), 121–129.

Jensen, P. S., Arnold, L. E., Swanson, J. M., Vitiello, B., Abikoff, H. B., Greenhill, L. L., . . . Conners, C. K. (2007). 3-year follow-up of the NIMH MTA study. *Journal of the American Academy of Child and Adolescent Psychiatry, 46*(8), 989–1002.

Jensen, P. S., Hinshaw, S. P., Kraemer, H. C., Lenora, N., Newcorn, J. H., Abikoff, H. B., . . . Elliott, G. R. (2001). ADHD comorbidity findings from the MTA study: Comparing comorbid subgroups. *Journal of the American Academy of Child and Adolescent Psychiatry, 40*(2), 147–158.

Jensen-Doss, A., Youngstrom, E. A., Youngstrom, J. K., Feeny, N. C., & Findling, R. L. (2014). Predictors and moderators of agreement between clinical and research diagnoses for children and adolescents. *Journal of Consulting and Clinical Psychology, 82*(6), 1151–1162.

Johnston, C., & Mash, E. J. (2001). Families of children with ADHD: Review and recommendations for future research. *Clinical Child and Family Psychology Review, 4*(3), 183–207.

Kamphaus, R. W., DiStefano, C., Dowdy, E., Eklund, K., & Dunn, A. R. (2010). Determining the presence of a problem: Comparing two approaches for detecting youth behavioral risk. *School Psychology Review, 39*(3), 395–408.

Kao, G. S., & Thomas, H. M. (2010). Test Review: C. Keith Conners Conners 3rd Edition. *Journal of Psychoeducational Assessment, 28*(6), 598–602.

Karpenko, V., Owens, J. S., Evangelista, N. M., & Dodds, C. (2009). Clinically significant symptom change in children with attention-deficit/hyperactivity disorder: Does it correspond with reliable improvement in functioning? *Journal of Clinical Psychology, 65*, 76–93.

Kent, K. M., Pelham, W. E., Molina, B. S., Sibley, M. H.,

Waschbusch, D. A., Yu, J., . . . Karch, K. M. (2011). The academic experience of male high school students with ADHD. *Journal of Abnormal Child Psychology, 39*(3), 451–462.

Klein, D. N., Dougherty, L. R., & Olino, T. M. (2005). Toward guidelines for evidence-based assessment of depression in children and adolescents. *Journal of Clinical Child and Adolescent Psychology, 34*(3), 412–432.

Klein, R. G., Mannuzza, S., Olazagasti, M. A. R., Roizen, E., Hutchison, J. A., Lashua, E. C., & Castellanos, F. X. (2012). Clinical and functional outcome of childhood ADHD 33 years later. *Archives of General Psychiatry, 69*, 1295–1303.

Kofler, M. J., Rapport, M. D., Sarver, D. E., Raiker, J. S., Orban, S. A., Friedman, L. M., & Kolomeyer, E. G. (2013). Reaction time variability in ADHD: A meta-analytic review of 319 studies. *Clinical Psychology Review, 33*(6), 795–811.

Kofler, M. J., Sarver, D. E., Harmon, S. L., Moltisanti, A., Aduen, P. A., Soto, E. F., & Ferretti, N. (2018). Working memory and organizational skills problems in ADHD. *Journal of Child Psychology and Psychiatry, 59*(1), 57–67.

Lahey, B. B., Pelham, W. E., Loney, J., Lee, S. S., & Willcutt, E. (2005). Instability of the DSM-IV subtypes of ADHD from preschool through elementary school. *Archives of General Psychiatry, 62*(8), 896–902.

Langberg, J. M., Dvorsky, M. R., & Evans, S. W. (2013). What specific facets of executive function are associated with academic functioning in youth with attention-deficit/hyperactivity disorder? *Journal of Abnormal Child Psychology, 41*(7), 1145–1159.

Langberg, J. M., Dvorsky, M. R., Molitor, S. J., Bourchtein, E., Eddy, L. D., Smith, Z. R., . . . Eadeh, H. M. (2018). Overcoming the research-to-practice gap: A randomized trial with two brief homework and organization interventions for students with ADHD as implemented by school mental health providers. *Journal of Consulting and Clinical Psychology, 86*(1), 39–55.

Langberg, J. M., Epstein, J. N., Girio-Herrera, E., Becker, S. P., Vaughn, A. J., & Altaye, M. (2011). Materials organization, planning, and homework completion in middle-school students with ADHD: Impact on academic performance. *School Mental Health, 3*(2), 93–101.

Langberg, J. M., Evans, S. W., Schultz, B. K., Becker, S. P., Altaye, M., & Girio-Herrera, E. (2016). Trajectories and predictors of response to the Challenging Horizons Program for adolescents with ADHD. *Behavior Therapy, 47*(3), 339–354.

Larsson, H., Chang, Z., D'Onofrio, B. M., & Lichtenstein, P. (2014). The heritability of clinically diagnosed ADHD across the lifespan. *Psychological Medicine, 44*(10), 2223–2229.

Larsson, H., Sariaslan, A., Långström, N., D'Onofrio, B., & Lichtenstein, P. (2014). Family income in early childhood and subsequent attention deficit/hyperactivity disorder: A quasi-experimental study. *Journal of Child Psychology and Psychiatry, 55*(5), 428–435.

Lawson, G. M., Nissley-Tsiopinis, J., Nahmias, A., McConaughy, S. H., & Eiraldi, R. (2017). Do parent and teacher report of ADHD symptoms in children differ by SES and racial status? *Journal of Psychopathology and Behavioral Assessment, 39*(3), 426–440.

Leth-Steensen, C., Elbaz, Z. K., & Douglas, V. I. (2000). Mean response times, variability, and skew in the responding of ADHD children: A response time distributional approach. *Acta Psychologica, 104*(2), 167–190.

Lindemann, C., Langner, I., Banaschewski, T., Garbe, E., & Mikolajczyk, R. T. (2017). The risk of hospitalizations with injury diagnoses in a matched cohort of children and adolescents with and without attention deficit/hyperactivity disorder in Germany: A database study. *Frontiers in Pediatrics, 5*, 220.

Loe, I. M., & Feldman, H. M. (2007). Academic and educational outcomes of children with ADHD. *Journal of Pediatric Psychology, 32*(6), 643–654.

Marshal, M. P., Molina, B. S., & Pelham, W. E., Jr. (2003). Childhood ADHD and adolescent substance use: An examination of deviant peer group affiliation as a risk factor. *Psychology of Addictive Behaviors, 17*(4), 293–302.

Martel, M. M., Schimmack, U., Nikolas, M., & Nigg, J. T. (2015). Integration of symptom ratings from multiple informants in ADHD diagnosis: A psychometric model with clinical utility. *Psychological Assessment, 27*(3), 1060–1071.

Massetti, G. M., Lahey, B. B., Pelham, W. E., Loney, J., Ehrhardt, A., Lee, S. S., & Kipp, H. (2008). Academic achievement over 8 years among children who met modified criteria for ADHD at 4–6 years of age. *Journal of Abnormal Child Psychology, 36*(3), 399–410.

Mathai, J., Anderson, P., & Bourne, A. (2004). Comparing psychiatric diagnoses generated by the Strengths and Difficulties Questionnaire with diagnoses made by clinicians. *Australian and New Zealand Journal of Psychiatry, 38*(8), 639–643.

McCart, M. R., & Sheidow, A. J. (2016). Evidence-based psychosocial treatments for adolescents with disruptive behavior. *Journal of Clinical Child and Adolescent Psychology, 45*(5), 529–563.

McConaughy, S. H., & Achenbach, T. M. (2009). *Manual for the ASEBA direct observation form.* Burlington: Research Center for Children, Youth, and Families, University of Vermont.

McConaughy, S. H., Harder, V. S., Antshel, K. M., Gordon, M., Eiraldi, R., & Dumenci, L. (2010). Incremental validity of test session and classroom observations in a multimethod assessment of ADHD. *Journal of Clinical Child and Adolescent Psychology, 39*(5), 650–666.

McConaughy, S. H., Volpe, R. J., Antshel, K. M., Gordon, M., & Eiraldi, R. B. (2011). Academic and social impairments of elementary school children with at-

tention deficit hyperactivity disorder. *School Psychology Review, 40*(2), 200–226.

Merikangas, K. R., He, J. P., Brody, D., Fisher, P. W., Bourdon, K., & Koretz, D. S. (2010). Prevalence and treatment of mental disorders among US children in the 2001–2004 NHANES. *Pediatrics, 125*(1), 75–81.

Miller, F. G., Crovello, N. J., & Chafouleas, S. M. (2017). Progress monitoring the effects of daily report cards across elementary and secondary settings using Direct Behavior Rating: Single Item Scales. *Assessment for Effective Intervention, 43*(1), 34–47.

Molina, B. S., Flory, K., Hinshaw, S. P., Greiner, A. R., Arnold, L. E., Swanson, J. M., . . . Pelham, W. E. (2007). Delinquent behavior and emerging substance use in the MTA at 36 months: Prevalence, course, and treatment effects. *Journal of the American Academy of Child and Adolescent Psychiatry, 46*, 1028–1040.

Molina, B. S., & Pelham, W. E., Jr. (2003). Childhood predictors of adolescent substance use in a longitudinal study of children with ADHD. *Journal of Abnormal Psychology, 112*(3), 497–507.

Molina, B. S. G., Pelham, W. E., Jr., Cheong, J., Marshal, M. P., Gnagy, E. M., & Curran, P. J. (2012). Childhood attention-deficit/hyperactivity disorder (ADHD) and growth in adolescent alcohol use: The roles of functional impairments, ADHD symptom persistence, and parental knowledge. *Journal of Abnormal Psychology, 121*(4), 922–935.

MTA Cooperative Group. (1999). A 14-month randomized clinical trial of treatment strategies for attention-deficit/hyperactivity disorder. *Archives General Psychiatry, 56*, 1073–1086.

Murray, D. W., Rabiner, D., Schulte, A., & Newitt, K. (2008). Feasibility and integrity of a parent–teacher consultation intervention for ADHD students. *Child and Youth Care Forum, 37*(3), 111–126.

Narad, M. E., Garner, A. A., Peugh, J. L., Tamm, L., Antonini, T. N., Kingery, K. M., . . . Epstein, J. N. (2015). Parent–teacher agreement on ADHD symptoms across development. *Psychological Assessment, 27*(1), 239–248.

Nigg, J. T., & Breslau, N. (2007). Prenatal smoking exposure, low birth weight, and disruptive behavior disorders. *Journal of the American Academy of Child and Adolescent Psychiatry, 46*(3), 362–369.

Norfolk, P. A., & Floyd, R. G. (2016). Detecting parental deception using a behavior rating scale during assessment of attention-deficit/hyperactivity disorder: An experimental study. *Psychology in the Schools, 53*(2), 158–172.

Nutt, D. J., Fone, K., Asherson, P., Bramble, D., Hill, P., Matthews, K., . . . Weiss, M. (2007). Evidence-based guidelines for management of ADHD in adolescents in transition to adult services and in adults: Recommendations from the British Association for Psychopharmacology. *Journal of Psychopharmacology, 21*(1), 10–41.

Owens, J. S., Evans, S. W., Coles, E. K., Himawan, L.

K., Holdaway, A. S., Mixon, C., & Egan, T. (2018). Consultation for classroom management and targeted interventions: Examining benchmarks for teacher practices that produce desired change in student behavior. *Journal of Emotional and Behavioral Disorders.* [Epub ahead of print]

Owens, J. S., Goldfine, M. E., Evangelista, N. M., Hoza, B., & Kaiser, N. M. (2007). A critical review of self-perceptions and the positive illusory bias in children with ADHD. *Clinical Child and Family Psychology Review, 10*(4), 335–351.

Owens, J. S., Holdaway, A. S., Serrano, V. J., Himawan, L. K., Watabe, Y., Storer, J., . . . Andrews, N. (2016). Screening for social, emotional, and behavioral problems at kindergarten entry: The utility of two teacher rating scales. *School Mental Health, 8*(3), 319–331.

Owens, J. S., Holdaway, A. S., Smith, J., Evans, S. W., Himawan, L. K., Coles, E. K., . . . Dawson, A. E. (2018). Rates of common classroom behavior management strategies and their associations with challenging student behavior in elementary school. *Journal of Emotional and Behavioral Disorders, 26*(3), 156–169.

Owens, J. S., Holdaway, A. S., Zoromski, A. K., Evans, S. W., Himawan, L. K., Girio-Herrera, E., & Murphy, C. E. (2012). Incremental benefits of a daily report card intervention over time for youth with disruptive behavior. *Behavior Therapy, 43*(4), 848–861.

Owens, J. S., Murphy, C. E., Richerson, L., Girio, E. L., & Himawan, L. K. (2008). Science to practice in underserved communities: The effectiveness of school mental health programming. *Journal of Clinical Child and Adolescent Psychology, 37,* 434–447.

Pelham, W. E., Jr. (2001). Are ADHD/I and ADHD/C the same or different?: Does it matter? *Clinical Psychology: Science and Practice, 8*(4), 502–506.

Pelham, W. E., Jr., Fabiano, G. A., & Massetti, G. M. (2005). Evidence-based assessment of ADHD in children and adolescents. *Journal of Clinical Child and Adolescent Psychology, 34*(3), 449–476.

Pelham, W. E., Jr., Fabiano, G. A., Waxmonsky, J. G., Greiner, A. R., Gnagy, E. M., Pelham, W. E., III, . . . Karch, K. (2016). Treatment sequencing for childhood ADHD: A multiple-randomization study of adaptive medication and behavioral interventions. *Journal of Clinical Child and Adolescent Psychology, 45*(4), 396–415.

Pelham, W. E., Jr., Gnagy, E. M., Greenslade, K. E., & Milich, R. (1992). Teacher ratings of DSM-III-R symptoms for the disruptive behavior disorders. *Journal of the American Academy of Child and Adolescent Psychiatry, 31*(2), 210–218.

Pelham, W. E., Greiner, A. R., & Gnagy, E. M. (2008). *Student behavior teacher response observation code manual.* Unpublished manual.

Pettersson, E., Sjölander, A., Almqvist, C., Anckarsäter, H., D'Oonofrio, B. M., Lichtenstein, P., & Larsson, H. (2015). Birth weight as an independent predictor of ADHD symptoms: A within-twin pair analysis. *Journal of Child Psychology and Psychiatry, 56*(4), 453–459.

Pliszka, S., & AACAP Work Group on Quality Issues. (2007). Practice parameter for the assessment and treatment of children and adolescents with ADHD. *Journal of the American Academy of Child and Adolescent Psychiatry, 46*(7), 894–921.

Polanczyk, G., de Lima, M. S., Horta, B. L., Biederman, J., & Rohde, L. A. (2007). The worldwide prevalence of ADHD: A systematic review and metaregression analysis. *American Journal of Psychiatry, 164,* 942–948.

Polanczyk, G. V., Willcutt, E. G., Salum, G. A., Kieling, C., & Rohde, L. A. (2014). ADHD prevalence estimates across three decades: An updated systematic review and meta-regression analysis. *International Journal of Epidemiology, 43*(2), 434–442.

Power, T. J., Watkins, M. W., Anastopoulos, A. D., Reid, R., Lambert, M. C., & DuPaul, G. J. (2017). Multi-informant assessment of ADHD symptom-related impairments among children and adolescents. *Journal of Clinical Child and Adolescent Psychology, 46*(5), 661–674.

Raiker, J. S., Freeman, A. J., Perez-Algorta, G., Frazier, T. W., Findling, R. L., & Youngstrom, E. A. (2017). Accuracy of Achenbach scales in the screening of ADHD in a community mental health clinic. *Journal of the American Academy of Child and Adolescent Psychiatry, 56*(5), 401–409.

Reinke, W. M., Lewis-Palmer, T., & Merrell, K. (2008). The classroom check-up: A classwide teacher consultation model for increasing praise and decreasing disruptive behavior. *School Psychology Review, 37*(3), 315–332.

Reynolds, C. R., Kamphaus, R. W., & Vannest, K. J. (2015). *BASC3: Behavior Assessment System for Children.* Bloomington, MN: Pearson.

Rieppi, R., Greenhill, L. L., Ford, R. E., Chuang, S., Wu, M., Davies, M., . . . Hechtman, L. (2002). Socioeconomic status as a moderator of ADHD treatment outcomes. *Journal of the American Academy of Child and Adolescent Psychiatry, 41*(3), 269–277.

Rimvall, M. K., Elberling, H., Rask, C. U., Helenius, D., Skovgaard, A. M., & Jeppesen, P. (2014). Predicting ADHD in school age when using the Strengths and Difficulties Questionnaire in preschool age: A longitudinal general population study, CCC2000. *European Child and Adolescent Psychiatry, 23*(11), 1051–1060.

Sanetti, L. M. H., Collier-Meek, M. A., Long, A. C., Kim, J., & Kratochwill, T. R. (2014). Using implementation planning to increase teachers' adherence and quality to behavior support plans. *Psychology in the Schools, 51*(8), 879–895.

Schatz, D. B., & Rostain, A. L. (2006). ADHD with comorbid anxiety: A review of the current literature. *Journal of Attention Disorders, 10*(2), 141–149.

Schmidt, M., Reh, V., Hirsch, O., Rief, W., & Christiansen, H. (2017). Assessment of ADHD symptoms and the issue of cultural variation: Are Conners 3 Rating Scales applicable to children and parents with migration background? *Journal of Attention Disorders*, *21*(7), 587–599.

Schuch, V., Utsumi, D. A., Costa, T. V. M. M., Kulikowski, L. D., & Muszkat, M. (2015). ADHD in the light of the epigenetic paradigm. *Frontiers in Psychiatry*, *6*, 126.

Shapiro, E. S. (2011). *Academic skills problems: Direct assessment and intervention.* New York: Guilford Press.

Shemmassian, S. K., & Lee, S. S. (2016). Predictive utility of four methods of incorporating parent and teacher symptom ratings of ADHD for longitudinal outcomes. *Journal of Clinical Child and Adolescent Psychology*, *45*(2), 176–187.

Sibley, M. H., Pelham, W. E., Jr., Molina, B. S., Gnagy, E. M., Waschbusch, D. A., Garefino, A. C., . . . Karch, K. M. (2012). Diagnosing ADHD in adolescence. *Journal of Consulting and Clinical Psychology*, *80*(1), 139–150.

Silverman, W. K., & Ollendick, T. H. (2005). Evidence-based assessment of anxiety and its disorders in children and adolescents. *Journal of Clinical Child and Adolescent Psychology*, *34*(3), 380–411.

Swanson, J. M. (1992). *School-based assessments and interventions for ADD students.* Independence, MO: K. C. Publishing.

Swanson, J., Baler, R. D., & Volkow, N. D. (2011). Understanding the effects of stimulant medications on cognition in individuals with ADHD: A decade of progress. *Neuropsychopharmacology*, *36*(1), 207–226.

Tannock, R., Frijters, J. C., Martinussen, R., White, E. J., Ickowicz, A., Benson, N. J., & Lovett, M. W. (2018). Combined modality intervention for ADHD with comorbid reading disorders: A proof of concept study. *Journal of Learning Disabilities*, *51*(1), 55–72.

Thompson, T., Lloyd, A., Joseph, A., & Weiss, M. (2017). The Weiss Functional Impairment Rating Scale—Parent Form for assessing ADHD: Evaluating diagnostic accuracy and determining optimal thresholds using ROC analysis. *Quality of Life Research*, *26*(7), 1879–1885.

Toplak, M. E., West, R. F., & Stanovich, K. E. (2013). Practitioner review: Do performance-based measures and ratings of executive function assess the same construct? *Journal of Child Psychology and Psychiatry*, *54*(2), 131–143.

Tracey, T. J., & Kokotovic, A. M. (1989). Factor structure of the working alliance inventory. *Psychological Assessment*, *1*(3), 207–210.

Tripp, G., Schaughency, E. A., & Clarke, B. (2006). Parent and teacher rating scales in the evaluation of ADHD: Contribution to diagnosis and differential diagnosis in clinically referred children. *Journal of Developmental and Behavioral Pediatrics*, *27*(3), 209–218.

Vaughn, A. J., & Hoza, B. (2013). The incremental utility of behavioral rating scales and a structured diagnostic interview in the assessment of ADHD. *Journal of Emotional and Behavioral Disorders*, *21*(4), 227–239.

Visser, S. N., Danielson, M. L., Bitsko, R. H., Holbrook, J. R., Kogan, M. D., Ghandour, R. M., . . . Blumberg, S. J. (2014). Trends in the parent-report of health care provider-diagnosed and medicated ADHD: United States, 2003–2011. *Journal of the American Academy of Child and Adolescent Psychiatry*, *53*(1), 34–46.

Volpe, R. J., DiPerna, J. C., Hintze, J. M., & Shapiro, E. S. (2005). Observing students in classroom settings: A review of seven coding schemes. *School Psychology Review*, *34*(4), 454–475.

Volpe, R. J., & Fabiano, G. A. (2013). *Daily behavior report cards: An evidence-based system of assessment and intervention.* New York: Guilford Press.

Vujnovic, R. K., Holdaway, A. S., Owens, J. S., & Fabiano, G. A. (2014). Response to intervention for youth with ADHD: Incorporating an evidence-based intervention within a multi-tiered framework. In M. D. Weist, N. A. Lever, C. P. Bradshaw, & J. S. Owens (Eds.), *Handbook of school mental health* (2nd ed., pp. 399–411). New York: Springer Science + Business Media.

Waschbusch, D. A., Cunningham, C. E., Pelham, W. E., Jr., Rimas, H. L., Greiner, A. R., Gnagy, E. M., . . . Scime, M. (2011). A discrete choice conjoint experiment to evaluate parent preferences for treatment of young, medication naive children with ADHD. *Journal of Clinical Child and Adolescent Psychology*, *40*(4), 546–561.

Waschbusch, D. A., & King, S. (2006). Should sex-specific norms be used to assess ADHD or oppositional defiant disorder? *Journal of Consulting and Clinical Psychology*, *74*(1), 179–185.

Watabe, Y., Owens, J. S., Serrano, V., & Evans, S. W. (2018). Is positive bias in children with ADHD a function of low competence or disorder status? *Journal of Emotional and Behavioral Disorders*, *26*(2), 79–92.

Weiss, M. D. (2000). *Weiss Functional Impairment Rating Scale (WFIRS) instructions.* Vancouver: University of British Columbia.

Weiss, M. D., McBride, N. M., Craig, S., & Jensen, P. (2018). Conceptual review of measuring functional impairment: Findings from the Weiss Functional Impairment Rating Scale. *Evidence-Based Mental Health*, *21*(4), 155–164.

Weyandt, L., DuPaul, G. J., Verdi, G., Rossi, J. S., Swentosky, A. J., Vilardo, B. S., . . . Carson, K. S. (2013). The performance of college students with and without ADHD: Neuropsychological, academic, and psychosocial functioning. *Journal of Psychopathology and Behavioral Assessment*, *35*(4), 421–435.

Wodka, E. L., Loftis, C., Mostofsky, S. H., Prahme, C., Larson, J. C. G., Denckla, M. B., & Mahone, E. M. (2008). Prediction of ADHD in boys and girls using the DKEFS. *Archives of Clinical Neuropsychology*, *23*(3), 283–293.

Wolraich, M. L., Bard, D. E., Neas, B., Doffing, M., & Beck, L. (2013). The psychometric properties of the Vanderbilt Attention-Deficit Hyperactivity Disorder Diagnostic Teacher Rating Scale in a community population. *Journal of Developmental and Behavioral Pediatrics*, *34*(2), 83–93.

Wolraich, M. L., Lambert, W., Doffing, M. A., Bickman, L., Simmons, T., & Worley, K. (2003). Psychometric properties of the Vanderbilt ADHD Diagnostic Parent Rating Scale in a referred population. *Journal of Pediatric Psychology*, *28*(8), 559–568.

Wymbs, F. A., Cunningham, C. E., Chen, Y., Rimas, H. M., Deal, K., Waschbusch, D. A., & Pelham, W. E., Jr. (2016). Examining parents' preferences for group and individual parent training for children with ADHD symptoms. *Journal of Clinical Child and Adolescent Psychology*, *45*(5), 614–631.

Xu, G., Strathearn, L., Liu, B., Yang, B., & Bao, W. (2018). Twenty-year trends in diagnosed ADHD among US children and adolescents, 1997–2016. *JAMA Network Open*, *1*(4), e181471.

Yeguez, C. E., & Sibley, M. H. (2016). Predictors of informant discrepancies between mother and middle school teacher ADHD ratings. *School Mental Health*, *8*(4), 452–460.

Youngstrom, E. A., Van Meter, A., Frazier, T. W., Hunsley, J., Prinstein, M. J., Ong, M. L., & Youngstrom, J. K. (2017). Evidence-based assessment as an integrative model for applying psychological science to guide the voyage of treatment. *Clinical Psychology: Science and Practice*, *24*(4), 331–363.

Zhou, X., Reynolds, C. R., Zhu, J., Kamphaus, R. W., & Zhang, O. (2018). Evidence-based assessment of ADHD diagnosis in children and adolescents. *Applied Neuropsychology: Child*, *7*(2), 150–156.

Zoromski, A. K., Evans, S. W., Gahagan, H. D., Serrano, V. J., & Holdaway, A. S. (2015). Ethical and contextual issues when collaborating with educators and school mental health professionals. In J. Sadler, C. W. van Staden & K. W. M. Fulford (Eds.), *Oxford handbook of psychiatric ethics* (Vol. 1, pp. 214–230). New York: Oxford University Press.

Zoromski, A. K., Owens, J. S., Evans, S. W., & Brady, C. E. (2015). Identifying ADHD symptoms most associated with impairment in early childhood, middle childhood, and adolescence using teacher report. *Journal of Abnormal Child Psychology*, *43*(7), 1243–1255.

CHAPTER 6

Conduct and Oppositional Disorders

Toni M. Walker, Paul J. Frick, and Robert J. McMahon

Preparation

Conduct problems (CPs) in youth have been a major focus of research and practice in child psychology for a number of reasons. First, serious and impairing CPs are relatively common in children and adolescents, with meta-analyses of epidemiological studies showing rates between 3 and 4% worldwide for children and adolescents ages 6–18 years old (Canino, Plancyz, Bauermeister, Rohde, & Frick, 2010). However, this prevalence rate varies across boys and girls, especially after early childhood; that is, boys and girls show very similar rates of CPs before age 5, but this changes to a 3:1 ratio, with boys showing higher prevalence of CPs in later childhood. In adolescence, girls tend to show increases in CPs, closing the gap to a 2:1 male:female ratio (Frick, 2016). Second, CPs are some of the most common reasons for referral to mental health services in children and adolescents

(Kazdin, Whitley, & Marciano, 2006; Kimonis, Frick, & McMahon, 2014), likely due to the fact that CPs can place a child at risk for peer rejection and school suspension or expulsion (Dodge & Pettit, 2003; Frick, 2012), as well as involvement with the legal system (Frick, Stickle, Dandreaux, Farrell, & Kimonis, 2005). As a result, the CPs prevalence rates in clinic-referred children range from 60 to 70% (Freeman, Youngstrom, Youngstrom, & Findling, 2016) and from 80 to 90% in incarcerated samples (Karnik et al., 2009; Livanou, Furtado, Winsper, Silvester, & Singh, 2019). Third, CPs may also have effects beyond childhood and adolescence, with research suggesting that CPs in childhood predict mental health (e.g., substance use), legal (e.g., being arrested), occupational (e.g., poor job performance), social (e.g., poor marital adjustment), and physical health (e.g., poor respiration) problems in adulthood (Odgers et al., 2007, 2008).

The substantial research on CPs has led to an increased understanding of the many processes that may be involved in the development of severe CPs (Frick & Viding 2009; Moffitt, 2017), with important implications for designing more effective interventions to prevent or treat these problems (Frick, 2012). Much less attention has been paid to the implications that this research may have for improving the methods for assessing children and adolescents with severe CPs (McMahon & Frick,

2005). However, if the field is to continue to improve its intervention outcomes by being guided by advances in research on the different causal processes that can lead to CPs, it is critical that assessment strategies used in practice also be informed by these research findings. Specifically, if treatment is to be tailored to the unique needs of children with CPs, clinical assessments must be able to measure these needs in psychometrically sound ways, and clinical assessors must be knowledgeable about the most current research in order to interpret the assessment results appropriately.

An exhaustive review of recent research on the many causal factors that can lead to CPs is not possible within the space limitations of this chapter. Therefore, we have chosen to focus on four findings from research that we think have the clearest, most direct, and most important implications for the evidence-based assessment of children with CPs. First, we focus on the well-documented *heterogeneity* in the types and severity of CPs that may be displayed by a child or adolescent. Second, we review research showing that severe CPs can lead to a host of *comorbid problems* in adjustment that may be important targets for treatment. Third, we review research on the *multiple risk factors*, both within the child and within his or her psychosocial context, that are associated with CPs. Fourth, we discuss research supporting the presence of several *causal pathways* that can lead a child to display CPs, each involving somewhat distinct risk factors and developmental processes, and each requiring a somewhat different approach to treatment. After reviewing this research, we discuss the implications of these findings for guiding clinical assessments for diagnosis (prediction), treatment planning (prescription), and outcome monitoring (process). Finally, we identify key methods and measures that we believe have the potential for contributing to the evidence-based assessment of CPs in each of these areas.

Heterogeneity in the Types and Severity of CPs

CPs constitute a broad spectrum of "acting-out" behaviors, ranging from relatively minor oppositional behaviors such as yelling, temper tantrums, and defiance to authority, to more serious forms of antisocial behavior that involve the violation of the rights of others (e.g., aggression, physical destructiveness, and stealing) or the violation of major societal norms (e.g., running away from home, truancy). A number of different ways have been proposed for differentiating within this broad

category of behavior. For example, based on a meta-analysis of over 60 published factor analyses, Frick and colleagues (1993) found that CPs can be described by two bipolar dimensions. The first is an overt–covert dimension. The overt pole includes directly confrontational behaviors such as oppositional defiant behaviors and aggression. In contrast, the covert pole includes behaviors that are nonconfrontational in nature, such as stealing and lying. The second dimension divides the overt behaviors into those that were overt–destructive (aggression) and those that are overt–nondestructive (oppositional), and it divides the covert behaviors into those that are covert–destructive (property violations) and those that are covert–nondestructive (status offenses involving behaviors that are illegal because of the child's or adolescent's age, such as truancy and running away from home).

Another method for differentiating the different types of CPs is to distinguish between those children who show primarily aggressive behaviors, defined as behaviors that directly harm another person, and those who show primarily nonaggressive or rule-breaking behavior (Burt, 2012). This method has some appeal for clinical assessments because the presence of aggression by definition identifies children in need of treatment because of the harm their behavior causes to others. However, these two forms of CPs tend to be fairly highly correlated. For example, in a comprehensive review, Burt reported that the average correlation between aggressive and nonaggressive CPs is .43 in nonreferred samples and .51 in clinical samples. Furthermore, when examining the same list of CPs across multiple large samples ($n = 27,861$), correlations between the two types of CPs were .68 for boys and .63 for girls (Burt et al., 2015).

One of the most common ways to differentiate between types of CPs is the distinction used by the fifth edition of the *Diagnostic and Statistical Manual of Mental Disorders* (DSM-5; American Psychiatric Association, 2013). In its broad category of Disruptive, Impulse Control, and Conduct Disorders, it distinguishes between oppositional defiant disorder (ODD) and conduct disorder (CD). ODD is defined as a pattern of vindictive (e.g., deliberately doing things that annoy other people, blaming others for own mistakes), argumentative/defiant (e.g., defying or not complying with grown-ups' rules or requests), and angry/irritable (e.g., losing one's temper) behaviors. To distinguish these CPs from behaviors shown to some degree in typically developing children (Frick &

Nigg, 2012), a child must have shown at least four of the behaviors over the preceding 6 months with a degree of persistence and frequency that exceeds what is normative for his or her age, sex, and culture. Also, the behavior must lead to substantial impairment for the child at home, at school, or with peers. In contrast, CD consists of more severe antisocial and aggressive behavior that involves serious violations of others' rights or deviations from major age-appropriate norms. The child must show at least three behaviors from four categories that largely fit within the covert–overt and destructive–nondestructive dimensions summarized earlier: aggressiveness to people and animals (e.g., bullying, fighting); property destruction (e.g., firesetting, other destruction of property); deceptiveness or theft (e.g., breaking and entering, stealing without confronting victim); and serious rule violations (e.g., running away from home, being truant from school before age 13).

Within the two categories of ODD and CD, DSM-5 includes specifiers to designate different levels of severity. Within the ODD category, children can range in severity from "mild" if the CPs is confined to one setting (e.g., only at home), to "moderate" if symptoms are present in two settings, and "severe" if the CPs are present in three or more settings (American Psychiatric Association, 2013). For CD, severity is determined by the number of symptoms present in excess of those required to meet criteria for the diagnosis (i.e., three) and the level of harm to others associated with the CPs. Specifically, a child is considered to have "mild" CD if he or she shows few, if any, additional symptoms beyond those required for the diagnosis and the CPs cause relatively minor harm to others. A "severe" rating is given if the child shows many symptoms in excess of those required for diagnosis and the CPs cause considerable harm to others, such as in the cases of rape or physical cruelty. There is also a "moderate" level of severity, which is a level of symptom severity and degree of harm in between mild and severe.

CPs and Multiple Problems in Adjustment

In addition to documenting the wide variety of behaviors displayed by children with CPs, another important research finding is that youth with CPs also are at increased risk for manifesting a variety of other adjustment problems. Attention-deficit/hyperactivity disorder (ADHD), which is defined as developmentally non-normative levels of inattention–disorganization and/or impulsiv-ity–hyperactivity, is the most common comorbid condition found in children with CPs. ADHD symptoms most often precede the development of CPs and signal the presence of a more severe and chronic form of CPs (see Waschbusch, 2002). In a meta-analytic study, Waschbusch reported that 36% of boys and 57% of girls with CPs had comorbid ADHD. The overlap appears to be even higher for those whose CPs start early in childhood compared to those in whom they start later in development (Frick & Viding, 2009).

Internalizing disorders, such as depression and anxiety, also co-occur with CPs at rates higher than expected by chance (Cunningham & Ollendick, 2010; Fanti & Henrich, 2010; Nock, Kazdin, Hiripi, & Kessler, 2006; Zoccolillo, 1992). However, unlike ADHD, CPs most often precede the onset of depressive and anxiety symptoms (Burke, Loeber, Lahey, & Rathouz, 2005; Hipwell et al., 2011; Loeber & Burke, 2011; Nock et al., 2006). This temporal pattern has led some to suggest that anxiety and depression may often develop as a consequence of the problems a child with CPs experiences at home, at school, and with peers (Frick, 2012). However, it also possible that the co-occurrence of internalizing disorders and CPs reflect common underlying problems in emotional regulation (Burke, Hipwell, & Loeber, 2010; Fergusson, Lynskey, & Horwood, 1996; Wolff & Ollendick, 2006). This is supported by the finding that internalizing problems are most common in children who present with the angry/irritable mood symptoms of ODD (Burke et al., 2010; Rowe, Costello, Arnold, Copeland, & Maughan, 2010; Stringaris & Goodman, 2009).

Importantly, these problems regulating mood in children with ODD tend to be chronic, which differentiates children with CPs from those who show episodic abnormal mood states associated with bipolar or major depressive disorders (Carlson, 2016). However, due to concerns that many children and adolescents with severe and chronic irritable mood were being diagnosed with a bipolar mood disorder and placed on medications with potentially serious side effects, DSM-5 added the diagnosis of disruptive mood dysregulation disorder (DMDD) to the chapter that describes depressive disorders (American Psychiatric Association, 2013). DMDD is defined by chronic, severe, persistent irritability characterized by frequent temper outbursts in persons whose mood is chronically angry and irritable between these outbursts (American Psychiatric Association, 2013). As would be expected given the overlap between the symptoms of this new disorder and the angry/irritable symptoms included in the ODD criteria, almost all persons diagnosed with DMDD also meet criteria for ODD (Freeman et al., 2016; Mayes, Waxmonsky, Calhoun, & Bixler, 2016). According to the DSM-5, these children would be diagnosed with DMDD only and not ODD. However, in the 11th edition of the *International Classification of Diseases*, published by the World Health Organization (2018), these children are classified as showing a subtype of ODD. Specifically, children can be diagnosed with ODD with persistent anger/irritability if:

- The persistent angry or irritable mood is independent of any apparent provocation.
- It is often accompanied by regularly occurring severe temper outbursts that are grossly out of proportion in intensity or duration to the provocation.
- The chronic irritability and anger are characteristic of the individual's functioning nearly every day.
- The chronic irritability and anger are observable across multiple settings or domains of functioning (e.g., home, school, social relationships).
- The chronic irritability and anger are not limited to occasional episodes or discrete periods (e.g., irritable mood in the context of manic or depressive episodes).

In addition to the overlap with mood problems, both longitudinal and cross-sectional studies have documented that CPs constitute a significant risk factor for substance use (e.g., Stone, Becker, Huber, & Catalano, 2012). The comorbidity between CPs and substance abuse is important because when youth with CPs also abuse substances, they tend to show an early onset of substance use and are more likely to abuse multiple substances (Lynskey & Fergusson, 1995). Although most of the research on the association between CPs and substance abuse prior to adulthood has been conducted with adolescents, the association between CPs and substance use may begin much earlier in development (Van Kammen, Loeber, & Stouthamer-Loeber, 1991).

CPs can also lead to a number of school-related problems. Approximately 20–25% of youth with CPs underachieve in school relative to a level predicted by their age and intellectual abilities (Frick et al., 1991). In addition, children with CPs are more likely to receive school discipline referrals beginning as early as the first grade (Pas, Bradashaw, & Mitchell, 2011; Rusby, Taylor, & Foster,

2007). This can perpetuate an escalating cycle in which discipline referrals lead to chronic school suspensions (Tobin & Sugai, 1999) and eventually lead to early school dropout, which can have longlasting consequences for the person's adjustment into adulthood (Conduct Problems Prevention Research Group, 2013; Odgers et al., 2007).

Multiple Risks Associated with CPs

Most researchers agree that CPs are the result of a complex interaction of multiple causal factors (Frick & Viding, 2009; Moffitt, 2017). Prior research has identified a large number of factors that may a play a role in development and/or maintenance of CPs (for reviews, see Dodge & Pettit, 2003; Frick & Viding, 2009; Kimonis, Frick, et al., 2014; Moffitt, 2017). They include dispositional risk factors, such as neurochemical (e.g., low serotonin) and autonomic (e.g., low resting heart rate) irregularities; neurocognitive deficits (e.g., deficits in executive functioning); deficits in social information processing (e.g., a hostile attributional bias); temperamental vulnerabilities (e.g., poor emotional regulation); and personality predispositions (e.g., impulsivity). In addition, they include risk factors in the child's prenatal environment (e.g., exposure to toxins); early child care (e.g., poor quality child care); and family (e.g., harsh and/or ineffective discipline), peer (e.g., association with deviant peers), and neighborhood (e.g., high levels of exposure to violence) environments.

Multiple Developmental Pathways to CPs

While research has been very successful in documenting the numerous risk factors that are associated with CPs, there has been extensive debate over the best way to integrate these factors into comprehensive causal models to explain the development of CPs. However, there are a few points of agreement (Frick, 2012, 2016).

1. To adequately explain the development of CP behavior, causal models must consider the potential role of multiple risk factors and not focus on any single causal variable.
2. Causal models must consider the possibility that subgroups of antisocial youth may have distinct causal mechanisms underlying their CP behaviors.
3. Causal models need to integrate research on the development of CP behavior with research on typically developing youth.

To illustrate this third point, research has suggested that the ability to adequately regulate emotions and behavior, and to feel empathy and guilt toward others, seems to play an important role in the development of CPs (Frick & Viding, 2009). As a result, understanding the processes involved in the typical development of these abilities is critical for understanding how they may go awry in some children and place them at risk for acting in an aggressive or antisocial manner.

Thus, current conceptualizations of CPs recognize that there are likely multiple causal pathways leading to these behavior problems, with each pathway involving multiple interacting risk factors. Furthermore, these risk factors disrupt critical developmental processes that make a child more likely to act in an antisocial and aggressive manner. Consideration of these pathways could be quite critical to clinical assessments because they might explain some of the variations in the type and severity of CPs, the co-occurring problems, and the multiple risk factors displayed by children with CPs. However, most importantly, these pathways could be critical for guiding individualized approaches to treating CPs (Frick, 2012).

The most widely accepted model for delineating distinct pathways in the development of CPs distinguishes between childhood-onset and adolescent-onset subtypes of CPs (see Fairchild, van Goozen, Calder, & Goodyer, 2013). DSM-5 (American Psychiatric Association, 2013) makes the distinction between youth who begin showing severe CP behaviors before age 10 (i.e., childhood onset) and those who do not show severe CPs before age 10 (i.e., adolescent onset). This distinction is supported by a substantial amount of research documenting important differences between these two groups of youth with CPs (for reviews, see Frick & Viding, 2009; Moffitt, 2017). Specifically, youth in the childhood-onset group show more severe CPs in childhood and adolescence, and are more likely to continue to show antisocial and criminal behavior into adulthood (Moffitt & Caspi, 2001; Odgers et al., 2007). More relevant to causal theory, most of the dispositional (e.g., temperamental risk, low intelligence) and contextual (e.g., family dysfunction) correlates that have been associated with CPs are more strongly associated with the childhood-onset subtype. This led Moffit (2017) to propose that youth in the childhood-onset group develop CPs through a transactional process involving a difficult and vulnerable child (e.g., impulsive, verbal deficits, difficult temperament) who experiences an inadequate rearing environment (e.g., poor parent supervision, poor quality schools). This dysfunctional transactional process disrupts the child's socialization, leading to poor social relations with persons both inside (i.e., parents and siblings) and outside (i.e., peers and teachers) the family, which further disrupts the child's socialization. These disruptions lead to enduring vulnerabilities that can negatively affect the child's psychosocial adjustment across multiple developmental stages. In contrast, Moffitt views youth on the adolescent-onset pathway as showing an exaggeration of the normative developmental process of identity formation that takes place in adolescence. Engagement in antisocial and delinquent behaviors is conceptualized as a misguided attempt to obtain a subjective sense of maturity and adult status in a way that is maladaptive (e.g., breaking societal norms) but encouraged by an antisocial peer group. Given that their behavior is viewed as an exaggeration of a process specific to adolescent development and not due to enduring vulnerabilities, this form of CPs is less likely to persist beyond adolescence. However, youth on the adolescent-onset pathway may still have impairments that persist into adulthood due to the consequences of their CPs (e.g., a criminal record, dropping out of school, substance abuse) (Moffitt, 2017).

More recently, there has been increasing recognition of another distinction that may be important for designating important developmental pathways to CPs. As noted earlier, childhood-onset CP is considered to be indicative of an enduring vulnerability that results from an interaction between dispositional traits in the child and problems in his or her rearing environment. However, there may be several different types of vulnerabilities within the childhood-onset group that reflect different developmental consequences of this interaction. In DSM-5, another specifier for CD was added that is labeled "with limited prosocial emotions" and is applied to persons who meet the criteria for CD and show a significant level of callous–unemotional (CU) traits in multiple relationships and settings (American Psychiatric Association, 2013). According to DSM-5, significant levels of CU traits are defined as two or more of the following characteristics that are shown by the child persistently (12 months or longer) and in multiple relationships or settings:

- Lack of remorse or guilt
- Callous lack of empathy

- Lack of concern about performance in important activities
- Shallow or deficient affect

Although only a minority of children and adolescents with CD show elevated rates of CU traits (Kahn, Frick, Youngstrom, Findling, & Youngstrom, 2012; Pardini, Stepp, Hipwell, Stouthamer-Loeber, & Loeber, 2012), research suggests that separating this group from other youth with CD is critical for both etiological theories and for designing individualized treatment in clinical practice. Specifically, Frick, Ray, Thornton, and Kahn (2014) reviewed over 200 published studies and found relatively consistent support for the potential role of CU traits in designating an important subgroup of youth who show serious antisocial behavior that is more stable, aggressive, and less responsive to typical treatments. Furthermore, they also reviewed research suggesting that these traits classify a group of youth with CPs who show very different genetic, cognitive, emotional, and social characteristics. These findings seem to suggest that the causes of CPs are different in those with and without CU traits. Frick and colleagues proposed that children with serious CPs and elevated CU traits, but not other children with serious CPs, have a temperament (i.e., fearless, insensitive to punishment, low responsiveness to cues of distress in others) that can interfere with the normal development of conscience and place the child at risk for a particularly severe and aggressive pattern of antisocial behavior. In contrast, children and adolescents with childhood-onset antisocial behavior with normative levels of CU traits do not typically show problems in empathy and guilt. In fact, they appear to be highly reactive to emotional cues in others and are highly distressed by the effects of their behavior on others (Frick & Viding, 2009). Thus, the CP behavior in this group does not seem to be easily explained by deficits in conscience development. Furthermore, they display higher levels of emotional reactivity to provocation from others (Frick & Morris, 2004). The CPs in this group are strongly associated with hostile/coercive parenting (Frick et al., 2014). As a result, children in this group seem to show a temperament characterized by strong emotional reactivity and inadequate socializing experiences that combine to make it difficult for them to develop the skills needed to adequately regulate their emotional reactivity (Frick & Morris, 2004). These emotional regulation problems can result in these children committing impulsive and unplanned aggressive and antisocial acts for which they may feel remorseful afterward but still have difficulty controlling in the future.

Prediction

Again, this review is not meant to be an exhaustive review of the phenomenology, course, and causes of CPs (see Frick, 2016). Instead, we have chosen to focus on a few key areas of research that we judge to be most critical for conducting an evidence-based assessment of children and adolescents with CPs. In this section, we discuss how these research findings can guide the multiple purposes for clinical assessments of children and adolescents with CPs. In Table 6.1, we provide a summary of the three primary purposes for which evidence-based assessments of CPs are typically conducted, and a summary of how the research reviewed earlier should guide the assessment in each area and provide examples of measures that can be used for each purpose. This list is not meant to be an exhaustive summary of all measures that may be used in the assessment of CPs; instead, it is designed to give specific examples of a "starter kit" that can be used by clinicians for the various assessment purposes. Furthermore, in Table 6.1 we differentiate between more time-efficient measures that can be used for screening or intake purposes in each area, as well more intensive measures that can be used for more comprehensive clinical assessments.

The first section in Table 6.1 focuses on prediction. This part of the assessment may also be described as the process of making a diagnosis. In the context of this chapter, "making a diagnosis" of a child with CPs is not synonymous with determining whether he or she meets DSM-5 criteria for a CP-related diagnosis, such as ODD or CD. Instead, we use a broader definition of "diagnosis" to refer to the determination of whether the child or adolescent is showing CPs to an extent that may warrant treatment. Several considerations are important for making this determination.

First, it is important to rule out the possibility of an inappropriate referral due to unrealistic parental or teacher expectations; that is, as noted previously, research has indicated that many CPs, especially those associated with ODD, are displayed to some degree in normally developing children (Frick & Nigg, 2012). Therefore, it is necessary to determine whether the youth is exhibiting CPs

TABLE 6.1. An Evidence-Based Assessment of Conduct Problems

Goals	Methods	Research basis
• Prediction: Does the child need treatment? • Assess a wide range of CPs. • Assess the amount of harm a child's behavior is causing to other individuals. • Assess the level of impairment that the child's behavior is causing in multiple situations and settings (e.g., home, school, work, and interpersonal relationships).	• Norm-referenced behavior rating scales from multiple informants who interact with the child in different settings • (e.g., ASEBA, BASC-3, ECBI, SESBI-R)[a] • Unstructured clinical interviews with the child and other adults who see the child in different settings[a] • Behavioral observations of the child interacting with adults and peers (e.g., BASC-SOS, BCS, or DPICS)[b] • Structured or semistructured diagnostic interviews with the child and other adults who see the child in different settings (e.g., DISC or K-SADS)[b]	• Children with CPs can vary greatly in the types and severity of their behaviors, especially in the amount of harm they cause others and in the degree of impairment that they cause the child.
• Prescription: What should be the most important targets of treatment? • Screen broadly for a wide range of common problems that often occur with CPs, including psychiatric disorders, self-harm, legal problems, education difficulties, and social problems. • Screen for a wide range of individual risk factors (see Table 6.2). • Screen for a wide range of contextual risk factors that could contribute to the child's CPs (see Table 6.2). • Obtain history of when the child's CPs first emerged (e.g., before or after age 10 years). • Assess for the presence of CU traits	• Norm-referenced behavior rating scales that cover a broad range of potential problems in adjustment (e.g., ASEBA or BASC-3)[a] • Rating scales assessing parenting and family conflict (e.g., APQ or BASC-3)[a] • Behavior rating scales assessing CU traits from child, parents, and other informants (e.g., CPTI or ICU)[a] • Unstructured clinical interviews with the child and other adults who know the child well and provide a history of the child's CPs[a] • Structured or semistructured diagnostic interviews with the child and other adults who know the child well (e.g., DISC or K-SADS)[b] • Observations of parent–child interactions (e.g., DPICS or BCS)[b] • Review of school records[b] • Standardized measure of academic achievement (e.g., WJ-IV-TA)[b]	• Children with CPs often have multiple comorbid disorders and/or problems in adjustment. • CPs often result from multiple risk factors both within the child and their context. • There can be multiple causal pathways to CPs, each involving somewhat distinct risk factors that could necessitate an individualized approach to treatment.
• Process: Is treatment leading to meaningful changes in the child's behavior and adjustment? • Monitor changes in the child's behavior over the course of treatment. • Monitor changes in parenting strategies over the course of treatment. • Assess parent and child satisfaction with the progress of treatment.	• Behavior rating scales that have proven sensitive to changes in behavior over time (ECBI, ICU)[a] • Behavior rating scales that assess parenting and that have proven sensitive to treatment (APQ)[a] • Use of consumer satisfaction surveys that assess satisfaction with treatment (PCSQ, TAI)[a] • Unstructured interviews to gather information on parent and child perceptions of treatment progress[a] • Behavioral observations of CPs and parenting behaviors (BCS or DPICS)[b]	• Research suggests that many interventions for CPs are ineffective and sometimes even harmful to the child.

Note. APQ, Alabama Parenting Questionnaire (*https://sites01.lsu.edu/faculty/pfricklab/apq*); ASEBA, Achenbach System of Empirically Based Assessment (*www.aseba.org*); BASC-3, Behavioral Assessment System for Children, Third Edition (*www.pearsonclinical.com*); BASC-3 SOS, BASC-3 Student Observation System (*www.pearsonclinical.com*); Behavioral Coding System (BCS; *www.guilford.com/books/helping-the-noncompliant-child/mcmahon-forehand/9781593852412*); CPs, conduct problems; CPTI, Child Problematic Traits Inventory (*www.oru.se/english/research/research-environments/hs/caps/cpti*); DISC, Diagnostic Interview Schedule for Children (*www.cdc.gov/nchs/data/nhanes/limited_access/interviewer_manual.pdf*); DPICS, Dyadic Parent–Child Coding System (*www.pcit.org/measures.html*); ECBI, Eyberg Child Behavior Inventory (*www.parinc.com*); ICU, Inventory of Callous–Unemotional Traits (*https://sites01.lsu.edu/faculty/pfricklab/icu*); K-SADS, Kiddie Schedule for Affective Disorders and Schizophrenia (*http://pediatricbipolar.pitt.edu/resources/instruments*); PCSQ, Parent's Consumer Satisfaction Questionnaire (*www.guilford.com/books/helping-the-noncompliant-child/mcmahon-forehand/9781593852412*); SESBI-R, Sutter–Eyberg Student Behavior Inventory—Revised (www.parinc.com); SDQ, Strengths and Difficulties Questionnaire (*www.sdqinfo.com*); TAI, Therapy Attitude Inventory (*www.pcit.org/measures.html*); WASI, Wechsler Abbreviated Scale of Intelligence (*www.pearsonclinical.com*); WISC-V, Wechsler Intelligence Scale for Children—Fifth Edition (*www.pearsonclinical.com*); WJ-IV-TA, Woodcock–Johnson IV Tests of Achievement (*www.hmhco.com*).

[a]Time-efficient screening measures

[b]Measures for more comprehensive clinical assessments, as indicated by screening.

levels that are atypical in type and frequency for his or her age. Second, it is important to assess the degree of impairment that is associated with the youth's CPs. As noted earlier, youth can vary greatly in the severity of their CPs, ranging from mild oppositional and defiant behaviors only at home to severe aggression that results in substantial harm to others in the community. Assessing the severity of the youth's behavior can determine not only whether the youth needs treatment but also the treatment intensity and the most appropriate treatment setting. In the following sections, we review methods that can be used for these assessment goals.

Behavior Rating Scales

Behavior rating scales are a core part of a battery for assessing children and adolescents with CPs, not just for making a diagnosis for all three assessment aims. However, a variety of rating scales are available and have useful specific characteristics for meeting diagnostic goals (Frick, Barry, & Kamphaus, 2010). Of primary importance, most behavior rating scales assess a range of CPs and can be completed by adults who observe the child or adolescent in important psychosocial contexts (i.e., parents and teachers) and by the youth him- or herself. Having multiple informants who see the child in different settings can provide important information on the pervasiveness of the youth's CPs, as well as help to detect potential biases in the report of any single informant. Although most behavior rating scales have similar content across different raters, such as the Achenbach System of Empirically Based Assessment (ASEBA; Achenbach & Rescorla, 2000, 2001) or Conners Rating Scales, Third Edition (CRS-3; Conners, 2008), a few scales assess for very different content across raters. For example, the Behavior Assessment System for Children, Third Edition (BASC-3; Reynolds & Kamphaus, 2015) has similar content for the teacher- and parent-report versions. However, the content of the self-report version is quite different. Specifically, the youth does not rate his or her own level of CPs, but the self-report provides more extended coverage of the youth's attitudes (e.g., toward parents and teachers), self-concept (e.g., self-esteem and sense of inadequacy), and social relationships.

Most of these measures are broad rating scales that cover many dimensions of child and adolescent adjustment, not just CPs. This breadth of coverage makes them useful for the second goal of clinical assessments, prescription, which is described below. However, this breadth of coverage means that these broad rating scales often only include a limited number of items regarding CPs behaviors. There are, however, several behavior rating scales that focus solely on CPs and provide more comprehensive coverage of various types of CPs. Examples of scales that have both parent- and teacher-report versions and focus specifically on CPs are the Eyberg Child Behavior Inventory (ECBI) and the Sutter–Eyberg Student Behavior Inventory—Revised (SESBI-R; Eyberg & Pincus, 1999). The ECBI is completed by parents and is intended for use with children ages 2–16. The 36 items describe specific CPs behaviors (primarily overt) and are scored on both a frequency-of-occurrence (Intensity) scale and a yes–no problem identification (Problem) scale. This latter focus on whether the behavior is a problem or not is particularly helpful for prediction because it directly assesses the level of impairment caused by the behavior. The SESBI is identical in format to the ECBI, with 36 items that are rated on both Intensity and Problem scales, although items on the ECBI that were not relevant to the school setting were replaced by 13 different items to measure behaviors in each setting independently (Caselman & Self, 2008; Funderburk, Eyberg, Rich, & Behar, 2003).

Rating scales provide some of the best norm-referenced data on youth behavior, which, again, is particularly relevant for prediction. Such information is critical for determining whether the youth's CPs are significantly greater relative to those of other youth of the same age and sex. For example, the standardization sample for the ASEBA (Achenbach & Rescorla, 2000, 2001) is representative of the 48 contiguous United States for socioeconomic status, sex, ethnicity, region, and urban–suburban–rural residence.

Interviews

In addition to determining whether a youth's behaviors are more severe than what is expected for his or her age, assessment of the level of impairment that the behavior problems cause is an important consideration for determining whether the child's CPs warrant a diagnosis; that is, it is important to determine the degree to which the child's behavior is causing problems for him or her, either by causing functional impairment (e.g., problems performing academically due to numerous detentions or suspensions; being rejected from peer groups due to problematic behavior) or emotional distress for the child, and the degree to which the behavior is causing problems for those around the child (e.g., physical harm to others; harm to others' property; distress in others, such as parents and teachers).

This information is most often obtained through interviews. Interviews can vary depending on their level of structure, ranging from unstructured clinical interviews that allow the clinician to tailor questions to the individual child and family to highly structured interviews, in which the questions are standardized and asked in the same way for all children and families. Semistructured interviews provide an intermediate level of structure, in which the clinician is provided with some key areas to assess but is also given flexibility in how the information is obtained (e.g., what questions are asked).

Unstructured and semistructured interviews with the parent provide a very time-efficient and individualized method for assessing the type, severity, and impairment associated with the youth's CPs, including how long the youth has displayed the problems and whether they have changed in frequency and severity over time. When the youth's CPs are being displayed at school, interviews with the youth's teachers are also helpful. Such interviews can help to determine the severity of the youth's CPs because children who show CPs outside the home often show a more severe and stable pattern relative to those whose behavior problems are largely confined to the home (Frick & Nigg, 2012). Also, interviews with the child's teachers can help in assessing contextual factors that can influence the youth's CPs, such as classroom rules of conduct, teacher expectations, and the behavior of other children in the classroom.

Because unstructured and semistructured interviews allow for highly individualized information about a specific child or adolescent, highly trained clinicians are required to conduct the interviews. Also, it is often difficult to obtain reliable information in these formats. As a result, *structured interview schedules* were developed to improve the reliability of the information obtained during a clinical interview by providing very clear and detailed questions that are to be asked in the interview. Two structured diagnostic interviews that are frequently used in the assessment of youth with CPs are the Diagnostic Interview Schedule for Children (DISC-IV; Shaffer, Fisher, Lucas, Dulcan, & Schwab-Stone, 2000) and the Diagnostic Interview for Children and Adolescents (DICA; Reich, 2000). These structured interviews provide a format for obtaining parent and youth reports on the symptoms that comprise the criteria for ODD and CD according to DSM-IV-TR (American Psychiatric Association, 2000). Thus, they provide the most direct method for assessing DSM criteria for these diagnoses. Both the DISC-IV and DICA are currently being updated to reflect the changes in criteria for the disorders included in the DSM-5 (American Psychiatric Association, 2013).

Structured interviews provide standardized question-and-answer formats that result in much higher reliability compared to unstructured clinical interviews. For example, a stem question is asked (e.g., "Does your child get into fights?"), and follow-up questions are only asked if the stem question is answered affirmatively (e.g., "Is this only with his or her brothers and sisters?" and "Does he or she usually start these fights?"). Most structured interviews assess many other types of problems in adjustment beyond CPs, such as ADHD, depressive disorders, and anxiety disorders. Thus, as we discuss below, they are often helpful for determining important targets for treatment. However, this can make structured interviews quite lengthy if a child has a large number of problems. As a result, administration time can range widely, from 45 minutes for children and adolescents with few problems to over 2 hours for youth with many adjustment problems (Frick et al., 2010). Thus, as noted in Table 6.1, such interviews typically are used only for more extended clinical assessments.

Thus, structured interviews provide several pieces of important information for determining whether a youth with CPs needs treatment; furthermore, they do so in a reliable manner. However, as noted earlier, structured interviews are time consuming. Also, they typically do not provide normative information as to whether the child is showing a level of CPs that is more severe than what is normative for a child's age. In addition, most structured interviews do not have formats for obtaining teacher information, and it is difficult to obtain reliable information on structured interviews using self-report for young children below the age of 9 (Frick et al., 2010). Of greatest concern, however, is that there is evidence that the number of reported symptoms declines within a structured interview schedule. Specifically, parents and youth tend to report more symptoms for disorders that are assessed early in the interview, regardless of which diagnoses are assessed first (Jensen, Watanabe, & Richters, 1999; Piacentini et al., 1999). This is likely due the stem/follow-up format that makes it increasingly clear to informants that the interview becomes longer the more symptoms that are endorsed. This is a crucial limitation given that CPs are often assessed last in most interview schedules and, as a result, may be underreported.

Behavioral Observation

Another critical assessment method that can be used to diagnose a youth with CPs is behavioral observation. Observing a child's or adolescent's behavior can provide important information for the assessment because that information is not filtered through the perception of an informant and, thus, can provide a method for documenting the severity of the child's CPs in a way that may be less susceptible to biases and/or unrealistic expectations. Two widely used observation procedures for assessing children with CP in younger (3–8 years) children are the Behavioral Coding System (BCS; Forehand & McMahon, 1981) and the Dyadic Parent–Child Interaction Coding System (DPICS; Eyberg, Nelson, Ginn, Bhuiyan, & Boggs, 2013). The BCS and the DPICS are modifications of the assessment procedure developed by Hanf (1970) that places the parent–child dyad in standard situations that vary in the degree to which parental control is required, ranging from a free-play situation to a parent-directed activity such as completing math problems or cleaning up toys. Each task typically lasts 5–10 minutes. The coding system scores a variety of parent and child behaviors, particularly parental antecedents to (e.g., commands) or consequences of (e.g., use of verbal hostility) the child's behavior. Scores from both the BCS and the DPICS have been shown to differentiate clinic-referred children with CPs from nonreferred children (Eyberg et al., 2013; Griest, Forehand, Wells, & McMahon, 1980).

It is important to note that most observations systems require very extensive training to achieve reliable coding of parent and child behaviors (e.g., 20–25 hours for the BCS). Such intensive training often limits the usefulness of these systems in many clinical settings (Frick et al., 2010). However, simplified versions of both the DPICS and the BCS that have been developed to reduce training demands are more useful for most clinical settings

(Eyberg, Bessmer, Newcomb, Edwards, & Robinson, 1994; McMahon & Estes, 1997).

Several behavioral observation systems have been developed for use in school settings (Nock & Kurtz, 2005). Both the BCS (Forehand & McMahon, 1981) and the DPICS (Eyberg et al., 2013) have been modified for use in the classroom to assess child behavior (Breiner & Forehand, 1981; Jacobs et al., 2000). An adaptation of the DPICS, the REDSOCS (Revised Edition of the School Observation Coding System) has been utilized in several samples of children (Bagner, Boggs, & Eyberg, 2010; Jacobs et al., 2000). REDSOCS coding is done in 10-second intervals, and several disruptive behaviors (e.g., whining, crying, yelling, showing aggression) are coded. Of most importance, noncompliant behavior is coded when a child does not initiate or attempt to comply with a teacher command (either direct or indirect) 5 seconds following the command.

The BASC-3 Student Observation System (SOS; Reynolds & Kamphaus, 2015) is similar to the REDSOCS in that it is a system for observing children's behavior in the classroom using a momentary time-sampling procedure. With the purchase of an application for a smartphone, tablet, or laptop, the observations can be entered directly into a digital database that can be integrated with the results of the parent and teacher ratings on the BASC-3. The SOS specifies 65 behaviors that are commonly displayed in the classroom and includes both adaptive (e.g., "follows directions" and "returns material used in class") and maladaptive behaviors, including a number of CPs (e.g., "teases others"). The observation period in the classroom is 15 minutes, which is divided into 30 intervals of 30 seconds each. The child's behavior is observed for 3 seconds at the end of each interval, and the observer codes all behaviors observed during this time window. Although the newest version of the SOS has not been extensively tested, scores from the earlier version of this observation system differentiated students with CPs from other children (Lett & Kamphaus, 1997).

One limitation of observational systems is the difficulty in obtaining an adequate sample of a child's behavior; that is, it is sometimes hard to know whether the child's behavior during the observation period is representative of his or her typical way of behaving. It is often hard to observe covert CPs (e.g., lying and stealing) and low-base-rate CPs (e.g., fighting) that are often the most severe and, as a result, the most critical for determining need for treatment. Furthermore, observations are subject to reactivity, such that a child's behavior can change because the child knows that he or she is being observed (Aspland & Gardner, 2003). To reduce problems with reactivity, parents can be trained to record a child's CPs. For example, the Parent Daily Report (PDR; Chamberlain & Reid, 1987), a parent observation measure, is typically administered during brief (5- to 10-minute) telephone interviews. Parents are asked during the interview which of a number of CPs has been displayed by the child over the past 24 hours.

Putting It into Practice

To illustrate this use of assessment to make a diagnosis, we provide the case of Andrew, an 11-year-old boy referred for evaluation because of his parents' concerns about behavior problems he displays at home and at school. In an unstructured intake interview, Andrew's parents report that he is inattentive, disruptive, and defiant during school, which has led to his retention in the fourth grade due to his refusal to complete schoolwork. He currently has behavior management plans in place at school, but they are not effective because Andrew reportedly does not feel bad or guilty for his misbehavior. His parents report that his behavior causes other students at school to dislike him; thus, Andrew does not have any friends. Again, based on the unstructured intake interview, Andrew's behavior problems are also present at home, with his parents reporting that he argues with them, deliberately defies their rules (e.g., watches TV past the time he is supposed to), and frequently lies. Prior to the intake session, Andrew, his parents, and his teacher completed the BASC-3. On the Conduct Problems and Aggression subscales of BASC-3, Andrew's CPs were rated above the 99th percentile for his age by both parents and his teacher. Thus, based on this information, it appears that Andrew's CPs are more severe than those of children his age and are causing problems for him in multiple settings.

This initial intake information was followed by a clinical session in which the DISC-IV was administered. On this structured interview, it was reported that Andrew has physically hurt an animal, destroyed others' property, threatens and intimidates other children, has been physically aggressive to other children, annoys others on purpose, and argues with adults. Andrew's mother reported during her interview that these behaviors have been occurring since kindergarten. In short, this information was enough to indicate that Andrew's

CPs are in need of treatment and that a diagnosis of CD is warranted.

Prescription

Once it is determined that a youth's CPs require treatment, it is then critical to determine what should be the most important targets of treatment (i.e., prescription). As noted in Table 6.1, a number of key research areas should guide this assessment goal. One key research finding is that children with CPs are at risk for host of other problems in adjustment that may need to be considered in developing a treatment plan. Another key research area for guiding treatment is the extensive evidence that CPs typically are caused by multiple risk factors. This requires a comprehensive assessment of the many dispositional and contextual risk factors that may have played a role in the development, maintenance, and course of the youth's CPs. Finally, interpreting such a comprehensive assessment can be aided by the research on the common developmental pathways that can lead to serious CPs in children and adolescents. As described earlier, youth with CPs can fall into childhood-onset or adolescent-onset pathways, depending on the age at which their significant antisocial and aggressive behavior started. Furthermore, important differences exist in the typical co-occurring problems that can be present with CPs and the risk factors that lead to the development or maintenance of CPs for children with and without elevated levels of CU traits (Frick et al., 2014). Knowledge of the characteristics of children on these different pathways can aid in treatment planning by providing a set of working hypotheses about the most likely causes of the youth's CPs and the most important targets of treatment (i.e., a case conceptualization; Frick, 2012).

A summary of this research that highlights important areas to assess across the different developmental pathways to CPs (see Table 6.2). As noted in Table 6.2, for youth whose serious CPs did not emerge until adolescence, based on the available research, it is reasonable to hypothesize that they may be less likely to be aggressive, have intellectual deficits and temperamental vulnerabilities, and have comorbid ADHD. However, the adolescent-onset youth's association with deviant peer groups, as well as factors that may contribute to the deviant peer group affiliation (e.g., lack of parental monitoring and supervision) would be important to assess for youth on this pathway. In contrast,

TABLE 6.2. Key Risk Factors for Conduct Problems across the Common Developmental Pathways

Developmental pathway	Key individual risk factors	Key contextual risk factors
Adolescent onset	• Rebelliousness • Rejection of rules and authority	• Association with antisocial peers • Poor parental monitoring and supervision
Childhood onset	• Executive functioning deficits • Cognitive deficits (especially low verbal intelligence) • Impulsivity–hyperactivity • Attention deficits • Emotion regulation problems, including anger, anxiety, and depression • Low self-esteem	• Family conflict/instability • Harsh and inconsistent parenting • Peer rejection/victimization
Childhood onset with limited prosocial emotions	• Insensitivity to distress or pain in others • Insensitivity to punishment • Instrumental and premeditated aggression • Fearlessness and thrill and adventure seeking	• Low parental warmth

for youth whose serious CPs began prior to adolescence, one would expect more cognitive and temperamental vulnerabilities, comorbid ADHD, and more serious problems in family functioning. For youth in this childhood-onset group who do not exhibit high levels of CU traits, verbal intelligence deficits would be more likely, as well as difficulties regulating emotions, leading to higher levels of anxiety, depression, and aggression involving anger. In contrast, for a youth with childhood-onset CPs who exhibits high levels of CU traits, the cognitive deficits are more likely to involve a lack of sensitivity to punishment, and the temperamental vulnerabilities are more likely to involve a preference for dangerous and novel activities and a failure to express many types of emotion. Assessing the level and severity of aggressive behavior, especially the presence of instrumental aggression, would be pivotal for children and adolescents in this group as well.

Most clinicians recognize that people do not fall neatly into the prototypes that are suggested by research. As such, these descriptions of prototypical youth within the three common developmental pathways to CPs are meant to help generate hypotheses around which to organize an evidence-based assessment and to develop a clear case conceptualization as to the most likely causes of the youth's CPs and the most effective targets for intervention (Frick, 2012). In the following sections, we summarize some the methods that can be used to address each of these areas to design a treatment plan for a child with CPs.

Assessing Common Co-occurring Problems

Based on research, the first part of designing a treatment plan is to determine whether the child or adolescent with CPs has significant problems in other areas of adjustment that should also be the focus of treatment. Most behavior rating scales provide a time-efficient method for screening a large number of important psychological domains that may be influenced by a youth's CPs, such as anxiety, depression, social problems, and family relationships. Furthermore, these rating scales typically provide some of the best information about whether any of these problems in adjustment are more severe than what would be expected given a child's age. Thus, rating scales can be very useful in providing a broad screening of some of the most common co-occurring problems that are displayed by children and adolescents with serious CPs.

It is important to note, however, that rating scales vary somewhat in how well they assess the various co-occurring conditions. For example, the ASEBA does not include separate depression and anxiety scales, nor does it include a hyperactivity scale. In a similar vein, rating scales vary in how well they map onto DSM definitions of children's emotional and behavioral problems. The ASEBA (Achenbach, 2013) and the Conners, Third Edition (Conners, 2008) standard subscales do not conform closely to DSM diagnoses but they both include scoring algorithms for supplementary DSM-5 oriented scales. However, rating scales developed by Gadow and Sprafkin (2002), such as the Child Symptom Inventory, Early Childhood

Inventory, and the Child and Adolescent Symptom Inventory were specifically developed to correspond closely to DSM criteria.

Interviews can also help in assessing co-occurring problems. Unstructured or semistructured interviews with the child and his or her parent can screen for the most common adjustment problems that often accompany CPs, especially those causing the most problems for the child. Any problem area that is of concern, based on these interviews or the behavior rating scales, can be assessed in more detail using structured interview schedules. From this information, it can be determined whether the child meets criteria for other disorders, in addition to ODD or CD.

Assessing Key Risk Factors

In Table 6.2, we include a summary of some of the most common risk factors associated with each of the developmental pathways to CPs. Many of these risk factors can be assessed through unstructured or semistructured interviews with the parent, teacher, or youth. Also, various risk factors can be assessed through some of the same behavior rating scales that are used to assess the level and severity of child's CPs. For example, the BASC-3 assesses attention problems and hyperactivity that would likely be common in youth with childhood-onset CPs, as well as anxiety and depression, which would be associated with CPs in youth who do not show significant levels of CU traits and who instead may show problems with emotional regulation. In addition, the BASC-3 assesses sensation seeking, which could be important for assessing children with CU traits, as well as relationships with parents and peers, which are important across all pathways (Reynolds & Kamphaus, 2015).

There are other behavior rating scales that specifically target some risk factors associated with CPs. For example, a 20-item child version of Carver and White's (1994) Behavioral Inhibition and Behavioral Activation System Scales (BIS/BAS) can be used to assess both impulsivity and fearlessness in children (Muris, Meesters, de Kanter, & Timmerman, 2005), as scores on the BIS/BAS are significantly associated with CPs and CU traits (Fanti, Panayiotou, Lazarou, Michael, & Georgiou, 2016). Frick, Cornell, Barry, Bodin, and Dane (2003) used the Thrill and Adventure Seeking subscale from the Sensation Seeking Scale for Children (Russo et al., 1993) to assess fearlessness and reported a significant association with CU traits.

One risk factor that deserves particular attention in the assessment of CPs is parenting practices. Parenting is important to the assessment processes for two main reasons. First, parenting plays a critical role in the development of CPs across the multiple developmental pathways to CP (Frick & Viding, 2009). Second, most successful treatment programs for CPs include a primary focus on changing parenting practices (McMahon & Frick, 2019).

Parenting is often assessed through unstructured and semistructured interviews and behavioral observations. For example, a clinical interview with a parent helps to assess stressors that may be occurring in the family (e.g., parental divorce, parental substance abuse) relative to the youth's CPs. In addition, semistructured interviews can assess typical parent–child interactions, especially interactions involving parental behaviors that may make the CPs more likely to occur (e.g., yelling at the child) and parental behaviors in response to the youth's behavior that either increase (i.e., give the child attention) or decrease (i.e., ignore) the likelihood that the CPs will reoccur. Finally, the clinical interview allows the parent to describe previous attempts to reduce the youth's CPs, both formally (e.g., seeking mental health counseling) and informally (e.g., change in discipline).

Many of the behavioral observation systems we reviewed in the previous section (e.g., BCS, DPICS) observe the child in interactions with his or her parents and other important persons in the immediate context. Thus, they provide important information on the potential role of parents and teachers in the development and maintenance of the child's CPs. For example, behavioral observations can indicate how others in the child's environment (e.g., home and school) respond to the child's behavior, which is important for identifying factors that may be maintaining or exacerbating these behaviors.

In addition, several behavior rating scales have also been specifically developed to assess parenting practices that are important for treatment planning for children and adolescents with CPs. Two examples that have significant psychometric support are the Parenting Scale (Arnold, O'Leary, Wolff, & Acker, 1993) and the Alabama Parenting Questionnaire (APQ; Shelton, Frick, & Wootton, 1996; see Morsbach & Prinz, 2006, for a summary of parent-report measures of parenting practices and suggestions for improving their validity).

The Parenting Scale (Arnold et al., 1993) consists of 30 items that describe parental discipline practices in response to child misbehavior. Each of the items includes a 7-point rating scale that is anchored by statements of effective and ineffective forms of a particular parenting behavior (e.g., "I coax or beg my child to stop" and "I firmly tell my child to stop"). Items are worded at a sixth-grade level or below, and the measure takes 5–10 minutes to complete. Scores on the Parenting Scale have been significantly related to CPs in community samples of children ranging from ages 3 to 12 years (Bor & Sanders, 2004; Lorber & Slep, 2015) and clinical samples ranging from ages 2 to 8 years (Sanders & Woolley, 2005). Parental harshness measured by the Parenting Scale has also been associated with CU traits in preschoolers (Waller et al., 2012).

The APQ (Shelton et al., 1996) was developed for use with parents of elementary school-aged children and adolescents (ages 6–17 years), although it has been used in samples as young as age 3 (Dadds, Maujean, & Fraser, 2003). It consists of 42 items assessing five dimensions of parenting that research has suggested are critical for the development of CPs: Involvement, Positive Reinforcement, Poor Monitoring/Supervision, Inconsistent Discipline, and Corporal Punishment. It also includes several items assessing "other discipline practices," such as time out or taking away privileges. The items are presented in both global report (i.e., questionnaire) and telephone interview formats, and there are separate versions of each format for parents and children. Thus, there are currently four different versions of the APQ. The questionnaire format employs a 5-point Likert-type frequency scale and asks the informant how frequently each of the various parenting practices typically occurs. Four telephone interviews are conducted, and the informant is asked to report the frequency with which each parenting practice has occurred over the previous 3 days.

A number of studies have shown that the APQ scales are associated with CPs in children in community (Crum, Waschbush, Bagner, & Coxe, 2015), clinic-referred (Hawes & Dadds, 2006; Muratori et al., 2015), and inpatient (Blader, 2004) samples, as well as in families with deaf children (Brubaker & Szakowski, 2000) and those with substance-abusing parents (Stanger, Dumenci, Kamon, & Burstein, 2004). Also, these studies have documented this relationship in samples as young as age 3 (de la Osa, Granero, Penelo, Domènech, & Expeleta, 2014; Hawes & Dadds, 2006) and as old as age 17 (Dandreaux & Frick, 2009; Frick, Christian, & Wootton, 1999). How-

ever, Frick and colleagues did demonstrate some differences in which dimensions of parenting were most strongly associated with CPs at different ages, with Inconsistent Discipline being most strongly associated with CPs in young children (ages 6–8), Corporal Punishment being most strongly associated with CPs in older children (ages 9–12), and Involvement and Poor Monitoring/Supervision being most strongly related to CPs in adolescents (ages 13–17). Also, this study raised concerns about the reliability of the child-report format in very young children (before age 9) (see also Shelton et al., 1996). Parental involvement and parental use of positive reinforcement, as measured by the APQ, also have been significantly associated with levels of CU traits in an ethnically diverse sample of kindergarten students (Clark & Frick, 2018) and in a sample of at-risk school-age youth (Pardini, Lochman, & Powell, 2007).

Assessing Age of Onset

As noted previously, the risk factors associated with CPs can vary depending on the age at which CPs first develop. Thus, another crucial piece of information for clinical assessments that can inform treatment planning is assessing the age at which the serious CPs were first displayed by the youth, which helps to determine whether the youth fits more with the childhood-onset or adolescent-onset pathway. This information is usually obtained through interviews. For example, most structured interviews include standard questions that assess the age at which a youth's behavioral difficulties began to emerge (onset) and how long (persistence) they have caused problems for the youth.

One complicating factor is that research has not been consistent about the exact age at which to distinguish between childhood and adolescent onset of CPs (Fairchild et al., 2013) or even whether this distinction should be based on chronological age or on the pubertal status of the child (Moffitt, 2006). For example, DSM-5 criteria for CD (American Psychiatric Association, 2013) make the distinction between children who begin showing severe CPs before age 10 (i.e., childhood onset) and those who do not show severe CP until age 10 or older (i.e., adolescent onset). However, other researchers have used age 11 (Robins, 1966) or age 14 (Patterson & Yoerger, 1993; Tibbetts & Piquero, 1999) to define adolescent onset. Thus, onset of severe CPs before age 10 clearly seems to be considered childhood onset, and onset after age

13 is clearly adolescent onset. However, classifying children whose severe CPs began between ages 11 and 13 is less clear and is likely dependent on the level of physical, cognitive, and social maturity of the child.

Another important issue when assessing age of onset of a child's CPs relates to the accuracy of parent and youth reports. Three research findings can help in interpreting such reports on the youth's history of CPs. First, the longer the time frame involved in the retrospective report (e.g., a parent of a 17-year-old reporting on preschool behavior vs. a parent of a 6-year-old reporting on preschool behavior), the less accurate the report is likely to be (Green, Loeber, & Lahey, 1991). Second, although parental report of the exact age of onset may not be very reliable over time, typical variations in years are usually small, and the relative rankings within symptoms (e.g., which symptom began first) and within a sample (e.g., which children exhibited the earliest onset of behavior) seem to be fairly stable (Green et al., 1991). Therefore, these reports should be viewed as rough estimates of the timing of onset and not as exact dating procedures. Third, there is evidence that combining informants (e.g., a parent or youth) or combining sources of information (e.g., self-report and school/clinical/police records), and taking the earliest reported age of onset from any source, provide an estimate that shows somewhat greater validity than any single source of information alone (Lahey et al., 1999).

Assessing CU Traits

In addition to age of onset of the child's CPs, the presence of elevated levels of CU traits is also important for treatment planning (Frick, 2012). As noted earlier, DSM-5 included in the diagnosis of CD a specifier called "with limited prosocial emotions" and the criteria for this specifier provide guidance for the clinical assessment of CU. These symptoms were selected for inclusion in the specifier, and the choice of the diagnostic cutoff used to designate elevated levels of these traits (i.e., two or more symptoms) was based on extensive secondary data analyses across several large samples of youth in different countries (Kimonis et al., 2015). Specifically, these four symptoms (lack of empathy, lack of guilt, lack of concern about performance in important activities, and shallow or deficient affect) consistently were the best indicators of the overall construct of CU traits in factor analyses across samples, and the presence of two or

more symptoms, if shown persistently, designated a more severely impaired group of antisocial youth across these samples.

CU traits can be assessed in unstructured clinical interviews. Also, because these traits correspond closely to the affective dimension of psychopathy (Hare & Neumann, 2008), measures for assessing psychopathic features in youth can be used to assess these traits, such as the Psychopathy Checklist: Youth Version (PCL-YV; Forth, Kosson, & Hare, 2003). The PCL-YV is a widely used clinician-rated checklist with a long history of use in largely forensic samples of adolescents (Kotler & McMahon, 2010). However, because it was designed largely for institutionalized adolescents, its utility for assessing children or for assessing children and adolescents in other mental health settings has not been firmly established. Furthermore, its format requires a highly trained clinician to administer and score the measure.

To overcome these limitations, the Antisocial Process Screening Device (APSD; Frick & Hare, 2001) was developed to assess the same content as the PCL-YV using a behavior rating scale format that is completed by parents and teachers. A self-report version is also available for older children and adolescents (Muñoz & Frick, 2007). Unfortunately, the APSD, like the PCL-YV, was developed to assess the broader construct of psychopathy; as a result, it includes only six items directly assessing CU traits. Furthermore, it only has three response options for rating the frequency of the behaviors. The small number of items, the limited range of response options, and the fact that ratings of CU traits are negatively skewed in most samples resulted in the CU subscale of the APSD showing poor internal consistency in many samples (Poythress, Dembo, Wareham, & Greenbaum, 2006). Options for assessing CU traits that include a broader assessment than the APSD but still include the other dimensions of psychopathy are the Youth Psychopathic Traits Inventory (YPI; Andershed, Kerr, Strattin, & Levander, 2002) and the Child Problematic Traits Inventory (CPTI; Colins et al., 2014).

Another option for assessing CU traits, the Inventory of Callous–Unemotional Traits (ICU; Kimonis et al., 2008), was developed specifically to provide a more extended assessment of CU traits, but in a way that is directly tied to the four items that are included in the "with limited prosocial emotions" specifier. Items were developed to have six items (three positively and three negatively worded items) to assess each of the four symptoms. These 24 items were then placed on a 4-point Likert scale that could be rated from 0 (*Not at all true*) to 3 (*Definitely true*). Parent, teacher, and self-report versions were developed to encourage multi-informant assessments. The ICU has a number of positive qualities for assessing CU traits. The larger number of items and its extended response format has resulted in a 24-item total score that is internally consistent in many samples, with Cronbach's alphas ranging between .77 and .89 (Cardinale & Marsh, 2020; Frick & Ray, 2015). Furthermore, there is a preschool version for use with children as young as age 3 (Ezpeleta, de la Osa, Granero, Penelo, & Domènech, 2013), and the ICU has been translated into over 20 languages, with substantial support for its validity across these translations (Ciucci, Baroncelli, Franchi, Golmaryami, & Frick, 2014; Fanti, Frick, & Georgiou, 2009; Kimonis et al., 2008). For example, in a meta-analyses of 75 papers with 115 samples and 27,947 participants, the average correlation between the ICU total score and measures of CPs was $r = .34$ ($n = 13,899$) and with measures of empathy was $r = -.42$ ($n = 2,575$; Kimonis, Fanti, & Singh, 2014). However, these positive qualities need to be weighed against the lack of a large and representative normative sample for the ICU and with empirically derived cutoffs available only for certain versions of the scale.

Putting It into Practice

Going back to the case of Andrew, after determining that he met criteria for CD, the clinician administered a number of rating scales to assess parenting. Andrew and his parents completed the APQ to assess the frequency and types of parenting practices on various domains. Andrew reported that his parents infrequently used positive reinforcement, and his parents reported that they were very inconsistent in how they used discipline. This was supported by reports from his mother on a clinical interview that Andrew frequently argued when disciplined, leaving his mother frustrated and resorting to coercion or letting him out of the punishments early.

Andrew and his mother also completed the ICU scale, in which a number of CU behaviors were reported. These were consistent with reports from his teacher on a clinical interview that Andrew reportedly does not feel bad or guilty when he does something wrong and does not care about others' feelings, but he does appears concerned about his school performance. Also, his parents reported that Andrew does not show any fear and will do dangerous things without thinking that he may get hurt. They also reported in a clinical interview that Andrew does not seem to care whether he gets punished. Therefore, in addition to the diagnosis of CD, Andrew was given the specifier "with limited prosocial emotions."

Process

As summarized in Table 6.1, the final important goal for clinical assessments of children and adolescents with CPs is treatment monitoring and outcomes assessment. This goal focuses on whether the intervention is leading to meaningful change in the child's or adolescent's adjustment, either for better or worse. This step is particularly important in the treatment of CPs given a number of documented cases in which treatment has led to increases, rather than decreases, in CPs (Dishion, McCord, & Poulin, 1999; Dodge, Dishion, & Lansford, 2007). Youth with elevated CU traits especially have been found to be a treatment challenge in that they fail to show as much improvement as other youth with CPs in response to many of the most commonly used mental health treatments (Frick et al., 2014; Hawes, Price, & Dadds, 2014; Wilkinson, Waller, & Viding, 2016).

Several of the previously mentioned rating scales assessing child behavior and parenting practices have demonstrated sensitivity to intervention outcomes. For example, the Parenting Scale has demonstrated changes in disruptive parenting following several types of interventions for children with CPs (Baker, Sanders, Turner, & Morawska, 2017; Joachim, Sanders, & Turner, 2010; Sanders, Baker, & Turner, 2012; Schmidt, Chomycz, Houlding, Kruse, & Franks, 2014). The APQ scales have also demonstrated significant postintervention improvements in parenting practices (e.g., Muratori et al., 2017).

One important consideration in treatment monitoring is the inclusion of ratings of the youth's behavior from other individuals who may not have been involved in the treatment or the use of behavioral observations of treatment effects, especially by an observer who is unaware that the youth and his or her parents are involved in treatment. This consideration is important because parent-report behavior rating scales can be influenced by expectancy results on the part of the parent, who may anticipate positive responses to treatment. The BCS and DPICS have been extensively used as outcome measures for parenting interventions for CPs and have demonstrated sensitivity to intervention effects (e.g., Furlong et al., 2012; Herschell, Calzado, Eyberg, & McNeil, 2002; McCabe & Yeh, 2009; McMahon, Long, & Forehand, 2010; Niec, Barnett, Prewett, & Shanley Chatham, 2016; Webster-Stratton & Hammond, 1997).

The assessment of treatment satisfaction is an additional component related to treatment–outcome measurement. This is a form of social validity that may be assessed in terms of satisfaction with the outcome of treatment, therapists, treatment procedures, and teaching format (McMahon & Forehand, 1983). The Therapy Attitude Inventory (TAI; Brestan, Jacobs, Rayfield, & Eyberg, 1999; Eyberg, 1993) and the Parent's Consumer Satisfaction Questionnaire (PCSQ; McMahon & Forehand, 2003; McMahon, Tiedemann, Forehand, & Griest, 1984) are examples of measures designed to evaluate parental satisfaction with parenting interventions for CPs (e.g., Funderburk & Eyberg, 2011; McMahon & Forehand, 2003). Importantly, these measures largely focus on *parental* satisfaction with treatment. Children and adolescents themselves have rarely been asked about their satisfaction with treatment, with the exception of some evaluations of multisystemic therapy (MST) with adolescents (Henggeler et al., 1999). Furthermore, there has been relatively little empirical assessment of these measures of treatment satisfaction (for exceptions, see Brestan et al., 1999; McMahon et al., 1984).

There are several important issues involved in developing measures suitable for treatment monitoring and outcome evaluation (McMahon & Metzler, 1998). First, the way questions on an interview or rating scale are framed can affect its sensitivity to change. For example, the response scale on a parent-report behavior rating scale may be too general (e.g., "never" vs. "sometimes" vs. "always") or the time interval for reporting the frequency of a parent behavior (e.g., the past 6 months) may not be discrete enough to detect changes brought about by treatment. Second, the degree to which the behaviors measured in assessment match the behaviors targeted in intervention can greatly affect sensitivity to change. For example, if major parenting constructs addressed by an intervention (e.g., limit setting, positive reinforcement, monitoring) are measured weakly or not at all in the assessment, then changes in these constructs as a function of intervention are not likely to be captured. Finally, assessment-by-

intervention interactions may occur. For example, as a function of intervention, parents may learn to become more effective monitors of their child's behavior and be more aware of their child's CPs. Comparison of parental reports of their child's behavior prior to and after the intervention may suggest that parents perceive deterioration in their children's behavior (i.e., a false iatrogenic effect), when, in reality, the parents have simply become more accurate reporters of such behavior (Dishion & McMahon, 1998).

Conclusion

In this chapter, we have summarized four areas of research that have direct and important implications for assessing youth with CPs. Specifically, research has documented (1) the heterogeneity in the types and severity of CPs, (2) the common presence of multiple comorbid conditions in children and adolescents with CP, (3) the multiple risk factors in the child or adolescent and his or her psychosocial context that can be associated with CPs, and (4) the multiple developmental pathways that can lead to CPs. For each of these domains, we discussed the implications of these research findings for making a diagnosis of CP (i.e., prediction), for developing treatments for children and adolescents with CP (i.e., prescription), and for assessing the success of treatment (i.e., process). We also have made a number of practical recommendations for assessment methods to meet each of these assessment goals. However, this discussion also results in a number of overarching issues that are important for an evidence-based assessment of a child or adolescent with CPs.

The first overarching issue is the need, in most cases, for a comprehensive assessment when evaluating youth with CPs. We have emphasized throughout this chapter that an adequate assessment of youth with CPs must make use of multiple methods (e.g., interviews, behavior rating scales, observation) completed by multiple informants (parents, teacher, youth) concerning multiple aspects of the child's or adolescent's adjustment (e.g., CPs, anxiety, learning problems) in multiple settings (e.g., home, school). However, because of issues of time, expense, and practicality, how best to acquire and interpret this large array of information become important issues. Thus, a multistage approach to assessment may prove to be cost-effective for conducting such comprehensive assessments, starting with more time-efficient measures (e.g., broad-band behavior rating scales, unstructured clinical interviews) that are then followed by more time-intensive measures (e.g., structured interviews, behavioral observations) when indicated (McMahon & Frick, 2005; Nock & Kurtz, 2005). Methods that can be used at each stage are listed in Table 6.1.

However, once these assessment data are collected, there are few clinician guidelines for how to integrate and synthesize the multiple pieces of information to make important clinical decisions at each stage of the assessment process. This endeavor is made more complicated by the fact that information from different informants (De Los Reyes & Kazdin, 2005) and from different methods (Barkley, 2013) often show only modest correlations with each other. As a result, after collecting information from multiple sources on a youth's adjustment, the clinician must make sense out of an array of often conflicting information. Several clinically oriented strategies for integrating and interpreting information from comprehensive assessments have been proposed elsewhere (Frick, Barry, & Kamphaus, 2010; McMahon & Forehand, 2003; Wakschlag & Danis, 2004).

As one example, Frick and colleagues (2010) outlined a multistage strategy for integrating results from a comprehensive assessment into a clear case conceptualization to guide treatment planning. At the first step, the clinician documents all clinically significant findings regarding the youth's adjustment (e.g., elevations on ratings scales, diagnoses from structured interviews, and problem behaviors from observations). At the second step, the clinician looks for convergent findings across these methods. At the third step, the assessor attempts to explain, using available research as much as possible, any discrepancies in the assessment results. At the fourth step, the clinician then develops a profile of the areas of most concern for the youth and develops a coherent explanation for the youth's CPs, again using existing research as much as possible. While such guides are a promising development for aiding clinicians in integrating information from a comprehensive evaluation, much more research is needed to inform this process.

Another area in need of more research is the disconnect between assessment concerning case conceptualization and treatment planning. For example, interventions for youth who are engaging primarily in covert forms of CPs (e.g., stealing, firesetting) are much less developed than those for more overt types of CPs, such as noncompli-

ance and aggression (McMahon, Wells, & Kotler, 2006). Similarly, subtype-specific interventions for the treatment of youth with and without CU traits are in the early stages of development. As one example, Kimonis and colleagues (2019) recently reported on an open trial of an adjunctive intervention to enhance an evidence-based parenting intervention for youth with CPs and elevated CU traits. Specifically, they adapted parent–child interaction therapy (PCIT; Zisser-Nathensen, Herschell, & Eyberg, 2017) to address limitations in the efficacy of the standard program for children with elevated CU traits. PCIT-CU, as this targeted intervention was called, differed from standard PCIT in three key ways:

1. It systematically and explicitly coaches parents to engage in warm, emotionally responsive parenting.
2. It shifts emphasis from punishment to reward to achieve effective discipline by systematically supplementing punishment-based disciplinary strategies (i.e., time out) with reward-based techniques (i.e., dynamic and individualized token economy).
3. It delivers an adjunctive module called *Coaching and Rewarding Emotional Skills* (CARES) to target the emotional deficits of children with both CP and CU symptoms.

In their open trial of 23 families of children ages 3–6 years who were referred to a mental health clinic for serious CPs with elevated CU traits, the intervention produced decreases in child CPs and CU traits, and produced increases in empathy, with "medium" to "huge" effect sizes (d's = 0.7–2.0) that were maintained at a 3-month follow-up. Finally, by 3 months posttreatment, 75% of treatment completers no longer showed clinically significant CPs relative to 25% of dropouts (Kimonis et al., 2019). While these results are quite promising, there is a clear need for randomized controlled tests of such modifications to existing interventions for subgroups of children and adolescents with CPs.

Another area that requires additional investigation is testing the sensitivity of measures to change. Much of the research on the assessment process has focused on making diagnostic decisions (e.g., determining whether a CP is severe and impairing enough to warrant treatment) and on treatment planning (e.g., determine what types of treatment may be needed by the child with CPs). However, an important third goal of the assessment process is intervention monitoring and evaluating treatment outcome (McMahon & Metzler, 1998). Evidence-based assessments should provide a means for testing whether interventions have brought about meaningful changes in the child's or adolescent's adjustment, either for better or worse. Relatedly, evidence-based assessment to evaluate both the parent's and child's satisfaction with treatment is also needed, including their satisfaction with the assessment procedures and measures themselves (e.g., Kazdin, 2005; Rhule-Louie, McMahon, & Vando, 2009).

Perhaps the most central issue for advancing evidence-based assessment is the need to have assessments guided by research on the different developmental pathways to CPs. This body of research may be the most important for understanding youth with CPs because it may explain many of the variations in severity, multiple co-occurring conditions, and the variety of risk factors associated with CP. This research could also be very important in the design of more individualized treatments for youth with CPs, especially older children and adolescents with more serious CPs (Frick, 2012). However, in order to translate research on developmental pathways into practice, it is critical to develop better assessment methods for reliably and validly designating youth in these pathways. This is especially the case for girls and for ethnically diverse youth. Furthermore, the causal processes and developmental mechanisms (e.g., lack of empathy and guilt, poor emotion regulation) that may be involved in the different pathways need to be assessed. To date, this typically has involved translating measures that have been used in developmental research into forms that are appropriate for clinical practice (Frick & Morris, 2004). This is perhaps the best illustration of how translating research into practice is critical for evidence-based assessments for CPs.

REFERENCES

Achenbach, T. M. (2013). *DSM-oriented guide for the Achenbach System of Empirically Based Assessment (ASEBA)*. Burlington: University of Vermont Research Center for Children, Youth, and Families.

Achenbach, T. M., & Rescorla, L. A. (2000). *Manual for the ASEBA preschool forms and profiles*. Burlington, VT: University of Vermont, Department of Psychiatry.

Achenbach, T. M., & Rescorla, L. A. (2001). *Manual for the ASEBA school-age forms and profiles*. Burlington, VT: University of Vermont, Research Center for Children, Youth, and Families.

American Psychiatric Association. (2000). *Diagnostic and statistical manual of mental disorders* (4th ed., text rev.). Washington, DC: Author.

American Psychiatric Association. (2013). *Diagnostic and statistical manual of mental disorders* (5th ed.). Arlington, VA: Author.

Andershed, H. A., Kerr, M., Stattin, H., & Levander, S. (2002). Psychopathic traits in non-referred youths: A new assessment tool. In E. Blaauw & L. Sheridan (Eds.), *Psychopathy: Current international perspectives* (pp. 131–158). Den Haag, the Netherlands: Elsevier.

Arnold, D. S., O'Leary, S. G., Wolff, L. S., & Acker, M. M. (1993). The Parenting Scale: A measure of dysfunctional parenting in discipline situations. *Psychological Assessment, 5*, 137–144.

Aspland, H., & Gardner, F. (2003). Observational measures of parent–child interaction: An introductory review. *Child and Adolescent Mental Health, 8*, 136–143.

Bagner, D. M., Boggs, S. R., & Eyberg, S. M. (2010). Evidence-based school behavior assessment of externalizing behavior in young children. *Education and Treatment of Children, 33*, 65–83.

Baker, S., Sanders, M. R., Turner, K. M., & Morawska, A. (2017). A randomized controlled trial evaluating a low-intensity interactive online parenting intervention, Triple P Online Brief, with parents of children with early onset conduct problems. *Behaviour Research and Therapy, 91*, 78–90.

Barkley, R. A. (2013). *Defiant children: A clinician's manual for assessment and parent training* (3rd ed.). New York: Guilford Press.

Blader, J. C. (2004). Symptom, family, and service predictors of children's psychiatric rehospitalization within one year of discharge. *Journal of the American Academy of Child and Adolescent Psychiatry, 43*, 440–451.

Bor, W., & Sanders, M. R. (2004). Correlates of self-reported coercive parenting of preschool-aged children at high risk for the development of conduct problems. *Australian and New Zealand Journal of Psychiatry, 38*, 738–745.

Breiner, J., & Forehand, R. (1981). An assessment of the effects of parent training on clinic-referred children's school behavior. *Behavioral Assessment, 3*, 31–42.

Brestan, E. V., Jacobs, J. R., Rayfield, A. D., & Eyberg, S. M. (1999). A consumer satisfaction measure for parent–child treatments and its relation to measures of child behavior change. *Behavior Therapy, 30*, 17–30.

Brubaker, R. G., & Szakowski, A. (2000). Parenting practices and behavior problems among deaf children. *Child and Family Behavior Therapy, 22*(4), 13–28.

Burke, J. D., Hipwell, A. E., & Loeber, R. (2010). Dimensions of oppositional defiant disorder as predictors of depression and conduct disorder in preadolescent girls. *Journal of the American Academy of Child and Adolescent Psychiatry, 49*, 484–492.

Burke, J. D., Loeber, R., Lahey, B. B., & Rathouz, P. J.

(2005). Developmental transitions among affective and behavioral disorders in adolescent boys. *Journal of Child Psychology and Psychiatry, 46*, 1200–1210.

Burt, S. A. (2012). How do we optimally conceptualize the heterogeneity within antisocial behavior?: An argument for aggressive versus non-aggressive behavioral dimensions. *Clinical Psychology Review, 32*, 236–279.

Burt, S. A., Rescorla, L. A., Achenbach, T. M., Ivanova, M. Y., Almqvist, F., Begovac, I., . . . Döpfner, M. (2015). The association between aggressive and non-aggressive antisocial problems as measured with the Achenbach System of Empirically Based Assessment: A study of 27,861 parent–adolescent dyads from 25 societies. *Personality and Individual Differences, 85*, 86–92.

Canino, G., Polanczyk, G., Bauermeister, J. J., Rohde, L. A., & Frick, P. J. (2010). Does the prevalence of CD and ODD vary across cultures? *Social Psychiatry and Psychiatric Epidemiology, 45*, 695–704.

Cardinale, E. M., & Marsh, A. A. (2020). The reliability and validity of the Inventory of Callous Unemotional Traits: A meta-analytic review. *Assessment, 27*, 57–71.

Carlson, G. A. (2016). Disruptive mood dysregulation disorder: Where did it come from and where is it going? *Journal of Child and Adolescent Psychopharmacology, 26*, 90–93.

Carver, C. S., & White, T. L. (1994). Behavioral inhibition, behavioral activation, and affective responses to impending reward and punishment: The BIS/BAS scales. *Journal of Personality and Social Psychology, 67*, 319–333.

Caselman, T. D., & Self, P. A. (2008). Assessment instruments for measuring young children's social–emotional behavioral development. *Children and Schools, 30*, 103–115.

Chamberlain, P., & Reid, J. B. (1987). Parent observation and report of child symptoms. *Behavioral Assessment, 9*, 97–109.

Ciucci, E., Baroncelli, A., Franchi, M., Golmaryami, F. N., & Frick, P. J. (2014). The association between callous–unemotional traits and behavioral and academic adjustment in children: Further validation of the Inventory of Callous–Unemotional Traits. *Journal of Psychopathology and Behavioral Assessment, 36*, 189–200.

Clark, J. E., & Frick, P. J. (2018). Positive parenting and callous–unemotional traits: Their association with school behavior problems in young children. *Journal of Clinical Child and Adolescent Psychology, 47*(Suppl. 1), S242–S254.

Colins, O. F., Andershed, H., Frogner, L., Lopez-Romero, L., Veen, V., & Andershed, A. K. (2014). A new measure to assess psychopathic personality in children: The Child Problematic Traits Inventory. *Journal of Psychopathology and Behavioral Assessment, 36*, 4–21.

Conduct Problems Prevention Research Group. (2013).

School outcomes of aggressive–disruptive children: Prediction from kindergarten risk factors and impact of the Fast Track prevention program. *Aggressive Behavior, 39*, 114–130.

Conners, C. K. (2008). *Conners' Comprehensive Rating Scales—3rd Edition.* Toronto: Multi-Health Systems.

Crum, K. I., Waschbusch, D. A., Bagner, D. M., & Coxe, S. (2015). Effects of callous–unemotional traits on the association between parenting and child conduct problems. *Child Psychiatry and Human Development, 46*, 967–980.

Cunningham, N. R., & Ollendick, T. H. (2010). Comorbidity of anxiety and conduct problems in children: Implications for clinical research and practice. *Clinical Child and Family Psychology Review, 13*, 333–347.

Dadds, M. R., Maujean, A., & Fraser, J. A. (2003). Parenting and conduct problems in children: Australian data and psychometric properties of the Alabama Parenting Questionnaire. *Australian Psychologist, 38*, 238–241.

Dandreaux, D. M., & Frick, P. J. (2009). Developmental pathways to conduct problems: A further test of the childhood and adolescent-onset distinction. *Journal of Abnormal Child Psychology, 37*, 375–385.

de la Osa, N., Granero, R., Penelo, E., Domènech, J. M., & Ezpeleta, L. (2014). Psychometric properties of the Alabama Parenting Questionnaire–Preschool Revision (APQ-PR) in 3-year-old Spanish preschoolers. *Journal of Child and Family Studies, 23*, 776–784.

De Los Reyes, A., & Kazdin, A. E. (2005). Informant discrepancies in the assessment of childhood psychology: A critical review, theoretical framework, and recommendations for further study. *Psychological Bulletin, 131*, 483–509.

Dishion, T. J., McCord, J., & Poulin, F. (1999). When interventions harm: Peer groups and problem behavior. *American Psychologist, 54*, 755–764.

Dishion, T. J., & McMahon, R. J. (1998). Parental monitoring and the prevention of child and adolescent problem behavior: A conceptual and empirical formulation. *Clinical Child and Family Psychology Review, 1*, 61–75.

Dodge, K. A., Dishion, T. J., & Lansford, J. E. (2007). *Deviant peer influences in programs for youth: Problems and solutions.* New York: Guilford Press.

Dodge, K. A., & Pettit, G. S. (2003). A biopsychosocial model of the development of chronic conduct problems in adolescence. *Developmental Psychology, 39*, 349–371.

Eyberg, S. (1993). Consumer satisfaction measures for assessing parent training programs. In L. VandeCreek, S. Knapp, & T. L. Jackson (Eds.), *Innovations in clinical practice: A source book* (Vol. 12, pp. 377–382). Sarasota, FL: Professional Resource Press/Professional Resource Exchange.

Eyberg, S., Bessmer, J., Newcomb, K., Edwards, D., & Robinson, E. (1994). *Dyadic Parent–Child Interaction Coding Scheme II: A manual.* Unpublished manuscript, University of Florida, Gainesville, FL.

Eyberg, S. M., Nelson, M. M., Ginn, N. C., Bhuiyan, N., & Boggs, S. R. (2013). *Dyadic Parent–Child Interaction Coding System: Comprehensive manual for research and training* (4th ed.). Gainesville, FL: PCIT International.

Eyberg, S. M., & Pincus, D. (1999). *The Eyberg Child Behavior Inventory and Sutter–Eyberg Student Behavior Inventory: Professional manual.* Lutz, FL: Psychological Assessment Resources.

Ezpeleta, L., de la Osa, N., Granero, R., Penelo, E., & Domènech, J. M. (2013). Inventory of Callous–Unemotional Traits in a community sample of preschoolers. *Journal of Clinical Child and Adolescent Psychology, 42*, 91–105.

Fairchild, G., van Goozen, S. H., Calder, A. J., & Goodyer, I. M. (2013). Research review: Evaluating and reformulating the developmental taxonomic theory of antisocial behaviour. *Journal of Child Psychology and Psychiatry, 54*, 924–940.

Fanti, K. A., Frick, P. J., & Georgiou, S. (2009). Linking callous–unemotional traits to instrumental and non-instrumental forms of aggression. *Journal of Psychopathology and Behavioral Assessment, 31*, 285–298.

Fanti, K. A., & Henrich, C. C. (2010). Trajectories of pure and co-occurring internalizing and externalizing problems from age 2 to age 12: Findings from the National Institute of Child Health and Human Development Study of Early Child Care. *Developmental Psychology, 46*, 1159–1175.

Fanti, K. A., Panayiotou, G., Lazarou, C., Michael, R., & Georgiou, G. (2016). The better of two evils?: Evidence that children exhibiting continuous conduct problems high or low on callous–unemotional traits score on opposite directions on physiological and behavioral measures of fear. *Development and Psychopathology, 28*, 185–198.

Fergusson, D. M., Lynskey, M. T., & Horwood, L. J. (1996). Origins of comorbidity between conduct and affective disorders. *Journal of the American Academy of Child and Adolescent Psychiatry, 35*, 451–460.

Forehand, R., & McMahon, R. J. (1981). *Helping the noncompliant child: A clinician's guide to parent training.* New York: Guilford Press.

Forth, A. E., Kosson, D., & Hare, R. D. (2003). *The Hare Psychopathy Checklist: Youth Version.* Toronto: Multi-Health Systems.

Freeman, A. J., Youngstrom, E. A., Youngstrom, J. K., & Findling, R. L. (2016). Disruptive mood dysregulation disorder in a community mental health clinic: Prevalence, comorbidity, and correlates. *Journal of Child and Adolescent Psychopharmacology, 26*, 123–130.

Frick, P. J. (2012). Developmental pathways to conduct disorder: Implications for future directions in research, assessment, and treatment. *Journal of Clinical Child and Adolescent Psychology, 41*, 378–389.

Frick, P. J. (2016). Current research on conduct disorder in children and adolescents. *South African Journal of Psychology, 46*, 160–174.

Frick, P. J., Barry, C. T., & Kamphaus, R. W. (2010).

Clinical assessment of child and adolescent personality and behavior (3rd ed.). New York: Springer.

Frick, P. J., Barry, C. T., & Kamphaus, R. W. (2020). *Clinical assessment of child and adolescent personality and behavior* (4th ed.). New York: Springer.

Frick, P. J., Christian, R. E., & Wootton, J. M. (1999). Age trends in the association between parenting practices and conduct problems. *Behavior Modification, 23*(1), 106–128.

Frick, P. J., Cornell, A. H., Barry, C. T., Bodin, S. D., & Dane, H. A. (2003). Callous–unemotional traits and conduct problems in the prediction of conduct problem severity, aggression, and self-report of delinquency. *Journal of Abnormal Child Psychology, 31*, 457–470.

Frick, P. J., & Hare, R. D. (2001). *Antisocial process screening device: APSD.* Toronto: Multi-Health Systems.

Frick, P. J., Kamphaus, R. W., Lahey, B. B., Loeber, R., Christ, M. A. G., Hart, E. L., & Tannenbaum, L. E. (1991). Academic underachievement and the disruptive behavior disorders. *Journal of Consulting and Clinical Psychology, 59*, 289–294.

Frick, P. J., Lahey, B. B., Loeber, R., Tannenbaum, L., Van Horn, Y., Christ, M. A. G., . . . Hanson, K. (1993). Oppositional defiant disorder and conduct disorder: A meta-analytic review of factor analyses and cross-validation in a clinic sample. *Clinical Psychology Review, 13*, 319–340.

Frick, P. J., & Morris, A. S. (2004). Temperament and developmental pathways to conduct problems. *Journal of Clinical Child and Adolescent Psychology, 33*, 54–68.

Frick, P. J., & Nigg, J. T. (2012). Current issues in the diagnosis of attention deficit hyperactivity disorder, oppositional defiant disorder, and conduct disorder. *Annual Review of Clinical Psychology, 8*, 77–107.

Frick, P. J., & Ray, J. V. (2015). Evaluating callous–unemotional traits as a personality construct. *Journal of Personality, 83*, 710–722.

Frick, P. J., Ray, J. V., Thornton, L. C., & Kahn, R. E. (2014). Can callous–unemotional traits enhance the understanding, diagnosis, and treatment of serious conduct problems in children and adolescents?: A comprehensive review. *Psychological Bulletin, 140*, 1–57.

Frick, P. J., Stickle, T. R., Dandreaux, D. M., Farrell, J. M., & Kimonis, E. R. (2005). Callous–unemotional traits in predicting the severity and stability of conduct problems and delinquency. *Journal of Abnormal Child Psychology, 33*, 471–487.

Frick, P. J., & Viding, E. M. (2009). Antisocial behavior from a developmental psychopathology perspective. *Development and Psychopathology, 21*, 1111–1131.

Funderburk, B. W., & Eyberg, S. (2011). Parent–child interaction therapy. In J. C. Norcross, G. R. VandenBos, & D. K. Freedheim (Eds.), *History of psychotherapy: Continuity and change* (pp. 415–420). Washington, DC: American Psychological Association.

Funderburk, B. W., Eyberg, S. M., Rich, B. A., & Behar,

L. (2003). Further psychometric evaluation of the Eyberg and Behar rating scales for parents and teachers of preschoolers. *Early Education and Development, 14,* 67–79.

Furlong, M., McGilloway, S., Bywater, T., Hutchings, J., Smith, S. M., & Donnelly, M. (2012). Cochrane Review: Behavioural and cognitive-behavioural group-based parenting programmes for early-onset conduct problems in children aged 3 to 12 years. *Cochrane Database of Systematic Reviews,* Issue 2, Article No. CD008225. doi: 10.1002/14651858.CD008225.pub2

Gadow, K. D., & Sprafkin, J. (2002). *CSI-4 screening manual.* Stony Brook, NY: Checkmate Plus.

Green, S. M., Loeber, R., & Lahey, B. B. (1991). Stability of mothers' recall of the age of onset of their child's attention and hyperactivity problems. *Journal of the American Academy of Child and Adolescent Psychiatry, 30,* 135–137.

Griest, D. L., Forehand, R., Wells, K. C., & McMahon, R. J. (1980). An examination of differences between nonclinic and behavior problem clinic-referred children. *Journal of Abnormal Psychology, 89,* 497–500.

Hanf, C. (1970). *Shaping mothers to shape their children's behavior.* Unpublished manuscript, University of Oregon Medical School, Eugene, OR.

Hare, R. D., & Neumann, C. S. (2008). Psychopathy as a clinical and empirical construct. *Annual Review of Clinical Psychology, 4,* 217–246.

Hawes, D. J., & Dadds, M. R. (2006). Assessing parenting practices through parent-report and direct observation during parenting-training. *Journal of Child and Family Studies, 15,* 555–568.

Hawes, D. J., Price, M. J., & Dadds, M. R. (2014). Callous–unemotional traits and the treatment of conduct problems in childhood and adolescence: A comprehensive review. *Clinical Child and Family Psychology Review, 17,* 248–267.

Henggeler, S. W., Rowland, M. D., Randall, J., Ward, D. M., Pickrel, S. G., Cunningham, P. B., . . . Santos, A. B. (1999). Home-based multisystemic therapy as an alternative to the hospitalization of youths in psychiatric crisis: Clinical outcomes. *Journal of the American Academy of Child and Adolescent Psychiatry, 38,* 1331–1339.

Herschell, A., Calzada, E., Eyberg, S. M., & McNeil, C. B. (2002). Clinical issues in parent–child interaction therapy: Clinical past and future. *Cognitive and Behavioral Practice, 9,* 16–27.

Hipwell, A. E., Stepp, S., Feng, X., Burke, J., Battista, D. R., Loeber, R., & Keenan, K. (2011). Impact of oppositional defiant disorder dimensions on the temporal ordering of conduct problems and depression across childhood and adolescence in girls. *Journal of Child Psychology and Psychiatry, 52,* 1099–1108.

Jacobs, J., Boggs, S. R., Eyberg, S. M., Edwards, D., Durning, P., Querido, J., . . . Funderburk, B. (2000). Psychometric properties and reference point data for the revised edition of the School Observation Coding System. *Behavior Therapy, 31,* 695–712.

Jensen, P. S., Watanabe, H. K., & Richters, J. E. (1999). Who's up first?: Testing for order effects in structured interviews using a counterbalanced experimental design. *Journal of Abnormal Child Psychology, 27,* 439–445.

Joachim, S., Sanders, M. R., & Turner, K. M. (2010). Reducing preschoolers' disruptive behavior in public with a brief parent discussion group. *Child Psychiatry and Human Development, 41,* 47–60.

Kahn, R. E., Frick, P. J., Youngstrom, E., Findling, R. L., & Youngstrom, J. K. (2012). The effects of including a callous–unemotional specifier for the diagnosis of conduct disorder. *Journal of Child Psychology and Psychiatry, 53,* 271–282.

Karnik, N. S., Soller, M., Redlich, A., Silverman, M., Kraemer, H. C., Haapanen, R., & Steiner, H. (2009). Prevalence of and gender differences in psychiatric disorders among juvenile delinquents incarcerated for nine months. *Psychiatric Services, 60,* 838–841.

Kazdin, A. E. (2005). Evidence-based assessment for children and adolescents: Issues in measurement development and clinical application. *Journal of Clinical Child and Adolescent Psychology, 34,* 548–558.

Kazdin, A. E., Whitley, M., & Marciano, P. L. (2006). Child–therapist and parent–therapist alliance and therapeutic change in the treatment of children referred for oppositional, aggressive, and antisocial behavior. *Journal of Child Psychology and Psychiatry, 47,* 436–445.

Kimonis, E. R., Fanti, K. A., Frick, P. J., Moffitt, T. E., Essau, C., Bijttebier, P., & Marsee, M. A. (2015). Using self-reported callous–unemotional traits to cross-nationally assess the DSM-5 "With Limited Prosocial Emotions" specifier. *Journal of Child Psychology and Psychiatry, 56,* 1249–1261.

Kimonis, E. R., Fanti, K. A., & Singh, J. P. (2014). Establishing cut-off scores for the parent-reported Inventory of Callous–Unemotional Traits. *Archives of Forensic Psychology, 1,* 27–48.

Kimonis, E. R., Fleming, G., Briggs, N., Brouwer-French, L., Frick, P. J., Hawes, D. J., . . . Dadds, M. (2019). Parent–child interaction therapy adapted for preschoolers with callous–unemotional traits: An open trial pilot study. *Journal of Clinical Child and Adolescent Psychology, 48*(Suppl. 1), S347–S361.

Kimonis, E. R., Frick, P. J., & McMahon, R. J. (2014). Conduct and oppositional defiant disorders. In E. J. Mash & R. A. Barkley (Eds.), *Child psychopathology* (3rd ed., pp. 145–179). New York: Guilford Press.

Kimonis, E. R., Frick, P. J., Skeem, J. L., Marsee, M. A., Cruise, K., Munoz, L. C., . . . Morris, A. S. (2008). Assessing callous–unemotional traits in adolescent offenders: Validation of the Inventory of Callous–Unemotional Traits. *International Journal of Law and Psychiatry, 31,* 241–252.

Kotler, J. S., & McMahon, R. J. (2010). Assessment of child and adolescent psychopathy. In R. T. Salekin & D. R. Lynam (Eds.), *Handbook of child and adolescent psychopathy* (pp. 79–109). New York: Guilford Press.

Lahey, B. B., Goodman, S. H., Waldman, I. D., Bird, H., Canino, G., Jensen, P., . . . Applegate, B. (1999). Relation of age of onset to the type and severity of child and adolescent conduct problems. *Journal of Abnormal Child Psychology, 27,* 247–260.

Lett, N. J., & Kamphaus, R. W. (1997). Differential validity of the BASC Student Observation System and the BASC Teacher Rating Scale. *Canadian Journal of School Psychology, 13,* 1–14.

Livanou, M., Furtado, V., Winsper, C., Silvester, A., & Singh, S. P. (2019). Prevalence of mental disorders and symptoms in incarcerated youth: A meta-analysis of 30 studies. *International Journal of Mental Health, 18*(4), 400–414.

Loeber, R., & Burke, J. D. (2011). Developmental pathways in juvenile externalizing and internalizing problems. *Journal of Research on Adolescence, 21,* 34–46.

Lorber, M. F., & Slep, A. M. S. (2015). Are persistent early onset child conduct problems predicted by the trajectories and initial levels of discipline practices? *Developmental Psychology, 51,* 1048–1061.

Lynskey, M. T., & Fergusson, D. M. (1995). Childhood conduct problems, attention deficit behaviors, and adolescent alcohol, tobacco, and illicit drug use. *Journal of Abnormal Child Psychology, 23,* 281–302.

Mayes, S. D., Waxmonsky, J. D., Calhoun, S. L., & Bixler, E. O. (2016). Disruptive mood dysregulation disorder symptoms and association with oppositional defiant and other disorders in a general population child sample. *Journal of Child and Adolescent Psychopharmacology, 26,* 101–106.

McCabe, K., & Yeh, M. (2009). Parent–child interaction therapy for Mexican-Americans: A randomized clinical trial. *Journal of Clinical Child and Adolescent Psychology, 38,* 753–759.

McMahon, R. J., & Estes, A. M. (1997). Conduct problems. In E. J. Mash & L. G. Terdal (Eds.), *Assessment of childhood disorders* (3rd ed., pp. 130–193). New York: Guilford Press.

McMahon, R. J., & Forehand, R. (1983). Consumer satisfaction in behavioral treatment of children: Types, issues, and recommendations. *Behavior Therapy, 14,* 209–225.

McMahon, R. J., & Forehand, R. L. (2003). *Helping the noncompliant child: Family-based treatment for oppositional behavior* (2nd ed.). New York: Guilford Press.

McMahon, R. J., & Frick, P. J. (2005). Evidence-based assessment of conduct problems in children and adolescents. *Journal of Clinical Child and Adolescent Psychology, 34,* 477–505.

McMahon, R. J., & Frick, P. J. (2019). Conduct and oppositional disorders. In M. J. Prinstein, E. A. Youngstrom, E. J. Mash, & R. A. Barkley (Eds.), *Treatment of disorders in childhood and adolescence* (4th ed., pp. 102–172). New York: Guilford Press.

McMahon, R. J., Long, N., & Forehand, R. L. (2010). Parent training for the treatment of oppositional behavior in young children: Helping the noncompliant child. In R. C. Murrihy, A. D. Kidman, & T. H. Ollendick (Eds.), *Clinical handbook of assessing and treating conduct problems in youth* (pp. 163–191). New York: Springer.

McMahon, R. J., & Metzler, C. W. (1998). Selecting parenting measures for assessing family-based preventive interventions. In R. S. Ashery, E. B. Robertson, & K. L. Kumpfer (Eds.), *Drug abuse prevention through family interventions* (NIDA Research Monograph No. 177, pp. 294–323). Rockville, MD: National Institute on Drug Abuse.

McMahon, R. J., Tiedemann, G. L., Forehand, R., & Griest, D. L. (1984). Parental satisfaction with parent training to modify child noncompliance. *Behavior Therapy, 15,* 295–303.

McMahon, R. J., Wells, K. C., & Kotler, J. S. (2006). Conduct problems. In E. J. Mash & R. A. Barkley (Eds.), *Treatment of childhood disorders* (3rd ed., pp. 137–268). New York: Guilford Press.

Moffitt, T. E. (2006). Life-course-persistent versus adolescence-limited antisocial behavior. In D. Cicchetti & D. J. Cohen (Eds.), *Developmental psychopathology* (pp. 570–598). New York: Wiley.

Moffitt, T. E. (2017). Adolescence-limited and life-course persistence offending: A complementary pair of developmental theories. In T. P. Thornberry (Ed.), *Developmental theories of crime and delinquency* (2nd ed., pp. 11–54). New York: Routledge.

Moffitt, T. E., & Caspi, A. (2001). Childhood predictors differentiate life-course persistent and adolescence-limited antisocial pathways in males and females. *Development and Psychopathology, 13,* 355–376.

Morsbach, S. K., & Prinz, R. J. (2006). Understanding and improving the validity of self-report of parenting. *Clinical Child and Family Psychology Review, 9,* 1–21.

Muñoz, L. C., & Frick, P. J. (2007). The reliability, stability, and predictive utility of the self-report version of the Antisocial Process Screening Device. *Scandinavian Journal of Psychology, 48,* 299–312.

Muratori, P., Milone, A., Manfredi, A., Polidori, L., Ruglioni, L., Lambruschi, F., . . . Lochman, J. E. (2017). Evaluation of improvement in externalizing behaviors and callous–unemotional traits in children with disruptive behavior disorder: A 1-year follow up clinic-based study. *Administration and Policy in Mental Health and Mental Health Services Research, 44,* 452–462.

Muratori, P., Milone, A., Nocentini, A., Manfredi, A., Polidori, L., Ruglioni, L., . . . Lochman, J. E. (2015). Maternal depression and parenting practices predict treatment outcome in Italian children with disruptive behavior disorder. *Journal of Child and Family Studies, 24,* 2805–2816.

Muris, P., Meesters, C., de Kanter, E., & Timmerman, P. E. (2005). Behavioural inhibition and behavioural activation system scales for children: Relationships with Eysenck's personality traits and psychopathological symptoms. *Personality and Individual Differences, 38,* 831–841.

Niec, L. N., Barnett, M. L., Prewett, M. S., & Shanley

Chatham, J. R. (2016). Group parent–child interaction therapy: A randomized control trial for the treatment of conduct problems in young children. *Journal of Consulting and Clinical Psychology, 84,* 682–698.

Nock, M. K., Kazdin, A. E., Hiripi, E., & Kessler, R. C. (2006). Prevalence, subtypes, and correlates of DSM-IV conduct disorder in the National Comorbidity Survey Replication. *Psychological Medicine, 36,* 699–710.

Nock, M. K., & Kurtz, S. M. S. (2005). Direct behavioral observation in school settings: Bringing science to practice. *Cognitive and Behavioral Practice, 12,* 359–370.

Odgers, C. L., Caspi, A., Broadbent, J. M., Dickson, N., Hancox, R. J., . . . Moffitt, T. E. (2007). Prediction of differential adult health burden by conduct problem subtypes in males. *Archives of General Psychiatry, 64,* 476–484.

Odgers, C. L., Moffitt, T. E., Broadbent, J. M., Dickson, N., Hancox, R. J., Harrington, H., . . . Caspi, A. (2008). Female and male antisocial trajectories: From childhood origins to adult outcomes. *Development and Psychopathology, 20,* 673–716.

Pardini, D. A., Lochman, J. E., & Powell, N. (2007). The development of callous–unemotional traits and antisocial behavior in children: Are there shared and/or unique predictors? *Journal of Clinical Child and Adolescent Psychology, 36,* 319–333.

Pardini, D., Stepp, S., Hipwell, A., Stouthamer-Loeber, M., & Loeber, R. (2012). The clinical utility of the proposed DSM-5 callous–unemotional subtype of conduct disorder in young girls. *Journal of the American Academy of Child and Adolescent Psychiatry, 51,* 62–73.

Pas, E. T., Bradshaw, C. P., & Mitchell, M. M. (2011). Examining the validity of office discipline referrals as an indicator of student behavior problems. *Psychology in the Schools, 48,* 541–555.

Patterson, G. R., & Yoerger, K. (2002). A developmental model for early and late-onset delinquency. In J. B. Reid, G. R. Patterson, & J. Snyder (Eds.), *Antisocial behavior in children and adolescents: A developmental analysis and model for intervention* (pp. 147–172). Washington, DC: American Psychological Association.

Piacentini, J., Roper, M., Jensen, P., Lucas, C., Fisher, P., Bird, H., . . . Dulcan, M. (1999). Informant-based determinants of symptom attenuation in structured child psychiatric interviews. *Journal of Abnormal Child Psychology, 27,* 417–428.

Poythress, N. G., Dembo, R., Wareham, J., & Greenbaum, P. E. (2006). Construct validity of the Youth Psychopathic Traits Inventory (YPI) and the Antisocial Process Screening Device (APSD) with justice-involved adolescents. *Criminal Justice and Behavior, 33,* 26–55.

Reich, W. (2000). Diagnostic Interview for Children and Adolescents (DICA). *Journal of the American Academy of Child and Adolescent Psychiatry, 39,* 59–66.

Reynolds, C. R., & Kamphaus, R. W. (2015). *Behavior Assessment System for Children—3rd Edition (BASC-3).* Bloomington, MN: Pearson Assessments.

Rhule-Louie, D. M., McMahon, R. J., & Vando, J. (2009). Acceptability and representativeness of standardized parent–child interaction tasks. *Behavior Therapy, 40,* 393–402.

Robins, L. N. (1966). *Deviant children grown up.* Baltimore: Williams & Wilkins.

Rowe, R., Costello, J., Angold, A., Copeland, W. E., & Maughan, B. (2010). Developmental pathways in oppositional defiant disorder and conduct disorder. *Journal of Abnormal Psychology, 119,* 726–738.

Rusby, J. C., Taylor, T. K., & Foster, E. M. (2007). A descriptive study of school discipline referrals in first grade. *Psychology in the Schools, 44,* 333–350.

Russo, M. F., Stokes, G. S., Lahey, B. B., Christ, M. A. G., McBurnett, K., Loeber, R., . . . Green, S. M. (1993). A sensation seeking scale for children: Further refinement and psychometric development. *Journal of Psychopathology and Behavioral Assessment, 15,* 69–86.

Sanders, M. R., Baker, S., & Turner, K. M. (2012). A randomized controlled trial evaluating the efficacy of Triple P Online with parents of children with early-onset conduct problems. *Behaviour Research and Therapy, 50,* 675–684.

Sanders, M. R., & Woolley, M. L. (2005). The relationship between maternal self-efficacy and parenting practices: Implications for parent training. *Child: Care, Health and Development, 31,* 65–73.

Schmidt, F., Chomycz, S., Houlding, C., Kruse, A., & Franks, J. (2014). The association between therapeutic alliance and treatment outcomes in a group Triple P intervention. *Journal of Child and Family Studies, 23,* 1337–1350.

Shaffer, D., Fisher, P., Lucas, C. P., Dulcan, M. K., & Schwab-Stone, M. E. (2000). NIMH Diagnostic Interview Schedule for Children Version IV (NIMH DISC-IV): Description, differences from previous versions, and reliability of some common diagnoses. *Journal of the American Academy of Child and Adolescent Psychiatry, 39,* 28–38.

Shelton, K. K., Frick, P. J., & Wootton, J. (1996). Assessment of parenting practices in families of elementary school-age children. *Journal of Clinical Child Psychology, 25,* 317–329.

Stanger, C., Dumenci, L., Kamon, J., & Burstein, M. (2004). Parenting and children's externalizing problems in substance-abusing families. *Journal of Clinical Child and Adolescent Psychology, 33,* 590–600.

Stone, A. L., Becker, L. G., Huber, A. M., & Catalano, R. F. (2012). Review of risk and protective factors of substance use and problem use in emerging adulthood. *Addictive Behaviors, 37,* 747–775.

Stringaris, A., & Goodman, R. (2009). Longitudinal outcome of youth oppositionality: Irritable, headstrong, and hurtful behaviors have distinct predictions. *Journal of the American Academy of Child and Adolescent Psychiatry, 48,* 404–412.

Tibbetts, S. G., & Piquero, A. R. (1999). The influence of gender, low birth weight, and disadvantaged environment in predicting early onset of offending: A test of Moffitt's interactional hypothesis. *Criminology, 37,* 843–878.

Tobin, T. J., & Sugai, G. M. (1999). Using sixth-grade school records to predict school violence, chronic discipline problems, and high school outcomes. *Journal of Emotional and Behavioral Disorders, 7,* 40–53.

Van Kammen, W. B., Loeber, R., & Stouthamer-Loeber, M. (1991). Substance use and its relationships to conduct problems and delinquency in young boys. *Journal of Youth and Adolescence, 20,* 399–413.

Wakschlag, L. S., & Danis, B. (2004). Assessment of disruptive behaviors in young children: A clinical-developmental framework. In R. Del Carmen & A. Carter (Eds.), *Handbook of infant and toddler mental health assessment* (pp. 421–440). New York: Oxford University Press.

Waller, R., Gardner, F., Hyde, L. W., Shaw, D. S., Dishion, T. J., & Wilson, M. N. (2012). Do harsh and positive parenting predict parent reports of deceitful–callous behavior in early childhood? *Journal of Child Psychology and Psychiatry, 53,* 946–953.

Waschbusch, D. A. (2002). A meta-analytic examination of comorbid hyperactive–impulsive–attention problems and conduct problems. *Psychological Bulletin, 128,* 118–150.

Webster-Stratton, C., & Hammond, M. (1997). Treating children with early-onset conduct problems: A comparison of child and parent training programs. *Journal of Consulting and Clinical Psychology, 65,* 93–109.

Wilkinson, S., Waller, R., & Viding, E. (2016). Practitioner review: Involving young people with callous unemotional traits in treatment–does it work?: A systematic review. *Journal of Child Psychology and Psychiatry, 57,* 552–565.

Wolff, J. C., & Ollendick, T. H. (2006). The comorbidity of conduct problems and depression in childhood and adolescence. *Clinical Child and Family Psychology Review, 9,* 201–220.

World Health Organization. (2018). *International classification of diseases, 11th revision (ICD-11).* Geneva, Switzerland: Author.

Zisser-Nathenson, A. R., Herschell, A. D., & Eyberg, S. M. (2017). Parent–child interaction therapy and the treatment of disruptive behavior disorders. In J. R. Weisz & A. E. Kazdin (Eds.), *Evidence-based psychotherapies for children and adolescents* (3rd ed., pp. 103–121). New York: Guilford Press.

Zoccolillo, M. (1992). Co-occurrence of conduct disorder and its adult outcomes with depressive and anxiety disorders: A review. *Journal of the American Academy of Child and Adolescent Psychiatry, 31,* 547–556.

PART III

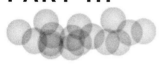

Internalizing Problems and Self-Harm

CHAPTER 7

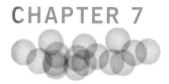

Depression

Benjamin L. Hankin and Joseph R. Cohen

Assessment is integral to all sciences, and assessment is fundamentally about measurement. The necessity of rigorous measurement is often most apparent when an error is made, such as when the Space Mountain roller coaster in Disneyland Tokyo suddenly broke and flew off the rails. An axle broke because of a measurement error in the design: English units were used instead of planned metric units. The incorrect sizing of the gap between axle and bearing (designed to be 0.2 mm, reality of over 1 mm) caused excessive stress and vibration that led the roller coaster to derail in 2003.

In the evidence-based assessment (EBA) movement, clinical decision making is expected to be grounded in a scientific literature. To date, much of the focus on measurement has centered around

reliability, and this emphasis on reproducibility is important—having clear, precise, reliable measurement (e.g., metric vs. U.S. customary units) is necessary to successfully and safely run a roller coaster. Equally important, though, is *what* is being measured. It is essential to have a clear connection between how something is being measured and the latent entity of what is measured as articulated in a conceptual model. The disaster of the Disneyland Space Mountain roller coaster was not a problem of the fundamental nature of *what* was being measured (i.e., metric vs. English units); rather, the problem was the translation of these instruments into practice (i.e., the how). In order to address the issue of depression assessment, it is critical for us to consider *what* pediatric depression is and *how* should we measure it.

This chapter comes at an important, interesting, and critical time in child clinical psychological science and allied mental health disciplines. Most past chapters and reviews of depression assessment since the DSM emerged as the dominant psychiatric classification starting with DSM-III in 1980, up to the present with the revised DSM-5, have had a clear and consistent view of depression. This chapter is situated in a potential historical inflection point, in that much of the knowledge that has been assumed and believed to be valid regarding depression and other psychiatric disorders has been questioned and critiqued (e.g., Krueger, 2018; Uher & Rutter, 2012). It is essential that any clinical researcher and applied practitioner be cognizant of the definition of depression, as there are various options to conceptualize what depression is (see Hankin, 2019). In addition to the familiar notion of DSM-defined depression as a categorical, episodic disorder, alternatives have been proposed for all psychopathologies (see Clark et al., 2017) and are receiving support. Recent structural models can organize depression and other psychopathologies from a hierarchical latent dimensional model (Caspi & Moffitt, 2018; Hankin, Snyder, Gulley, et al., 2016; Kotov et al., 2017; Lahey, Krueger, Rathouz, Waldman, & Zald, 2017). As we discuss throughout the chapter, we urge researchers and practitioners to think carefully about what they are measuring because the selection of a depression measure depends on the conceptual notion of what depression is and will inform various decision in the assessment process.

We hope that this chapter illuminates the steps in the assessment process to assist with EBA that clearly meets the needs of the clinical scientist and applied practitioner. The first part of this chapter reviews *what* depression is as a construct to be assessed. We discuss in the second half of the chapter *how* to choose different methods used for depression assessment and how to leverage these tools to guide EBA. We also review measures and procedures to evaluate depression outcomes and monitor change related to depression interventions. Throughout, we consider practical decision points that face both clinical researchers and applied practitioners.

Definitions, Conceptualizations, and Models of Depression

We provide a brief summary of taxonic approaches typically used to define *what* depression is (e.g., Compas, Ey, & Grant, 1993). We briefly discuss the first two dimensional options, then elaborate on the final categorical diagnostic approach that is most commonly used. Of the simple dimensional perspectives, first is depressed *mood*. Here, one conceptualizes depression from an affective, mood-based perspective, including phenomenology such as unhappiness, sadness, feeling down or blue, and so forth. Depressed mood is typically assessed via youth self-reported checklists. On the basis of adolescents' self-reports, approximately 20–35% of boys and 25–40% of girls report depressed mood (Petersen et al., 1993). Second, depression can also be considered as a "syndrome," which is defined

as an empirically determined grouping of emotions (e.g., depressed mood), behaviors, thoughts, and symptoms that statistically cohere in multivariate analyses (e.g., factor analysis). Here, depression is conceived as quantitative deviations in a set of symptoms (e.g., feeling lonely, nervous, unloved, guilty, sad; needing to be perfect; crying) that vary on a continuum. Depression as a syndrome is most frequently assessed via checklists that multiple informants (e.g., youth, parent, clinician, teacher) can complete (e.g, the Achenbach System of Empirically Based Assessment [ASEBA] set of instruments that can provide an assessment of the anxious–depressed syndrome; Achenbach & Recorla, 2001). Under a syndrome view, depression varies continuously, so cutoff scores are applied to arrive at base rates and prevalence estimates.

Categorically, depression is defined as a *diagnosis* within a psychiatric nosological system. Currently, DSM-5 represents the most dominant perspective on whether a child/adolescent *is* or *is not* depressed. The most common forms of depression diagnoses within this taxonomy are major depressive disorder (MDD), dysthymia, or other specified or underspecified disorder. For MDD, certain symptoms (i.e., depressed mood, irritability, or anhedonia) are deemed essential to qualify an individual child for a depression diagnosis, whereas other symptoms (e.g., feelings of worthlessness, suicidality, eating problems, sleep problems) can be, but need not be, present. The individual must endorse at least five symptoms, one of which must be an essential criterial symptom, and these symptoms must last "most of the day, nearly every day" for a minimum of 2 weeks. Regarding dysthymia, at least two out of six symptoms must be endorsed "more often than not" for at least 1 year in youth. Cross-sectionally ascertained base rates of a DSM-based diagnosis (MDD or dysthymia) from a large U.S. national sample of adolescents (ages 13–18) find a lifetime prevalence of 11.7%, and these prevalence rates increase with age. Longitudinal studies of youth from the general community who have been repeatedly interviewed over time likewise show surges in depression diagnoses from childhood into late adolescence (e.g., around 3% in early adolescence, rising to around 17% by age 18; Hankin et al., 1998, 2015).

An *unspecified depressive disorder* is defined as a form of depression that causes impairment but does not meet the threshold for MDD or dysthymia. For example, a child or adolescent presenting with depressed mood, sleep problems, and fatigue (i.e., three symptoms), but not other symptoms or diagnoses, may be diagnosed with a depressive disorder with the insufficient symptoms specifier. Thus, even within categorical frameworks of depression, there is an ability to incorporate some dimensional perspectives concerning the nature of depression.

Outside the context of DSM-5, the *International Statistical Classifications of Diseases* (ICD-11), represents the other dominant classification perspective relevant to depression diagnoses. Changes from ICD-10 to ICD-11, however, result in the two classification systems being fairly similar across the two disorders (e.g., five symptoms are necessary in both, with at least one being depressed mood, irritability, or anhedonia). The main difference is that consistent across versions of and disorders within ICD-11, there are more formal depression clusters (e.g., neurovegetative cluster) that can be labeled within this taxonomy (Chakrabarti, 2018).

Neither DSM-5 nor ICD-11 necessarily make official claims that a depression diagnosis is qualitatively discrete from normality (i.e., the categorical vs. dimensional classification debate). In other words, the categorical approach functions as a heuristic and is based on pragmatic needs: It is an efficient way to summarize and communicate information in putatively reliable ways that could inform decision making, treatment, reimbursement, and policy. For DSM-5, the practical need is typically for practitioners to have a diagnosis to guide treatment planning and routine assessment, while for ICD-11, it is typically to understand the prevalence of disorders from a public health perspective. We assume that for readers of this chapter, the DSM-5 definition of MDD may be the most relevant framework for defining *what* depression is, so we provide more context on this depression definition below.

Assumptions and Questions Regarding DSM-Defined Depression

It is important to note that there are strengths, as well as significant assumptions and concerns, related to a categorically based diagnostic approach. There is positive value in having a categorical diagnostic label that serves a useful heuristic purpose for practical clinical needs, such as quickly summarizing and communicating symptom information about a child in a possibly reliable manner that improves decision making, treatment planning, symptom monitoring, forecasting, and policy. Still, there are well-documented concerns (e.g., Berenbaum, 2013; Kendell & Jablensky,

2003; Kendler, 2012; Lilienfeld, Smith, & Watts, 2013; Rutter, 2013; Uher & Rutter, 2012; Widiger & Clark, 2000). Most notably from an EBA-perspective, there are concerns about reliability and validity of a DSM-based conceptualization of depression. Regarding reliability, the most recent DSM-5 field trials showed surprisingly low levels of reliability for diagnosing MDD (Freedman et al., 2013): interrater reliability kappas of .28 for adults and children. Contributing to challenges in reliability, there are an astoundingly high number of combinations of symptoms (e.g., up to 1,030 unique symptom profile combinations that can be diagnosed under MDD; Fried & Nesse, 2015) that can yield an MDD diagnosis, suggesting that a DSM-oriented MDD diagnosis is a highly heterogeneous and fuzzy category. Typically, reliability is seen as necessary to establish validity, and this level of interrater agreement is problematic.

Regarding validity, Uher and Rutter (2012) concluded the following about the scientific foundation for modern psychiatric classifications: "Most published psychiatric research is predicated on the validity of classification. . . . (The lack of validity) is the most important reason why most published research is uninformative. . . . Psychiatric research must discard the false assumptions that current classification is valid" (p. 601). Thus, many may presently choose to use a categorical approach to depression, such as that defined by DSM, for practical reasons (e.g., you work in a health care setting that requires diagnostic codes). At the same time, the conceptual and empirical foundation, based on its reliability and validity, is questionable. There are different options for optimal and most valid classification approaches to psychopathology (Clark et al., 2017), and depression specifically (Hankin, 2019). But given the current dominance of DSM-5 classification in assessment, especially for practical reasons, we necessarily proceed under this perspective, while highlighting that conceptual models undergirding the definition of depression could change and thus affect assessment practice in the future.

A long-standing debate concerns whether a depressive episode, as diagnosed via MDD, is categorical or dimensional in nature. The preponderance of research using taxometric analyses shows that depression, even when conceptualized taxonically as a diagnosis using DSM-based criteria, is dimensionally distributed (Hankin, Fraley, Lahey, & Waldman, 2005; Liu, 2016). As such, assessments ideally should ascertain the presence of milder forms of depression with enduring symptom presentations that do not formally meet official DSM-based criteria for a MDD diagnosis (e.g., other specified or underspecified disorder). Note that the research shows that depression is dimensional *at the latent trait*; an arbitrary categorical cutoff can be applied to an actual dimensional measure for practical, clinical purposes and thus debates about where these cutoff points should be made (e.g., Child Depression Inventory [CDI] > 15; Child Behavior Checklist [CBCL] *T*-score > 70).

There exists strong overlap between depression and other psychiatric diagnoses. Angold, Costello, and Erklani (1999), in their meta-analytic review, demonstrated substantial, significant concurrent co-occurrence between pairs of single psychiatric disorder classes, including between depression and anxiety disorders (median odds ratio [OR] = 8.2) behavioral disorders (OR = 6.6), and attention-deficit/hyperactivity disorder (ADHD; OR = 5.5). These and other reviewers (e.g., Avenevoli, Stolar, Li, Dierker, & Ries Merikangas, 2001; Garber & Weersing, 2010; Yorbik, Birmaher, Axelson, Williamson, & Ryan, 2004) estimate that 15–75% of depressed youth carry a comorbid diagnosis. These comorbidity patterns are important to take into account when conducting an assessment, as the individual presenting with depressed mood, loss of interest, or other common symptoms will likely need to be evaluated for other, co-occurring behavioral and emotional problems; one should not assume that depression is the sole or primary problem.

How Measurement Models Affect Assessment

We know that you as the reader are sorely tempted to bypass and skip over this section; eyes most likely glaze over upon seeing the words "psychometrics" and "measurement models," and the desire to skim is alluring. Our aim here is to illustrate the importance of how different measurement models can affect clinical researchers' and applied practitioners' selection and interpretation of depression measurement tools. The ensuing results and data from the depression assessment enterprise and process are grounded in one's conceptualization of what depression is and how one defines its meaning, as discussed earlier, as well as how accurately the measurement model of an assessment tool matches the conceptual construct of that definition. Unfortunately, researchers and applied practitioners (including the authors of this chapter for many years!) frequently assume that published and commonly used depression measures must be

reliable and valid enough to use, and besides, what big difference would it make anyway? In graduate training, everyone learns about the usual reliability indicators showing that a measure is acceptable to use (e.g., decent internal consistency with coefficient alpha > .70, moderate test–retest reliability, reasonable criterion validity). So long as these traditional psychometric thresholds are met, the measure is frequently deemed reliable and valid for assessment.

But it is not so simple. Here we summarize main concerns from psychometrics that affect traditional, routine depression assessment. In short, just as the designers of the Disneyland Space Mountain roller coaster assumed that their measurement model was accurate (metric vs. English units), the lack of a clear and deliberate consideration of a precise measurement model that reflects the intended purpose can unknowingly yield poor results and unintended consequences. The underlying measurement model optimally needs to reflect the core theoretical notion of what depression is; poor connection between the measurement model and depression conceptualization may yield data and results that are not what the clinical researcher and applied practitioner meant or intended to obtain from the assessment procedure. Borsboom (2006) articulated primary psychometric considerations in measurement and how these can affect what psychologists do in research and clinical assessment. He cautions that "measurement problems abound in psychology" (p. 425), and "the daily practice of psychological measurement is plagued by highly questionable interpretations of psychological test scores" (p. 426).

First, any measure (e.g., self-report of depressive symptoms, such as the CDI) is not fully equivalent with the theoretical attribute (e.g., construct of depression). Instead, there is a measurement model that relates the observable scores on a test (CDI) with the theoretical construct (depression). In other words, pure operationalism, or the notion that the "CDI equals depression" is incorrect and problematic. Second, most psychologists learn about classical test theory (CTT) in introductory research methods and assessment classes. Central to CTT is the idea of a test having a true score and error; *true score* on a test is defined as the expectation of a test score over a series of many observations and repeated administrations, and *error* is observations that are inconsistent with the true score. The primary concern with sole emphasis on CTT for depression measurement is that CTT implicitly equates the theoretical attribute with expected test scores. The result of unknowingly accepting CTT as the measurement model for depression assessments is that the clinical scientist or applied practitioner accepts an individual's observed scores on a traditional depression measure (e.g., CDI score of 19) as equaling that adolescent's true depression amount (i.e., level of "depression"). Additionally, CTT is based on particular assumptions that likely do not hold for a heterogeneous, fuzzy construct such as depression. In particular, CTT assumes that (1) there is a single latent variable that produces the manifest depression item scores, (2) all of the disparate symptom items on a depression scale are interchangeable and measure the same singular latent variable, and (3) this latent variable is unidimensional. Frequently, practitioners using a depression scale believe they can simply add up the items to get a single score. However, considerable psychometric work shows that this easy approach of adding up manifest depression items on a scale does not hold because depression scale measures are not unidimensional, and depression severity cannot be reflected in one singular sum score (Fried et al., 2016).

These formal measurement models are not only academic but also essential: The Disneyland Tokyo Space Mountain designers have the advantage over psychologists of working from a suitable theoretical model of *what* length is, but they still need an accurate and replicable measurement model for *how* to assess length using a consistent unit (English vs. metric) to make the roller coaster work. As Borsboom (2006, p. 435) summarizes, the problem is that "the crucial decisions in psychological measurement are made on the basis of pragmatic or conventional grounds, instead of substantive considerations." For an EBA approach to depression to advance, clinical research needs to continue investigating what the latent construct of depression is, whether it is a unitary construct (as is often assumed in our measurement models and everyday assessments), how is depression best structured and organized (e.g., categorical diagnosis or as dimensional latent construct), and whether the construct and measurement of depression changes or is relatively invariant across development.

Developmental Considerations in Depression Conceptualizations

Information on continuity across time and age-related expression of depressive symptoms has important implications for assessment. If depression varies across the developmental lifespan, than targeted assessments of the most salient symptoms based on age are needed. However, it is common-

place for similar diagnostic interviews and rating/questionnaire methods to be used across many developmental levels and ages (e.g., ages 8–18). Overall, little research has systematically examined reliability, validity, and clinical utility of common depression assessments across different age groups. Most clinical researchers and applied practitioners assume that depression can be assessed with the most frequently used instruments equivalently across wide age ranges; there is not an evidence-based developmental adjustment or differential scoring applied given different developmental levels.

Regarding continuity of depression from adolescence into young adulthood, considerable research indicates that adolescent-onset depression forecasts later depression into adulthood in both community (e.g., Lewinsohn, Rohde, Klein, & Seeley, 1999; Pine, Cohen, Gurley, Brook, & Ma, 1998) and clinical (Weissman et al., 1999) samples. The degree of continuity from childhood into adolescence, however, is less consistent. There appears to be a subset of individuals with childhood-onset depression, such as those with recurrent depression during childhood or with a family history (Weissman et al., 1999), who progress to experience depression later in adulthood. Other longitudinal research suggests that a majority of childhood-onset depression is discontinuous (Cohen, Andrews, Davis, & Rudolph, 2018) and may signal other externalizing patterns of psychopathology and adjustment problems later in life (e.g., Harrington, Fudge, Rutter, Pickles, & Hill, 1990).

In addition to these results, the pattern of when the sex difference in depression emerges further suggests that there may be relatively greater discontinuity from childhood depression into adolescence. Prior to early adolescence or middle puberty, prevalence rates of depression are relatively equal between boys and girls, but then the well-known sex difference in depression (twice as many females compared to males) skyrockets in adolescents and adults (Hankin & Abramson, 2001; Hankin et al., 1998, 2015; Salk, Hyde, & Abramson, 2017). Taken together, such findings have been interpreted as implying that certain childhood-onset depressive disorders, such as those comorbid with disruptive behavioral disorders, may represent a different expression of depression than individuals with adolescent- or adult-onset depression.

A significant line of research in the last 10–15 years has focused on investigating preschool depression, and the impressive, expanding body of accumulated literature shows that depression among preschoolers can be reliably identified and assessed (Luby, 2010; Luby et al., 2002). Validity for the existence of preschool depression derives from research documenting various risk factors (e.g., negative and positive emotionality, dysregulated cortisol, cortical thickness, neural circuitry; Dougherty, Klein, Olino, Dyson, & Rose, 2009; Gaffrey, Barch, Singer, Shenoy, & Luby, 2013; Luby et al., 2016; Shankman et al., 2011), recognizing the longitudinal course of homotypic continuity and recurrence (Bufferd, Dougherty, Carlson, Rose, & Klein, 2012; Luby, Gaffrey, Tillman, April, & Belden, 2014; Luby, Si, Belden, Tandon, & Spitznagel, 2009), and establishing negative outcomes, impairment, and features (linked with depressive symptoms at this age) (Bufferd et al., 2014; Whalen, Sylvester, & Luby, 2017).

A key issue for assessment is whether symptom expressions of depression are the same across development. If not, then different assessment measures (e.g., interviews, rating scales, or questionnaires) are needed that more carefully map onto the symptom manifestations typical of a particular age group. DSM-5 generally asserts that there are not major age-related effects on the course or treatment of MDD, or in the symptom presentation, although the diagnostic guide suggests hypersomnia and excessive eating are more likely in younger individuals (ages not specified), whereas melancholia and psychomotor disturbances are more common in older individuals. The diagnostic system permits irritable mood to count as a criterial mood symptom instead of sad/depressed mood for MDD; DSM-5 allows a shorter duration (1 year) for dysthymia as opposed to minimum duration of 2 years in adults. Still, other descriptive developmental phenomenological research suggests that adolescents are more likely than children to report hopelessness, anhedonia, vegetative (e.g., sleeping and eating) and motivational symptoms, and younger children are more likely to appear sad and express somatic complaints (Weiss & Garber, 2003). At present, there is not a clear and consistent picture regarding possible age-related systematic symptom expressions in MDD. DSM-5, as the official classification system, predominantly asserts that the symptom picture is similar in children, adolescents, and adults, with the allowable exception of irritability as a mood symptom for youth.

Measurement Overview

Recent years have brought an emphasis on EBAs within the context of mental health (e.g., Hunsley, 2015; Hunsley & Mash, 2007; Jensen-Doss, 2015; Stiffler & Dever, 2015; Youngstrom, Halverson, Youngstrom, Lindhiem, & Findling, 2017), including focused reviews on best practices for assessing depression (e.g., Klein, Dougherty, & Olino, 2005; Mash & Barkley, 2007; Rudolph & Lambert, 2007; Siu et al., 2016). Yet few reviewers discuss how the assessment protocol may vary as a function of definitional differences of depression, the setting, and the ultimate aim of that specific protocol. Furthermore, only recently has a literature base emerged around evidence-based decision making, including the use of multiple assessment strategies (e.g., De Los Reyes, 2013; Martel, Markon, & Smith, 2017). Below, we review the state of the science on different assessment protocols for depression in youth. We then contextualize these different assessment protocols within specific clinical and research settings. We conclude by discussing qualitative rubrics and quantitative algorithms that can be used to leverage the strengths of different assessment methods, and bring the promise of EBA strategies to larger depression prevention and intervention initiatives.

Diagnostic Interviews

Diagnostic interviews have long been seen as the "gold standard" for child and adolescent depression assessment (Klein et al., 2005). Diagnostic interviews can be dichotomized into "unstructured" and "structured" approaches. Unstructured diagnostic interviews are idiosyncratic methods that vary by clinician for determining whether someone is presenting with or is at risk for depression. Temporal, educational, and financial resources have all been stated reasons why unstructured diagnostic assessments may be more commonly used in depression assessment compared to structured or semistructured approaches (D'Angelo & Augenstein, 2012). Yet as these approaches are less reliable and valid (Angold & Costello, 2000; Lauth, Levy, Júlíusdóttir, Ferrari, & Pétursson, 2008; Zimmerman, 2003) due to their susceptibility to biases, their use is incongruent with an EBA.

"Structured interviews" are defined as standardized protocols in which the presence or absence of a depression diagnosis (based on specific criteria; e.g., DSM diagnoses) is determined via a set of predetermined questions and probes. Diagnostic interviews often include contextual information on specific symptoms endorsed, duration, and past history of depression (Angold, Costello, Messer, & Pickles, 1995; Kaufman et al., 1997). The majority of structured interview protocols include both parent and child self-report versions that should ideally be administered to both the youth and caregiver within a single protocol. Structured interviews are not only reliable but can also facilitate dissemination and collaboration by providing a shared language among treatment teams (Ely, Graber, & Croskerry, 2011; Leffler, Riebel, & Hughes, 2015).

The broad category of structured interviews can be further separated into semistructured and fully structured interviews. Semistructured interviews, also referred to as "interviewer based," because the interviewer is responsible for determining whether the criteria for a given symptom or diagnosis reaches the predetermined threshold, provide the most flexibility within an assessment protocol. To make a symptom or diagnostic-based decision, the interviewer uses all information at his or her disposal, and when needed, asks additional questions to clarify discrepant or vague responses. Fully structured interviews, sometimes referred to as "respondent based," limit the interviewer to the predetermined list of questions.

A further (and related) distinction is made between "filtered" and "unfiltered" interview administrations. A "filtered" approach assesses for other disorders beyond depression and includes lifetime mental health history. "Filtered" approaches can be either semistructured or structured in nature. Meanwhile, an "unfiltered" approach focuses solely on whether a depression symptom is present or not, regardless of comorbid diagnoses or lifetime history; these approaches are fully structured (Findling et al., 2010; Yee et al., 2015).

Typically, mental health professionals or technicians/students, performing tasks under supervision of a licensed mental health professional, conduct semistructured and filtered interviews. Meanwhile, structured and unfiltered diagnostic interviews can be used within a public health or primary care setting when the availability of trained mental health professionals may be limited (e.g., Angold & Costello, 2000). Semistructured approaches may be especially valuable when evaluating depression with members of a population who possess limited insight into their thoughts, feelings, and behaviors (e.g., when working with younger children; Klein et al., 2005). For clinical and diagnostic purposes, we recommend a "filtered" approach that queries about other, potentially comorbid childhood diagnoses (e.g., anxiety, ADHD) given the strong co-occurrence of depression with other emotional and behavioral diagnoses. On the other hand, if using a more dimensional approach, an "unfiltered" approach can provide

a more rapid assessment of impairing internalizing symptoms regardless of diagnostic classification.

To date, the five most commonly used structured diagnostic interviews for children and adolescents (see Table 7.1)v include the Child and Adolescent Psychiatric Assessment (CAPA; Angold & Costello, 2000), the Schedule for Affective Disorders and Schizophrenia for School-Age Children (K-SADS; Kaufman et al., 1997), the Children's Interview for Psychiatric Syndromes (ChIPS; Weller, Fristad, Weller, & Rooney, 1999), the Diagnostic Interview Schedule for Children (DISC; Shaffer, Fisher, Lucas, Dulcan, & Schwab-Stone, 2000), and the Mini-International Neuropsychiatric Interview for Children and Adolescents (MINI-KID; Sheehan, Shytle, Milo, Janavs, & Lecrubier, 2009) (see Leffler et al., 2015, for a review of these diagnostic assessments). All include unipolar depression modules and other diagnostic modules to assess co-occurring symptoms and disorders. Overall, there is little evidence to suggest that one diagnostic interview is superior to another when making diagnoses in youth (Costello, Egger, & Angold, 2005). Instead, selection of any given interview relies on weighing the pros and cons of each interview based on the objective and setting for the given protocol. Next, we review two of the more widely used interviews, which are also free to download and use if specific degree requirements are met.

The K-SADS, the most commonly used depression assessment within research contexts (Klein et al., 2005), is a semistructured, interviewer-driven measure that allows some flexibility in how depressive episodes are probed and coded (Kaufman et al., 1997). The most thorough version of the K-SADS is the Present and Lifetime version (K-SADS-PL), although versions that focus only on the present episode (e.g., KSADS-PE) or one's lifetime (K-SADS-E) exist for other purposes (e.g., the K-SADS-E is designed for epidemiological research) (Leffler et al., 2015). Both caretaker and child are often interviewed to ascertain depression diagnoses. In addition to being psychometrically sound and free to use, the K-SADS has significant advantages to assess depression. First, it covers a wide range of mental health diagnoses within a large age range (6–18 years), so that diagnostic symptom specificity can be assessed reliably and validly across ages. Second, as a semistructured interview, one can tailor the questions to assess potentially challenging symptoms in youth (e.g., anhedonia). Relatedly, the flexibility inherent in the interview makes it easier to assess for depression in a more dimension-

TABLE 7.1. Review of Diagnostic Interviews

	Informant	Parent version (age)	Youth version (age)	Format of item administration	Format of response style	Cost and access	Administration time (for full interview in minutes)	Rater qualifications and training
CAPA	Parent and child	9–18	9–18	Structured with the option for additional semistructured inquires	Closed-ended (Y/N), mix of closed-ended (Likert) and open-ended	Information available through the Developmental Epidemiology Center at Duke University	60–120 min	Bachelor's degree plus required training by individuals trained on this interview
ChIPS	Parent or child	6–18	6–18	Structured with the option for additional semistructured inquires	Closed-ended (Y/N)	Approximately $90; available through various retailers	20–50 min	Trained layperson supervised by a licensed clinician; administration manual includes training materials
DISC-IV	Parent or child	6–17	9–17	Structured	Closed-ended (Y/N)	Ranges from $150 to $2,000 per computer installation; charge for paper version is minimal to cover copying and mailing expenses; e-mail disc@worldnet.att.net	90–120 min	Layperson supervised by a licensed clinician; training is strongly recommended; details on training available by contacting disc@worldnet.att.net
K-SADS-PL 2009	Parent and child	6–18	6–18	Semistructured	Closed-ended (Likert) and open-ended	Free for download and use if specific criteria are met	90 min	Trained professional; training is required
MINI-KIDS	Parent or child	6–17	13–17	Structured	Closed-ended (Y/N)	Free for download and use if specific criteria are met	15–50 min	Trained layperson supervised by a licensed clinician; training by licensed clinician is recommended

Note. CAPA, Child and Adolescent Psychiatric Assessment (Angold & Costello, 2000); ChIPS, Children's Interview for Psychiatric Syndromes (Weller et al., 2000); DISC-IV, NIMH Diagnostic Interview Schedule for Children–IV (Shaffer et al., 2000); K-SADS-PL, Schedule for Affective Disorders and Schizophrenia for School-Age Children—Present and Lifetime Version (Kaufman et al., 1997); MINI-KIDS, Mini-International Neuropsychiatric Interview for Children and Adolescents (Sheehan et al., 2009).

al manner. For instance, inclusion of "minor depression," or the DSM-5 diagnosis of other specific depressive disorder, can easily be assessed with the K-SADS depression module. The biggest limitation to using the K-SADS is the significant time burden. The interview, when administered in its totality with all diagnostic modules, can take up to 3 hours to complete with both parent and youth as informants (Leffler et al., 2015). Using an "unfiltered" approach (i.e., only asking about current depression symptoms), or asking about symptoms for specific disorders within fewer modules (e.g., social anxiety or oppositional defiant disorder) can substantially reduce the time burden.

The MINI-KID is a structured, respondent-driven interview that can be used with youth between ages 6 and 17 years. Similar to the K-SADS-PL, the depression module includes questions about symptoms occurring in the past 2 weeks, as well as over one's lifetime, and includes options for both parent and youth report (Sheehan et al., 2009). The MINI-KID also includes a structured, 14-item suicide interview following the depression section. The structured nature of the interview lends itself to settings in which quicker administrations and less-intensive training are needed, for instance, in settings in which beginning trainees conduct the majority of the assessments. In total, it has been estimated that the MINI-KID takes between 15 and 50 minutes to complete based on individuals' responses to the introductory screening questions for each diagnostic module (Leffler et al., 2015). The limitations include the brief structured interview that limits decision making on severity of certain symptoms and reduces the chance of a thorough diagnostic evaluation, including assessment of potentially comorbid psychiatric disorders.

One option is pairing the MINI-KID with an intensive depressive symptom rating scale. For instance, the Children's Depression Rating Scale—Revised (CDRS-R; Poznanski & Mokros, 1996) has become a popular option for assessing severity of depression and change in depressive symptoms, especially in psychopharmacological and psychotherapy randomized clinical trials with youth (Myers & Winters, 2002; Varigonda et al., 2015). As a structured interview of 17 items, trained mental health clinicians administer the CDRS-R; there are caretaker and youth versions. It shows reliability and validity in indicating depression diagnostic status (Mayes, Bernstein, Haley, Kennard, & Emslie, 2010). The CDRS-R is not free and does not assess for symptoms other than depression. Therefore, the CDRS-R is typically included with

another diagnostic interview or used when comorbid diagnoses may be less of a concern.

Questionnaire Symptom Scales

Due to their convenience, the most common manner for assessing depression is via questionnaire-based rating scales (Myers & Winters, 2002; Rudolph & Lambert, 2007). Rating scales are reliable and valid markers of depression symptom severity over time for both research and clinical purposes (Brooks & Kutcher, 2001; Myers & Winters, 2002; Stockings et al., 2015). Still, despite their widespread use, the limitations of using rating scales for depression assessments are well documented. Research shows mixed results for using questionnaires as index tests (i.e., predictors in a protocol) to ascertain depression diagnostic status (Fristad, Emery, & Beck, 1997; Stockings et al., 2015). For example, past research indicates that over 80% of depressed patients will be missed when using published cutoffs on the CDI for MDD (Matthey & Petrovski, 2002). Although some have recommended that using lower cutoffs will improve the validity of these symptoms scales (Cohen, So, Young, Hankin, & Lee, 2019; Timbremont, Braet, & Dreessen, 2004) issues with sensitivity (i.e., correctly identifying a youth as depressed) and specificity (i.e., properly classifying a youth as nondepressed) persist.

Another criticism of traditionally used rating scales is that the inventories typically measure facets of depression (e.g., academic impairment, behavioral problems at school, anxiety symptoms) that are not formally part of DSM-5's official diagnostic criteria for MDD. Depending on the objective of the assessment, this may be a strength or limitation. For example, for a dimensional perspective of depression, inclusion of comorbid symptoms or correlated impairment may identify youth at higher severity of depression. Alternatively, within a categorical perspective, inclusion of these items introduces contamination into measurement, possibly contributing to issues of using rating scales as an index of depression diagnostic status (Fristad et al., 1997). A second criticism is that most depression rating scales do not directly measure key timing facets of depression (e.g., duration of a potential depressive episode; persistence of symptoms); rather, most questionnaires ask about experience of symptoms in a circumscribed time window (e.g, the past 2 weeks). These contextual data, which are integrated into diagnostic interviews, may be key to accurately ascertaining whether someone is depressed. Thus, rating scales may best be viewed as a marker of depression severity (within a dimensional perspective) for a circumscribed time period. Next, we review some of the more common methods for assessing depression with rating scales (see Table 7.2). Similar to diagnostic interviews, there is little evidence that any given scale is superior, and selection of an inventory depends on the assessment purpose and resources of the setting.

The ASEBA (Achenbach & Rescorla, 2001) represents the most common symptom scale used in child and adolescent mental health research and services (De Los Reyes et al., 2015; Rosanbalm et al., 2016). The rating scales include the Youth Self-Report (YSR), the CBCL, and the Teacher Report Form (TRF) to provide a multi-informant perspective on internalizing and externalizing psychopathology in children and adolescents. The measure can be used with youth between ages 6 and 18. Relevant to depression, there is both a DSM-oriented subscale (Affective Disorders) and three syndrome subscales (Withdrawn/Depressed, Anxious/Depressed, and Somatic Symptoms) that together form the Internalizing Subscale related to the disorder. The Anxious/Depressed subscale has the most robust support as an assessment for MDD. Area under the curves (AUCs) and diagnostic likelihood ratios (DLRs) for different cutoff scores have been published in the literature across both clinical and community populations, facilitating its use as a depression assessment tool (for up-to-date psychometric information, see https://en.wikiversity.org/wiki/Evidence-based_assessment/Depression_in_youth). A limitation is length, as each informant scale (YSR, CBCL, and TRF) includes over 100 items.

The Strengths and Difficulties Questionnaire (SDQ) is comparable to the ASEBA. Moreover, it is briefer and measures impairment (Goodman, 2001). The SDQ Internalizing subscale performs similarly to the CBCL Internalizing subscales for detecting symptoms of broad, general emotional distress (Goodman & Scott, 1999). Another advantage of the SDQ is that it is free to use, unlike the ASEBA system. At the same time, the SDQ Emotional Symptoms subscale only contains five items and likely lacks discriminant validity for depression versus co-occurring anxiety problems; this limitation potentially necessitates pairing the SDQ with a more depression-centric self-report measure for a more thorough assessment.

The most common rating scale used in the depression literature is the CDI (Myers & Winters,

2002; Stockings et al., 2015). Different than the AESBA scales, the CDI was designed to function as a measure specifically for depressive symptoms in childhood and adolescence (7- to 18-year-olds). The CDI-2, the newest version, includes self-, parent-, and teacher-report versions with recommended cutoff scores (Kovacs, 2010). The CDI-2 also includes subscales that puport to assess specific symptom clusters related to depression (i.e., Negative Mood, Interpersonal Problems, Ineffectiveness, Anhedonia, and Negative Self-Esteem), which may be useful for individuals assessing depression within an ICD-11 framework.[1] In the past, the CDI has been criticized as a self-report measure because it includes questions outside DSM symptom criteria for MDD (Cole, Truglio, & Peeke, 1997; Craighead, Smucker, Wilcoxon Craighead, & Ilardi, 1998), and having relatively weak reliability for discriminating between DSM-based depressed and nondepressed youth (Fristad et al., 1997; Matthey & Petrovski, 2002; Saylor, Finch, Spirito, & Bennett, 1984). Yet in a recent review, the relation between the CDI and a diagnostic interview was similar to the Beck Depression Inventory (BDI; the adult version of the CDI), the Center for Epidemiological Studies Depression Scale (CES-D), and the Reynolds Adolescent Depression Scale (RADS; Stockings et al., 2015). A reasonable, free alternative to the CDI is using the CES-D (Radloff, 1977). The 10-item version of the CES-D can adequately identify depressive impairment (Haroz, Ybarra, & Eaton, 2014).

Increasingly, governmental and professional agencies are encouraging that universal depression screening begin at age 12. It is likely with increasing research that this recommendation will be extended downward to younger populations (Siu et al., 2016). Along with substance use, this makes depression the only pediatric psychiatric/psychological disorder in which universal screening is recommended by the U.S. Preventive Services Task Force (USPSTF). The CBCL, SDQ, CDI, and CES-D can be used, and have been recommended for this purpose (Siu et al., 2016; Stockings et al., 2015). However, others have suggested a multigated approach to screening, in which even briefer depression screening inventories are used

---

[1] We note that a number of proposed cutoff scores and symptom subscales reported in the literature are not included in the official CDI manual. Furthermore, the Anhedonia subscale included in the manual contains eight items, while the subscale commonly used in research only has six items. Consideration of these differences is necessary when making comparisons across clinical and research settings.

TABLE 7.2. Rating Scales for Depression

	Reporter	Age	Minutes to complete	Test–retest reliability	Construct validity	Content validity	AUC and DLRs available?	Cost and access
Mood and Feelings Questionnaire	Youth	6–17	5–10 min	Adequate	Good	Adequate	No	Free to download
Children's Depression Inventory (CDI and CDI-2)	Youth and parent	7–17	15–20 min	Adequate	Good	Adequate	Yes	Pricing varies, available at *www.pearsonassessments.com*
Revised Children's Anxiety and Depression Scale	Youth	6–18	12 min	Adequate	Good	Adequate	No	Free, available at *www.corc.uk.net/outcome-experience-measures/revised-childrens-anxiety-and-depression-scale-and-subscales*
Strength and Difficulties Questionnaire	Youth and parent	4–17	5–10 min	Good	Adequate	Adequate	Yes	Free, *available at www.sdqinfo.com*
Patient Health Questionnaire–9 (modified for adolescents)	Youth	12–17	3–5 min	Good	Good	Good	Yes	Free to download
Achenbach Scales (YSR/CBCL)	Youth (YSR) and parent (CBCL)	6–18	15–30 min	Good	Adequate	Adequate	Yes	Pricing varies, at *https://aseba.org/aseba-overview*

Note. For further information on these rating scales, see *https://en.wikiversity.org/wiki/Evidence-based_assessment/Depression_in_youth.*

in pediatric and school contexts (Lavigne, Feldman, & Meyers, 2016; Stiffler & Dever, 2015). As such, two items from the Patient Health Questionnaire–2 (PHQ-2) represent a reliable and valid approach. More commonly used with adults, the PHQ-2, which consists of two questions for depressed mood and anhedonia, respectively, has also been shown to be relatively reliable and valid for predicting adolescent diagnostic status measured via a clinical interview (Richardson et al., 2010). Yet it is important to note that the longer nine-item version of the PHQ represents a statistically superior screening measure (as indexed by measures of sensitivity and specificity; e.g., AUC) compared to the briefer two-item version (Allgaier, Pietsch, Frühe, Sigl-Glöckner, & Schulte-Körne, 2012). Thus, as with all decisions within assessment, a balance between predictive superiority and temporal resources is required.

Novel Assessment Strategies

Diagnostic assessment and questionnaire-based rating scales represent the two methods most commonly used in a depression assessment. Yet for decades, best practices have advocated for a multimethod approach that integrates "subjective" and "objective" assessment strategies (Hunsley & Mash, 2007; Klein et al., 2005). A wide array of proposed biological and behavioral risk factors have been examined and suggested for pediatric depression (Carvalho et al., 2014; Hankin, 2012; Slavich & Irwin, 2014; Woody & Gibb, 2015). In recent years, for example, psychophysiological assessments have become increasingly popular in the child assessment literature (Bylsma, Mauss, & Rottenberg, 2016; De Los Reyes et al., 2015) for several reasons. First, empirical literature has amassed to the point that psychophysiological indicators are reliable and incrementally valid indicators of pediatric depression (e.g., heart rate variability: Bylsma, Morris, & Rottenberg, 2008; Koenig, Kemp, Beauchaine, Thayer, & Kaess, 2016; event-related potentials: Moran, Schroder, Kneip, & Moser, 2017; pupilometry: Cohen, Thakur, Burkhouse, & Gibb, 2019). Second, technological advancements enable low-cost assessment of depression-related cardiac and psychophysiological indicators (De Los Reyes et al., 2015; Youngstrom & De Los Reyes, 2015). Third, technology allows for interpretation of the information gathered by these devices by individuals without significant training. These developments include publicly available devices (e.g., sensors in smartphone applications; Mohr, Zhang,

& Schueller, 2017) and software that can calculate risk indicators from raw psychophysiological data (De Los Reyes et al., 2015; Thomas, Aldao, & De Los Reyes, 2012).

An alternative to biological and behavioral markers is self-reported risk factors such as cognitive and interpersonal vulnerabilities. "Cognitive vulnerabilities" are enduring, depressogenic ways of thinking that precede the emergence of depression and include dysfunctional attitudes, negative cognitive style, and rumination. Self-reported "interpersonal vulnerabilities" include interpersonal styles (e.g., reassurance seeking), interpersonal interactions (e.g., rejection), and relationship quality (e.g., level of support and conflict within relationships) (Coyne, 1976; Joiner, Alfano, & Metalsky, 1992; Stewart & Harkness, 2017). Youth can be identified at heightened risk for depression by using cutoffs on both cognitive and interpersonal vulnerabilities that predict future onset of depressive episodes (Hankin, Young, Gallop, & Garber, 2018). Cognitive vulnerabilities can be used for evidence-based screening that provides incremental validity above and beyond traditional depression rating scales. Assessing for cognitive risks directly measures hypothesized mechanisms of risk targeted by an intervention (e.g., cognitive-behavioral therapy [CBT]), so there is a more seamless transition from assessment to treatment. Also, cognitive vulnerabilities exist before onset of a depressive episode (e.g., Hankin et al., 2009; Hankin, Snyder, & Gulley, 2016), so they can be used to identify youth at risk and thus enhance early intervention efforts and improve pediatric outcomes. For example, rumination and depressogenic inferential styles predict prospective and recurrent episodes of depression, and rumination was the only index test that uniquely forecasted future onset of depressive episodes (Cohen et al., 2018). In addition, a short, 13-item Rumination Scale better discriminated between currently depressed and nondepressed individuals than the CDI as the standard screening instrument (Cohen et al., 2018).

Last, technological advancements in sensors and mobile technology have paved the way for *digital phenotyping* (Insel, 2017; Mohr et al., 2017; Torous et al., 2018), which refers to data collected via smartphone sensors, keyboard interaction, and voice and speech analysis. Limited empirical research at present evaluates this approach for pediatric depression. Investigators speculate on its potential as the ability to readily collect data via smartphone technology, and meaningfully processing the digital phenotyping information (e.g., via machine learning and other quantitative approaches) will lead to a paradigm shift in assessing for depression (Torous et al., 2018).

Assessing psychophysiological, self-reported cognitive and interpersonal risk factors, and digital phenotyping, all represent promising avenues for improving the ability to assess for depression across dimensional and categorical definitions. In the coming years, it will be critical to use these methods within a clinical setting to demonstrate their feasibility with recommended evidence-based depression assessment and screening protocol (Siu et al., 2016). Additionally, a translational analytic approach (see Youngstrom et al., 2017) that demonstrates sensitive cutoffs and incremental validity above and beyond traditional assessment efforts is necessary (see Cohen, Thakur, et al., 2019, for an example). Thus, it is our hope that in the coming years, the use of a multimethod approach to assessing depression is feasible across clinical and research settings.

Assessment Starter Kit: Recommendations and Practical Issues

Often, individuals who are interested in conducting depression assessments have one simple question: So what should I use to assess for depression? As frustrating as this may be, there is no simple or correct answer to this question. Forming a depression assessment battery is a delicate calculation of costs and benefits based on the resources and aims of the given assessment's purpose and context. In this next section, we attempt to address some practical concerns investigators or practitioners may differentially value within an assessment context. Based on forming answers and opinions on these questions, one can begin selecting an evidence-based depression assessment protocol.

The first practical obstacle for choosing between EBA options is resources. With regard to cost, the K-SADS and MINI-KID diagnostic interviews, and the CES-D rating scale, represent widely used and well-established assessments that are freely available (Klein et al., 2005; Leffler et al., 2015; Stocking et al., 2015). The Patient-Reported Outcomes Measurement Information System (PROMIS) measures, the product of a National Institute of Mental Health (NIMH) initiative, also offer free, evidence-based screening measures for pediatric depression (Irwin et al., 2010). Depression is a multifaceted construct, and these assessment protocols

map onto the distinctions described earlier. For instance, the K-SADS is best seen as an assessment tool for a DSM-5-based diagnosis of depression, the CBCL can be used to measure the syndrome of depression, and the PHQ-2 can be used to screen for depressed mood. Some of these measures can assess more than one conceptualization of depression simultaneously. For example, the CDRS-R is seen as a valid measure of depressed mood, depressive symptoms/syndrome, and diagnostic status (Mayes et al., 2010; Poznanski & Mokros, 1996). Thus, when building an assessment battery, one must ensure that the criterion most related to one's ultimate goal is being measured.

Below, we discuss assessments in outpatient mental health and screening for pediatric primary care as two different scenarios in which one may be tasked with building a depression assessment protocol outside the context of ongoing therapy (which we discuss later) and the unique considerations for each of these contexts. We emphasize the importance of tailoring an assessment battery for depression, and related mental health problems, that depends on the context as opposed to using a "one-size-fits-all" approach.

Assessment Starter Kit for Outpatient Mental Health

Currently, most insurance plans and models for reimbursement require a medically based diagnosis (DSM, ICD). As diagnostic interviews can robustly discriminate between clinically depressed and nondepressed youth, these interviews should be the cornerstone of any depression assessment conducted within a clinical setting. At the same time, these are the most time-intensive assessment strategies. Thus, a reasonable first option is using a broad-band measure of internalizing and externalizing symptoms (e.g., the Achenbach scales) to help "rule out" certain diagnoses prior to the diagnostic assessment. This can significantly reduce the number of modules administered within the diagnostic interview if time is of concern, by allowing the clinician to develop hypotheses concerning potential diagnoses. It also helps demonstrate "medical necessity" for the subsequent interview, changing its reimbursability. The degree to which diagnostic specificity is required in a clinic can also affect whether additional inventories are paired with the initial broad-band measures. Specifically, if preliminarily distinguishing between depression and anxiety could be especially helpful during the screening stage (e.g., anxiety and depression subclinics have separate intakes), pairing the broad-band measures with brief depression inventories (e.g., the PHQ-9) could be advantageous. In a recent meta-analysis, the PHQ-9, and other depression-specific measures, was better equipped to discriminate between internalizing disorders compared to the Achenbach subscales (E. A. Youngstrom, personal communication, March 1, 2020).

The importance of fidelity concerning a DSM-5 depression diagnosis should also impact which diagnostic assessment is subsequently chosen following the initial screening stage. In clinics in which a specific diagnosis of DSM-5 MDD and separating other comorbid disorders is required, using filtered, semistructured interviews (e.g., the K-SADS; Kaufman et al., 1997) that provide flexibility to distinguish between disorders are advised. However, as transdiagnostic intervention protocols for broad emotional and internalizing disorders become more common with increasing evidence for validity and utility (e.g., Ehrenreich-May et al., 2017; Kennedy, Bilek, & Ehrenreich-May, 2018), some clinical settings may not require rigid diagnostic specificity. Within these contexts, the use of unfiltered, structured interviews (e.g., MINI-KID) may be reasonable to determine whether the patient crosses a clinical severity threshold for a more general emotional disorder, as opposed to arriving at a putatively sensitive and specific MDD diagnosis that rules out alternative disorders. Following the diagnostic interview, it may be advised to administer a depression-specific measure in order to (1) provide an index of depression severity (Fristad et al., 1997), (2) provide a baseline marker of depressive symptoms that should be routinely assessed during the intervention (Youngstrom et al., 2017), and (3) provide a multimethod perspective on the depression diagnosis (Hunsley & Mash, 2007).

A second issue that is worthy of consideration is impairment. Depression impairment can be conceptualized in terms of both functional (e.g., academic difficulties, physical health/limitations; Judd, Paulus, Wells, & Rapaport, 1996) and social (e.g., isolation and conflict; Hammen, 1991) domains. The impact within different domains may vary between individuals (McKnight & Kashdan, 2009). That noted, it is regrettable that less than 20% of assessment inventories assess functional impairment (Kamenov, Cabello, Coenen, & Ayuso-Mateos, 2015). The lack of regular assessment of impairment in depression measures is particularly problematic because there is only a moderate correlation between depressive symptoms and functional impairment (McKnight & Kashdan, 2009), so symptoms of distress and indicators of impairment can be conceptually distinguished and need to be assessed separately. Thus, it is strongly recommended to include an explicit measure of functional impairment (Kaemnov et al., 2015). Some of the measures already reviewed include explicit questions related to impairment. For example, the SDQ includes a supplement to address school, social, and functional impairment, in addition to emotional distress. Relatedly, the PROMIS measures include a structured measure of peer relationships (DeWalt et al., 2013) which can be used as an index of social impairment in adolescence. Explicitly measuring both distress (depressive symptom severity) and impairment can enable selection of an intervention and tracking of progress across these two separable aspects of pediatric depression.

Assessment Starter Kit for Screening in Primary Care

The USPSTF recommends screening for primary depression in youth older than age 12 (Siu et al., 2016). This recommendation has led to a flurry of interest concerning best practices to achieve this public health aim (e.g., Fallucco, Seago, Cuffe, Kraemer, & Wysocki, 2015; Gadomski et al., 2015; Zuckerbrot et al., 2018). Whereas a diagnostic assessment typically takes place in a specialty clinic, or at the very least is administered by a mental health professional in an integrated health or school setting, screening is meant to detect current distress or impairment in an unselected or at-risk sample, and often those who administer the screening protocol do not have specialty training in pediatric mental health, let alone depression specifically (Fallucco et al., 2015; Siu et al., 2016; Wissow et al., 2013). Screenings also have to be conducted within the context of other, competing needs (Harris, 2015). Therefore, screening protocols tend to be brief and easily interpreted by providers who may not have extensive training in assessment of depression. Given such exigencies of the screening context, the PHQ-2, the two-item questionnaire that assesses depressed mood and anhedonia, has emerged as a leading candidate for depression screening initiatives due to its brevity and simplicity (Richardson et al., 2010). Despite being 15 questions shorter, the PHQ-2 has similar capabilities to correctly identify depressed youth as more traditional screening inventories, such as the

Patient Symptom Checklist–17 (Gardner, Lucas, Kolko, & Campo, 2007). Yet the PHQ-2 is limited in that two self-report items may not adequately capture the diversity of depression-related distress and impairment. It does not address suicidality, an important reason for depression screening. The PHQ-2 may be used as part of a multigated screening protocol (Lavigne et al., 2016), and if an adolescent answers "yes" to either item on the PHQ-2, then a longer depression rating scale is administered, such as the PHQ-9.

Considerations for "Putting It into Practice"

Demographic Considerations in Base Rate

Within an evidence-based medicine approach, elevated risk due to demographic differences corresponds to a heightened risk (Youngstrom, Halverson, et al., 2018). In other words, identical results from a rating scale may lead to different clinical decisions within an assessment context. Let us use an example to illustrate this point. Consider that population A has a 10% lifetime prevalence rate of depression, while population B has a 30% lifetime prevalence rate of depression. As part of our initial screening battery, we administer the CBCL and notice that youth from both populations report a raw score above 9 on the Anxious/Depressed subscale. Consulting the Wikiversity pages for EBA of depression in youth, we see that this corresponds to a DLR of 1.49. First we convert the prevalence of depression in both populations from percentages (10%, 30%) to odds (e.g., .30/(1 − .30) = .43). Now, we can simply multiply our pretest odds by our DLR (e.g., 1.49 × .43 = 0.64), and convert this number back to a percentage (.64/1.64 = .39). Once we have factored in the pretest prevalence, we see quite a difference in how we would interpret that score on the rating scale. For an individual from Population A, there is a 14% chance he or she has depression, whereas for the person from Population B there is a 39% chance. Thus, one may want to include a depression module in the diagnostic assessment for the youth from Population B, but including this module for the youth from Population A may need to be based on other contextual information.

Here we consider gender and race/ethnicity as two broad demographic, compositional diversity influences that have been most studied with respect to reported levels of depression and potential measurement invariance to assess a latent depression construct across demographic groups. Understanding depression disparities across these two demographic variables can help practitioners form decision rules within depression screening and assessment protcols.

Gender Differences

One of the most well-established and replicated findings is the emergence of the gender difference in depression, as assessed across DSM diagnosis and dimensional syndromes (e.g., for reviews, see Hankin, Wetter, & Cheely, 2008; Salk et al., 2017). Starting in early adolescence (around ages 12–14) or middle puberty (e.g., Hankin et al., 1998, 2015), approximately twice as many girls relative to boys receive a categorical diagnosis of depression (OR = 1.94), and more girls than boys report depressed mood or a dimensional depressive syndrome (Cohen's d for effect size = 0.27; Salk et al., 2017). Numerous theoretical models have been proposed to explain the emergence of this gender differences (e.g., Cyranowski, Frank, Young, & Shear, 2000; Hankin & Abramson, 2001; Keenan & Hipwell, 2005; Nolen-Hoeksema & Girgus, 1994; Taylor et al., 2000). More directly pertinent to assessment of depression is measurement invariance: Do boys and girls respond to depression measures (and the different items on them) equivalently, or is there gender bias in the measurement of depression that affects manifest scores and prevalence effects? Few studies have directly addressed measurement invariance (e.g., Santor, Ramsay, & Zuroff, 1994; Wang, Conrad, Hankin, & Huang, 2005). Evidence suggests little bias in depression measurement between genders, although girls are more willing to endorse distorted body image and crying. Still, adjusting for these few items has little effect on the established mean-level gender difference in depression. In summary, this means that scores on a depression measure likely are assessing the same latent construct for girls and boys.

Racial and Ethnic Differences

Other demographic factors may also be important to consider for depression assessment. Findings have been mixed as to whether African Americans experience more or fewer depressive symptoms compared to European Americans after researchers control for socioeconomic disparities (e.g., Angold et al., 2002; Kistner, David-Ferdon, Lopez, & Dunkel, 2007). Meanwhile, more robust findings document elevated levels of depressive symptoms in Hispanic youth (Céspedes & Huey,

2008; McDonald et al., 2005), in particular Latina adolescents (McLaughlin, Hilt, & Nolen-Hoeksema, 2007). Equivalent symptoms are observed in Asian-American youth compared to European-American peers (Anderson & Mayes, 2010). With respect to assessment using diagnostic interviews and rating scales, the factor structure for the presentation of depression is similar across racial and ethnic child and adolescent populations (Banh et al., 2012; Kessler et al., 2012; Umaña-Taylor et al., 2014). This suggests that traditional depression diagnostic interview assessment batteries can be used efficaciously across racial and ethnic groups.

Yet it is important to note that sole reliance on racial/ethnic categories to understand cultural differences is problematic for any outcome, including depression. Ethnic identity (Hughes, Kiecolt, Keith, & Demo, 2015), acculturative stress (Hovey & King, 1996), and experiences with racism and discrimination (Hammack, 2003; Nyborg & Curry, 2003) are some of the cultural processes linked to depression that may offer insight into racial/ethnic differences in depression (Rudolph & Lambert, 2007). Thus, given the state of the science, we suggest that threshold depression scores may confer increased risk for Latina adolescents, but otherwise, similar instruments and decision rules are acceptable for depression assessment protocols across diverse adolescent samples.

Integrating Multiple Depression Assessments

An agreed-upon assessment principle is that investigators use a multi-informant, multimethod approach for assessing depression (De Los Reyes et al., 2015; Klein et al., 2005). Youth report tends to better index current depressive symptoms (Cohen, So, et al., 2019; Lewis et al., 2012). Parent and/or teacher reports can be useful for identifying behavioral forms of distress and impairment (De Los Reyes et al., 2015; Thapar et al., 2016). Furthermore, parental reports may be necessary when conducting depression assessments in younger populations (e.g., preadolescent children) that may lack insight or a sufficient descriptive vocabulary to articulate various depressive symptoms (Luby et al., 2002). Relatedly, using multiple informants can identify depression-related distress and impairment by providing incrementally valid perspectives across subjective, behavioral, and biological levels of functioning.

At the same time, assessments that use multiple informants involve notable challenges to interpreting the results. In particular, discrepancies between multiple informants/methods are the rule rather than the exception. Having a system to integrate across informants and the multiple tests is necessary. While new quantitative frameworks are being developed to address informant differences (Martel et al., 2017; Youngstrom et al., 2017), traditionally, over the years, several logical approaches have been proposed to resolve such disagreements, especially when using clinical interviews to arrive at a depression diagnosis. A dominant approach in the field is simply pooling or adding together scores across informants, in order to form an "average." Adding or averaging usually improves the reliability of the composite, which indirectly may improve validity (Youngstrom, Findling, & Calabrese, 2003). Although valid when there is no reason to believe one predictor is better than the other, its use has been discouraged due to several conceptual and methodological limitations within a multi-informant assessment perspective when self- or parent reports may carry more weight (Horton & Fitzmaurice, 2004).

Another, potentially better, approach advocates the use of "or" rules (i.e., diagnosing if any single test from an informant indicates depression) or "and" rules (i.e., all tests across informants must indicate a diagnosis) that can be used to make depression diagnoses that systematically incorporate multiple informants (Horton & Fitzmaurice, 2004; Kraemer et al., 2003; Martel et al., 2017). With "or" rules, a clinician counts a positive result from any source as a reason to proceed further with assessment or treatment. For example, if the parent, the youth, the teacher, or clinical observation indicated depression, then the clinician would treat the youth as having depression. "Or" maximizes diagnostic sensitivity, but it tends to have low specificity (Youngstrom et al., 2003). "And," or multiple gating, behaves the opposite way. By requiring the youth to clear multiple hurdles (e.g., high scores on both the self-report *and* the parent report), the pool of positive results gets filtered more, raising the specificity, but at the cost of ruling out true cases and thus lowering specificity. In other words, the "or" rules are vulnerable to false-positive decisions, and the "and" rules are likely to result in too many false-negative decisions (Guion, 2011).

Finally, in practice, using "best estimate" procedures may be the optimal approach presently available to resolve potential discrepancies across informants. Specifically, this means evaluating the perceived quality, accuracy, and believability across informants (e.g., both the caretaker and child) who provide diagnostic symptom information on the child, then evaluating which informant provides greater clarity (Youngstrom et al., 2011). Best-estimate procedures can be performed at a global level or for different symptoms (Hankin et al., 2015; Klein et al., 2005; Polanczyk, Salum, Sugaya, Caye, & Rohde, 2015), such as counting the child's report of particular emotional or cognitive symptoms (e.g, sadness, crying, worthlessness) while using the caretaker's report for certain vegetative or behaviorally observable symptoms (e.g., sleeping and eating changes). Best-estimate procedures are recommended and are fairly reliable in clinical and applied research studies (Klein et al., 2005), although use of the best estimate can introduce subjectivity and idiosyncratic decision making into the diagnostic process. However, the use of existing qualitative algorithms and models, such as the operations triad model (OTM; De Los Reyes, Lerner, Thomas, Daruwala, & Goepel, 2013), can be used to help ensure best-estimate procedures remain evidence based.

Selecting Tests and Decision Rules

The choice of which assessments to select, as well as the procedures and rules to use in order to make evidence-based clinical decisions, is affected by the system in which one works. Broadly speaking, individuals' options for selecting tests and making decisions based on particular EBA algorithms depend on whether one works in a large *systemwide* setting or a smaller *practitioner-based* context.

In a systemwide approach, an individual operates within a large system, such as a sizable medical setting or insurance system, in which the organization has sufficient resources and available data to create decision rules based on empirically based algorithms that are directly grounded and relevant for that system. Typically, the system has data culled from existing medical records, and such systems-level data are used to determine how different sources of data relate to depression as the outcome of interest. Then the extensive systemwide data can be analyzed via advanced statistical procedures, such as actuarial tools derived from machine learning (Mohr et al., 2017) or recursive partitioning (Strobl, Malley, & Tutz, 2009). For instance, Walsh, Riberio, and Franklin (2017) used machine learning to build a decision algorithm based on data found in hospital medical records covering over 600 unique data sources to identify a prognostic algorithm for prospective suicide attempts. Future research can use these and related forecasting methods with data collected from large

pediatric systems to refine and advance empirically based assessment protocols and decision rules to predict depression, although it will be important to check generalizability, as algorithms get transported to new settings that may differ substantially in terms of demographics or clinical features (Konig et al., 2007; Youngstrom, Halverson, et al., 2018).

On the other hand, use of these systemwide algorithms may be limited in smaller, lower resourced pediatric settings in which extensive databases may not be available. For these practitioner-based practices, it may not be realistic for an individual in private practice to have the resources to examine and interpret many data sources to develop and use an empirically based algorithm specific to the local practitioner's setting. Instead, for the vast majority of individuals in local practitioner practices, evidence-based decision making can be accomplished using available reliable, valid assessments that are interpreted, and via a receiver operator characteristic (ROC) framework to quantify whether an individual youth is depressed (Youngstrom, 2014). The defining feature of an ROC approach is the AUC statistic, which provides insight into the sensitivity (i.e., how well the index test correctly identifies positive depression cases) and specificity (i.e., how well the index test correctly identifies nondepressed cases) associated with a given cutoff score on that assessment test. Individual practitioners can use DLRs, which can be obtained for various depression assessment tests, and apply an ROC approach to help quantify how likely an individual youth is to present with depression (DLR+) or not (DLR–) given the individual child's risk profile, as obtained via various assessments (Straus, Glasziou, Richardson, & Haynes, 2011). Using DLRs has the advantage of providing an empirical framework for systematically combining assessment tests in an understandable and straightforward manner. Recent studies have applied an ROC approach using DLRs to demonstrate the incremental validity of certain measures (e.g., social support, cognitive vulnerabilities) when using multiple assessments to predict depression in youth following a natural disaster (Cohen et al., 2016) and within a school sample (Cohen et al., 2018). At the end of this section, we demonstrate how DLRs can be used to make evidence-based decisions in a case study of an individual child. The DLR approach may generalize to a wider range of clinical settings than might a more complicated model (see Youngstrom, Halverson, et al., 2018, for a model comparison across multiple settings and discussion).

Translating and Linking Methods and Measures

Thus far, we have summarized many commonly used depression scales and interviews, and this review shows that no one single measure is optimal to recommend widespread use for all EBA. Most likely, different clinical researchers and applied practitioners will continue to use particular and different measures for select goals and purposes. This raises the question of how to compare and translate across different depression assessment measures in an empirical manner and how best to use different measures to assess the range of depression severity across different samples using a similar latent metric. Item response theory (IRT) linking procedures enable clinical researchers to "go between" different depression measures and translate scores from one assessment approach (e.g., CDI) to another (CES-D) by placing items and scores from these disparate measures onto a common scale of latent trait severity (see Reise & Waller, 2009, for method details). Linking methods can be especially helpful if different assessment tools are used at different times for various assessment goals, such as using the K-SADS for a baseline diagnostic evaluation, then using the CDI to track progress and symptom severity over time. Additionally, computerized adaptive testing (CAT; Reise & Waller, 2009), using IRT approaches, can decrease the number of items needed for optimal assessment of the latent trait of depression severity and automate the IRT analytics for a clinician in the office to track severity over time, even if using different assessments. To date, a few studies have demonstrated the utility and EBA practice of linking via IRT in pediatric depression (e.g., Choi, Schalet, Cook, & Cella, 2014; Olino et al., 2013).

Clinical Case Example

The following is a realistic referral one might receive while working in an outpatient psychology clinic (see Table 7.3). Below, we distill some of the theory and practical knowledge disseminated in this chapter, and show how it can be used clinically, so that a practicing psychologist can make an evidence-based method (EBM)-informed decision. We discuss this vignette within two constraints typical of this setting: (1) A DSM/ICD diagnosis is necessary to engage in treatment, and (2) the assessment needs to take place within the context of typical time limits (e.g., a single 90-minute assessment appointment). We rely on traditional assessment measures (e.g., self-reports and diagnostic interviews) and methods for integrating different sources of information (i.e., a combined pooling approach and "best estimate" approach) to make the example apply to as broad an audience as possible. Furthermore, we use an EBM approach to demonstrate how practitioners can quantify the likelihood of a disorder, and how this may be useful in making challenging decisions regarding diagnosis.

As a practicing clinician at an outpatient psychology clinic, you receive a referral from a primary care physician (PCP) concerning a 12-year-old girl. As part of your clinic's triage process, as the staff psychologist, you are informed that the child seems "more irritable than usual," and her mother reports increased school refusal and arguments with her siblings and father at home, both of which are new behaviors. The PCP states in the referral that neither the PCP nor the mother are certain whether intervention is necessary, and they are interested in an assessment with consultation and recommendations regarding possible intervention.

You begin by sending the ASEBA home to the family, including the CBCL for the caretaker and the YSR for the adolescent girl to complete because these query informants about a wide range of psychopathological symptoms and syndromes. Based on responses on different subscales on the Achenbach scales, you can decide which modules to include in your 90-minute appointment. This can be done in several ways: prioritizing the highest T-scores reported by both parent and youth; focusing on areas of agreement first, then prioritizing internalizing reports from the girl and discrepant reports from caregiver; or using an EBM-approach (as modeled in the demographic section), in which you multiply the DLRs (which can be obtained from the Wikiversity EBA assessment websites) by her pretest prevalence (as modeled below).

Upon receiving the completed CBCL/YSR forms, you are able to rule out several behavioral/externalizing syndromes. For instance, both the CBCL Attention Problems and Aggression subscale scores were 54. These scores suggest a decreased likelihood for a diagnosis of ODD/CD given that the DLR is approximately 0.35 (Hudziak, Copeland, Stanger, & Wadsworth, 2004), and one can be "moderately certain" the child does not have ADHD (DLR = 0.23; Raiker et al., 2017) using Straus and colleagues' (2011) benchmarks. Parent report of youth externalizing symptoms is preferred to youth report for behavioral problems (De Los Reyes et al., 2015), so you conclude that

TABLE 7.3. Example of an Outpatient Psychology Clinical Referral

	Depression	Anxiety
Pretest probability	7%	14%
Pretest prevalence (based on female gender)	10%	14%
T-score from YSR	62	65
Diagnostic likelihood ratio (DLR) from YSR	0.52	0.98
Revised probability	5%	14%
T-score from CBCL	71	72
DLR from CBCL	3.78	1.51
Posterior probability	19%	19%
Action step	Based on her Achenbach profile, she is nearly twice as likely to be suffering from depression compared to her gender base rate. Include depression in the diagnostic assessment.	Based on her Achenbach profile, she is approximately 50% more likely to be suffering from an anxiety disorder compared to her peers. Note that her risk of anxiety is equivalent to her risk for depression. Diagnostic interviews with both parent and youth should be conducted to determine which diagnosis(es) may best capture her distress and impairment.

Note. For depression, *T*-scores and DLRs are derived from the Anxious/Depressed subscale for depression and the broad-band Internalizing subscale for anxiety-based recommendations (Thakur & Cohen, 2019; Van Meter et al., 2014). Given that base rates of gender disorders vary based on subtype, we did not calculate different prevalence estimates for females compared to the general population, consistent with past research (Van Meter et al., 2014). DLRs for the vignette were taken from Thakur and Cohen (2019) for depression and Van Meter and colleagues (2014) for anxiety. DLRs vary between studies, and selection of DLRs should be based on population for the assessment (e.g., community vs. outpatient clinic), as well as one's conceptualization of depression. These methodological factors could also have an impact on selection of pretest prevalence. For more explanation on the calculation of posterior probability, please see the clinical case example and consult Straus and colleagues (2011) for more details on how to compute posterior probability.

diagnostic interviews for externalizing disorders are unnecessary.

For the internalizing disorders, you can consider either the broad Internalizing scale or the three individual subscales (Anxious/Depressed, Withdrawn, and Somatic) from the ASEBA measures. For depression, the Anxious/Depressed subscale is the most robust predictor of diagnostic status across the CBCL and the YSR (Thakur & Cohen, 2019), whereas the broad internalizing subscale is most commonly used for anxiety (Van Meter, Youngstrom, Ollendick, Demeter, & Findling, 2014). Research on informant gradients suggest that youth-reports are preferred to parent reports for current depression, although both are valid indicators of depression (Cohen, So, et al., 2019), while for anxiety disorders, informants are equivalent (Van Meter et al., 2014). On the YSR,

the youth reports below the subthreshold range on the Anxious/Depressed subscale (*T* = 62) and in the subthreshold range of the Internalizing scale (*T* = 65); the parent reports above the threshold range on the Anxious/Depressed subscale of the CBCL (*T* = 71) and Internalizing scale (*T* = 72). As discussed previously, in order to make the most informed decision concerning diagnostic likelihood for depression, we use a "best estimate" approach, first interpreting the YSR Anxious/Depressed subscale, followed by the CBCL Anxious/Depressed subscale. Taken together, these findings suggest that this youth is experiencing depression somewhere on the continuum of mild-to-moderate (as indicated by the YSR) to more moderate (as indicated by the CBCL), and further assessment is necessary. A similar conclusion can be drawn concerning anxiety.

Following administration of the Achenbach scales, the practitioner may still have questions about whether it is necessary to do a diagnostic interview for both and *which* disorder to prioritize within the assessment. To help inform this decision, an EBM approach may be helpful. Therefore, once again we return to the literature to gather the necessary data. Our first step for calculating the posterior probability (i.e., the likelihood the youth has depression based on her Achenbach scores) is to calculate the pretest probability. For youth depression, one can consult recent epidemiological studies (e.g., Avenevoli, Swendsen, He, Burstein, & Merikangas, 2015), or visit the Wikiverse. Similarly, the investigator can decide which demographics to include in establishing pretest probability. As reviewed earlier, differentiating between female and male prevalence estimates may be particularly relevant for depression. Recent estimates report the 12-month prevalence to be 10.7% for adolescent girls and 4.6% for adolescent boys (Avenevoli et al., 2015). Meanwhile, for anxiety, EBA methods in the past have not distinguished between girls and boys for pretest probability; prevalence rates suggest that approximately 14% of youth present with an anxiety disorder.

Based on these estimates and ASEBA *T*-scores, the posterior probability can now be calculated. Similar to pretest prevalence rates, a range of DLRs can be identified in the literature for the AESBA (e.g., Thakur & Cohen, 2019) or using the Wikiversity. As we did earlier (see "Demographic Considerations in Base Rate") we convert the percentage of youth with depression into pretest odds. Next, we multiply the DLRs (taken from Thakur & Cohen, 2019, in this case, as it provides subthreshold and threshold levels on the YSR and CBCL), which is 0.52 for the subthreshold YSR score and 3.78 for the threshold CBCL score. Using a naive Bayesian approach, we can now utilize a widely available nomogram to "connect the dots" (see Van Meter et al., 2014) or multiply the odds together to derive the posterior odds, and subsequent probability. Based on this calculation, this girl's estimated probability for depression is 19%, approximately twice as likely as her pretest estimate. As for a possible anxiety disorder, the DLR for youth report is 0.98 and that for parent report is 1.51 (Van Meter et al., 2014). Based on this information, the girl's estimated probability of presenting with an anxiety disorder is 19%, nearly 50% higher than her pretest probability of 14%, and nearly identical to the likelihood of depression.

Based on these ASEBA measures collected prior to the in-person assessment and the EBA calculations with DLRs, you decide that a more in-depth diagnostic assessment focused on ascertaining potential depression and anxiety disorders is warranted in this case. As this approach did not dictate which disorder may be more likely, you decide to speak to the adolescent girl to build rapport, and first ask about depressive symptoms, as the informant gradient suggests that she is the best informant of these symptoms (Cohen, So, et al., 2019). For the interview, you use the K-SADS as your diagnostic interview and decide to conduct the in-person assessment using only the Depression and Anxiety modules given the time constraints (a 90-minute appointment). Furthermore, you have the parent and youth complete the CDI and a standard child anxiety measure (e.g., the Multidimensional Anxiety Scale for Children [MASC]; for more information, see Fleischer, Crane, & Kendall, Chapter 10, this volume). During the diagnostic interview, the girl reports experiencing significant peer stress since transitioning into the sixth grade; she endorses increased irritability and feelings of worthlessness. She states that these symptoms are impairing and have lasted the majority of each day, every day, for the past 2 months, but she does not endorse the minimum of five symptoms necessary for a MDD diagnosis according to DSM-5. Meanwhile, the caregiver reports a significant change in her daughter's mood over the past month but does not understand the source. The caregiver reports increased irritability, decreased appetite, and hypersomnia, and these symptoms are impairing. Yet these do not reach the minimum of five symptoms. Using a best-estimate approach that integrates across informants, the girl met the following four depressive symptoms: irritability and worthlessness (self-report for more internal symptoms), as well as reduced appetite and hypersomnia (parent report for vegetative, externally observable symptoms). Using best-estimate procedures from the interview suggests that the girl meets DSM-5 criteria for unspecified depressive disorder. With respect to any DSM-5-based anxiety disorder, neither the girl nor the caregiver report any impairment related to anxiety symptoms.

Additionally, you consult the self-report forms that the youth and parent completed. On the youth's CDI report, a raw score of 10 was reported, which falls within the "moderate" range. Meanwhile, the parent report on the CDI was 16, suggesting elevated symptoms. Alternatively, scores on the MASC fall within the normative range. Overall, these findings are congruent with the diagnostic interview, and you determine the most appropriate diagnosis at this time to be unspecified depressive disorder, with the specifier "insufficient symptoms," because only four symptoms were endorsed across observers using a best-estimate procedure. You plan to initiate treatment to relieve the girl's distress and depression-related impairment. Her scores on the CDI provide important benchmarks prior to the intervention concerning depression severity.

Tracking Treatment Progress in Depression Interventions

Commonly Used Measures

There exists no single measure that is universally deemed optimal for assessing depression. As a field intent on practicing evidence-based mental health interventions to reduce distress and suffering, we are supposed to consult and be guided by randomized controlled trials (RCTs) to make informed choices for intervention on youth depression. As such, it follows that clinicians would consult this literature to use appropriate depression instruments to assess for and evaluate change in depression severity based on these RCTs. So, what assessments are most suitable to make evidence-based practice decisions and track progress in intervention? To address which measures are most commonly used as the EBAs of depression in randomized clinical trials of depression, we consulted major meta-analytic reviews for various intervention modalities to reduce depression, including (1) psychosocial depression treatments (Weersing, Jeffreys, Do, Schwartz, & Bolano, 2017), (2) depression psychopharmacological treatments (Cipriani et al., 2016), (3) psychosocial depression preventions (Seeley, Stice, & Rohde, 2009), and (4) prevention of depression in offspring of depressed parents (Loechner et al., 2018).

In their meta-analytic review and update of evidence-based psychosocial interventions to reduce depression, Weersing and colleagues (2017) summarized data from RCTs, and the following illustrates the frequency with which particular depression outcome measures were used to calculate effect sizes for diagnostic interviews: K-SADS (one) and CDRS-R (six), and for symptom measures: CES-D (three), Mood and Feelings Questionnaire (MFQ) (four), CDI (three), Clinical Global Impressions (CGI) (one), and BDI (four). (Note that for these meta-analyses of intervention effects, some studies used more than one depression assessment, so the frequencies may not uniquely add up.) For depression psychopharmacology interventions, Cipriani and colleagues (2016) reviewed 34 trials and reported that the CDRS-R, as a clinician rating scale, or the BDI or CDI were the most commonly used self-reported depressive symptom measures to calculate effect sizes for antidepressant medication efficacy. Regarding prevention of adolescent depression, Stice, Shaw, Bohon, Marti, and Rohde (2009) meta-analyzed prevention programs; some of the effect sizes were based on diagnostic interviews to ascertain depression diagnosis (three with K-SADS, one SCID, one DISC); 22 of the effect sizes were based on the CDI, seven on the BDI, eight with the CES-D, and four with the RADS or Reynolds Child Depression Scale (RCDS). Last, in their meta-analytic review of preventing depression in offspring of depressed parents, Loechner and colleagues (2018) included the following outcome measures: diagnostic or clinician interview of the K-SADS (four), the Hamilton Rating Scale for Depression (HAM-D) (one), and the CDRS-R (one), and depressive symptoms scales including Achenbach scales (YSR/CBCL; three), CES-D (three), MFQ (one), SDQ (one), and CDI (one).

This brief summary of meta-analytic reviews of major interventions to reduce depression in youth reveals that many of the instruments reviewed earlier, including the K-SADS and CDRS as clinician-rated interviews, as well as the CDI or ASEBA suite (e.g., YSR/CBCL) as questionnaires, are most commonly used to assess and monitor pediatric depression. Although there is not a systematic consensus choice for a depression assessment that is consistently used in the evidence-based intervention literature, knowing which depression instruments are most frequently used for evaluation and tracking of progress for certain interventions (e.g., psychosocial or pharmacological treatments; prevention efforts) can help the practicing clinician to use a similar measure and more directly track patient progress against the data reported in a particular RCT.

Measuring and Evaluating Changes in Depression

The topic of ascertaining change in depression over time is clearly an important one for EBA of depression, as knowing whether an individual has clearly exhibited clinically significant change in levels of depression is an essential goal in EBA and evidence-based medicine. Did this adolescent improve as a result of an intervention? Is a different intervention option needed because the child has not improved sufficiently (e.g., lack of sufficient change given time for a particular intervention)? Several definitional, conceptual, statistical, and analytic issues need to be considered thoughtfully when interpreting change in depression over time.

Ideally, the clinician using evidence-based principles will repeatedly administer measures to assess a depression construct before, during, and after a depression intervention. A primary consideration here for EBA of tracking progress and monitoring potential change that may be the result of interventions designed to reduce depression is knowing the prototypic and expected trajectory of depression. A key issue, then, is knowing what the modal course of depression looks like, so that the clinician can evaluate whether clinically meaningful change in reductions of depressive symptoms has occurred beyond any decrement in depression expected normatively with the passage of time (e.g., potential regression to the mean effects). How much change should be expected in depression scores over time? How do the clinical researcher and the health practitioner then use this information to analyze individual clients' depression scores to ascertain that some degree of clinically relevant change has occurred?

In making such decisions from an evidence-based perspective via assessment of change over time, the following need to be considered, as these knotty points complicate any easy evaluation and interpretation of change: (1) attenuation effects in mean-level depressive symptom scores, (2) rank-order stability of depression scores over time, and (3) methods used in the evidence-based research literature to analyze change in depression-relevant constructs for individuals as a way to track and monitor intervention progress.

Attenuation Effect in Depressive Symptoms

Many likely expect normative, mean levels of depression (symptoms or episodes) to *increase* across time and development, based on the usual developmental epidemiological picture that we reviewed earlier in the chapter. For example, DSM-based diagnoses of depression increase as a function of age, with an approximate sixfold increase in rates of MDD from early to middle (2–3% rate) to late (17% rate) adolescence (e.g., Hankin et al., 1998). Yet this developmental picture of average prevalence rates across many years is different from the pattern of change in depressive symptoms that

might be expected when depressive symptoms are repeatedly assessed over relatively shorter time frames (i.e., weeks to months), as is the case with an intervention. Knowing this modal pattern of depressive symptoms change is highly relevant for EBA practice when a clinician is tracking intervention effects and monitoring progress across the course of a depression intervention.

Research on longitudinal administration of self-report questionnaire measures of depression shows an *attenuation, or repeated measures, effect*. This means that clinical professionals should expect a decrease in reported symptom levels across the first few successive assessments of depression (Angold & Costello, 1995; Klein et al., 2005; Sharpe & Gilbert, 1998; Twenge & Nolen-Hoeksema, 2002) regardless of the intervention. Also known as the Hawthorne effect, the number of time points for which this decrease in repeated measures should be expected ranges from two to six. Our most recent work, in which we tracked a large sample of youth repeatedly—every 3 months across 3 years, for a total of 13 assessments of CDI-measured depressive symptoms—showed a substantial attenuation effect and decline in scores across the first two assessments; then depression scores stabilized, starting with the third assessment and thereafter slowly began to increase over the remaining time points (Long, Young, & Hankin, 2019). The reasons why self-reported depression scores decline for the first few administrations are unclear and represent an important topic for further research. In summary, clinicians should expect a substantial decline in self-reported symptoms for at least the first two assessments for the average youth, and this decrement in depression scores likely does not reflect change in depression due to intervention; change in depression may be expected after the third time point, when the repeated measures pattern has stabilized.

Stability and Change in Depression

The attenuation effect describes the pattern of how much mean scores on depression measures decline for samples on average, but this does not address the degree of rank-order continuity (or test–retest stability) in depression measures over time. Repeated measures work on rank-order stability shows that average test–retest stability correlation of depressive symptoms is moderately high. Mean test–retest r's center around .70, and this high stability estimate is obtained regardless of whether a relatively short follow-up time frame (e.g., every 5 weeks; Hankin, 2008) or a longer evaluation window (e.g., every 6 months; Tram & Cole, 2006) is used. To put these rank-order stability estimates in context, these mean differential stability effects for depressive symptoms ($r \sim .70$) can be compared to the magnitude of rank-order stabilities obtained in research on stability of temperament and personality trait measures. For instance, a meta-analysis estimated the population test–retest stability of personality traits as $r = .43$ for ages 6–18 (Roberts & DelVecchio, 2000). Other longitudinal studies of trait stability show moderately high continuity (e.g., $r = .69$ for parent-reported emotional instability traits for children ages 12–13 years; De Fruyt et al., 2006). Interestingly, most define temperament and personality traits as individual differences that are relatively stable across time and situation, and such moderately high rank-order stability estimates are often taken as *prima facie* evidence that temperament and personality traits are stable. Yet depressive symptom scores show comparable or higher levels of rank-order stability between individuals than is observed with personality traits.

These findings are particularly notable because depression, especially as defined by DSM-5 as a categorical disorder, is traditionally believed to be episodic (i.e., a child is currently depressed or mentally healthy), and symptoms are expected to exhibit considerable change and fluctuations over time. When monitoring depression scores and tracking the degree of potential change that may result from intervention, it is useful to keep in mind that depressive symptoms among youth (especially adolescents) exhibit strong rank-order stability between individuals across time, and a majority of this enduring stability in depression is explained by trait-like forces (Cole & Martin, 2005). Thus, parsing trait- and state-like aspects of depression reports is an important area for future translational research to improve EBA practices for youth depression.

Most clinical researchers and applied practitioners inherently are interested in "how much *this particular individual* changes over time." Yet the majority of research, including the evidence just reviewed regarding mean-level depression scores over time and test–retest stability patterns, uses between-subjects analytic approaches that provide an estimate for the average child. To answer how much a specific child changes over time, it is essential to separate between-person from within-person effects when evaluating and interpreting change in depression over time. The findings from between-person data analytic methods cannot be automatically and uncritically translated to infer individual level change (Fisher, Medaglia, & Jeronimus, 2018). Analyzing and interpreting both within-person and between-persons change over time can provide a more accurate representation of tracking symptom change over time; this represents an important area for future research (see Piccirillo & Rodebaugh, 2019, for a discussion of idiographic assessment methods).

Analyzing and Monitoring Symptom Change

This section considers three options to track, then analyze, individuals' progress as a result of any intervention. The first is change according to an absolute level, such as no longer meeting official DSM-5 diagnostic criteria or falling below threshold cutoff on a dimensional symptom profile. Second is analyzing individuals' decreases on scores for clinically reliable and meaningful change, such as through the reliable change index (RCI). Last is an idiographic top-problems approach of assessing specific symptoms as the primary focus of change.

First is change according to an absolute level. In their meta-analysis of psychosocial interventions for youth depression, Weersing and colleagues (2016) noted a "defining response" as the "absence of current depression diagnosis," and this was defined in variable ways. Clinicians commonly use certain absolute metrics to decide that an individual has improved during the course of intervention, such as a 50% change or a decrease of 5 points or more on the sum score of the PHQ-9, which covers the nine MDD symptoms of DSM. Another classic, traditional approach to defining change by an absolute level is determining that a specific child no longer meets diagnostic criteria for a DSM-defined depressive episode. But there are clear problems with using *absolute change* approaches. Take the example, for instance, of an adolescent who has five major depressive episode (MDE) symptoms for 1 month then drops one symptom; now this adolescent has four MDE symptoms and no longer officially meets DSM criteria for MDD. How effective was the intervention? On the other hand, a child who initially had nine symptoms present for a month and after intervention only met criteria for five symptoms, would still be diagnosed with depression. But is this not the child who conceivably benefited most from therapy? Thus, even if one has to use a categorical approach for diagnoses at the beginning of treatment for practical reasons (e.g., insurance reimbursement), there is little reason why clinicians would be unable to use a more nuanced, dimensional approach when attempting to determine progress within the context of a depression intervention.

The RCI attempts to quantify whether there is meaningful change across an individual's continuum of symptoms based on an initial assessment. Briefly, Jacobson and Truax (1991) developed RCI as an analysis to determine whether individuals have demonstrated clinically significant change, and not just group-level statistical change. Traditionally, in evaluating change via the RCI, sum scores on a depression measure (e.g., CDI) from preintervention assessment are compared to postintervention, and this difference score is adjusted by the standard error of the measure to ensure that the change score for the individual is reliably different beyond chance of measurement error. The RCI has clear advantages over an absolute threshold analysis of change and takes into account whether the clinical change from pre- to postassessment is still within the zone of a scale's standard error of measurement, and therefore, not representing meaningful change. However, examining change scores from an initial assessment to later, after intervention, even with RCI, can be especially problematic on "quasi-traits" (a unipolar construct that is relevant in one direction and in which variation at the low end of the scale provides less information; Reise & Waller, 2009). Depression is a classic example of a quasi-trait, as the low end of a depression scale is not happiness but lack of depression. Furthermore, as we discussed earlier, deciding which assessment point to count as the "pre" baseline measure during the course of intervention is complicated by the attenuation effects observed with the first two to three assessments; depression scores will be higher to start due to the Hawthorne effect, and the expected decline after these first few measurements can challenge real assessment and evaluation of pre- to post-change via the RCI approach. Freeman and Young (Chapter 4, this volume) go into more detail about the Jacobson approach, including discussion of normative benchmarks and some more technical alternatives. More information is also available on the Process section of Wikiversity (*https://en.wikiversity.org/wiki/Evidence-based_assessment/Process_phase*).

A final method to evaluate intervention progress and monitoring change is the top-problems approach, in which clients generate up to three primary problems and goals for which help in therapy is requested. The top-problems approach is idiographic and has demonstrated reliability and validity (Weisz et al., 2011). Focusing on specific symptoms or problems to remediate for individual clients is consistent with view that depression, defined typically by DSM and syndrome measurements, is heterogeneous, and two particular clients may share no symptoms in common. A top-problems approach may focus on specific symptoms that are commonly observed in depressed youth, such as crying, loss of energy, early morning insomnia, irritability, anger, thoughts about being humiliated or embarrassed in social situations, feeling nervous, behaviorally withdrawing from friends, self-harming, feeling sad, losing interest in specific activities, or not succeeding in school. Note these are not all traditional symptoms of a DSM-5 MDD diagnosis. Conducting repeated assessments of such specific problems and symptoms that are most concerning and distressing to a particular individual before, during, and after intervention is consistent with traditional behavioral roots of psychology and with some calls for personalized, individualized approaches to treatment. Repeated (e.g., daily, weekly) tracking of symptoms requiring clinical attention can be used to monitor individuals' specific symptoms across time during and after intervention. This approach does not require sophisticated psychometrics of full depression scales or fancy statistical analyses; it is easily, quickly and efficiently completed by the client; and it can be scored and plotted by the therapist to have immediate understanding and impact regarding intervention success (or stalled treatment requiring a different approach). Using a top-problems approach can be a powerful EBA method to track individual progress for a specific intervention focused on certain target symptoms that may not represent the full hetereogeneous spectrum of a DSM MDD diagnosis or a traditionally used depression syndrome questionnaire or clinical scale. For tools and examples, see *https://en.wikiversity.org/wiki/Evidence-based_assessment/Idiographic_progress_assessment*.

Summary and Future Directions

In this chapter we have reviewed EBA considerations and procedures for measuring depression in children and adolescents. Almost all of the questionnaires, rating scales, and interviews that are used to make diagnostic decisions and to track intervention progress are based on the assumed conceptualization of depression as a singular syndrome or disorder. For several decades, most mental health research, including risk factors, etiological mechanisms, assessment, treatment and prevention, as well as the training of most mental health practitioners and researchers, have all been grounded in the assumptions that (1) depression exists as a discrete entity and (2) psychiatric disorders are defined appropriately and validly by modern psychiatric nosologies, such as DSM-5. As such, the knowledge that undergirds many systems of care and programs of research is based on these organizing principles, and it is therefore important to have a firm grasp of how to assess this conceptualization of depression.

While we have necessarily organized this chapter around the existing literature that forms the basis for EBA, it bears noting that how a clinical researcher or applied practitioner chooses to conduct any particular depression assessment is essentially based on his or her beliefs about "what depression is." As noted earlier, the validity of DSM-5 as a psychiatric classification system has been seriously questioned (Uher & Rutter, 2012), and the reliability of MDD diagnoses is relatively poor (Freedman et al., 2013). There are recently proposed alternatives to conceptualizing depression and co-occurring emotional (e.g., anxiety) and behavioral (e.g., conduct and attention) problems from a latent dimensional perspective that can represent these symptoms across hierarchies (e.g., Hankin, Snyder, et al., 2016; Kotov et al., 2017). Evidence for these alternative approaches to organize and structure depression and other psychopathologies is growing (e.g., Caspi & Mofitt, 2018; Hankin, 2019; Krueger, 2018; Lahey et al., 2017). As these newer structural models potentially gain an evidentiary basis and validity, future research can translate the latent factors identified in these structural models of psychopathology to provide clinical assessments that can measure this latent construct of depression across hierarchical levels (cf. Ruggero et al., 2019).

As child mental health researchers and clinicians continue to advance knowledge in and practice EBA of depression in youth, future research will need to evaluate the most optimal manner to define depression. This will enable the most accurate EBA of depression that can be used to more precisely characterize and identify depression in initial assessment protocols, then track and monitor progress throughout intervention. As we noted at the start, assessment is about measurement, and this requires an accurate and clear definition of *what* is being measured. There can be EBA of depression, as the technology and procedures for *how*

to measure depression are reasonably understood; the key task is being clear and knowing *what* pediatric depression is.

REFERENCES

Achenbach, T. M., & Rescorla, L. A. (2001). *Manual for the Achenbach system of empirically based assessment school-age forms profiles.* Burlington: University of Vermont.

Allgaier, A.-K., Pietsch, K., Frühe, B., Sigl-Glöckner, J., & Schulte-Körne, G. (2012). Screening for depression in adolescents: Validity of the patient health questionnaire in pediatric care. *Depression and Anxiety, 29*(10), 906–913.

American Psychiatric Association. (2013). *Diagnostic and statistical manual of mental disorders* (5th ed.). Arlington, VA: Author.

Anderson, E. R., & Mayes, L. C. (2010). Race/ethnicity and internalizing disorders in youth: A review. *Clinical Psychology Review, 30*(3), 338–348.

Angold, A., & Costello, E. J. (1995). A test–retest reliability study of child-reported psychiatric symptoms and diagnoses using the Child and Adolescent Psychiatric Assessment (CAPA-C). *Psychological Medicine, 25*(4), 755–762.

Angold, A., & Costello, E. J. (2000). The Child and Adolescent Psychiatric Assessment (CAPA). *Journal of the American Academy of Child and Adolescent Psychiatry, 39*(1), 39–48.

Angold, A., Costello, E. J., & Erkanli, A. (1999). Comorbidity. *Journal of Child Psychology and Psychiatry, 40*(1), 57–87.

Angold, A., Costello, E. J., Messer, S. C., & Pickles, A. (1995). Development of a short questionnaire for use in epidemiological studies of depression in children and adolescents. *International Journal of Methods in Psychiatric Research, 5*(4), 237–249.

Angold, A., Erkanli, A., Farmer, E. M., Fairbank, J. A., Burns, B. J., Keeler, G., & Costello, E. J. (2002). Psychiatric disorder, impairment, and service use in rural African American and white youth. *Archives of General Psychiatry, 59*(10), 893–901.

Avenevoli, S., Stolar, M., Li, J., Dierker, L., & Ries Merikangas, K. (2001). Comorbidity of depression in children and adolescents: Models and evidence from a prospective high-risk family study. *Biological Psychiatry, 49*(12), 1071–1081.

Avenevoli, S., Swendsen, J., He, J.-P., Burstein, M., & Merikangas, K. (2015). Major depression in the National Comorbidity Survey—Adolescent Supplement: Prevalence, correlates, and treatment. *Journal of the American Academy of Child and Adolescent Psychiatry, 54*(1), 37–44.

Banh, M. K., Crane, P. K., Rhew, I., Gudmundsen, G., Stoep, A. V., Lyon, A., & McCauley, E. (2012). Measurement equivalence across racial/ethnic groups of the Mood and Feelings Questionnaire for Childhood

Depression. *Journal of Abnormal Child Psychology, 40*(3), 353–367.

Berenbaum, H. (2013). Classification and psychopathology research. *Journal of Abnormal Psychology, 122*(3), 894–901.

Borsboom, D. (2006). The attack of the psychometricians. *Psychometrika, 71*(3), 425–440.

Brooks, S. J., & Kutcher, S. (2001). Diagnosis and measurement of adolescent depression: A review of commonly utilized instruments. *Journal of Child and Adolescent Psychopharmacology, 11*(4), 341–376.

Bufferd, S. J., Dougherty, L. R., Carlson, G. A., Rose, S., & Klein, D. N. (2012). Psychiatric disorders in preschoolers: Continuity from ages 3 to 6. *American Journal of Psychiatry, 169*(11), 1157–1164.

Bufferd, S. J., Dougherty, L. R., Olino, T. M., Dyson, M. W., Laptook, R. S., Carlson, G. A., & Klein, D. N. (2014). Predictors of the onset of depression in young children: A multi-method, multi-informant longitudinal study from ages 3 to 6. *Journal of Child Psychology and Psychiatry and Allied Disciplines, 55*(11), 1279–1287.

Bylsma, L. M., Mauss, I. B., & Rottenberg, J. (2016). Is the divide a chasm?: Bridging affective science with clinical practice. *Journal of Psychopathology and Behavioral Assessment, 38*(1), 42–47.

Bylsma, L. M., Morris, B. H., & Rottenberg, J. (2008). A meta-analysis of emotional reactivity in major depressive disorder. *Clinical Psychology Review, 28*(4), 676–691.

Carvalho, A. F., Rocha, D. Q. C., McIntyre, R. S., Mesquita, L. M., Köhler, C. A., Hyphantis, T. N., . . . Berk, M. (2014). Adipokines as emerging depression biomarkers: A systematic review and meta-analysis. *Journal of Psychiatric Research, 59*, 28–37.

Caspi, A., & Moffitt, T. E. (2018). All for one and one for all: Mental disorders in one dimension. *American Journal of Psychiatry, 175*(9), 831–844.

Céspedes, Y. M., & Huey, S. J. (2008). Depression in Latino adolescents. *Cultural Diversity and Ethnic Minority Psychology, 14*(2), 168–172.

Chakrabarti, S. (2018). Mood disorders in the International Classification of Diseases–11: Similarities and differences with the Diagnostic and *Statistical Manual of Mental Disorders 5* and the *International Classification of Diseases–10*. *Indian Journal of Social Psychiatry, 34*, 17–22.

Choi, S. W., Schalet, B., Cook, K. F., & Cella, D. (2014). Establishing a common metric for depressive symptoms: Linking the BDI-II, CES-D, and PHQ-9 to PROMIS Depression. *Psychological Assessment, 26*(2), 513–527.

Cipriani, A., Zhou, X., Del Giovane, C., Hetrick, S. E., Qin, B., Whittington, C., . . . Xie, P. (2016). Comparative efficacy and tolerability of antidepressants for major depressive disorder in children and adolescents: A network meta-analysis. *Lancet, 388*(10047), 881–890.

Clark, L. A., Cuthbert, B., Lewis-Fernández, R., Narrow, W. E., & Reed, G. M. (2017). Three approaches to understanding and classifying mental disorder: ICD-11, DSM-5, and the National Institute of Mental Health's Research Domain Criteria (RDoC). *Psychological Science in the Public Interest, 18*(2), 72–145.

Cohen, J. R., Adams, Z. W., Menon, S. V., Youngstrom, E. A., Bunnell, B. E., Acierno, R., . . . Danielson, C. K. (2016). How should we screen for depression following a natural disaster?: An ROC approach to post-disaster screening in adolescents and adults. *Journal of Affective Disorders, 202*, 102–109.

Cohen, J. R., Andrews, A. R., Davis, M. M., & Rudolph, K. D. (2018). Anxiety and depression during childhood and adolescence: Testing theoretical models of continuity and discontinuity. *Journal of Abnormal Child Psychology, 46*, 1295–1308.

Cohen, J. R., So, F. K., Young, J. F., Hankin, B. L., & Lee, B. A. (2019). Youth depression screening with parent and self-reports: Assessing current and prospective depression risk. *Child Psychiatry and Human Development, 50*, 647–660.

Cohen, J. R., Thakur, H., Burkhouse, K. L., & Gibb, B. E. (2019). A multimethod screening approach for pediatric depression onset: An incremental validity study. *Journal of Consulting and Clinical Psychology, 87*, 184–197.

Cole, D. A., & Martin, N. C. (2005). The longitudinal structure of the Children's Depression Inventory: Testing a latent trait–state model. *Psychological Assessment, 17*(2), 144–155.

Cole, D. A., Truglio, R., & Peeke, L. (1997). Relation between symptoms of anxiety and depression in children: A multitrait–multimethod–multigroup assessment. *Journal of Consulting and Clinical Psychology, 65*(1), 110–119.

Compas, B. E., Ey, S., & Grant, K. E. (1993). Taxonomy, assessment, and diagnosis of depression during adolescence. *Psychological Bulletin, 114*(2), 323–344.

Costello, E. J., Egger, H., & Angold, A. (2005). 10-year research update review: The epidemiology of child and adolescent psychiatric disorders: I. Methods and public health burden. *Journal of the American Academy of Child and Adolescent Psychiatry, 44*(10), 972–986.

Coyne, J. C. (1976). Depression and the response of others. *Journal of Abnormal Psychology, 85*(2), 186–193.

Craighead, W. E., Smucker, M. R., Craighead, L. W., & Ilardi, S. S. (1998). Factor analysis of the Children's Depression Inventory in a community sample. *Psychological Assessment, 10*(2), 156–165.

Cyranowski, J. M., Frank, E., Young, E., & Shear, M. K. (2000). Adolescent onset of the gender difference in lifetime rates of major depression: A theoretical model. *Archives of General Psychiatry, 57*(1), 21–27.

D'Angelo, E. J., & Augenstein, T. M. (2012). Developmentally informed evaluation of depression:

Evidence-based instruments. *Child and Adolescent Psychiatric Clinics of North America, 21*(2), 279–298.

De Fruyt, F., Bartels, M., Van Leeuwen, K. G., De Clercq, B., Decuyper, M., & Mervielde, I. (2006). Five types of personality continuity in childhood and adolescence. *Journal of Personality and Social Psychology, 91*(3), 538–552.

De Los Reyes, A. (2013). Strategic objectives for improving understanding of informant discrepancies in developmental psychopathology research. *Development and Psychopathology, 25*(3), 669–682.

De Los Reyes, A., Augenstein, T. M., Wang, M., Thomas, S. A., Drabick, D. A. G., Burgers, D. E., & Rabinowitz, J. (2015). The validity of the multi-informant approach to assessing child and adolescent mental health. *Psychological Bulletin, 141*(4), 858–900.

De Los Reyes, A., Lerner, M. D., Thomas, S. A., Daruwala, S., & Goepel, K. (2013). Discrepancies between parent and adolescent beliefs about daily life topics and performance on an emotion recognition task. *Journal of Abnormal Child Psychology, 41*(6), 971–982.

DeWalt, D. A., Thissen, D., Stucky, B. D., Langer, M. M., DeWitt, E. M., Irwin, D. E., . . . Varni, J. W. (2013). PROMIS Pediatric Peer Relationships Scale: Development of a peer relationships item bank as part of social health measurement. *Health Psychology, 32*(10), 1093–1103.

Dougherty, L. R., Klein, D. N., Olino, T. M., Dyson, M., & Rose, S. (2009). Increased waking salivary cortisol and depression risk in preschoolers: The role of maternal history of melancholic depression and early child temperament. *Journal of Child Psychology and Psychiatry and Allied Disciplines, 50*(12), 1495–1503.

Ehrenreich-May, J., Kennedy, S. M., Sherman, J. A., Bilek, E. L., Buzzella, B. A., Bennett, S. M., & Barlow, D. H. (2017). *Unified protocols for transdiagnostic treatment of emotional disorders in children and adolescents: Therapist guide.* New York: Oxford University Press.

Ely, J. W., Graber, M. L., & Croskerry, P. (2011). Checklists to reduce diagnostic errors. *Academic Medicine, 86*(3), 307–313.

Fallucco, E. M., Seago, R. D., Cuffe, S. P., Kraemer, D. F., & Wysocki, T. (2015). Primary care provider training in screening, assessment, and treatment of adolescent depression. *Academic Pediatrics, 15*(3), 326–332.

Findling, R. L., Youngstrom, E. A., Fristad, M. A., Birmaher, B., Kowatch, R. A., Arnold, L. E., . . . Horwitz, S. M. (2010). Characteristics of children with elevated symptoms of mania: The Longitudinal Assessment of Manic Symptoms (LAMS) study. *Journal of Clinical Psychiatry, 71*(12), 1664–1672.

Fisher, A. J., Medaglia, J. D., & Jeronimus, B. F. (2018). Lack of group-to-individual generalizability is a threat to human subjects research. *Proceedings of the National Academy of Sciences of the USA, 115*(27), E6106–E6115.

Freedman, R., Lewis, D. A., Michels, R., Pine, D. S., Schultz, S. K., Tamminga, C. A., . . . Yager, J. (2013). The initial field trials of DSM-5: New blooms and old thorns. *American Journal of Psychiatry, 170*(1), 1–5.

Fried, E. I., & Nesse, R. M. (2015). Depression is not a consistent syndrome: An investigation of unique symptom patterns in the STAR*D study. *Journal of Affective Disorders, 172*, 96–102.

Fried, E. I., van Borkulo, C. D., Epskamp, S., Schoevers, R. A., Tuerlinckx, F., & Borsboom, D. (2016). Measuring depression over time . . . Or not?: Lack of unidimensionality and longitudinal measurement invariance in four common rating scales of depression. *Psychological Assessment, 28*(11), 1354–1367.

Fristad, M. A., Emery, B. L., & Beck, S. J. (1997). Use and abuse of the Children's Depression Inventory. *Journal of Consulting and Clinical Psychology, 65*(4), 699–702.

Gadomski, A. M., Fothergill, K. E., Larson, S., Wissow, L. S., Winegrad, H., Nagykaldi, Z. J., . . . Roter, D. L. (2015). Integrating mental health into adolescent annual visits: Impact of previsit comprehensive screening on within-visit processes. *Journal of Adolescent Health, 56*(3), 267–273.

Gaffrey, M. S., Barch, D. M., Singer, J., Shenoy, R., & Luby, J. L. (2013). Disrupted amygdala reactivity in depressed 4–6-year-old children. *Journal of the American Academy of Child and Adolescent Psychiatry, 52*(7), 737–746.

Garber, J., & Weersing, V. R. (2010). Comorbidity of anxiety and depression in youth: Implications for treatment and prevention. *Clinical Psychology: Science and Practice, 17*(4), 293–306.

Gardner, W., Lucas, A., Kolko, D. J., & Campo, J. V. (2007). Comparison of the PSC-17 and alternative mental health screens in an at-risk primary care sample. *Journal of the American Academy of Child and Adolescent Psychiatry, 46*(5), 611–618.

Goodman, R. (2001). Psychometric properties of the Strengths and Difficulties Questionnaire. *Journal of the American Academy of Child and Adolescent Psychiatry, 40*(11), 1337–1345.

Goodman, R., & Scott, S. (1999). Comparing the Strengths and Difficulties Questionnaire and the Child Behavior Checklist: Is small beautiful? *Journal of Abnormal Child Psychology, 27*(1), 17–24.

Guion, R. M. (2011). *Assessment, measurement, and prediction for personnel decisions* (2nd ed.). Hillsdale, NJ: Erlbaum.

Hammack, P. L. (2003). Toward a unified theory of depression among urban African American youth: Integrating socioecologic, cognitive, family stress, and biopsychosocial perspectives. *Journal of Black Psychology, 29*(2), 187–209.

Hammen, C. (1991). Generation of stress in the course of unipolar depression. *Journal of Abnormal Psychology, 100*(4), 555–561.

Hankin, B. L. (2012). Future directions in vulnerability to depression among youth: Integrating risk factors and processes across multiple levels of analysis. *Journal of Clinical Child and Adolescent Psychology, 41,* 695–718.

Hankin, B. L. (2019). A choose your own adventure story: Conceptualizing depression in children and adolescents from traditional DSM and alternative latent dimensional approaches. *Behaviour Research and Therapy, 118,* 94–100.

Hankin, B. L., & Abramson, L. Y. (2001). Development of gender differences in depression: An elaborated cognitive vulnerability-transactional stress theory. *Psychological Bulletin, 127*(6), 773–796.

Hankin, B. L., Abramson, L. Y., Moffitt, T. E., Silva, P. A., McGee, R., & Angell, K. E. (1998). Development of depression from preadolescence to young adulthood: Emerging gender differences in a 10-year longitudinal study. *Journal of Abnormal Psychology, 107*(1), 128–140.

Hankin, B. L., Fraley, R. C., Lahey, B. B., & Waldman, I. D. (2005). Is depression best viewed as a continuum or discrete category?: A taxometric analysis of childhood and adolescent depression in a population-based sample. *Journal of Abnormal Psychology, 114*(1), 96–110.

Hankin, B. L., Oppenheimer, C., Jenness, J., Barrocas, A., Shapero, B. G., & Goldband, J. (2009). Developmental origins of cognitive vulnerabilities to depression: Review of processes contributing to stability and change across time. *Journal of Clinical Psychology, 65*(12), 1327–1338.

Hankin, B. L., Snyder, H. R., & Gulley, L. D. (2016). Cognitive risks in developmental psychopathology. In D. Cicchetti (Ed.), *Developmental psychopathology* (3rd ed., pp. 312–385). Hoboken, NJ: Wiley.

Hankin, B. L., Snyder, H. R., Gulley, L. D., Schweizer, T. H., Bijtebier, P., Nelis, S., . . . Vasey, M. W. (2016). Understanding comorbidity among internalizing problems: Integrating latent structural models of psychopathology and risk mechanisms. *Development and Psychopathology, 28*(4, Pt. 1), 987–1012.

Hankin, B. L., Wetter, E., & Cheely, C. (2008). Sex differences in child and adolescent depression: A developmental psychopathological approach. In J. R. Z. Abela & B. L. Hankin (Eds.), *Handbook of depression in children and adolescents* (pp. 377–414). New York: Guilford Press.

Hankin, B. L., Young, J. F., Abela, J. R. Z., Smolen, A., Jenness, J. L., Gulley, L. D., . . . Oppenheimer, C. W. (2015). Depression from childhood into late adolescence: Influence of gender, development, genetic susceptibility, and peer stress. *Journal of Abnormal Psychology, 124*(4), 803–816.

Hankin, B. L., Young, J. F., Gallop, R., & Garber, J. (2018). Cognitive and interpersonal vulnerabilities to adolescent depression: Classification of risk profiles for a personalized prevention approach. *Journal of Abnormal Child Psychology, 46*(7), 1521–1533.

Haroz, E. E., Ybarra, M. L., & Eaton, W. W. (2014). Psychometric evaluation of a self-report scale to measure adolescent depression: The CESDR-10 in two national adolescent samples in the United States. *Journal of Affective Disorders, 158,* 154–160.

Harrington, R., Fudge, H., Rutter, M., Pickles, A., & Hill, J. (1990). Adult outcomes of childhood and adolescent depression: I. Psychiatric status. *Archives of General Psychiatry, 47*(5), 465–473.

Harris, S. K. (2015). Making time for mental health: Computerized previsit screening in primary care. *Journal of Adolescent Health, 56*(3), 257–258.

Horton, N. J., & Fitzmaurice, G. M. (2004). Regression analysis of multiple source and multiple informant data from complex survey samples. *Statistics in Medicine, 23*(18), 2911–2933.

Hovey, J. D., & King, C. A. (1996). Acculturative stress, depression, and suicidal ideation among immigrant and second-generation Latino adolescents. *Journal of the American Academy of Child and Adolescent Psychiatry, 35*(9), 1183–1192.

Hudziak, J. J., Copeland, W., Stanger, C., & Wadsworth, M. (2004). Screening for DSM-IV externalizing disorders with the Child Behavior Checklist: A receiver-operating characteristic analysis. *Journal of Child Psychology and Psychiatry and Allied Disciplines, 45*(7), 1299–1307.

Hughes, M., Kiecolt, K. J., Keith, V. M., & Demo, D. H. (2015). Racial identity and well-being among African Americans. *Social Psychology Quarterly, 78*(1), 25–48.

Hunsley, J. (2015). Translating evidence-based assessment principles and components into clinical practice settings. *Cognitive and Behavioral Practice, 22*(1), 101–109.

Hunsley, J., & Mash, E. J. (2007). Evidence-based assessment. *Annual Review of Clinical Psychology, 3*(1), 29–51.

Insel, T. R. (2017). Digital phenotyping: Technology for a new science of behavior. *Journal of the American Medical Association, 318*(13), 1215–1216.

Irwin, D. E., Stucky, B., Langer, M. M., Thissen, D., DeWitt, E. M., Lai, J.-S., . . . DeWalt, D. A. (2010). An item response analysis of the pediatric PROMIS anxiety and depressive symptoms scales. *Quality of Life Research, 19*(4), 595–607.

Jacobson, N. S., & Truax, P. (1991). Clinical significance: A statistical approach to defining meaningful change in psychotherapy research. *Journal of Consulting and Clinical Psychology, 59,* 12–19.

Jensen-Doss, A. (2015). Practical, evidence-based clinical decision making: Introduction to the special series. *Cognitive and Behavioral Practice, 22*(1), 1–4.

Johnston, C., & Murray, C. (2003). Incremental validity in the psychological assessment of children and adolescents. *Psychological Assessment, 15,* 496–507.

Joiner, T. E., Alfano, M. S., & Metalsky, G. I. (1992). When depression breeds contempt: Reassurance seeking, self-esteem, and rejection of depressed college students by their roommates. *Journal of Abnormal Psychology, 101*(1), 165–173.

Judd, L. L., Paulus, M. P., Wells, K. B., & Rapaport, M. H. (1996). Socioeconomic burden of subsyndromal depressive symptoms and major depression in a sample of the general population. *American Journal of Psychiatry, 153*(11), 1411–1417.

Kamenov, K., Cabello, M., Coenen, M., & Ayuso-Mateos, J. L. (2015). How much do we know about the functional effectiveness of interventions for depression?: A systematic review. *Journal of Affective Disorders, 188,* 89–96.

Kaufman, J., Birmaher, B., Brent, D., Rao, U., Flynn, C., Moreci, P., . . . Ryan, N. (1997). Schedule for Affective Disorders and Schizophrenia for School-Age Children—Present and Lifetime version (K-SADS-PL): Initial reliability and validity data. *Journal of the American Academy of Child and Adolescent Psychiatry, 36,* 980–988.

Keenan, K., & Hipwell, A. E. (2005). Preadolescent clues to understanding depression in girls. *Clinical Child and Family Psychology Review, 8*(2), 89–105.

Kendell, R., & Jablensky, A. (2003). Distinguishing between the validity and utility of psychiatric diagnoses. *American Journal of Psychiatry, 160*(1), 4–12.

Kendler, K. (2012). The dappled nature of causes of psychiatric illness: Replacing the organic–functional/hardware–software dichotomy with empirically based pluralism. *Molecular Psychiatry, 17*(4), 377–388.

Kennedy, S. M., Bilek, E. L., & Ehrenreich-May, J. (2019). A randomized controlled pilot trial of the unified protocol for transdiagnostic treatment of emotional disorders in children. *Behavior Modification, 43,* 330–360.

Kessler, R. C., Avenevoli, S., McLaughlin, K. A., Green, J. G., Lakoma, M. D., Petukhova, M., . . . Merikangas, K. R. (2012). Lifetime co-morbidity of DSM-IV disorders in the US National Comorbidity Survey Replication Adolescent Supplement (NCS-A). *Psychological Medicine, 42*(9), 1997–2010.

Kistner, J. A., David-Ferdon, C. F., Lopez, C. M., & Dunkel, S. B. (2007). Ethnic and sex differences in children's depressive symptoms. *Journal of Clinical Child and Adolescent Psychology, 36*(2), 171–181.

Klein, D. N., Dougherty, L. R., & Olino, T. M. (2005). Toward guidelines for evidence-based assessment of depression in children and adolescents. *Journal of Clinical Child and Adolescent Psychology, 34*(3), 412–432.

Koenig, J., Kemp, A. H., Beauchaine, T. P., Thayer, J. F., & Kaess, M. (2016). Depression and resting state heart rate variability in children and adolescents—A systematic review and meta-analysis. *Clinical Psychology Review, 46,* 136–150.

Konig, I. R., Malley, J. D., Weimar, C., Diener, H. C., & Ziegler, A. (German Stroke Study Collaboration). (2007). Practical experiences on the necessity of external validation. *Statistics in Medicine, 26,* 5499–5511.

Kotov, R., Waszczuk, M. A., Krueger, R. F., Forbes, M. K., Watson, D., Clark, L. A., . . . Zimmerman, M. (2017). The hierarchical taxonomy of psychopathology (HiTOP): A dimensional alternative to traditional nosologies. *Journal of Abnormal Psychology, 126*(4), 454–477.

Kovacs, M. (2010). *Children's Depression Inventory 2 (CDI 2).* North Tonawanda. NY: Multi-Health Systems.

Kraemer, H. C., Measelle, J. R., Ablow, J. C., Essex, M. J., Boyce, W. T., & Kupfer, D. J. (2003). A new approach to integrating data from multiple informants in psychiatric assessment and research: Mixing and matching contexts and perspectives. *American Journal of Psychiatry, 160*(9), 1566–1577.

Krueger, R. F. (2018). Taking the next steps in the science of clinical personality psychology. *European Journal of Personality, 32*(5), 525–624.

Lahey, B. B., Krueger, R. F., Rathouz, P. J., Waldman, I. D., & Zald, D. H. (2017). A hierarchical causal taxonomy of psychopathology across the life span. *Psychological Bulletin, 143*(2), 142–186.

Lauth, B., Levy, S. R. A., Júlíusdóttir, G., Ferrari, P., & Pétursson, H. (2008). Implementing the semi-structured interview Kiddie-SADS-PL into an in-patient adolescent clinical setting: Impact on frequency of diagnoses. *Child and Adolescent Psychiatry and Mental Health, 2,* 14.

Lavigne, J. V., Feldman, M., & Meyers, K. M. (2016). Screening for mental health problems: Addressing the base rate fallacy for a sustainable screening program in integrated primary care. *Journal of Pediatric Psychology, 41*(10), 1081–1090.

Leffler, J. M., Riebel, J., & Hughes, H. M. (2015). A review of child and adolescent diagnostic interviews for clinical practitioners. *Assessment, 22*(6), 690–703.

Lewinsohn, P. M., Rohde, P., Klein, D. N., & Seeley, J. R. (1999). Natural course of adolescent major depressive disorder: I. Continuity into young adulthood. *Journal of the American Academy of Child and Adolescent Psychiatry, 38*(1), 56–63.

Lewis, K. J., Mars, B., Lewis, G., Rice, F., Sellers, R., Thapar, A. K., . . . Thapar, A. (2012). Do parents know best?: Parent-reported vs. child-reported depression symptoms as predictors of future child mood disorder in a high-risk sample. *Journal of Affective Disorders, 141*(2–3), 233–236.

Lilienfeld, S. O., Smith, S. F., & Watts, A. L. (2013). Issues in diagnosis: Conceptual issues and controversies. In W. E. Craighead, D. J. Miklowitz, & L. W. Craighead (Eds.), *Psychopathology: History, diagnosis, and empirical foundations* (pp. 1–35). Hoboken, NJ: Wiley.

Liu, R. T. (2016). Taxometric evidence of a dimensional latent structure for depression in an epidemiological sample of children and adolescents. *Psychological Medicine, 46*(6), 1265–1275.

Loechner, J., Starman, K., Galuschka, K., Tamm, J., Schulte-Körne, G., Rubel, J., & Platt, B. (2018). Preventing depression in the offspring of parents with depression: A systematic review and meta-analysis of randomized controlled trials. *Clinical Psychology Review, 60,* 1–14.

Long, E. E., Young, J. F., & Hankin, B. L. (2019). Separating within-person from between-person effects in the longitudinal co-occurrence of depression and different anxiety syndromes in youth. *Journal of Research in Personality, 81,* 158–167.

Luby, J. L. (2010). Preschool depression: The importance of identification of depression early in development. *Current Directions in Psychological Science, 19*(2), 91–95.

Luby, J. L., Belden, A. C., Jackson, J. J., Lessov-Schlaggar, C. N., Harms, M. P., Tillman, R., . . . Barch, D. M. (2016). Early childhood depression and alterations in the trajectory of gray matter maturation in middle childhood and early adolescence. *JAMA Psychiatry, 73*(1), 31–38.

Luby, J. L., Gaffrey, M. S., Tillman, R., April, L. M., & Belden, A. C. (2014). Trajectories of preschool disorders to full DSM Depression at school age and early adolescence: Continuity of preschool depression. *American Journal of Psychiatry, 171*(7), 768–776.

Luby, J. L., Heffelfinger, A. K., Mrakotsky, C., Hessler, M. J., Brown, K. M., & Hildebrand, T. (2002). Preschool major depressive disorder: Preliminary validation for developmentally modified DSM-IV criteria. *Journal of the American Academy of Child and Adolescent Psychiatry, 41*(8), 928–937.

Luby, J. L., Si, X., Belden, A. C., Tandon, M., & Spitznagel, E. (2009). Preschool depression. *Archives of General Psychiatry, 66*(8), 897–905.

Martel, M. M., Markon, K., & Smith, G. T. (2017). Research review: Multi-informant integration in child and adolescent psychopathology diagnosis. *Journal of Child Psychology and Psychiatry and Allied Disciplines, 58*(2), 116–128.

Mash, E. J., & Barkley, R. A. (Eds.). (2007). *Assessment of childhood disorders* (4th ed.). New York: Guilford Press.

Matthey, S., & Petrovski, P. (2002). The Children's Depression Inventory: Error in cutoff scores for screening purposes. *Psychological Assessment, 14*(2), 146–149.

Mayes, T. L., Bernstein, I. H., Haley, C. L., Kennard, B. D., & Emslie, G. J. (2010). Psychometric properties of the Children's Depression Rating Scale–Revised in adolescents. *Journal of Child and Adolescent Psychopharmacology, 20*(6), 513–516.

McDonald, E. J., McCabe, K., Yeh, M., Lau, A., Garland, A., & Hough, R. L. (2005). Cultural affiliation and self-esteem as predictors of internalizing symptoms among Mexican American adolescents. *Journal of Clinical Child and Adolescent Psychology, 34*(1), 163–171.

McKnight, P. E., & Kashdan, T. B. (2009). The importance of functional impairment to mental health outcomes: A case for reassessing our goals in depression treatment research. *Clinical Psychology Review, 29*(3), 243–259.

McLaughlin, K. A., Hilt, L. M., & Nolen-Hoeksema, S. (2007). Racial/ethnic differences in internalizing and externalizing symptoms in adolescents. *Journal of Abnormal Child Psychology, 35*(5), 801–816.

Mohr, D. C., Zhang, M., & Schueller, S. M. (2017). Personal sensing: Understanding mental health using ubiquitous sensors and machine learning. *Annual Review of Clinical Psychology, 13*(1), 23–47.

Moran, T. P., Schroder, H. S., Kneip, C., & Moser, J. S. (2017). Meta-analysis and psychophysiology: A tutorial using depression and action-monitoring event-related potentials. *International Journal of Psychophysiology, 111,* 17–32.

Myers, K., & Winters, N. C. (2002). Ten-year review of rating scales: II. Scales for internalizing disorders. *Journal of the American Academy of Child and Adolescent Psychiatry, 41*(6), 634–659.

Nolen-Hoeksema, S., & Girgus, J. S. (1994). The emergence of gender differences in depression during adolescence. *Psychological Bulletin, 115*(3), 424–443.

Nyborg, V. M., & Curry, J. F. (2003). The impact of perceived racism: Psychological symptoms among African American boys. *Journal of Clinical Child and Adolescent Psychology, 32*(2), 258–266.

Olino, T. M., Yu, L., McMakin, D. L., Forbes, E. E., Seeley, J. R., Lewinsohn, P. M., & Pilkonis, P. A. (2013). Comparisons across depression assessment instruments in adolescence and young adulthood: An item response theory study using two linking methods. *Journal of Abnormal Child Psychology, 41*(8), 1267–1277.

Petersen, A. C., Compas, B. E., Brooks-Gunn, J., Stemmler, M., Ey, S., & Grant, K. E. (1993). Depression in adolescence. *American Psychologist, 48*(2), 155–168.

Piccirillo, M. L., & Rodebaugh, T. L. (2019). Foundations of idiographic methods in psychology and applications for psychotherapy. *Clinical Psychology Review, 71,* 90–100.

Pine, D. S., Cohen, P., Gurley, D., Brook, J., & Ma, Y. (1998). The risk for early-adulthood anxiety and depressive disorders in adolescents with anxiety and depressive disorders. *Archives of General Psychiatry, 55*(1), 56–64.

Polanczyk, G. V., Salum, G. A., Sugaya, L. S., Caye, A., & Rohde, L. A. (2015). Annual research review: A meta-analysis of the worldwide prevalence of mental disorders in children and adolescents. *Journal of Child Psychology and Psychiatry and Allied Disciplines, 56*(3), 345–365.

Poznanski, E. O., & Mokros, H. B. (1996). *Children's Depression Rating Scale, Revised (CDRS-R).* Los Angeles: Western Psychological Services.

Radloff, L. S. (1977). The CES-D Scale: A self-report depression scale for research in the general population. *Applied Psychological Measurement, 1*(3), 385–401.

Raiker, J. S., Freeman, A. J., Perez-Algorta, G., Frazier, T. W., Findling, R. L., & Youngstrom, E. A. (2017).

Accuracy of Achenbach scales in the screening of attention-deficit/hyperactivity disorder in a community mental health clinic. *Journal of the American Academy of Child and Adolescent Psychiatry, 56*(5), 401–409.

Reise, S. P., & Waller, N. G. (2009). Item response theory and clinical measurement. *Annual Review of Clinical Psychology, 5*, 27–48.

Richardson, L. P., Rockhill, C., Russo, J. E., Grossman, D. C., Richards, J., McCarty, C., . . . Katon, W. (2010). Evaluation of the PHQ-2 as a brief screen for detecting major depression among adolescents. *Pediatrics, 125*(5), e1097–e1103.

Roberts, B. W., & DelVecchio, W. F. (2000). The rank-order consistency of personality traits from childhood to old age: A quantitative review of longitudinal studies. *Psychological Bulletin, 126*(1), 3–25.

Rosanbalm, K. D., Snyder, E. H., Lawrence, C. N., Coleman, K., Frey, J. J., van den Ende, J. B., & Dodge, K. A. (2016). Child wellbeing assessment in child welfare: A review of four measures. *Children and Youth Services Review, 68*, 1–16.

Rudolph, K., & Lambert, S. (2007). Child and adolescent depression. In E. J. Mash & R. A. Barkley (Eds.), *Assessment of childhood disorders* (4th ed., pp. 213–252). New York: Guilford Press.

Ruggero, C. J., Kotov, R., Hopwood, C. J., First, M., Clark, L. A., Skodol, A. E., . . . Zimmerman, J. (2019). Integrating a dimensional hierarchical taxonomy of psychopathology into clinical practice. *Journal of Consulting and Clinical Psychology, 87*, 1069–1084.

Rutter, M. (2013). Annual research review: Resilience—clinical implications. *Journal of Child Psychology and Psychiatry and Allied Disciplines, 54*(4), 474–487.

Salk, R. H., Hyde, J. S., & Abramson, L. Y. (2017). Gender differences in depression in representative national samples: Meta-analyses of diagnoses and symptoms. *Psychological Bulletin, 143*(8), 783–822.

Santor, D. A., Ramsay, J. O., & Zuroff, D. C. (1994). Nonparametric item analyses of the Beck Depression Inventory: Evaluating gender item bias and response option weights. *Psychological Assessment, 6*(3), 255–270.

Saylor, C. F., Finch, A. J., Spirito, A., & Bennett, B. (1984). The Children's Depression Inventory: A systematic evaluation of psychometric properties. *Journal of Consulting and Clinical Psychology, 52*(6), 955–967.

Seeley, J. R., Stice, E., & Rohde, P. (2009). Screening for depression prevention: Identifying adolescent girls at high risk for future depression. *Journal of Abnormal Psychology, 118*(1), 161–170.

Shaffer, D., Fisher, P., Lucas, C. P., Dulcan, M. K., & Schwab-Stone, M. E. (2000). NIMH Diagnostic Interview Schedule for Children Version IV (NIMH DISC-IV): Description, differences from previous versions, and reliability of some common diagnoses. *Journal of the American Academy of Child and Adolescent Psychiatry, 39*(1), 28–38.

Shankman, S. A., Klein, D. N., Torpey, D. C., Olino, T. M., Dyson, M. W., Kim, J., . . . Tenke, C. E. (2011). Do positive and negative temperament traits interact in predicting risk for depression?: A resting EEG study of 329 preschoolers. *Development and Psychopathology, 23*(2), 551–562.

Sharpe, J. P., & Gilbert, D. G. (1998). Effects of repeated administration of the Beck Depression Inventory and other measures of negative mood states. *Personality and Individual Differences, 4*(24), 457–463.

Sheehan, D., Shytle, D., Milo, K., Janavs, J., & Lecrubier, Y. (2009). *Mini International Neuropsychiatric Interview for Children and Adolescents, English version 6.0.* Tampa: University of South Florida.

Siu, A. L., Bibbins-Domingo, K., Grossman, D. C., Baumann, L. C., Davidson, K. W., Ebell, M., . . . Pignone, M. P. (2016). Screening for depression in adults: US Preventive Services Task Force Recommendation Statement. *Journal of the American Medical Association, 315*(4), 380–387.

Slavich, G. M., & Irwin, M. R. (2014). From stress to inflammation and major depressive disorder: A social signal transduction theory of depression. *Psychological Bulletin, 140*(3), 774–815.

Stewart, J. G., & Harkness, K. L. (2017). Testing a revised interpersonal theory of depression using a laboratory measure of excessive reassurance seeking: Depression, ERS, and romantic relationships. *Journal of Clinical Psychology, 73*(3), 331–348.

Stice, E., Shaw, H., Bohon, C., Marti, C. N., & Rohde, P. (2009). A meta-analytic review of depression prevention programs for children and adolescents: Factors that predict magnitude of intervention effects. *Journal of Consulting and Clinical Psychology, 77*(3), 486–503.

Stiffler, M. C., & Dever, B. V. (2015). *Mental health screening at school: Instrumentation, implementation, and critical issues.* Cham, Switzerland: Springer International.

Stockings, E., Degenhardt, L., Lee, Y. Y., Mihalopoulos, C., Liu, A., Hobbs, M., & Patton, G. (2015). Symptom screening scales for detecting major depressive disorder in children and adolescents: A systematic review and meta-analysis of reliability, validity and diagnostic utility. *Journal of Affective Disorders, 174*, 447–463.

Straus, S. E., Glasziou, P., Richardson, W. S., & Haynes, R. B. (2011). *Evidence-based medicine: How to practice and teach EBM* (4th ed.). New York: Churchill Livingstone.

Strobl, C., Malley, J., & Tutz, G. (2009). An introduction to recursive partitioning: Rationale, application and characteristics of classification and regression trees, bagging and random forests. *Psychological Methods, 14*(4), 323–348.

Taylor, S. E., Klein, L. C., Lewis, B. P., Gruenewald, T. L., Gurung, R. A. R., & Updegraff, J. A. (2000). Biobehavioral responses to stress in females: Tend-and-befriend, not fight-or-flight. *Psychological Review, 107*(3), 411–429.

Thakur, H., & Cohen, J. R. (2019). Depression screening in trauma-exposed youth: Multi-informant algorithms for the child welfare setting. *Psychological Assessment, 31,* 1028–1039.

Thapar, A. K., Hood, K., Collishaw, S., Hammerton, G., Mars, B., Sellers, R., . . . Rice, F. (2016). Identifying key parent-reported symptoms for detecting depression in high risk adolescents. *Psychiatry Research, 242,* 210–217.

Thomas, S. A., Aldao, A., & De Los Reyes, A. (2012). Implementing clinically feasible psychophysiological measures in evidence-based assessments of adolescent social anxiety. *Professional Psychology: Research and Practice, 43*(5), 510–519.

Timbremont, B., Braet, C., & Dreessen, L. (2004). Assessing depression in youth: Relation between the Children's Depression Inventory and a structured interview. *Journal of Clinical Child and Adolescent Psychology, 33*(1), 149–157.

Torous, J., Larsen, M. E., Depp, C., Cosco, T. D., Barnett, I., Nock, M. K., & Firth, J. (2018). Smartphones, sensors, and machine learning to advance real-time prediction and interventions for suicide prevention: A review of current progress and next steps. *Current Psychiatry Reports, 20*(7), 51.

Tram, J. M., & Cole, D. A. (2006). A multimethod examination of the stability of depressive symptoms in childhood and adolescence. *Journal of Abnormal Psychology, 115*(4), 674–686.

Twenge, J. M., & Nolen-Hoeksema, S. (2002). Age, gender, race, socioeconomic status, and birth cohort difference on the Children's Depression Inventory: A meta-analysis. *Journal of Abnormal Psychology, 111,* 578–588.

Uher, R., & Rutter, M. (2012). Basing psychiatric classification on scientific foundation: Problems and prospects. *International Review of Psychiatry, 24*(6), 591–605.

Umaña-Taylor, A. J., Quintana, S. M., Lee, R. M., Cross, J. W., Rivas-Drake, D., Schwartz, S. J., . . . Seaton, E. (2014). Ethnic and racial identity during adolescence and into young adulthood: An integrated conceptualization. *Child Development, 85*(1), 21–39.

Van Meter, A., Youngstrom, E. A., Ollendick, T., Demeter, C., & Findling, R. L. (2014). Clinical decision-making about child and adolescent anxiety disorders using the Achenbach system of empirically based assessment. *Journal of Clinical Child and Adolescent Psychology, 43*(4), 552–565.

Varigonda, A. L., Jakubovski, E., Taylor, M. J., Freemantle, N., Coughlin, C., & Bloch, M. H. (2015). Systematic review and meta-analysis: Early treatment responses of selective serotonin reuptake inhibitors in pediatric major depressive disorder. *Journal of the American Academy of Child and Adolescent Psychiatry, 54*(7), 557–564.

Walsh, C. G., Ribeiro, J. D., & Franklin, J. C. (2017). Predicting risk of suicide attempts over time through machine learning. *Clinical Psychological Science, 5*(3), 457–469.

Wang, Z., Conrad, K. J., Hankin, B. L., & Huang, Z. (2005). Comparison and co-calibration of the Mood and Anxiety Symptom Questionnaire and the Beck Depression Inventory using Rasch analysis. In N. Bezruczko (Ed.), *Rasch measurement in health sciences* (pp. 334–362). Maple Grove, MN: JAM Press.

Weersing, V. R., Jeffreys, M., Do, M.-C. T., Schwartz, K. T. G., & Bolano, C. (2017). Evidence base update of psychosocial treatments for child and adolescent depression. *Journal of Clinical Child and Adolescent Psychology, 53, 46*(1), 11–43.

Weersing, V. R., Shamseddeen, W., Garber, J., Hollon, S. D., Clarke, G. N., Beardslee, W. R., . . . Brent, D. A. (2016). Prevention of depression in at-risk adolescents: Predictors and moderators of acute effects. *Journal of the American Academy of Child and Adolescent Psychiatry, 55*(3), 219–226.

Weiss, B., & Garber, J. (2003). Developmental differences in the phenomenology of depression. *Development and Psychopathology, 15*(2), 403–430.

Weissman, M. M., Wolk, S., Goldstein, R. B., Moreau, D., Adams, P., Greenwald, S., . . . Wickramaratne, P. (1999). Depressed adolescents grown up. *Journal of the American Medical Association, 281*(18), 1707–1713.

Weisz, J. R., Chorpita, B. F., Frye, A., Ng, M. Y., Lau, N., Bearman, S. K., . . . Hoagwood, K. E. (2011). Youth top problems: Using idiographic, consumer-guided assessment to identify treatment needs and to track change during psychotherapy. *Journal of Consulting and Clinical Psychology, 79*(3), 369–380.

Weller, E. B., Fristad, M. A., Weller, R. A., & Rooney, M. T. (1999). *Children's Interview for Psychiatric Syndromes: ChIPS.* Washington, DC: American Psychiatric Association.

Whalen, D. J., Sylvester, C. M., & Luby, J. L. (2017). Depression and anxiety in preschoolers: A review of the past 7 years. *Child and Adolescent Psychiatric Clinics, 26*(3), 503–522.

Widiger, T. A., & Clark, L. A. (2000). Toward DSM-V and the classification of psychopathology. *Psychological Bulletin, 126*(6), 946–963.

Wissow, L. S., Brown, J., Fothergill, K. E., Gadomski, A., Hacker, K., Salmon, P., & Zelkowitz, R. (2013). Universal mental health screening in pediatric primary care: A systematic review. *Journal of the American Academy of Child and Adolescent Psychiatry, 52*(11), 1134–1147.

Woody, M. L., & Gibb, B. E. (2015). Integrating NIMH Research Domain Criteria (RDoC) into depression research. *Current Opinion in Psychology, 4,* 6–12.

Yee, A. M., Algorta, G. P., Youngstrom, E. A., Findling, R. L., Birmaher, B., . . . LAMS Group. (2015). Unfiltered administration of the YMRS and CDRS-R in a clinical sample of children. *Journal of Clinical Child and Adolescent Psychology, 44*(6), 992–1007.

Yorbik, O., Birmaher, B., Axelson, D., Williamson, D. E., & Ryan, N. D. (2004). Clinical characteristics of depressive symptoms in children and adolescents with major depressive disorder. *Journal of Clinical Psychiatry, 65*(12), 1654–1659.

Youngstrom, E. A. (2014). A primer on receiver operating characteristic analysis and diagnostic efficiency statistics for pediatric psychology: We are ready to ROC. *Journal of Pediatric Psychology, 39*(2), 204–221.

Youngstrom, E. A., & De Los Reyes, A. (2015). Commentary: Moving toward cost-effectiveness in using psychophysiological measures in clinical assessment: Validity, decision making, and adding value. *Journal of Clinical Child and Adolescent Psychology, 44*(2), 352–361.

Youngstrom, E. A., Findling, R. L., & Calabrese, J. R. (2003). Who are the comorbid adolescents?: Agreement between psychiatric diagnosis, parent, teacher, and youth report. *Journal of Abnormal Child Psychology, 31*, 231–245.

Youngstrom, E. A., Halverson, T. F., Youngstrom, J. K., Lindhiem, O., & Findling, R. L. (2018). Evidence-based assessment from simple clinical judgments to statistical learning: Evaluating a range of options using pediatric bipolar disorder as a diagnostic challenge. *Clinical Psychological Science, 6*(2), 243–265.

Youngstrom, E. A., Van Meter, A., Frazier, T. W., Hunsley, J., Prinstein, M. J., Ong, M. L., & Youngstrom, J. K. (2017). Evidence-based assessment as an integrative model for applying psychological science to guide the voyage of treatment. *Clinical Psychology: Science and Practice, 24*(4), 331–363.

Youngstrom, E. A., Van Meter, A., Frazier, T. W., Youngstrom, J. K., & Findling, R. L. (2020). Developing and validating short forms of the Parent General Behavior Inventory Mania and Depression scales for rating youth mood symptoms. *Journal of Clinical Child and Adolescent Psychology, 49*(2), 162–177.

Youngstrom, E. A., Youngstrom, J. K., Freeman, A. J., De Los Reyes, A., Feeny, N. C., & Findling, R. L. (2011). Informants are not all equal: Predictors and correlates of clinician judgments about caregiver and youth credibility. *Journal of Child and Adolescent Psychopharmacology, 21*, 407–415.

Zimmerman, M. (2003). What should the standard of care for psychiatric diagnostic evaluations be? *Journal of Nervous and Mental Disease, 191*(5), 281–286.

Zuckerbrot, R. A., Cheung, A., Jensen, P. S., Stein, R. E. K., & Laraque, D. (2018). Guidelines for Adolescent Depression in Primary Care (GLAD-PC): Part I. Practice preparation, identification, assessment, and initial management. *Pediatrics, 141*, e20174081.

CHAPTER 8

Bipolar Spectrum Disorders

Eric A. Youngstrom, Emma E. Morton, and Greg Murray

The tremendous amount of research on bipolar spectrum disorders (BSD) in children and adolescents over the past two decades has done much to address myths and controversies surrounding the diagnosis. While the phenomenology, prevalence, and treatment of BSD has historically been debated, an accumulation of good, large-scale data has informed the consensus that, while rare, BSD does indeed present in children and adolescents, and that differences between pediatric and adult BSD are likely overstated (B. Goldstein et al., 2017). Clinicians should remain cautious in their approach to assessment given the rarity of the condition before puberty, difficulty in disentangling mood symptoms from developmentally appropri-

ate behavior, or problems due to more common conditions, such as attention-deficit/hyperactivity disorder (ADHD) or unipolar depression, and frequent comorbidity, further obscuring the clinical presentation. Thoughtful and careful assessment for BSD contributes to clinical care by *predicting* meaningful outcomes, *prescribing* interventions (or contraindicating other approaches), or measuring *processes* that are related to successful intervention.

BSD is associated with higher risk for poorer educational, family, and social functioning outcomes, as well as substance use and suicidality (Birmaher et al., 2006; Geller, Tillman, Craney, & Bolhofner, 2004; Lewinsohn, Klein, & Seeley, 2000). Early identification and treatment may not only reduce poor outcomes but also enable use of less intense treatment to change illness trajectory. A bipolar case formulation alerts a clinician to a set of potential concerns that extend beyond management of anger, impulse control, and internalizing problems—although these issues are also likely to be part of the presenting problem. A BSD diagnosis should trigger a focus on sleep hygiene, activity scheduling, management of both positive and negative events, and a plan to support adherence to treatment (Fristad & MacPherson, 2014). A growing body of high-quality research can guide the selection of appropriate pharmacological and psychosocial treatments for BSD, as well as approaches less likely to help (B. Goldstein et al., 2017). Besides routine evaluation of internalizing and externalizing symptoms, a BSD formulation requires more systematic tracking of mood and energy levels. Unlike unipolar depression (see Hankin & Cohen, Chapter 7, this volume), BSD needs more systematic monitoring of both highs and lows of mood and energy, as well as periods of irritability. Relapse prevention becomes an important formal component of treatment, so identification of "triggers" and early warning signs of mood destabilization ("roughening" of mood; Sachs, Guille, & McMurrich, 2002) becomes paramount. Finally, good evaluation improves detection of individuals with BSD (i.e., raising the diagnostic "sensitivity"), while also recognizing when the problem is not BSD (i.e., bettering the diagnostic "specificity"). Correct diagnosis of nonbipolar illnesses connects to a much larger evidence base for treatment and avoids unnecessarily exposing children to potentially iatrogenic pharmacological agents (Correll, 2008; McClellan, Kowatch, & Findling, 2007; Ray et al., 2019)

Doing a good job assessing potential BSD pushes us to better understand the needs and nuances of most families, not just those who actually have BSD.

Preparing to Assess Potential BSD

To get ready to evaluate an individual who might have BSD, we want to have the diagnostic criteria in front of us and make sure that we understand nuances, such as what rapid cycling or a mixed state would look like. We also want to know what are the common comorbidities, as well as how BSD might affect dimensions of functioning and symptomatology. It also is crucial to have a sense of the clinical epidemiology—the base rates in different settings, and a good sense of how demographic and cultural factors might influence presentation and course. We pull all of this contextual information together in this section and on the preparation portion of the Wikiversity page. Table 8.1 also lists a potential "starter kit" of measures and interviews to have on hand, depending on the age of the client.

Diagnostic Criteria

In order to do a good job assessing mood disorders, it is crucial to understand the wide range of how they can appear and how they affect people. What does bipolar disorder look like? It might look like wide-eyed, fast talking person on a mission-to-save-the-world, with pacing, sleepless psychosis (psychotic mania). It might be a wise-cracking, playful, creative person, experimenting with new things; or it might one who is impulsive, risk-taking, irritable, and aggressive when challenged (both could be hypomania). It might also mean one is seriously and suicidally depressed; or the person might be fine, experiencing only ordinary ups and downs in a given week. All of these states may be experienced by the same individual at different times in the course of the same bipolar illness! Confused? The first step is to have the criteria ready at hand, and to understand how the pieces fit together to build the case for a particular mood diagnosis.

Diagnostic Categories

The challenges of assessing BSD begin with the diagnostic criteria themselves. The DSM-5 currently delineates three different diagnoses that are commonly conceptualized as a bipolar spectrum: bipolar I, bipolar II, and cyclothymic disorder, in addition to four other specified bipolar and related disorders (OSBRD; American Psychiatric Association, 2013). Furthermore, diagnosing a mood disorder first requires gathering information about the lifetime history of mood *states*. Different *diagnoses* require different combinations of mood *states*, introducing a level of complexity not found with most other diagnoses.

The mood states that must be assessed in order to correctly ascertain a DSM-5 diagnosis of mood disorder include manic episode, major depressive episode, hypomanic episode, dysthymic episode, and dysthymia with superimposed hypomanic symptoms. Although the last mood state is not formally distinguished in DSM-5, it is needed in order to diagnose cyclothymic disorder (which requires marked hypomanic *symptoms* but not necessarily hypomanic *episodes* with duration of 4 or more days). Table 8.2 reviews the symptoms and criteria for a DSM-5 diagnosis of manic or hypomanic episodes. Hankin and Cohen (Chapter 7, this volume) review the criteria for unipolar depressive disorders. Depression is the more common phase of bipolar illnesses, so correct diagnosis hinges on whether there is any history of hypomania or mania.

There are some additional complexities in the diagnosis of BSD. Bipolar II disorder requires both a major depressive episode and a hypomanic episode at some point in the person's life. Cyclothymic disorder, on the other hand, involves depres-

TABLE 8.1. Recommended Starter Kits for Assessing Potential BSD

Tool	Identified patient age			Adult client or parent about self
	School age (5–10 years)	Adolescent (11–18 years)	Parent about youth	
Anchor probability	Very rare in general population	Uncommon	Uncommon	Uncommon
Bipolar spectrum benchmark probability	~1% general; ~5% clinical (<1% bipolar I)	~4% general population; ~10% clinical	Use age of youth to pick	~4% general population; ~20% of clinical
Broad screen	N/A (reading level)	YSR, BASC, SDQ, or ASI	CBCL, BASC, CSI, or SDQ	YASR
Follow-up measures	PPDS (puberty) N/A for self-report questionnaires (reading level)	PPDS (puberty); GBI-10M or 7 Up	PPDS (puberty); PGBI-10M or CMRS10; FIRM	FIRM; HCL, BSDS, MDQ, or ISS
Diagnostic interview	MINI-KID	MINI-KID or MINI	MINI	MINI
Severity	Interview: KMRS, KDRS; rating scale: none (reading)	Interview: KMRS, KDRS; rating scale: GBI10M, GBI10Da/Db	Interview: KMRS, KDRS; rating scale: PGBI10M, PGBI10Da/Db	Interview: YMRS, HDRS; rating scale: Altman
Global functioning	CGAS (1 to 100)	CGAS (1 to 100)	CGAS (1 to 100)	GAF
Quality of life	Kiddy KINDL	KINDL	Parent KINDL	QoL.BSD
Sleep	See Meltzer (Chapter 23, this volume)	See Meltzer (Chapter 23)	PGBI-Sleep; see Meltzer (Chapter 23)	Chronotype (SMEQ); sleep problems (PSQI)
Mood change	N/A	Mood charting app	Mood charting app	Mood charting app

Note. Bipolar disorder is extremely rare before the age of 5; do not consider as a possible diagnosis except under highly extenuating circumstances. YSR, Youth Self-Report (Achenbach & Rescorla, 2001); BASC, Behavior Assessment Scale for Children (Reynolds & Kamphaus, 2015); SDQ, Strengths and Difficulties Questionnaire (Goodman, Ford, Simmons, Gatward, & Meltzer, 2003), ASI, Adolescent Symptom Inventory (Gadow & Sprafkin, 1997); CSI, Child Symptom Inventory (Gadow & Sprafkin, 1994); YASR, Young Adult Self-Report (Achenbach, 1997); PPDS, Petersen Pubertal Developmental Screen (Petersen et al., 1988); FIRM, Family Index of Risk for Mood Disorders (Algorta et al., 2013); GBI, General Behavior Inventory (Depue et al., 1981); 7 Up, 7 Up 7 Down (Youngstrom et al., 2013); PGBI-10M, 10Da, 10Db, 10-item forms of parent-reported GBI (Youngstrom, Van Meter, et al., 2018); HCL, Hypomania Checklist (Angst et al., 2010); BSDS, Bipolar Spectrum Diagnostic Scale (Ghaemi et al., 2005); MDQ, Mood Disorder Questionnaire (Hirschfeld et al., 2000); ISS, Internal States Scale (Bauer et al., 1991); MINI, Mini-International Neuropsychiatric Interview (Sheehan et al., 1998); MINI-KID, MINI for Children and Adolescents (Sheehan et al., 2010); KMRS, K-SADS Mania Rating Scale (Axelson et al., 2003); KDRS, K-SADS Depression Rating Scale (Demeter et al., 2013); YMRS, Young Mania Rating Scale (Young et al., 1978); HDRS, Hamilton Depression Rating Scale (Hamilton, 1967); CGAS, Children's Global Assessment Scale (Shaffer et al., 1983); GAF, Global Assessment of Functioning (Hall, 1995); KINDL, quality-of-life scale (not an acronym) (Ravens-Sieberer & Bullinger, 2000); QoL.BSD, Quality of Life for Bipolar Disorder (Michalak et al., 2010); PGBI Sleep, sleep scale carved from parent GBI (Meyers & Youngstrom, 2008); SMEQ, Student Morningness–Eveningness Questionnaire (Košćec, Radošević-Vidaček, & Kostović, 2001); PSQI, Pittsburgh Sleep Quality Index (Buysse, Reynolds, Monk, Berman, & Kupfer, 1989).

TABLE 8.2. Criteria for Manic or Hypomanic Episode

A. A distinct period of abnormally and persistently elevated, expansive, or irritable mood, clearly different from usual mood; increased energy
   Duration: At least 1 week (unless treatment cuts it short) for mania; at least 4 days for hypomanic episode (though data suggest that 2-day periods are more common and still impairing)

B. During the mood episode, at least three of the following symptoms are also present to a significant degree (four or more if mood is mostly irritable):
   1. Inflated self-esteem or grandiosity
   2. Decreased need for sleep (e.g., feeling rested with only 3 hours of sleep)
   3. Pressured speech or more talkative than usual
   4. Flight of ideas or racing thoughts
   5. Distractibility
   6. Increased goal-directed activity or psychomotor agitation
   7. Excessive activities with a high risk for painful or damaging consequences

C. *Mania:* Causes marked impairment in school, at home, or with peers; may also require hospitalization to prevent harm to self or others; may also have psychotic features
   Hypomania: An unequivocal change in functioning from what is typical for person when not symptomatic, observable by others; but *not* severe enough to cause marked impairment, and with no psychotic features

D. Rule out symptoms due to physiological effects of a substance (including stimulant or antidepressant medication), or symptoms due to a general medical condition

Note. Data from ICD-11 (World Health Organization, 2018) and International Society for Bipolar Disorders (ISBSD) Child Diagnosis Task Force (Youngstrom, Birmaher, & Findling, 2008). The DSM-5 criteria are similar (American Psychiatric Association, 2013).

sive and hypomanic symptoms that are insufficient in severity to qualify for a full-blown major depressive, hypomanic, or manic episode, at least during the first year of mood disturbance in children or adolescents—yet they clearly mark a change from typical functioning. A diagnosis of bipolar I disorder can be based on a single manic episode. In the DSM scheme, one need never be depressed to be diagnosed with what used to be called "manic–depression"!

The *International Classification of Diseases* (ICD-11; World Health Organization, 2018) uses similar categories for bipolar disorder; diagnosis of a manic episode requires that mood be predominantly elevated, expansive, or irritable—unlike DSM-5, increased goal-directed activity is not a

gate criterion. ICD-11 criteria harmonize with DSM-5 by adding bipolar II disorder, allowing diagnosis of bipolar I disorder based on a single manic or mixed episode, and including increased activity as core manic symptom. Both systems offer little additional guidance for assessment of mood disorders in children or adolescents. Besides noting that irritable mood may be more common than sad mood in children's depression, DSM-5 does not make any developmental modifications of the symptom criteria for diagnosing any of the previously mentioned mood states. The only developmental modification to the durational criteria is to accept a 1-year instead of 2-year duration for dysthymic and cyclothymic episodes (which ICD-11 does not appear to mention). Without good normative developmental data, it is difficult to tell whether these minimal adjustments are adequate. Research has concentrated on validating the extant diagnostic criteria in youth, then proposing incremental modifications for depression and mania.

The following descriptions provide an overview of the criteria, along with a discussion of the strengths and limitations of the current DSM framework, especially as applied to youth.

Bipolar I Disorder

Often considered the most serious form of bipolar illness, a bipolar I diagnosis requires the presence of at least one manic episode during a person's lifetime. Once a manic episode has occurred, the DSM–ICD nosology considers the individual to have a lifetime diagnosis of bipolar I disorder. If the individual is currently functioning well, then the classification is bipolar I "in remission." If the person develops classic major depression, even years after the mania, then the correct diagnosis is "bipolar I, current episode: depressed." Mania requires that the behavior be a change from typical functioning for the individual, and that the behavior cause impairment (even though it may not cause distress to the person experiencing the mood disturbance). The mood disturbance must either occur much of the day for most days over a period of at least 1 week, or else the mood is so extreme as to result in psychiatric hospitalization, in which case the 1-week duration requirement is waived. Although a person need never become depressed in order to be diagnosed with bipolar I, it appears that depression is the more common phase of illness, at least in adults; it often is the first phase of the illness to come to clinical attention in teens

(Hillegers et al., 2005), and depression appears to impose more burden than mania over the course of illness (Judd et al., 2005).

Bipolar II Disorder

A diagnosis of bipolar II requires at least two lifetime mood states: Both a major depressive episode and a hypomanic episode are necessary. Although often considered less severe than bipolar I, bipolar II may be associated with higher risk of suicide (Berk & Dodd, 2005; Rihmer & Kiss, 2002). Bipolar II is also much more difficult to diagnose than bipolar I because hypomania by definition is more subtle and less impairing than mania. In addition, affected individuals are much more likely to seek treatment during the depressed phase of the illness, and neither they nor the interviewing clinician are likely to disclose or assess for the hypomanic episodes that would distinguish a bipolar II illness from unipolar depression. Furthermore, bipolar II has rarely been systematically evaluated in clinical or research settings with children (Jensen-Doss, Youngstrom, Youngstrom, Feeny, & Findling, 2014; Youngstrom, Youngstrom, & Starr, 2005).

Clinicians are most likely to encounter persons with bipolar II during the depressed phase of the illness (Mesman et al., 2016). It is important to recognize the bipolar–unipolar distinction given its implications for suicide risk, substance use, choice of pharmacological agent, and possibly choice of strategies for psychotherapy. Being alert to bipolar II presentation is particularly important in youth: unfortunately, individuals affected with bipolar II tend to first present clinically in the depressed phase of the illness, and early-onset depression may be a marker for BSD, with depressive symptoms occurring in childhood or adolescence in more than half of cases (Kessler, Berglund, Demler, Jin, & Walters, 2005; Perlis et al., 2004). Many children and young adolescents afflicted with what appears to be depression might actually be experiencing the depressed phase of a bipolar illness. Applying a "bipolar" label to depressed presentations in youth has been fraught with controversy. Some clinical features may suggest a need to be more attentive to the possibility of BSD in clinical assessment: Depressions that has early onset, acute instead of gradual onset, have atypical features (e.g., lethargy, hypersomnia, increased appetite or weight gain, and rejection sensitivity), recur, respond poorly to antidepressants, or happen in the context of a family history of BSD all

are at higher risk of being depressed phases of what ultimately proves to be a bipolar illness (Birmaher, Arbelaez, & Brent, 2002; Kessler, Avenevoli, & Merikangas, 2001; Luby & Mrakotsky, 2003).

Cyclothymic Disorder

The diagnosis of cyclothymic disorder requires a period of mood disturbance that lasts at least 1 year (2 years in adults), with no more than 2 months free of symptoms. The mood disturbance represents a clear change from the individual's typical pattern of behavior (distinguishing it from temperament) that is observable by others. The mood involves depressive or dysthymic symptoms, along with periods of hypomanic symptoms that do not meet criteria for a hypomanic episode. During this index period, the depressive symptoms cannot become sufficiently severe to meet criteria for a major depressive episode (or else the diagnosis changes to unipolar depression, or perhaps bipolar II disorder), nor can the hypomanic symptoms become too impairing (or else the diagnosis changes to bipolar I disorder). It is possible to meet criteria for both cyclothymia and bipolar I disorder (much as it is possible to meet criteria for dysthymia and major depression over the course of lifetime)—provided that the cyclothymic or dysthymic episode precede the onset of the more severe mood state. This is analogous to the "double depression" in which dysthymia/persistent depressive disorder preceded the first major depression, and it may signal a more pernicious course.

Cyclothymia is especially slippery to assess (Van Meter, Youngstrom, & Findling, 2012). The long duration of the mood disturbance makes it hard to discern between temperamental traits and cyclothymic episodes, particularly for children. A year represents a long portion of a young child's life (blurring the boundary between episode and trait), and assessors need to rely more on collateral informants such as parents or teachers to identify changes in mood and energy. Cyclothymia has rarely been diagnosed in youth in clinical practice, even in the United States (Van Meter et al., 2012; Youngstrom, Meyers, et al., 2005). Past research has sometimes lumped these clinical presentations into a "bipolar not otherwise specified" category instead (Birmaher et al., 2006). Pediatric cyclothymia shows high levels of impairment (Findling, Youngstrom, et al., 2005; Lewinsohn, Seeley, Buckley, & Klein, 2002; Van Meter, Burke, et al., 2016; Van Meter, Youngstrom, Demeter, & Findling, 2013; Van Meter, Youngstrom, Freeman,

Feeny, Youngstrom, & Findling, 2016; Van Meter, Youngstrom, Youngstrom, Feeny, & Findling, 2011), yet also often shows spontaneous remission or a lack of progression to more severe forms of mood disorder (Axelson et al., 2011; Lewinsohn et al., 2002).

Other Specified Bipolar and Related Disorders

Other specified bipolar and related disorders (OSBRD; previously referred to as "bipolar not otherwise specified," or bipolar NOS, in DSM-IV) is a residual category used to describe clinical presentations that appear to be on the bipolar spectrum but do not fit into any of the three previously mentioned categories. DSM-5 gives several examples of possible presentations for OSBRD. These include repeated episodes of hypomania without lifetime history of manic or depressive episodes— a presentation that is unlikely to come to clinical attention but has been described in studies of nonclinical adolescents and young adults (Depue, Krauss, Spoont, & Arbisi, 1989) and in family studies.

Another prototype has an insufficient number of "Criterion B" symptoms. This could take the form of a manic episode without enough symptoms to pass the formal threshold, or a hypomanic episode with a lifetime history of major depressive episodes, again falling short on the symptom count. The "not enough symptoms" operational definition has been studied in several large samples because it is easy for researchers to investigate with cross-sectional data (Van Meter, Moreira, & Youngstrom, 2019).

A third operational definition is based on inadequate duration to meet established criteria for a diagnosis. Mania lasting less than a week (without hospitalization) or hypomanias lasting less than 4 days would both be examples. The 4-day threshold for hypomania was set in DSM-IV without data being available to guide the decision. Now both epidemiological and longitudinal studies suggest that 2-day hypomanias are the modal length, yet DSM-5 retained the 4-day threshold due to concerns that setting the bar at 2 days would make it too easy to diagnose bipolar disorders (Angst et al., 2012; Bschor et al., 2012; Hoertel, Le Strat, Angst, & Dubertret, 2013; Merikangas et al., 2012; Youngstrom, Birmaher, & Findling, 2008). DSM-5 added cyclothymia with insufficient duration as another prototype, with 6+ months as the threshold mentioned in the example (American Psychiatric Association, 2013). In addition, different research groups have used different operational definitions of OSBRD (see Table 8.3).

OSBRD is linked to substantial clinical impairment, including poor functioning academically and interpersonally, high rates of service utilization and suicide risk, and substantial mood disturbance, whether defined as insufficient number of symptoms (Lewinsohn, Seeley, & Klein, 2003), insufficient duration (Findling, Youngstrom, et al., 2005), or a combination of the two (Axelson et al., 2011). OSBRD appears to show patterns of familial risk (Findling, Youngstrom, et al., 2005) and symptom severity that would be consistent with it being on the bipolar spectrum, and almost half of individuals with cyclothymic disorder or OSBRD progress to more fully syndromal bipolar presentations (i.e., meeting criteria for bipolar I or II disorder) within 5 years of initially being diagnosed (Axelson et al., 2011; Hafeman et al., 2016).

Substance-Induced Hypomania or Mania

Manic-like symptoms can be induced by not only street drugs such as cocaine but also prescription drugs, including corticosteroids. Worries that stimulant medications (Carlson & Mick, 2003; DelBello, Soutullo, et al., 2001), tricyclic antidepressants (Geller, Fox, & Fletcher, 1993), or selective serotonin reuptake inhibitors (SSRIs; Ghaemi, Hsu, Soldani, & Goodwin, 2003; Papolos, 2003; Reichart & Nolen, 2004) might induce manic symptoms tend not to be verified in clinical trials and carefully controlled analyses (Joseph, Youngstrom, & Soares, 2009). It is hard to tell whether the appearance of manic symptoms while taking a medication represents (1) the spontaneous emergence of mania in someone already at risk, independent of the effects of the medication; (2) a side effect of the medication, irrelevant to the person's true status with regard to bipolar illness; (3) an "unmasking" of a previously undetected bipolar illness in someone already genetically at risk; or (4) an iatrogenic effect of medication that changes the nervous system in a way that individuals not carrying genes of risk still become at risk of manifesting bipolar behaviors, even after medication is discontinued (a "scar hypothesis"). Stimulants appear to be well tolerated when used in the treatment for BSD in conjunction with mood stabilizing compounds (Findling, McNamara, et al., 2005; Scheffer, Kowatch, Carmody, & Rush, 2005). For all these reasons, it is appropriate to follow the DSM recommendation to diagnose these cases as having "substance-induced mania" rather than

TABLE 8.3. Definitions of Bipolar Disorder, BSD, and Research Definitions of Pediatric Bipolar Subtypes

Definition (source)	Comment
Bipolar I	• Requires lifetime presence of a manic episode (can be mixed); mood disturbance duration of 7 days or until hospitalization • DSM: No requirement of depression—ever • ICD-10 required multiple episodes in order to be confident of diagnosis; only "provisional" with single episode, even in adults
Bipolar II	• Requires lifetime combination of a major depressive episode and at least one hypomanic episode (of at least 4 days' duration) (either can be mixed)
Cyclothymia (DSM-IV-TR)	• Technically not considered a type of "bipolar NOS" in DSM • Rarely diagnosed in children or adolescents in research or clinical settings • Many research groups lump cyclothymic disorder with other specified bipolar and related disorders (e.g., Birmaher et al., 2006) • Difficult to disentangle from normal development, temperament, and comorbid conditions • Possible to diagnose reliably, and associated with significant impairment (Findling, Youngstrom, et al., 2005; Van Meter et al., 2013; Van Meter, Youngstrom, et al., 2011, 2016)
Repeated hypomanias in the absence of lifetime mania or depression (DSM-5—other specified bipolar and related disorders [OSBRD])	• Unlikely to be impairing enough to lead to treatment seeking; thus, they are not seen clinically • Challenging to differentiate from normal behavior
Insufficient duration of mood episodes (DSM-5 OSBRD; Leibenluft et al. [2003] further distinguish between cases with elated mood and/or grandiosity versus those with only irritability as mood disturbance, following Geller et al., 2002b)	• Common BSD presentation (Axelson et al., 2006; Findling, Youngstrom, et al., 2005) • Often high impairment (Angst et al., 2003) • May include cases with mood severity that would otherwise warrant a diagnosis of manic, mixed, or depressive state • May include mixed states with polarity shifts • Note that DSM-5 specifically added insufficient duration of cyclothymic "episode" as another prototype, with 6+ months as the duration in example
Insufficient number of manic symptoms (Leibenluft et al. [2003] include "irritable hypomania" and "irritable mania" as another "intermediate" phenotype, even if accompanied by four or more other manic symptoms)	• More prevalent than bipolar I or II, both in adolescents (Van Meter et al., 2019) and adults (Moreira et al., 2017) • Possible to meet criteria with only nonspecific symptoms (e.g., irritable mood plus distractibility, high motor activity, and rapid speech) • Research designs typically have not documented episodicity of symptoms • High rates of impairment and service utilization (Galanter et al., 2003; Hazell, Carr, Lewin, & Sly, 2003)
Severe mood dysregulation (SMD), previously referred to as a "broad phenotype" (Leibenluft et al. [2003] definition)	• Research criteria: Abnormal mood (anger or sadness) present at least half the day most days; accompanied by "hyperarousal" (insomnia,* agitation, distractibility, racing thoughts/flight of ideas; pressured speech, or social intrusiveness*); also shows increased reactivity to negative emotional stimuli compared to peers*; onset before age 12; duration at least 12 months; symptoms severe in at least one setting (*Symptom is not part of DSM-IV or DSM-5 criteria for mania) • Rule outs: Elated mood, grandiosity, or episodically decreased need for sleep; distinct episodes of 4+ days' duration; meeting criteria for schizophreniform, schizophrenia, pervasive developmental disorder, or posttraumatic stress disorder; or meeting criteria for a substance use disorder in the past 3 months; or IQ < 80; or symptoms are attributable to a medication or general medical condition.

(continued)

TABLE 8.3. *(continued)*

Definition (source)	Comment
Severe mood dysregulation *(continued)*	• Comments: The *exclusion* of episodicity and of several symptoms more specific to BSD are both intended to exclude bipolar cases. The inclusion of chronic presentations and sensitive but nonspecific symptoms is likely to include many cases with presentations that are not on the bipolar spectrum. This category may blend different etiologies and mechanisms as a result.
Disruptive mood dysregulation disorder (DMDD)	• Fewer exclusions than the SMD research definition • Symptoms overlap entirely with ODD • DSM-5 put in "Depressive Disorders" chapter • ICD-11 did not add diagnosis; treats as ODD modifier (Evans et al., 2017) • We recommend conceptualizing as a disruptive behavior disorder and treating first with behavioral parenting-oriented interventions, combined with careful assessment of response • Episodic presentation would suggest reconceptualizing as a mood disorder
Bipolar not otherwise specified—Research criteria from "Course and Outcomes of Bipolar Youth" Study (NIMH R01 MH059929) (Axelson et al., 2006; Birmaher et al., 2006; Horwitz et al., 2010)	• Requires "core positive"—presence of distinct period of abnormally elevated, expansive, or irritable mood • Minimum of two other "B criteria" symptoms if mood is mostly elated; at least three "B criteria" if irritable • Requires clear change from individual's typical functioning (consistent with DSM-IV and ICD guidelines for hypomania) • Requires 4+ hours of irritable mood within a 24-hour period to be counted as an index "day" of disturbance • Requires 4+ days at a minimum over the course of a lifetime to diagnose bipolar NOS; nonconsecutive days are acceptable • Beginning to garner empirical support (Axelson et al., 2006) • Needs replication in other samples/research groups but overlaps substantially with "insufficient duration" and "insufficient number of B criterion symptoms" definitions of bipolar NOS
Child Behavior Checklist proxy diagnosis (after Mick, Biederman, Pandina, & Faraone, 2003); often operationally defined as parent-reported *T*-scores of 70+ on Aggressive Behavior, Attention Problems, and Anxious/Depressed scales. Not recommended for clinical use (Althoff et al., 2010)	• Pros: • Convenient to use for large sample studies • Avoids problems of rater training and anchoring effects • Cons: • Focuses on symptoms that are likely to be "shared" with other disorders at a genetic level • Items overlap with Posttraumatic Stress Disorder scale (You et al., 2017) • Prone to factors that might bias parent report • Does not capture diagnostically specific symptoms; instead concentrates on sensitive symptoms that might also have high false-positive rate • Agreement with clinical or research-interview-derived (K-SADS) diagnoses of bipolar spectrum might be modest (Althoff et al., 2010)

"unmasked" bipolar I or bipolar II illness. DSM-5 stipulates that the diagnosis can change to a bipolar disorder if the episode continues after discontinuation of the medication.

The "Broad Phenotype" and Disruptive Mood Dysregulation Disorder

The "broad phenotype" of bipolar illness, a presentation of chronic irritability and mood lability *without* distinct episodes with marked changes in mood or energy (Leibenluft, Charney, Towbin, Bhangoo, & Pine, 2003), is no longer supported for inclusion on the bipolar spectrum. Although irritability is commonly present in youth with BSD, a BSD diagnosis only is warranted when irritability begins or increases significantly in conjunction with manic symptoms (B. Goldstein et al., 2017). The DSM-5 diagnosis of disruptive mood dysregulation disorder (DMDD) grew out of the research on the "broad phenotype." The original proposed definition of "severe mood dysregulation" included several exclusion criteria that were dropped from the DSM-5 definition, making it important to pay attention to the operational definition used in each study. DMDD does not appear to be on the bipolar spectrum based on cross-sectional correlates (Freeman, Youngstrom, Youngstrom, & Findling, 2016), treatment studies (Waxmonsky et al., 2016), or reanalyses of longitudinal data (Copeland, Shanahan, Egger, Angold, & Costello, 2014; Dougherty et al., 2016; Kessel et al., 2016).

DSM-5 considers DMDD a form of unipolar depressive disorder. In contrast, ICD-11 considers it an externalizing disorder and has an emotional dysregulation specifier that can be coded on top of oppositional defiant disorder (Evans et al., 2017). Based on the treatment outcome data for using antidepressants with oppositional defiant disorder (Boylan & Kim, 2016; Pappadopulos et al., 2006), as well as the emerging treatment data for DMDD (Stringaris, Vidal-Ribas, Brotman, & Leibenluft, 2018; Tourian et al., 2015; Waxmonsky et al., 2016), we agree that DMDD is probably better conceptualized as an externalizing disorder and treated first with interventions that address externalizing problems (see Walker, Frick, & McMahon, Chapter 6, this volume, for assessment recommendations).

Rapid Cycling: Relapse versus Mood Lability

BSD has a high relapse rate. Whereas some people are able to go for periods of years, or even decades, between episodes of pathological mood disturbance (Goodwin & Jamison, 2007), most people have more frequent relapses into mood states. "Rapid cycling" means that a person shows at least four distinct mood episodes over the course of a year (American Psychiatric Association, 2013). Recognizing this pattern is vital: Rapid cycling shows a more chronic course of illness, with greater comorbidity, less responsiveness to lithium, and higher risk of mortality (Coryell et al., 2003).

Note that the term "rapid cycling" refers to the number of episodes, not to mood instability. A more descriptive name would be "rapid relapsing" or "prone to recurrent episodes" (Youngstrom, 2009). Use of the term "ultradian" cycling to describe polarity switches (e.g., from mania to depression) in the course of the same day has created confusion about the rate of cycling for youth, with some estimates of yearly rates in the tens of thousands (Geller et al., 1995). However, polarity switches often occur within a single mood episode (Kraepelin, 1921); thus, the apparent discrepancies between adult and pediatric BSD are due to slippage in the definition of terms. The "ultradian" cycling label applied sometimes with youth is therefore likely to a synonym for an overarching mixed *state* involving rapid polarity switches with brief durations at either extreme (Youngstrom, Joseph, & Greene, 2008). If the clinical picture is the same, it would be better to use consistent terminology, so we recommend using *mixed* instead of *ultradian* to describe this presentation.

Mixed States and the Mixed Specifier

Mixed states involve showing manic and depressive symptoms during the same mood episode. According to DSM-5, if full criteria for a (hypo)manic or depressive episode are met, the mixed-features specifier may be applied if there are an adequate number of symptoms of the opposite polarity present "during the majority of days of the current or most recent episode" (American Psychiatric Association, 2013). "Majority of days" could entail having both manic and depressive symptoms in a single, homogeneous mood state. Kay Jamison (1995) has described this as a "black mania," combining the hopelessness, low self-esteem, pathological guilt, and despair of depression with the high energy, racing thoughts, and impulsivity of mania. The result is a high-energy mood state with a negative valence. The depressive and manic features have blended together to form a qualitatively different experience, much as milk and chocolate syrup mix together to form chocolate milk (Youngstrom et al., 2008). Not surprisingly, such a mood state presents a high risk for suicide (Goodwin & Jamison, 2007).

An alternative mixed presentation has mood shifting rapidly between depressed and manic states, perhaps within the same day. Kraepelin (1921) noted unstable and shifting moods, and these have been documented in adults with BSD using clinical observation (Kramlinger & Post, 1996), as well as prospective "life charting" of mood and energy (Denicoff et al., 1997) and objective markers of physical activity (Faurholt-Jepsen et al., 2015). This unstable, labile form of "mixed state" is what has been described by some as "ultradian cycling" in children (Geller & Cook, 2000). The picture can look similar to the mood instability characteristic of borderline personality disorder in adults (cf. Zimmerman, Ruggero, Chelminski, & Young, 2010). Because there may be patches of depressed or hypomania presentation mixed together in a conglomerate episode, we can think of this as a "fudge ripple" ice-cream presentation instead of a homogeneous "chocolate milk" one (Youngstrom et al., 2008).

It appears relatively rare for children or adolescents to experience multiple remissions of their mixed state and then multiple relapses within the same year (Birmaher et al., 2006; Geller et al., 2004), particularly when remission is defined as a period of 2 months free of impairing symptoms (Findling et al., 2001; Frank et al., 1991). Thus, "rapid cycling" in the strictest sense appears uncommon in children, and there appears to be a high rate of oscillating mixed states instead.

DSM-5 abolished mixed episodes as a distinct category of mood episode and instead created a specifier that could apply to hypomanic or depressive episodes, not just to manic ones. This aligns with data and clinical observations that hypomanias often can be irritable or negative valence but high energy, as well as evidence that there is not a categorical boundary between mania, hypomania, and ordinary behavior (Prisciandaro & Roberts, 2011; Prisciandaro & Tolliver, 2015). Using the mixed specifier with depressive episodes theoretically could help detect and track bipolar II and also alert the clinician to possible differences in treatment response (Pacchiarotti et al., 2013). However, the specifier only works if clinicians use it, and it is unlikely that practicing clinicians will change their habits without external reminders and support, particularly because the specifiers are not tied to billing. The DSM-5 operational definition is also complicated, as it tries to exclude overlapping symptoms between mania and depression; it is unlikely that people will be able to implement the criteria consistently without checklists or other decision support tools. Some have suggested that a simpler way of thinking would be to ask, "How bipolar is this person's illness?" rather than "Which category or type of mood disorder do they have?" (Sachs, 2004). Thinking dimensionally, in terms of degree of bipolarity, aligns with the data and simplifies the formulation.

Comorbidity

BSD has tremendously high rates of comorbidity with other mental disorders and substance use. The most common comorbidities identified in youth meeting criteria for BSD are ADHD, oppositional defiant disorder, conduct disorder, substance abuse or dependence, and anxiety disorders (Birmaher, Axelson, Goldstein, et al., 2009; Kowatch, Youngstrom, Danielyan, & Findling, 2005; Mesman et

al., 2016). Similar rates of comorbidity have been observed in adult populations (Birmaher et al., 2006; Van Meter, Burke, Youngstrom, et al., 2016).

Although high rates of comorbidity between ADHD and BSD persist across the lifespan, the degree of comorbidity between ADHD and BSD has led some to question whether these are in fact independent conditions. The much higher rate of coincidence could be due to the pronounced overlap in diagnostic criteria. ADHD often involves distractibility, high motor activity, talkativeness, irritability, and impulsive behavior that all could readily look like manic behaviors, or indeed, vice versa (Youngstrom, Arnold, & Frazier, 2010). Thus, apparent comorbidity might be inflated by research interviews or clinicians not sufficiently determining whether the symptom is most attributable to a mood disorder versus an additional condition. The clinical correlates and family aggregation of BSD and ADHD differ (Birmaher & Axelson, 2006; Findling, Youngstrom, et al., 2005; Fristad et al., 2012), making it useful to conceptualize these as distinct disorders. It is important to assess for ADHD alongside BSD, as youth with this comorbidity often show greater impairment and a worse course, and may warrant adjustments to treatment (McClellan et al., 2007).

Comorbid anxiety disorders are open to similar discussion: Rates of comorbidity vary too widely to be due merely to chance sampling differences (Kowatch, Youngstrom, et al., 2005). Higher comorbidity estimates may partially be due to diagnosing anxiety disorders on the basis of anxious symptoms reported during the course of a mood episode. Again, "comorbid" anxiety is associated with greater impairment and a worse course—but it is unclear whether this is due to the comorbidity, or whether the perceived "comorbidity" is another way of describing the person as experiencing a greater number of total problems in the context of the illness (Wagner, 2006).

Clinically, we can expect to see "pure" bipolar presentations only rarely. It also makes sense to assess for attention problems and anxiety, as well as substance use and other antisocial behavior, when confronted with potential BSD. What are sometimes considered patterns of comorbidity may also prove to be useful "endophenotypes" (Hasler, Drevets, Gould, Gottesman, & Manji, 2006)—dimensional biobehavioral features that cut across or underpin the recognized binary diagnoses—as they may reflect the activity of particular genes that are not uniformly present in all cases meeting DSM criteria for either disorder. For example, cases with bipolar and generalized anxiety disorder (GAD) may involve genes related to the behavioral inhibition system that are not present in other cases with BSD, and they will also have genes affecting mood dysregulation that are not present in most individuals meeting criteria for GAD. The Research Domain Criteria (RDoC) approach is another way to reconceptualize mood disorders (Cuthbert & Insel, 2013).

Major Symptom Dimensions and Associated Features

The categorical diagnoses emphasized thus far are valuable pragmatic terms to improve communication and simplify our task of working with complex, poorly understood phenomenology. However, we can expect clinicians' expertise to also include a deeper understanding of the likely nature of these clusters of presenting symptoms; this nature is likely neither binary nor unidimensional (Hickie, 2014).

The two major symptom dimensions involved in bipolar illness are depressive symptoms and manic symptoms (Youngstrom, Freeman, & Jenkins, 2009). Counterintuitively, depression and mania do not appear to be opposite poles of a single dimension. Instead, they are two distinct sets of symptoms that can occur independently of each other or overlap. This is consistent with the RDoC matrix having separate domains for positive valence (e.g., mania) and negative valence (depression and anxiety) phenomenology. Mixed states would involve high levels of both depressed and manic symptoms (Youngstrom & Izard, 2008). A dimensional model resolves many of the problems noted with the current categorical classification system, including the large number of cases with "mixed hypomanias" or "anger attacks" in the context of depression, or agitated depressive presentations. Rather than requiring a proliferation of subcategories, these clinical presentations could be conceptualized as the simultaneous elevation of multiple problem dimensions. A two-dimensional model fits better with the data, and it also is elegant in accommodating clinical presentations when the DSM system has gaps, such as mild (vs. major) depressive episodes, or mixed dysthymias. Figure 8.1 shows how the different mood episodes would map onto this two-dimensional space. Sometimes people use thresholds and rules of thumb to demarcate "hypomanic range" from "manic range" scores, or depressed versus not depressed, on severity scales (e.g., Duax, Youngstrom, Calabrese, & Findling, 2007). These thresholds do not have a strong psychometric foundation, and looking at Figure 8.1, it is clear that there is no sharp dividing line, or even bimodal tendencies, in the scores. It is worth thinking in terms of two dimensions because there may be different risk factors associated with triggering depressive versus hypomanic or manic symptoms (Johnson & Roberts, 1995), as well as distinct genetic factors (Hickie, 2014). A major clinical implication is that assessment should include measures of both hypomanic–manic and depressed symptoms not only at intake but also as outcome measures, due to the potential for new mood symptoms emerging, including those of a different polarity than the presenting problem.

Mania and depression can be linked to major motivational systems, such as Gray's behavioral inhibition system (BIS) and behavioral activation system (BAS) (Fowles, 1994; Gray & McNaughton, 1996), or Depue's behavioral facilitation system (BFS; Depue & Iacono, 1989). RDoC include BIS in the negative valence domain, and BAS in the positive valence domain, since earlier formulations (www.nimh.nih.gov/research/research-funded-by-nimh/rdoc/constructs/rdoc-matrix.shtml). These models put anxiety, depression, and mania within a larger evolutionary and neurobehavioral framework, in which the clinical disorders are pathologically extreme or situationally inappropriate expressions of systems that otherwise serve important roles in the development of personality and healthy functioning (Youngstrom & Izard, 2008). These models suggest linkages between mania and dopaminergic systems related to reward, extraversion, and approach-oriented behaviors (Alloy & Nusslock, 2019; Depue & Collins, 1999). BIS and BAS models also predict a high degree of overlap between anxious and depressive symptoms because both anxiety and depression involve high levels of BIS activation, also conceptualized as high levels of "negative affectivity" (Tellegen, Watson, & Clark, 1999).

According to the "tripartite model" of depression and anxiety, negative affect or high BIS activity is a shared component of both anxiety and depression, whereas physiological hyperarousal is specific to anxiety, and low positive affect (or low BAS) is a specific marker for depression (Watson et al., 1995). The tripartite model's description of depressed states, as well as negative affect as a shared component of anxiety and depression, has

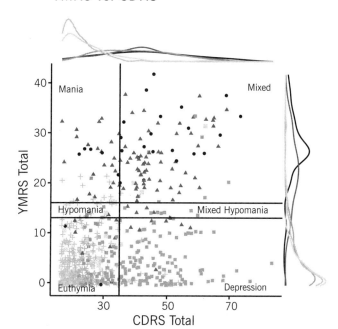

FIGURE 8.1. Mapping severity of manic (YMRS Total) and depressive (CDRS Total) symptoms to DSM mood states. These are YMRS and CRDS-R scores for youth seeking outpatient mental health services. The ratings were based on direct interview of the youth and caregiver. The suggested thresholds are based research conventions (Duax et al., 2007), not on strong psychometric or normative data. Copyright © 2019 Youngstrom and Langfus CC-BY 4.0.

been replicated in multiple child and adolescent samples (Chorpita, 2002; Chorpita, Albano, & Barlow, 1998; Chorpita & Daleiden, 2002; Lonigan, Phillips, & Hooe, 2003). Although there are measures of BIS and BAS that include nonclinical behaviors (e.g., Carver & White, 1994), it is not clear that these instruments offer incremental value to clinical assessment. Instead, the clinical value of BIS and BAS models might primarily lie in the identification of "subsyndromal" or adaptive behaviors falling along the same dimension as mania or depression. Awareness of these behaviors might help normalize and depathologize some aspects, and also might be helpful in monitoring warning signs that presage the return of more severe mood disturbance. The BIS and BAS models also contribute a potential explanation for the frequent co-occurrence of anxious and depressive symptoms, which might otherwise be perceived as "comorbidity" of multiple disorders (Alloy & Nusslock, 2019).

A third model of the dimensions of illness was first proposed by Kraepelin (1921), who described three clusters of symptoms involved in mood disorder: *Cognitive or intellective*, including racing thoughts and heightened creativity at one extreme, and slowed thinking or dulled perceptions at the other; *vegetative*, including motor agitation and heightened energy at one extreme and fatigue or psychomotor retardation at the other; and finally an *affective* component ranging from manic excitement, expansiveness, and grandiosity down to depressive hopelessness and despair. This dimensional model elegantly accounts for both classic mania and depression (high or low levels across all three clusters, respectively), as well as mixed states such as agitated depression (high levels of the motor activity cluster of symptoms while remaining low on the affective and cognitive dimensions). This framework would also provide a means for integrating neuropsychological performance into a broader conceptual model of mood disorder.

However, little recent work on neuropsychological performance in children or adolescents has included this historical model.

A fourth major dimension would be sleep. Thinking of sleep as a dimension or system of functioning rather than a symptom of depression or mania helps us reconceptualize mood problems along a construct that has clear biological and environmental inputs (Alloy & Nusslock, 2019; Cuthbert & Insel, 2013; Harvey, Murray, Chandler, & Soehner, 2011). Focusing on sleep also unlocks a treasure trove of assessment strategies that can be helpful for monitoring treatment progress and outcomes (see Meltzer, Chapter 23, this volume). Good sleep hygiene plays a key role in maintenance of recovery, and in navigating developmental transitions such as leaving home and going to college.

Domains of Impairment

BSD is not simply associated with disturbances of mood and activation. The depressed phase of the illness brings with it all of the impairment and burden associated with unipolar depression (Judd et al., 2005). Manic episodes involve externalizing behaviors, along with the increased motor activity and poor concentration often typical of ADHD. Extreme mood states degrade executive function and cognitive performance, although it does not appear that these deficits are specific to BSD (Walshaw, Alloy, & Sabb, 2010). Both depression and mania are associated with academic underachievement, poor educational attainment, peer rejection, abuse, and family conflict (Du Rocher Schudlich et al., 2015; Du Rocher Schudlich, Youngstrom, Calabrese, & Findling, 2008; Geller et al., 2000, 2004; Perez Algorta, MacPherson, et al., 2018; Siegel, La Greca, Freeman, & Youngstrom, 2015). BSD is also linked with increased use of alcohol and street drugs (B. Goldstein et al., 2008), and the combination of substance use and other impulsive behaviors (Stewart et al., 2012) also greatly increases the risk that youth with BSD will come into contact with the justice system (Pliszka, Sherman, Barrow, & Irick, 2000). BSD is a well-established risk factor for suicide (Algorta et al., 2011; Esposito-Smythers et al., 2010; T. Goldstein, 2009; T. Goldstein et al., 2005), and earlier age of onset is related to elevated risk of suicide and of violent behavior in general (Perlis et al., 2004). Overall, BSD involves pervasive impairment across most social, emotional, cognitive, and vocational/educational areas of functioning, producing larger reductions in functioning and quality of life than most other mental health or pediatric medical conditions (Freeman et al., 2009). Without proper management, BSD puts an individual at higher risk of incarceration, academic and occupational failure, or suicide. These are all excellent reasons for better assessment and titrated intervention earlier in the course.

Epidemiology: Base Rates, Age of Onset, Clinical Incidence, and Long-Term Outcomes

Epidemiological Data

Base rates of BSD give us benchmarks to use as a starting point in our assessments. Epidemiological estimates convey a sense of the relative prevalence or rarity of different conditions, and how much rates vary by age or other demographic features. A meta-analysis identified 19 studies, comprising $N = 56,103$ youth between ages 5 and 18 years, drawn from the United States (seven studies), Central and South America, and Europe (Van Meter et al., 2019). The average rate of mania was 6 per 1,000 youth in the general population, and the rate of BSD was 39 per 1,000 (3.9%). The meta-analysis found no evidence that the rates were higher in the United States than the other countries, nor was there any indication that rates have been increasing in the general population over a period of three decades (Van Meter, Moreira, & Youngstrom, 2011; Van Meter et al., 2019). These findings rebut the perception that BSD is limited to the United States or absent from other countries. The lack of regional differences is reassuring inasmuch as it suggests that the diagnosis is not an artifact of one region's local diagnostic practices. A similar meta-analysis of adult epidemiological studies did find significantly lower rates in Asia and Africa (Moreira, Van Meter, Genzlinger, & Youngstrom, 2017), which did not contribute any studies to the literature on youth. Regional differences could become evident with more research.

There are several causes for caution in interpreting epidemiological results. One is that most instruments used in youth-oriented epidemiological studies were written at a time when the prevailing wisdom was that mania does not occur in children, and only rarely in adolescents. As a result, there was little training about recognizing manic behavior, and there were no attempts to modify descriptions or anchors to be developmentally appropriate. Subsequent experience has revealed that some instruments, such as the Diagnostic Interview Schedule for Children (DISC; Shaffer et al., 1996), appear less sensitive to mania as a result (Galanter, Hundt, Goyal, Le, & Fisher, 2012). Second, epidemiological studies, with few exceptions, have not systematically assessed for hypomania. Without careful assessment of hypomania, only bipolar I illness can be diagnosed (see earlier discussion). As a result, most epidemiological studies have not tracked bipolar II, cyclothymia, or bipolar not otherwise specified (NOS). Furthermore, bipolar II illness would be misdiagnosed as depression. However, when hypomania and cyclothymia have been assessed, these other bipolar spectrum diagnoses appear to be at least five times as common as bipolar I disorder (Judd & Akiskal, 2003; Lewinsohn et al., 2002), consistent with the difference between rates of bipolar I disorder versus the full spectrum in the meta-analysis (Van Meter et al., 2019). Adding systematic assessment of just bipolar II disorder raises the estimated lifetime prevalence of BSD in the adult U.S. population to 3.9% (Kessler et al., 2005). Although these other diagnoses have flown "under the radar" of most epidemiological studies, they are still associated with substantial burden and impairment (Fletcher, Tan, Scott, & Murray, 2018; Van Meter et al., 2012). Third, some of the epidemiological studies have relied solely on self-report, particularly those that focused solely on adolescents or young adults. It will become evident in later sections of this chapter that self-report often underestimates the occurrence and severity of manic and particularly hypomanic symptoms. Due to these concerns, epidemiological studies are not definitive yet.

Evidence of a balanced interpretation might suggest that BSD is rare in children, somewhat more common in adolescents, and yet more common in adults; at the same time, the "fuzzy" spectrum presentations will outnumber clear cases of bipolar I disorder at all ages. The data at this point also establish that bipolar disorder is more common than autism spectrum disorders or early-onset schizophrenia, and substantially less common than ADHD, unipolar depression, or oppositional defiant disorder in children and teens. These are helpful bookends for clinical practice. Unless we are working at a specialty clinic, bipolar disorder will be a more likely explanation of psychosis than schizophrenia in youth, but it will be important to be able to tease apart from the usual suspects that are more likely causes of high motor activity, moodiness, or irritability.

Age of Onset

Not surprisingly, the age of onset of BSD is also controversial. Adult retrospective reporting about the onset of mood symptoms indicates that more than 50% of adults with BSD had their first mood symptoms before age 18 (Kessler, Rubinow, Holmes, Abelson, & Zhao, 1997), and often before the age of 16 (Perlis et al., 2004; Post et al., 2011). Surveys of adult consumers indicate median delays of between 11 and 19 years when mood symptoms begin versus when treatment is sought and a correct diagnosis is made (Calabrese et al., 2001; Hirschfeld, Lewis, & Vornik, 2003; Lish, Dime-Meenan, Whybrow, Price, & Hirschfeld, 1994). Studies with youth indicate substantial lags between first mood problems and clinical diagnoses as well (Drancourt et al., 2013; Marchand, Wirth, & Simon, 2006). The disconnect between onset and clinical detection is large, and retrospective report is imperfect at best; but it still is clear that bipolar disorder is not limited to adults, and better assessment has plenty of room to improve detection.

Most epidemiological studies do not consistently measure age of onset. More recent epidemiological studies suggest that the median age of onset currently is around age 16 years (Kessler et al., 2005; Merikangas & Pato, 2009). However, there are data suggesting a secular trend with earlier ages of onset of mood disorder, and higher rates of mood disorder, in each generation since World War II in the United States (Post, Leverich, Xing, & Weiss, 2001; Weissman et al., 1984). The National Comorbidity Survey—Revised (NCS-R) found that the youngest age cohort surveyed showed at least four times the lifetime hazard of developing BSD (with an estimated prevalence of 6% by age 75) compared to the rate in the oldest age cohort (with a 1.5% lifetime prevalence). Onset in the United States also appears to be significantly younger than that in Europe, based on both self-report measures and on clinical interviews (Post et al., 2011). Apparent earlier onset in the United States may be linked with higher rates of risk factors, including more familial history of mood disorder, higher familial rates of suicide, and greater exposure to childhood physical and sexual abuse (Mesman et al., 2016).

Age of onset is an important prognostic variable: Earlier age of onset predicts higher rates of comorbidity with anxiety disorder and substance abuse, more rapid cycling, more chronic impairment, and more days in poor mood state and greater risk of suicide or violence (Masi et al., 2006; Perlis et al., 2004), and possibly less responsiveness to lithium monotherapy (Duffy et al., 2002). "Take-home messages" for clinicians are that the age of onset often appears to be younger than conventional wisdom would indicate, and also that early onset predicts a more challenging course of illness, requiring different forms of pharmacotherapy (and possibly other forms of psychosocial intervention) (Van Meter, Burke, Kowatch, Findling, & Youngstrom, 2016).

Clinical Incidence

Information about clinical incidence is even more useful to practicing clinicians than general population epidemiological figures. Ideally, clinicians would have accurate statistics documenting the base rate of bipolar illness at their own setting. Failing that, it would be helpful to have estimates from similar clinical settings to use as benchmarks, which can serve as "base rates" or starting probabilities for assessment. Table 8.4 represents a broad sampling of published estimates from different clinical settings. There are important caveats to consider for any of these estimates. Referral patterns can vary dramatically between settings. Artifacts of the assessment process also generate highly discrepant estimates: Clinical diagnoses are more prone to the effects of heuristics than are semistructured diagnostic interviews (Jensen-Doss, Patel, Casline, & McLeod, Chapter 3, this volume), but interviews also involve varying degrees of clinical judgment (Garb, 1998). Differing conceptualizations of bipolar illness also influence the apparent rate. Estimates based on strict bipolar I disorder are much lower than estimates including other diagnoses on the bipolar spectrum. Estimates including parent report are more sensitive to BSD (see below), but they may also increase the rate of false-positive diagnoses—both contributing to higher rates. All of these issues apply with equal force to estimates derived from one's own clinical practice. Thus, Table 8.4 offers an opportunity to compare the effects of different definitions and assessment methodologies, and to reflect on how one's own assessment methods might compare.

Table 8.4 justifies three overarching conclusions: (1) Rates can be highly variable, even within the same setting, but (2) BSD is occurring in clinical settings, and (3) rates in clinical settings are higher than those in the general population, roughly corresponding to the intensity of services offered at the setting. Similar to the epidemiological rates from the general population, the rates fall in between the lower bookend of rates of schizophrenia or autistic spectrum disorders, and the higher bookend of rates for ADHD, depression, or oppositional/conduct problems (Rettew, Lynch, Achenbach, Dumenci, & Ivanova, 2009).

Demographic and Cultural Issues in Assessment

The epidemiological data reviewed earlier indicate that bipolar disorder occurs around the world, so it is not a culture-limited phenomenon. However, there are large differences in attitudes and beliefs around mental health and illness, and around mania and depression in particular (Oedegaard et al., 2016). There also may be differences in the distribution of genetic risk factors, and differences in diet, lifestyle, and exposure to risk factors all may influence prevalence, course, and support-seeking behavior.

Sex Differences

Bipolar I disorder occurs equally often in men and women (Goodwin & Jamison, 2007; Kessler et al., 1997). Pediatric data indicate no sex differences in the diagnosis of bipolar I disorder after adjusting for the fact that more young males present to clinics for externalizing problems in general (Biederman et al., 2004; Demeter et al., 2013; Duax et al., 2007; Youngstrom, Youngstrom, et al., 2005).

Apparent sex differences in BSD are complicated by comorbid diagnoses such as ADHD, ODD, and conduct disorder (Kowatch, Youngstrom, et al., 2005). In particular, ADHD has repeatedly shown higher rates of comorbidity in young males versus young females with BSD (Biederman et al., 2004). Externalizing disorders are more common among boys than girls (Costello et al., 1996), potentially leading to greater rates of boys also being diagnosed with BSD. It is still important for clinicians to recognize subtler symptoms of BSD, so that children and adolescents seeking treatment for depressive symptoms, particularly females, do not go misdiagnosed or mismanaged. Although separate sex norms or diagnostic criteria for BSD are probably unnecessary (Biederman et al., 2004), clinicians need to be more vigilant about BSD in females, whose presentation is less likely to show pure mania or hypomania.

Racial and Cultural Differences

Little is known about racial or cultural differences in the prevalence or phenomenology of BSD.

TABLE 8.4. Base Rates of BSD in Different Clinical Settings

Setting (reference)	Base rate	Demography	Diagnostic method
Rates of bipolar disorders in general population	0.6%	Bipolar I in youth ages 5–18 years	Meta-analysis of epidemiological studies, 19 samples, N = 56,103 participants (Van Meter et al., 2019)
Rates of BPS (I, II, cyclothymia, NOS) in general population	3.9%	Bipolar spectrum in youth age 5–18 years	Metaregression estimate (Van Meter et al., 2019)
High school epidemiological (Lewinsohn et al., 2000)	0.6%	Northwestern U.S. high school	KSADS-PL[y]
Community mental health center (Youngstrom et al., 2005)	6%	Midwestern urban, 80% nonwhite, low-income	Clinical interview and treatment[p,y]
General outpatient clinic (Geller, Zimerman, Williams, Delbello, Frazier, et al., 2002)	6–8%	Urban academic research centers	WASH-U-K-SADS[p,y]
County wards (DCFS) (Naylor, Anderson, Kruesi, & Stoewe, 2002)	11%	State of Illinois	Clinical interview and treatment[y]
Specialty outpatient service (Biederman et al., 1996)	15–17%	New England	K-SADS-E[p,y (only p young)]
Incarcerated adolescents (Teplin, Abram, McClelland, Dulcan, & Mericle, 2002)	2%	Midwestern urban	DISC[y]
Incarcerated adolescents (Pliszka et al., 2000)	22%	Texas	DISC[p,y]
Acute psychiatric hospitalizations in 2002–2003—*adolescents* (Blader & Carlson, 2007)	21%	All of U.S.	Centers for Disease Control and Prevention survey of discharge diagnoses
Inpatient service (Carlson & Youngstrom, 2003)	30% manic symptoms, <2% strict BP I	New York City metro region	DICA; KSADS[p,y]
Acute psychiatric hospitalizations in 2002–2003—*children* (Blader & Carlson, 2007)	40%	All of U.S.	Centers for Disease Control and Prevention survey of discharge diagnoses
Psychiatric outpatient clinic (Ghanizadeh, Mohammadi, & Yazdanshenas, 2006)	16–17%	Iran	K-SADS-PL (Farsi)
Inpatient and partial hospitalization programs at a psychiatric treatment center (Pellegrini et al., 1986)	Mania (0%), hypomania (6%)	Richmond, VA	DISC

Note. K-SADS-PL, Kiddie Schedule for Affective Disorders and Schizophrenia—Present and Lifetime version; WASH-U, Washington University version, -E, Epidemiological version of the K-SADS; DISC, Diagnostic Interview Schedule for Children; DICA, Diagnostic Interview for Children and Adolescents. Table modified from Wikiversity.
[p]Parent interviewed as component of diagnostic assessment; [y]youth interviewed as part of diagnostic assessment.

However, minority youth with a mood disorder are more likely to be misdiagnosed with conduct disorder or schizophrenia (DelBello, Lopez-Larson, Soutullo, & Strakowski, 2001), and more likely to be treated with older and/or depot antipsychotic medications (Arnold et al., 2004; DelBello, Soutullo, & Strakowski, 2000). Clinicians should assess systematically for mood disorder with patients from ethnic minorities, particularly when the presenting problem involves aggressive behavior or psychosis. Clinicians should also be alert to the potential for racial bias in diagnosis when gathering family history (Garb, 1998). Rather than taking family members' historical diagnoses at face value, it would be prudent to gather family history at the symptom level whenever possible.

Racial bias on the part of the clinician may not be the biggest issue. One study presented clinicians with vignettes to look at their case formulation and randomly manipulated whether the cases were presented as black or white; there was no significant difference in the formulations based on race, even though the study had sufficient statistical power to detect $r > .2$, and found large effects for changing other cognitive debiasing strategies (Jenkins & Youngstrom, 2016). In contrast, a medical anthropologist who watched several dozen clinical interviews was struck by the very different language that families used to describe their children's problems. White, middle-class families who had a child with bipolar disorder (per the research interview) were more likely to describe worries about "mood swings," and intake clinicians were more likely to explore and confirm hypotheses about mood disorders. Black families, on the other hand, typically described the issues in terms of behaviors—"Sometimes, he or she goes off the hook, and he or she is out of control . . ." Even when the youth would meet full criteria for a bipolar disorder based on a semistructured diagnostic interview, a clinician doing an unstructured interview was likely to frame the issue as a conduct problem, then confirm a diagnosis of ODD or conduct disorder, without ever exploring potential mood issues as a competing hypothesis (Carpenter-Song, 2009). Differences in how families conceptualize the problem and cultural differences in the language used created a different set of initial hypotheses, and then cognitive heuristics took over. Confirmation bias, failure to look for disconfirming evidence, and search-satisficing (calling off the search as soon as one hypothesis is confirmed) led to large discrepancies in diagnoses and treatment plans (Jenkins & Youngstrom, 2016).

Young Adult Outcomes

Multiple longitudinal studies have generated data on stability, course, and outcome up to 8 years after the initial assessment identifying BSD (Geller, Tillman, Bolhofner, & Zimerman, 2008; Hafeman et al., 2017; Youngstrom & Algorta, 2014). These findings have been cross-validated by a more recent multisite study: 70% of patients recovered within an average follow-up period of 2 years, but 50% relapsed within the same time frame, and syndromal or subsyndromal mood symptoms were present during at least 60% of weeks during the follow-up period (Birmaher et al., 2006). Roughly half of those with cyclothymic/NOS at baseline had progressed to bipolar I or II disorder by 5 years later, whereas about one-third continued to show the cyclothymic pattern of "subsyndromal" mood disturbance (Axelson et al., 2011). Unfortunately, not "progressing" to bipolar I or II disorder did not necessarily mean that they were doing better: Those persons also showed worse outcomes on most measures of functioning than did youth with more "classic, syndromal" presentations (Axelson et al., 2011; Birmaher et al., 2006). These findings appear similar to results from the follow-up waves of a longitudinal study of an epidemiological sample (Lewinsohn et al., 2000). Taken together, findings suggest that there are two subtypes—a more episodic version of mood disorder, conforming to classic definitions, and having a less chronic although still highly impairing course and a more chronic pattern of mood dysregulation that does not meet full criteria for bipolar I or II disorder but tends to show developmental continuity and remain highly impairing. See Youngstrom and Algorta (2014) for a more detailed review of more than a dozen longitudinal cohorts.

Perhaps the most intriguing development from longitudinal studies is evidence that at least some people may achieve remission or long-term recovery. The largest epidemiological studies with prospective follow-up in the United States find that roughly one-third of those with hypomanic or manic episodes by adolescence have no recurrence of mood episode within 5 years of follow-up (Cicero, Epler, & Sher, 2009; Shankman et al., 2009). Similarly, a portion of youth seeking services for bipolar disorders in childhood or adolescence achieve long-term remission with treatment over later years (Birmaher et al., 2014). This does not undermine the severity of the illness during active episodes, but it does offer more than a glimmer of hope that good identification and early intervention could alter the trajectory for the better.

The Prediction Phase: Evidence-Based Assessment of Potential BSD

Clinical Base-Rate Benchmarks

In the evidence-based assessment model (Youngstrom, 2013), the first piece of information to consider is the "base rate," or how common BSD is likely to be at a given setting. A practitioner working in an inpatient unit is likely to see more cases with BSD than would a school psychologist working in a regular educational setting. The base rate provides an excellent foundation for the integration of additional information. Knowing that the base rate of BSD is around 5% in many outpatient clinics, for example, suggests, on the one hand, that bipolar disorder is a diagnosis that should be considered and carefully assessed in some cases. On the other hand, a 5% prevalence reminds the practitioner that the diagnosis is likely to be rare, and other problems (including those with similar clinical presentations; e.g., ADHD or unipolar depression) are likely to be more common. This anchoring helps avoid over- or underdiagnosis due to availability heuristics that could be unduly influenced by the faddishness of a diagnosis (Davidow & Levinson, 1993). Clinicians can either rely on their own archival records to estimate the rate of BSD or use published estimates from similar clinical settings to provide a ballpark estimate. Table 8.4 provides some published estimates for calibration purposes, along with some comments about the design of each study. If computerized abstract databases are available, then it would be even better to search for newer benchmark estimates using keywords such as "prevalence or incidence" and "bipolar disorder," along with terms describing the clinical context of interest (Youngstrom & Duax, 2005). Practitioners relying on local diagnoses should be aware that clinical diagnoses tend to underestimate the amount of comorbidity present in cases, and also may be particularly inaccurate in the case of BSD (Rettew et al., 2009).

Whether using local estimates or published values, we should reflect on how those benchmark diagnoses were made and consider the possible sources of bias that might influence the estimates. A more thorough dissection of the validity of an estimate can be accomplished by comparing the design features to the 25 recommendations in the STAndardized Reporting of Diagnostic tests

(STARD) Criteria (Bossuyt et al., 2003), or by evaluating the applicability of the findings to the individual patient in question (Jaeschke, Guyatt, & Sackett, 1994). Meta-analyses of the epidemiological rates and the diagnostic accuracy of rating scales have coded the quality of the studies, and the scores are included in tables (Moreira et al., 2017; Van Meter et al., 2019; Youngstrom, Egerton, et al., 2018; Youngstrom, Genzlinger, Egerton, & Van Meter, 2015).

Even when initial estimates of the base rate are flawed, they still can lessen the impact of other factors that undermine the accuracy of the assessment process. Furthermore, if the practitioner follows other recommendations for evidence-based assessment, then periodically reevaluates the base rate of disorders, there is the potential for the process to become self-correcting. Reevaluation of base rates in one's own clinical setting is also good practice because changes in public awareness and other external factors can also change the referral pattern over time.

Busy clinicians are hard pressed to regularly update their knowledge of the epidemiological literature to find useful base rate estimates to inform case assessment decisions. Table 8.4 covers that content, and the Wikiversity page on bipolar disorder in the Evidence-Based Assessment site has updates and additional information.

Risk Factors

Pubertal Status

The risk of mood disorders doubles or triples with puberty (Cyranowski et al., 2000; Van Meter et al., 2019). The diagnosis of bipolar disorder is less controversial in adolescents, too. However, puberty arrives, often earlier than we would expect. Epidemiological studies suggest that 20% of 8-year-old girls may be starting the transition to puberty, and some achieve menarche before age 10 (Ullsperger & Nikolas, 2017). The secular trend for earlier age of onset for puberty may be related to the increasing rate of obesity or to other dietary or environmental factors. Although the mechanism of association is not yet understood, pubertal status is clearly relevant to the case formulation when mood disorder might be involved (Peper & Dahl, 2013). Puberty changes not only the risk of bipolar disorder but also the potential consequences of impulsive behavior, including sexual debut, pregnancy, sexual assault, and exposure to sexually transmitted illnesses (Stewart et al., 2012).

For psychologists, the easiest method for assessing pubertal status is probably using the Petersen Pubertal Development Screen (PPDS; Petersen, Crockett, Richards, & Boxer, 1988). There are both parent and youth self-report versions. The PPDS is widely used in research, is available for free on Wikiversity, and it is reasonably well calibrated against the "gold standard" physical examination. Table 8.5 lists several other risk factors that should also increase the amount of clinical attention focused on evaluating potential bipolar disorder.

Early-Onset Depression

Several lines of evidence suggest that depression in youth should trigger evaluation for potential bipolar disorder: The potential for depression to be the first episode of bipolar disorder that comes to clinical attention (Duffy, Alda, Hajek, & Grof, 2009), the high rate of depressive episodes over the course of illness, and a high rate of conversion from early-onset depression to bipolar disorder over the course of a person's life (Angst et al., 2011) all suggest that clinicians working with youth with depression would do well to consider the possibility of a bipolar disorder. In fact, the U.S. Food and Drug Administration has suggested language for antidepressant medications to include in the package insert, saying that anyone who is going to prescribe or take an antidepressant to treat depression should consider whether there is any history of hypomania or mania, or whether there is a family history of bipolar disorder.

Family History

A meta-analysis reviewed more than 100 articles discussing more than 30 different risk factors potentially associated with BSD. Only family history of BSD has been robust enough to merit clinical interpretation (Tsuchiya, Byrne, & Mortensen, 2003). Another found that, on average, 5% of children with a biological parent affected by BSD already met criteria for a BSD themselves at the time of the research assessment (Hodgins, Fau-

TABLE 8.5. Red Flags That Should Trigger Thorough Evaluation of Possible BSD

Red flag	Description	References
Early-onset depression	Variously described as onset before age 15, or prepubertal	Duffy et al. (2009); Hillegers et al. (2005); Kowatch, Youngstrom, et al. (2005); Youngstrom & Algorta (2014)
Psychotic features	True delusions or hallucinations occurring in the context of mood	Kowatch, Youngstrom, et al. (2005); Van Meter, Burke, Kowatch, et al. (2016)
Episodic aggressive behavior (including high parent reports of externalizing behavior)	Not specific to bipolar, but most bipolar cases will show this; more episodic should trigger evaluation to rule out	Axelson et al. (2012); Hunt et al. (2009)
Family history of BSD	Fivefold increase in risk for first-degree relative; 2.5× for second-degree or "fuzzy" bipolar	Algorta et al. (2013); Fristad et al. (2012); Hodgins et al. (2002)
Atypical depression	Hypersomnia (vs. insomnia), increased appetite and weight gain (vs. decreased), decreased energy, and interpersonal rejection sensitivity	Benazzi & Rihmer (2000); Birmaher et al. (1996)
Early onset of puberty	Puberty doubles or triples risk of mood disorder. Early-onset depression may be more likely to follow a bipolar course.	Peper & Dahl (2013); Ullsperger & Nikolas (2017)
Sleep disturbance	Especially decreased sleep without fatigue or combined with increased energy. Need to differentiate from insomnia with depression, or passive staying up with electronics	Algorta et al. (2013); Harvey (2008); Perez Algorta et al. (2018); Phelps (2008)

cher, Zarac, & Ellenbogen, 2002). Conversely, no children in the "low-risk" comparison groups developed bipolar spectrum illness in any of the studies reviewed. Having a bipolar parent also doubled the children's risk of developing psychopathology in general, and tripled the risk of mood disorders (not just bipolar spectrum illness). When interpreting the 5% rate of bipolar illness, we should remember that (1) family history of bipolar illness increases risk of psychopathology, and especially BSD; (2) the vast majority of children who have a parent with diagnosed BSD will still not have BSD themselves; (3) they often will show other, nonbipolar behavioral problems; and (4) the youth participating in the studies were not followed into middle age, so it is impossible to know how many of them later developed full-blown bipolar illness.

Besides conveying information about the degree of bipolar risk for the youth, family history also reveals the family's strengths and challenges that could impinge on therapy. Having a family member already obtaining treatment for mood disorder provides prior experience that shapes the family's attitudes toward intervention. If prior treatment went well, then the family member offers a powerful role model and excellent potential social support for the youth. If prior experiences were negative, then it is crucial to find out the family's perceptions of what was suboptimal, so that alternative recommendations can be pursued, or other strategies may be used to help address the challenges and resistance. An adult's undiagnosed or poorly managed mood disorder often magnifies the chaos and conflict in a family, reducing the chances of good treatment adherence for the child. Family history can be informative about the likely course of illness for the youth and also has prescriptive value in shaping treatment selection. Children of parents with lithium-responsive BSD tend to show better premorbid functioning, more distinct mood episodes, better interepisode functioning, and better response to lithium themselves (Duffy, Alda, Kutcher, Fusee, & Grof, 1998). Conversely, children whose parents had earlier onset, more rapid-cycling bipolar illness (which tends to be less lithium responsive) themselves are more likely to show a refractory and more chronically impaired course of illness (Duffy et al., 2002; Masi et al., 2006).

Integrating Family History into a Risk Assessment Model

The more systematic and structured the interview, the more cost is added to the evaluation process,

and the more burden imposed on families. For these reasons, there need to be clear benefits before deciding to do more than the routine amount of clinical assessment of family history. The differential diagnosis of BSD is a situation in which the potential gains justify some increased time and burden. Accurate evaluation of familial history tells us about the child's risk and also informs case formulation and treatment strategies. Given how prone "historical" diagnoses are to error, simply asking whether anyone in the family has been diagnosed with BSD is unlikely to be an adequate shortcut to evaluating family history.

One practical approach might be to ask the parents to fill out a brief screening measure, such as the Mood Disorder Questionnaire (MDQ; Hirschfeld et al., 2000), the Bipolar Spectrum Diagnostic Scale (BSDS; Ghaemi et al., 2005), or the Hypomania Checklist (HCL; Angst et al., 2005) about themselves. These are all short, with a low required reading level, yet they fared best in terms of diagnostic accuracy in a meta-analysis (Youngstrom, Egerton, et al., 2018). If the parent reports a history of depression, it would definitely be worthwhile administer one of these measures as a way of checking for potential bipolar disorder.

If a lifetime diagnosis of BSD is found in a first-degree relative (e.g., biological mother, biological father, or a full biological sibling), then the child's risk of having BSD increases by a factor of at least five (Youngstrom & Algorta, 2014). This risk estimate is based on 5% of biological at-risk youth manifesting BSD (Hodgins et al., 2002), compared to a rough estimate of 1% of the general population of youth having any bipolar spectrum illness. We can use this as an effect size to update the probability that a person has bipolar disorder. This would be a diagnostic likelihood ratio (DLR) of 5, which we could use in a probability nomogram or calculator (Van Meter, Chapter 2, this volume).

What if a second-degree relative, such as an aunt, uncle, grandparent, or half-sibling, has a bipolar illness? On average, these relatives share half as many genes with the youth in question, as compared to a first-degree relative. Thus the youth is half as likely to share the genes of risk, and the risk of BSD would increase by half as much, or a factor of 2.5.

Family history of mood disorder (including depression) also increases the risk of the child developing BSD, roughly doubling the risk (Hodgins et al., 2002). "Fuzzy" presentations suggestive of possible BSD, such as moodiness and alcoholism, or "schizophrenia" diagnosed in an individual from an ethnic minority with a history of impulsivity and depression, might also be treated as a "fuzzy" bipolar diagnosis, increasing the risk—but much less so than a confirmed bipolar diagnosis would (Fristad et al., 2012; Youngstrom & Algorta, 2014).

It rarely is possible to directly interview all of the family members to get a sense of their history and functioning. The Family Index of Risk for Mood Disorders (FIRM), a free, brief, systematic means to collect clinically meaningful information about family history of mood disorders and related conditions (Algorta et al., 2013), is a table of 25 questions about established risk factors related to bipolar disorder (e.g., mania, depression, suicide, hospitalizations, or substance use) across several relatives (caregiver's grandparents, parents, aunts/uncles, or children), which can be combined to present a total risk score or separated by type of problem (e.g., family history of mania). High FIRM scores are associated with BSD diagnoses, are not significantly associated with ADHD, ODD, or conduct disorder diagnoses, and add incremental predictive validity after controlling for other family-informant screening measures such as the Child Behavior Checklist (CBCL; Algorta et al., 2013).

The FIRM can provide a fast and free scouting report. We can treat it as a risk estimate, with a DLR of 2.5 for scores of 8+, and .31 for scores less than 8 (Algorta et al., 2013). It also creates an opportunity for clinical exploration, asking the family to share details about the different relatives and their story. This is an opportunity to dig and sometimes uncover inaccurate past diagnoses, particular when working with members of underrepresented minority groups who may have been particularly likely to be misdiagnosed in the past. It also helps to reveal attitudes toward different treatment options: Talking through the FIRM is a chance to learn more about patient preferences (evidence-based assessment model step).

Another tool that can be helpful and engaging is to draw a genogram to diagram the family (McGoldrick & Gerson, 1985). The genogram also can organize notes about relationships, points of conflict, and developmental and medical history. Several case examples on the Wikiversity website include genograms, including Arlene, Christopher, Deshawn, Lea, and Tamika, as well as Ty. Pairing the FIRM and the genogram could be an effective way of unpacking the details from the FIRM to enrich the picture of the family history and systems on the genogram.

Behavior Checklists and Mood Rating Scales

Many researchers have worked on validating rating scales and checklists for bipolar disorder, culminating in two meta-analyses of all studies that used semistructured or structured diagnostic interviews as a criterion. One focused on the diagnostic accuracy of all available scales when completed by adults (Youngstrom, Egerton, et al., 2018), and the other included caregiver- and teacher-completed scales, as well as youth self-report about the youth's mood symptoms (Youngstrom et al., 2015). These meta-analyses provide a set of clear guides for clinical use:

Broad measures can rule out bipolar disorder. A low score on the Externalizing scale on a broad-band measure such as the CBCL decreases the probability of bipolar disorder. Caregiver ratings of externalizing behavior are highly sensitive to bipolar disorder, which means that most individuals who truly have bipolar disorder will get high scores. Combined with bipolar disorder being uncommon in most clinical settings (with the exception of hospitals and residential treatment), low scores on a sensitive test effectively rule the diagnosis out (the SnNOut [on a highly Sensitive test, a Negative result rules the diagnosis Out] heuristic) (Straus, Glasziou, Richardson, & Haynes, 2011). Although no peer-reviewed research has been published yet with most other broad-band scales, the content is similar enough that the SnNOut principle would work similarly for them as well.

Broad measures cannot rule in bipolar disorder. High scores on externalizing problems can occur for myriad reasons besides bipolar disorder. ODD, conduct disorder, and ADHD all are associated with high-average externalizing scores. More subtly, depression and anxiety disorders can also raise externalizing scores: DSM lists "irritability" as a symptom of both. Irritability and moodiness are associated features of most child psychopathology. Efforts to use extremely high externalizing scores as a warning flag for bipolar disorder have failed to show statistical validity (Kahana, Youngstrom, Findling, & Calabrese, 2003; Youngstrom, Findling, Calabrese, et al., 2004), and attempts to select items that might be indicative of bipolar disorder also fail to show diagnostic specificity (Youngstrom, Meyers, Youngstrom, Calabrese, & Findling, 2006a, 2006b), overlapping considerably with symptoms putatively measuring posttraumatic stress disorder (You, Youngstrom, Feeny,

Youngstrom, & Findling, 2017). What used to be mooted as the "bipolar profile" has been renamed the "mood dysregulation profile" instead (Althoff, Ayer, Rettew, & Hudziak, 2010).

Across all measures, caregiver report of manic symptoms has higher discriminative validity than youth or teacher report on the same scales (Youngstrom et al., 2015; see Figure 8.2). The greater validity is partly due to parents being in a better position to observe some of the more diagnostically specific symptoms (e.g., decreased need for sleep) than teachers, who also have difficulty distinguishing between hypomania and ADHD symptoms in the classroom (Youngstrom et al., 2008). Youth also are likely to have less insight into their behavior than adults might, as suggested by the larger validity coefficients for the same

scales when completed by adults instead of teens (Youngstrom, Egerton, et al., 2018). The same symptoms may be more annoying or noticeable by the parent than the youth at earlier stages of the episode or at milder levels (Freeman, Youngstrom, Freeman, Youngstrom, & Findling, 2011). For all of these reasons, a good rule of thumb is to get a caregiver report whenever possible when working with mood disorder to help decide whether one is dealing with unipolar or bipolar disorder.

The meta-analyses also identify a handful of scales that have four or more published studies that produce top-tier results. For assessment of children or teenagers, the parent-rated General Behavior Inventory, the MDQ, and Child Mania Rating Scale (CMRS) are three that are free and perform best. The parent GBI (P-GBI) has the highest reading

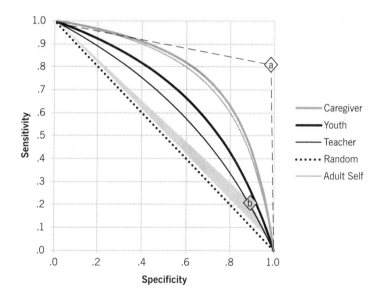

FIGURE 8.2. Plot of diagnostic accuracy of five different ways of assessing for potential bipolar disorder. The figure plots sensitive (percentage of true cases identified) as a function of specificity (percentage of noncases correctly identified). The figure is known as a receiver operating characteristic (ROC) curve, and the corresponding effect size for accuracy is the area under the curve (AUC). The diagonal line represents chance performance (50% AUC). The current best-case scenario would to base the diagnosis on a semistructured diagnostic interview with carefully trained interviewers, then review the case in a consensus meeting that adds additional clinical considerations such as family history or prior treatment; this might push accuracy to a kappa ~.85 and an AUC of .925 for 10% prevalence. At the other end, accuracy of unstructured clinical interviews <b> is slightly better than chance (AUC = .55 based on kappa ~.1 and prevalence of ~.1) (see (Jensen-Doss et al., 2014; Rettew et al., 2009). The typical accuracy of teacher report is significantly better than chance, but youth self-report is better; parent report about the youth and adult self-report provide the best accuracy of any of the rating scale options, with virtually identical AUCs. Note that all of these estimates are based on meta-analyses, using mixed-effect regressions to estimate accuracy under clinically realistic conditions (Youngstrom, Egerton, et al., 2018; Youngstrom et al., 2015) for details. Copyright © 2019 Youngstrom CC-BY 4.0.

level, and the MDQ is easiest, but the MDQ does not gather information about severity. In contrast, the GBI also can serve as a severity or outcome measure. To reduce burden, there are 10-item short forms of the CMRS (Henry, Pavuluri, Youngstrom, & Birmaher, 2008) and P-GBI for mania, as well as two alternative 10-item depression forms (Youngstrom, Van Meter, Frazier, Youngstrom, & Findling, 2020). All three of the best free instruments are available on Wikipedia and the Wikiversity page for bipolar assessment. The P-GBI 10-item forms are recommended for use in research as part of the PhenX Toolkit, and they have been translated into more than two dozen languages for use in clinical trials. Another promising scale is the parent report on the Child and Adolescent Symptom Inventory (CASI; Gadow & Sprafkin, 1994, 1999), which has parent, youth, and teacher report forms, each covering the DSM symptoms of different disorders. Unlike the Achenbach System of Empirically Based Assessment (ASEBA), the CASI includes all of the symptoms of mania, along with depression and several anxiety and disruptive behavior disorders. The CASI Mania scale looks promising in one study (Ong et al., 2016), but this needs replication, as well as investigation of the youth report. Still, the CASI has the advantages of covering multiple disorders and mapping directly to multiple DSM diagnoses, albeit without normative data about typical levels of endorsement at different ages.

For adult self-report (e.g., assessing parents about themselves), the HCL, the BSDS, the MDQ, and the Internal States Scale are all top-tier, free options available on Wiki (Youngstrom, Egerton, et al., 2018). The GBI also performed well, but its reading level and length make it less suited for routine clinical use, and the short forms need additional validation in adults before being recommended for widespread adoption (Youngstrom, Murray, Johnson, & Findling, 2013); see Figure 8.2.

In adolescents, the MDQ and several short forms of the GBI (A-GBI) also show validity across a range of samples, performing better than the Achenbach scales (Youngstrom et al., 2015), albeit not as well as the parent report (or self-report in adults). These, too, are available on the Wiki pages.

Teacher report is not sufficiently accurate to warrant clinical use for diagnostic assessment (B. Goldstein et al., 2017). The scales can produce statistically significant discrimination in large samples and in the meta-analysis, but the effect sizes are too small to inform decisions about individual cases (e.g., the DLRs are close to 1 across the range of scores) (Youngstrom et al., 2008). Teacher perspectives still can be helpful for treatment planning, and definitely for educational planning, but they are not helpful for diagnosis per se.

The specialized mania scales tend to produce higher diagnostic specificity than the broadband measures. However, they are still not accurate enough, and bipolar disorder is not common enough, to recommend using them for universal screening. In schools or other settings drawing from the general population—as opposed to treatment-seeking settings—the base rate is low enough that even high-risk scores only yield moderate probabilities of youth having bipolar disorder. In other words, if interpreted in a black or white way, the majority of the high scorers would still be "false positives." The scales are useful additions but not something that would be part of the default core battery in many settings.

Revising Probabilities Based on Assessments and Risk Factors

It is possible to do much better than relying on rules of thumb or eyeball estimates to combine the information gathered so far. Using the Bayesian methods advocated by evidence-based measurement (EBM; Straus et al., 2011) and evidence-based assessment (EBA; Youngstrom, 2013), we can quickly use risk factors and assessment findings to update the probability of bipolar disorder for an individual client. Van Meter (Chapter 2, this volume) walks through the mechanics. Table 8.4 provides base rates in different settings that serve as a menu for us to select a benchmark starting probability. The case examples on Wikiversity all were seen at community outpatient clinics, so we used 6% as a starting probability estimate. Family history is a well-established risk factor. High scores on the FIRM would have a DLR of 2.6. Combining that DLR with a 6% prior probability in a calculator provides a revised probability of 14%. If we interviewed the family instead and felt more confident about the bipolar diagnosis of the relative, then we could use a DLR of 5 for first-degree relatives (i.e., a biological mother, father, or full sibling of the person we are assessing), or 2.5 for a second-degree relative (e.g., grandparent, aunt/uncle, or half sibling). We could use the FIRM as the basis for a semistructured clinical interview to discuss the family history and refine our formulation (and the associated DLR).

Scores on a broad-band measure, such as the Externalizing score on the CBCL, would be another data source at this stage. Low scores have potent DLRs for decreasing the probability of BSD in youth. They are more than enough to cancel out the effect of a bipolar relative on the probability estimate. Conceptually, the algebra is telling us that even though the youth has a risky family history, the low level of behavior problems noted by the caregiver makes it unlikely that he or she has developed BSD. High scores, on the other hand, increase the probability moderately (e.g., DLR values ~3, roughly tripling the odds). In an outpatient clinic, this would raise the probability to between 50 and 60%. We would consider this the "yellow zone" and want to add more assessment techniques focused on confirming or disconfirming the bipolar hypothesis. If the family insisted on treatment before we had a more decisive evaluation, then we would want to start with broad-spectrum, low-risk interventions such as psychotherapy, skills building, improved sleep hygiene—all things that would be at least somewhat helpful if the person has BSD, but also potentially helpful and unlikely to harm if the problem is actually something else. Table 8.6 lists the diagnostic accuracy and the likelihood ratios (DLRs) for some of the recommended scales. More comprehensive details are in the meta-analysis (Youngstrom et al., 2015).

When we are in the "yellow zone" is a great time to add one of the best validated, free mood scales. The minimum would be to add one of the 10-item mania scales, either the CMRS-10 or the PGBI-10M. There is not any clear value added by doing both, and the Internalizing scales on the Achenbach or a similar scale may provide enough information about depressive symptoms for this stage. We can frame the delivery by telling the family that we do not ask everyone to do this type of instrument, but it will be helpful in their case because it can clarify why the youth is getting irritable and moody. Often families ask to do the full-length version rather than a short form when they see how the results directly inform their child's care. Once we have the results from this more mood-focused instrument, we look up the DLR for the score, and replace the DLR from the CBCL with it. We only want to use one DLR per informant per hypothesis, as explained in the introductory chapters. If we have a youth report on a similar scale, we can include it by finding the associated DLR and adding it to the risk calculator, or working through the probability nomogram again.

The combination of base rate and parent report on an externalizing scale is enough to rule out bipolar disorder for most cases in an outpatient setting with a high degree of accuracy (e.g., the negative predictive value would be >99%). For the ones that have high externalizing scores, following up with the FIRM and CMRS-10 adds no cost, 1.5 pages to the paperwork for the caregiver, and will be sufficient to move the probability down (into the "green zone," where bipolar is considered "ruled out" for the time being) or up into the "yellow zone," where bipolar is one of the candidates that is the focus of more detailed assessment.

The Prescription Phase: Establishing Diagnoses, Case Formulation, and Treatment Plan

All of the assessment tools covered so far can be completed by the family before the first appointment. They can be mailed or e-mailed ahead of time, done in the waiting room, or completed online. A collaboration between several divisions of the American Psychological Association and a nonprofit organization, Helping Give Away Psychological Science (hgaps.org), has built online versions of several of these scales, with automated scoring that can be used for free. The goal is to improve the dissemination of the best free tools and make them easier to use.

If nothing in the results so far suggests BSD (i.e., if the updated probability is in the "green zone," <5% chance), then the interview and case formulation should concentrate on other issues. If the family members sought an evaluation because they suspected BSD, then we need to be ready to respectfully walk them through the evidence gathered that makes BSD unlikely. Done well, this should not feel dismissive or invalidating to the family. The metamessages are "Good news! It probably is not bipolar disorder that is the problem!" and "We agree that there definitely is something that needs to be addressed, and we are closing in together on what the (nonbipolar) factors are." If a family is strongly attached to the bipolar label, it may be helpful to point out that the field has a lot more experience, and bigger evidence base guiding treatment, for most other problems that are likely to be the culprit.

For cases that are in the "yellow zone" at this stage, the next step is to do a thorough interview to decide whether BSD is part of the clinical picture.

TABLE 8.6. Feature Comparison of Measures that are Free to Use, Including Discriminative Performance

Feature	Adult about self (including parent about self)		
	MDQ	BSDS	HCL
Length			
Maximum	15	20	32
Shortest	12	19	16
Reading level[a]	7.3	10.0	7.2
Languages	13+[b]	7+[c]	18+[d]
Projected d	1.00	1.05	0.95
Projected AUC (95% CI)	.76 (.68–.83)	.77 (.69–.84)	.75 (.67–.82)
Sensitivity at Sp = .9	.41	.43	.38
DLR+	4.1	4.3	3.8
Time frame	Lifetime	Lifetime	Lifetime

Feature	Teen about self			Any mood
	MDQ	GBI-10M	7 Up	GBI-10Da
Length				
Maximum	15	79	79	79
Shortest	12	10	7	10
Reading level[a]	7.3	11.1	11.1	11.1
Languages	13+[b]	25+[e]	4+[e]	25+[e]
Projected d	0.40	0.43	0.36	
Projected AUC (95% CI)	.61 (.54–.67)	.62 (.58–.67)	.60 (.56–.65)	.66 (.62–.70)
Sensitivity at Sp = .9	.20	.22	.20	.23
DLR+	2.0 raw 9+	2.2 raw 19+	2.0 raw 11+	2.3 raw 16+
Time frame	Lifetime	Past year	Past year	Past year

Feature	Parent about youth			Any mood
	PGBI-10M	CMRS	FIRM	PGBI-10Da
Length				
Maximum	79	21	1-page grid	79
Shortest	10	10	1 page	10
Reading level[a]	11.1	6.5	7.6	11.1
Languages	25+[e]	5[f]	2[g]	25+[e]
Projected d	1.30	0.87	0.47	1.30
Projected AUC (95% CI)	.82 (.80–.84)	.73 (.66–.80)	.63 (.54–.72)	.82 (.80–.84)
Sensitivity at Sp = .9	.47	.21	.28	.52
DLR+	4.7 raw 15.5+	2.1 raw 12+	2.8 raw 8+	5.2 raw 10+
Time frame	Past year	Lifetime	Lifetime (family history)	Past year

Note. Estimates based on saturated regression model for studies from 2000 and later, with 2016 as reference year (Youngstrom, Egerton, et al., 2018). AUC, area under curve from receiver operating characteristic analysis; estimate assumes parametric distribution. Sensitivity for specificity = .90 uses same assumptions. DLR+ is the diagnostic likelihood ratio associated with scoring above the threshold attached to a specificity of .90; note that this might not be the most discriminating region of performance on a given test. The Wikiversity pages have more details, including multilevel DLRs. DLRs of 1 indicate that the test result did not change impressions at all. DLRs larger than 10 or smaller than .10 are frequently clinically decisive; DLRs of 5.0 or .20 are helpful, and DLRs between 2.0 and .5 are small enough that they rarely result in clinically meaningful changes of formulation (Sackett et al., 2000). English versions of all measures are available on Wikipedia.
[a]Flesch–Kincaid grade level, estimated on the combination of instructions and items.
[b]MDQ available in English, Spanish, Chinese, Danish, Dutch, Farsi/Persian, Finnish, French, German, Italian, Japanese, Korean, Portuguese.
[c]BSDS available in English (U.S. and U.K.), Arabic, Chinese, Japanese, Korean, Persian, Portuguese, Spanish.
[d]HCL available in English, Arabic, Croatian, Danish, Dutch, Flemish, French, German, Greek, Hungarian, Italian, Japanese, Polish, Portuguese (Portuguese and Brazilian), Russian, Spanish, Turkish.
[e]GBI available in English, Spanish, Portuguese, Korean in full length and 7 Up 7 Down versions; available in 20 other languages for 10-M and 10-Da versions.
[f]CMRS available in English, Spanish, Chinese, Arabic, Portuguese.
[g]FIRM available in English and Spanish.

Diagnostic Interviews

One of the most powerful tools available for establishing a diagnosis is diagnostic interviews. These run the gamut from unstructured clinical interviews guided by the intuition and experience of the clinician, all the way to fully structured interviews that provide a rigid framework and clear scripting of the questions and probes. There are advantages and drawbacks to either extreme (see Jensen-Doss et al., Chapter 3, this volume).

Most clinicians prefer to do unstructured interviews, despite the evidence that interrater reliability is abysmal (Rettew et al., 2009), the content covered is highly variable, and the interviews are susceptible to a wide range of cognitive biases (Croskerry, 2003; Jenkins & Youngstrom, 2016). Appeals to professional autonomy do not hold water when the reliability and validity are low. Fears that more structured approaches would damage rapport or overburden clients are allayed by surveys that indicate clients prefer more structured, systematic approaches because they feel that they are more thorough (Suppiger et al., 2009). It would be a bad idea, verging on irresponsible, to make decisions about bipolar disorder on the basis of an unstructured interview—especially given how prone we can be to overdiagnosing or underdiagnosing it due to differences in training and cognitive heuristics. The Harvard surgeon Atul Gawande (2010) convincingly makes the case in *The Checklist Manifesto* that a good checklist reduces error and improves outcomes in virtually any complex human activity. If a checklist makes a Harvard professor a better surgeon, we can certainly use some checklists to make our high-stakes diagnoses more accurate.

The MINI-KID is probably the most widely used fully structured interview that covers BSD in child and adolescent age groups. The MINI-KID was built as a faster, easier-to-train competitor to the Structured Clinical Interview for DSM Disorders (SCID) (Sheehan et al., 2010). It has reasonable interrater and retest reliability for adults; less work has been done with the MINI-KID version. The current licensing makes the MINI-KID free for personal use, with a fee attached for grant- or industry-funded research. Unfortunately, there are no published data pertaining to psychometrics specifically with BSD in youth. In fact, at the moment, there is no fully structured diagnostic interview that has demonstrated good validity for diagnosing BSD. Some instruments have failed to detect any cases of BSD in epidemiological studies (Costello et al., 1996; Shaffer et al., 1996), raising concerns about their sensitivity to bipolar diagnoses (Galanter et al., 2012).

Most published research on BSD has relied one of the several different versions of the Kiddie Schedule for Affective Disorders and Schizophrenia (K-SADS). However, the K-SADS requires considerable training and supervision to learn to administer it reliably. Even though it is free, this is not something that one should just download, then use with a client. The K-SADS is also cumbersome. The core module of the Present and Lifetime (PL) version is nearly 200 pages long (Kaufman et al., 1997), with five additional supplements, and the Washington University (WASH-U) version is even longer (Geller et al., 2001). The complete K-SADS interview with parent and child takes anywhere from 2 to 6 hours. Thus, training, expense, and burden on the family all mitigate against routine clinical use of the K-SADS. A Wikipedia page has gathered details about different variations and links to PDF versions. A new DSM-5 version is based on the PL, and probably would be the most practical as well as updated option.

A practical compromise might be to print and use the criteria for mood episodes and disorders as a checklist to guide the interview in a semistructured manner. Photocopying or printing out the criteria for depression, dysthymia, mania, hypomania, and the half-dozen mood disorders would be less than a dozen pages. We would not read them to the client, but we would use them as a guide to make sure we had explored enough details to be confident in a diagnostic decision. A variation on this idea would be to print copies of the K-SADS Mania Rating Scale and Depression Rating Scale (Axelson et al., 2003). These cover all of the DSM and ICD symptoms of mania and depression, and have stems and anchors designed to be more developmentally appropriate than the older, interview-based scales. They would provide good material for a systematic evaluation, and would just need questions about duration and impairment to be sufficient to cover the same ground as much longer interviews.

Cognitive Debiasing Strategies

Cognitive psychology has identified a variety of shortcuts and heuristics that our brains use to process complex information quickly. These "fast and frugal" algorithms automatically guide interpretation without conscious cognitive control (Gigerenzer, 2001; Kahneman, 2011). By learning how these predictable approaches fail, we can build in habits and compensating tactics to make more accurate decisions.

More than 30 different cognitive heuristics and associated errors have been documented and examined in different medical settings (Croskerry, 2003). Several of these are likely to have a big influence on our diagnostic decisions with regard to bipolar disorder. These include the availability heuristic, confirmation bias, anchoring, and search satisficing (Jenkins & Youngstrom, 2016). *Availability* refers to when the concept is cognitively salient, such as when a diagnosis becomes trendy or is prominent in the news, or when a family includes it in their description of the presenting problem. High availability can feed into a tendency to overdiagnose. *Confirmation bias* refers to a documented proclivity for humans to look for evidence that supports their idea, and to discount or ignore inconsistent evidence. *Anchoring* refers to a tendency to make a global initial impression, then to make only minor adjustments to move away from the cognitive "anchor." *Search satisficing* describes the tendency to call off the search for explanations or diagnoses once one is confirmed. In addition to the usual cognitive tendency to stop at the first confirmed hypothesis, our reimbursement system is tied to having at least one diagnosis, and there is no incentive to be thorough and document comorbid conditions (Rettew et al., 2009).

If we know about these potential pitfalls, they are relatively easy to avoid. Using the base rate as a starting probability combats the availability heuristic, using data to guide our starting point regardless of whether a diagnosis is in or out of vogue. Anchoring then becomes a virtue, so that we begin at a well-calibrated starting point. Using the DLRs would build on this by giving objective weights to each new piece of information. We can combat confirmation bias by writing down more than one hypothesis that could be consistent with the presenting problem, then look for both confirming and disconfirming evidence for everything on our list. In essence, we are changing the game from "shooting from the hip" to "Case Formulation Survivor," where we have a set of plausible contestants who are competing to not get voted off the island (in this case, demoted to the "green zone" of low probability—where they still could make a return appearance in a new season if the ratings change!). The way to avoid search satisficing is to remember that comorbidity is the rule, and not the exception, in most mental health

settings—so it is possible to have more than one diagnosis get confirmed as part of the formulation. Jenkins and Youngstrom (2016) showed that teaching practicing clinicians this set of strategies, plus one more rule of thumb—when a person mentions depression, make sure to ask about past hypomania or mania, as they do not always spontaneously volunteer this—took less than 15 minutes to learn and produced large improvements in accuracy and consistency of assessments and treatment plans across a range of clinical vignettes. Installing these good habits will improve our decision making whether we are using semistructured or unstructured interviews.

Concentrate on "Handle" Symptoms

When interviewing about mood disorders, it is essential to ask about all of the DSM symptoms of mania or hypomania. However, the symptoms are not equally useful indicators of potential BSD (see Table 8.7). Many symptoms commonly seen in mania or hypomania (Birmaher, Axelson, Strober, et al., 2009; Kowatch, Youngstrom, et al., 2005; Van Meter, Burke, Kowatch, Findling, & Youngstrom, 2016; Van Meter, Burke, Youngstrom, et al., 2016) also frequently occur in other conditions besides BSD (Carlson, Danzig, Dougherty, Bufferd, & Klein, 2016; Youngstrom et al., 2010). Irritable mood, poor concentration, and high levels of motor activity are examples of symptoms that are highly sensitive but not specific to BSD. Their high sensitivity means that the *absence* of the symptom may be helpful in ruling out BSD (SnNOut at the symptom level), but the presence of such symptoms by itself is ambiguous. Irritability is analogous to the "fever" or "pain" of child mental health—it indicates that something is wrong but does not provide as much guidance in deciding what is wrong. These also are often symptoms that the parent will notice sooner than the youth, both in terms of catching them at a milder level of severity, as well as finding them annoying faster (Freeman et al., 2011).

Other symptoms are more helpful in getting a "handle" on whether BSD is present. Episodes of abnormally elated and expansive mood are one such symptom. Although elated mood is not the most impairing symptom associated with BSD and rarely is high on the list of presenting problems, it is present in more than 80% of cases with BSD (Kowatch, Youngstrom, et al., 2005; Van Meter, Burke, Kowatch, et al., 2016). Furthermore, elated mood that is noticeably more frequent, more intense, or longer in duration than would be developmentally appropriate rarely occurs in other child mental health syndromes (Kowatch, Fristad, et al., 2005). Grandiosity also appears to be fairly common in BSD but less frequent in ADHD (Geller, Zimerman, Williams, DelBello, Bolhofner, et al., 2002). However, chronic grandiosity or an inflated but brittle sense of self-esteem is associated with conduct disorder (which was excluded from earlier studies of BSD), undermining the specificity of this symptom in settings where antisocial behavior might occur.

Decreased need for sleep is not present in all cases, but it is highly specific to BSD. Decreased need for sleep can be challenging to assess clinically for many reasons: Self-report is not always accurate about the onset and offset of sleep periods (cf. Meltzer, Chapter 23, this volume) and parents may not know when the child is falling asleep or waking (especially if the parent is asleep at the time). In addition, sleep disturbance is more suggestive of BSD when the person is not sleeping because he or she has too much energy or is getting less sleep than usual yet still feels energetic the following day, rather than lying in bed watching movies or TV. This should be distinguished from the insomnia often seen with unipolar depression, in which the person wants to sleep but has difficulty falling asleep despite low energy due to stress and rumination about problems. See Meltzer (Chapter 23, this volume) for practical strategies for evaluating sleep clinically.

Hypersexuality is another symptom that deserves comment. Most cases of BSD will not show hypersexuality (see Table 8.7). However, hypersexuality is rarely present in prepubertal children outside of the context of either sexual abuse (Milojevich & Wolfe, Chapter 18, this volume) or mood disorder. Thus, hypersexual behavior should trigger careful assessment of both possibilities.

Clinicians have noticed many other features that tend to occur with mood episodes. Table 8.7 (adapted from Youngstrom et al., 2008, and Wikiversity) lists DSM and ICD symptoms of mania, along with some of these clinically associated features. Where available, sensitivity estimates for the symptom or sign are provided. Quantitative estimates of specificity are rarer, and the few published estimates are unlikely to be clinically generalizable because of the inclusion and exclusion criteria used. Table 8.7 also offers brief comments about aspects of clinical presentation that would be more indicative of bipolar versus nonbipolar diagnoses.

For all of these symptoms, the case for BSD is most compelling when the symptoms occur together in episodes that are a distinct shift from the person's typical functioning. Although not all authorities agree about the importance of distinct episodes, episodicity increases confidence in the diagnosis of mood disorders, particularly when mood episodes have recurred. The presence of episodes even when symptoms are prodromal or subthreshold also predicts later BSD (Egeland, Hostetter, Pauls, & Sussex, 2000). Careful assessment of episodicity or fluctuations in symptom presentation also may help clarify otherwise ambiguous symptoms. ADHD is associated with chronically high energy and poor concentration, for example. Hearing about periods of a week or two at a time in which the person suddenly had more energy than usual, and had difficulty staying focused on tasks at the same time, sounds more like a mood disorder and less like ADHD. Careful evaluation of temperament and developmental history are vital to establish the backdrop against which these changes in functioning can be detected (Quinn & Fristad, 2004).

Methods Not Yet Diagnostically Informative

Many widely used assessment procedures have not yet demonstrated validity for the assessment of BSD. Some have not been systematically investigated, and others have some preliminary data available but nothing adequate to draw inferences about the diagnostic validity of the tool when applied in clinical settings. There have been no published evaluations of projective techniques such as the Rorschach, Thematic Apperception Test, or kinetic family drawing, despite a clinical lore that BSD might be associated with gory content (Popper, 1990). There also are no published studies with objective personality inventories. Without rigorous research, it is impossible to tell how helpful assessment results on any of these instruments might be in determining a bipolar diagnosis. Even face-valid results might be frequent enough in nonbipolar cases to undermine the diagnostic value, much as the ubiquity of irritable mood offsets its high sensitivity to BSD.

Other tests have shown statistically significant differences between bipolar and nonbipolar groups, including some neuropsychological and affective processing tasks (for meta-analysis and review, see Joseph, Frazier, Youngstrom, & Soares, 2008; Robinson et al., 2006; Walshaw et al., 2010). Recent meta-analyses have confirmed

TABLE 8.7. Symptoms and Associated Features of BSD Based on Meta-Analysis

Symptom	Sensitivity to BSD[a]	Specificity to BSD	Features suggesting BSD	Features suggesting other diagnoses	Recommendation
Handle symptoms (high specificity)					
A.1. Elated, expansive, euphoric mood	$M_{weighted}$ = 64% (95% CI: 53–75%); 19 studies	High	Extreme, causes impairment, situationally inappropriate, extreme duration	Transient, more responsive to redirection, more situationally driven; substance abuse	Highly specific feature—presence helps rule-in diagnosis. Assess even though family may not consider it part of presenting problem
A.2. Irritable mood	77% (64–88%); 17 studies	Low	Irritability in context of other mood symptoms; high- versus low-energy irritability	Chronic oppositional behavior in absence of changes in mood or energy; might be unipolar depression	Assess via collateral informant—self-report underestimates; if collaterals deny irritability, effectively rule out BSD because of high sensitivity; embed in context of changes in mood and energy
B.1. Grandiosity	57% (44–69%); 19 studies	Moderately high—much lower if conduct disorder is included	Episodic quality, and should fluctuate with mood; periods of grandiosity contrasted with low self-esteem, feelings of worthlessness	More chronic, arrogant, not associated with mood is suggestive of CD/APD or adolescent overconfidence; substance abuse	Worth emphasizing, but probably not specific enough to elevate to required feature; fluctuations a key feature in discerning from CD/APD
Increased energy	79% (61–93%); 8 studies; highest sensitivity in meta-analysis	Low for "high energy," which is also common in ADHD; *episodic periods of high energy would be more specific to mood disorder*	Higher if ask about fluctuation or change; low if ask about chronic (b/c common feature with ADHD)	Chronic high motor activity	Need to assess as change in functioning from youth's typical behavior; episodic quality is more specific to bipolar illness; focus on *energy* versus motor activity for self-report (Geller et al., 2002b); *change* in motor activity for collaterals
Nonspecific symptoms (in descending order of sensitivity to BSD)					
Pressured speech	63% (49–77%); 18 studies	Unclear. Carlson (2002) raises issue of expressive language problems; but not evaluated yet in published samples	Episodic quality, change from typical for youth; set against slowed or impoverished speech during depression	Chronically "chatty" or talkative is more suggestive of ADHD	Emphasize changes from typical functioning embedded in shifts of mood or energy

Racing thoughts	61% (45–76%); 15 studies	Good if embedded in mood context	Ask about imagery, as well as words	Distinguish from expressive language disorder; substance abuse, meds	
Decreased need for sleep	56% (46–67%); 19 studies	High if framed as decreased need, not insomnia. Low if just focus on trouble falling asleep.	High energy, actively engaged in activities, does not miss sleep the next day	Decreased sleep due to stimulant use (ADHD), use of substances or medications; difficulty falling asleep with unipolar depression (vs. decreased need for sleep). Depressed persons want to sleep, but cannot	Emphasize decreased need for sleep, as distinct from difficulty falling asleep (particularly due to stress or rumination); high energy, little diminution of energy despite decreased sleep
Mood swings/lability	76% (55–95%); 6 studies	High—based on PGBI, CBCL, Conners items	Frequent, intense, with periods of long duration	May be induced by substance abuse, medications, medical/neurological illnesses, borderline personality traits, disruptive disorders	Parent report highly sensitive. BSD unlikely if parent denies. Specificity appears promising, based on multiple scales; conceptualize as mixed state with volatile mood
Hypersexuality	32% (23–42%); 12 studies	High—typically either pediatric BSD or sexual abuse	Hypersexuality is not characteristic, embedded in episodes of energy/mood; has pleasure-seeking quality	Sexual abuse—linked to trauma, perhaps more seductive/reenacting quality than sensation seeking; pornography exposure; actual sex	Insensitive to BSD, so absence not informative; highly specific: Presence should trigger careful assessment of BSD and abuse (recognize that they could co-occur)
Distractibility	74% (61–85%); 17 studies	Low—ADHD, unipolar, anxiety, PTSD, and low cognitive functioning all show this, too	Higher if ask about change from typical, embed in context of mood	Chronic problems much more suggestive of ADHD or neurological impairment	Probably important to assess via collateral instead of self-report; high sensitivity could make negative collateral helpful at ruling out bipolar illness
Poor judgment	61% (45–76%); 17 studies	Moderate	Episodic, embedded in mood/energy	Impulsive or accident-prone, clumsy	Episodic, sensation seeking may be most specific presentation
Flight of ideas	54% (42–66%); 12 studies	Moderate		(Speech problems again) substance abuse, medication-induced	
Increased sociability/people seeking/overfamiliarity (ICD-10, p. 113); added to WASH-U KSADS	41% (27–56%); 7 studies	Unknown	Could be the positive affect, could be sensation seeking		Needs investigation

[a]Sensitivity estimates from Van Meter, Burke, Kowatch, et al. (2016) meta-analysis.

that youth at familial risk for developing bipolar disorder show small decrements in general cognition (weighted $d = 0.29$) and social cognition ($d = 0.23$; Bora & Ozerdem, 2017); and neurocognitive deficits also persist even when youths with bipolar disorder are euthymic (Hedges's g .76–.99; Elias et al., 2017). Despite the enthusiasm for having more "objective" performance tests or biomarkers, these are not yet ready for clinical use for several reasons. First, the effect sizes are often only moderate. Although statistically significant, they fall short of being large enough to classify individuals with reasonable accuracy. For example, a cognitive test that delivered Cohen's d values of ~0.73 (the weighted average across four studies using the Tower of London, meta-analyzed by Walshaw et al., 2010) would translate to an area under the curve (AUC) in ROC analysis of .70, and a DLR+ of 2.4 at a cutoff score that had .80 specificity. These are algebraic transformations that can be verified using some of the calculators on Wikiversity. A second caveat is that most of these studies use healthy controls as the comparison group (e.g., Couzin, 2008; Rocha-Rego et al., 2014; Woodruff, El-Mallakh, & Thiruvengadam, 2012). Similar deficits are likely to occur in association with other pathology. Walshaw and colleagues (2010) reviewed the literature about the same neurocognitive tasks in ADHD, and found that $d = 0.38$ for ADHD versus controls, which suggests that the bipolar effect size would be cut in half trying to separate bipolar from ADHD. This is the much more clinically relevant scenario. In contrast, the best free validated checklists would all deliver AUCs >.95 separating cases with bipolar versus healthy controls, and they maintain clinically useful discriminating power when also tested with clinically meaningful comparison groups (Youngstrom et al., 2006b). A third caveat is that most articles are not reporting effect sizes, such as DLRs, that would make it easier to apply to clinical cases. It is possible for savvy users to convert the effect sizes (again, using the Wiki tools is an option).

The bottom line for now is that neurocognitive performance, imaging, and biomarker studies obtain effect sizes smaller than would be needed to classify individuals accurately based on test results, especially when they have used tight inclusion and exclusion criteria that increase internal validity (which is important for these novel investigations). Clinicians attempting to use the same tools in clinical settings, with fewer inclusion and exclusion criteria, will obtain even more modest results, further weakening the chances of a test

contributing accurately to diagnostic formulation. Given the current evidence base:

1. There is no value added by administering any of these tests to aid in the differential diagnosis of BSD. Although many of these tools might demonstrate validity in future studies, at present they can only be considered unproven.
2. If these tests already have been given as part of an assessment battery, they should not be interpreted as changing the diagnostic formulation with regard to BSD.
3. These tests should only be added to an assessment battery for youth diagnosed with BSD if the test serves some other, additional clinical purpose, such as ascertaining an appropriate educational placement (Youngstrom & De Los Reyes, 2015).

Implications of Cross-Informant Agreement for Impairment and Treatment Planning

In outpatient clinics, a common scenario is for the parent to report significantly more problems than youth or teachers endorse on similar scales. This situation is due to a combination of two well-established psychometric facts: modest agreement between informants and regression to the mean. It is the rare child or teenager who is worried about his or her own mental health, schedules an appointment with a clinic, then gets the parent to consent and bring him or her. Instead, at most private practices and outpatient clinics, we see the subset of youth whose parents are highly concerned. Essentially, our setting has selection bias for high scores on parent-reported measures.

Regression to the mean dictates that when scores are extremely high on one variable, they will be above average on other, positively correlated variables, but closer to the average score. The degree of shrinkage is a function of the size of the correlation. The typical agreement between parent and youth, based on multiple meta-analyses, is r ~.3, and between parent and teacher is r ~.25 (Achenbach, McConaughy, & Howell, 1987; De Los Reyes et al., 2015). On a scale using T-scores, the correlation means that for every 10 points (= 1 SD) that the mom is more worried, the average response for the youth with be ~3 points higher, and for the teacher about 2.5 points higher. Thus, the typical scenario when a parent endorses a T-score of 70 ("clinically elevated") would be for the youth to report a score around 56, and teachers around a 55. In large samples, these would be statistically significant associations, but at the level of the individual case, they are underwhelming.

The disagreement is not due to poor reliability. It reflects differences in access to information about symptoms and behaviors, and differences in perspective that can change motivation for treatment. Clinicians are frequently worried that the parent might be hypervigilant or have unrealistic expectations about appropriate behavior, that ineffective parenting styles might be creating behavior problems that otherwise are well managed in the classroom and other settings, or that the parent's anxiety or depression might be biasing his or her reports about the child's behavior (Richters, 1992). When parent and youth perceptions differ, then clinicians tend to give more weight to youth report about internalizing problems because youth have direct access to their own feelings (Loeber, Green, & Lahey, 1990). Part of the discrepancy between caregiver and child relates to the thresholds at which informants report various symptoms: A study of adolescent–caregiver pairs showed that parents report irritability at lower thresholds of mania than adolescents, while adolescents endorse increased energy and hyperactivity at lower severities than do caregivers (Freeman et al., 2011).

With regard to bipolar disorder, the low level of parent–youth or parent–teacher agreement sometimes has raised concerns about both the accuracy of parent report and the stability of behavior across settings (Thuppal, Carlson, Sprafkin, & Gadow, 2002). There was debate about whether to require evidence of clinically concerning levels of manic symptoms in multiple settings to corroborate a diagnosis of bipolar disorder, similar to what is done with ADHD. Despite these concerns, results have consistently demonstrated that parent appraisals of mood and behavior do significantly better at identifying bipolar cases than do self-report or teacher report, even when predicting research diagnoses made on the basis of direct interviews of both the parent and child, as well as clinical observation (Youngstrom et al., 2015). The greater validity of parent report persists in spite of high rates of mood disorder in the reporting parent in many of these samples, and in spite of the high levels of parents' own reported distress (Youngstrom, Findling, & Calabrese, 2004). In addition, parent–youth agreement about mood symptoms is significantly higher in youth with bipolar disorder than in youth with other diagnoses (Youngstrom et al., 2006b), further allaying concerns that it might often be a figment of a worried caregiver's imagination. Especially with younger children, clinical interviewers also perceive the caregiver as the more credible informant (Youngstrom et al., 2011).

Despite concerns to the contrary, agreement among informants about cases with BSD is actually higher than typical: According to both themselves and their teachers, affected youth experience more behavior problems than would be expected based on the level of problems described by the parent (Youngstrom et al., 2006a). Interrater agreement appears to be even higher when focusing on mood symptoms in particular instead of behavior problems generally (Youngstrom, Findling, & Calabrese, 2004; Youngstrom, Van Meter, et al., 2020), so there is likely to be even more cross-situational consistency than broad-band measures reveal. When manic symptoms are reported by more informants and in more settings, global functioning and objective measures of behavior on an inpatient unit all indicate progressively more severe impairment (Carlson & Youngstrom, 2003).

The lower validity of teacher versus parent report (Youngstrom et al., 2008) appears to be due partly to the tendency of teachers to focus on increased motor activity and poor concentration, then to attribute these behaviors to ADHD (Abikoff, Courtney, Pelham, & Koplewicz, 1993). The school setting is also not amenable to observing sleep disturbance or disrupted family functioning, which are important both to the differential diagnosis and to case formulation for treatment.

Considerations about Validity of Youth Report

At least four factors challenge the validity of youth self-report: (1) Children and adolescents are often less cognitively capable of completing questionnaires, and less psychologically minded than adults; (2) social desirability effects might make youth minimize endorsement of irritable mood or hypersexuality; (3) mania and hypomania tend to be more distressing to people around the affected person than to the person him- or herself (Carlson & Youngstrom, 2011); and (4) mood symptoms often are associated with a reduction in insight into one's own behavior (Dell'Osso et al., 2002; Pini, Dell'Osso, & Amador, 2001; Youngstrom, Findling, & Calabrese, 2004). Clinicians often perceive youth as less credible sources of information about externalizing problems, although they do give more weight to youth who acknowledge some of these behaviors in themselves (Youngstrom et al., 2011).

Treatment Moderators

The distinction between unipolar and bipolar depression is important to make. Although the symptoms and presenting complaints of bipolar depression may appear similar to those in unipolar depression, the treatment response can be quite different. Antidepressant medications may be overactivating in BSD, triggering mania or possibly increasing suicide risk (Carlson, 2003; Geller et al., 1993; Kowatch, Fristad, et al., 2005). Similarly, cognitive strategies or social activation strategies need to be qualified to avoid the risk of the person not just lifting the depression but triggering mania (Newman, Leahy, Beck, Reilly-Harrington, & Gyulai, 2002). Besides avoiding unintended harmful effects, recognition that it is a bipolar depression also suggests positive strategies that can be effective, including improved sleep hygiene and avoidance of self-medication of symptoms (Danielson, Feeny, Findling, & Youngstrom, 2004; Perez Algorta, Van Meter, et al., 2018). It also is worth monitoring for treatment-emergent hypomania in teens taking antidepressants for depression (Joseph et al., 2009; Pacchiarotti et al., 2013).

Comorbidity also may change the treatment plan. If there is comorbid ADHD, shown by symptoms that persist outside of the mood episodes or continuing even after the mood symptoms respond to treatment, then adding stimulant medication may be warranted (McClellan et al., 2007). Comorbid substance misuse may require additional intervention to prevent it undermining other treatment. Suicidal or nonsuicidal self-injurious behaviors are important to assess directly, and each requires additional components of risk management and treatment.

EBA of Process, Progress, and Outcomes

There has been much debate around the conceptualization of meaningful outcomes for bipolar disorders in adult populations. Commonly, and not surprisingly, researchers and clinicians have focused on symptom remission or reduced severity as primary outcomes. There are a range of measures and options for definitions and tracking. A recent systematic review summarizes the self-report and interview-based options (Cerimele, Goldberg, Miller, Gabrielson, & Fortney, 2019).

Families want more than just reduction of problem behaviors, though. They want youth to achieve positive outcomes as well. Some therapeutic contexts can aim to influence the impact of symptoms on an individual's ability to function and lead a meaningful and fulfilling life. The recovery movement, which has been informed by people with lived experience of severe mental health difficulties, has emphasized the importance of functional and personal recovery, in which the focus has shifted to the extent to which an individual is able to contribute and to lead a meaningful life despite any ongoing symptoms. These issues have received less attention in the pediatric context, partly because the long-term trajectory of the disorder in a given young person is confounded with developmental change, and partly because personal autonomy may not be on the minds of younger children. Still, the use of functioning and quality-of-life measures has a place in the outcome assessment in pediatric bipolar disorder.

Symptom Reduction

There are many rating instruments that can measure symptoms during the course of treatment. Some are better suited for baseline and outcome evaluation, and shorter versions are more suitable for monitoring progress during the course of treatment. The life chart methodology (Denicoff et al., 1997) or session-by-session checkups on mood and energy are cases in point. These are unlikely to be primary outcome measures in research studies, but they provide helpful weekly feedback about progress and setbacks in the course of treatment.

Mood and Energy Checkups

Tracking daily mood and energy over the course of treatment quickly shows whether there are fluctuations suggestive of a mood disorder. Rather than the traditional assessment model used to bunch measurement at the beginning of treatment, a "dental model" of scheduling regular mood and energy checkups will clarify mood diagnosis and treatment response in ways that a single panel of assessment cannot. These checkups may be as basic as asking about changes in mood and energy at each appointment, or they could use brief checklists. Brevity is crucial to minimize burden and increase cooperation. Many instruments that are good choices for an initial assessment battery are poor options for the repetitions needed to get prospective information.

At the extreme, the "life charting method" boils questions down to a bare minimum of two or three items (one rating energy, another rating mood, and possibly distinguishing irritability from "up" or "down" moods) but then has the patient or parent rate the items several times a day for several weeks or months (Denicoff et al., 1997). The life charting method provides extremely detailed information about shifts in mood and energy, and it can be a powerful tool for identifying triggers that exacerbate mood disturbance. Several excellent examples of life charts are available at no charge on the Internet (a Google search for "bipolar life chart" provides multiple hits). Some families take readily to the life charting methodology. Others find it too burdensome.

Another option would be to do ecological momentary assessment (EMA) using a smartphone app to ask a handful of questions at different times in the day or week. EMA used to be the province of social-psychological research, but now mental health apps have the functionality built in. Some might blend the function of a calendar with activity scheduling, and tracking whether or not the activity occurred. There is not yet a clear front runner, but PsyberGuide and other review websites will help to select among the best current options.

Clinician-Rated Measures of Symptom Severity

For clinical trials, the primary outcome measures are clinician-rated assessments of the severity of manic and depressive symptoms. The industry standards have been the Young Mania Rating Scale (YMRS; Young, Biggs, Ziegler, & Meyer, 1978) and the Children's Depression Rating Scale—Revised (CDRS-R; Poznanski, Miller, Salguero, & Kelsh, 1984). The YMRS was originally designed for use with adults on an inpatient unit, with ratings completed by staff nurses based on direct observation of behavior over an 8-hour shift. With children and adolescents, YMRS ratings are typically based on clinician interviews with the child and the primary caregiver, and the reference period is usually extended to cover the past 2 weeks instead of 8 hours. Although the item anchors and weights were developed for use with inpatient adults, no adaptations have been made to the anchors to make them more developmentally appropriate for children or adolescents. The scoring, which doubles the weight given to irritability and aggression because they were rare to observe on the unit with adult patients (Young et al., 1978), is not psychometrically sound and lacks even conceptual justification with youth. The YMRS also includes some items covering behav-

iors that are not DSM symptoms of mania, and it omits other core symptoms (e.g., grandiosity or increased engagement in pleasurable but risky acts).

In spite of these shortcomings, the YMRS has demonstrated considerable evidence of validity in youth (Fristad, Weller, & Weller, 1992, 1995; Youngstrom, Danielson, Findling, Gracious, & Calabrese, 2002). Two of the 11 items on the YMRS are weak enough to lower the internal consistency of an already short scale (Demeter et al., 2013). One of these is the "bizarre appearance" item, and the other is the item rating "lack of insight." Both items are also problematic in parent-report versions of the YMRS (Gracious, Youngstrom, Findling, & Calabrese, 2002; Youngstrom, Gracious, Danielson, Findling, & Calabrese, 2003). Using a nine-item version would likely be shorter, less confusing, yet no less accurate. The calibration of YMRS scores across sites may also be different, such that similar clinical presentations earn widely divergent scores (Mackin, Targum, Kalali, Rom, & Young, 2006; Youngstrom et al., 2003).

The K-SADS Mania Rating Scale (KMRS) is an alternative that addresses several of the shortcomings of the YMRS (Axelson et al., 2003). It covers all of the DSM symptoms of mania, provides a more consistent set of anchors, and was designed for use with children and adolescents, so the examples and anchors are more developmentally appropriate. The KMRS shows strong interrater reliability and internal consistency, and excellent convergent validity (Yee et al., 2015). The KMRS is available for free online, with links in the Wikiversity EBA pages.

For rating depression, the CDRS-R was developed specifically for use with children and adolescents (Poznanski et al., 1984), and it includes 17 items rated on scales of either 1–5 or 1–7 points, with higher scores signaling greater severity. Ratings are based on interviews with both the caregiver and the youth, with three items rated entirely on the basis of direct observation during the course of the youth interview. Strengths of the CDRS-R include (1) being designed specifically for youth, with developmentally appropriate anchors and validation samples; (2) high internal consistency (alphas often exceed .90); and (3) sensitivity to treatment effects. Limitations of the CDRS-R include not covering all DSM symptoms of depression and failure to distinguish between psychomotor agitation and retardation, not assessing hypersomnia as well as insomnia (a big problem, inasmuch as hypersomnia might denote bipolar depression), and that scores also might depend substantially on the rater rather than the severity of depression.

There is a K-SADS Depression Rating Scale, analogous to the KMRS. It provides complete coverage of the DSM symptoms of depression, uses more consistent anchors than the CDRS-R, and also shows strong psychometrics (Demeter et al., 2013; Yee et al., 2015). It, too, is available for free use, linked to the Wikiversity pages for bipolar assessment.

The degree to which clinician ratings are susceptible to variations in clinical judgment poses a major challenge for not only for multisite trials but also independent clinicians attempting to use the measures in their own practice. Without using standardized videos or training vignettes, clinicians have no means of knowing whether their sense of mood severity corresponds with other clinicians' perceptions. A study using video recordings found large effect sizes for differences between the scores assigned by American, Indian, and British psychiatrists (in descending order of average ratings; Mackin et al., 2006). The fact that so much variance in scores depends on the rater and not the diagnosis or the severity of illness hides potential similarities across sites and studies. We should not put great faith in commonly used rules of thumb, such as YMRS scores of 13 or higher connoting hypomania, or scores of 16 and higher designating moderate mania. No clinician-rated instrument will resolve the problems associated with rater effects (e.g., different calibration across sites or raters) without requiring calibration against a standard set of training tapes.

Parent-Rated Measures of Severity and Outcome

Parent checklists are much easier to deploy across sites and clinics than clinician-rated instruments. Training costs are lower, and susceptibility to idiosyncratic clinical interpretations of behaviors is also lessened. As yet, there is no established front-runner for parent-reported symptom outcome measures.

The most promising include the 10-item mania and depression short forms from the P-GBI (Youngstrom, Van Meter, et al., 2020). The P-GBI has proven highly sensitive to treatment effects (Cooperberg, 2001), showing large effects on both the manic/mixed and the depression scales. However, the reading level (roughly 11th grade) and the burden imposed by the GBI (10 pages of questions in 12-point font) hinder its utility as an outcome measure in clinical settings. The 10-item short

forms retain excellent content coverage, a substantial reduction in burden (although the reading level remains high), and they are as sensitive to treatment effects as doing a 45-minute CDRS and YMRS interview, based on effect sizes in a large, double-blind randomized trial (Youngstrom et al., 2013). The short forms, as well as other versions of the GBI, are all on Wikiversity.

Other contenders all have limitations. The CMRS-10 (Henry et al., 2008) is promising in terms of brevity, strong psychometrics, and measuring severity, but to our knowledge it has not been used as an outcome measure in a published trial, so there are no data showing sensitivity to treatment effects yet. It still might be the better choice than the P-GBI when reading level is an issue. The CBCL often shows little improvement over the course of treatment, possibly because ratings cover a 6-month window. The CBCL may also be hampered by the lack of scales with content specific to mood disorders. The MDQ focuses on symptoms of mania, but it uses a simple present–absent format, so it does not get enough information about severity to be sensitive to treatment effects. Parent-rated YMRS scores are less sensitive to treatment effects than other measures in head-to-head comparisons, in part due to the lower reliability of the instrument and also because many of the items are not specific to bipolar disorder.

Youth Self-Report Measures

As documented earlier, youth self-report is not efficient from a diagnostic perspective for identifying BSD. Youth might seek treatment for the depressed phase of illness, but they are very unlikely to self-refer for treatment during manic, hypomanic, or mixed phases of illness. As a result, treatment referrals are often made by a concerned adult instead of the adolescent. It follows that the baseline levels of symptoms typically are lower when assessed via self-report than via collateral informants because referrals are usually driven by the adult collateral perspective. The youth's lack of initial insight and lower baseline self-rated severity limit the room for improvement during therapy, making self-report a less sensitive method for quantifying outcomes (Cooperberg, 2001; Youngstrom et al., 2013).

There still is value in gathering youth-reported measures. If the parent is not available, or if the youth initiated the referral, then the youth may be the most convenient or only rater perspective available. When both youth and parent ratings are feasible, then comparing them will show points of agreement and disagreement, and also suggest how motivated the youth is for treatment. "Finding the pain" and measuring things that the youth finds irritating or distressing will help with engagement (see the idiographic assessment sections).

For psychometric scales, the 7 Up 7 Down Inventory (Youngstrom, Murray, et al., 2013) and the 10-item P-GBI Mania and Depression scales (Youngstrom, Van Meter, et al., 2020), all carved from the full length GBI, offer a reasonable compromise in terms of reduced burden while still having good reliability and discrimination, and probably similar sensitivity to treatment effects. Self-report on the YMRS performed badly on several criteria and is not recommended for clinical use. No other scales have had their sensitivity to treatment effects evaluated yet.

Other Collateral Informants

Although there is a broad spectrum of possible informants about psychosocial functioning in youth, including siblings, peers, and teachers, among others, relatively little has been done to date in terms of collecting outcome data. Based on the low discriminating power of teacher report in a diagnostic context, it is unlikely that it would be a helpful outcome measure: If the scores do not go up significantly in the presence of a bipolar diagnosis, they are unlikely to show the loss of diagnosis with successful treatment.

Outcome Benchmarks

Ongoing assessment of BSD in the context of an 8- to 10-week period of care, typical of North American treatment centers, shows parallels with teaching. In order to evaluate student/patient progress, a series of brief weekly tests may provide a coarse overview of progress or a narrow focus on changes in a key symptom. In comparison, "midterms" and "final exams" can use longer measures that have demonstrated sensitivity to treatment effects and may be most useful when normative data are used to make nomothetic comparisons (Youngstrom et al., 2017). If the "midterm" looks bad, this should prompt reevaluation of treatment approaches and goals. A comprehensive "final exam" should have a broad focus on the different goals of the treatment period, including nomothetic benchmarks for symptom reduction, as well as personal goals and improved functioning. Nomothetic benchmarks provide a means for clinicians to interpret the clinical significance of progress on these "mid-

terms" and "final exams." In clinical settings in which treatment of BSD has no predefined endpoint, ongoing assessment may take the form of a "dental model" in which regular "checkups" help both to monitor progress toward agreed-upon goals and to identify any areas in need of more targeted intervention.

"Social validation" involves confirming with parents, teachers, peers, or other significant individuals in the youth's life that they see observable improvement in the symptoms or functioning (Kazdin, 1977). Social validation emphasizes ecologically valid indicators of functioning. For BSD, these indicators might include improved school attendance, better grades, fewer disciplinary incidents, increases in the number of friends, or similar social, educational, or vocational gains, or even improvements on scores of quality-of-life measures.

A complementary system for measuring clinically significant change developed by Jacobson and colleagues has gained popularity among research-oriented clinicians (Jacobson, Roberts, Berns, & McGlinchey, 1999; Jacobson & Truax, 1991). Jacobson's approach to clinical significance involves using a relevant psychometric measure, then showing (1) that the scores change by enough to be confident that an individual patient really is improving given the precision of the instrument and (2) that the scores have moved past a benchmark compared to clinical and nonclinical score distributions. The advantages of this approach to clinical significance include feasibility, its strong psychometric underpinnings, and its reliance on empirically defined benchmarks (Jacobson et al., 1999). It also clearly focuses on whether treatment is helping each individual patient, versus the way that effect sizes describe the average outcome for an aggregate of cases. The big drawback to Jacobson's approach is that it requires psychometric information that is typically not reported in technical manuals or articles. Specifically, determination of "reliable change" requires knowledge of the standard error of the difference score for the measure. With regard to the three benchmarks, setting the threshold for getting the patient away from the clinical distribution requires having norms for a clinical population, or at least a mean and standard deviation for a representative clinical sample. Similarly, it is only possible to determine if a patient has moved back into the nonclinical range of functioning (defined here as scoring within two standard deviations of the nonclinical mean) by having nonclinical norms available. The third threshold, crossing closer to the nonclinical than clinical mean, requires information about both the clinical and nonclinical distributions to calculate a weighted average.

To make it more practical for clinicians to apply Jacobson's approach, Cooperberg meta-analyzed studies with relevant data on measures frequently used with BSD, pooling estimates of the mean and standard deviation for each measure in samples of youths with and without BSD. Table 8.8 presents the standard error of the difference, allowing calculation of Jacobson's reliable change index,

and for convenience it also presents the number of points change needed to be 90 or 95% confident (two-tailed) that the patient is improving. For most clinicians, the critical scores will be more useful, as they do not require computation. Table 8.8 also presents the benchmark values for moving away from the clinical distribution ("A"), back into the nonclinical range ("B"), or moving closer to the nonclinical than the clinical average ("C"). The Wikiversity site has an online tool that compares a client's scores to these thresholds.

TABLE 8.8. Clinically Significant Change Benchmarks with Common Instruments and Mood Rating Scales

Measure	Cutoff scores			Critical change (unstandardized scores)			MID
	A	B	C	95%	90%	$SE_{difference}$	$d \sim 0.5$
Benchmarks based on published norms							
CBCL T-scores (2001 norms)							
Externalizing	49	70	58	7	6	3.4	5
Internalizing	n/a	70	56	9	7	4.5	5
Attention Problems	n/a	66	58	8	7	4.2	5
TRF T-scores (2001 norms)							
Externalizing	n/a	70	56	6	5	3.0	5
Internalizing	n/a	70	55	9	7	4.4	5
Attention Problems	n/a	66	57	5	4	2.3	5
YSR T-scores (2001 norms)							
Externalizing	n/a	70	54	9	8	4.6	5
Internalizing	n/a	70	54	9	8	4.8	5
Benchmarks based on outpatient samples							
P-GBI-10M[a]	1	9	6	6	5	3.2	3
CMRS 10[b]	—	6	4	5	4	2.3	2
P-GBI-10Da[a]	—	7	4	6	5	3.0	3
P-GBI-10Db[a]	—	7	4	6	5	2.9	3
A-GBI-10M[c]	—	14	7	6	5	3.1	3
A-GBI-10Da[c]	—	18	7	6	5	3.2	3
A-GBI-10Db[c]	—	16	7	6	5	2.9	4
7 Up[c]	—	8	4	4	4	2.2	3
7 Down[c]	—	12	5	5	4	2.3	3
KMRS[b]	19	19	19	3	3	1.6	3
KDRS[b]	12	19	18	5	4	2.4	3
CDRS-R Total[a]	—	24	22	6	5	2.9	5
YMRS Total[a]	4	3	3	3	3	1.8	3

Note. A, away from the clinical range; B, back into the nonclinical range; C, closer to the nonclinical than the clinical mean. The outpatient samples use all cases with BSD for the clinical reference group for mania measures, and any mood disorder as the reference for depression measures. MID, minimally important difference.
[a]Data from Youngstrom, Van Meter, et al. (2018).
[b]Data from Youngstrom et al. (2005).
[c]Data from Youngstrom, Halverson, et al. (2018).

Other areas of medicine have proposed using the minimally important difference (MID) as a simple way of deciding whether the person is improving (Streiner, Norman, & Cairney, 2015). The original concept was to ask patients in focus groups or surveys what would be the smallest change in a symptom rating scale that would represent a meaningful improvement in their lives. The goal was to bridge the gap between symptom reduction, which has relatively well-developed measurement strategies, and consumer perceptions of meaningful benefit. Because gathering feedback entails doing a separate study in its own right, researchers have also tested different statistical definitions and approximations (Thissen et al., 2016). Norman and colleagues suggest a rule of thumb of Cohen's d ~0.5 as a proxy definition of MID when no better research evidence is available (Streiner et al., 2015). They based this on a combination of reviewing more than 30 studies looking at MID in different medical issues and alluding to psychophysical thresholds for "just noticeable differences" in a range of stimuli (Streiner et al., 2015). For the Achenbach, Behavior Assessment System for Children (BASC), and similar measures using T-scores, the rule of thumb indicates that a 5-point improvement would be a simple and practical definition of MID. We have added $d = 0.5$ definitions to our outcome benchmark table so that the reader can use them for other scales and see how they compare to more psychometrically sophisticated definitions, which tend to be more conservative.

Functioning, Quality of Life, and Positive Outcomes

There is growing recognition that treatment should attend to improving quality of life (QOL) and positive aspects of functioning rather than focusing on symptom reduction (Butcher et al., 2019). Though "normal" functioning is difficult to define, it is often conceptualized as an individual's ability to perform daily activities required for maintaining him- or herself in the real world (encompassing daily living skills, and social and occupational skills). With children and adolescents, it is important to promote social and educational development, in addition to ameliorating problem behaviors. Improvements in symptoms do not directly map onto improvements in functioning; therefore, separate assessment of functioning is necessary to comprehensively capture treatment outcomes. Common measures of different areas of functioning in bipolar disorder include the Chil-

dren's Global Assessment Scale (CGAS; Shaffer et al., 1983), Global Assessment of Functioning (GAF; Hall, 1995), and Clinical Global Impressions (CGI; Guy, National Institute of Mental Health, Psychopharmacology Research, & Early Clinical Drug Evaluation, 1976). All of these are global ratings that use a single number to convey the level of the person's functioning, collapsing across life domains and time periods. High scores reflect better functioning. They are quick, single-item scales, with all the limitations these usually entail; they also are highly feasible and much better than nothing. They can be considered the bare minimum of functional tracking in the sense that we should not do less than one of these, and we may want to do more.

There are rating scales that address the related construct quality of life (QOL). Broadly, "quality of life," as referred to in health literature, is a multidimensional concept relating to the impact of a disease and treatment on domains of physical, psychological, and social functioning, and the resulting degree of satisfaction with these areas (Morton, Michalak, & Murray, 2017). Generic measures of health-related QOL have been used to characterize functioning in youth with bipolar disorders (Freeman et al., 2009; Horwitz et al., 2010). While there is some argument for the use of disorder-specific measures, these have not yet been developed for pediatric bipolar disorder (Michalak, Murray, & Collaborative Research Team to Study Psychosocial Issues in Bipolar Disorder, 2010).

The KINDL (not an acronym; Ravens-Sieberer & Bullinger, 2000, 2006) is probably the best option if we want to add a formal QOL scale to the assessment package for bipolar disorder. It was developed in Germany, with parent and youth report versions adapted for three different age groups. The KINDL has been used in a wide range of medical conditions and is available for free use in more than a dozen languages. The KIDSCREEN (Ravens-Sieberer et al., 2008) is a successor to the KINDL, but we are not aware of any research using the KIDSCREEN with bipolar disorder.

Whether a formal QOL measure is used or not, clinicians should assess peer relationships, family functioning, and academic performance. There are brief measures of peer relations that are free and show differences in youth with bipolar versus other conditions (Siegel et al., 2015). These might be interesting to use as the basis for discussion in treatment, although they have not been used as outcome measures per se. Grades are easy to track via report cards, if we remember to ask. Family functioning assessments can include the Family Assessment Device (Byles, Byrne, Boyle, & Offord, 1988), which measures communication and problem solving, as well as general functioning, or measures of perceived criticalness and expressed negative emotion (Hooley & Richters, 1991). Bipolar illness tends to have a detrimental effect on all of these areas of functioning, and interventions that address these deficits have a tremendous impact on both reducing the burden and improving the prognosis.

Idiographic Outcome Measures for Case-Formulation-Driven Work

When the goals of treatment are based around an individualized case formulation rather than a diagnosis, monitoring of improvement correspondingly moves from nomothetic to idiographic. In the case of pediatric bipolar disorder, for example, engagement and motivation toward therapy are potentially enhanced by encouraging the client to characterize positive change in terms that are personally meaningful: Improved relationships with peers, increased school attendance, and calmer family dinner times may be more valid and engaging goals than decreased hypo/mania. Cognitive-behavioral therapy (CBT), for example, is a case-formulation-based approach to psychotherapy for BSD that aims to impact bipolar disorder in its full biopsychosocial context (e.g., recognizing comorbidities, strengths, personality issues, interpersonal issues) while being cognizant of the specific mechanisms of relevance to the binary diagnosis of bipolar disorder.

The Youth Top Problems is a general method for selecting idiographic (personalized) goals and tracking them frequently (typically by session, or weekly) (Weisz et al., 2011). The heart of the method is that patients pick a few (usually three) items that they care about, then rates them on a 0- to 10-point scale. The power of the method is its simplicity, personalization, and brevity—which allows for more frequent repetition than longer psychometric scales. Repeating this over a period of weeks yields data about trends over time. A researcher could model changes in slope (Speer & Greenbaum, 1995); clinicians and patients care about the simple visual trends.

The various life charting and mood charting methods also are ways of tracking changes in mood and energy on a daily basis. These are much more fine-grained than the other scales and, again, the brevity makes more intense repetition

tolerable. The original versions were paper-and-pencil diaries that are still available for free online. Now there are websites and apps that automate the charting and are much more visually appealing, as well as more engaging for teens. Going to the app store and searching for "mood charting" will find options complete with consumer reviews.

In a similar way, apps are adapting the ecological momentary assessment strategy and turning it into a tool for monitoring clinical progress (Trull & Ebner-Priemer, 2013). This type of method only becomes feasible with a smartphone, and research studies have found that there are considerable barriers to implementation when participants all use different phones and operating systems. The more practical approaches at present are likely to be using tools that are Web-based and that can push the questions as e-mail or small messaging service (SMS) surveys rather than relying on an app installed on the phone. The alternative may be to browse the app store in session with the client and select a tool that will work on his or her phone and give the clinician helpful information.

Passive Tracking

A more recent development has been to use smartphones and wearables to gather information about the person's sleep, activity, and behavior passively (Faurholt-Jepsen et al., 2015; Matthews et al., 2016). The passive aspect means that the method takes no additional effort from the person; it runs in the background or takes advantage of behavioral traces left by the daily use of the device. Looking at time of first and last text or messaging can be a good indirect measure of sleep and wake times for some teens. The phone or Fitbit provides a consumer-grade (vs. research-grade) measure of actigraphy. Preliminary data show that geotracking can discern between people with and without depression based on the range and diversity of places they go (Pratap et al., 2019; Saeb, Lattie, Schueller, Kording, & Mohr, 2016). Websites and apps are starting to passively monitor search terms and activity, with algorithms to provide support resources if it looks like the person is searching for ways to hurt him- or herself. These sound like science fiction, but they are already available. In the words of William Gibson, "The future is already here—it's just not very evenly distributed" (*https://en.wikiquote.org/wiki/william_gibson*). To this we would add that it also is not always validated under clinically realistic conditions, and we may not have sorted through all of the ethical issues yet. Passive monitoring is still at the stage of comparing sick versus well, not differentiating between types of clinical problems. It also raises issues of informed consent and privacy. On the other hand, it also addresses many problems in terms of reducing missing data due to forgetting or lack of motivation, and it provides an objective perspective. The best way to proceed is probably on a case-by-case basis, discussing the pros and cons, and making sure that the client and family understand what would be tracked, how it would be measured, and how it could improve care and outcomes.

Adherence

Nonadherence to treatment is a major issue when working with BSD in children and adolescents, as well as adults. Patients frequently refuse to take medications, or take them inconsistently, due to attitudes about illness and treatment, concern about the side effects of the medications, or a lack of understanding about the recurrent nature of the illness. Consistent attendance at therapy appointments is also difficult, with the chaotic family environment often creating obstacles to compliance. It is crucial that practitioners monitor adherence to treatment recommendations, which includes checking in on homework and skills exercises, as well as tracking kept appointments. Psychoeducation about the nature of BSD, the potential benefits of medication and other treatment components, as well as potential side effects to monitor, have been demonstrated to substantially improve adherence and therefore improve overall outcomes (Fristad, Gavazzi, & Mackinaw-Koons, 2003; Fristad, Goldberg-Arnold, & Gavazzi, 2003).

Monitoring for Relapse

Once the case conceptualization includes a mood disorder, then repeated assessments become a valuable means of monitoring progress and identifying "triggers" that can worsen mood and functioning. Although there are many generic triggers, such as stress or sleep disruption, others are subtle or unique to the individual. These assessments are also valuable in learning the signs that indicate potential "roughening" or relapse (Sachs, 2004). A promising line of research is to look at developing risk calculators that estimate an individual person's risk of relapse, as well as predicting whether the person is more likely to have a hypomanic/manic or depressive episode (e.g., Hafeman et al., 2017). As these get refined and externally validat-

ed, they will be increasingly useful clinical tools for the long-term management of mood disorders.

When treating the youth, clinicians also need to be alert to the frequent lack of insight into behavior, and the frequent differences in perspective between the parent and youth in bipolar illness. Many youth are not self-referred for treatment, and if their behaviors are driven by manic or mixed states, they may perceive the problem as being other people's, not theirs. What appears to be irritable mood to observers may seem more like parents and teachers are "hassling," "nagging," or otherwise provoking the youth. Sometimes it may be possible to increase insight, but this is more often accomplished after the mood states are stabilized.

Conclusion

BSD in adolescence and childhood has been a controversial topic. Practitioners should be cautiously open to the possibility diagnosing it and look for convincing data. The degree of skepticism should go down rapidly with increasing age of the youth. Families are not well served by misdiagnosis in either direction.

Assessment of BSD presents numerous challenges, such as a fluctuating presentation, complicated diagnostic criteria, and high rates of comorbidity. The hurdles to accurate recognition grow only higher with younger cases. At the same time, there is now extensive research in terms of demonstrating the validity of the diagnosis, understanding the associated burden, and learning about the prognosis over at least 8 years of follow-up (B. Goldstein et al., 2017; Youngstrom & Algorta, 2014). The field has also made gains in the number and quality of assessment tools available for diagnosing and measuring progress and outcomes with children and adolescents.

The assessment model advocated in this chapter is heavily influenced by the recommendations of evidence-based medicine (Guyatt & Rennie, 2002; Sackett, Straus, Richardson, Rosenberg, & Haynes, 2000), and represents a different perspective than traditional approaches to psychological assessment. The information about the relative performance of tests and the clinical features associated with BSD are valuable regardless of whether practitioners adopt the other innovations, such as using the nomogram for estimating risk. There also are clear take-home messages, including some that counter conventional wisdom about assessment, such as the importance of involving a parent or other familiar adult in the assessment of manic symptoms, versus the relatively lower validity of self-report or teacher report.

Using the evidence-based methods described here makes the best use of the assessment tools available to make more accurate formulations, build better treatment plans, and improve treatment processes and outcomes. EBA also helps strike the balance between being open to the possibility of BSD while also avoiding overdiagnosis of an uncommon yet sometimes popularized condition. By using a sequenced approach to assessment, it is possible to work smarter and not harder, getting better results without increasing the cost to the clinician or the family.

ACKNOWLEDGMENTS

This work was supported in part by Grant No. NIH 5R01 MH066647 (Eric Youngstrom, Principal Investigator). We thank Guillermo Perez Algorta, PhD, for comments, and Joshua Langfus, BS, for programming visualizations and other technical assistance.

REFERENCES

Abikoff, H., Courtney, M., Pelham, W. E., & Koplewicz, H. S. (1993). Teachers' ratings of disruptive behaviors: The influence of halo effects. *Journal of Abnormal Child Psychology, 21*, 519–533.

Achenbach, T. M. (1997). *Manual for the Young Adult Self-Report and Young Adult Behavior Checklist.* Burlington: University of Vermont, Department of Psychiatry.

Achenbach, T. M., McConaughy, S. H., & Howell, C. T. (1987). Child/adolescent behavioral and emotional problems: Implication of cross-informant correlations for situational specificity. *Psychological Bulletin, 101*, 213–232.

Achenbach, T. M., & Rescorla, L. A. (2001). *Manual for the ASEBA School-Age Forms and Profiles.* Burlington: University of Vermont.

Algorta, G. P., Youngstrom, E. A., Frazier, T. W., Freeman, A. J., Youngstrom, J. K., & Findling, R. L. (2011). Suicidality in pediatric bipolar disorder: Predictor or outcome of family processes and mixed mood presentation? *Bipolar Disorders, 13*, 76–86.

Algorta, G. P., Youngstrom, E. A., Phelps, J., Jenkins, M. M., Youngstrom, J. K., & Findling, R. L. (2013). An inexpensive family index of risk for mood issues improves identification of pediatric bipolar disorder. *Psychological Assessment, 25*, 12–22.

Alloy, L. B., & Nusslock, R. (2019). Future directions for understanding adolescent bipolar spectrum disorders: A reward hypersensitivity perspective. *Journal of Clinical Child and Adolescent Psychology, 48*, 669–683.

Althoff, R. R., Ayer, L. A., Rettew, D. C., & Hudziak, J. J. (2010). Assessment of dysregulated children using the Child Behavior Checklist: A receiver operating characteristic curve analysis. *Psychological Assessment, 22*, 609–617.

American Psychiatric Association. (2013). *Diagnostic and statistical manual of mental disorders* (5th ed.). Arlington, VA: Author.

Angst, J., Adolfsson, R., Benazzi, F., Gamma, A., Hantouche, E., Meyer, T. D., . . . Scott, J. (2005). The HCL-32: Towards a self-assessment tool for hypomanic symptoms in outpatients. *Journal of Affective Disorders, 88*, 217–233.

Angst, J., Azorin, J. M., Bowden, C. L., Perugi, G., Vieta, E., Gamma, A., & Young, A. H. (2011). Prevalence and characteristics of undiagnosed bipolar disorders in patients with a major depressive episode: The BRIDGE study. *Archives of General Psychiatry, 68*, 791–798.

Angst, J., Gamma, A., Benazzi, F., Ajdacic, V., Eich, D., & Rossler, W. (2003). Toward a re-definition of subthreshold bipolarity: Epidemiology and proposed criteria for bipolar-II, minor bipolar disorders and hypomania. *Journal of Affective Disorders, 73*, 133–146.

Angst, J., Gamma, A., Bowden, C. L., Azorin, J. M., Perugi, G., Vieta, E., & Young, A. H. (2012). Diagnostic criteria for bipolarity based on an international sample of 5,635 patients with DSM-IV major depressive episodes. *European Archives of Psychiatry and Clinical Neuroscience, 262*, 3–11.

Angst, J., Meyer, T. D., Adolfsson, R., Skeppar, P., Carta, M., Benazzi, F., . . . Gamma, A. (2010). Hypomania: A transcultural perspective. *World Psychiatry, 9*, 41–49.

Arnold, L. M., Strakowski, S. M., Schwiers, M. L., Amicone, J., Fleck, D. E., Corey, K. B., & Farrow, J. E. (2004). Sex, ethnicity, and antipsychotic medication use in patients with psychosis. *Schizophrenia Research, 66*, 169–175.

Axelson, D. A., Birmaher, B. J., Brent, D., Wassick, S., Hoover, C., Bridge, J., & Ryan, N. (2003). A preliminary study of the Kiddie Schedule for Affective Disorders and Schizophrenia for School-Age Children mania rating scale for children and adolescents. *Journal of Child and Adolescent Psychopharmacology, 13*, 463–470.

Axelson, D. A., Birmaher, B., Strober, M., Gill, M. K., Valeri, S., Chiappetta, L., . . . Keller, M. (2006). Phenomenology of children and adolescents with bipolar spectrum disorders. *Archives of General Psychiatry, 63*, 1139–1148.

Axelson, D. A., Birmaher, B., Strober, M. A., Goldstein, B. I., Ha, W., Gill, M. K., . . . Hunt, J. I. (2011). Course of subthreshold bipolar disorder in youth: Diagnostic progression from bipolar disorder not otherwise specified. *Journal of the American Academy of Child and Adolescent Psychiatry, 50*, 1001–1016.

Axelson, D., Findling, R. L., Fristad, M. A., Kowatch, R. A., Youngstrom, E. A., McCue Horwitz, S., . . . Birmaher, B. (2012). Examining the proposed disruptive mood dysregulation disorder diagnosis in children in the Longitudinal Assessment of Manic Symptoms study. *Journal of Clinical Psychiatry, 73,* 1342–1350.

Bauer, M. S., Crits-Christoph, P., Ball, W. A., Dewees, E., McAllister, T., Alahi, P., . . . Whybrow, P. C. (1991). Independent assessment of manic and depressive symptoms by self-rating: Scale characteristics and implications for the study of mania. *Archives of General Psychiatry, 48,* 807–812.

Benazzi, F., & Rihmer, Z. (2000). Sensitivity and specificity of DSM-IV atypical features for bipolar II disorder diagnosis. *Psychiatry Research, 93,* 257–262.

Berk, M., & Dodd, S. (2005). Bipolar II disorder: A review. *Bipolar Disorders, 7,* 11–21.

Biederman, J., Faraone, S., Mick, E., Wozniak, J., Chen, L., Ouellette, C., . . . Lelon, E. (1996). Attention-deficit hyperactivity disorder and juvenile mania: An overlooked comorbidity? *Journal of the American Academy of Child and Adolescent Psychiatry, 35,* 997–1008.

Biederman, J., Kwon, A., Wozniak, J., Mick, E., Markowitz, S., Fazio, V., & Faraone, S. V. (2004). Absence of gender differences in pediatric bipolar disorder: Findings from a large sample of referred youth. *Journal of Affective Disorders, 83,* 207–214.

Birmaher, B., Arbelaez, C., & Brent, D. (2002). Course and outcome of child and adolescent major depressive disorder. *Child and Adolescent Psychiatric Clinics of North America, 11,* 619–638.

Birmaher, B., & Axelson, D. (2006). Course and outcome of bipolar spectrum disorder in children and adolescents: A review of the existing literature. *Development and Psychopathology, 18,* 1023–1035.

Birmaher, B., Axelson, D., Goldstein, B., Strober, M., Gill, M. K., Hunt, J., . . . Keller, M. (2009). Four-year longitudinal course of children and adolescents with bipolar spectrum disorders: The Course and Outcome of Bipolar Youth (COBY) study. *American Journal of Psychiatry, 166,* 795–804.

Birmaher, B., Axelson, D., Strober, M., Gill, M. K., Valeri, S., Chiappetta, L., . . . Keller, M. (2006). Clinical course of children and adolescents with bipolar spectrum disorders. *Archives of General Psychiatry, 63,* 175–183.

Birmaher, B., Axelson, D., Strober, M., Gill, M. K., Yang, M., Ryan, N., . . . Leonard, H. (2009). Comparison of manic and depressive symptoms between children and adolescents with bipolar spectrum disorders. *Bipolar Disorders, 11,* 52–62.

Birmaher, B., Gill, M. K., Axelson, D. A., Goldstein, B. I., Goldstein, T. R., Yu, H., . . . Keller, M. B. (2014). Longitudinal trajectories and associated baseline predictors in youths with bipolar spectrum disorders. *American Journal of Psychiatry, 171,* 990–999.

Birmaher, B., Ryan, N. D., Williamson, D. E., Brent, D. A., Kaufman, J., Dahl, R. E., . . . Nelson, B. (1996). Childhood and adolescent depression: A review of the past 10 years: Part I. *Journal of the American Academy of Child and Adolescent Psychiatry, 35,* 1427–1439.

Blader, J. C., & Carlson, G. A. (2007). Increased rates of bipolar disorder diagnoses among U.S. child, adolescent, and adult inpatients, 1996–2004. *Biological Psychiatry, 62,* 107–114.

Bora, E., & Ozerdem, A. (2017). A meta-analysis of neurocognition in youth with familial high risk for bipolar disorder. *European Psychiatry, 44,* 17–23.

Bossuyt, P. M., Reitsma, J. B., Bruns, D. E., Gatsonis, C. A., Glasziou, P. P., Irwig, L. M., . . . de Vet, H. C. W. (2003). Towards complete and accurate reporting of studies of diagnostic accuracy: The STARD initiative. *British Medical Journal, 326,* 41–44.

Boylan, K., & Kim, S. (2016). Effectiveness of antidepressant medications for symptoms of irritability and disruptive behaviors in children and adolescents. *Journal of Child and Adolescent Psychopharmacology, 28,* 1–11.

Bschor, T., Angst, J., Azorin, J. M., Bowden, C. L., Perugi, G., Vieta, E., . . . Kruger, S. (2012). Are bipolar disorders underdiagnosed in patients with depressive episodes?: Results of the multicenter BRIDGE screening study in Germany. *Journal of Affective Disorders, 142,* 45–52.

Butcher, N. J., Monsour, A., Mew, E. J., Szatmari, P., Pierro, A., Kelly, L. E., . . . Offringa, M. (2019). Improving outcome reporting in clinical trial reports and protocols: Study protocol for the Instrument for reporting Planned Endpoints in Clinical Trials (InsPECT). *Trials, 20,* Article No. 161.

Buysse, D. J., Reynolds, C. F., III, Monk, T. H., Berman, S. R., & Kupfer, D. J. (1989). The Pittsburgh Sleep Quality Index: A new instrument for psychiatric practice and research. *Psychiatry Research, 28,* 193–213.

Byles, J., Byrne, C., Boyle, M. H., & Offord, D. R. (1988). Ontario Child Health Study: Reliability and validity of the General Functioning subscale of the McMaster Family Assessment Device. *Family Process, 27,* 97–104.

Calabrese, J. R., Shelton, M. D., Bowden, C. L., Rapport, D. J., Suppes, T., Shirley, E. R., . . . Caban, S. J. (2001). Bipolar rapid cycling: Focus on depression as its hallmark. *Journal of Clinical Psychiatry, 62*(Suppl. 14), 34–41.

Carlson, G. A. (2002). Bipolar disorder in children and adolescents: A critical review. In D. Shaffer & B. Waslick (Eds.), *The many faces of depression in children and adolescents* (Vol. 21, pp. 105–128). Washington, DC: American Psychiatric Association.

Carlson, G. A. (2003). The bottom line. *Journal of Child and Adolescent Psychopharmacology, 13,* 115–118.

Carlson, G. A., Danzig, A. P., Dougherty, L. R., Bufferd, S. J., & Klein, D. N. (2016). Loss of temper and irritability: The relationship to tantrums in a community and clinical sample. *Journal of Child and Adolescent Psychopharmacology, 26,* 114–122.

Carlson, G. A., & Mick, E. (2003). Drug induced disinhibition in psychiatrically hospitalized children. *Journal of Child and Adolescent Psychopharmacology, 13*, 153–163.

Carlson, G. A., & Youngstrom, E. A. (2003). Clinical implications of pervasive manic symptoms in children. *Biological Psychiatry, 53*, 1050–1058.

Carlson, G. A., & Youngstrom, E. A. (2011). Two opinions about one child—What's the clinician to do? *Journal of Child and Adolescent Psychopharmacology, 21*, 385–387.

Carpenter-Song, E. (2009). Caught in the psychiatric net: Meanings and experiences of ADHD, pediatric bipolar disorder and mental health treatment among a diverse group of families in the United States. *Culture, Medicine, and Psychiatry, 33*, 61–85.

Carver, C. S., & White, T. L. (1994). Behavioral inhibition, behavioral activation, and affective responses to impending reward and punishment: The BIS/BAS Scales. *Journal of Personality and Social Psychology, 67*, 319–333.

Cerimele, J. M., Goldberg, S. B., Miller, C. J., Gabrielson, S. W., & Fortney, J. C. (2019). Systematic review of symptom assessment measures for use in measurement-based care of bipolar disorders. *Psychiatric Services, 70*, 396–408.

Chorpita, B. F. (2002). The tripartite model and dimensions of anxiety and depression: An examination of structure in a large school sample. *Journal of Abnormal Child Psychology, 30*, 177–190.

Chorpita, B. F., Albano, A. M., & Barlow, D. H. (1998). The structure of negative emotions in a clinical sample of children and adolescents. *Journal of Abnormal Psychology, 107*, 74–85.

Chorpita, B. F., & Daleiden, E. L. (2002). Tripartite dimensions of emotion in a child clinical sample: Measurement strategies and implications for clinical utility. *Journal of Consulting and Clinical Psychology, 70*, 1150–1160.

Cicero, D. C., Epler, A. J., & Sher, K. J. (2009). Are there developmentally limited forms of bipolar disorder? *Journal of Abnormal Psychology, 118*, 431–447.

Cooperberg, M. (2001). *Clinically significant change for outcome measures used with pediatric bipolar disorders.* Doctoral dissertation, Case Western Reserve University, Cleveland, OH.

Copeland, W. E., Shanahan, L., Egger, H., Angold, A., & Costello, E. J. (2014). Adult diagnostic and functional outcomes of DSM-5 disruptive mood dysregulation disorder. *American Journal of Psychiatry, 171*, 668–674.

Correll, C. U. (2008). Assessing and maximizing the safety and tolerability of antipsychotics used in the treatment of children and adolescents. *Journal of Clinical Psychiatry, 69*(Suppl. 4), 26–36.

Coryell, W., Solomon, D., Turvey, C., Keller, M., Leon, A. C., Endicott, J., . . . Mueller, T. (2003). The long-term course of rapid-cycling bipolar disorder. *Archives of General Psychiatry, 60*, 914–920.

Costello, E. J., Angold, A., Burns, B. J., Stangl, D. K., Tweed, D. L., Erkanli, A., & Worthman, C. M. (1996). The Great Smoky Mountains Study of youth: Goals, design, methods, and the prevalence of DSM-III-R disorders. *Archives of General Psychiatry, 53*, 1129–1136.

Couzin, J. (2008). Science and commerce. Gene tests for psychiatric risk polarize researchers. *Science, 319*, 274–277.

Croskerry, P. (2003). The importance of cognitive errors in diagnosis and strategies to minimize them. *Academic Medicine, 78*, 775–780.

Cuthbert, B. N., & Insel, T. R. (2013). Toward the future of psychiatric diagnosis: The seven pillars of RDoC. *BMC Medicine, 11*, 126.

Cyranowski, J. M., Frank, E., Young, E., & Shear, K. (2000). Adolescent onset of the gender difference in lifetime rates of major depression. *Archives of General Psychiatry, 57*, 21–27.

Danielson, C. K., Feeny, N. C., Findling, R. L., & Youngstrom, E. A. (2004). Psychosocial treatment of bipolar disorders in adolescents: A proposed cognitive-behavioral intervention. *Cognitive and Behavioral Practice, 11*, 283–297.

Davidow, J., & Levinson, E. M. (1993). Heuristic principles and cognitive bias in decision making: Implications for assessment in school psychology. *Psychology in the Schools, 30*, 351–361.

De Los Reyes, A., Augenstein, T. M., Wang, M., Thomas, S. A., Drabick, D. A., Burgers, D. E., & Rabinowitz, J. (2015). The validity of the multi-informant approach to assessing child and adolescent mental health. *Psychological Bulletin, 141*, 858–900.

DelBello, M. P., Lopez-Larson, M. P., Soutullo, C. A., & Strakowski, S. M. (2001). Effects of race on psychiatric diagnosis of hospitalized adolescents: A retrospective chart review. *Journal of Child and Adolescent Psychopharmacology, 11*, 95–103.

DelBello, M. P., Soutullo, C. A., Hendricks, W., Niemeier, R. T., McElroy, S. L., & Strakowski, S. M. (2001). Prior stimulant treatment in adolescents with bipolar disorder: Association with age at onset. *Bipolar Disorders, 3*, 53–57.

DelBello, M. P., Soutullo, C. A., & Strakowski, S. M. (2000). Racial differences in treatment of adolescents with bipolar disorder. *American Journal of Psychiatry, 157*, 837–838.

Dell'Osso, L., Pini, S., Cassano, G. B., Mastrocinque, C., Seckinger, R. A., Saettoni, M., . . . Amador, X. F. (2002). Insight into illness in patients with mania, mixed mania, bipolar depression and major depression with psychotic features. *Bipolar Disorders, 4*, 315–322.

Demeter, C. A., Youngstrom, E. A., Carlson, G. A., Frazier, T. W., Rowles, B. M., Lingler, J., . . . Findling, R. L. (2013). Age differences in the phenomenology of pediatric bipolar disorder. *Journal of Affective Disorders, 147*, 295–303.

Denicoff, K. D., Smith-Jackson, E. E., Disney, E. R., Suddath, R. L., Leverich, G. S., & Post, R. M. (1997). Preliminary evidence of the reliability and validity of the prospective life-chart methodology (LCM-p). *Journal of Psychiatric Research, 31,* 593–603.

Depue, R. A., & Collins, P. F. (1999). Neurobiology of the structure of personality: Dopamine, facilitation of incentive motivation, and extraversion. *Behavioral and Brain Sciences, 22,* 491–569.

Depue, R. A., & Iacono, W. G. (1989). Neurobehavioral aspects of affective disorders. *Annual Review of Psychology, 40,* 457–492.

Depue, R. A., Krauss, S., Spoont, M. R., & Arbisi, P. (1989). General Behavior Inventory identification of unipolar and bipolar affective conditions in a nonclinical university population. *Journal of Abnormal Psychology, 98,* 117–126.

Depue, R. A., Slater, J. F., Wolfstetter-Kausch, H., Klein, D. N., Goplerud, E., & Farr, D. A. (1981). A behavioral paradigm for identifying persons at risk for bipolar depressive disorder: A conceptual framework and five validation studies. *Journal of Abnormal Psychology, 90,* 381–437.

Dougherty, L. R., Smith, V. C., Bufferd, S. J., Kessel, E. M., Carlson, G. A., & Klein, D. N. (2016). Disruptive mood dysregulation disorder at the age of 6 years and clinical and functional outcomes 3 years later. *Psychological Medicine, 46,* 1103–1114.

Drancourt, N., Etain, B., Lajnef, M., Henry, C., Raust, A., Cochet, B., . . . Bellivier, F. (2013). Duration of untreated bipolar disorder: Missed opportunities on the long road to optimal treatment. *Acta Psychiatrica Scandinavica, 127,* 136–144.

Du Rocher Schudlich, T. D., Youngstrom, E. A., Calabrese, J. R., & Findling, R. L. (2008). The role of family functioning in bipolar disorder in families. *Journal of Abnormal Child Psychology, 36,* 849–863.

Du Rocher Schudlich, T., Youngstrom, E. A., Martinez, M., Kogos Youngstrom, J., Scovil, K., Ross, J., . . . Findling, R. L. (2015). Physical and sexual abuse and early-onset bipolar disorder in youths receiving outpatient services: Frequent, but not specific. *Journal of Abnormal Child Psychology, 43,* 453–463.

Duax, J. M., Youngstrom, E. A., Calabrese, J. R., & Findling, R. L. (2007). Sex differences in pediatric bipolar disorder. *Journal of Clinical Psychiatry, 68,* 1565–1573.

Duffy, A., Alda, M., Hajek, T., & Grof, P. (2009). Early course of bipolar disorder in high-risk offspring: Prospective study. *British Journal of Psychiatry, 195,* 457–458.

Duffy, A., Alda, M., Kutcher, S., Cavazzoni, P., Robertson, C., Grof, E., & Grof, P. (2002). A prospective study of the offspring of bipolar parents responsive and nonresponsive to lithium treatment. *Journal of Clinical Psychiatry, 63,* 1171–1178.

Duffy, A., Alda, M., Kutcher, S., Fusee, C., & Grof, P. (1998). Psychiatric symptoms and syndromes among adolescent children of parents with lithium-responsive or lithium-nonresponsive bipolar disorder. *American Journal of Psychiatry, 155,* 431–433.

Egeland, J. A., Hostetter, A. M., Pauls, D. L., & Sussex, J. N. (2000). Prodromal symptoms before onset of manic-depressive disorder suggested by first hospital admission histories. *Journal of the American Academy of Child and Adolescent Psychiatry, 39,* 1245–1252.

Elias, L. R., Miskowiak, K. W., Vale, A. M., Kohler, C. A., Kjaerstad, H. L., Stubbs, B., . . . Carvalho, A. F. (2017). Cognitive impairment in euthymic pediatric bipolar disorder: A systematic review and meta-analysis. *Journal of American Academy of Child and Adolescent Psychiatry, 56,* 286–296.

Esposito-Smythers, C., Goldstein, T., Birmaher, B., Goldstein, B., Hunt, J., Ryan, N., . . . Keller, M. (2010). Clinical and psychosocial correlates of nonsuicidal self-injury within a sample of children and adolescents with bipolar disorder. *Journal of Affective Disorders, 125,* 89–97.

Evans, S. C., Burke, J. D., Roberts, M. C., Fite, P. J., Lochman, J. E., de la Pena, F. R., & Reed, G. M. (2017). Irritability in child and adolescent psychopathology: An integrative review for ICD-11. *Clinical Psychology Review, 53,* 29–45.

Faedda, G. L., Baldessarini, R. J., Glovinsky, I. P., & Austin, N. B. (2004). Pediatric bipolar disorder: Phenomenology and course of illness. *Bipolar Disorders, 6,* 305–313.

Faurholt-Jepsen, M., Vinberg, M., Frost, M., Christensen, E. M., Bardram, J. E., & Kessing, L. V. (2015). Smartphone data as an electronic biomarker of illness activity in bipolar disorder. *Bipolar Disorders, 17,* 715–728.

Findling, R. L., Gracious, B. L., McNamara, N. K., Youngstrom, E. A., Demeter, C., & Calabrese, J. R. (2001). Rapid, continuous cycling and psychiatric co-morbidity in pediatric bipolar I disorder. *Bipolar Disorders, 3,* 202–210.

Findling, R. L., McNamara, N. K., Youngstrom, E. A., Stansbrey, R., Gracious, B. L., Reed, M. D., & Calabrese, J. R. (2005). Double-blind 18-month trial of lithium versus divalproex maintenance treatment in pediatric bipolar disorder. *Journal of the American Academy of Child and Adolescent Psychiatry, 44,* 409–417.

Findling, R. L., Youngstrom, E. A., McNamara, N. K., Stansbrey, R. J., Demeter, C. A., Bedoya, D., . . . Calabrese, J. R. (2005). Early symptoms of mania and the role of parental risk. *Bipolar Disorders, 7,* 623–634.

Fletcher, K., Tan, E. J., Scott, J., & Murray, G. (2018). Bipolar II disorder: The need for clearer definition and improved management. *Australian and New Zealand Journal of Psychiatry, 52,* 598–599.

Fowles, D. C. (1994). A motivational theory of psychopathology. In W. D. Spaulding (Ed.), *Integrative views of motivation, cognition, and emotion* (Vol. 41, pp. 181–238). Lincoln: University of Nebraska Press.

Frank, E., Prien, R. F., Jarrett, R. B., Keller, M. B., Kupfer, D. J., Lavori, P. W., . . . Weissman, M. M. (1991). Conceptualization and rationale for consensus definitions of terms in major depressive disorder: Remission, recovery, relapse, and recurrence. *Archives of General Psychiatry, 48,* 851–855.

Freeman, A. J., Youngstrom, E. A., Freeman, M. J., Youngstrom, J. K., & Findling, R. L. (2011). Is caregiver–adolescent disagreement due to differences in thresholds for reporting manic symptoms? *Journal of Child and Adolescent Psychopharmacology, 21,* 425–432.

Freeman, A. J., Youngstrom, E. A., Michalak, E., Siegel, R., Meyers, O. I., & Findling, R. L. (2009). Quality of life in pediatric bipolar disorder. *Pediatrics, 123,* e446–e452.

Freeman, A. J., Youngstrom, E. A., Youngstrom, J. K., & Findling, R. L. (2016). Disruptive mood dysregulation disorder in a community mental health clinic: Prevalence, comorbidity and correlates. *Journal of Child and Adolescent Psychopharmacology, 26,* 123–130.

Fristad, M. A., Frazier, T. W., Youngstrom, E. A., Mount, K., Fields, B. W., Demeter, C., . . . Findling, R. L. (2012). What differentiates children visiting outpatient mental health services with bipolar spectrum disorder from children with other psychiatric diagnoses? *Bipolar Disorders, 14,* 497–506.

Fristad, M. A., Gavazzi, S. M., & Mackinaw-Koons, B. (2003). Family psychoeducation: An adjunctive intervention for children with bipolar disorder. *Biological Psychiatry, 53,* 1000–1008.

Fristad, M. A., Goldberg-Arnold, J. S., & Gavazzi, S. M. (2003). Multi-family psychoeducation groups in the treatment of children with mood disorders. *Journal of Marital and Family Therapy, 29,* 491–504.

Fristad, M. A., & MacPherson, H. A. (2014). Evidence-based psychosocial treatments for child and adolescent bipolar spectrum disorders. *Journal of Clinical Child and Adolescent Psychology, 43,* 339–355.

Fristad, M. A., Weller, E. B., & Weller, R. A. (1992). The Mania Rating Scale: Can it be used in children?: A preliminary report. *Journal of the American Academy of Child and Adolescent Psychiatry, 31,* 252–257.

Fristad, M. A., Weller, R. A., & Weller, E. B. (1995). The Mania Rating Scale (MRS): Further reliability and validity studies with children. *Annals of Clinical Psychiatry, 7,* 127–132.

Gadow, K. D., & Sprafkin, J. (1994). *Child Symptom Inventories manual.* Stony Brook, NY: Checkmate Plus.

Gadow, K. D., & Sprafkin, J. (1997). *Adolescent Symptom Inventory: Screening manual.* Stony Brook, NY: Checkmate Plus.

Gadow, K. D., & Sprafkin, J. (1999). *Youth's Inventory–4 Manual.* Stony Brook, NY: Checkmate Plus.

Galanter, C., Carlson, G., Jensen, P., Greenhill, L., Davies, M., Li, W., . . . Swanson, J. (2003). Response to methylphenidate in children with attention deficit hyperactivity disorder and manic symptoms in the Multimodal Treatment Study of children with Attention Deficit Hyperactivity Disorder Titration Trial. *Journal of Child and Adolescent Psychopharmacology, 13,* 123–136.

Galanter, C. A., Hundt, S. R., Goyal, P., Le, J., & Fisher, P. W. (2012). Variability among research diagnostic interview instruments in the application of DSM-IV-TR criteria for pediatric bipolar disorder. *Journal of the American Academy of Child and Adolescent Psychiatry, 51,* 605–621.

Garb, H. N. (1998). *Studying the clinician: Judgment research and psychological assessment.* Washington, DC: American Psychological Association.

Gawande, A. (2010). *The checklist manifesto.* New York: Penguin.

Geller, B., Bolhofner, K., Craney, J. L., Williams, M., DelBello, M. P., & Gundersen, K. (2000). Psychosocial functioning in a prepubertal and early adolescent bipolar disorder phenotype. *Journal of the American Academy of Child and Adolescent Psychiatry, 39,* 1543–1548.

Geller, B., & Cook, E. H., Jr. (2000). Ultradian rapid cycling in prepubertal and early adolescent bipolarity is not in transmission disequilibrium with val/met COMT alleles. *Biological Psychiatry, 47,* 605–609.

Geller, B., Fox, L. W., & Fletcher, M. (1993). Effect of tricyclic antidepressants on switching to mania and on the onset of bipolarity in depressed 6- to 12-year-olds. *Journal of the American Academy of Child and Adolescent Psychiatry, 32,* 43–50.

Geller, B., Sun, K., Zimerman, B., Luby, J., Frazier, J., & Williams, M. (1995). Complex and rapid-cycling in bipolar children and adolescents: A preliminary study. *Journal of Affective Disorders, 34,* 259–268.

Geller, B., Tillman, R., Bolhofner, K., & Zimerman, B. (2008). Child bipolar I disorder: Prospective continuity with adult bipolar I disorder; characteristics of second and third episodes; predictors of 8-year outcome. *Archives of General Psychiatry, 65,* 1125–1133.

Geller, B., Tillman, R., Craney, J. L., & Bolhofner, K. (2004). Four-year prospective outcome and natural history of mania in children with a prepubertal and early adolescent bipolar disorder phenotype. *Archives of General Psychiatry, 61,* 459–467.

Geller, B., Zimerman, B., Williams, M., Bolhofner, K., Craney, J. L., DelBello, M. P., & Soutullo, C. (2001). Reliability of the Washington University in St. Louis Kiddie Schedule for Affective Disorders and Schizophrenia (WASH-U-KSADS) mania and rapid cycling sections. *Journal of the American Academy of Child and Adolescent Psychiatry, 40,* 450–455.

Geller, B., Zimerman, B., Williams, M., Delbello, M. P., Bolhofner, K., Craney, J. L., . . . Nickelsburg, M. J. (2002a). DSM-IV mania symptoms in a prepubertal and early adolescent bipolar disorder phenotype compared to attention-deficit hyperactive and normal controls. *Journal of Child and Adolescent Psychopharmacology, 12,* 11–25.

Geller, B., Zimerman, B., Williams, M., Delbello, M. P., Frazier, J., & Beringer, L. (2002b). Phenomenology of prepubertal and early adolescent bipolar disorder: Examples of elated mood, grandiose behaviors, decreased need for sleep, racing thoughts and hyper-sexuality. *Journal of Child and Adolescent Psychopharmacology, 12,* 3–9.

Ghaemi, S. N., Hsu, D. J., Soldani, F., & Goodwin, F. K. (2003). Antidepressants in bipolar disorder: The case for caution. *Bipolar Disorders, 5,* 421–433.

Ghaemi, S. N., Miller, C. J., Berv, D. A., Klugman, J., Rosenquist, K. J., & Pies, R. W. (2005). Sensitivity and specificity of a new bipolar spectrum diagnostic scale. *Journal of Affective Disorders, 84,* 273–277.

Ghanizadeh, A., Mohammadi, M. R., & Yazdanshenas, A. (2006). Psychometric properties of the Farsi translation of the Kiddie Schedule for Affective Disorders and Schizophrenia—Present and Lifetime Version. *BMC Psychiatry, 6,* 10.

Gigerenzer, G. (2001). The adaptive toolbox: Toward a darwinian rationality. *Nebraska Symposium on Motivation, 47,* 113–143.

Goldstein, B. I., Birmaher, B., Carlson, G. A., DelBello, M. P., Findling, R. L., Fristad, M., . . . Youngstrom, E. A. (2017). The International Society for Bipolar Disorders Task Force report on pediatric bipolar disorder: Knowledge to date and directions for future research. *Bipolar Disorders, 19,* 524–543.

Goldstein, B. I., Strober, M. A., Birmaher, B., Axelson, D. A., Esposito-Smythers, C., Goldstein, T. R., . . . Keller, M. B. (2008). Substance use disorders among adolescents with bipolar spectrum disorders. *Bipolar Disorders, 10,* 469–478.

Goldstein, T. R. (2009). Suicidality in pediatric bipolar disorder. *Child and Adolescent Psychiatric Clinics of North America, 18,* 339–352.

Goldstein, T. R., Birmaher, B., Axelson, D., Ryan, N. D., Strober, M. A., Gill, M. K., . . . Keller, M. (2005). History of suicide attempts in pediatric bipolar disorder: Factors associated with increased risk. *Bipolar Disorders, 7,* 525–535.

Goodman, R., Ford, T., Simmons, H., Gatward, R., & Meltzer, H. (2003). Using the Strengths and Difficulties Questionnaire (SDQ) to screen for child psychiatric disorders in a community sample. *International Review of Psychiatry, 15,* 166–172.

Goodwin, F. K., & Jamison, K. R. (2007). *Manic–depressive illness* (2nd ed.). New York: Oxford University Press.

Gracious, B. L., Youngstrom, E. A., Findling, R. L., & Calabrese, J. R. (2002). Discriminative validity of a parent version of the Young Mania Rating Scale. *Journal of the American Academy of Child and Adolescent Psychiatry, 41,* 1350–1359.

Gray, J. A., & McNaughton, N. (1996). The neuropsychology of anxiety: Reprise. In D. A. Hope (Ed.), *Perspectives in anxiety, panic and fear* (Vol. 43, pp. 61–134). Lincoln: University of Nebraska Press.

Guy, W., National Institute of Mental Health, Psychopharmacology Research Branch, & Division of Extramural Research Programs. (1976). *ECDEU assessment manual for psychopharmacology.* Rockville, MD: U.S. Department of Health, Education, and Welfare, Public Health Service, Alcohol, Drug Abuse, and Mental Health Administration.

Guyatt, G. H., & Rennie, D. (Eds.). (2002). *Users' guides to the medical literature.* Chicago: AMA Press.

Hafeman, D. M., Merranko, J., Axelson, D., Goldstein, B. I., Goldstein, T., Monk, K., . . . Birmaher, B. (2016). Toward the definition of a bipolar prodrome: Dimensional predictors of bipolar spectrum disorders in at-risk youths. *American Journal of Psychiatry, 173,* 695–704.

Hafeman, D. M., Merranko, J., Goldstein, T. R., Axelson, D., Goldstein, B. I., Monk, K., . . . Birmaher, B. (2017). Assessment of a person-level risk calculator to predict new-onset bipolar spectrum disorder in youth at familial risk. *JAMA Psychiatry, 74,* 841–847.

Hall, R. C. W. (1995). Global assessment of functioning: A modified scale. *Psychosomatics, 36,* 267–275.

Hamilton, M. (1967). Development of a rating scale for primary depressive illness. *British Journal of Social and Clinical Psychology, 6,* 278–296.

Harvey, A. G. (2008). Insomnia, psychiatric disorders, and the transdiagnostic perspective. *Current Directions in Psychological Science, 17,* 299–303.

Harvey, A. G., Murray, G., Chandler, R. A., & Soehner, A. (2011). Sleep disturbance as transdiagnostic: Consideration of neurobiological mechanisms. *Clinical Psychology Review, 31,* 225–235.

Hasler, G., Drevets, W. C., Gould, T. D., Gottesman, I. I., & Manji, H. K. (2006). Toward constructing an endophenotype strategy for bipolar disorders. *Biological Psychiatry, 60,* 93–105.

Hazell, P. L., Carr, V., Lewin, T. J., & Sly, K. (2003). Manic symptoms in young males with ADHD predict functioning but not diagnosis after 6 years. *Journal of the American Academy of Child and Adolescent Psychiatry, 42,* 552–560.

Henry, D. B., Pavuluri, M. N., Youngstrom, E., & Birmaher, B. (2008). Accuracy of brief and full forms of the Child Mania Rating Scale. *Journal of Clinical Psychology, 64,* 368–381.

Hickie, I. B. (2014). Evidence for separate inheritance of mania and depression challenges current concepts of bipolar mood disorder. *Molecular Psychiatry, 19,* 153–155.

Hillegers, M. H., Reichart, C. G., Wals, M., Verhulst, F. C., Ormel, J., & Nolen, W. A. (2005). Five-year prospective outcome of psychopathology in the adolescent offspring of bipolar parents. *Bipolar Disorders, 7,* 344–350.

Hirschfeld, R. M., Lewis, L., & Vornik, L. A. (2003). Perceptions and impact of bipolar disorder: How far have we really come? Results of the National Depressive and Manic–Depressive Association 2000 survey of individuals with bipolar disorder. *Journal of Clinical Psychiatry, 64,* 161–174.

Hirschfeld, R. M., Williams, J. B. W., Spitzer, R. L., Calabrese, J. R., Flynn, L., Keck, P. E. J., . . . Zajecka, J.

(2000). Development and validation of a screening instrument for bipolar spectrum disorder: The Mood Disorder Questionnaire. *American Journal of Psychiatry, 157,* 1873–1875.

Hodgins, S., Faucher, B., Zarac, A., & Ellenbogen, M. (2002). Children of parents with bipolar disorder: A population at high risk for major affective disorders. *Child and Adolescent Psychiatric Clinics of North America, 11,* 533–553.

Hoertel, N., Le Strat, Y., Angst, J., & Dubertret, C. (2013). Subthreshold bipolar disorder in a U.S. national representative sample: Prevalence, correlates and perspectives for psychiatric nosography. *Journal of Affective Disorders, 146,* 338–347.

Hooley, J. M., & Richters, J. E. (1991). Alternative measures of expressed emotion: A methodological and cautionary note. *Journal of Abnormal Psychology, 100,* 94–97.

Horwitz, S. M., Demeter, C. A., Pagano, M. E., Youngstrom, E. A., Fristad, M. A., Arnold, L. E., . . . Findling, R. L. (2010). Longitudinal Assessment of Manic Symptoms (LAMS) study: Background, design, and initial screening results. *Journal of Clinical Psychiatry, 71,* 1511–1517.

Hunt, J., Birmaher, B., Leonard, H., Strober, M., Axelson, D., Ryan, N., . . . Keller, M. (2009). Irritability without elation in a large bipolar youth sample: Frequency and clinical description. *Journal of the American Academy of Child and Adolescent Psychiatry, 48,* 730–739.

Jacobson, N. S., Roberts, L. J., Berns, S. B., & McGlinchey, J. B. (1999). Methods for defining and determining the clinical significance of treatment effects: Description, application, and alternatives. *Journal of Consulting and Clinical Psychology, 67,* 300–307.

Jacobson, N. S., & Truax, P. (1991). Clinical significance: A statistical approach to defining meaningful change in psychotherapy research. *Journal of Consulting and Clinical Psychology, 59,* 12–19.

Jaeschke, R., Guyatt, G. H., & Sackett, D. L. (1994). Users' guides to the medical literature: III. How to use an article about a diagnostic test: B. What are the results and will they help me in caring for my patients? *Journal of the American Medical Association, 271,* 703–707.

Jamison, K. R. (1995). *An unquiet mind: A memoir of moods and madness.* New York: Vintage Books.

Jenkins, M. M., & Youngstrom, E. A. (2016). A randomized controlled trial of cognitive debiasing improves assessment and treatment selection for pediatric bipolar disorder. *Journal of Consulting and Clinical Psychology, 84,* 323–333.

Jensen-Doss, A., Youngstrom, E. A., Youngstrom, J. K., Feeny, N. C., & Findling, R. L. (2014). Predictors and moderators of agreement between clinical and research diagnoses for children and adolescents. *Journal of Consulting and Clinical Psychology, 82,* 1151–1162.

Johnson, S. L., & Roberts, J. E. (1995). Life events and bipolar disorder: Implications from biological theories. *Psychological Bulletin, 117,* 434–449.

Joseph, M., Frazier, T. W., Youngstrom, E. A., & Soares, J. C. (2008). A quantitative and qualitative review of neurocognitive performance in pediatric bipolar disorder. *Journal of Child and Adolescent Psychopharmacology, 18,* 595–605.

Joseph, M., Youngstrom, E. A., & Soares, J. C. (2009). Antidepressant-coincident mania in children and adolescents treated with selective serotonin reuptake inhibitors. *Future Neurology, 4,* 87–102.

Judd, L. L., & Akiskal, H. S. (2003). The prevalence and disability of bipolar spectrum disorders in the US population: Re-analysis of the ECA database taking into account subthreshold cases. *Journal of Affective Disorders, 73,* 123–131.

Judd, L. L., Akiskal, H. S., Schettler, P. J., Endicott, J., Leon, A. C., Solomon, D., . . . Keller, M. (2005). Psychosocial disability in the course of bipolar I and II disorders: A prospective, comparative, longitudinal study. *Archives of General Psychiatry, 62,* 1322–1330.

Kahana, S. Y., Youngstrom, E. A., Findling, R. L., & Calabrese, J. R. (2003). Employing parent, teacher, and youth self-report checklists in identifying pediatric bipolar spectrum disorders: An examination of diagnostic accuracy and clinical utility. *Journal of Child and Adolescent Psychopharmacology, 13,* 471–488.

Kahneman, D. (2011). *Thinking, fast and slow.* New York: Farrar, Straus & Giroux.

Kaufman, J., Birmaher, B., Brent, D., Rao, U., Flynn, C., Moreci, P., . . . Ryan, N. (1997). Schedule for Affective Disorders and Schizophrenia for School-Age Children—Present and Lifetime version (K-SADS-PL): Initial reliability and validity data. *Journal of the American Academy of Child and Adolescent Psychiatry, 36,* 980–988.

Kazdin, A. E. (1977). Assessing the clinical or applied importance of behavior change through social validation. *Behavior Modification, 1,* 427–452.

Kessel, E. M., Dougherty, L. R., Kujawa, A., Hajcak, G., Carlson, G. A., & Klein, D. N. (2016). Longitudinal associations between preschool disruptive mood dysregulation disorder symptoms and neural reactivity to monetary reward during preadolescence. *Journal of Child and Adolescent Psychopharmacology, 26,* 131–137.

Kessler, R. C. (1998). Sex differences in DSM-III-R psychiatric disorders in the United States: Results from the National Comorbidity Survey. *Journal of American Medical Women's Association, 53,* 148–158.

Kessler, R. C., Avenevoli, S., & Merikangas, K. R. (2001). Mood disorders in children and adolescents: An epidemiologic perspective. *Biological Psychiatry, 49,* 1002–1014.

Kessler, R. C., Berglund, P., Demler, O., Jin, R., & Walters, E. E. (2005). Lifetime prevalence and age-of-onset distributions of DSM-IV disorders in the National

Comorbidity Survey Replication. *Archives of General Psychiatry, 62*, 593–602.

Kessler, R. C., Rubinow, D. R., Holmes, C., Abelson, J. M., & Zhao, S. (1997). The epidemiology of DSM-III-R bipolar I disorder in a general population survey. *Psychological Medicine, 27*, 1079–1089.

Koščec, A., Radošević-Vidaček, B., & Kostović, M. (2001). Morningness–eveningness across two student generations: Would two decades make a difference? *Personality and Individual Differences, 31*, 627–638.

Kowatch, R. A., Fristad, M. A., Birmaher, B., Wagner, K. D., Findling, R. L., & Hellander, M. (2005). Treatment guidelines for children and adolescents with bipolar disorder. *Journal of the American Academy of Child and Adolescent Psychiatry, 44*, 213–235.

Kowatch, R. A., Youngstrom, E. A., Danielyan, A., & Findling, R. L. (2005). Review and meta-analysis of the phenomenology and clinical characteristics of mania in children and adolescents. *Bipolar Disorders, 7*, 483–496.

Kraepelin, E. (1921). *Manic–depressive insanity and paranoia.* Edinburgh, UK: Livingstone.

Kramlinger, K. G., & Post, R. M. (1996). Ultra-rapid and ultradian cycling in bipolar affective illness. *British Journal of Psychiatry, 168*, 314–323.

Leibenluft, E., Charney, D. S., Towbin, K. E., Bhangoo, R. K., & Pine, D. S. (2003). Defining clinical phenotypes of juvenile mania. *American Journal of Psychiatry, 160*, 430–437.

Lewinsohn, P. M., Klein, D. N., & Seeley, J. (2000). Bipolar disorder during adolescence and young adulthood in a community sample. *Bipolar Disorders, 2*, 281–293.

Lewinsohn, P. M., Seeley, J. R., Buckley, M. E., & Klein, D. N. (2002). Bipolar disorder in adolescence and young adulthood. *Child and Adolescent Psychiatric Clinics of North America, 11*, 461–476.

Lewinsohn, P. M., Seeley, J. R., & Klein, D. N. (2003). Bipolar disorder in adolescents: Epidemiology and suicidal behavior. In B. Geller & M. P. DelBello (Eds.), *Bipolar disorder in childhood and early adolescence* (pp. 7–24). New York: Guilford Press.

Lish, J. D., Dime-Meenan, S., Whybrow, P. C., Price, R. A., & Hirschfeld, R. M. (1994). The National Depressive and Manic–Depressive Association (DMDA) survey of bipolar members. *Journal of Affective Disorders, 31*, 281–294.

Loeber, R., Green, S. M., & Lahey, B. B. (1990). Mental health professionals' perception of the utility of children, mothers, and teachers as informants on childhood psychopathology. *Journal of Clinical Child Psychology, 19*, 136–143.

Lonigan, C. J., Phillips, B., & Hooe, E. (2003). Relations of positive and negative affectivity to anxiety and depression in children: Evidence from a latent variable longitudinal study. *Journal of Consulting and Clinical Psychology, 71*, 465–481.

Luby, J. L., & Mrakotsky, C. (2003). Depressed preschoolers with bipolar family history: A group at high risk for later switching to mania? *Journal of Child and Adolescent Psychopharmacology, 13*, 187–197.

Mackin, P., Targum, S. D., Kalali, A., Rom, D., & Young, A. H. (2006). Culture and assessment of manic symptoms. *British Journal of Psychiatry, 189*, 379–380.

Marchand, W. R., Wirth, L., & Simon, C. (2006). Delayed diagnosis of pediatric bipolar disorder in a community mental health setting. *Journal of Psychiatric Practice, 12*, 128–133.

Masi, G., Perugi, G., Toni, C., Millepiedi, S., Mucci, M., Bertini, N., & Akiskal, H. S. (2006). The clinical phenotypes of juvenile bipolar disorder: Toward a validation of the episodic–chronic distinction. *Biological Psychiatry, 59*, 603–610.

Matthews, M., Abdullah, S., Murnane, E., Voida, S., Choudhury, T., Gay, G., & Frank, E. (2016). Development and evaluation of a smartphone-based measure of social rhythms for bipolar disorder. *Assessment, 23*, 472–483.

McClellan, J., Kowatch, R., & Findling, R. L. (2007). Practice parameter for the assessment and treatment of children and adolescents with bipolar disorder. *Journal of the American Academy of Child and Adolescent Psychiatry, 46*, 107–125.

McGoldrick, M., & Gerson, R. (1985). *Genograms in family assessment.* New York: Norton.

Merikangas, K. R., Cui, L., Kattan, G., Carlson, G. A., Youngstrom, E. A., & Angst, J. (2012). Mania with and without depression in a community sample of US adolescents. *Archives of General Psychiatry, 69*, 943–951.

Merikangas, K. R., & Pato, M. (2009). Recent developments in the epidemiology of bipolar disorder in adults and children: Magnitude, correlates, and future directions. *Clinical Psychology: Science and Practice, 16*, 121–133.

Mesman, E., Birmaher, B. B., Goldstein, B. I., Goldstein, T., Derks, E. M., Vleeschouwer, M., . . . Hillegers, M. H. (2016). Categorical and dimensional psychopathology in Dutch and US offspring of parents with bipolar disorder: A preliminary cross-national comparison. *Journal of Affective Disorders, 205*, 95–102.

Meyers, O. I., & Youngstrom, E. A. (2008). A Parent General Behavior Inventory subscale to measure sleep disturbance in pediatric bipolar disorder. *Journal of Clinical Psychiatry, 69*, 840–843.

Michalak, E. E., Murray, G., & Collaborative Research Team to Study Psychosocial Issues in Bipolar Disorder (CREST.BD). (2010). Development of the QoL.BD: A disorder-specific scale to assess quality of life in bipolar disorder. *Bipolar Disorders, 12*, 727–740.

Mick, E., Biederman, J., Pandina, G., & Faraone, S. V. (2003). A preliminary meta-analysis of the child behavior checklist in pediatric bipolar disorder. *Biological Psychiatry, 53*, 1021–1027.

Moreira, A. L. R., Van Meter, A., Genzlinger, J., & Youngstrom, E. A. (2017). Review and meta-analysis of epidemiologic studies of adult bipolar disorder. *Journal of Clinical Psychiatry, 78*, e1259–e1269.

Morton, E., Michalak, E. E., & Murray, G. (2017). What does quality of life refer to in bipolar disorders research?: A systematic review of the construct's definition, usage and measurement. *Journal of Affective Disorders, 212,* 128–137.

Naylor, M. W., Anderson, T. R., Kruesi, M. J., & Stoewe, M. (2002, October). *Pharmacoepidemiology of bipolar disorder in abused and neglected state wards.* Paper presented at the national meeting of the American Academy of Child and Adolescent Psychiatry, San Francisco, CA.

Newman, C. F., Leahy, R. L., Beck, A. T., Reilly-Harrington, N. A., & Gyulai, L. (2002). *Bipolar disorder: A cognitive therapy approach.* Washington, DC: American Psychological Association.

Oedegaard, C. H., Berk, L., Berk, M., Youngstrom, E. A., Dilsaver, S. C., Belmaker, R. H., . . . Engebretsen, I. M. (2016). An ISBD perspective on the sociocultural challenges of managing bipolar disorder. *Australian and New Zealand Journal of Psychiatry, 50,* 1096–1103.

Ong, M. L., Youngstrom, E. A., Chua, J. J., Halverson, T. F., Horwitz, S. M., Storfer-Isser, A., . . . LAMS Group. (2016). Comparing the CASI-4R and the PGBI-10 M for differentiating bipolar spectrum disorders from other outpatient diagnoses in youth. *Journal of Abnormal Child Psychology, 45,* 611–623.

Pacchiarotti, I., Bond, D. J., Baldessarini, R. J., Nolen, W. A., Grunze, H., Licht, R. W., . . . Vieta, E. (2013). The International Society for Bipolar Disorders (ISBD) Task Force report on antidepressant use in bipolar disorders. *American Journal of Psychiatry, 170,* 1249–1262.

Papolos, D. F. (2003). Switching, cycling, and antidepressant-induced effects on cycle frequency and course of illness in adult bipolar disorder: A brief review and commentary. *Journal of Child and Adolescent Psychopharmacology, 13,* 165–171.

Pappadopulos, E., Woolston, S., Chait, A., Perkins, M., Connor, D. F., & Jensen, P. S. (2006). Pharmacotherapy of aggression in children and adolescents: Efficacy and effect size. *Journal of the Canadian Academy of Child and Adolescent Psychiatry, 15,* 27–39.

Pellegrini, D., Kosisky, S., Nackman, D., Cytryn, L., McKnew, D. H., Gershon, E., . . . Cammuso, K. (1986). Personal and social resources in children of patients with bipolar affective disorder and children of normal control subjects. *American Journal of Psychiatry, 143,* 856–861.

Peper, J. S., & Dahl, R. E. (2013). The teenage brain: Surging hormones—brain–behavior interactions during puberty. *Current Directions in Psychological Science, 22,* 134–139.

Perez Algorta, G., MacPherson, H. A., Youngstrom, E. A., Belt, C. C., Arnold, L. E., Frazier, T. W., . . . Fristad, M. A. (2018). Parenting stress among caregivers of children with bipolar spectrum disorders. *Journal of Clinical Child and Adolescent Psychology, 47*(Suppl. 1), S306–S320.

Perez Algorta, G., Van Meter, A., Dubicka, B., Jones, S.,

Youngstrom, E., & Lobban, F. (2018). Blue blocking glasses worn at night in first year higher education students with sleep complaints: A feasibility study. *Pilot Feasibility Studies, 4,* 166.

Perlis, R., Miyahara, S., Marangell, L. B., Wisniewski, S. R., Ostacher, M., DelBello, M. P., . . . Nierenberg, A. A. (2004). Long-term implications of early onset in bipolar disorder: Data from the first 1000 participants in the systematic treatment enhancement program for bipolar disorder (STEP-BD). *Biological Psychiatry, 55,* 875–881.

Petersen, A. C., Crockett, L., Richards, M., & Boxer, A. (1988). A self-report measure of pubertal status: Reliability, validity, and initial norms. *Journal of Youth and Adolescence, 17,* 117–133.

Phelps, J. (2008). Dark therapy for bipolar disorder using amber lenses for blue light blockade. *Medical Hypotheses, 70,* 224–229.

Pini, S., Dell'Osso, L., & Amador, X. F. (2001). Insight into illness in schizophrenia, schizoaffective disorder, and mood disorders with psychotic features. *American Journal of Psychiatry, 158,* 122–125.

Pliszka, S. R., Sherman, J. O., Barrow, M. V., & Irick, S. (2000). Affective disorder in juvenile offenders: A preliminary study. *American Journal of Psychiatry, 157,* 130–132.

Popper, C. W. (1990). Diagnostic gore in children's nightmares. *American Academy of Child and Adolescent Psychiatry Newsletter, 17,* 3–4.

Post, R. M., Leverich, G. S., Altshuler, L. L., Frye, M. A., Suppes, T., Keck, P. E., . . . Rowe, M. (2011). Differential clinical characteristics, medication usage, and treatment response of bipolar disorder in the US versus the Netherlands and Germany. *International Clinical Psychopharmacology, 26,* 96–106.

Post, R. M., Leverich, G. S., Xing, G., & Weiss, S. R. B. (2001). Developmental vulnerabilities to the onset and course of bipolar disorder. *Development and Psychopathology, 13,* 581–598.

Poznanski, E. O., Miller, E., Salguero, C., & Kelsh, R. C. (1984). Preliminary studies of the reliability and validity of the Children's Depression Rating Scale. *Journal of the American Academy of Child Psychiatry, 23,* 191–197.

Pratap, A., Atkins, D. C., Renn, B. N., Tanana, M. J., Mooney, S. D., Anguera, J. A., & Areán, P. A. (2019). The accuracy of passive phone sensors in predicting daily mood. *Depression and Anxiety, 36,* 72–81.

Prisciandaro, J. J., & Roberts, J. E. (2011). Evidence for the continuous latent structure of mania in the Epidemiologic Catchment Area from multiple latent structure and construct validation methodologies. *Psychological Medicine, 41,* 575–588.

Prisciandaro, J. J., & Tolliver, B. K. (2015). Evidence for the continuous latent structure of mania and depression in out-patients with bipolar disorder: Results from the Systematic Treatment Enhancement Program for Bipolar Disorder (STEP-BD). *Psychological Medicine, 45,* 2595–2603.

Quinn, C. A., & Fristad, M. A. (2004). Defining and identifying early onset bipolar spectrum disorder. *Current Psychiatry Reports, 6*, 101–107.

Ravens-Sieberer, U., & Bullinger, M. (2000). KINDL: Questionnaire for measuring health-related quality of life in children and adolescents. Retrieved from *www.kindl.org/english/information.*

Ravens-Sieberer, U., Erhart, M., Wille, N., Wetzel, R., Nickel, J., & Bullinger, M. (2006). Generic health-related quality-of-life assessment in children and adolescents: Methodological considerations. *Pharmacoeconomics, 24*, 1199–1220.

Ravens-Sieberer, U., Gosch, A., Rajmil, L., Erhart, M., Bruil, J., Power, M., . . . KIDSCREEN Group. (2008). The KIDSCREEN-52 quality of life measure for children and adolescents: Psychometric results from a cross-cultural survey in 13 European countries. *Value in Health, 11*, 645–658.

Ray, W. A., Stein, C. M., Murray, K. T., Fuchs, D. C., Patrick, S. W., Daugherty, J., . . . Cooper, W. O. (2019). Association of antipsychotic treatment with risk of unexpected death among children and youths. *JAMA Psychiatry, 76*, 162–171.

Reichart, C. G., & Nolen, W. A. (2004). Earlier onset of bipolar disorder in children by antidepressants or stimulants?: An hypothesis. *Journal of Affective Disorders, 78*, 81–84.

Rettew, D. C., Lynch, A. D., Achenbach, T. M., Dumenci, L., & Ivanova, M. Y. (2009). Meta-analyses of agreement between diagnoses made from clinical evaluations and standardized diagnostic interviews. *International Journal of Methods in Psychiatric Research, 18*, 169–184.

Reynolds, C. R., & Kamphaus, R. (2015). *Behavior Assessment System for Children (BASC)* (3rd ed.). Bloomington, MN: Pearson Clinical Assessment.

Richters, J. E. (1992). Depressed mothers as informants about their children: A critical review of the evidence for distortion. *Psychological Bulletin, 112*, 485–499.

Rihmer, Z., & Kiss, K. (2002). Bipolar disorders and suicidal behaviour. *Bipolar Disorders, 4*, 21–25.

Robinson, L. J., Thompson, J. M., Gallagher, P., Goswami, U., Young, A. H., Ferrier, I. N., & Moore, P. B. (2006). A meta-analysis of cognitive deficits in euthymic patients with bipolar disorder. *Journal of Affective Disorders, 93*, 105–115.

Rocha-Rego, V., Jogia, J., Marquand, A. F., Mourao-Miranda, J., Simmons, A., & Frangou, S. (2014). Examination of the predictive value of structural magnetic resonance scans in bipolar disorder: A pattern classification approach. *Psychological Medicine, 44*, 519–532.

Sachs, G. S. (2004). Strategies for improving treatment of bipolar disorder: Integration of measurement and management. *Acta Psychiatrica Scandinavica, 422*, 7–17.

Sachs, G. S., Guille, C., & McMurrich, S. L. (2002). A clinical monitoring form for mood disorders. *Bipolar Disorders, 4*, 323–327.

Sackett, D. L., Straus, S. E., Richardson, W. S., Rosenberg, W., & Haynes, R. B. (2000). *Evidence-based medicine: How to practice and teach EBM* (2nd ed.). New York: Churchill Livingstone.

Saeb, S., Lattie, E. G., Schueller, S. M., Kording, K. P., & Mohr, D. C. (2016). The relationship between mobile phone location sensor data and depressive symptom severity. *PeerJ, 4*, e2537.

Scheffer, R. E., Kowatch, R. A., Carmody, T., & Rush, A. J. (2005). Randomized, placebo-controlled trial of mixed amphetamine salts for symptoms of comorbid ADHD in pediatric bipolar disorder after mood stabilization with divalproex sodium. *American Journal of Psychiatry, 162*, 58–64.

Shaffer, D., Fisher, P., Dulcan, M. K., Davies, M., Piacentini, J., Schwab-Stone, M. E., . . . Regier, D. A. (1996). The NIMH Diagnostic Interview Schedule for Children Version 2.3 (DISC-2.3): Description, acceptability, prevalence rates, and performance in the MECA Study: Methods for the Epidemiology of Child and Adolescent Mental Disorders Study. *Journal of the American Academy of Child and Adolescent Psychiatry, 35*, 865–877.

Shaffer, D., Gould, M. S., Brasic, J., Ambrosini, P., Fisher, P., Bird, H., & Aluwahlia, S. (1983). A children's global assessment scale (CGAS). *Archives of General Psychiatry, 40*, 1228–1231.

Shankman, S. A., Lewinsohn, P. M., Klein, D. N., Small, J. W., Seeley, J. R., & Altman, S. E. (2009). Subthreshold conditions as precursors for full syndrome disorders: A 15-year longitudinal study of multiple diagnostic classes. *Journal of Child Psychology and Psychiatry and Allied Disciplines, 50*, 1485–1494.

Sheehan, D. V., Lecrubier, Y., Sheehan, K. H., Amorim, P., Janavs, J., Weiller, E., . . . Dunbar, G. C. (1998). The Mini-International Neuropsychiatric Interview (M.I.N.I.): The development and validation of a structured diagnostic psychiatric interview for DSM-IV and ICD-10. *Journal of Clinical Psychiatry, 59*, 22–33.

Sheehan, D. V., Sheehan, K. H., Shytle, R. D., Janavs, J., Bannon, Y., Rogers, J. E., . . . Wilkinson, B. (2010). Reliability and validity of the Mini International Neuropsychiatric Interview for Children and Adolescents (MINI-KID). *Journal of Clinical Psychiatry, 71*, 313–326.

Siegel, R., La Greca, A., Freeman, A. J., & Youngstrom, E. A. (2015). Peer relationship difficulties in adolescents with bipolar disorder. *Child and Youth Care Forum, 44*, 355–375.

Speer, D. C., & Greenbaum, P. E. (1995). Five methods for computing significant individual client change and improvement rates: Support for an individual growth curve approach. *Journal of Consulting and Clinical Psychology, 63*, 1044–1048.

Stewart, A. J., Theodore-Oklota, C., Hadley, W., Brown, L. K., Donenberg, G., DiClemente, R., & Project Style Study Group. (2012). Mania symptoms and HIV-risk behavior among adolescents in mental health treatment. *Journal of Clinical Child and Adolescent Psychology, 41,* 803–810.

Straus, S. E., Glasziou, P., Richardson, W. S., & Haynes, R. B. (2011). *Evidence-based medicine: How to practice and teach EBM* (4th ed.). New York: Churchill Livingstone.

Streiner, D. L., Norman, G. R., & Cairney, J. (2015). *Health measurement scales: A practical guide to their development and use* (5th ed.). New York: Oxford University Press.

Stringaris, A., Vidal-Ribas, P., Brotman, M. A., & Leibenluft, E. (2018). Practitioner review: Definition, recognition, and treatment challenges of irritability in young people. *Journal of Child Psychology & Psychiatry, 59,* 721–739.

Suppiger, A., In-Albon, T., Hendriksen, S., Hermann, E., Margraf, J., & Schneider, S. (2009). Acceptance of structured diagnostic interviews for mental disorders in clinical practice and research settings. *Behavior Therapy, 40,* 272–279.

Tellegen, A., Watson, D., & Clark, L. A. (1999). On the dimensional and hierarchical structure of affect. *Psychological Science, 10,* 297–303.

Teplin, L. A., Abram, K. M., McClelland, G. M., Dulcan, M. K., & Mericle, A. A. (2002). Psychiatric disorders in youth in juvenile detention. *Archives of General Psychiatry, 59,* 1133–1143.

Thissen, D., Liu, Y., Magnus, B., Quinn, H., Gipson, D. S., Dampier, C., . . . DeWalt, D. A. (2016). Estimating minimally important difference (MID) in PROMIS pediatric measures using the scale-judgment method. *Quality of Life Research, 25,* 13–23.

Thuppal, M., Carlson, G. A., Sprafkin, J., & Gadow, K. D. (2002). Correspondence between adolescent report, parent report, and teacher report of manic symptoms. *Journal of Child and Adolescent Psychopharmacology, 12,* 27–35.

Tourian, L., LeBoeuf, A., Breton, J. J., Cohen, D., Gignac, M., Labelle, R., . . . Renaud, J. (2015). Treatment options for the cardinal symptoms of disruptive mood dysregulation disorder. *Journal of the Canadian Academy of Child and Adolescent Psychiatry, 24,* 41–54.

Trull, T. J., & Ebner-Priemer, U. (2013). Ambulatory assessment. *Annual Review of Clinical Psychology, 9,* 151–176.

Tsuchiya, K. J., Byrne, M., & Mortensen, P. B. (2003). Risk factors in relation to an emergence of bipolar disorder: A systematic review. *Bipolar Disorders, 5,* 231–242.

Ullsperger, J. M., & Nikolas, M. A. (2017). A meta-analytic review of the association between pubertal timing and psychopathology in adolescence: Are there sex differences in risk? *Psychological Bulletin, 143,* 903–938.

Van Meter, A., Moreira, A. L., & Youngstrom, E. A. (2011). Meta-analysis of epidemiological studies of pediatric bipolar disorder. *Journal of Clinical Psychiatry, 72,* 1250–1256.

Van Meter, A., Moreira, A. L. R., & Youngstrom, E.

(2019). Updated meta-analysis of epidemiologic studies of pediatric bipolar disorder. *Journal of Clinical Psychiatry, 80.* [Epub ahead of print]

Van Meter, A., Youngstrom, E. A., Demeter, C., & Findling, R. L. (2013). Examining the validity of cyclothymic disorder in a youth sample: Replication and extension. *Journal of Abnormal Child Psychology, 41,* 367–378.

Van Meter, A., Youngstrom, E., Freeman, A., Feeny, N., Youngstrom, J. K., & Findling, R. L. (2016). Impact of irritability and impulsive aggressive behavior on impairment and social functioning in youth with cyclothymic disorder. *Journal of Child and Adolescent Psychopharmacology, 26,* 26–37.

Van Meter, A., Youngstrom, E. A., Youngstrom, J. K., Feeny, N. C., & Findling, R. L. (2011). Examining the validity of cyclothymic disorder in a youth sample. *Journal of Affective Disorders, 132,* 55–63.

Van Meter, A. R., Burke, C., Kowatch, R. A., Findling, R. L., & Youngstrom, E. A. (2016). Ten-year updated meta-analysis of the clinical characteristics of pediatric mania and hypomania. *Bipolar Disorders, 18,* 19–32.

Van Meter, A. R., Burke, C., Youngstrom, E. A., Faedda, G. L., & Correll, C. U. (2016). The bipolar prodrome: Meta-analysis of symptom prevalence prior to initial or recurrent mood episodes. *Journal of the American Academy of Child and Adolescent Psychiatry, 55,* 543–555.

Van Meter, A. R., Youngstrom, E. A., & Findling, R. L. (2012). Cyclothymic disorder: A critical review. *Clinical Psychology Review, 32,* 229–243.

Wagner, K. D. (2006). Bipolar disorder and comorbid anxiety disorders in children and adolescents. *Journal of Clinical Psychiatry, 67,* 16–20.

Walshaw, P. D., Alloy, L. B., & Sabb, F. W. (2010). Executive function in pediatric bipolar disorder and attention-deficit hyperactivity disorder: In search of distinct phenotypic profiles. *Neuropsychology Review, 20,* 103–120.

Watson, D., Clark, L. A., Weber, K., Assenheimer, J. S., Strauss, M. E., & McCormick, R. A. (1995). Testing a tripartite model: II. Exploring the symptom structure of anxiety and depression in student, adult, and patient samples. *Journal of Abnormal Psychology, 104,* 15–25.

Waxmonsky, J. G., Waschbusch, D. A., Belin, P., Li, T., Babocsai, L., Humphery, H., . . . Pelham, W. E. (2016). A randomized clinical trial of an integrative group therapy for children with severe mood dysregulation. *Journal of American Academy of Child and Adolescent Psychiatry, 55,* 196–207.

Weissman, M. M., Wickramaratne, P., Merikangas, K. R., Leckman, J. F., Prusoff, B. A., Caruso, K. A., . . . Gammon, G. D. (1984). Onset of major depression in early adulthood: Increased familial loading and specificity. *Archives of General Psychiatry, 41,* 1136–1143.

Weisz, J. R., Chorpita, B. F., Frye, A., Ng, M. Y., Lau, N.,

Bearman, S. K., . . . Hoagwood, K. E. (2011). Youth Top Problems: Using idiographic, consumer-guided assessment to identify treatment needs and to track change during psychotherapy. *Journal of Consulting and Clinical Psychology, 79*, 369–380.

Woodruff, D. B., El-Mallakh, R. S., & Thiruvengadam, A. P. (2012). Validation of a diagnostic screening blood test for bipolar disorder. *Annals of Clinical Psychiatry, 24*, 135–139.

World Health Organization. (2018). *International classification of diseases for mortality and morbidity statistics* (11th rev.). Geneva: Author.

Yee, A. M., Algorta, G. P., Youngstrom, E. A., Findling, R. L., Birmaher, B., Fristad, M. A., & Group, L. (2015). Unfiltered Administration of the YMRS and CDRS-R in a clinical sample of children. *Journal of Clinical Child and Adolescent Psychology, 44*, 992–1007.

You, S. D., Youngstrom, E. A., Feeny, N. C., Youngstrom, J. K., & Findling, R. L. (2017). Comparing the diagnostic accuracy of five instruments for detecting posttraumatic stress disorder in youth. *Journal of Clinical Child and Adolescent Psychology, 46*, 511–522.

Young, R. C., Biggs, J. T., Ziegler, V. E., & Meyer, D. A. (1978). A rating scale for mania: Reliability, validity, and sensitivity. *British Journal of Psychiatry, 133*, 429–435.

Youngstrom, E. A. (2009). Definitional issues in bipolar disorder across the life cycle. *Clinical Psychology: Science and Practice, 16*, 140–160.

Youngstrom, E. A. (2013). Future directions in psychological assessment: Combining evidence-based medicine innovations with psychology's historical strengths to enhance utility. *Journal of Clinical Child and Adolescent Psychology, 42*, 139–159.

Youngstrom, E. A., & Algorta, G. P. (2014). Pediatric bipolar disorder. In E. J. Mash & R. A. Barkley (Eds.), *Child psychopathology* (3rd ed., pp. 264–316). New York: Guilford Press.

Youngstrom, E. A., Arnold, L. E., & Frazier, T. W. (2010). Bipolar and ADHD comorbidity: Both artifact and outgrowth of shared mechanisms. *Clinical Psychology: Science and Practice, 17*, 350–359.

Youngstrom, E. A., Birmaher, B., & Findling, R. L. (2008). Pediatric bipolar disorder: Validity, phenomenology, and recommendations for diagnosis *Bipolar Disorders, 10*, 194–214.

Youngstrom, E. A., Danielson, C. K., Findling, R. L., Gracious, B. L., & Calabrese, J. R. (2002). Factor structure of the Young Mania Rating Scale for use with youths ages 5 to 17 years. *Journal of Clinical Child and Adolescent Psychology, 31*, 567–572.

Youngstrom, E. A., & De Los Reyes, A. (2015). Commentary: Moving toward cost-effectiveness in using psychophysiological measures in clinical assessment: Validity, decision making, and adding value. *Journal of Clinical Child and Adolescent Psychology, 44*, 352–361.

Youngstrom, E. A., & Duax, J. (2005). Evidence based

assessment of pediatric bipolar disorder: Part 1. Base rate and family history. *Journal of the American Academy of Child and Adolescent Psychiatry, 44*, 712–717.

Youngstrom, E. A., Egerton, G. A., Genzlinger, J., Freeman, L. K., Rizvi, S. H., & Van Meter, A. (2018). Improving the global identification of bipolar spectrum disorders: Meta-analysis of the diagnostic accuracy of checklists. *Psychological Bulletin, 144*, 315–342.

Youngstrom, E. A., Findling, R. L., & Calabrese, J. R. (2004). Effects of adolescent manic symptoms on agreement between youth, parent, and teacher ratings of behavior problems. *Journal of Affective Disorders, 82*, S5–S16.

Youngstrom, E. A., Findling, R. L., Calabrese, J. R., Gracious, B. L., Demeter, C., DelPorto Bedoya, D., & Price, M. (2004). Comparing the diagnostic accuracy of six potential screening instruments for bipolar disorder in youths aged 5 to 17 years. *Journal of the American Academy of Child and Adolescent Psychiatry, 43*, 847–858.

Youngstrom, E. A., Freeman, A. J., & Jenkins, M. M. (2009). The assessment of children and adolescents with bipolar disorder. *Child and Adolescent Psychiatric Clinics of North America, 18*, 353–390.

Youngstrom, E. A., Genzlinger, J. E., Egerton, G. A., & Van Meter, A. R. (2015). Multivariate meta-analysis of the discriminative validity of caregiver, youth, and teacher rating scales for pediatric bipolar disorder: Mother knows best about mania. *Archives of Scientific Psychology, 3*, 112–137.

Youngstrom, E. A., Gracious, B. L., Danielson, C. K., Findling, R. L., & Calabrese, J. R. (2003). Toward an integration of parent and clinician report on the Young Mania Rating Scale. *Journal of Affective Disorders, 77*, 179–190.

Youngstrom, E. A., Halverson, T. F., Youngstrom, J. K., Lindhiem, O., & Findling, R. L. (2018). Evidence-based assessment from simple clinical judgments to statistical learning: Evaluating a range of options using pediatric bipolar disorder as a diagnostic challenge. *Clinical Psychological Science, 6*, 234–265.

Youngstrom, E. A., & Izard, C. E. (2008). Functions of emotions and emotion-related dysfunction. In A. J. Elliot (Ed.), *Handbook of approach and avoidance motivation* (pp. 367–384). New York: Psychology Press.

Youngstrom, E. A., Joseph, M. F., & Greene, J. (2008). Comparing the psychometric properties of multiple teacher report instruments as predictors of bipolar disorder in children and adolescents. *Journal of Clinical Psychology, 64*, 382–401.

Youngstrom, E. A., Meyers, O. I., Demeter, C., Kogos Youngstrom, J., Morello, L., Piiparinen, R., . . . Calabrese, J. R. (2005). Comparing diagnostic checklists for pediatric bipolar disorder in academic and community mental health settings. *Bipolar Disorders, 7*, 507–517.

Youngstrom, E. A., Meyers, O. I., Youngstrom, J. K., Calabrese, J. R., & Findling, R. L. (2006a). Comparing the effects of sampling designs on the diagnostic accuracy of eight promising screening algorithms for pediatric bipolar disorder. *Biological Psychiatry, 60,* 1013–1019.

Youngstrom, E. A., Meyers, O. I., Youngstrom, J. K., Calabrese, J. R., & Findling, R. L. (2006b). Diagnostic and measurement issues in the assessment of pediatric bipolar disorder. *Development and Psychopathology, 18,* 989–1021.

Youngstrom, E. A., Murray, G., Johnson, S. L., & Findling, R. L. (2013). The 7 Up 7 Down Inventory: A 14-item measure of manic and depressive tendencies carved from the General Behavior Inventory. *Psychological Assessment, 25,* 1377–1383.

Youngstrom, E. A., Van Meter, A., Frazier, T. W., Hunsley, J., Prinstein, M. J., Ong, M.-L., & Youngstrom, J. K. (2017). Evidence-based assessment as an integrative model for applying psychological science to guide the voyage of treatment. *Clinical Psychology: Science and Practice, 24,* 331– 363.

Youngstrom, E. A., Van Meter, A., Frazier, T. W., Youngstrom, J. K., & Findling, R. L. (2020). Developing and validating short forms of the Parent General Behavior Inventory Mania and Depression Scales for rating youth mood symptoms. *Journal of Clinical Child and Adolescent Psychology, 49*(2), 162–177.

Youngstrom, E. A., Youngstrom, J. K., Freeman, A. J., De Los Reyes, A., Feeny, N. C., & Findling, R. L. (2011). Informants are not all equal: Predictors and correlates of clinician judgments about caregiver and youth credibility. *Journal of Child and Adolescent Psychopharmacology, 21,* 407–415.

Youngstrom, E. A., Youngstrom, J. K., & Starr, M. (2005). Bipolar diagnoses in community mental health: Achenbach CBCL profiles and patterns of comorbidity. *Biological Psychiatry, 58,* 569–575.

Youngstrom, E. A., Zhao, J., Mankoski, R., Forbes, R. A., Marcus, R. M., Carson, W., . . . Findling, R. L. (2013). Clinical significance of treatment effects with aripiprazole versus placebo in a study of manic or mixed episodes associated with pediatric bipolar I disorder. *Journal of Child and Adolescent Psychopharmacology, 23,* 72–79.

Zimmerman, M., Ruggero, C. J., Chelminski, I., & Young, D. (2010). Clinical characteristics of depressed outpatients previously overdiagnosed with bipolar disorder. *Comprehensive Psychiatry, 51,* 99–105.

CHAPTER 9

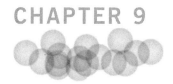

Self-Injurious Thoughts and Behaviors

Alexander J. Millner and Matthew K. Nock

Self-injurious thoughts and behaviors (SITB) in youth are among the largest public health concerns. Suicide is a leading cause of death globally for both children and adolescents (Kassebaum et al., 2017). Rates of nonlethal SITB among children and adolescents are approximately 4–12%, with some higher end estimates reaching above 20% (Brunner et al., 2014; Nock, Borges, Bromet, Cha, et al., 2008; Nock et al., 2013). Overall, SITB among youth are prevalent and have the potential to result in death. Therefore, clinicians should thoroughly assess these behaviors with instruments that have substantial empirical grounding.

There have been several advances in the measurement of SITB since the publication of the prior edition of this chapter (Goldston & Comp-

ton, 2007), including the introduction of multiple validated instruments that focus exclusively on measuring SITB outcomes, as well as research that focuses on accurate measurement of SITB. We begin this chapter by providing basic information regarding SITB definitions, classification and measurement issues, and the goals and complexities of assessing SITB. We also provide the prevalence statistics of SITB for youth. Following this basic background information, we suggest a "starter kit" of potential assessments suitable for assessing the presence and characteristics of SITB outcomes, case formulation and treatment planning, and progress monitoring and goal evaluation. We then provide a more comprehensive review of the empirical evidence supporting instruments used to assess SITB among youth. Many instruments assess a subset of SITB outcomes; therefore, we take care to specify which thoughts and behaviors each measure assesses.

For those interested in an analogous review focused on adults and youth, we recently wrote a similar chapter in A *Guide to Assessments that Work* (Millner & Nock, 2018). Before continuing, we note an important distinction between the assessment of SITB history, the focus of this chapter, and the assessment of future risk of SITB, particularly suicide risk. The presence and severity of prior SITB increases the likelihood of future SITB (Ribeiro et al., 2016); thus, instruments discussed here are relevant for risk assessment. However, risk assessment includes other considerations, such as factors associated with SITB (e.g., a history of child abuse, family disturbances or sexual orientation of the youth (Shaffer & Pfeffer, 2001)) and other risk factors (e.g., hopelessness, mental disorders) that are beyond the scope of this chapter.

Background

Classification and Measurement

SITB are thoughts and behaviors that entail imagined or actual intentional physical injury to one's body and extend to more passive desires, such as wishing one were dead. Historically, research and clinical practice dealing with SITB have been hampered by classification issues. For instance, researchers commonly used overly broad categories that combined disparate forms of SITB, such as "deliberate self-harm," which did not distinguish between suicidal and nonsuicidal forms of self-injury, and "suicidality," which referred to any suicidal thought or action. Over the past two decades, there has been a focus on establishing taxonomies to aid classification and measurement, with several articles seeking to establish a nomenclature for SITB (O'Carroll et al., 1996; Silverman, Berman, Sanddal, O'Carroll, & Joiner, 2007) and U.S. government agencies implementing classification systems for clinical care and research (the U.S. Food and Drug Administration [FDA], the Centers for Disease Control and Prevention, and the Department of Defense) (Brenner et al., 2011; Posner, Oquendo, Gould, Stanley, & Davies, 2007; U.S. Food and Drug Administration & U.S. Department of Health and Human Services, 2012). There continue to be outstanding issues and disagreements in the classification of SITB (Hasley et al., 2008; Matarazzo, Clemans, Silverman, & Brenner, 2013; Silverman & De Leo, 2016), particularly in terms of how granular classification systems should be (Sheehan, Giddens, & Sheehan, 2014a); however, there has been clear advancement in this area.

Generally, consensus classification distinguishes between SITB that are *suicidal*, in which the person has some intent (i.e., nonzero) or wish to die from his or her behavior and SITB that are *nonsuicidal*, in which people injure themselves or think about injuring themselves with no intent to die. There are three major categories within suicidal SITB: *suicidal ideation*, which is thoughts about engaging in a behavior to end one's life; a *suicide plan*, which refers to thinking about how

(i.e., method) and where (i.e., place) to engage in a suicidal act; and a *suicide attempt*, which is engaging in a potentially harmful or lethal behavior with some intention of dying from the behavior.

More recent research has also begun to measure a broader array of SITB thoughts and behaviors that are suicidal or approximately suicidal in nature: *passive suicidal ideation*, which is concerning thoughts about death, such as wishing one were dead; *preparatory behaviors*, which are actions to prepare for a suicide attempt (e.g., obtaining a gun) or for the consequences of one's death (e.g., preparing a will); an *aborted attempt*, which is defined as starting to take steps to attempt suicide but stopping oneself prior to engaging in a potentially harmful or lethal behavior; and an *interrupted attempt*, which is identical to an aborted attempt except someone or something prevents a person from attempting suicide. Another, related behavior that is considered nonsuicidal is a *suicide gesture*, in which a person does something to give the appearance of a suicide attempt for some purpose other than dying (e.g., to communicate pain) and actually has zero intention of dying.

Despite the establishment of consensus definitions for most suicidal behaviors, one important behavior has not been clearly defined: a suicide plan. Despite the intuitive understanding of a "plan," it is unclear whether tentative thoughts about how to kill oneself are sufficient to constitute a plan or, instead, a person needs to have selected the method, place, and even the time to try to kill him- or herself in order to meet the definition of a plan. One instrument assesses a "specific plan," defined as "details of a plan fully or partially worked out," but there is no precise operationalization (Posner et al., 2011), and it is unclear how this is different than a regular plan.

When a construct does not have a clear definition, assessment relies on respondents' interpretation of the term or question, which can differ and result in inconsistent measurement. Research has suggested that this may be a problem for questions regarding the presence of a suicide plan (Millner, Lee, & Nock, 2015). Inconsistent measurement might also be the result of respondents, clinicians, or interviewers not clearly understanding the definition of the behavior in question. Thus, for example, even though researchers have a consensus definition for the term "suicide attempt," respondents may not know this definition and provide inconsistent responses. Indeed, research has shown that 10–40% incorrectly endorse making a prior attempt (Hom, Joiner, & Bernert, 2015;

Millner et al., 2015; Nock & Kessler, 2006; Plöderl, Kralovec, Yazdi, & Fartacek, 2011) and, in hospital settings, medical notes incorrectly label a behavior as a suicide attempt 6% of the time and fail to identify a suicide attempt 18% of the time (Brown, Currier, Jager-Hyman, & Stanley, 2015). These studies were all among adults, but the problem of ensuring that respondents understand the definition of the construct being asked is presumably a similar or larger issue among youth, who may be more prone to misunderstand unfamiliar terms or constructs (Velting, Rathus, & Asnis, 1998).

One way to reduce inconsistent measurement is to increase the *clarity* of the question by embedding the definition in the question and to increase the *coverage* by providing several thoughts or behaviors that people can choose. Coverage can reduce misclassification that occurs when people endorse the wrong outcome because the behavior in which they actually engaged is not listed (e.g., a person who engages in an aborted attempt endorses a suicide attempt because an aborted attempt was not an option). Accurate classification also relies on interviewers who are well trained in the definitions of SITB outcomes, so that they can accurately classify reported behaviors. Training for SITB definitions can be obtain through some government agencies that have established SITB classification systems and some instruments, such as the Columbia–Suicide Severity Rating Scale (Posner et al., 2011), which offers free, Web-based training (*http://cssrs.columbia.edu*). The prior section on classification and measurement also provides an introduction to these topics. One crucial area is assessing what took place during a suicidal action to determine whether the behavior constitutes a suicide attempt. For example, a person who walks to a bridge, strongly considers jumping off, but does not may classify this episode as a "suicide attempt"; however, this behavior would be classified as an aborted attempt. Similarly, people may deny a suicide attempt by claiming that an action that appeared to be a suicide attempt was actually a "cry for help." If the person engaged in an action that was potentially harmful or lethal and had any (nonzero) intent to die from this action, it should be categorized as a suicide attempt. Thus, categorization of a suicide attempts revolves around whether the person engaged in a harmful action and had any intent to die from the action at the time, and it is important to thoroughly assess these topics, both for research and clinical purposes.

Overall, research into misclassification and its reduction is very recent and only relates to adults.

Difficulties with interpretation and misclassification may be different among youth depending on whether instruments take more care to explain concepts rather than assume respondents understand the terms in question. However, barring increased explanations or carefully worded questions, problems with interpretations and misclassification are likely to be just as problematic among youth (Velting et al., 1998). Continued work in this area, including the best way to pose questions to allow for understanding and reduce misclassification, particularly among youth, will help improve the validity and reliability of the assessment of SITB.

Prevalence and Conditional Probability

When assessing SITB, it is important to consider the prevalence of different behaviors. In a study with a large-scale representative sample of youth ages 13–18 years, Nock and colleagues (2013) found that the prevalence of suicide ideation, plans, and attempts within the United States are 12.1, 4.0, and 4.1%, respectively. Based on retrospective age-of-onset reports, it is rare for any of these outcomes to occur among children younger than 10 years of age (<1% prevalence for each outcome). Given that most people who attempt suicide report having thought of suicide at some prior point in time, it is useful to understand the proportion of people who transition from ideation to suicide attempts. Approximately one-third of youth who report ideation go on to attempt suicide. Among ideators who attempt suicide, around 60% endorse a plan at the same age or an earlier age as their attempt. However, as we discussed earlier, given that these data are retrospective and no definition or criteria for a plan is provided, many youth who attempt suicide may be more likely to endorse a plan simply because they attempted suicide, not necessarily because it was carried out with extensive planning and premeditation. Like adults, most youth that transition from ideation to an attempt do so within a year of the onset of ideation. It is worth noting that, like adults, the prevalence of nearly all nonlethal suicidal behaviors is greater among females, compared with males. In addition, non-Hispanic black youth also have lower prevalence of suicidal thoughts and attempts.

The prevalence of nonsuicidal self-injury (NSSI) among youth is unknown because representative epidemiological studies have not included this behavior. Rates of NSSI also are affected by how it is measured with checklists of different behaviors eliciting higher rates than a single-item question regarding the presence of any lifetime NSSI (Muehlenkamp, Claes, Havertape, & Plener, 2012; Swannell, Martin, Page, Hasking, & St John, 2014). A recent cross-national meta-analysis of studies with nonclinical samples, which attempted to correct for measurement approach, as well as other methodological factors, found a prevalence of 17.2% among adolescents (Swannell et al., 2014). A study of more than 500 middle schoolers (ages 10–14 years) found a lower rate of 7.5% (Hilt, Nock, Lloyd-Richardson, & Prinstein, 2008), which is consistent with studies showing that age of onset for NSSI occurs between ages 12 and 14 years (Jacobson & Gould, 2007). Other studies of adolescents have found different rates. For example, a study across 11 European countries found an NSSI rate of 27.6%; however, only 7.8% reported repetitive NSSI, with the remaining 19.7% of participants reporting occasional NSSI (Brunner et al., 2014). Another study with large samples ($n > 350$) of adolescents from two European countries and the United States found NSSI rates of 22–26% when looking within each sample (Giletta, Scholte, Engels, Ciairano, & Prinstein, 2012). Importantly, no prior studies have contained truly representative samples, limiting their ability to provide estimates representative of the population of adolescents.

Purposes of Assessment

In the fifth edition of the *Diagnostic and Statistical Manual of Mental Disorders* (DSM-5; American Psychiatric Association, 2013), certain SITB are included among criteria of some diagnoses, such as major depressive disorder and borderline personality disorder, but there are no official diagnoses with criteria that include only SITB. However, DSM-5 has proposed two SITB-related disorders, suicidal behavior disorder and NSSI, as conditions that require further study. In addition, researchers have put forward acute suicide affective disorder, which is a hypothesized disorder associated with increased intent to act on suicidal thoughts (Rogers et al., 2017; Tucker, Michaels, Rogers, Wingate, & Joiner, 2016). A small number of researchers has started to investigate the clinical utility and validity of these disorders and to develop instruments containing the respective criteria (Tucker et al., 2016; Victor, Davis, & Klonsky, 2016; Washburn, Juzwin, Styer, & Aldridge, 2010), but, currently, the purpose of assessment is not to diagnose a particular disorder. Instead, assessment is intended to determine (1) the presence or absence of each SITB; (2) characteristics of SITB, such as frequency and severity; and (3) whether SITB have changed over time. Thus, for this chapter, we focus on scales that primarily assess SITB or aspects of SITB (e.g., frequency, severity, functions) rather than those that assess SITB and several other constructs (e.g., depressive symptoms). For example, we have omitted measures such as the Suicide Probability Scale, which has been used in studies with adolescents (Larzelere, Smith, Batenhorst, & Kelly, 1996); although it has six items assessing suicidal ideation, it also has 30 items assessing risk factors, such as hopelessness and hostility. It is important to thoroughly assess SITB outcomes, and we focus on the several instruments that provide this ability.

Assessing SITB

We recommend that all patients, even those who appear low risk or nonsuicidal, receive a comprehensive clinical interview (e.g., intake or discharge interview) that directly assesses SITB. There is a temptation for clinicians to rely on symptom severity to infer suicidal status without direct assessment; however, those who do not appear to be at high risk may still engage in SITB. Among patients known to be suicidal, there is a similar temptation to use ancillary "warning signs," such as giving things away, to infer risk (Rudd et al., 2006). We do not recommend this practice and instead encourage clinicians to obtain direct expression of SITB or self-injurious intentions. In some cases, such as with young children, it might be beneficial to begin with softer language, such as asking whether the person has thought about not wanting to be alive or has thoughts of hurting him- or herself, before probing more serious suicidal thoughts and behaviors.

There is a common perception that directly assessing SITB increases proximate risk of SITB or cause increased distress. However, multiple randomized controlled trials, including one among adolescents, suggest that directly assessing SITB does not result in harmful effects, such as increased suicidal ideation or suicide risk (Gould et al., 2005; Harris & Goh, 2016; Law et al., 2015). Still, SITB topics require appropriate sensitivity, particularly if patient and clinician or interviewer are unacquainted. We recommend that clinicians begin with less severe thoughts and behaviors, such as symptoms of depression, before assessing SITB.

Starter Kit

Depending on the clinical environment, the first assessment may include a self-report scale to provide a quick, brief assessment of SITB severity. For more in-depth, thorough assessment of SITB, two instruments directly and comprehensively assess SITB that are both suicidal and nonsuicidal in nature. First, the *Columbia–Suicide Severity Rating Scale* (C-SSRS; Posner et al., 2011; *http://cssrs.columbia.edu*), which has been validated in an adolescent sample (Posner et al., 2011) and has a version for young children, assesses all suicidal outcomes (passive and active ideation, suicide plan, suicide attempt, as well as aborted and interrupted attempts), NSSI, and intensity of ideation and explicit suicide intent. Second, the *Self-Injurious Thoughts and Behaviors Interview* (SITBI; Nock, Holmberg, Photos, & Michel, 2007; *https://nock-lab.fas.harvard.edu/tasks*), which also been validated in an adolescent sample, assesses the same suicidal outcomes as the C-SSRS (albeit in a different question order) and NSSI. The SITBI also assesses the presence of a suicide gesture and several characteristics (severity, frequency, recency, reasons for engaging in the SITB) of each outcome. An updated version of the SITBI is forthcoming. This new version assesses a range of passive problematic thoughts (e.g., "I wish I was never born") and specific planning steps rather than just asking about the presence of a "plan." Both the C-SSRS and the new version of the SITBI have been validated in self-report online versions, although this may be of more use in research settings. The main difference between the two instruments is that whereas the C-SSRS collects a complete but brief overview of SITB, the SITBI collects more information but takes longer to administer. If SITB are of particular concern within a patient population, then perhaps the SITBI is more appropriate, whereas if SITB are less severe among typical patients, then the C-SSRS might be more applicable. In addition to being available through the respective developers' websites, these interviews, as well as individual modules (e.g., suicidal ideation only) are available at the Phnx Toolkit website (*www.phenxtoolkit.org*; search "suicide" or "nonsuicidal self-injury"), a website of freely available, recommended measurement protocols.

If initial assessment results in the presence of SITB, it is clinically useful to determine patients' views on factors that influence engagement in SITB events for case conceptualization. The SITBI can be used for this purpose because for each outcome, the SITBI assesses several reasons or circumstances preceding an SITB (e.g., for suicidal ideation, respondents are asked to rate on a scale of 1–4, "How much did problems with your romantic relationships lead to these thoughts?"). If one prefers a stand-alone assessment to determine reasons for engaging in SITB, there are separate scales available to assess reasons for attempting suicide, such as the *Inventory of Motivations for Suicide Attempts* (IMSA; May & Klonsky, 2013), and reasons for engaging in NSSI, such as the *Functional Assessment of Self-Mutilation* (FASM; Lloyd, Kelley, & Hope, 1997; available at *https://osf.io/qps3v*). Case conceptualization may also be helped by determining protective factors for SITB, such as reasons for living assessed by the *Reasons for Living for Adolescents* (RFL-A; Osman et al., 1998; available at *www.phenxtoolkit.org*; search "RFL-A"). Finally, both the SITBI and C-SSRS can be used for progress monitoring and treatment outcomes. Both the young child and regular versions of the C-SSRS have a "since last visit" version, although it is nearly identical to the baseline scale. The SITBI does not have an explicit version for progress monitoring but it can be used in this way if the interviewer asks the items in regards to the intervening period. We now review the wide array of instruments to assess the presence of SITB among youth.

Screening and Predicting Suicide

Predicting suicidal behaviors is extremely difficult. Because SITB have such low base rates, particularly suicide attempts and suicide death, odds ratios (ORs) for predictors need to be extremely high (e.g., for death or suicide attempts, ORs > 20 at the minimum) to impact any clinical decisions (Franklin et al., 2017). A recent meta-analysis of 50 years of research on prospective predictors of suicidal SITB failed to find any strong predictors (none had an OR > 5; Franklin et al., 2017). Recent prospective studies among psychiatric adolescents using SITB assessments, such as the C-SSRS, also have found statistically significant but clinically insignificant predictors (ORs < 5; Gipson, Agarwala, Opperman, Horwitz, & King, 2015; Horwitz, Czyz, & King, 2015). Importantly, these studies, including the aforementioned meta-analysis, revealed that the strongest predictors of SITB were prior SITB or outcomes associated with prior

SITB, such as psychiatric hospitalization. These findings represent part of the rationale behind the main goal of assessment, which is to clearly identify prior instances and characteristics (e.g., recency, frequency, severity) of SITB. However, this goal is accompanied by the caveat that although assessments are unlikely to provide precise information on how likely a person is to attempt suicide within the next month, for example, they still provide important information when gauging SITB risk. We begin with self-report instruments that have relatively short administration times and empirical support assessing SITB among youth.

Self-Report Measures

The *Beck Scale for Suicidal Ideation* (BSI; Beck & Steer, 1991) is a self-report scale that assesses characteristics of past week suicidal thoughts and actions, including the presence, frequency, and severity of suicidal thoughts, as well as reasons for suicide, planning, and the presence and intent of prior attempts. It contains 21 items, with each item rated on a scale of 0–3. The BSI has been found to have excellent internal consistency, good construct validity (Steer, Kumar, & Beck, 1993), and strong psychometric properties among adolescent psychiatric inpatient (Kim et al., 2015; Kumar & Steer, 1995) and outpatient (Rathus & Miller, 2002) samples.

The *Self-Harm Behavior Questionnaire* (SHBQ; Gutierrez, Osman, Barrios, & Kopper, 2001) contains 32 items that assess the presence and characteristics (e.g., age of onset, frequency, lethality, method, and intent) of four self-injurious behaviors: nonsuicidal self-harm, suicidal ideation, suicide attempts, and suicide threats. The validity and reliability of the SBHQ have been supported in youth (Muehlenkamp, Cowles, & Gutierrez, 2009), and the SBHQ has been used across ethnically and racially diverse adolescent samples (Andrews, Martin, Hasking, & Page, 2013; Brausch & Gutierrez, 2010; Muehlenkamp et al., 2009; Muehlenkamp & Gutierrez, 2004).

The *Suicidal Behaviors Questionnaire* (SBQ; Linehan, 1981) assesses the presence and frequency of suicidal ideation, attempts and NSSI. Scores from the full 34-item SBQ have shown excellent reliability among adolescents (Watkins & Gutierrez, 2003), but the measure has been infrequently tested among youth. A four-item derivation of the SBQ, the *SBQ—Revised* (SBQ-R), has also demonstrated strong psychometric properties within

adolescent samples (Glenn, Bagge, & Osman, 2013; Osman et al., 2001).

The *Suicidal Ideation Questionnaire* (SIQ; Reynolds, 1988) and *Suicidal Ideation Questionnaire Junior* (SIQ-JR; Reynolds, 1987) were developed specifically for use in grades 10–12 and 7–9, respectively. The SIQ has 30 items, whereas the SIG-JR has 15 items. Scores on both scales have shown strong psychometric properties (Gutierrez & Osman, 2009; Huth-Bocks, Kerr, Ivey, Kramer, & King, 2007; Pinto, Whisman, & McCoy, 1997; Reynolds & Mazza, 1999).

The *Harkavy–Asnis Suicide Scale* (HASS; Harkavy-Friedman & Asnis, 1989) assesses demographic information, the presence and characteristics (age of onset, recency) of suicidal thoughts and plans, and suicide attempts, as well as substance abuse history and exposure to suicidal behavior. Scores on the HASS have shown strong psychometric properties in studies with high school students (Harkavy Friedman & Asnis, 1989) and psychiatric outpatient adolescents (Wetzler et al., 1996), a treatment study (Rathus & Miller, 2002), and in a pediatric emergency department (Asarnow, McArthur, Hughes, Barbery, & Berk, 2012).

Cross-Informant Agreement

There has been very little work examining cross-informant work within the context of SITB. The few studies that have examined agreement between parent and adolescent assessment have found poor agreement (Klimes-Dougan, 1998; Prinstein, Nock, Spirito, & Grapentine, 2001). When adolescents report SITB on self-report measures, they generally endorse higher rates of SITB than do parents or clinicians. In a recent unpublished study examining adolescents and their parents' reports on adolescents' depressive symptoms, Augenstein and colleagues (2018) found that adolescents' reports of their depression were more concurrently predictive of their self-reported suicidal thoughts than were parents' reports of the adolescents' depressive symptoms. The outcome most predictive of prospective suicidal thoughts occurred when the teen reported high levels of depression but the parent disagreed and said the adolescent had low levels of depression. Thus, knowing that a parent may not fully appreciate his or her child's level of depression may be predictive of suicidal ideation, but parents in this study did not provide clinically useful information that their child omitted. Parent's lack of knowledge regarding their child's SITB could contribute to the discrepant reports. Alternatively, in a different study, Van Meter and colleagues (2018) found that parents' reports were actually better at classifying previous suicidal behaviors (based on a structured interview with the child) than the child's own self-report. The authors suggest that this may have been due to the child's hesitancy to disclose the suicidal behavior. Overall, it might be helpful to assess both the parent and the child, and even to do so across different formats (e.g., interview style, self-report questionnaire) to probe for the presence of SITB, then discuss discrepancies between formats or between child and parent.

There also has been little research examining agreement between clinician and patient reports of SITB among adolescents. Research on adults has found substantial disagreement between patient and clinician reports of SITB (Gao et al., 2015; Joiner, Rudd, & Rajab, 1999; Malone, Szanto, Corbitt, & Mann, 1995; Yigletu, Tucker, Harris, & Hatlevig, 2004). Joiner and colleagues (1999) found that baseline patient reports were more corroborative of their future reports than were clinicians. In one study of adolescents, Prinstein and colleagues (2001) found that clinicians provided reports that were more consistent with adolescents' reports than with parents' reports, but there was still substantial disagreement. An important stipulation, however, is that in this study, adolescents themselves provided discordant responses when reporting SITB on self-report versus interview formats. Therefore, the disagreement across different informants or formats could also be due in part to method variance (Prinstein et al., 2001). Velting and colleagues (1998) found that half of participants gave discrepant responses between self-report and interview SITBI outcomes. The reasons for discrepancies had to do with various problems with interpretation of operational definitions, intentional minimization of suicidal behaviors, careless responding, misunderstanding instructions, and the authors being unsure about the reason for discrepancy. Overall, the more formats and the more informants that can be utilized when assessing SITB, the better.

Protective Factors

The most relevant protective factor for suicidal SITB are people's reasons for living. These reasons differ by age. For example, a scale that asks about whether children are a reason for staying alive will not pertain to most adolescents. This has led to the development of several age-specific derivations of the original Reasons for Living Inventory.

The *Reasons for Living Inventory* (RFL; Linehan, Goodstein, Nielsen, & Chiles, 1983) is a 48-item scale (with an expanded 72-item version) to assess various reasons people might have for living or for not attempting suicide. The RFL has six factor-analytically derived subscales: Survival and Coping Beliefs, Responsibility to Family, Child Concerns, Fear of Suicide, Fear of Social Disapproval, and Moral Objections (to suicide). Although, the vast majority of studies using the RFL have been with adults, the scale has received psychometric support among adolescents. For example, one study of psychiatric hospitalized adolescents found a similar different factor structure for the RFL (although the original factor structure did not provide a good fit). Overall, the RFL scores have showed strong psychometric properties with good-to-excellent internal consistency and convergent validity across multiple studies (Cole, 1989; Pinto, Whisman, & Conwell, 1998), although these studies removed Child Concerns items from the scale because, as we mentioned earlier, most adolescents do not have children. Osman and colleagues (1996) also administered the RFL to a sample of psychiatric inpatient adolescents and pared it down to 14 items, which they referred to as the *Brief Reasons for Living—Adolescent* (BRFL-A) scale. The authors then collected a second sample, which provided psychometric support for the BRFL-A (Osman et al., 1996).

The RFL-A (Osman et al., 1998) is a 32-item scale that assesses five factors: Future Optimism, Suicide-Related Concerns, Family Alliance, Peer Acceptance and Support, and Self-Acceptance. Of note, none of the items overlap with the original RFL. The RFL-A scores have shown good reliability and predictive validity with both high school students (Gutierrez, Osman, Kopper, & Barrios, 2000; Osman et al., 1998) and psychiatric inpatient adolescents (Osman et al., 1998).

Assessment for Case Formulation and Treatment Planning

Self-report measures provide efficient assessment of SITB but in some cases result in arbitrary scores (Blanton & Jaccard, 2006; e.g., a score of 15 on the BSI) and do not allow for follow-up questions to clarify what actually took place during an SITB event. Several interviews, however, overcome both of these limitations by assessing the presence of actual SITB outcomes and nonarbitrary characteristics, such as the number of weeks out of the past year a person has thought about suicide. Most interviews also permit follow-up questions to clarify the details of SITB occurrences.

Structured and Semistructured Interviews

Many of the interviews we review are referred to as structured interviews (Linehan, Comtois, Brown, Heard, & Wagner, 2006; Nock et al., 2007); however, these instruments' instructions permit interviewers to ask unstructured follow-up questions to accurately classify a behavior in question (e.g., classify a behavior as an aborted attempt vs. an actual attempt). Given the availability of these unstructured follow-up questions, we do not differentiate between structured and semistructured interviews.

The SITBI (Nock et al., 2007), a structured interview with long (169-item) and short (72-item) forms, provides a comprehensive assessment of SITB, including suicidal ideation, plans, and attempts, aborted and interrupted attempts, NSSI, and knowledge of others with a history of suicidal behaviors. For each outcome endorsed, the SITBI also assesses several characteristics, such as age of onset, frequency, severity, method used (for behaviors), self-reported reason for engaging in the SITB, the presence of external and internal stressors, use of alcohol or drugs, and experience of pain during SITB engagement. Questions on the SITBI are to be read as worded, but interviewers may ask clarifying ad hoc questions to accurately classify the behavior. Thus, like several of the other measures, it is important that interviewers be trained to know precise definitions of each SITB to provide accurate classification. It takes between 3 and 75 minutes to administer the SITBI, depending on the modules administered.

Nock and colleagues (2007) tested the reliability and validity of scores on the SITBI among adolescents and young adults (ages 12–19 years) and reported excellent interrater reliability and adequate test–retest reliability for the presence of each self-injurious outcome assessed over a 6-month period. Scores on the SITBI also showed good concurrent validity among a sample of adolescents in a psychiatric inpatient setting (Venta & Sharp, 2014) and has been used to assess SITB in children as young as 7 years old (Barrocas, Hankin, Young, & Abela, 2012). As of the writing of this chapter,

an updated version of the SITBI has been tested and an article is now available online (Fox, Harris, Millner, & Nock, 2020). The recent changes include adding several passive suicidal ideation items (the original version did not ask about passive ideation) and removing a question about the presence of a "suicide plan" in favor of questions regarding specific planning steps. Also, the validity and reliability of scores on the aborted and interrupted attempts sections were tested for the first time (these constructs were added to the original instrument after the initial validation study). Finally, an online version of the updated SITBI was validated. Overall, responses on the updated SITBI were found to have strong psychometric properties, similar to the original version. One limitation of this recent study, as it pertains to assessing youth, is that it was conducted with adults, whereas the first validation study was mainly with adolescents. However, given that the majority of the updated instrument was identical to the original version, the updated version would likely continue to show strong psychometric properties among youth, although it has not been fully tested yet.

The *Suicide Attempt Self-Injury Interview* (SASII; Linehan, Comtois, Brown, et al., 2006) is a 31-item structured interview that assesses detailed characteristics of and motivations for a self-injurious action (or "clusters" of actions). For a given self-injurious event, such as a suicide attempt or NSSI, the SASII assesses the following: the intent and expected outcome (e.g., death); the method used to injure; the extent to which the act was impulsive; medical and life consequences of the action; whether self-injurious intent was communicated; context, function and other mental characteristics (e.g., being "disconnected from feelings"); and other circumstances occurring when the action took place. The SASII is used to assess in-depth characteristics of instances when actual self-injury occurred and therefore does not assess suicidal thoughts or suicide planning unconnected to a self-injurious event, interrupted or aborted attempts, or suicide gestures. In addition to the SASII, there is an abbreviated L-SASII, that measures lifetime self-injurious actions and their characteristics. Scores on both measures have shown good concurrent validity and sensitivity to change in studies with adolescents (Crowell et al., 2012; Kaufman et al., 2018; McCauley et al., 2018).

Given that SASII is intended to assess a high level of detail about every self-injurious event, it may be time-intensive for respondents with a longer history of self-injury. An alternative is that the measure permits the interviewer to focus on self-injurious events within a given time period. Scores on the SASII show excellent interrating reliability and adequate validity metrics. As with the SITBI, interviewers should be trained in SITBI definitions and categorization because, although they are instructed to state the interview questions as worded, they should use unstructured follow-up questions to gather additional details or clarify responses (Bland & Murray-Gregory, 2006).

The C-SSRS (Posner et al., 2011) is a semistructured interview that assesses the presence of lifetime SITB and characteristics of ideation. There are three sections that assess (1) ideation, plans and intent together in increasing severity (ranging from passive ideation to ideation with a specific plan and intent), (2) characteristics of ideation (frequency, intensity, controllability, and deterrents of suicidal ideation, as well as reasons for ideation), and (3) presence and frequency of self-injurious actions (suicide attempts, NSSI, interrupted and aborted attempts, preparatory actions). When a suicide attempt is endorsed, follow-up questions assess the actual and potential lethality of the attempt. The first section is rated on a 1- to 5-point scale, depending on the most severe combination of ideation, plans, and intent.

A study of the reliability and validity of the C-SSRS found scores with excellent internal consistency and moderate-to-good convergent validity for each section among adolescents (Posner et al., 2011). The "since last visit" version (which was used in studies assessing SITB outcomes every 4–6 weeks and is nearly identical to the baseline version) also had scores with strong convergent validity, sensitivity to change, and predictive validity among adolescents (Gipson et al., 2015; Horwitz et al., 2015; Posner et al., 2011). There also is a pediatric version of the C-SSRS, although it has not been evaluated, and we could find no study that has used it. The phrasing of the pediatric version is identical to the original scale with one exception: The pediatric version uses the phrase "make yourself not alive anymore" (e.g., "Have you thought about doing something to make yourself not alive anymore?") instead of "kill yourself." As mentioned, the creators of the C-SSRS have established several options for training on C-SSRS administration, including Web-based videos and tutorials. Furthermore, the measure itself contains definitions for several constructs. The instructions state that the questions included are intended to be guidelines and do not have to be asked. Instead, like the other interviews, interviewers should focus on collecting information to accurately classify the behavior in question. There is also an electronic version of the C-SSRS (eC-SSRS; Mundt et al., 2010) that has scores with adequate reliability and good convergent and predictive validity (Greist, Mundt, Gwaltney, Jefferson, & Posner, 2014; Mundt et al., 2013). The C-SSRS takes between 5 and 11 minutes to administer (Sheehan, Alphs, et al., 2014). Finally, of note, FDA and other government agencies support the C-SSRS as a scale for SITB assessment in clinical trials.

The *Sheehan–Suicide Tracking Scale* (S-STS; Sheehan, Giddens, & Sheehan, 2014b) is a 16-item structured interview that assesses a range of SITB, including "accidental" overdoses, several forms of passive ideation (within a single question), active ideation, suicidal command hallucinations, specific planning steps, intent to act on suicidal thoughts, intent to die from the act itself, an impulse to kill oneself, preparatory actions, NSSI, and suicide attempts. Items are either rated on a scale of 0–4 (ranging from *not at all* to *extremely*) or collect frequency information. Interrupted and aborted attempts are not assessed; however, they can be inferred to some degree (although imprecisely; see Youngstrom et al., 2015) if a person endorses having selected a time to attempt suicide and taking active steps to prepare for an attempt but never actually engaging in a suicide attempt. There also is a self-report version of S-STS that is identical to the interview. Some studies with the S-STS have used a computerized self-report scale and clinician interview that alerts the clinician to deviations between the interview and self-reported ratings. This gives the clinician an opportunity to reconcile discrepant items with the patient (Sheehan, Alphs, et al., 2014; Sheehan, Giddens, & Sheehan, 2014b). To create pediatric versions of the S-STS, the authors consulted with reading specialists and used empirically derived graded vocabulary lists. The result of this work was three different "linguistically validated" versions of the S-STS for youth: one for children ages 6–8 years, another for children ages 9–12 years, and one for adolescents ages 13–17 (Amado, Beamon, & Sheehan, 2014). However, none of these versions has received psychometric evaluation.

The only study that evaluated the psychometric properties of the S-STS used a sample of young Italian adults, who were mostly undergraduate students. An early version of the S-STS was tested; it therefore contained only eight items rather than the 16 items in the more recent version (Preti et al., 2013; Sheehan, Giddens, & Sheehan, 2014b).

Outcomes for suicidal behaviors had acceptable internal consistency but moderate-to-poor test–retest reliability. Scores on each S-STS section showed acceptable convergent and criterion validity. Like the other interviews, the authors recommend that interviewers be trained in the definitions of suicidal behaviors and encourage the use of additional information to improve classification accuracy. The S-STS has a patient-rated version, a clinician-rated version, a "clinically meaningful change measure" version, and can be adapted for use over any time period (e.g., since the last visit). The administration time is 4–13 minutes for the S-STS self-report scale, 3–15 minutes for the S-STS interview, and 1.5–3.5 minutes for the reconciliation form (Sheehan, Alphs, et al., 2014).

The *Scale for Suicide Ideation* (SSI; Beck, Kovacs, & Weissman, 1979) is a semistructured interview with 21 items to assess characteristics of past week suicidal thoughts and actions, including the presence, frequency, and severity of suicidal thoughts, as well as reasons for suicide, planning, and the presence and intent of prior attempts. Items are on a 2-point scale (0–2). A total score is calculated by summing the first 19 items. Items regarding prior suicide attempts are excluded from the total score. It takes approximately 10 minutes to administer the SSI. Scores on the SSI have shown good-to-excellent internal consistency, and multiple studies have supported their validity among psychiatric inpatient children and adolescents (Allan, Kashani, Dahlmeier, Taghizadeh, & Reid, 1997; Nock & Kazdin, 2002) as well as outpatient adolescents (Holi et al., 2005).

The *Suicide Behaviors Interview* (SBI; Reynolds, 1990) is a 22-item semistructured interview that assesses suicidal behaviors among adolescents. Items are rated on scales of 0–2 or 0–4. The first section assesses risk factors for suicidal behaviors, including major negative life events, chronic and acute stress, and social support. The second section assesses suicidal SITB, suicidal ideation, suicide planning, and suicide attempts, as well as characteristics of the most recent attempt, such as the confidence that one would die. Scores on the SBI have good internal consistency and excellent interrater reliability, as well as adequate content and good convergent validity (Reynolds, 1990; Reynolds & Mazza, 1999).

The *Child Suicide Potential Scales* (CSPS; Pfeffer, Conte, Plutchik, & Jerrett, 1979) include a semistructured interview with eight scales, only one of which measures suicidal behavior (ranging from nonsuicidal to "serious" attempts on a 5-point spectrum). Other sections assess precipitating events, family background, one's concept of death, ego functioning (emotion regulation) and ego defense (e.g., denial). Finally, there are two sections that assess emotional states and behaviors, one in the previous 6 months and one more than 6 months prior. The psychometric properties of the CSPS are relatively strong, with excellent to adequate internal consistency for all but one scale (Precipitating Events), excellent interrater reliability (Ofek, Weizman, & Apter, 1998; Pfeffer et al., 1979) and concurrent validity demonstrated in numerous studies across both clinical and typical populations (Pfeffer, Conte, Plutchik, & Jerrett, 1980; Pfeffer, Newcorn, Kaplan, Mizruchi, & Plutchik, 1988; Pfeffer, Solomon, Plutchik, Mizruchi, & Weiner, 1982; Pfeffer, Zuckerman, Plutchik, & Mizruchi, 1984).

Summary

There is a large assortment of interviews to assess SITB (see Table 9.1); however, the instruments assess many different of characteristics of SITB. Therefore, the selection of an instrument should be based on the purpose and focus of the assessment. For example, some instruments collect in-depth characteristics (e.g., presence and frequency) of an array of SITB (e.g., SITBI, SASII, C-SSRS, STS), others collect only the presence of several outcomes, as well as other factors (CSPS). The reader should consider the goals of assessment and the outcomes of interest when selecting an assessment instrument. Within clinical settings, we recommend that each form of SITB be comprehensively assessed. The denial of some SITB (e.g., a suicide plan) may not preclude the presence of more severe forms of SITB (e.g., a suicide attempt). In addition, many SITB co-occur, and the presence of less severe SITB outcomes predict more severe SITB.

Assessment of Aspects of SITB

During case conceptualization or treatment planning, it is important to assess factors that individual patients report as influencing the occurrence of each SITB. These patient-reported factors might be related to risk factors associated with SITB, although, as noted previously, a recent meta-analysis suggests that most risk factors are weak prospective predictors of SITB (Franklin et al., 2017) potentially because risk factors for SITB vary for

TABLE 9.1. Ratings of Instruments to Assess SITB in Youth

Instrument	NSSI			Suicidal ideation				Suicide plans				Aborted and interrupted attempts		Suicide attempts					Reasons for SITB
	Presence	Frequency	Methods	Presence	Frequency	Severity/intensity	Passive suicidal ideation	Presence	Frequency	Details/specific methods	Preparation	Presence	Frequency	Presence	Frequency	Method used	Circumstances	Medical consequences	
Self-report																			
Beck Scale for Suicidal Ideation (BSI)				y	*	y	y	y	*		*			y	*				
Self-Harm Behavior Questionnaire (SHBQ)	y	y		y	*			y		y				y	y	y	y	y	
Suicidal Behaviors Questionnaire (SBQ)	y	y	y	y	*			y		y				y	y	y	y	y	
SBQ–Revised (SBQ-R)				y				y						y					
Suicidal Ideation Questionnaire (SIQ)				y	y	*	y	y	y		*								
Suicidal Ideation Questionnaire–JR (SIQ-JR)				y	y	*	y	y	y		*								
Harkavy–Asnis Suicide Scale (HASS)				y	y	y	y	y						y	y	y	y	y	y
Interviews																			
Self-Injurious Thoughts and Behaviors Interview (SITBI)	y	y	y	y	y	y	y	y	y	y		y	y	y	y	y	y	y	y
Suicide Attempt Self-Injury (SASII)	y	y	y	y	*			y			*		y	y	*	y	y	y	y
Columbia–Suicide Severity Rating Scale (C-SSRS)				y	y	y	y	y			y	y	y	y	y	y	y	y	y
Sheehan–Suicide Tracking Scale (S-STS)				y			y	y				y	y	y	y				
Scale for Suicide Ideation (SSI)				y	*	y	y	y	*		*			y	*				
Suicide Behaviors Interview (SBI)	y			y	y	y	y	y			*								
Child Suicide Potential Scales (CSPS)				y										y				y	

Note. "y" indicates that yes, the instrument covers this content; *indicates that the SITB characteristic was specified on a rating scale or within the question (i.e., a specific form of preparation).

different people. Therefore, individual patients' specific reasons and circumstances that precede SITB events are important to assess and may provide information for treatment targets. Several instruments that can help with the assessment of reasons for engaging in SITB are described below.

Although it is not possible to determine definitively an individuals' risk of engaging in a future SITB, there are a few factors worth considering. First, all forms of suicidal SITB are associated with the presence of mental disorders (Nock, Borges, Bromet, Alonso, et al., 2008). However, disorders that are the largest cross-sectional predictors of suicidal ideation, such as major depressive disorder, differ from disorders that provide the strongest prediction of suicide attempts among ideators (Nock, Hwang, Sampson, & Kessler, 2010; Nock, Hwang, et al., 2009). Thus, it is important to identify a patient's SITB history and his or her current state and how risk factors may change depending on the severity of the recent SITB.

Two interviews that can be used to determine the presence or absence of SITB, the SITBI and the SASII, also assess information regarding an individual's reasons for engaging in SITB and situational conditions during SITB, such as stressors or triggers. In addition, there are several stand-alone measures for this purpose.

The *Reasons for Suicide Attempt Questionnaire* (RASQ; Holden, Kerr, Mendonca, & Velamoor, 1998) contains 14 items that assess motivations for attempting suicide across two subscales: Extrapunitive/Manipulative Reasons (eight items) and Internal Perturbation Based Motivations (six items). The RASQ has shown good psychometric properties within several populations (Holden & Delisle, 2006; Holden et al., 1998; Holden & Kroner, 2003), but we know of no studies among youth conducted with this instrument.

The FASM (Lloyd et al., 1997) is an interview to assess characteristics and functions of NSSI. As such, the FASM does not assess any suicidal behaviors. It provides 12 NSSI methods that respondents can endorse. For each endorsed method, the respondent is asked to relate how often this method was used (i.e., frequency) and how often medical treatment was required. In addition, several characteristics of general NSSI are assessed, including when NSSI started (i.e., age of onset), how impulsively the individual engaged in NSSI, history of substance use, and the amount of pain one feels during NSSI. The FASM also assesses 22 different reasons for engaging in NSSI. Among adolescent samples, scores on the FASM have shown excellent-to-adequate internal consistency (Guertin, Lloyd-Richardson, Spirito, Donaldson, & Boergers, 2001; Klonsky, May, & Glenn, 2013) and excellent convergent validity with the SITBI (Nock et al., 2007).

Prior studies using factor analyses of FASM items (Nock & Prinstein, 2004) or theoretically derived subscales on the SASII (Brown, Comtois, & Linehan, 2002) suggest a four-function model of self-injury. The functions followed a 2×2 pattern whereby NSSI is negatively or positively reinforced (i.e., to terminate a negative experience or trigger a positive experience), crossed with being intrapersonal (i.e., carried out to affect one's own emotions) or interpersonal (i.e., to affect others). These functions have received empirical support in several studies, including among adolescents (Bentley, Nock, & Barlow, 2014).

The *Inventory of Statements about Self-Injury* (ISAS; Klonsky & Glenn, 2009) assesses reasons for engaging in NSSI and is has considerable overlap with the FASM. The ISAS assesses 12 NSSI methods that mostly overlap with those assessed in the FASM: age of onset, impulsiveness of the behaviors, experience of physical pain, and reasons for engaging in self-injury, some of which are the behavioral functions served by the behavior. The ISAS aims to assess 13 behavioral functions of NSSI, but factor analysis suggests that it captures only two functions: the interpersonal and intrapersonal functions of NSSI (Klonsky & Glenn, 2009). This finding was replicated among a sample of mostly adolescents (Klonsky, Glenn, Styer, Olino, & Washburn, 2015). Scores on the ISAS among adolescents have shown strong psychometric properties (Bildik, Somer, Kabukçu Başay, Başay, & Özbaran, 2013; Klonsky et al., 2015).

The IMSA (May & Klonsky, 2013) contains 40 items for 10 separate scales that assess self-reported reasons for attempting suicide, including Hopelessness, Psychache, Escape, Burdensomeness, Low Belongingness, Fearlessness, Help Seeking, Interpersonal Influence, Problem Solving, and Impulsivity. This scale is intended to assess a wider array of reasons for attempting suicide than the RSAQ. A study with adolescents found a two-factor solution for the functions, which consisted of internal motivations (e.g., hopelessness) and communicative motivations (e.g., interpersonal influence) and found favorable psychometric properties (May, O'Brien, Liu, & Klonsky, 2016).

The *Multi-Attitude Suicide Tendency Scale for Adolescents* (MAST; Orbach et al., 1991) contains 30 items that examines four components: attraction and repulsion to both life and death. Scores on the MAST have demonstrated adequate to excellent reliability (Orbach et al., 1991; Osman et al., 1994) and concurrent validity (Cotton & Range, 1993; Muehlenkamp & Gutierrez, 2004) in youth samples.

Summary

There are several measures for assessing people's reasons for engaging in suicidal or NSSI SITB. These measures can assist in case conceptualization and suggest potential treatment targets. For example, if a patient reports attempting suicide because of painful emotions, then implementing emotion regulation or distress tolerance skills might be an effective treatment. If, on the other hand, SITB are intended to communicate the severity of psychological distress to others, then interpersonal effectiveness might be a useful skill to address this issue. An important limitation, however, is that although it may make sense to use a functional approach to selecting treatment targets, no research has tested whether the aforementioned scales assessing various functions for SITB actually enhance case conceptualization or improve treatment outcomes.

Treatment Progress and Outcome Measurement

A recent review of treatments for SITB among youth found generally little empirical support for interventions to reduce SITB (Glenn, Esposito, Porter, & Robinson, 2019). At the time of this review, one treatment approach, dialectical behavior therapy (DBT), qualified as a well-established treatment (based on standards set forth by the *Journal of Clinical Child and Adolescent Psychology*). Some interventions were rated as "probably" or "possibly efficacious," but most were only supported by a single study. Overall, there is modest support for treatments aimed at reducing SITB in youth (Brent et al., 2009; Glenn et al., 2019).

Given that the foci of treatment monitoring and outcome evaluation are to track the presence, frequency, and severity of SITB, many of the instruments described in this chapter can be used for these purposes. It should be noted, however, that only a single study has provided psychometric support for instruments assessing changes in SITB among youth over time (Posner et al., 2011). Clearly, it is important to assess a period of time that corresponds to the time between assessments.

Assessing SITB over a period longer than the time between assessments could result in SITB being recorded in both the current and past assessments (i.e., doubly counted). Alternatively, if the assessment is shorter than the time between assessments, some SITB might be mistakenly omitted. Several instruments, including the C-SSRS, S-STS and SASII, allow for flexible assessments time periods in their instructions (Bland & Murray-Gregory, 2006; Posner et al., 2011; Sheehan, Giddens, & Sheehan, 2014b); however, this is an arbitrary decision that could be applied to other scales, such as the SITBI, that do not explicitly provide this flexibility. The C-SSRS provides a "since last visit" version, with the only difference being that it says "since last visit" rather than "lifetime" where one circles the responses. This C-SSRS "since last visit" scale was tested among adolescents for sensitivity to change by correlating C-SSRS outcomes with SITB outcomes assessed with other measures (Posner et al., 2011). Several studies have used the SASII to monitor progress and evaluate outcomes (Linehan, Comtois, Murray, et al., 2006; Linehan et al., 2015; McMain et al., 2009), although only one such study has been among adolescents (McCauley et al., 2018). Other relatively untested versions of instruments for treatment monitoring and outcome evaluation are abbreviated C-SSRS screeners for assessment of past month or "since last contact" SITBI and a "clinically meaningful change" version of the S-STS that assesses purported SITB risk factors, the severity of self-injurious thoughts, and the capacity not to engage in SITB (Sheehan, Giddens, & Sheehan, 2014b). Overall, several measures are appropriate for treatment progress and outcome measurement, in that they measure the presence and characteristics of SITB, which are the focus of treatment. However, as mentioned, there is little evidence supporting their use for such cases.

Summary

There are several instruments with psychometric support for cross-sectional evaluation of the presence, frequency, and characteristics of SITB and, presumably, these instruments can be used to assess SITB to monitor treatment progress and evaluate treatment outcomes. However, nearly all instruments lack psychometric evidence showing that they validly assess changes in SITB over time, leaving open the possibility that repeated assessment adversely affects precise measurement. In general, we recommend that SITB are evaluated as rigorously and comprehensively as possible, to inform treatment planning and risk assessment. This may require well-trained interviewers and further questioning to ascertain the actual series of events that occurred during a reported SITB (e.g., did the person actually swallow the pills or just get very close to doing so?). We also recommend that SITB be routinely assessed to inform treatment modifications and continuous risk monitoring. Finally, it is assumed that the use of instruments with empirical support provide enhanced clinical care and decision making; however, this assumption is untested. Future research should examine whether assessment instruments have clinical utility for treatment planning, monitoring, and outcomes.

Conclusions and Future Directions

We have provided an overview of a relatively large number of instruments available for assessing SITB and their characteristics among youth. We have also reviewed research indicating that some SITB measurement approaches can lead to misclassification, both within research and clinical settings (Brown et al., 2015; Hom et al., 2015; Millner et al., 2015; Plöderl et al., 2011). Given that adolescents and children may have less understanding of operational definitions, this problem may be more acute among youth (Velting et al., 1998). Therefore, we emphasize the importance of having interviewers be well trained in the classification of SITB and ensuring that youth understand terms describing outcomes of interest, such as a suicide attempt. We also reiterate that when selecting which instruments to use, one should carefully consider the purpose and goals of assessment.

There are several future directions for improving the assessment of SITB among youth. First, as we mentioned earlier, in a study that assessed a range of SITB-related outcomes, adolescents were asked to explain discrepancies between SITB outcomes on interview and self-report forms. Fifty percent of the sample provided discrepant results, and there were several different explanations for the discrepancies, including a lack of understanding of operational definition of particular terms, intentional minimization of SITB, carelessness, misunderstanding of instructions, or for unknown reasons (Velting et al., 1998). These each represent threats to valid measurement of SITB. Future studies should replicate this study with larger samples and report the percentage of each cause

of discrepant reporting to better understand the magnitude of each. In addition, research should focus on understanding approaches to minimize these discrepancies to provide more accurate and valid measurement. For example, providing definitions and examples could help increase youth participants' understanding of operational definitions for SITB terms measured. Research could also test prompts that perhaps reduce stigma or help participants feel more comfortable answering questions about SITB to reduce intentional minimization or nondisclosure. Finally, research could examine incentives or other efforts to combat careless responding. Overall, research seeking to understand the causes of SITB and effectively treat and prevent SITB relies on accurate measurement of these outcomes. Therefore, it is critical that researchers work toward increasing the validity of SITB assessments.

Second, it is worth noting that advanced computational and statistical approaches, such as machine learning, are now being used to predict SITB. Recent studies have produced compelling classification characteristics regarding who attempted suicide over different periods of time by applying advanced statistics to, for example, electronic health records or military administrative records (Barak-Corren et al., 2017; Kessler et al., 2015; McCarthy et al., 2015; Walsh, Ribeiro, & Franklin, 2017). These powerful techniques could potentially identify outcomes that are most relevant to assess (i.e., which outcomes to ask the patient about) in terms of risk and to use a wide range of variables to increase the precision of risk prediction. Currently, these approaches have yet to be integrated into everyday health care practices. However, it is possible that in the ensuing decades they will transform our approach to assessing risk and treatment of SITB for both youth and adults.

Third, there are several future directions that would advance the understanding of SITB. First, there is a lack of basic descriptions of many important SITB processes, particularly how these processes operate on a short-term basis (i.e., within hours or days). For example, there is little information on (1) the degree to which SITB, such as NSSI and suicidal ideation, fluctuate throughout a day, week or month (Armey, Crowther, & Miller, 2011; Kleiman et al., 2017; Nock, Prinstein, & Sterba, 2009), (2) the trajectory of problematic behaviors (e.g., alcohol use) and SITB in the hours or days prior to an attempt (Bagge, Glenn, & Lee, 2013; Bagge, Lee, et al., 2013; Bagge, Littlefield, Conner, Schumacher, & Lee, 2014) and, relatedly, (3) when thinking and planning steps occur prior to a suicide attempt (Bagge, Littlefield, & Lee, 2013; Millner, Lee, & Nock, 2017). Collecting information on these outcomes involve assessments that differ from those described in this chapter. For example, Millner and colleagues (2017) introduced an instrument called the Pathway to Suicide Action Interview (PSAI), which assesses the timing of different planning steps and decision points just prior to a suicide attempt. This instrument assesses specific details that are best recounted around the time of a suicide attempt; otherwise, the information is likely imprecise due to memory. Furthermore, the PSAI has not received formal psychometric testing. Another SITB assessment approach not included here is the use of ecological momentary assessment (EMA; i.e., in which participants report current thoughts, behaviors, or feelings on a mobile device), which allows researchers to gain insight into short-term (i.e., within hours) changes in SITB. These assessments are usually in the form of single items, and there has been little psychometric work done on EMA or the SITB items used in this approach. Some researchers have started to use EMA to collect information on the basic description of short-term SITB processes that can help inform the understanding of when and why people think about and try to kill themselves. Another exciting and novel but untested approach is to provide participants with wearable technology, such as smart watches, that can collect passive psychophysiological and movement data (Onnela & Rauch, 2016). Other *in vivo* data that can now be collected with mobile devices include voice samples (to extract voice characteristics, such as prosody; Pestian et al., 2017) and number of incoming and outgoing texts or phone calls to approximate social interactions. Finally, some researchers have found that outcomes on reaction time-based behavioral tasks prospectively predict suicidal outcomes (Nock et al., 2010; Nock & Banaji, 2007; Randall, Rowe, Dong, Nock, & Colman, 2013); however, more research is required. The ultimate goal is to use advanced statistics and computational approaches to identify the most relevant outcomes across self-report, passive and active monitoring, and behavioral task outcomes for predicting SITB and to combine them in predictive models that can greatly improve efforts to predict and prevent SITB. Until that time, this chapter provides information on several instruments that can be used by researchers and clinicians to assess SITB.

REFERENCES

Allan, W. D., Kashani, J. H., Dahlmeier, J., Taghizadeh, P., & Reid, J. C. (1997). Psychometric properties and clinical utility of the Scale for Suicide Ideation with inpatient children. *Journal of Abnormal Child Psychology, 25*(6), 465–473.

Amado, D. M., Beamon, D. A., & Sheehan, D. V. (2014). Linguistic validation of the pediatric versions of the Sheehan Suicidality Tracking Scale (S-STS). *Innovations in Clinical Neuroscience, 11*(9–10), 141–163.

American Psychiatric Association. (2013). *Diagnostic and statistical manual of mental disorders* (5th ed.). Arlington, VA: Author.

Andrews, T., Martin, G., Hasking, P., & Page, A. (2013). Predictors of continuation and cessation of nonsuicidal self-injury. *Journal of Adolescent Health, 53*(1), 40–46.

Armey, M. F., Crowther, J. H., & Miller, I. W. (2011). Changes in ecological momentary assessment reported affect associated with episodes of nonsuicidal self-injury. *Behavior Therapy, 42*(4), 579–588.

Asarnow, J., McArthur, D., Hughes, J., Barbery, V., & Berk, M. (2012). Suicide attempt risk in youths: Utility of the Harkavy–Asnis Suicide Scale for monitoring risk levels. *Suicide and Life-Threatening Behavior, 42*(6), 684–698.

Augenstein, T. M., Visser, K. H., Gallagher, K., De Los Reyes, A., D'Angelo, E. J., & Nock, M. K. (2018). *Multi-informant reports of depressive symptoms and explicit suicidal ideation among adolescent inpatients.* Unpublished manuscript, University of Rochester, Rochester, NY.

Bagge, C. L., Glenn, C. R., & Lee, H.-J. (2013). Quantifying the impact of recent negative life events on suicide attempts. *Journal of Abnormal Psychology, 122*(2), 359–368.

Bagge, C. L., Lee, H.-J., Schumacher, J. A., Gratz, K. L., Krull, J. L., & Holloman, G. (2013). Alcohol as an acute risk factor for recent suicide attempts: A case-crossover analysis. *Journal of Studies on Alcohol and Drugs, 74*(4), 552–558.

Bagge, C. L., Littlefield, A. K., Conner, K. R., Schumacher, J. A., & Lee, H.-J. (2014). Near-term predictors of the intensity of suicidal ideation: An examination of the 24h prior to a recent suicide attempt. *Journal of Affective Disorders, 165*, 53–58.

Bagge, C. L., Littlefield, A. K., & Lee, H.-J. (2013). Correlates of proximal premeditation among recently hospitalized suicide attempters. *Journal of Affective Disorders, 150*(2), 559–564.

Barak-Corren, Y., Castro, V. M., Javitt, S., Hoffnagle, A. G., Dai, Y., Perlis, R. H., . . . Reis, B. Y. (2017). Predicting suicidal behavior from longitudinal electronic health records. *American Journal of Psychiatry, 174*(2), 154–162.

Barrocas, A. L., Hankin, B. L., Young, J. F., & Abela, J. R. Z. (2012). Rates of nonsuicidal self-injury in youth:

Age, sex, and behavioral methods in a community sample. *Pediatrics, 130*(1), 39–45.

Beck, A. T., Kovacs, M., & Weissman, A. (1979). Assessment of suicidal intention: The Scale of Suicide Ideation. *Journal of Consulting and Clinical Psychology, 47*(2), 343–352.

Beck, A. T., & Steer, R. A. (1991). *Manual for the Beck Scale for Suicide Ideation.* San Antonio, TX: Psychological Corporation.

Bentley, K. H., Nock, M. K., & Barlow, D. H. (2014). The four-function model of nonsuicidal self-injury key directions for future research. *Clinical Psychological Science, 2*(5), 638–656.

Bildik, T., Somer, O., Kabukçu Başay, B., Başay, Ö., & Özbaran, B. (2013). The validity and reliability of the Turkish version of the inventory of statements about self-injury. *Turkish Journal of Psychiatry, 24*(1), 49–57.

Bland, S., & Murray-Gregory, A. (2006, September 28). Instructions for use of Suicide Attempt Self-Injury Interview. Retrieved from *http://depts.washington.edu/brtc/files/SASII%20Instructions.pdf.*

Blanton, H., & Jaccard, J. (2006). Arbitrary metrics redux. *American Psychologist, 61*(1), 62–71.

Brausch, A. M., & Gutierrez, P. M. (2010). Differences in non-suicidal self-injury and suicide attempts in adolescents. *Journal of Youth and Adolescence, 39*(3), 233–242.

Brenner, L. A., Breshears, R. E., Betthauser, L. M., Bellon, K. K., Holman, E., Harwood, J. E. F., . . . Nagamoto, H. T. (2011). Implementation of a suicide nomenclature within two VA healthcare settings. *Journal of Clinical Psychology in Medical Settings, 18*(2), 116–128.

Brent, D. A., Greenhill, L. L., Compton, S., Emslie, G., Wells, K., Walkup, J. T., . . . Turner, J. B. (2009). The Treatment of Adolescent Suicide Attempters study (TASA): Predictors of suicidal events in an open treatment trial. *Journal of the American Academy of Child and Adolescent Psychiatry, 48*(10), 987–996.

Brown, G. K., Currier, G. W., Jager-Hyman, S., & Stanley, B. (2015). Detection and classification of suicidal behavior and nonsuicidal self-injury behavior in emergency departments. *Journal of Clinical Psychiatry, 76*(10), 1397–1403.

Brown, M. Z., Comtois, K. A., & Linehan, M. M. (2002). Reasons for suicide attempts and nonsuicidal self-injury in women with borderline personality disorder. *Journal of Abnormal Psychology, 111*(1), 198–202.

Brunner, R., Kaess, M., Parzer, P., Fischer, G., Carli, V., Hoven, C. W., . . . Wasserman, D. (2014). Life-time prevalence and psychosocial correlates of adolescent direct self-injurious behavior: A comparative study of findings in 11 European countries. *Journal of Child Psychology and Psychiatry, 55*(4), 337–348.

Cole, D. A. (1989). Validation of the reasons for living inventory in general and delinquent adolescent samples. *Journal of Abnormal Child Psychology, 17*(1), 13–27.

Cotton, C. R., & Range, L. M. (1993). Suicidality, hopelessness, and attitudes toward life and death in children. *Death Studies, 17*(2), 185–191.

Crowell, S. E., Beauchaine, T. P., Hsiao, R. C., Vasilev, C. A., Yaptangco, M., Linehan, M. M., & McCauley, E. (2012). Differentiating adolescent self-injury from adolescent depression: Possible implications for borderline personality development. *Journal of Abnormal Child Psychology, 40*(1), 45–57.

Fox, K. R., Harris, J. A., Wang., S. B., Millner, A. J., Deming, C. A., & Nock, M. K. (2020). Self-Injurious Thoughts and Behaviors Interview-Revised: Development, reliability, and validity. *Psychological Assessment.* [Epub ahead of print]

Franklin, J. C., Ribeiro, J. D., Fox, K. R., Bentley, K. H., Kleiman, E. M., Huang, X., . . . Nock, M. K. (2017). Risk factors for suicidal thoughts and behaviors: A meta-analysis of 50 years of research. *Psychological Bulletin, 143*(2), 187–232.

Gao, K., Wu, R., Wang, Z., Ren, M., Kemp, D. E., Chan, P. K., . . . Calabrese, J. R. (2015). Disagreement between self-reported and clinician-ascertained suicidal ideation and its correlation with depression and anxiety severity in patients with major depressive disorder or bipolar disorder. *Journal of Psychiatric Research, 60,* 117–124.

Giletta, M., Scholte, R. H. J., Engels, R. C. M. E., Ciairano, S., & Prinstein, M. J. (2012). Adolescent non-suicidal self-injury: A cross-national study of community samples from Italy, the Netherlands and the United States. *Psychiatry Research, 197*(1), 66–72.

Gipson, P. Y., Agarwala, P., Opperman, K. J., Horwitz, A., & King, C. A. (2015). Columbia–Suicide Severity Rating Scale: Predictive validity with adolescent psychiatric emergency patients. *Pediatric Emergency Care, 31*(2), 88–94.

Glenn, C. R., Bagge, C. L., & Osman, A. (2013). Unique associations between borderline personality disorder features and suicide ideation and attempts in adolescents. *Journal of Personality Disorders, 27*(5), 604–616.

Glenn, C. R., Esposito, E. C., Porter, A. C., & Robinson, D. J. (2019). Evidence base update of psychosocial treatments for self-injurious thoughts and behaviors in youth. *Journal of Clinical Child and Adolescent Psychology, 48*(3), 357–392.

Glenn, C. R., Franklin, J. C., & Nock, M. K. (2015). Evidence-based psychosocial treatments for self-injurious thoughts and behaviors in youth. *Journal of Clinical Child and Adolescent Psychology, 44*(1), 1–29.

Goldston, D. B., & Compton, J. S. (2007). Adolescent suicidal and nonsuicidal self-harm behaviors and risk. In E. J. Mash & R. A. Barkley (Eds.), *Assessment of childhood disorders* (4th ed., pp. 305–345). New York: Guilford Press.

Gould, M. S., Marrocco, F. A., Kleinman, M., Thomas, J. G., Mostkoff, K., Cote, J., & Davies, M. (2005). Evaluating iatrogenic risk of youth suicide screening programs: A randomized controlled trial. *Journal of the American Medical Association, 293*(13), 1635–1643.

Greist, J. H., Mundt, J. C., Gwaltney, C. J., Jefferson, J. W., & Posner, K. (2014). Predictive value of baseline electronic Columbia–Suicide Severity Rating Scale (eC–SSRS) assessments for identifying risk of prospective reports of suicidal behavior during research participation. *Innovations in Clinical Neuroscience, 11*(9–10), 23–31.

Guertin, T., Lloyd-Richardson, E., Spirito, A., Donaldson, D., & Boergers, J. (2001). Self-mutilative behavior in adolescents who attempt suicide by overdose. *Journal of the American Academy of Child and Adolescent Psychiatry, 40*(9), 1062–1069.

Gutierrez, P. M., & Osman, A. (2009). Getting the best return on your screening investment: An analysis of the Suicidal Ideation Questionnaire and Reynolds Adolescent Depression Scale. *School Psychology Review, 38*(2), 200–217.

Gutierrez, P. M., Osman, A., Barrios, F. X., & Kopper, B. A. (2001). Development and initial validation of the Self-Harm Behavior Questionnaire. *Journal of Personality Assessment, 77*(3), 475–490.

Gutierrez, P. M., Osman, A., Kopper, B. A., & Barrios, F. X. (2000). Why young people do not kill themselves: The Reasons for Living Inventory for Adolescents. *Journal of Clinical Child Psychology, 29*(2), 177–187.

Harkavy-Friedman, J. M. H., & Asnis, G. M. (1989). Assessment of suicidal behavior: A new instrument. *Psychiatric Annals, 19*(7), 382–387.

Harris, K. M., & Goh, M. T.-T. (2017). Is suicide assessment harmful to participants?: Findings from a randomized controlled trial. *International Journal of Mental Health Nursing, 26,* 181–190.

Hasley, J. P., Ghosh, B., Huggins, J., Bell, M. R., Adler, L. E., & Shroyer, A. L. W. (2008). A review of "suicidal intent" within the existing suicide literature. *Suicide and Life-Threatening Behavior, 38*(5), 576–591.

Hilt, L. M., Nock, M. K., Lloyd-Richardson, E. E., & Prinstein, M. J. (2008). Longitudinal study of nonsuicidal self-injury among young adolescents rates, correlates, and preliminary test of an interpersonal model. *Journal of Early Adolescence, 28*(3), 455–469.

Holden, R. R., & Delisle, M. M. (2006). Factor structure of the Reasons for Attempting Suicide Questionnaire (RASQ) with suicide attempters. *Journal of Psychopathology and Behavioral Assessment, 28*(1), 1–8.

Holden, R. R., Kerr, P. S., Mendonca, J. D., & Velamoor, V. R. (1998). Are some motives more linked to suicide proneness than others? *Journal of Clinical Psychology, 54*(5), 569–576.

Holden, R. R., & Kroner, D. G. (2003). Differentiating suicidal motivations and manifestations in a forensic sample. *Canadian Journal of Behavioural Science, 35*(1), 35–44.

Holi, M. M., Pelkonen, M., Karlsson, L., Kiviruusu, O., Ruuttu, T., Heilä, H., . . . Marttunen, M. (2005). Psy-

chometric properties and clinical utility of the Scale for Suicidal Ideation (SSI) in adolescents. *BMC Psychiatry, 5*(1), Article 8.

Hom, M. A., Joiner, T. E., & Bernert, R. A. (2015). Limitations of a single-item assessment of suicide attempt history: Implications for standardized suicide risk assessment. *Psychological Assessment, 28*(8), 1026–1030.

Horwitz, A. G., Czyz, E. K., & King, C. A. (2015). Predicting future suicide attempts among adolescent and emerging adult psychiatric emergency patients. *Journal of Clinical Child & Adolescent Psychology, 44*(5), 751–761.

Huth-Bocks, A. C., Kerr, D. C. R., Ivey, A. Z., Kramer, A. C., & King, C. A. (2007). Assessment of psychiatrically hospitalized suicidal adolescents: Self-report instruments as predictors of suicidal thoughts and behavior. *Journal of the American Academy of Child and Adolescent Psychiatry, 46*(3), 387–395.

Jacobson, C. M., & Gould, M. (2007). The epidemiology and phenomenology of non-suicidal self-injurious behavior among adolescents: A critical review of the literature. *Archives of Suicide Research, 11*(2), 129–147.

Joiner, T. E., Jr., Rudd, M. D., & Rajab, M. H. (1999). Agreement between self- and clinician-rated suicidal symptoms in a clinical sample of young adults: Explaining discrepancies. *Journal of Consulting and Clinical Psychology, 67*(2), 171–176.

Kassebaum, N., Kyu, H. H., Zoeckler, L., Olsen, H. E., Thomas, K., Pinho, C., . . . Vos, T. (2017). Child and adolescent health from 1990 to 2015: Findings from the Global Burden of Diseases, Injuries, and Risk Factors 2015 Study. *JAMA Pediatrics, 171*(6), 573–592.

Kaufman, E. A., Crowell, S. E., Coleman, J., Puzia, M. E., Gray, D. D., & Strayer, D. L. (2018). Electroencephalographic and cardiovascular markers of vulnerability within families of suicidal adolescents: A pilot study. *Biological Psychology, 136,* 46–56.

Kessler, R. C., Warner, C. H., Ivany, C., Petukhova, M. V., Rose, S., Bromet, E. J., . . . Ursano, R. J. (2015). Predicting suicides after psychiatric hospitalization in US Army soldiers: The Army Study to Assess Risk and Resilience in Servicemembers (Army STARRS). *JAMA Psychiatry, 72*(1), 49–57.

Kim, K. L., Galvan, T., Puzia, M. E., Cushman, G. K., Seymour, K. E., Vanmali, R., . . . Dickstein, D. P. (2015). Psychiatric and self-injury profiles of adolescent suicide attempters versus adolescents engaged in nonsuicidal self-injury. *Suicide and Life-Threatening Behavior, 45*(1), 37–50.

Kleiman, E. M., Turner, B. J., Fedor, S., Beale, E. E., Huffman, J. C., & Nock, M. K. (2017). Examination of real-time fluctuations in suicidal ideation and its risk factors: Results from two ecological momentary assessment studies. *Journal of Abnormal Psychology, 126*(6), 726–738.

Klimes-Dugan, B. (1998). Screening for suicidal ideation in children and adolescents: Methodological considerations. *Journal of Adolescence, 21*(4), 435–444.

Klonsky, E. D., & Glenn, C. R. (2009). Assessing the functions of non-suicidal self-injury: Psychometric properties of the Inventory of Statements about Self-injury (ISAS). *Journal of Psychopathology and Behavioral Assessment, 31*(3), 215–219.

Klonsky, E. D., Glenn, C. R., Styer, D. M., Olino, T. M., & Washburn, J. J. (2015). The functions of non-suicidal self-injury: Converging evidence for a two-factor structure. *Child and Adolescent Psychiatry and Mental Health, 9*(1), 44.

Klonsky, E. D., May, A. M., & Glenn, C. R. (2013). The relationship between nonsuicidal self-injury and attempted suicide: Converging evidence from four samples. *Journal of Abnormal Psychology, 122*(1), 231–237.

Kumar, G., & Steer, R. A. (1995). Psychosocial correlates of suicidal ideation in adolescent psychiatric inpatients. *Suicide and Life-Threatening Behavior, 25*(3), 339–346.

Larzelere, R. E., Smith, G. L., Batenhorst, L. M., & Kelly, D. B. (1996). Predictive validity of the Suicide Probability Scale among adolescents in group home treatment. *Journal of the American Academy of Child and Adolescent Psychiatry, 35*(2), 166–172.

Law, M. K., Furr, R. M., Arnold, E. M., Mneimne, M., Jaquett, C., & Fleeson, W. (2015). Does assessing suicidality frequently and repeatedly cause harm?: A randomized control study. *Psychological Assessment, 27*(4), 1171–1181.

Linehan, M. M. (1981). *Suicide Behaviors Questionnaire.* Unpublished manuscript, University of Washington, Seattle, WA.

Linehan, M. M., Comtois, K. A., Brown, M. Z., Heard, H. L., & Wagner, A. (2006). Suicide Attempt Self-Injury Interview (SASII): Development, reliability, and validity of a scale to assess suicide attempts and intentional self-injury. *Psychological Assessment, 18*(3), 303–312.

Linehan, M. M., Comtois, K. A., Murray, A. M., Brown, M. Z., Gallop, R. J., Heard, H. L., . . . Lindenboim, N. (2006). Two-year randomized controlled trial and follow-up of dialectical behavior therapy vs therapy by experts for suicidal behaviors and borderline personality disorder. *Archives of General Psychiatry, 63*(7), 757–766.

Linehan, M. M., Goodstein, J. L., Nielsen, S. L., & Chiles, J. A. (1983). Reasons for staying alive when you are thinking of killing yourself: The Reasons for Living Inventory. *Journal of Consulting and Clinical Psychology, 51*(2), 276–286.

Linehan, M. M., Korslund, K. E., Harned, M. S., Gallop, R. J., Lungu, A., Neacsiu, A. D., . . . Murray-Gregory, A. M. (2015). Dialectical behavior therapy for high suicide risk in individuals with borderline personality disorder: A randomized clinical trial and component analysis. *JAMA Psychiatry, 72*(5), 475–482.

Lloyd, E. E., Kelley, M. L., & Hope, T. (1997). *Self-mu-tilation in a community sample of adolescents: Descriptive characteristics and provisional prevalence rates.* Presented at the 18th annual meeting of the Society for Behavioral Medicine, New Orleans, LA.

Malone, K. M., Szanto, K., Corbitt, E. M., & Mann, J. J. (1995). Clinical assessment versus research methods in the assessment of suicidal behavior. *American Journal of Psychiatry, 152*(11), 1601–1607.

Matarazzo, B. B., Clemans, T. A., Silverman, M. M., & Brenner, L. A. (2013). The Self-Directed Violence Classification System and the Columbia Classification Algorithm for suicide assessment: A crosswalk. *Suicide and Life-Threatening Behavior, 43*(3), 235–249.

May, A. M., & Klonsky, E. D. (2013). Assessing motivations for suicide attempts: Development and psychometric properties of the Inventory of Motivations for Suicide Attempts. *Suicide and Life-Threatening Behavior, 43*(5), 532–546.

May, A. M., O'Brien, K. H. M., Liu, R. T., & Klonsky, E. D. (2016). Descriptive and psychometric properties of the Inventory of Motivations for Suicide Attempts (IMSA) in an inpatient adolescent sample. *Archives of Suicide Research, 20*(3), 476–482.

McCarthy, J. F., Bossarte, R. M., Katz, I. R., Thompson, C., Kemp, J., Hannemann, C. M., . . . Schoenbaum, M. (2015). Predictive modeling and concentration of the risk of suicide: Implications for preventive interventions in the US Department of Veterans Affairs. *American Journal of Public Health, 105*(9), 1935–1942.

McCauley, E., Berk, M. S., Asarnow, J. R., Adrian, M., Cohen, J., Korslund, K., . . . Linehan, M. M. (2018). Efficacy of dialectical behavior therapy for adolescents at high risk for suicide: A randomized clinical trial. *JAMA Psychiatry, 75*, 777–785.

McMain, S. F., Links, P. S., Gnam, W. H., Guimond, T., Cardish, R. J., Korman, L., & Streiner, D. L. (2009). A randomized trial of dialectical behavior therapy versus general psychiatric management for borderline personality disorder. *American Journal of Psychiatry, 166*(12), 1365–1374.

Millner, A. J., Lee, M. D., & Nock, M. K. (2015). Single-item measurement of suicidal behaviors: Validity and consequences of misclassification. *PLOS ONE, 10*(10), e0141606.

Millner, A. J., Lee, M. D., & Nock, M. K. (2017). Describing and measuring the pathway to suicide attempts: A preliminary study. *Suicide and Life-Threatening Behavior, 47*(3), 353–369.

Millner, A. J., & Nock, M. K. (2018). Self-injurious thoughts and behavior. In E. J. Mash & J. Hunsley (Eds.), *A guide to assessments that work* (2nd ed., pp. 193–215). New York: Oxford University Press.

Muehlenkamp, J. J., Claes, L., Havertape, L., & Plener, P. L. (2012). International prevalence of adolescent non-suicidal self-injury and deliberate self-harm. *Child and Adolescent Psychiatry and Mental Health, 6*(1), 10.

Muehlenkamp, J. J., Cowles, M. L., & Gutierrez, P. M.

(2009). Validity of the Self-Harm Behavior Questionnaire with diverse adolescents. *Journal of Psychopathology and Behavioral Assessment, 32*(2), 236–245.

Muehlenkamp, J. J., & Gutierrez, P. M. (2004). An investigation of differences between self-injurious behavior and suicide attempts in a sample of adolescents. *Suicide and Life-Threatening Behavior, 34*(1), 12–23.

Mundt, J. C., Greist, J. H., Gelenberg, A. J., Katzelnick, D. J., Jefferson, J. W., & Modell, J. G. (2010). Feasibility and validation of a computer-automated Columbia-Suicide Severity Rating Scale using interactive voice response technology. *Journal of Psychiatric Research, 44*(16), 1224–1228.

Mundt, J. C., Greist, J. H., Jefferson, J. W., Federico, M., Mann, J. J., & Posner, K. (2013). Prediction of suicidal behavior in clinical research by lifetime suicidal ideation and behavior ascertained by the electronic Columbia-Suicide Severity Rating Scale. *Journal of Clinical Psychiatry, 74*(9), 887–893.

Nock, M. K., & Banaji, M. R. (2007). Prediction of suicide ideation and attempts among adolescents using a brief performance-based test. *Journal of Consulting and Clinical Psychology, 75*(5), 707–715.

Nock, M. K., Borges, G., Bromet, E. J., Alonso, J., Angermeyer, M., Beautrais, A., . . . Williams, D. (2008). Cross-national prevalence and risk factors for suicidal ideation, plans and attempts. *British Journal of Psychiatry, 192*(2), 98–105.

Nock, M. K., Borges, G., Bromet, E. J., Cha, C. B., Kessler, R. C., & Lee, S. (2008). Suicide and suicidal behavior. *Epidemiologic Reviews, 30*(1), 133–154.

Nock, M. K., Green, J. G., Hwang, I., McLaughlin, K. A., Sampson, N. A., Zaslavsky, A. M., & Kessler, R. C. (2013). Prevalence, correlates, and treatment of lifetime suicidal behavior among adolescents: Results from the National Comorbidity Survey Replication Adolescent Supplement. *JAMA Psychiatry, 70*(3), 300–310.

Nock, M. K., Holmberg, E. B., Photos, V. I., & Michel, B. D. (2007). Self-Injurious Thoughts and Behaviors Interview: Development, reliability, and validity in an adolescent sample. *Psychological Assessment, 19*(3), 309–317.

Nock, M. K., Hwang, I., Sampson, N. A., & Kessler, R. C. (2010). Mental disorders, comorbidity and suicidal behavior: Results from the National Comorbidity Survey Replication. *Molecular Psychiatry, 15*(8), 868–876.

Nock, M. K., Hwang, I., Sampson, N., Kessler, R. C., Angermeyer, M., Beautrais, A., . . . Williams, D. R. (2009). Cross-national analysis of the associations among mental disorders and suicidal behavior: Findings from the WHO World Mental Health Surveys. *PLOS Medicine, 6*(8), e1000123.

Nock, M. K., & Kazdin, A. E. (2002). Examination of affective, cognitive, and behavioral factors and suicide-related outcomes in children and young adoles-

cents. *Journal of Clinical Child and Adolescent Psychology, 31*(1), 48–58.

Nock, M. K., & Kessler, R. C. (2006). Prevalence of and risk factors for suicide attempts versus suicide gestures: Analysis of the National Comorbidity Survey. *Journal of Abnormal Psychology, 115*(3), 616–623.

Nock, M. K., Park, J. M., Finn, C. T., Deliberto, T. L., Dour, H. J., & Banaji, M. R. (2010). Measuring the suicidal mind: Implicit cognition predicts suicidal behavior. *Psychological Science, 21*(4), 511–517.

Nock, M. K., & Prinstein, M. J. (2004). A functional approach to the assessment of self-mutilative behavior. *Journal of Consulting and Clinical Psychology, 72*(5), 885–890.

Nock, M. K., Prinstein, M. J., & Sterba, S. K. (2009). Revealing the form and function of self-injurious thoughts and behaviors: A real-time ecological assessment study among adolescents and young adults. *Journal of Abnormal Psychology, 118*(4), 816–827.

O'Carroll, P. W., Berman, A. L., Maris, R. W., Moscicki, E. K., Tanney, B. L., & Silverman, M. M. (1996). Beyond the tower of Babel: A nomenclature for suicidology. *Suicide and Life-Threatening Behavior, 26*(3), 237–252.

Ofek, H., Weizman, T., & Apter, A. (1998). The child Suicide Potential Scale: Inter-rater reliability and validity in Israel in-patient adolescents. *Israel Journal of Psychiatry and Related Sciences, 35*(4), 253–261.

Onnela, J.-P., & Rauch, S. L. (2016). Harnessing smartphone-based digital phenotyping to enhance behavioral and mental health. *Neuropsychopharmacology, 41*(7), 1691–1696.

Orbach, I., Milstein, I., Har-Even, D., Apter, A., Tiano, S., & Elizur, A. (1991). A Multi-Attitude Suicide Tendency Scale for adolescents. *Psychological Assessment, 3*(3), 398–404.

Osman, A., Bagge, C. L., Gutierrez, P. M., Konick, L. C., Kopper, B. A., & Barrios, F. X. (2001). The Suicidal Behaviors Questionnaire—Revised (SBQ-R): Validation with clinical and nonclinical samples. *Assessment, 8*(4), 443–454.

Osman, A., Barrios, F. X., Panak, W. F., Osman, J. R., Hoffman, J., & Hammer, R. (1994). Validation of the Multi-Attitude Suicide Tendency scale in adolescent samples. *Journal of Clinical Psychology, 50*(6), 847–855.

Osman, A., Downs, W. R., Kopper, B. A., Barrios, F. X., Baker, M. T., Osman, J. R., . . . Linehan, M. M. (1998). The Reasons for Living Inventory for Adolescents (RFL-A): Development and psychometric properties. *Journal of Clinical Psychology, 54*(8), 1063–1078.

Osman, A., Kopper, B. A., Barrios, F. X., Osman, J. R., Besett, T., & Linehan, M. M. (1996). The Brief Reasons for Living Inventory for Adolescents (BRFL-A). *Journal of Abnormal Child Psychology, 24*(4), 433–443.

Pestian, J. P., Sorter, M., Connolly, B., Bretonnel Cohen, K., McCullumsmith, C., Gee, J. T., . . . STM Research Group. (2017). A machine learning approach to identifying the thought markers of suicidal subjects: A prospective multicenter trial. *Suicide and Life-Threatening Behavior, 47*(1), 112–121.

Pfeffer, C. R., Conte, H. R., Plutchik, R., & Jerrett, I. (1979). Suicidal behavior in latency-age children: An empirical study. *Journal of the American Academy of Child Psychiatry, 18*(4), 679–692.

Pfeffer, C. R., Conte, H. R., Plutchik, R., & Jerrett, I. (1980). Suicidal behavior in latency-age children: An outpatient population. *Journal of the American Academy of Child Psychiatry, 19*(4), 703–710.

Pfeffer, C. R., Newcorn, J., Kaplan, G., Mizruchi, M. S., & Plutchik, R. (1988). Suicidal behavior in adolescent psychiatric inpatients. *Journal of the American Academy of Child Psychiatry, 27*(3), 357–361.

Pfeffer, C. R., Solomon, G., Plutchik, R., Mizruchi, M. S., & Weiner, A. (1982). Suicidal behavior in latency-age psychiatric inpatients: A replication and cross validation. *Journal of the American Academy of Child Psychiatry, 21*(6), 564–569.

Pfeffer, C. R., Zuckerman, S., Plutchik, R., & Mizruchi, M. S. (1984). Suicidal behavior in normal school children: A comparison with child psychiatric inpatients. *Journal of the American Academy of Child Psychiatry, 23*(4), 416–423.

Pinto, A., Whisman, M. A., & Conwell, Y. (1998). Reasons for living in a clinical sample of adolescents. *Journal of Adolescence, 21*(4), 397–405.

Pinto, A., Whisman, M. A., & McCoy, K. J. M. (1997). Suicidal ideation in adolescents: Psychometric properties of the Suicidal Ideation Questionnaire in a clinical sample. *Psychological Assessment, 9*(1), 63–66.

Plöderl, M., Kralovec, K., Yazdi, K., & Fartacek, R. (2011). A closer look at self-reported suicide attempts: False positives and false negatives. *Suicide and Life-Threatening Behavior, 41*(1), 1–5.

Posner, K., Brown, G. K., Stanley, B., Brent, D. A., Yershova, K. V., Oquendo, M. A., . . . Shen, S. (2011). The Columbia-Suicide Severity Rating Scale: Initial validity and internal consistency findings from three multisite studies with adolescents and adults. *American Journal of Psychiatry, 168*(12), 1266–1277.

Posner, K., Oquendo, M., Gould, M., Stanley, B., & Davies, M. (2007). Columbia Classification Algorithm of Suicide Assessment (C-CASA): Classification of suicidal events in the FDA's pediatric suicidal risk analysis of antidepressants. *American Journal of Psychiatry, 164*(7), 1035–1043.

Preti, A., Sheehan, D. V., Coric, V., Distinto, M., Pitanti, M., Vacca, I., . . . Petretto, D. R. (2013). Sheehan Suicidality Tracking Scale (S-STS): Reliability, convergent and discriminative validity in young Italian adults. *Comprehensive Psychiatry, 54*(7), 842–849.

Prinstein, M. J., Nock, M. K., Spirito, A., & Grapentine, W. L. (2001). Multimethod assessment of suicidality in adolescent psychiatric inpatients: Preliminary results. *Journal of the American Academy of Child and Adolescent Psychiatry, 40*(9), 1053–1061.

Randall, J. R., Rowe, B. H., Dong, K. A., Nock, M. K., & Colman, I. (2013). Assessment of self-harm risk using implicit thoughts. *Psychological Assessment, 25*(3), 714–721.

Rathus, J. H., & Miller, A. L. (2002). Dialectical behavior therapy adapted for suicidal adolescents. *Suicide and Life-Threatening Behavior, 32*(2), 146–157.

Reynolds, W. M. (1987). *Suicidal Ideation Questionnaire Junior.* Odessa, FL: Psychological Assessment Resources.

Reynolds, W. M. (1990). Development of a semistructured clinical interview for suicidal behaviors in adolescents. *Psychological Assessment, 2*(4), 382–390.

Reynolds, W. M., & Mazza, J. J. (1999). Assessment of suicidal ideation in inner-city children and young adolescents: Reliability and validity of the Suicidal Ideation Questionnaire-JR. *School Psychology Review, 28*(1), 17–30.

Ribeiro, J. D., Franklin, J. C., Fox, K. R., Bentley, K. H., Kleiman, E. M., Chang, B. P., & Nock, M. K. (2016). Self-injurious thoughts and behaviors as risk factors for future suicide ideation, attempts, and death: A meta-analysis of longitudinal studies. *Psychological Medicine, 46*(2), 225–236.

Rogers, M. L., Chiurliza, B., Hagan, C. R., Tzoneva, M., Hames, J. L., Michaels, M. S., . . . Joiner, T. E. (2017). Acute suicidal affective disturbance: Factorial structure and initial validation across psychiatric outpatient and inpatient samples. *Journal of Affective Disorders, 211*, 1–11.

Rudd, M. D., Berman, A. L., Joiner, T. E., Nock, M. K., Silverman, M. M., Mandrusiak, M., . . . Witte, T. (2006). Warning signs for suicide: Theory, research, and clinical applications. *Suicide and Life-Threatening Behavior, 36*(3), 255–262.

Shaffer, D., & Pfeffer, C. R. (2001). Practice parameter for the assessment and treatment of children and adolescents with suicidal behavior. *Journal of the American Academy of Child and Adolescent Psychiatry, 40*(7, Suppl.), 24S–51S.

Sheehan, D. V., Alphs, L. D., Mao, L., Li, Q., May, R. S., Bruer, E. H., . . . Williamson, D. J. (2014). Comparative validation of the S-STS, the ISST-Plus, and the C-SSRS for assessing the suicidal thinking and behavior FDA 2012 suicidality categories. *Innovations in Clinical Neuroscience, 11*(9–10), 32–46.

Sheehan, D. V., Giddens, J. M., & Sheehan, K. H. (2014a). Current assessment and classification of suicidal phenomena using the FDA 2012 draft guidance document on suicide assessment: A critical review. *Innovations in Clinical Neuroscience, 11*(9–10), 54–65.

Sheehan, D. V., Giddens, J. M., & Sheehan, I. S. (2014b). Status update on the Sheehan-Suicidality Tracking Scale (S-STS) 2014. *Innovations in Clinical Neuroscience, 11*(9–10), 93–140.

Silverman, M. M., Berman, A. L., Sanddal, N. D., O'Carroll, P. W., & Joiner, T. E. (2007). Rebuilding the tower of Babel: A revised nomenclature for the study of suicide and suicidal behaviors: Part 2.

Suicide-related ideations, communications, and behaviors. *Suicide and Life-Threatening Behavior, 37*(3), 264–277.

Silverman, M. M., & De Leo, D. (2016). Why there is a need for an international nomenclature and classification system for suicide. *Crisis: Journal of Crisis Intervention and Suicide Prevention, 37*(2), 83–87.

Steer, R. A., Kumar, G., & Beck, A. T. (1993). Self-reported suicidal ideation in adolescent psychiatric inpatients. *Journal of Consulting and Clinical Psychology, 61*(6), 1096–1099.

Swannell, S. V., Martin, G. E., Page, A., Hasking, P., & St John, N. J. (2014). Prevalence of nonsuicidal self-injury in nonclinical samples: Systematic review, meta-analysis and meta-regression. *Suicide and Life-Threatening Behavior, 44*(3), 273–303.

Tucker, R. P., Michaels, M. S., Rogers, M. L., Wingate, L. R., & Joiner, T. E. (2016). Construct validity of a proposed new diagnostic entity: Acute Suicidal Affective Disturbance (ASAD). *Journal of Affective Disorders, 189*, 365–378.

U.S. Food and Drug Administration, United States Department of Health and Human Services. (2012). *Guidance for industry: Suicidal ideation and behavior: Prospective assessment of occurrence in clinical trials, draft guidance*. Silver Spring, MD: Author.

Van Meter, A. R., Algorta, G. P., Youngstrom, E. A., Lechtman, Y., Youngstrom, J. K., Feeny, N. C., & Findling, R. L. (2018). Assessing for suicidal behavior in youth using the Achenbach system of empirically based assessment. *European Child and Adolescent Psychiatry, 27*(2), 159–169.

Velting, D. M., Rathus, J. H., & Asnis, G. M. (1998). Asking adolescents to explain discrepancies in self-reported suicidality. *Suicide and Life-Threatening Behavior, 28*(2), 10.

Venta, A., & Sharp, C. (2014). Extending the concurrent validity of the Self-Injurious Thoughts and Behaviors Interview to inpatient adolescents. *Journal of Psychopathology and Behavioral Assessment, 36*(4), 675–682.

Victor, S. E., Davis, T., & Klonsky, E. D. (2017). Descriptive characteristics and initial psychometric properties of the Non-Suicidal Self-Injury Disorder Scale. *Archives of Suicide Research, 21*, 265–278.

Walsh, C. G., Ribeiro, J. D., & Franklin, J. C. (2017). Predicting risk of suicide attempts over time through machine learning. *Clinical Psychological Science, 5*(3), 457–469.

Washburn, J. J., Juzwin, K. R., Styer, D. M., & Aldridge, D. (2010). Measuring the urge to self-injure: Preliminary data from a clinical sample. *Psychiatry Research, 178*(3), 540–544.

Watkins, R. L., & Gutierrez, P. M. (2003). The relationship between exposure to adolescent suicide and subsequent suicide risk (2002 Student Award Address). *Suicide and Life-Threatening Behavior, 33*(1), 21–32.

Wetzler, S., Asnis, G. M., Hyman, R. B., Virtue, C., Zimmerman, J., & Rathus, J. H. (1996). Characteristics of suicidality among adolescents. *Suicide and Life-Threatening Behavior, 26*(1), 37–45.

Yigletu, H., Tucker, S., Harris, M., & Hatlevig, J. (2004). Assessing suicide ideation: Comparing self-report versus clinician report. *Journal of the American Psychiatric Nurses Association, 10*(1), 9–15.

Youngstrom, E. A., Hameed, A., Mitchell, M. A., Van Meter, A. R., Freeman, A. J., Algorta, G. P., . . . Meyer, R. E. (2015). Direct comparison of the psychometric properties of multiple interview and patient-rated assessments of suicidal ideation and behavior in an adult psychiatric inpatient sample. *Journal of Clinical Psychiatry, 76*(12), 1676–1682.

PART IV

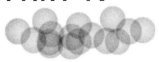

Anxiety Disorders and Obsessive–Compulsive Disorder

CHAPTER 10

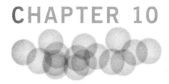

Anxiety Disorders

Nicole Fleischer, Margaret E. Crane, and Philip C. Kendall

This chapter documents evidence-based assessment (EBA) for anxiety disorders in youth. We address (1) prediction, (2) prescription, and (3) process approaches to assessing anxiety in youth, and differentiate it from other internalizing and externalizing disorders. We first consider features of anxiety that define the various anxiety disorders in youth, then explore various assessment approaches. We acknowledge that private practice and community mental health facilities may not have full resources, so we emphasize usable assessments within an application of EBA through the following case example (referred to throughout the chapter).

Daniel, a 14-year-old black male referred to a community mental health center in an urban setting, has not attended school for the past 2 weeks due to anxiety. The referral information suggests that he worries excessively about his grades and

what his peers think of him. Daniel stated that he has trouble paying attention at school. His mother reported that he has few friends and rarely spends time with his peers outside of school. Even prior to his absences, Daniel's grades were slipping due to his refusal to turn in homework assignments because he felt they were not done "well enough" for his own standards.

Preparation

Identify Whether Presentation Is Consistent with an Anxiety Disorder

Anxiety disorders are very common in youth (Beesdo, Knappe, & Pine, 2009). These disorders are characterized by a maladaptive fear or worry in response to a situation or object (Barlow, 2000). Although different anxiety disorders affect children and adolescents, the anxiety disorders share similarities. Youth with anxiety disorders often feel increased somatic sensations, including headaches, stomachaches, and difficulty breathing. They also avoid (or have intense fear reactions to) fear-provoking situations or stimuli. Even endurance of the anxiety-provoking situation is often met with avoidance (e.g., closing eyes, hiding behind hands).

These disorders have overlapping symptoms and presentations, but differential diagnosis can be determined by understanding the central theme of the worries (Crozier, Gillihan, & Powers, 2011). Anxiety disorders have common themes: avoidance of anxiety-producing situations and interfering cognitive or physical distress. Anxiety disorders in youth interfere with their functioning at home, at school, or in social situations (Cohen, Mychailyszyn, Settipani, Crawley, & Kendall, 2011; Swan & Kendall, 2016). The most common anxiety disorders in youth are separation anxiety disorder (SEP), social anxiety disorder (SOC), specific phobias (animal, natural environment, blood–injection–injury, situational, and other), and generalized anxiety disorder (GAD).

SEP is an anxiety disorder most commonly present during childhood. Children affected by SEP are anxious about separating from a caregiver (American Psychiatric Association, 2013). Their worries may encompass something negative happening to the caregiver when separated (e.g., accident, death), or something happening to themselves when separated. Children with SEP may experience school refusal or tantrums in response to situations in which they are separated from the caregiver. These children may also have difficulty spending time with friends or going to sleepovers. Their anxious distress is out of proportion to the likelihood of occurrence (e.g., parent has never been in a car accident).

Another common anxiety is GAD (American Psychiatric Association, 2013), characterized by excessive and persistent worrying that is often difficult to stop. Youth may worry about their performance in school, something happening to their family (e.g., divorce), safety concerns (e.g., burglaries, natural disasters), and/or new situations or a change in plans. According to diagnostic criteria, youth must be experiencing at least one physical symptom (e.g., muscle tension, sleep disturbance, headaches), but data suggest that youth with GAD experience a wide variety of physical symptoms, including shakiness, restlessness, and racing hearts (Cohen et al., 2011).

Youth also experience SOC, which consists of persistent fear of evaluative situations. They are overly concerned about being embarrassed when doing something in front of their peers, and they think their actions are being scrutinized. Youth with SOC avoid participating in group activities, initiating friendships or relationships, and even attending school. SOC is associated with long-term negative consequences such as adult anxiety (Aschenbrand, Kendall, Webb, Safford,

& Flannery-Schroeder, 2003), mood disorders, or substance use (Crozier et al., 2011).

Panic disorder is less likely in childhood but may occur in late childhood or early adolescence. Panic disorder involves unexpected and recurrent panic attacks, characterized by physical symptoms such as racing heart, stomachaches, hyperventilation, sweating, shaking, and dizziness, among many others (American Psychiatric Association, 2013). Youth with panic disorder often develop a fear of experiencing these panic attacks (fear of the experience of fear; Chambless, Caputo, Bright, & Gallagher, 1984) and may avoid situations that they believe could trigger a panic attack, or places where they would be unable to seek help if they had a panic attack (e.g., public transportation).

Agoraphobia, also less prevalent, may present in youth and can coincide with panic disorder (American Psychiatric Association, 2013). Agoraphobia is classified as intense fear of being in certain physical locations (e.g., public transpiration, open fields, malls, lines or crowds) and youth fear that they may require help or become ill in these situations and not be able to receive help. As characterized in anxiety, youth with agoraphobia avoid places or situations that increase anxiety or refuse to go out unless a friend or family member accompanies them. The avoidance or distress interferes with the youth's adjustment and family life (e.g., unable to leave the house).

Specific phobias, which are prevalent in youth, involve intense fear regarding a specific object or situation (e.g., dogs, spiders, visit to a physician). Children may throw tantrums (e.g., getting a shot) or avoid places where they may encounter the anxiety-provoking stimulus (e.g., a park where dogs may be off-leash). The distress is out of proportion with the threat (e.g., extreme fear in response to a friendly dog), and the fears are not developmentally appropriate.

Despite the features of specific disorders, (1) avoidance or intense fear reaction in response to the anxiety and (2) physical symptoms are consistent across the anxiety disorders. The level of avoidance depends on the intensity of anxiety when presented with the cues or triggers (Barlow, 2000). Youth with anxiety disorders either avoid the anxiety-provoking situations or endure them with extreme duress. Youth may avoid school projects, parties, camps, and new situations.

Somatic symptoms are often reported by youth suffering from anxiety disorders (Cohen et al., 2011; Kendall & Pimentel, 2003). These youth report headaches, muscle tension, restlessness, and stomachaches. Physical symptoms are often linked to increased anxiety sensitivity and impairment (Cohen et al., 2011). Perhaps due to their developmental level, youth may misinterpret their physical symptoms, thinking that something more serious is occurring instead of anxious arousal (Pilecki & McKay, 2011). Research has shown that children with GAD, social phobia, and separation anxiety exhibit the same frequency of somatic complaints despite the different themes in their worries (Hofflich, Hughes, & Kendall, 2006).

Consider the Base Rate of Anxiety Disorders

Anxiety disorders are the most prevalent mental health condition affecting children, and 25% of adolescents will suffer from an anxiety disorder within their lifetime (Anxiety and Depression Association of America, 2017). Within one year, it is estimated that 13% of youth will meet criteria for an anxiety disorder (Wilmhurst, 2015).

According to DSM-5, prevalence rates vary by diagnosis (American Psychiatric Association, 2013). SEP presents in about 2% of children, but this decreases as the children get older. Specific phobias affect approximately 5% of children, increasing to 15% in adolescence. Approximately 7% of children meet criteria for social phobia every year, but this rate increases with age. Panic disorder rates are lower in younger children (less than 0.4%), but increase in adolescents (2–3%). GAD is estimated to occur in 3% of children but 1% in adolescents (American Psychiatric Association, 2013).

Comorbidities

Children with an anxiety disorder are at risk for additional psychological problems (Beesdo et al., 2009). More common than not, anxiety is comorbid with other anxiety disorders (Kendall et al., 2010). As children mature, their risk of developing comorbid anxiety disorders increases, which may be related to the chronic nature of anxiety disorders (Beesdo et al., 2009). In many youth, especially those presenting in clinical settings, it is rare to meet criteria for only one anxiety disorder.

Anxiety disorders in youth may be comorbid with other conditions (Beesdo et al., 2009; Palitz et al., 2018). Youth with anxiety may present with mood disorders, specifically major depressive disorder and persistent depressive disorder (Costello,

Mustillo, Erkanli, Keeler, & Angold, 2003; Cummings, Caporino, & Kendall, 2014). Anxious youth may also present with attention-deficit/hyperactivity disorder (ADHD) (Larson, Russ, Kahn, & Halfon, 2011) and/or oppositional defiant disorder (ODD) (Boylan, Vaillancourt, Boyle, & Szatmari, 2007).

Presence in Mental Health Settings

Anxiety is highly prevalent in mental health settings. Merikangas and colleagues (2010) reported that 8% of adolescents with anxiety disorders exhibit severe impairment. In these cases, not surprisingly, youth with more severe and impairing anxiety are more likely to present for treatment. Researchers estimate anxiety disorder prevalence near 35% in mental health settings (Ollendick, Jarrett, Grills-Taquechel, Hovey, & Wolff, 2008). Despite the interference, anxiety symptoms may go unreported due to the stigma and negative associations of mental disorders (Kessler, Berglund, Demler, Jin, & Walters, 2005). Youth may meet criteria for an anxiety disorder but remain undiagnosed due to the negative associations of presenting for treatment. Comorbidities complicate the assessment, and the task is often to disentangle anxiety disorders from each other and from other conditions.

Starter Kit

An assessment battery ("Starter Kit") to guide the assessment process for anxiety disorders is presented in Table 10.1. The measures in this starter-kit are free, with two exceptions: Achenbach System of Empirically Based Assessment (ASEBA) Child Behavior Checklist and Youth Self-Report (CBCL/YSR; Achenbach, 1991) and the Anxiety Disorders Interview Schedule for Children, child and parent versions (ADIS; Albano & Silverman, 2015). For the prediction phase, we gave preference to measures with data on their reliability, validity, discriminate power, specificity, and sensitivity. We recommend using the CBCL/YSR and the Screen for Child Anxiety and Related Disorders (SCARED; Birmaher et al., 1997) for all children who may have an anxiety disorder. Although the CBCL/YSR is not free, it assesses a breadth of emotional and behavioral problems to provide clinicians with an overview of potential comorbidities. For example, returning to our case example, it is not initially clear whether Daniel's difficulty

TABLE 10.1. Anxiety Assessment Starter Kit

Prediction	Prescription	Process
ASEBA Child Behavior Checklist/Youth Self-Report	Anxiety Disorders Interview Schedule for Children, Child and Parent versions	Coping Questionnaire, Child and Parent versions
Screen for Child Anxiety Related Emotion Disorders	Child Anxiety Impact Scale	Clinical Global Impressions Scale—Improvement
	Clinical Global Impression Scale—Severity	

concentrating is ADHD or symptoms of GAD or SOC. Of the free measures of youth anxiety, the SCARED has the best support for its discriminate validity (see below). It assesses SEP, SOC, GAD, somatic/panic, and school phobia. For the prescription phase, the ADIS is the most commonly used semistructured interview. Although not free, it has the strongest psychometric support for anxiety disorders. The Child Anxiety Impact Scale (Langley, Bergman, McCracken, & Piacentini, 2004) and the Clinical Global Impression—Severity scale (Shaffer et al., 1983) assess the impact of anxiety on children's functioning. To evaluate treatment process and outcomes, we recommend using the Coping Questionnaire, Child and Parent versions (CQ-C/P; Crane & Kendall, 2018; Kendall, 1994), which assesses youth's perceived ability to cope in anxiety-provoking situations. Additionally, the Clinical Global Impression—Improvement scale (CGI-I) can be helpful in tracking the therapist's perception of client progress. Professionals may add or subtract measures based on the needs and resources; for example, low-resource settings could use the anxiety section of the Diagnostic Interview Schedule for Children—Revised (DISC-R; Shaffer et al., 1993), a free interview.

Prediction

Evaluate Risk and Protective Factors

Given the volume of research on risk and protective factors for youth anxiety, our coverage is illustrative rather than exhaustive (see Beesdo et al., 2009; Pahl, Barrett, & Gullo, 2012). That being said, several risk factors increase a child's likelihood of developing one or more anxiety disorders. Biological, environmental, and temperamental factors contribute to the increased risk of developing an anxiety disorder.

Genetic research involving both parents and twins suggests that multiple genes (but not a single gene) may contribute to a predisposition for de-

veloping anxiety (Beesdo et al., 2009; Ehringer, Rhee, Young, Corley, & Hewitt, 2006). Indeed, no specific gene has been linked to childhood anxiety, but genes are said to contribute to the diathesis of anxiety disorders. Risks for anxiety disorders increase when both parents present with an anxiety disorder, or at least one parent has a severe mental illness (Schreier, Wittchen, Höfler, & Lieb, 2008). Increased vulnerability has been linked to earlier presentation of anxiety symptoms (Arnold & Taillefer, 2011). However, the impact of genes on the development of anxiety disorders is often dependent on environmental interactions.

Several temperamental and environmental factors have been identified as being connected to anxiety disorder development: learning, cognitive vulnerabilities, and parental factors. Learning plays an important role in the development of anxiety in youth (Barlow, 2000). Classical conditioning may explain the development of specific anxiety disorders, as children learn to associate feared responses with previously neutral stimuli or body sensations. SOC (Heimberg & Magee, 2014), and GAD (Roemer & Orsillo, 2014) may also develop through classical conditioning. Children can develop anxiety from observing others (modeling) as well, whether parents, siblings, or peers. Learning experiences may increase a child's predisposition for anxiety based on his or her temperamental vulnerabilities.

Anxiety sensitivity (AS) has been linked to an increased rate of anxiety disorders in children, especially in relation to somatic complaints and panic-like symptoms (Reiss, Peterson, Gursky, & McNally, 1986). As evidenced by the tripartite model of emotion (Clark & Watson, 1991), negative affectivity (NA) and physiological hyperarousal (PH) may act as predecessors for anxiety in children. Specifically, research has demonstrated the role the tripartite model may have in anxiety and depression in children, leading to distinct assessment protocols for these concepts. We explore AS, NA, and PH further later in this chapter.

Parental factors contribute to increased anxiety (Pahl et al., 2012). Research indicates that parental psychopathology affects the parent's relationship with his or her child. Research has also demonstrated that parent factors such as parenting style and accommodation of anxiety avoidance contribute to the anxiety disorder (Kagan, Frank, & Kendall, 2017; Lebowitz et al., 2013; Pahl et al., 2012). Parents attempt to reduce their child's anxiety by removing the child from the situation (accommodation). An insecure parent–child attachment is linked to anxiety-related problems (Kerns & Brumariu, 2013), and parent modeling of anxious behaviors also increases the learning of anxious responses in children (Barlow, 2000).

Children with behavioral inhibition are more likely to develop anxiety (Degnan, Almas, & Fox, 2010). Pahl and colleagues (2012) demonstrated that many of the characteristics of the behavioral observation of "inhibition" (e.g., avoidance, withdrawal, hypervigilant attention to the environment) overlap with anxiety disorder symptoms.

Several protective factors may reduce a child's risk of developing anxiety disorders, including support systems, peer relationships, self-efficacy, and perceived control (Muris, 2006; Smokowski et al., 2014). Peer support has been associated with lower rates of internalizing symptoms in youth (Smokowski et al., 2014), and family support helps youth adapt to different settings (e.g., school, social). A child's sense of self-efficacy further reduces the risk of developing an anxiety disorder. For a full review, see Smokowski and colleagues (2014).

Putting It into Practice

During the brief phone interview of our case example, Daniel's mother reported that she had a history of anxiety in her family and is currently being treated for anxiety herself. Daniel and his mother provided multiple examples throughout the intake of parental accommodation, including letting Daniel stay home from school and at times completing his assignments for him. To reduce her own, as well as her son's, anxious arousal, she would accommodate (give in to) his complaints. However, Daniel claimed that he had a very supportive extended family, including his aunts and grandmother, who lived in his neighborhood and always offered positive encouragement to Daniel. What Daniel perceived as supportive was a relationship that tolerated avoidance.

Treatment Moderators

Are there factors that affect treatment outcome for youth with anxiety? Research suggests that there are no single factors that uniformly moderate for the effects of treatment (i.e., age, gender, IQ, symptom duration, diagnosis, and social functioning; Herres, Cummings, Swan, Makover, & Kendall, 2015; Nilsen, Eisemann, & Kvernmo, 2013). Yet practioners should be aware of the effects that age, maturity, and cognitive functioning have on a child's understanding of cognitive strategies. However, in one examination of moderating variables, Compton and colleagues (2014) reported that severe anxiety, caregiver strain, and social phobia are associated with less successful outcomes in treatment. Ollendick and Benoit (2012) postulated that moderating factors may interact with each other to provide a complex relationship between moderating variables and treatment outcomes. Clinicians should be aware of the various potential factors, but, at present, several of the hypothesized factors do not moderate treatment outcomes.

Comorbidity has been speculated to have an effect on treatment progression. As discussed, comorbidity of other psychological disorders is the rule and not the exception when assessing youth with anxiety. Not surprisingly, researchers have examined the role of comorbidity in the outcomes for principal anxiety disorder diagnoses. Current findings do not suggest that comorbidity acts as a significant moderating variable for anxiety disorder treatment (Ollendick et al., 2008), although teens with social anxiety who also evidence some depression have been reported to have less favorable 1-year follow-ups (Puleo, Conner, Benjamin, & Kendall, 2011). Comorbidities may not reduce the effectiveness of anxiety disorder treatment, but treatment may impact the various comorbidities.

Revise Probabilities Based on Intake Assessments

An important part of EBA is the use of questionnaires to calculate an initial probability that a client has a disorder. Intake questionnaires, completed at home or in the clinic, provide scores that indicate the likelihood that a client has a disorder. EBA provides more precise information about a client's risk of a disorder based on his or her score and the accuracy of the questionnaire. EBA can eliminate biases (i.e., geographic, training, clinic) that can mislead diagnoses. For instance, a bias that can emerge may be linked to the type of clinic in which a youth is seen: whether to attribute inattention to anxiety or to ADHD. An ADHD clinic may have a different view than an anxiety clinic. EBA standardizes the interpretation of questionnaires, thus increasing the consistency of diagnoses across settings.

Behavioral and physiological assessments, although often very informative in a research setting, are underutilized in practice. Systematic behavioral assessments are often cost prohibitive in a clinic, and there is no standard observation task for various anxiety disorders. The tasks that have been used lack norms and cutoff values. Physiological indices of anxiety, such as heart rate variability, cortisol levels, and galvanic skin response, have been studied (Beidel, 1988; Thayer, Åhs, Fredrikson, Sollers, & Wager, 2012; Weems, Zakem, Costa, Cannon, & Watts, 2005), but these indices also lack meaningful/useful norms. Physiological assessment also requires technology that is not routinely found in mental health clinics. Consequently, clinical assessment of anxiety disorders is generally limited to self-report from questionnaires and interviews (Craske, 2012; Silverman & Ollendick, 2005).

Measure Overview

Questionnaires are useful to screen for youth anxiety disorders. They enable a quick assessment of the severity of a youth's anxiety and of the specific situations in which the anxiety is experienced. When determining which questionnaires to use, consider factors that include cost, administration, and scoring time and, importantly, the psychometric properties of a measure. Table 10.2 summarizes commonly used questionnaires to assess youth anxiety. Anxiety questionnaires can be divided into three categories: multidimensional questionnaires, disorder-specific questionnaires, and questionnaires that assess specific characteristics of anxiety.

Multidimensional questionnaires include the CBCL/YSR (Achenbach, 1991), the Multidimensional Anxiety Scale for Children (MASC; March, Parker, Sullivan, Stallings, & Conners, 1997), the Pediatric Anxiety Rating Scale (PARS; Research Units on Pediatric Psychopharmacology Anxiety Study Group [RUPP], 2002), the Revised Child Anxiety and Depression Scale (RCADS; Chorpita, Yim, Moffitt, Umemoto, & Francis, 2000), the SCARED (Birmaher et al., 1997), the Spence Children's Anxiety Scale (SCAS; Spence, 1998), and the Youth Anxiety Measure for DSM-5 (YAM-5; Muris et al., 2016). With the exception

of the MASC and the CBCL/YSR, the multidimensional questionnaires examine youth anxiety according to DSM criteria. The PARS a clinician-rated measure rather than a parent and/or child report.

Disorder-specific questionnaires include the Fear Survey Schedule for Children—Revised (FSSC-R; Ollendick, 1983), the Leibowitz Social Anxiety Scale for Children and Adolescents (LSAS-CA; Masia-Warner et al., 2003), the Social Anxiety Scale for Children—Revised (SASC-R; La Greca & Stone, 1993), and the Social Phobia and Anxiety Inventory for Children (SPAIC; Beidel, Turner, & Morris, 1995, 1999). The FSSC-R assesses specific phobias, and the LSAS-CA, SASC-R, and SPAIC assess social anxiety.

Questionnaires that assess specific characteristics of anxiety include the State–Trait Anxiety Inventory for Children (STAIC; Spielberger, 1973), the Revised Children's Manifest Anxiety Scale (RCMAS; Reynolds & Richmond, 1978), Penn State Worry Questionnaire for Children (PSWQ-C; Brown, Antony, & Barlow, 1992), the Negative Affectivity Self-Statement Questionnaire (NASSQ; Ronan, Kendall, & Rowe, 1994), the Intolerance of Uncertainty Scale for Children (IUSC; Comer et al., 2009), and the Childhood Anxiety Sensitivity Index (CASI; Silverman, Fleisig, Rabian, & Peterson, 1991). The STAIC and the RCMAS are trait anxiety measures that have been used for over 40 years. The PSWQ-C and NASSQ assess worry and negative self-talk, respectively, two constructs associated with all anxiety disorders. Although intolerance of uncertainty, which is evaluated by the IUSC, is seen across anxiety disorders, it appears to be more related to GAD (Read, Comer, & Kendall, 2013). Similarly, AS (CASI; akin to trait anxiety) may reflect a response to panic, as well as a sensitivity to physiological sensations of anxiety across disorders.

Psychometric Properties

For a measure to be useful, it must have acceptable reliability and validity metrics. Table 10.3 summarizes the data for 17 measures. For reliability, we focus on internal consistency (Cronbach's alpha) and retest reliability (Pearson correlation or intraclass correlation coefficient [ICC]). We summarize validity metrics in two ways: convergent validity (Pearson's correlation; Table 10.3) and discriminant validity/diagnostic accuracy (receiver operator characteristics, sensitivity, and specify; see Table 10.4).

TABLE 10.2. Questionnaires: Descriptive Information of Selected Youth Anxiety Measures

Measure	No. of Items	Description	Time to complete (min)	Age	Reporter	Cost	Where to obtain
ASEBA Child Behavior Checklist (CBCL)/Youth Self-Report (YSR)	CBCL:118; YSR: 112	Respondents rate how true positive and problem behaviors are for the youth. Yields two broad-band subscales (Internalizing and Externalizing), eight narrow-band subscales (e.g., Anxious/Depressed, Withdrawn/Depressed, Somatic Complaints), and six DSM-oriented subscales (e.g, Anxiety, Affective Problems).	10–15	CBCL: 6–18; YSR: 11–18	Parent, child	Yes	*http://store.aseba.org*
Childhood Anxiety Sensitivity Index (CASI)	18	Respondents rate how aversively the youth views anxiety symptoms. Yields a total score and four subscales (Disease, Unsteady, Mental Incapacitation, and Social Concerns).	5–11	6–17	Child	Yes	*www.anxietysensitivityindex.com*
Fear Survey Schedule for Children (FSSC-R)	80	Respondents rate the amount of fear elicited by each object or situation listed. Yields a total score and five fear subscales (Failure and Criticism, The Unknown, Danger and Death, Medical, and Small Animals).	15–20	7–18	Child	No	*tho@vt.edu*
Intolerance of Uncertainty Scale for Children (IUSC)	27	Respondents rate how much statements about tolerating uncertainty apply to them. Yields a total score.	5–10	7–17	Child and parent	No	*https://doi.org/10.1037/a0016719*
Leibowitz Social Anxiety Scale (LSAS-CA)	24	Respondents rate each item for anxiety severity and frequency of avoidance. Yields seven scores (total LSAS-CA; Total Anxiety, Social Interaction Anxiety, and Performance Anxiety; and Total Avoidance, Avoidance of Social Interaction, and Avoidance of Performance Situations).	10	7–18	Clinician	No	*carrie.masia@nyumc.org*

(continued)

TABLE 10.2. *(continued)*

Measure	No. of Items	Description	Time to complete (min)	Age	Reporter	Cost	Where to obtain
Multidimensional Anxiety Scale for Children (MASC)	39	Respondents rate how true each item is for them. Yields a total score and four subscales (Separation Anxiety, Social Anxiety, Harm Avoidance, and Physical Symptoms).	10	8–19	Child and parent	Yes	*www.mhs.com/mhs-assessment?prodname=masc2*
Negative Affectivity Self-Statement Questionnaire (NASSQ)	70	Respondents rate the frequency with which they think of each negative self-statement. Yields a total score and three subscales (Anxiety, Depression, and Negative Affect).	20–30	7–15	Child	No	*pkendall@temple.edu*
Pediatric Anxiety Rating Scale (PARS)	50	Respondents rate anxiety symptoms and interference. Yields six symptom subscales (SEP, SOC, GAD, SP, Physical Signs and Symptoms, and Other), seven severity subscales (Number of Symptoms, Frequency of Symptoms, Distress, Interference at Home, Interference Out of Home, Severity of Physical Symptoms, and Avoidance), and a Total Interference score.	30	6–17	Clinician	No	*https://doi.org/10.1097/00004583-200209000-00006*
Penn State Worry Questionnaire for Children (PSWQ-C)	14	Respondents rate how much they agree with statements about the youth's worry. Yields a total score.	4	7–17	Child	No	*www.childfirst.ucla.edu/resources*
Revised Children's Anxiety and Depression Scale (RCADS, RCADS-P)	47	Respondents rate how often statements about anxiety apply to the youth. Yields a total score, total anxiety score, and six subscales related to DSM disorders (SEP, SOC, GAD, PD, OCD, and MDD).	12	8–18	Child and parent	No	*www.childfirst.ucla.edu/resources*
Revised Children's Manifest Anxiety Scale (RCMAS)	37	Respondents indicate whether they experience a symptom. Yields a total anxiety score, a lie score, and three subscales (Physiological Anxiety, Worry/Oversensitivity, and Social Concerns/Concentration).	5–15	6–19	Child	Yes	*www.mhs.com/mhs-assessment?prodname=rcmas2*

Measure	No. of items	Description	Time (min)	Age	Informant	Fee	Website
Screen for Child Anxiety Related Emotion Disorders (SCARED)	41	Respondents rate severity of the youth's anxiety and school refusal symptoms over the past three months. Yields five subscales (Separation Anxiety, Social Anxiety, General Anxiety, Somatic/Panic, and School Phobia).	10	6–19	Child and parent	No	www.pediatricbipolar.pitt.edu/resources/instruments
Social Anxiety Scale for Children and Adolescents (SAS-C/A)	C: 26; A: 22	Respondents rate how true each statement about social anxiety is for the youth. Yields three subscales (Fear of Negative Evaluation, Social Avoidance and Distress in New Situations, and General Social Avoidance and Distress).	15	8–18	Child; adolescent	Yes	alagreca@miami.edu
Social Phobia and Anxiety Inventory for Children (SPAI-C)	26	Respondents rate the degree of distress the youth exhibits in various social situations. Yields three subscales (Assertiveness/General Conversation, Traditional Social Encounters, and Public Performance).	20–30	8–17	Child	Yes	www.mhs.com/mhs-assessment?prodname=spai
Spence Children's Anxiety Scale (SCAS)	44	Respondents rate the frequency the youth experiences each symptom. Yields six subscales (SEP, SOC, GAD, OCD, PD/Agoraphobia, and Fears of Physical Injury).	11	7–19	Child and parent	Maybe (permission needed for commercial use)	www.scaswebsite.com
State–Trait Anxiety Inventory for Children (STAIC)	20	Respondents rate the frequency the youth experiences each symptom. Yields two subscales (Trait Anxiety and State Anxiety).	5–10	6–18	Child and parent	Yes	www.mindgarden.com/146-state-trait-anxiety-inventory-for-children#horizontalTab2
Youth Anxiety Measure for DSM-5 (YAM-5)	50	Respondents rate the frequency the youth experiences each anxiety symptom. Yields separation 10 subscales (SEP, SOC, GAD, PD, Selective Mutism, Specific Phobia–Animal Type, Natural Environment Type, Blood–Injection–Injury Type, Situational Type/Agoraphobia, and Other).	15	8–18	Child and parent	No	https://doi.org/10.1016/j.paid.2017.04.058

Note. SEP, separation anxiety disorder; SOC, social anxiety disorder; GAD, generalized anxiety disorder; PD, panic disorder; OCD, obsessive–compulsive disorder; MDD, major depressive disorder.

TABLE 10.3. Psychometric Properties of Youth Anxiety Questionnaires

Measure	References	Internal consistency (alpha)	Retest reliability (r)	Parent–child agreement (r)	Convergent validity (r)
ASEBA Child Behavior Checklist/Youth Self-Report[b]	Achenbach (1991); Achenbach & Rescorla (2001); Ebesutani et al. (2010, 2011); Monga et al. (2000); RUPP (2002); Southam-Gerow et al. (2003); Spence (1998)	.61–90	.68–91	.01–.28	.07–65
Childhood Anxiety Sensitivity Index	Silverman et al. (1991); Weems et al. (2008)	.87–89	.76–79	.16	.12–74
Fear Survey Schedule for Children	Muris et al. (2002); Ollendick (1983); Weems et al. (2008)	.94–95	.55–87	.30	-.69[a]–72
Intolerance of Uncertainty Scale for Children	Comer et al. (2009); Read et al. (2013)	.91–96	No data available	.16	.11–75
Leibowitz Social Anxiety Scale	Masia-Warner et al. (2003)	.83–97	ICC = .89–.94	n/a	-.68[a]–75
Multidimensional Anxiety Scale for Children	Anderson et al. (2009); Baldwin & Dadds (2007); March et al. (1997, 1999); RUPP (2002); Villabø et al. (2012); Wei et al. (2014)	.69–90	.70–93; ICC = .76–.92	-.04–.40	.22–84
Negative Affectivity Self-Statement Questionnaire	Ronan et al. (1994)	$r = .87$–.94	.78–96	n/a	.47–75
Pediatric Anxiety Rating Scale	RUPP (2002)	.64	ICC = .37–.59	n/a	.22–61
Penn State Worry Questionnaire for Children	Brown et al. (1992); Chorpita et al. (1997)	.83–93	.64–92	n/a	-.52[a]–.54

Measure	References				
Revised Children's Anxiety and Depression Scale	Chorpita et al. (2000); Ebesutani et al. (2012); Muris et al. (2003)	.71–.83	.65–.80	.17–.51	.49–.68
Revised Children's Manifest Anxiety Scale	Chorpita et al. (1996); Hodges (1990); Muris et al. (2002); Reynolds & Richmond (1978, 1985); Spence et al. (2003); Weems et al. (2008)	.64–.84	.64–.76	.26–.82	.13–.88
Screen for Child Anxiety Related Emotion Disorders	Birmaher et al. (1997, 1999); Monga et al. (2000); Muris et al. (2004); Rappaport et al. (2017); RUPP (2002)	.61–.94	ICC = .70–.90	–.06–.74	–.21[a]–.73
Social Anxiety Scale for Children and Adolescents	Kristensen & Torgersen (2006); La Greca et al. (1988); La Greca & Lopez (1998); La Greca & Stone (1993); Storch et al. (2004)	.69–.91	.69–.86	.46	–.48[a]–.84
Social Phobia and Anxiety Inventory for Children	Beidel et al. (1995, 1999); Storch et al. (2004)	.92–.95	.63–.86	.34–.40	–.33[a]–.84
Spence Children's Anxiety Scale	Brown-Jacobsen et al. (2011); Nauta et al. (2004); Reardon et al. (2018); Spence (1998); Spence et al. (2003)	.60–.92	.45–.69	.23–.66	.32–.76
State–Trait Anxiety Inventory for Children	Chorpita et al. (1996); Monga et al. (2000); Southam-Gerow et al. (2003); Spielberger (1973); Strauss (1987)	.78–.90	.65–.71	.13–.25	.06–.73
Youth Anxiety Measure for DSM-5	Fuentes-Rodriguez et al. (2018); Muris et al. (2016)	.35–.91	No data available	.42–.73	.28–.89

Note. alpha, Cronbach's alpha; r, Pearson correlation; ICC, intraclass correlation coefficient; RUPP, Research Units on Pediatric Psychopharmacology Anxiety Study Group.
[a]Predicted to correlate negatively.[b]psychometrics for the CBCL/YSR only include only data from the Internalizing subscale, the Anxious/Depressed subscale, and the DSM-Oriented Anxiety subscales.

TABLE 10.4. Receiver Operator Characteristics of Youth Anxiety Measures

Scale	References	Receiver operator characteristics (AUC)	Median cutoff score	Median LR+	Median LR−
ASEBA Child Behavior Checklist/Youth Self-Report	Aschenbrand et al. (2010); Ebesutani et al. (2010); Ferdinand (2008); Monga et al. (2000); Pauschardt et al. (2010); Van Meter et al. (2014)	Internalizing Problems = .52–.94 Anxious/Depressed = .64–.94 Withdrawn/Depressed = .55–.86 Somatic Complaints = .57–.77 Social Problems = .58–.82 Thought Problems = .57–.63 Attention Problems = .53–.64 DSM Anxiety Problems = .60–.84 DSM Affective Problems = .60–.63	T = 55	Internalizing Problems = 4.31 Anxious/Depressed = 7.71 Withdrawn/Depressed = 4.62 Somatic Complaints = 1.62 Social Problems = 3.63	Internalizing Problems = 0.20 Anxious/Depressed = 0.21 Withdrawn/Depressed = 0.39 Somatic Complaints 0.58 Social Problems = 0.50
Intolerance of Uncertainty Scale for Children	Comer et al. (2009)	IUSC = .60–.75	IUSC = 53	IUSC = 4.00	IUSC = 0.40
Leibowitz Social Anxiety Scale	Garcia-Lopez et al. (2015); Masia-Warner et al. (2003)	LSAS = .86–.99	LSAS = 26	LSAS = 5.39	LSAS = 0.07
Multidimensional Anxiety Scale for Children	Anderson et al. (2009); Dierker et al. (2001); Skarphedinsson et al. (2015); Thaler et al. (2010); van Gastel & Ferdinand (2008); Viana et al. (2008); Villabø et al. (2012); Wei et al. (2014); Wood et al. (2002)	MASC = .64–.75 SOC = .61–.89 SEP = .69–.80 Harm Avoidance = .52–.68 Physical Symptoms = .81–.84	MASC = 48 SOC = 13.5 SEP = 11 Harm Avoidance = 19 Physical Symptoms = 18	MASC = 2.77 SOC = 2.29 SEP = 2.17 Harm Avoidance = 2.50 Physical Symptoms = 3.44	MASC = 0.20 SOC = 0.31 SEP = 0.30 Harm Avoidance = 0.36 Physical Symptoms = 0.29
Negative Affectivity Self-Statement Questionnaire	Sood & Kendall (2007)	Anxiety scale = .85	Anxiety scale = 49	Anxiety scale = 4.00	Anxiety scale = 0.30

Scale	References	Reliability	Cutoff	LR+	LR−
Revised Children's Anxiety and Depression Scale	Chorpita et al. (2005)	No data available	SOC = 10 GAD = 7 SEP = 5 PD = 12	SOC = 1.64 GAD = 2.46 SEP = 2.35 PD = 9.75	SOC = 0.64 GAD = 0.43 SEP = 0.39 PD = 0.24
Revised Children's Manifest Anxiety Scale	Dierker et al. (2001); Hodges (1990)	No data available	RCMAS = $T > 60$	RCMAS = 1.39	RCMAS = 0.24
Screen for Child Anxiety Related Emotion Disorders	Birmaher et al. (1997, 1999); Canals et al. (2012); DeSousa et al. (2012); Kerns et al. (2015); Monga et al. (2000); Rappaport et al. (2017); Van Meter et al. (2016)	SCARED = .58–.86 SCARED-5 = n/a SEP = .80–.89 SOC = .70–.79 GAD = .64–.86 Somatic/panic = .74–.89 School phobia = n/a	SCARED = 22 SCARED-5 = 3 SEP = 7 SOC = 6.5 GAD = 8 Somatic/panic = 6 School phobia = 3	SCARED = 2.29 SCARED-5 = 2.66 SEP = 3.80 SOC = 3.24 GAD = 3.43 Somatic/panic = 4.88 School phobia = 1.60	SCARED = 0.46 SCARED-5 = 0.40 SEP = 0.30 SOC = 0.41 GAD = 0.35 Somatic/panic = 0.26 School phobia = 0.57
Social Anxiety Scale for Children and Adolescents	Garcia-Lopez et al. (2015); Inderbitzen-Nolan et al. (2004)	SAS-A = .92	SAS-A = 49	SAS-A = 3.36	SAS-A = 0.48
Social Phobia and Anxiety Inventory for Children	Bunnell et al. (2015); Garcia-Lopez et al. (2015); Inderbitzen-Nolan et al. (2004); Pina et al. (2013); Viana et al. (2008)	SPAIC = .65–.91 SPAIC, 16-item = .86 SPAIC, 11-item = .74–.94	SPAIC = 16.5 SPAIC, 16-item = 26.45 SPAIC, 11-item = 11	SPAIC = 4.10 SPAIC, 16-item = 12.29 SPAIC, 11-item = 4.95	SPAIC = 0.34 SPAIC, 16-item = 0.15 SPAIC, 11-item = 0.21
Spence Children's Anxiety Scale	Brown-Jacobsen et al. (2011); Nauta et al. (2004); Reardon et al. (2018); Zainal et al. (2014)	SCAS = n/a SCAS-8 = .70–.86	SCAS = $T \geq 62.5$ SCAS-8 = 6.5 SEP = $T \geq 65$ SOC = $T \geq 65$ GAD = $T \geq 65$ SP = $T \geq 65$ OCD = $T \geq 65$	SCAS = 1.79 SCAS-8 = 2.59 SEP = 1.54 SOC = 1.94 GAD = 1.18 SP = 1.91 OCD = 2.14	SCAS = 0.48 SCAS-8 = 0.41 SEP = 0.31 SOC = 0.52 GAD = 0.69 SP = 0.81 OCD = 0.23
State–Trait Anxiety Inventory for Children	Hishinuma et al. (2001); Hodges (1990); Monga et al. (2000)	STAI-S = .54 STAI-T = .61	STAI-S = 1 STAI-T = 2	STAI-S = 4.46 STAI-T = 6.02	STAI-S = 0.44 STAI-T = 0.24
Youth Anxiety Measure for DSM-5	Fuentes-Rodriguez et al. (2018)	SOC = 1.00	SOC = 4	SOC = 25.00	SOC = 0.00

Note. LR+, the likelihood ratio for a test score above the cutoff value; LR−, the likelihood ratio for a test score below the cutoff value. The analyses in this table represent a comparison either between the full-scale score and any anxiety disorder or between a subscale score and the corresponding anxiety disorder. In the analyses for the social anxiety measures (LSAS, SAS, and SPAI), the full-scale score is compared with social anxiety. The MASC Harm Avoidance subscale is used to assess GAD, and the MASC Physical Symptoms subscale is used to assess panic disorder/agoraphobia.

Overall, youth anxiety questionnaires possess strong support for internal consistency. The multidimensional nature of some scales indicates that internal consistency would be strong for both the total scale and the subscales. Cronbach's alpha was higher for the total scales than for subscales, which may be because Cronbach's alpha increases as the number of items in a scale increases. The extreme ends of the internal consistency ranges warrant a closer look. On the lower end, most of the YAM-5 Specific Phobia subscales (animal type, natural environment type, situational type/ agoraphobia, and other type) had Cronbach alpha coefficients lower than .60 (Muris et al., 2016). However, this may be more indicative of the nature of specific phobias: A person who is afraid of dogs, for example, is not necessarily afraid of other animals, so we would not expect a correlation between all items within a subscale. The shorter length of these subscales also may have contributed to the lower alpha coefficients (each subscale only included three to six items). On the upper end, many measures had Cronbach alpha coefficients higher than .90, which may indicate item redundancy (Streiner, 2003), which increases the amount of time it takes for respondents to complete measures and may offer diminishing returns in many clinical applications.

Retest reliability indicates how stable a measure is, in the absence of any intervention. Temporal stability was supported for all youth anxiety questionnaires (see Table 10.3). Most studies examined retest reliability for the full scales. To our knowledge, retest reliability has not been examined in the IUSC or the YAM-5, two relatively new measures. Retest reliability was generally strong, with coefficients great than .50. Unsurprisingly, the retest reliability was higher for shorter periods of time than it was for longer periods of time (Ollendick, 1983). The longer retest period may explain the low retest coefficients for the SCAS ($r = .45$ over a 6-month retest period). It is unclear whether a lower retest coefficient reflects poor retest reliability or a shift in anxiety over the retest period. The PARS also had low retest reliability (ICC = .37 to .59), although the authors noted that participants received psychoeducation during the 1- to 4-week retest period (RUPP, 2002).

Convergent validity was supported for all measures of youth anxiety, with questionnaires correlating in the expected directions. There were some instances in which the correlations were weak (Southam-Gerow, Flannery-Schroeder, & Kendall, 2003), but this lack of correlation may indicate that the constructs being compared are not significantly related. Studies generally used other questionnaires to examine convergent validity, although some studies used severity ratings from diagnostic interviews (March et al., 1997). Most evidence for convergent validity compared the total score of questionnaires rather than specific subscales. Shared method variance may account for some the significant correlations (Campbell & Fiske, 1959), a reason for encouraging measures from both parent and youth.

Most important to the prediction phase of EBA is the accuracy of a measure: the ability of the measure to discriminate between disorders (Youngstrom et al., 2017). Historically, studies have reported questionnaires' accuracy with effect sizes comparing the difference between scores of anxious and nonanxious youth (Youngstrom, Choukas-Bradley, Calhoun, & Jensen-Doss, 2015). Such studies have suggested that questionnaires are better at discriminating anxious youth from youth with externalizing disorders, but not other affective disorders (Muris, Merckelbach, Ollendick, King, & Bogie, 2002; Seligman, Ollendick, Langley, & Baldacci, 2004). Although such data are informative, it is not readily apparent how they could help a clinician assess whether a youth, like Daniel, has a specific anxiety disorder.

Recent research examines youth anxiety measures' accuracy using receiver operator analyses: sensitivity (accuracy in identifying true positives) and specificity (accuracy in identifying true negatives). Sensitivity and specificity ratings are based on cutoff scores and can be used to form a diagnostic likelihood ratio (DLR), which indicates the increased likelihood that a person has a disorder given a score above or below a cutoff score. Using the nomogram described by Van Meter (Chapter 2, this volume; or an online posttest probability calculator), clinicians can combine the pretest probability (often the base rate) with the DLR to produce a posttest probability. The posttest probability indicates the likelihood that a client has a disorder, based on the information gathered.

Table 10.4 summarizes the receiver operator characteristics and diagnostic likelihood ratios of youth anxiety measures. We focused this analysis on studies that used semistructured interviews in the receiver operator analyses, and we chose to report the area under the curve (AUC), which is not dependent on the cutoff score, and DLRs, which are not dependent on local prevalence rates. Some commonly used measures, such as the RCADS and the RCMAS, lack receiver operator analyses, and others, such as the PSWQ and the FSSC-R, lack receiver operator and sensitivity/specificity analyses. Many measures have a range of diagnostic accuracies reported. For example, studies indicate that the Internalizing Problems subscale of the CBCL has an AUC ranging from .52 (Monga et al., 2000) to .94 (Aschenbrand, Angelosante, & Kendall, 2010). In general, the diagnostic accuracy was lower in samples with learning disabilities (Thaler, Kazemi, & Wood, 2010) and autism (Kerns et al., 2015; Zainal et al., 2014). Diagnostic accuracy and optimal cutoff scores varied by study, by gender (Reardon, Spence, Hesse, Shakir, & Creswell, 2018; Storch, Masia-Warner, Dent, Roberti, & Fisher, 2004), by ethnicity (Pina, Little, Wynne, & Beidel, 2013), and by age (Wei et al., 2014). Although optimal cutoff scores based on parent and child report varied within each study, when information from all studies was combined, there was little difference between reporters. Additionally, one study specifically found no difference in discriminant validity for the CBCL between research and community clinics (Van Meter et al., 2014). Overall, and not surprisingly, measures fared worse when discriminating among specific anxiety disorders than when discriminating between youth with and without *any* anxiety disorder (Aschenbrand et al., 2010; Viana, Rabian, & Beidel, 2008), and youth with anxiety disorders and those with other internalizing disorders (Birmaher et al., 1997). Briefer measures had similar discriminate validities as their longer counterparts (e.g., the SPAIC), suggesting that briefer measures, which reduce assessment burden, are useful. Although Fuentes-Rodriguez, Sáez-Castillo, and Garcia-Lopez (2018) reported that the YAM-5, Social subscale had perfect diagnostic accuracy, this study had a small sample size, limiting its power to detect variations. Further investigation on the sensitivity and specificity of the YAM is warranted. The CBCL/YSR, MASC, and SCARED had the best support for discriminate validity, with the majority of studies reporting AUC values above .60.

Putting It into Practice

Select the measures and subscales that are relevant for the presenting problem. EBA uses a Bayesian framework that assumes assessment tools are not correlated: Youngstrom and colleagues (2017) suggest only including measures with correlations below 0.3. Daniel completed the YSR and the SCARED—Child version (SCARED-C). His

clinician chose to focus on the YSR, Attention Difficulty subscale to evaluate Daniel's attention problems and the SCARED-C, Social Anxiety and Generalized Anxiety subscales to evaluate his anxiety. Daniel's scores are reported in Table 10.5. For a client whose initial presentation appears to be limited to social anxiety, a clinician could substitute the SCARED-C with a measure specific to social anxiety, such as the SPAIC. If a client's initial presentation is less clear (e.g., attention problems), a clinician could begin with the YSR to screen for internalizing and externalizing problems, and if the YSR Anxiety/Depression subscales are elevated, they could use the SCARED-C to further probe for specific types of anxiety. Next, select the cutoff scores and DLRs from Table 10.4 to use in the posttest probability analysis. Use the nomogram to combine DLRs based on the intake assessment with the clinic base rates calculated in Step 2. As shown in Table 10.5, Daniel's posterior probability of having SOC is 71%, of having GAD is 24%, and of having ADHD is 1%. There is a wide range of probabilities for SOC and GAD because studies have indicated a range of sensitivity and specificity values for the SCARED.

Gather Collateral, Cross-Informant Perspectives

When assessing youth anxiety, it is considered best practice to collect information from both parents and youth (Comer & Kendall, 2004; De Los Reyes & Kazdin, 2005; De Los Reyes, Thomas, Goodman, & Kundey, 2013). Anxious youth may not disclose their feelings fully (Dadds, Perrin, & Yule, 1998), and younger children may have less emotional awareness to accurately report their symptoms (Southam-Gerow & Kendall, 2002). Younger children also report fewer overall symptoms than do their parents (Schniering, Hudson, & Rapee, 2000). Parents, too, have slants/biases that impact their reporting, such as attributing their child's symptoms to the child's personality rather than to external circumstances (De Los Reyes & Kazdin, 2005). Krain and Kendall (2000) found that parental depression predicted parent-reported child anxiety, even after they controlled for parental anxiety. For these reasons, the majority of measures of youth anxiety include versions for both parent and child report (see Table 10.2). Researchers have found a statistically significant increase in diagnostic accuracy when adding parent report to youth report (Van Meter et al., 2014; Villabø, Gere, Torgersen, March, & Kendall, 2012).

TABLE 10.5. Scores and Interpretive Information for Applying EBA to the Case of Daniel

Common diagnostic hypotheses (Step 1)	Starting probability (Step 2)	Broad measure (Step 4)			Cross-informant (Step 5)				Treatment phase		
		Scale and Score	DLR	Revised probability	Next test score	DLR	Revised probability	Confirmation (Step 6)	Process (Step 10)	Outcome (Step 11)	Maintenance (Step 12)
Social anxiety disorder	19%	SCARED-C/ SOC = 14	3.24	43%	SCARED-P/ SOC = 13	3.24	71%	ADIS-C/P	CQ-C/P SOC = 2	SCARED/ SOC = 6	Monitor avoidance of social situations
Generalized anxiety disorder	21%	SCARED-C/ GAD = 15	3.43	48%	SCARED-P/ GAD = 3	0.35	24%	ADIS-C/P	CQ-C/P GAD = 1	SCARED/ GAD = 7	Monitor homework procrastination
ADHD	10%	YSR T Attention = 61	0.86	9%	CBCL T Attention = 68	1.41	12%	ADIS-C/P	Not a primary focus		

Note. SCARED-C/P, Screen for Child Anxiety Related Emotion Disorders—Child/Parent report; SCARED/SOC, SCARED, Social Anxiety subscale; SCARED/GAD, SCARED, Generalized Anxiety subscale; YSR Attention, Youth Self-Report, Attention Problems subscale; ADIS-C/P, Anxiety Disorders Interview Schedule—Child and Parent versions; CQ-C/P, Coping Questionnaire—Child and Parent versions; DLR, diagnostic likelihood ratio; DLR for the YSR/CBCL were reported in Raiker et al. (2017).

Discrepancies between parent and youth reports are considered the norm and do not necessarily indicate that one report is more or less accurate than the other. Each reporter offers a unique perspective, and integrating many pieces of information improves diagnostic decision making (De Los Reyes et al., 2015). A meta-analysis of multiple-informant agreement found that the average correlation between parent- and child-reported internalizing symptoms was .26, and that age did not influence this effect (De Los Reyes et al., 2015). Additionally, there were low levels of agreement between parents: The average correlation between mothers and fathers was .48 (De Los Reyes et al., 2015). As shown in Table 10.3, parent–child agreement on questionnaires was generally less than .50. Parent–child agreement is higher for observable symptoms than for unobservable symptoms (Comer & Kendall, 2004; De Los Reyes et al., 2015). In practice, clinicians tend to favor parent-reported symptoms, even though parent report is not inherently more accurate than youth report about anxiety problems (De Los Reyes et al., 2015). Although discrepancies between informant reports complicate the diagnostic process, they can reveal factors that are important for the treatment process. Lower levels of youth-reported symptoms may indicate difficulty involving the youth in treatment (symptom denial), and lower parent-reported symptoms may suggest that the parent would benefit from psychoeducation about the youth's symptoms.

Although less common in assessment of youth anxiety, teacher report provides a useful prospective because teachers see youth in many different situations, such as separating from their parents in the morning, interacting with peers, and completing assignments and activities. Teachers' experiences with a range of youth enable them to compare a specific youth to similar-age youth based on what is age appropriate. The ASEBA CBCL/YSR has a teacher version: the Teacher Report Form (Achenbach & Rescorla, 2001). However, research suggests that teacher report is less valid for internalizing symptoms (De Los Reyes et al., 2015), with one study indicating that the TRF did no better than chance at predicting internalizing symptoms (Van Meter et al., 2014). Teacher reports pose difficulties because they are less accessible during the summer. The consensus is that teachers are not as useful to include in the assessment phase for youth anxiety (De Los Reyes et al., 2015; Loeber, Green, & Lahey, 1990).

Putting It into Practice

EBA offers a way to combine information from parent and youth reports. Youngstrom and Van Meter (2016) recommend including only one parent-report measure and one child-report measure per diagnostic issue to avoid problems with shared method variance. Because there are low levels of agreement between reporters, including assessments from parents and youth does not introduce bias into the Bayesian framework. Integrating information from different informants follows the same process as integrating any piece of assessment information. As with youth report, clinicians choose the most relevant scores based on the diagnostic issue and identify the associated cutoff scores and DLR. The posterior probability from the previous step becomes the starting probability for the nomogram. It is also possible to combine multiple pieces of assessment into one step by multiplying the DLRs from each piece of information.

Daniel's parents completed the CBCL and the SCARED—Parent version (SCARED-P). The clinician focused on the CBCL Attention Difficulty subscale and the SCARED-P Social Anxiety and Generalized Anxiety subscales. As shown in Table 10.5, Daniel's clinician combined the revised probability from Step 4 with the DLR corresponding to each measure. As is common with youth psychopathology, Daniel's parents reported more externalizing symptoms than he did, while Daniel reported more internalizing symptoms (Grills & Ollendick, 2002). In Daniel's case, both he and his parents reported scores above the cutoff score for the SCARED Social Anxiety subscale, but only Daniel reported scores above the cutoff score for the SCARED Generalized Anxiety subscale, and only his parents reported scores above the cutoff score for the CBCL/YSR Attention Difficulty subscale. Using the EBA method enabled the clinician to give equal weight to the parent and child reports when combining these discrepancies: The posterior probability is lower for GAD and ADHD than it would be if both Daniel and his parents reported scores in the clinical range, but higher than it would be if both had reported scores below the clinical range. After combining parent and child report with the clinic prevalence rate, the posterior probability of Daniel having SOC is 71%, of having GAD is 24%, and of having ADHD is 12%. Because the measures bring Daniel above the test–treat threshold or below the test–wait threshold, Daniel's clinician will continue the assessment process.

Prescription

Use Semistructured or Structured Interviews to Finalize Diagnoses

Using the posterior probabilities from the intake assessment, the clinician can determine which disorders to focus on in a clinical interview. Some clinicians may be tempted to skip the prediction phase and begin the intake assessment with a diagnostic interview; we caution against this urge. Intake questionnaires are brief to administer and interpret, and they provide a context to interpret symptoms reported during the diagnostic interview. The intake questionnaires guide the clinician on which diagnostic interview to select, and which supplementary modules can be used for particular clients. For example, for youth who may have an anxiety disorder, the Anxiety Disorders Interview Schedule, Child and Parent versions (ADIS-C/P) is the preferred diagnostic tool (Silverman & Ollendick, 2005). The aim of the clinical interview is to finalize the diagnosis. In addition to being necessary for insurance billing, diagnoses help the clinician conceptualize the case and create a treatment plan. For instance, cognitive-behavioral therapy (CBT) includes exposure and cognitive change strategies, and an understanding of the specific nature of the youth's anxiety enables the clinician to effectively plan both exposures (behavioral experiments) and cognitive interventions.

Semistructured diagnostic interviews are considered the "gold standard" when diagnosing people with a mental health disorder (e.g., Kendall & Flannery-Schroeder, 1998; McClellan & Werry, 2000). Semistructured interviews aim to reduce variability in both wording and interpretation of client responses, and in responses elicited by a specific diagnostician, and also to allow the diagnostician to flexibly gather information to make a diagnosis based on his or her clinical judgment (McClellan & Werry, 2000). By providing a standard set of questions for all clients, semistructured interviews reduce cognitive biases in diagnosis, such as the availability heuristic, confirmation bias, representativeness, search satisfying (Croskerry, 2003; Galanter & Patel, 2005). Within the context of youth anxiety disorders, semistructured interviews provide clinicians with a framework both to assess whether behaviors are age- or culturally appropriate (e.g., sleeping in a parent's bed), and to consider alternative diagnoses for common symptoms (e.g., attention difficulties in anxiety vs. ADHD).

Unfortunately, the use of diagnostic interviews is rare in community clinics, with one study group estimating that only 15% of clinicians use diagnostic interviews with their patients (Bruchmüller, Margraf, Suppiger, & Schneider, 2011). Clinicians may incorrectly think that diagnostic interviews damage rapport (Bruchmüller et al., 2011), or that they take too long to complete, and that insurance will not reimburse the cost of the assessment appointment. Two studies, however, indicate that patients viewed semistructured diagnostic interviews favorably (Suppiger et al., 2009). Although diagnostic interviews may require a longer initial session, they enable the clinician to immediately begin treatment planning based on a reliable diagnosis, which reduces the overall length of treatment and increases the likelihood that the clinician will provide effective treatment.

Table 10.6 summarizes the diagnostic interviews most commonly used to assess youth anxiety. Given that interrater reliability is an important metric for evaluating diagnostic interviews (Youngstrom et al., 2017), we include a summary of reliability coefficients. The authors of the ADIS-C/P, the National Institute of Mental Health (NIMH) Diagnostic Interview Schedule for Children (DISC), the Child and Adolescent Psychiatric Assessment (CAPA), and the Schedule for Affective Disorders and Schizophrenia for School-Age Children (K-SADS) are in the process of finalizing and evaluating new versions of the interviews to match DSM-5 criteria. Given that most of the content of the new interviews mirror DSM-IV versions, we suspect that similar psychometric properties will be reported. Relative to other youth diagnostic interviews, the ADIS-C/P is considered to be advantageous for diagnosing anxiety disorders given its focus on anxiety disorders and robust psychometric properties (Brooks & Kutcher, 2003; Kendall & Flannery-Schroeder, 1998; Langley, Bergman, & Piacentini, 2002; Schniering et al., 2000; Silverman & Ollendick, 2005). Therefore, we focus the bulk of our discussion on the ADIS-C/P. This said, there are certain instances in which it would be preferable to use a diagnostic interview other than the ADIS-C/P. For example, the CAPA and the DISC are structured interviews that require less clinical interpretation and can be administered by mental health workers with less training. Additionally, unlike the ADIS-C/P, the CAPA, DISC, and K-SADS are all free and therefore cheaper to administer. Nonetheless, we recommend using the ADIS-C/P for diagnosing youth anxiety.

TABLE 10.6. Structured and Semistructured Interviews for Diagnosing Anxiety Disorders in Youth

Diagnostic interview	References	Ages (years)	Versions	Structured or semistructured?	Time to complete (min)	Reliability of anxiety diagnoses	Where to obtain	Cost
Anxiety Disorders Interview Schedule for DSM-IV: Child and Parent Versions	Lyneham et al. (2007); Rapee et al. (1994); Silverman & Nelles (1988); Wood et al. (2002)	6–18	C/P	SS	60–90	kappa = .59–1.0 r = .74–.77	https://global.oup.com/academic/category/science-and-mathematics/psychology/clinical-psychology	Yes
Child and Adolescent Psychiatric Assessment	Angold & Costello (1995)	9–18	C/P	S	90	ICC = .60–.80	http://devepi.duhs.duke.edu/capa.html	No
NIMH Diagnostic Interview Schedule for Children Version IV	Shaffer et al. (1993)	9–17	C/P	S	70–120	kappa = .66–1.0	www.cdc.gov/nchs/data/nhanes/limited_access/interviewer_manual.pdf	No
Schedule for Affective Disorders and Schizophrenia for School-Age Children	Ambrosini (2000)	6–18	C/P	SS	90	kappa = .64–.85	www.kennedykrieger.org/sites/default/files/community_files/ksads-dsm-5-screener.pdf	No

Note. C, child; P, parent; A, adolescent; S, structured; SS, semistructured; SEP, separation anxiety disorder; SOC, social phobia; SP, specific phobia; GAD, generalized anxiety disorder; OAD, overanxious disorder; NIMH, National Institute of Mental Health.

The ADIS-C/P (Silverman & Albano, 1996) is a semistructured diagnostic interview that assesses anxiety, mood, and externalizing disorders in accordance with DSM-IV criteria (American Psychiatric Association, 1994). It is for youth ages 6–17 years (Silverman & Albano, 1996) and is modeled off the ADIS-IV Lifetime version (ADIS-IV-L), which is used for adults age 18 years and older (Brown, Barlow, & DiNardo, 1994). Parents and youth are interviewed separately. The ADIS-C and ADIS-P are nearly identical, except that the ADIS-P assesses for conduct disorder and ODD. The interview begins with an overview of school refusal, the child's social background, and other situational factors related to anxiety (Silverman & Albano, 1996). The ADIS-C/P provides screening questions and skips others, such that the diagnostician only asks questions for the full section if the parent or child endorse the initial symptoms. The ADIS-C/P is unique in that it includes dimensional ratings for severity, intensity, uncontrollability, avoidance, and interference at the both symptom and syndrome levels. Diagnosticians also provide a clinical severity rating (CSR) using a 9-point scale ranging from 0 (*no impairment*) to 8 (*severe impairment*), in which "impairment" is defined as affecting many domains of life or causing significant distress. Higher CSR scores indicate greater impairment, and a CSR ≥ 4 indicates meeting diagnostic criteria.

The psychometric properties of the ADIS-C/P have been evaluated (Table 10.6). Interrater reliability, for independent diagnosticians, on the ADIS-C/P ranged from kappa = .92 for principle diagnoses, kappa = .80–1.0 for individual anxiety disorders, and kappa = .65–.77 for comorbid disorders (Lyneham, Abbott, & Rapee, 2007). Interrater agreement for CSR for positive diagnoses of SEP, SOC, GAD, and panic disorder ranged from r = .74–.77 (Wood, Piacentini, Bergman, McCracken, & Barrios, 2002). Although the ADIS-C/P cannot be used to formally diagnosis ADHD, it has been found to be a reliable tool for identifying ODD (Anderson & Ollendick, 2012). The ADIS-C/P has demonstrated test–retest reliability, with stability coefficients of anxiety disorders ranging from .78 to .95 and of externalizing disorders ranging from .62 to 1.00 (Silverman, Saavedra, & Pina, 2001). As with questionnaires, research has demonstrated low levels of parent–child agreement on the ADIS-C/P (Choudhury, Pimentel, & Kendall, 2003; Comer & Kendall, 2004; Grills & Ollendick, 2002)—one reason why the ADIS-C/P provides separate interviews for both parents and youth.

As a diagnostic interview, the ADIS-C/P is often used to demonstrate convergent validity of questionnaires measuring anxiety symptoms. Youth who meet criteria for an anxiety disorder score higher on self-report measures of anxiety, including the SCAS (Nauta et al., 2004), the CBCL (Achenbach, McConaughy, & Howell, 1987), the MASC (March et al., 1997; March, Sullivan, & Parker, 1999), and the RCADS (Chorpita et al., 2000; Chorpita, Moffitt, & Gray, 2005). The ADIS-C/P also has demonstrated discriminant validity, with specific anxiety disorder diagnoses corresponding to specific subscales of each of these measures (Aschenbrand et al., 2010; Chorpita et al., 2005; Nauta et al., 2004; Villabø et al., 2012; Wood et al., 2002).

Although construct validity has not been formerly examined, McClellan and Weery (2000) noted that diagnostic interviews are only as valid as the diagnostic criteria for the disorder the interview purports to measure. In a study examining the validity of DSM criteria for anxiety disorders, Schniering and colleagues (2000) found only partial support for differentiation between specific anxiety disorders. A similar study that used the ADIS-C/P to answer this question found that worry differentiated youth with GAD from those other anxiety disorders (Tracey, Chorpita, Douban, & Barlow, 1997). The discriminant validity of the ADIS-C/P also has not been examined. However, the high rate of comorbidities between anxiety disorders (Kendall et al., 2010) no doubt contributes to limited discriminant validity. Given that many youth anxiety treatments address anxiety transdiagnostically (e.g., Coping Cat; Kendall & Hedtke, 2006), identifying a more global anxiety factor may provide enough resolution for treatment planning.

The ADIS-C/P is the recommended diagnostic interview in part due to its superior prescriptive validity. It is more comprehensive than other semistructured diagnostic interviews (Brooks & Kutcher, 2003; Kendall & Flannery-Schroeder, 1998; Schniering et al., 2000; Silverman & Ollendick, 2005). The ADIS-C/P expands on many DSM criteria by inquiring about situations that are commonly anxiety provoking for youth (e.g., being called on by the teacher in class). As such, the ADIS-C/P provides the clinician with numerous examples of anxiety-provoking situations that can become targets for treatment. Treatment outcome studies indicate that the ADIS-C/P has sensitivity to change (Silverman et al., 1999; Walkup et al., 2008). The ADIS-C/P is the most commonly used diagnostic interview on clinical trials of youth anxiety (Silverman & Ollendick, 2005).

Putting It into Practice

Based on posterior probabilities from Daniel's intake assessment, his clinician decided to administer an ADIS-C/P to Daniel and his parents. During the interview, both Daniel and his parents endorsed that Daniel feels anxious in many situations involving interactions with his peers and has concerns about achieving high standards in school. They also endorsed that Daniel worries about the uncertainty of his academic future, including whether he will be able to attend college. When conducting the diagnostic interview, it is important to be aware of "confirmation bias": looking for instances that confirm the posterior probabilities from the intake assessment. Diagnostic interviews enable clinicians to probe the symptoms reported on the intake assessment as they diagnose the client. During the ADIS-C/P, Daniel's clinician was able to clarify that he has difficulty concentrating, but only when he is feeling anxious. The clinician interpreted the elevated CBCL Attention Problems subscale as being related to Daniel's anxiety.

There may be instances in which the diagnostic interview conflicts with the intake assessments. Social desirability and other demand characteristics may cause youth to under- or overreport symptoms. For example, some youth endorse suicidal ideation on a questionnaire but not during a diagnostic interview. Such a situation typically requires additional information gathering.

Overall, Daniel's and his parents' reports during the interview were consistent with their responses on the intake questionnaires. Daniel's clinician diagnosed him with having SOC and GAD. The clinician also ruled out ADHD, as it appeared the attentional difficulties were better associated with his anxiety. Although the diagnostic interview generally occurs at the beginning of treatment, diagnoses can evolve throughout treatment as the clinician gains information about the client. After finalizing Daniel's diagnoses, his clinician entered them into the clinic database. This enables the clinic to have an up-to-date record of local prevalence rates.

Case Formulation Considerations

Assessment of anxiety in youth is best when guided by theoretically supported conceptualizations that help rule out other potentially differential conditions. Despite anxiety's frequent comorbidity with other conditions, anxiety disorders have specific characteristics and predictive factors that differentiate them from other psychopathologies. Assessment can help differentiate anxiety disorders in situations in which presenting symptoms may overlap with other internalizing disorders. Therefore, incorporating assessment tools specific to theoretical formulation can help clinicians separate the prevalence of anxiety disorders from other potential psychopathological hypotheses.

The tripartite model of anxiety and depression is helpful in differentiating not only internalizing and externalizing disorders but also anxiety and depression (Clark & Watson, 1991; De Bolle & De Fruyt, 2010). This model presents researchers and clinicians with the constructs and characteristics that are frequently observed in youth with anxiety, specifically NA and PH. Previous research has demonstrated that NA is a significant risk factor for the development of internalizing disorders in children (Brown, Chorpita, & Barlow, 1998). NA presenting with a distinct construct of PH separates many of the anxiety disorders from depression. This necessitates developing and using assessment tools to differentiate internalizing disorders (Chorpita, Albano, & Barlow, 1998).

In addition to NA and PH, children with anxiety disorders often report AS and intolerance of uncertainty (IU). AS is the fear of physiological sensations, typically with the idea that these sensations will result in negative consequences (e.g., physical harm, going crazy; Reiss et al., 1986). AS, while akin to trait anxiety and mostly associated with panic disorder, can increase the risk of comorbidity among anxiety disorders. Similarly, IU is a child's inability to cope with the absence of typically key information about upcoming events or situations, whether certain or hypothetical (Carleton, 2016). Children with increased IU view any potential negative events as threatening or unacceptable, despite whether the event will occur (Carleton, Sharpe, & Asmundson, 2007). Children with IU also often view ambiguous situations as threatening (Carleton et al., 2007). Figure 10.1 illustrates the relationship between IU, AS, NA, and PH, and the anxiety disorders commonly seen in childhood (Boelen & Carleton, 2012; Boelen, Reijntjes, & Carleton, 2014; Brown et al., 1998; Carleton, Collimore, & Asmundson, 2010; Carleton et al., 2014; Clark & Watson, 1991; Dugas & Ladouceur, 2000; Gentes & Ruscio, 2011; Ladouceur, Gosselin, & Dugas, 2000; Reiss et al., 1986). Carleton and colleagues (2007) demonstrated that

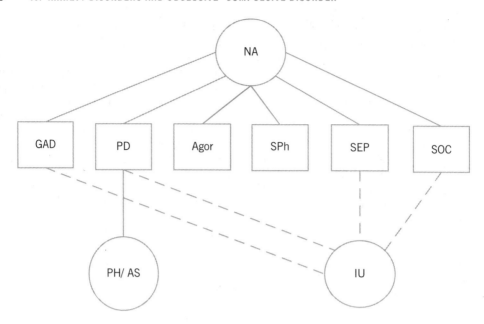

FIGURE 10.1. The relation of theoretical constructs to various anxiety disorders. This figure illustrates how negative affectivity (NA), physiological hyperarousal (PH), anxiety sensitivity (AS), and intolerance of uncertainty (IU) relate to the common childhood anxiety disorders. Agor, agoraphobia; SPh, specific phobia; SEP, separation anxiety; SOC, social anxiety disorder.

AS and IU are highly correlated, demonstrating the importance of assessing for both in children with anxiety disorders. However, these constructs are considered relatively independent of one another and may not be characteristic of every youth with an anxiety disorder. The purpose of identifying IU and AS is to help narrow down a clinician's list of potential diagnoses.

To assess for these common constructs in children and adolescents with potential anxiety disorders, clinicians can refer to measures previously mentioned in the prescription process. The NASSQ may provide insight into a child's self-talk, differentiating between anxious self-talk and depressive self-talk. Clinicians can use the CASI to assess the child's level of sensitivity to anxious arousal and the IUSC can be used to determine how much a child can tolerate unfamiliarity or uncertainty. Using these questionnaires helps develop hypotheses about specific anxiety disorders and treatment needs.

Putting It into Practice

After examining the questionnaires completed by Daniel and his mother, the clinician noted high scores on Daniel's NASSQ, especially regarding anxious self-talk. Daniel endorsed lower levels of AS but scored high on IU. Accordingly, the clinician hypothesized GAD, SEP, and SOC based on these preliminary predictive scores.

During the clinical assessment process, Daniel reported NA and increased PH. He stated that he was often critical of his performance in school and did not see himself as a good student, despite his mother indicating that he performs well when he attends school. In addition to his lower mood states, Daniel reported that he often experiences stomachaches, headaches, and difficulty breathing when he feels anxious. Daniel further stated that he often worries about his academic future and feels intimidated by the thoughts of college and a career. He said that the uncertainty of his future is scary.

Addressing Multicultural Issues

In addition to assessing anxiety, clinicians are wise to be aware of various cultural presentations and identities. In an increasingly diverse world, various cultural factors may influence assessment and treatment. Clinicians may include multicultural assessment questions to understand more about the child's background and how such factors may interplay with different treatment modalities (Youngstrom et al., 2015). A brief biopsychosocial assessment can be included as part of the semistructured interview to incorporate information regarding the youth's cultural identity, medical history, and social environment. Specifically, the ADDRESSING framework outlined by Hays (2016) can be helpful in organizing a youth's cultural information and comparing it to the cultural identity of the clinician. For an example using the case of Daniel, refer to Table 10.7.

Putting It into Practice

Given Daniel's background, factors were considered that may be contributing to or maintaining his anxiety. During the interview, Daniel stated that his family did not have enough money to send him to college, and that an academic scholarship was the only way he would be able to afford an engineering education. Daniel reported not having the same interests as many of his peers. He stated that he is often nervous that his peers will think he is weird because of his interests, and this causes him to isolate himself. These features of Daniel's life experience flavor his experience of anxiety and can be used to improve the likelihood of effective intervention.

Assess for Treatment Plan and Goal Setting

Using the assessment methods previously presented, a clinician can establish measurable and operationalized goals. The assessments help formulate the treatment plan and the goals associated with the specific presentation. The Coping Questionnaire (CQ), for example, details the youth's specific worries and his or her ability to tolerate and cope with them. The CQ is initially completed with collaboration between the assessor/clinician, the youth, and parent(s). Goals can be directed by the CQ content, and this content is directed by input from (1) the youth, (2) the parent(s), and (3) the therapist. This measure has demonstrated sensitivity to treatment, making it a useful measure for collaborative goal setting (Crane & Kendall, 2018). Understanding the context of the youth's anxiety can be helpful in formulating goals (Youngstrom & Van Meter, 2016). The clinician's role is to integrate objective information regarding the anxiety (e.g., anxiety scores, level of interference, avoidance) with information from the youth and parents (e.g., youth's interests and personal goals, family expectations). For example, if a youth's social anxiety is interfering with making friends, the clinician and youth may agree on a long-term goal of "making two new friends this school year."

It is important for the collaborative goals to be measurable and objective in nature. The purpose

TABLE 10.7. ADDRESSING Multicultural Issues Framework

ADDRESSING framework	Daniel	Clinician
Age (years)	14	33
Developmental or . . .	Normal development	Normal development
Other disability	Normal development but experiences seasonal allergies	Normal development
Religion and spiritual orientation	Nondenominational Christian	Nonreligious
Ethnic and racial identity	African American	European American
Socioeconomic status	Low SES	Middle class
Sexual orientation	Heterosexual	Heterosexual
Indigenous heritage	Non-Indigenous	Non-Indigenous
National origin	U.S. born	U.S. born
Gender	Male	Female

of these goals is to document progress throughout treatment. Goal measurement includes duration and frequency of desired behaviors. The assessment measures can be helpful in creating measurable goals. For example, the SCARED can be used to set and monitor goals regarding a youth's anxiety (i.e., Daniel's anxiety will reduce from a 32 on the SCARED to a 16 on the SCARED after 16 sessions). Additionally, goals are best when attainable: Outlandish and unreachable goals hint toward discouragement.

The youth, parents, and therapist are active participants in goal setting. The assessment process provides objective data, and collaboration with parents helps address how these problems interfere with daily lives. Youth integrate their own personal goals into their treatment plans, providing information on how they can reach their own goals.

Putting It into Practice

Following the initial assessment, Daniel and his parents were eager to come up with treatment goals. Daniel stated that he struggled with turning in school assignments and wanted help with reducing anxiety that would help his grades to be at a competitive level for academic recognition. Daniel's mother stated that his current school-related anxiety caused difficulty with her job, as they often spent an hour in the morning arguing about his school attendance. This has made her late to work on multiple occasions, resulting in her boss threatening probation. Daniel, his mother, and the therapist collaborated and agreed on the following initial goals:

1. Daniel will learn to manage anxiety with developmentally appropriate coping skills and be better able to perform at school with decreased avoidance.
2. Daniel will attend school 90% of the time (allowing for sick days) after 2 months of treatment.
3. Daniel will hand in 95% of schoolwork by the end of 2 months.

Solicit and Integrate Client Preferences

A portion of the assessment process incorporates rapport building and getting to know aspects of the youth aside from symptoms. During the assessment process, efforts are made to learn about the youth's interests, hobbies, and supports. Asking questions such as "What are some activities you enjoy?" or "What type of music do you listen to?" helps the clinician learn about the child. Additionally, questions can be inserted into various sections of the semistructured interview. For example, when asking about school performance or refusal, the clinician can pose the questions "What are some things you enjoy about school?" and "Do you have a favorite teacher?"

In addition to building rapport, knowing about the youth can help guide treatment. Incorporating the youth's interests into treatment makes the sessions more entertaining, and the youth may be more motivated to attend and put in the effort. Session material may pull from examples relevant to the child, forgoing generic examples to which the youth may not relate. A youth interested in comic books may be invested in the session when asked to draw comics about anxiety-provoking situations. Understanding interests can also help reward youth for completing tasks, especially difficult tasks or exposure tasks. A teenager who enjoys video games may be more motivated to complete an exposure task and homework task when earning points toward a new game.

Putting It into Practice

During the semistructured interview, the therapist asked questions about Daniel's experiences other than anxiety.

THERAPIST: So, Daniel, what is something you enjoy about school?

DANIEL: Well, there's one teacher I really like. He's been my favorite teacher throughout the semester.

THERAPIST: What do you like about him?

DANIEL: He really cares about history, and really tries to make it interesting for us. He'll try to incorporate music or make up a rap about whatever era we're in. A lot of the other kids think it's lame, but I really like how he teaches it. You can tell he's really interested in history and is trying to pass on his energy.

THERAPIST: So, you really like this teacher because of his passion and incorporation of music into lessons?

DANIEL: Yeah, pretty much.

During treatment, Daniel and his therapist incorporated songs and music into their sessions.

Daniel created a "cognitive distortions" rap, talking about the different distortions he experiences, and how he can "fight" them. He also later performed this rap in front of other clinicians as part of an exposure task.

Process

Chart Progress and Outcome

Measurable and objective goals help to motivate and track treatment progress. Each goal has assigned milestones and outcome expectations. Scores from the assessments provide benchmarks for treatment progress. Benchmark scores vary based on the instrument being used. For example, some measures may indicate clinical versus subclinical scores, while others indicate normal scores, at-risk scores, and clinical score levels. For example, the MASC can be used to measure remission rates in children with various level of anxiety (Palitz et al., 2018). A 35% reduction in MASC scores predicts remission from SOC. These measurements can be used to inform goals. Milestones can be set up based on percentage, with a long-term goal reaching for a 35% reduction compared to baseline MASC scores. We explore more on remission and treatment response later in this section.

It is helpful to note the differences that indicate a significant change for each of the measures. Questionnaires can be long and tedious, especially with repetition (Weisz et al., 2011), but programs such as the Patient-Reported Outcomes Measurement Information System (PROMIS; Cella et al., 2007) allow measures to be completed online and are stored for comparison in an electronic health record (EHR). Measures can then be compared to determine the magnitude of change, which can help develop milestones and outcome goals.

Measures of Progress

Various therapist-, youth-, and parent-report measures can be used to track progress. A recent meta-analysis on EBA demonstrated that the SCARED, the RCADS, and the SCAS are effective questionnaires for measuring progress in treatment. Beidas and colleagues (2015) reported that the SCARED, the RCADS, and the SCAS are sensitive to change in anxiety symptom severity. Additionally, Palitz and colleagues (2018) demonstrated that the MASC is sensitive to change in separation and social anxiety symptoms. Therapists can

use these measures to track changes: administered a few minutes before sessions weekly, or every few weeks as appropriately established by the therapist (e.g., once every four sessions). Additionally, forms such as the CQ-C/P allow youth input into the stated goals. This questionnaire measures progress of a child's ability to manage anxiety symptoms with the self-described main worries. These worries (main anxious concerns) are identified before treatment and incorporated into treatment goals. The CQ-C/P has demonstrated sensitivity to treatment (Kendall et al., 1997).

The therapist can provide updates to their client's treatment response through therapist-based measures. The Child Global Assessment Scale (CGAS) is a one-item rating completed by the therapist (Shaffer et al., 1983). This item measures level of functioning and is easy to fill out at a midpoint and at the end of treatment. Additionally, the therapist can use the Clinical Global Impression Scale (CGI) to measure progress (Guy, 1976). The CGI Improvement scale (CGI-I) is useful for rating how the client has improved since the last assessment. Both the CGI-I and the CQ allow quick implementation of a progress measure during treatment.

Putting It into Practice

Daniel and his therapist agreed on biweekly measures, including the SCARED, the RCADS, and the CQ-C/P, which Daniel and his mother filled out before the sessions. Throughout treatment, the therapist observed that Daniel's decreased SCARED and CQ scores, evidencing a meaningful decrease in scores by Session 12. Daniel's mother's scores were also consistent with decreased anxiety, and the therapist CGI Severity (CGI-S) and CGI-I tracked Daniel's improvement. These scores were evidence that Daniel's anxiety severity was decreasing.

Moderators of Treatment

What factors may moderate anxiety treatments? Although researchers have examined potential moderators, findings are largely inconsistent. One emerging theme is that severity, social anxiety, age, and depressive presentation, when all together, are linked to less favorable long-terms gains. Practitioners may include measures that address symptom severity, such as the SCARED (Birmaher et al., 1999), and/or depressed mood to monitor these factors. However, the data do not clearly indicate treatment moderators, so clinicians may have difficulty establishing appropriate measures of treatment moderators.

Mediators during Treatment

What has been identified as a mediator of the gains from treatment for anxiety in youth? Successful treatment of anxiety in youth involves increasing their ability to cope. Decreasing avoidance of feared situations and increasing a youth's ability to cope when faced with anxiety are central to reducing anxious arousal, anxious avoidance, and anxiety symptomatology. Indeed, change in coping (CQ) was identified as a significant mediator in an evaluation of beneficial treatment outcomes (Kendall et al., 2016). Tracking coping throughout treatment (e.g., using the CQ) is informative. The therapist can incorporate both the parent responses (CQ-P) and the youth's responses (CQ-C). This allows multiple perspectives in determining improvement; the CQ-C/P is sensitive to treatment and demonstrates improvement in coping over time (Kendall et al., 2016). Additionally, it provides a quick assessment that can be completed at the beginning of sessions.

Putting It into Practice

Daniel and his mother filled out the CQ-C and CQ-P weekly. The questionnaires were available for them to complete in the waiting room before a session. As treatment progressed, Daniel and his mother reported that Daniel was increasingly able to cope with his worries about school assignments, about interacting with peers, and about being evaluated on a presentation. Once Daniel began exposure tasks, his scores dropped even further, indicating that he was not only learning how to cope with anxiety but also was able to put into practice.

Evaluate the Therapeutic Process

Homework compliance can be important for improvement in anxiety disorder treatment (LeBeau, Davies, Culver, & Craske, 2013). The therapist stresses homework quality over quantity (Kazantzis, Deane, & Ronan, 2004). For example, having a client attempt and complete one meaningful exposure task may be more important than completing multiple low-ranking, low-impact exposure tasks. Homework and exposures can be ranked collaboratively by the therapist and child.

Homework, at times, may be difficult to remember, to complete. One of the therapist's roles is to find effective ways to increase the youth's motivation for completing homework, especially with tasks such as exposures.

Use rewards! Youth respond to prizes and rewards in return for completing various tasks in session, at home, and at school. Behavior charts can be used to encourage youth to complete homework. Parents can also track tasks. Reward charts vary based on the age and motivation of the youth. Younger children may require more frequent rewards, whereas adolescents may be more eager to earn points toward a larger reward in the future. Collaborating with the family and youth, the clinician creates a list of rewards relevant to the youth's interests. Therapists, however, should note that little research has been conducted on effective ways to assess and monitor homework.

Overall, homework can be tracked in a way that increases understanding and outlines expectations for the youth. Reward charts can be completed weekly in session, with the week's homework written down in steps. Exposures and psychoeducation tasks are best when written in measurable ways, so that parents, youth, and therapist agree on what it takes to complete the assignment. For example, a homework assignment may be written as "Daniel will attend 3 full days of school this week." This homework assignment outlines exactly what is expected, and the chart allows for documentation of completion (or attempt).

Session content can be measured in a variety of ways, including workbook pages, reward charts, and documenting anxiety levels (subjective units of distress [SUDS] scores) during exposure tasks. Earlier psychoeducation sessions may involve the use of workbooks pages to help track the information taught. Workbooks provide an organized approach to assessing the work completed. For example, the *Coping Cat* workbook includes a session-by-session breakdown of session goals, allowing the therapist to track task completion each session (Kendall & Hedtke, 2006). Additionally, the workbook includes reward charts and weekly homework trackers that facilitate keeping track.

Reward charts help track progress (e.g., for an example of a reward chart, see Figure 10.2). Children and adolescents are often motivated by rewards. Assigning points to session goals not only increases motivation for completing work during session but also assesses and tracks what tasks are accomplished in the session. These reward charts are especially beneficial for tracking exposure

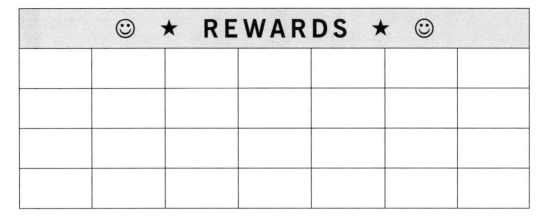

FIGURE 10.2. An example of a reward chart. A quick Google search for "reward charts" can yield results that not only appeal to children's individual tastes but such charts can also be made using Microsoft programs.

tasks: Having a tracker demonstrating how much progress was made helps the benefits of exposure.

Assessing SUDS tracks a youth's level of anxiety throughout the session (Benjamin et al., 2010; Wolpe, 1958). When conducting exposure sessions, SUDS provide brief communication of anxiety between therapist and youth, while still maintaining the integrity of the exposure. Typically, SUDS are rated on a scale of either 0–10 or 0–8, with 0 being the lowest level of anxiety. SUDS ratings allow the therapist to track a youth's habituation/change relative to the anxiety provoking stimulus. The youth's SUDS rating is measured during the exposure, so the therapist can use the information to determine whether the exposure is an adequate challenge for the youth, or whether the exposure needs to be adjusted to be more or less challenging.

Putting It into Practice

Before starting exposure tasks, Daniel and his therapist discussed potential rewards for completing exposures. Daniel stated that he likes anime and manga. His mother agreed that he could earn money toward a new manga book by completing exposures. Additionally, in session, Daniel worked toward being rewarded snacks, including candy bars.

During one of Daniel's initial exposure tasks, he and his therapist agreed that Daniel would present a short, prepared speech in front of the therapist and another staff member. Just before the exposure started, the therapist checked with Daniel about his anxiety.

THERAPIST: All right, we're getting ready to do our first challenge. What is your number on the SUDS scale?

DANIEL: I'm actually at about a 1 right now.

THERAPIST: You're at a 1! So, this exposure isn't making you anxious right now. What can we do to make it a little more challenging for you?

DANIEL: Well, I think I would be a little more anxious if I didn't have my notes during the presentation.

THERAPIST: OK. What do you think? Let's do the presentation without notes. What number are you now on the SUDS scale?

DANIEL: I'm about a 3 right now.

THERAPIST: OK. A 3 is a great place to start for our first challenge. I'll check back in afterwards to see your SUDS, and how you're feeling after the challenge.

Working Alliance

A strong working alliance is often considered important to the successful outcomes, and this is also true for treating anxiety disorders in youth (Anderson et al., 2012). Exposure tasks in therapy can often be difficult for youth and a stronger collaboration (alliance) helps when designing and encouraging youth to try and to complete exposures. It may be pertinent for the therapist to check in with the youth to make sure they are working toward the same goals. A questionnaire such as the short form of the Working Alliance Inventory (WAI-S; Tracey & Kokotovic, 1989) increases communication about the degree to which there is agreement on goals and tasks. The WAI-S may be completed quickly discussed as part of a check-in. The WAI-S can be used to assess the strength of the relationship before beginning exposures, allowing the therapist to address any needs or resolve issues with collaboration.

Monitor Maintenance and/or Relapse

Posttreatment Monitoring

As treatment progresses, the therapist needs to be aware of when the youth is ready for termination (Youngstrom et al., 2017), and weekly monitoring of improvement helps this determination. Progress measures can be monitored to track the improvement. A child's SUDS ratings in session provide information on how he or she is changing when facing challenging situations. As SUDS decrease despite increasingly challenging situations, they demonstrate that the youth is learning how to tolerate and manage anxiety. Using SUDS data, the therapist can determine the degree to which a youth is able to handle anxious situations on his or her own, without further assistance from therapy. For younger children, assistance from parents may be intermittent as developmentally appropriate to help cope and deal with emerging anxious situations.

Therapists can make decisions about termination based on outcome measures. Outcome mea-sures can be administered to assess whether the youth has improved meaningfully since the beginning of treatment (Youngstrom & Van Meter, 2016). Table 10.8 provides the current information on empirically based cutoff scores for determining clinically significant symptom reduction or disorder remission. Importantly, this is EBA near its best—using assessments that are easy to administer to make informed decisions about the magnitude of change that would have otherwise taken hours of structured diagnostic time to assess. To date, information on empirically determined cutoff scores is available for the MASC, PARS, SCARED, and SCAS. These scales can effectively predict disorder remission and treatment response for youth with previously diagnosed anxiety disorders.

The CGI-I is useful in tracking child improvement. The therapist's scores on the CGI-I is likely correlated with measures such as the MASC and the SCARED (McGuire et al., 2018). However, agreement between therapist and others appears to be highest with parents. Combined use of parent, youth, and therapist reports is helpful in determining treatment response and potential termination.

Putting It into Practice

Daniel demonstrated meaningful improvements on his SCARED scores after the 18th treatment session. Both Daniel's and his mother's reports in-

TABLE 10.8. Scores for Using Questionnaire Cutoffs to Determine Treatment Response and Remission

Measure	References	Cutoff for clinically significant reduction/ remission	Notes
Multidimensional Anxiety Scale for Children (MASC)	Palitz et al. (2018)	30% reduction—SEP; 35% reduction—SOC; 42 overall score	Overall score compared to ADIS-defined remission
Pediatric Anxiety Rating Scale (PARS)	Caporino et al. (2017)	35% reduction—treatment response; 50% reduction—anxiety remission	Raw scores of 8 and 10 fvor anxiety remission
Screen for Child Anxiety Related Emotion Disorders (SCARED)	Caporino et al. (2017)	55% reduction—parent; 50% reduction—child	Parent and child score cutoffs vary slightly depending on a child or adolescent presenting for treatment (see McGuire et al., 2019)
Spence Children's Anxiety Scale (SCAS)	Evans et al. (2017)	22—child; 18—parent	Cutoff scores indicate absence of anxiety disorder; cutoffs for recovery from various disorders may be higher (see Evans et al., 2017)

dicated a SCARED improvement of 60 and 65%, respectively. Additionally, the therapist rated Daniel's improvement as a 2 on the CGI-I. Daniel and his mother stated that he had significantly improved in his ability to tolerate uncertainty, especially regarding school assignments. The therapist noted that his SUDS ratings were lower for his in-session exposures, and he was completing his at-home exposures with little to no hesitation per reports from Daniel and his mother. After a review of the scores, Daniel, his mother, and the therapist agreed that they would wind down to termination.

Relapse Prevention

When a youth has completed anxiety treatment, he or she is ready to move on to a posttreatment life. Although many youth continue to thrive posttreatment, some may relapse. How do the therapist and family work together to reduce relapse? There are some factors that may predict recurrence of anxiety symptoms in youth, including initial trait anxiety and anxiety sensitivity (Taylor, Jakubovski, & Bloch, 2015). Youth with social anxiety, greater severity, and depressed presentation are more likely to experience less favorable maintenance of gains (Puleo et al., 2011). Difficult family situations (Schleider et al., 2015) and limited social support have been associated with anxiety symptom relapse. Appropriate plans can be implemented when a youth has indications of risk of relapse.

Relapse prevention plans include a brief review of the skills learned in therapy (Scott & Feeny, 2006) and associated applause for the youth's efforts. The plan can reference workbook pages used in treatment, online resources for additional worksheets, and resources for the family to encourage the practice of facing fears, being brave, and being nonavoidant. These resources are best when similar to those provided during treatment. Examples may include body drawings for physical symptoms, feelings thermometers, an illustration of the therapy model, and examples of self-talk. Relapse prevention plans identify specific stressors that may increase a youth's anxiety or susceptibility to anxiety, and it helps when the therapist and youth think about and plan for likely developmental challenges that lie ahead. The youth who is entering a new school can anticipate situations that may increase anxiety, and the therapist and youth can brainstorm ways to manage the anxiety.

The relapse prevention plan incorporates the coping skills that the youth learned and embraced (Scott & Feeny, 2006). Youth respond in different ways to the various coping skills they learn throughout treatment. The relapse prevention activity can be interactive, creating a coping skills "map" or drawing, or more practical for older children and adolescents (e.g., creating a coping skills list). The relapse prevention plan includes noting any resources that can be used (e.g., friend or relative who would be a social support).

Overall, relapse prevention includes an overview of the treatment as was customized for the child or adolescent. Coping skills information can give the youth a resource for times when he or she may have difficulty with anxious arousal. Finally, the relapse plan should anticipate and identify potential stressors and how to effectively implement coping skills in response. An effective relapse prevention plan reminds the youth of his or her progress and gains, and helps the youth adjust to new stressors as they emerge.

Putting It into Practice

In the closing sessions, a relapse prevention plan was created with Daniel and his mother. Daniel and his therapist reviewed what he learned in treatment and created a folder of worksheets and resources that he had found useful. This folder included a thought record, a list of positive coping thoughts, a list of relaxation techniques and online relaxation prompts, and a review of the cognitive-behavioral model of anxiety. The folder also included a list of additional coping skills and their rationale, including problem solving and cognitive restructuring. Daniel and his therapist created a list of potential upcoming stressors that may increase anxiety. Stressors included applying for college, meeting new people, and difficult assignments. Daniel left his last session with a packet labeled his "relapse prevention plan."

Conclusion

EBA has a valuable place within the treatment of anxiety in youth—measuring anxiety before, during, and after treatment. We have provided in this chapter several recommendations for approaching EBA for anxiety in youth, and each service-providing setting can use the information to adopt a practical yet efficient protocol for assessing anxiety disorders in youth. Several resources presented in this chapter are available at no cost for use during assessment and treatment. Additional materials may be purchased. Research encourages the use of the prediction, prescription, and processing approach to anxiety assessment in youth (Youngstrom et al., 2017), and therapists can adapt each step to the resources available at their clinic.

Future Directions

EBA of youth anxiety is a relatively new addition to evidence-informed treatment. Much has been done and much has been learned: The next challenge is to evaluate the degree to which EBA improves the treatment of youth. Future research might examine whether youth whose therapists follow EBA experience greater treatment gains than those whose therapists do not. Such studies could examine the importance of specific aspects of the EBA process, such as intake questionnaires or diagnostic interviews. As we move to embrace the NIMH Research Domain Criteria (RDoC), questionnaires may emerge that tap symptoms along RDoC units of analysis (Craske, 2012). Such measures warrant analyses within the EBA framework.

Given that EBA is an evolving area of scientific inquiry, there are many opportunities for research on the existing EBA measures. For example, some questionnaires do not have information regarding sensitivity and specificity. Studies are needed, especially in diverse samples, to inform the utility of these measures. Meta-analyses will help to summarize the existing data.

Advances in assessment technology provide exciting opportunities for EBA. Although there is little research regarding the treatment utility of physiological measures of youth anxiety, the advent of wearable measures such as Fitbit, and heart rate monitors on smartphones, such assessment is more accessible for clinical settings. Such technology could be used to monitor functioning between sessions, or heart rate during exposures. Smartphones can be used to complete ecological momentary assessments (Shiffman, Stone, & Hufford, 2008).

Preliminary research illustrates the use of smartphone applications (apps) in conjunction with CBT for youth with anxiety. These apps can serve to encourage youth and can measures progress. The SmartCAT app provides notifications to remind youth to complete exposure tasks and/or skill building tasks (Pramana, Pramanto, Kendall, & Silk, 2014). Additionally, the SmartCAT app encourages the youth to engage in *in vivo* exposures and encourages repetition of the exposures, leading to increased habituation/new learning. The application tracks the frequency of the youth's homework completion and allows the therapist to send reminders and secure messages to encourage the youth's involvement in tasks outside the session.

Initial and follow-up research has demonstrated that both therapists and youth find the aesthetics and feasibility of the app favorable for motivating and monitoring CBT tasks in between sessions (Pramana et al., 2014, 2018). Applications such as the SmartCAT app can help monitor homework in conjunction with weekly sessions. Recent research also indicates that adding game-like elements to the apps can increase use. Apps can also expand assessment topics: Research could examine sleep and daily functioning by tracking these constructs (Wallace et al., 2017). Although research is needed on smartphone app use for youth anxiety treatment, initial findings are promising for using this tool as a predictive and process measure.

Summary

EBA can increase the effectiveness of quick and accurate measurement of anxiety and anxiety disorder diagnoses in youth. Using the (1) prediction, (2) prescription, and (3) progress approach, practitioners and researchers alike can better understand anxiety presentations in youth. The prediction approach helps with the use of measures to predict the prevalence of general anxiety and the potential prevalence of specific anxiety disorders. After forming hypotheses regarding potential problems, use of prescription measures, such as the ADIS-V, helps to diagnose specific anxiety disorders. The progress step incorporates various measures and tools to determine the youth's response to treatment, including symptom reduction and homework compliance. Ultimately, progress measures inform therapists and researchers when youth symptom reduction indicates treatment completion. At this time, therapists and youth can collaborate to inform maintenance and a relapse prevention plan to increase the effectiveness of treatment. EBA allows professionals to make informed hypotheses about diagnosis of youth with anxiety, and EBA facilitates assessments throughout treatment.

REFERENCES

Achenbach, T. M. (1991). *Manual for the Child Behavior Checklist 4–18 and 1991 Profile.* Burlington: University of Vermont.

Achenbach, T. M., McConaughy, S. H., & Howell, C. T. (1987). Child/adolescent behavioral and emotional problems: Implications of cross-informant correlations for situational specificity. *Psychological Bulletin, 101,* 213–232.

Achenbach, T. M., & Rescorla, L. A. (2001). *Manual for the ASEBA School-Age Forms Profiles: An integrated system of multi-informant assessment.* Burlington, VT: ASEBA.

Albano, A. M., & Silverman, W. K. (2015). *Anxiety Disorders Interview Schedule for DSM-5: Child and Parent Versions.* New York: Oxford University Press.

Ambrosini, P. J. (2000). Historical development and present status of the Schedule for Affective Disorders and Schizophrenia for School-Age Children (K-SADS). *Journal of the American Academy of Child and Adolescent Psychiatry, 39,* 49–58.

American Psychiatric Association. (1994). *Diagnostic and statistical manual of mental disorders* (4th ed.). Washington, DC: Author.

American Psychiatric Association. (2013). *Diagnostic and statistical manual of mental disorders* (5th ed.). Arlington, VA: Author.

Anderson, E. R., Jordan, J. A., Smith, A. J., & Inderbitzen-Nolan, H. M. (2009). An examination of the MASC Social Anxiety scale in a non-referred sample of adolescents. *Journal of Anxiety Disorders, 23,* 1098–1105.

Anderson, R. E., Spence, S. H., Donovan, C. L., March, S., Prosser, S., & Kenardy, J. (2012). Working alliance in online cognitive behavior therapy for anxiety disorders in youth: Comparison with clinic delivery and its role in predicting outcome. *Journal of Medical Internet Research, 14,* e88.

Anderson, S. R., & Ollendick, T. H. (2012). Diagnosing oppositional defiant disorder using the Anxiety Disorders Interview Schedule for DSM-IV: Parent Version and the Diagnostic Interview Schedule for Children. *Journal of Psychopathology and Behavioral Assessment, 34,* 467–475.

Angold, A., & Costello, E. J. (1995). A test–retest reliability study of child-reported psychiatric symptoms and diagnoses using the Child and Adolescent Psychiatric Assessment (CAPA-C). *Psychological Medicine, 25,* 755–762.

Anxiety and Depression Association of America. (2017). Facts and statistics. Retrieved from *https://adaa.org/about-adaa/press-room/facts-statistics.*

Arnold, P. D., & Taillefer, S. (2011). Genetics of childhood and adolescent anxiety. In D. McKay & E. A. Storch (Eds.), *Handbook of child and adolescent anxiety disorders* (pp. 49–73). New York: Springer.

Aschenbrand, S. G., Angelosante, A. G., & Kendall, P.

C. (2010). Discriminant validity and clinical utility of the CBCL with anxiety-disordered youth. *Journal of Clinical Child and Adolescent Psychology, 34,* 735–746.

Aschenbrand, S., Kendall, P. C., Webb, A., Safford, S., & Flannery-Schroeder, E. (2003). Is childhood separation anxiety disorder a predictor of adult panic disorder and agoraphobia?: A seven-year longitudinal study. *Journal of the American Academy of Child and Adolescent Psychiatry, 42,* 1478–1485.

Baldwin, J. S., & Dadds, M. R. (2007). Reliability and validity of parent and child versions of the Multidimensional Anxiety Scale for Children in community samples. *Journal of the American Academy of Child and Adolescent Psychiatry, 46,* 252–260.

Barlow, D. H. (2000). Unraveling the mysteries of anxiety and its disorders from the perspective of emotion theory. *American Psychologist, 55,* 1247–1263.

Beesdo, K., Knappe, S., & Pine, D. S. (2009). Anxiety and anxiety disorders in children and adolescents: Developmental issues and implications for DSM-V. *Psychiatric Clinics of North America, 32,* 483–524.

Beidas, R. S., Stewart, R. E., Walsh, L., Lucas, S., Downey, M. M., . . . Mandell, D. S. (2015). Free, brief, and validated: Standardized instruments for low-resource mental health settings. *Cognitive Behavioral Practice, 22*(1), 5–19.

Beidel, D. C. (1988). Psychophysiological assessment of anxious emotional states in children. *Journal of Abnormal Psychology, 97,* 80–82.

Beidel, D. C., Turner, S. M., & Morris, T. L. (1995). A new inventory to assess childhood social anxiety and phobia: The Social Phobia and Anxiety Inventory for Children. *Psychological Assessment, 7,* 73–79.

Beidel, D. C., Turner, S. M., & Morris, T. L. (1999). Psychopathology of childhood social phobia. *Journal of the American Academy of Child and Adolescent Psychiatry, 38,* 643–650.

Benjamin, C. L., O'Neil, K. A., Crawley, S. A., Beidas, R. S., Coles, M., & Kendall, P. C. (2010). Patterns and predictors of subjective units of distress in anxious youth. *Behavioural and Cognitive Psychotherapy, 38,* 497–504.

Birmaher, B., Brent, D. A., Chiappetta, L., Bridge, J., Monga, S., & Baugher, M. (1999). Psychometric properties of the Screen for Child Anxiety Related Emotional Disorders (SCARED): A replication study. *Journal of the American Academy of Child and Adolescent Psychiatry, 38,* 1230–1236.

Birmaher, B., Khetarpal, S., Brent, D., Cully, M., Balach, L., Kaufman, J., & Neer, S. M. (1997). The Screen for Child Anxiety Related Emotional Disorders (SCARED): Scale construction and psychometric characteristics. *Journal of the American Academy of Child and Adolescent Psychiatry, 36,* 545–553.

Boelen, P. A., & Carleton, R. N. (2012). Intolerance of uncertainty, hypochondriacal concerns, obsessive–compulsive symptoms, and worry. *Journal of Nervous and Mental Disease, 200,* 208–213.

Boelen, P. A., Reijntjes, A., & Carleton, R. N. (2014). Intolerance of uncertainty and adult separation anxiety. *Cognitive Behaviour Therapy, 43,* 133–144.

Boylan, K., Vaillancourt, T., Boyle, M., & Szatmari, P. (2007). Comorbidity of internalizing disorders in children with oppositional defiant disorder. *European Child and Adolescent Psychiatry, 16,* 484–494.

Brooks, S. J., & Kutcher, S. (2003). Diagnosis and measurement of anxiety disorder in adolescents: A review of commonly used instruments. *Journal of Child and Adolescent Psychopharmacology, 13,* 351–400.

Brown, T. A., Antony, M. M., & Barlow, D. H. (1992). Psychometric properties of the Penn State Worry Questionnaire in a clinical anxiety disorders sample. *Behaviour Research and Therapy, 30,* 33–37.

Brown, T. A., Barlow, D. H., & DiNardo, P. A. (1994). *Anxiety Disorders Interview Schedule for DSM-IV.* New York: Oxford University Press.

Brown, T. A., Chorpita, B. F., & Barlow, D. H. (1998). Structural relationships among dimensions of the DSM-IV anxiety and mood disorders and dimensions of negative affect, positive affect, and autonomic arousal. *Journal of Abnormal Psychology, 107*(2), 179–192.

Brown-Jacobsen, A. M., Wallace, D. P., & Whiteside, S. P. H. (2011). Multimethod, multi-informant agreement, and positive predictive value in the identification of child anxiety disorders using the SCAS and ADIS-C. *Assessment, 18,* 382–392.

Bruchmüller, K., Margraf, J., Suppiger, A., & Schneider, S. (2011). Popular or unpopular?: Clinicians' use of structured interviews and their estimation of patient acceptance. *Behavior Therapy, 42,* 634–643.

Bunnell, B. E., Beidel, D. C., Liu, L., Joseph, D. L., & Higa-McMillan, C. K. (2015). The SPAIC-11 and SPAICP-11: Two brief child- and parent-rated measures of social anxiety. *Journal of Anxiety Disorders, 36,* 103–109.

Campbell, D. T., & Fiske, D. W. (1959). Convergent and discriminant validation by the multitrait–multimethod matrix. *Psychological Bulletin, 56,* 81–105.

Canals, J., Hernández-Martínez, C., Cosi, S., & Domènech, E. (2012). Examination of a cutoff score for the Screen for Child Anxiety Related Emotional Disorders (SCARED) in a non-clinical Spanish population. *Journal of Anxiety Disorders, 26,* 785–791.

Caporino, N. E., Sakolsky, D., Brodman, D. M., McGuire, J. F., Piacentini, J., . . . Birmaher, B. (2017). Establishing clinical cutoffs for response and remission on the Screen for Child Anxiety Related Emotional Disorders (SCARED). *Journal of the American Academy of Child and Adolescent Psychiatry, 56*(8), 696–702.

Carleton, R. N. (2016). Into the unknown: A review and synthesis of contemporary models involving uncertainty. *Journal of Anxiety Disorders, 28,* 463–470.

Carleton, R. N., Collimore, K. C., & Asmundson, G. J. (2010). "It's not just the judgements—It's that I don't know": Intolerance of uncertainty as a predictor of social anxiety. *Journal of Anxiety Disorders, 24*(2), 189–195.

Carleton, R. N., Duranceau, S., Freeston, M. H., Boelen, P. A., McCabe, R. E., & Antony, M. M. (2014). "But it might be a heart attack": Intolerance of uncertainty and panic disorder symptoms. *Journal of Anxiety Disorders, 28*(5), 463–470.

Carleton, R. N., Norton, M. A. P. J., & Asmundson, G. J. G. (2007). Fearing the unknown: A short version of the Intolerance of Uncertainty Scale. *Journal of Anxiety Disorders, 21,* 105–117.

Carleton, R. N., Sharpe, D., & Asmundson, G. J. (2007). Anxiety sensitivity and intolerance of uncertainty: Requisites of the fundamental fears? *Behaviour Research and Therapy, 45*(10), 2307–2316.

Cella, D., Yount, S., Rothrock, N., Gershon, R., Cook, K., Reeve, B., . . . Rose, M. (2007). The Patient-Reported Outcomes Measurement Information System (PROMIS): Progress of an NIH Roadmap cooperative group during its first two years. *Medical Care, 45*(5, Suppl. 1), S3–S11.

Chambless, D. L., Caputo, G. C., Bright, P., & Gallagher, R. (1984). Assessment of fear in agoraphobics: The Body Sensations Questionnaire and the Agoraphobic Cognitions Questionnaire. *Journal of Consulting and Clinical Psychology, 52*(6), 1090–1097.

ChoreTell. (2019). Dots reward charts: Potty training and more [Blog post]. Retrieved from *http://choretell.com/kids-5–12/special-needs/dots-reward-charts-potty-training-more.*

Chorpita, B. F., Albano, A. M., & Barlow, D. H. (1996). Child Anxiety Sensitivity Index: Considerations for children with anxiety disorders. *Journal of Clinical Child Psychology, 25,* 77–82.

Chorpita, B. F., Albano, A. M., & Barlow, D. H. (1998). The structure of negative emotions in a clinical sample of children and adolescents. *Journal of Abnormal Psychology, 107*(1), 74–85.

Chorpita, B. F., Moffitt, C. E., & Gray, J. (2005). Psychometric properties of the Revised Child Anxiety and Depression Scale in a clinical sample. *Behaviour Research and Therapy, 43,* 309–322.

Chorpita, B. F., Tracey, S. A., Brown, T. A., Collica, T. J., & Barlow, D. H. (1997). Assessment of worry in children and adolescents: An adaptation of the Penn State Worry Questionnaire. *Behaviour Research and Therapy, 35,* 569–581.

Chorpita, B. F., Yim, L., Moffitt, C., Umemoto, L. A., & Francis, S. E. (2000). Assessment of symptoms of DSM-IV anxiety and depression in children: A revised child anxiety and depression scale. *Behaviour Research and Therapy, 38,* 835–855.

Choudhury, M. S., Pimentel, S. S., & Kendall, P. C. (2003). Childhood anxiety disorders: Parent–child (dis)agreement using a structured interview for the DSM-IV. *Journal of the American Academy of Child and Adolescent Psychiatry, 42,* 957–964.

Clark, L. A., & Watson, D. (1991). Tripartite model of anxiety and depression: Psychometric evidence and taxonomic implications. *Journal of Abnormal Psychology, 100*(3), 316–336.

Cohen, J., Mychailyszyn, M., Settipani, C., Crawley, S., & Kendall, P. C. (2011). Issues in differential diagnosis among anxious youth: Considering generalized anxiety disorder, obsessive–compulsive disorder, and post-traumatic stress disorder. In D. McKay & E. Storch (Eds.), *Handbook of child and adolescent anxiety disorders* (pp. 23–37). New York: Springer.

Comer, J. S., & Kendall, P. C. (2004). A symptom-level examination of parent–child agreement in the diagnosis of anxious youths. *Journal of the American Academy of Child and Adolescent Psychiatry, 43,* 878–886.

Comer, J. S., Roy, A. K., Furr, J. M., Gotimer, K., Beidas, R. S., Dugas, M. J., & Kendall, P. C. (2009). The Intolerance of Uncertainty Scale for Children: A psychometric evaluation. *Psychological Assessment, 21,* 402–411.

Compton, S. N., Peris, T. S., Almirall, D., Birmaher, B., Sherrill, J., . . . Albano, A. M. (2014). Predictors and moderators of treatment response in childhood anxiety disorders: Results from the CAMS trial. *Journal of Consulting and Clinical Psychology, 82*(2), 212–224.

Costello, E. J., Mustillo, S., Erkanli, A., Keeler, G., & Angold, A. (2003). Prevalence and development of psychiatric disorders in childhood and adolescence. *Archives of General Psychiatry, 60,* 837–844.

Crane, M. E., & Kendall, P. C. (2018). *Psychometric Evaluation of the Child and Parent Versions of the Coping Questionnaire.* Manuscript in preparation.

Craske, M. G. (2012). The R-DOC initiative: Science and practice. *Depression and Anxiety, 29,* 253–256.

Croskerry, P. (2003). The importance of cognitive errors in diagnosis and strategies to minimize them. *Academic Medicine, 78,* 775–780.

Crozier, M., Gillihan, S. J., & Powers, M. B. (2011). Issues in differential diagnosis: Phobias and phobic conditions. In D. McKay & E. A. Storch (Eds.), *Handbook of child and adolescent anxiety disorders* (pp. 7–22). New York: Springer.

Cummings, C., Caporino, N., & Kendall, P. C. (2014). Comorbidity of anxiety and depression in children and adolescents: 20 years after. *Psychological Bulletin, 140,* 816–845.

Dadds, M. R., Perrin, S., & Yule, W. (1998). Social desirability and self-reported anxiety in children: An analysis of the RCMAS lie scale. *Journal of Abnormal Child Psychology, 26,* 311–317.

De Bolle, M., & De Fruyt, F. (2010). The tripartite model in childhood and adolescence: Future directions for developmental research. *Child Development Perspectives, 4,* 174–180.

De Los Reyes, A., Augenstein, T. M., Wang, M., Thomas, S. A., Drabick, D. A. G., Burgers, D. E., & Rabinowitz, J. (2015). The validity of the multi-informant approach to assessing child and adolescent mental health. *Psychological Bulletin, 141,* 858–900.

De Los Reyes, A., & Kazdin, A. E. (2005). Informant discrepancies in the assessment of childhood psychopathology: A critical review, theoretical framework, and recommendations for further study. *Psychological Bulletin, 131,* 483–509.

De Los Reyes, A., Thomas, S. A., Goodman, K. L., & Kundey, S. M. A. (2013). Principles underlying the use of multiple informants' reports. *Annual Review of Clinical Psychology, 9,* 123–149.

Degnan, K. A., Almas, A. N., & Fox, N. A. (2010). Temperament and the environment in the etiology of childhood anxiety. *Journal of Child Psychology and Psychiatry, 51,* 497–517.

DeSousa, D. A., Salum, G. A., Isolan, L. R., & Manfro, G. G. (2012). Sensitivity and specificity of the Screen for Child Anxiety Related Emotional Disorders (SCARED): A community-based study. *Child Psychiatry and Human Development, 44,* 391–399.

Dierker, L. C., Albano, A. M., Clarke, G. N., Heimberg, R. G., Kendall, P. C., Merikangas, K. R., . . . Kupfer, D. J. (2001). Screening for anxiety and depression in early adolescence. *Journal of the American Academy of Child and Adolescent Psychiatry, 40,* 929–936.

Dugas, M. J., & Ladouceur, R. (2000). Treatment of GAD targeting intolerance of uncertainty in two types of worry. *Behavior Modification, 24,* 635–657.

Ebesutani, C., Bernstein, A., Chorpita, B. F., & Weisz, J. R. (2012). A transportable assessment protocol for prescribing youth psychosocial treatments in real-world settings: Reducing assessment burden via self-report scales. *Psychological Assessment, 24,* 141–155.

Ebesutani, C., Bernstein, A., Martinez, J. I., Chorpita, B. F., & Weisz, J. R. (2011). The Youth Self Report: Applicability and validity across younger and older youths. *Journal of Clinical Child and Adolescent Psychology, 40,* 338–346.

Ebesutani, C., Bernstein, A., Nakamura, B. J., Chorpita, B. F., Higa-McMillan, C. K., Weisz, J. R., & Research Network on Youth Mental Health. (2010). Concurrent validity of the Child Behavior Checklist DSM-oriented scales: Correspondence with DSM diagnoses and comparison to syndrome scales. *Journal of Psychopathology and Behavioral Assessment, 32,* 373–384.

Ehringer, M. A., Rhee, S. H., Young, S., Corley, R., & Hewitt, J. K. (2006). Genetic and environmental contributions to common psychopathologies of childhood and adolescence: A study of twins and their siblings. *Journal of Abnormal Child Psychology, 34,* 1–17.

Evans, R., Thirlwall, K., Cooper, P., & Creswell, C. (2017). Using symptom and interference questionnaires to identify recovery among children with anxiety disorders. *Psychological Assessment, 29*(7), 835–843.

Ferdinand, R. F. (2008). Validity of the CBCL/YSR DSM-IV Scales Anxiety Problems and Affective Problems. *Journal of Anxiety Disorders, 22,* 126–134.

Fuentes-Rodriguez, G., Sáez-Castillo, A. J., & Garcia-Lopez, L.-J. (2018). Psychometric properties of the social anxiety subscale of the Youth Anxiety Measure for DSM-5 (YAM-5-I-SAD) in a clinical sample of Spanish-speaking adolescents. *Journal of Affective Disorders, 235,* 68–71.

Galanter, C. A., & Patel, V. L. (2005). Medical decision making: A selective review for child psychiatrists and psychologists. *Journal of Child Psychology and Psychiatry, 46,* 675–689.

Garcia-Lopez, L. J., Sáez-Castillo, A. J., Beidel, D., & La Greca, A. M. (2015). Brief measures to screen for social anxiety in adolescents. *Journal of Developmental and Behavioral Pediatrics, 36,* 562–568.

Gentes, E. L., & Ruscio, A. M. (2011). A meta-analysis of the relation of intolerance of uncertainty to symptoms of generalized anxiety disorder, major depressive disorder, and obsessive–compulsive disorder. *Clinical Psychology Review, 31,* 923–933.

Grills, A. E., & Ollendick, T. H. (2002). Issues in parent–child agreement: The case of structured diagnostic interviews. *Clinical Child and Family Psychology Review, 5,* 57–83.

Guy, W. (1976). *ECDEU assessment manual for psychopharmacology.* Rockville, MD: U.S. Department of Health, Education, and Welfare.

Hays, P. A. (2016). *Addressing cultural complexities in practice: Assessment, diagnosis, and therapy* (3rd ed.). Washington, DC: American Psychological Association.

Heimberg, R. G., & Magee, L. (2014). Social anxiety disorder. In D. H. Barlow (Ed.), *Clinical handbook of psychological disorders: A step-by-step treatment manual* (pp. 114–154). New York: Guilford Press.

Herres, J., Cummings, C., Swan, A., Makover, H., & Kendall, P. C. (2015). Moderators and mediators of the treatment for youth with anxiety. In M. Maric, P. J. M. Prins, & T. H. Ollendick (Eds.), *Moderators and mediators of youth treatment outcomes* (pp. 20–40). New York: Oxford University Press.

Hishinuma, E. S., Miyamoto, R. H., Nishimura, S. T., Goebert, D. A., Yuen, N. Y. C., Makini, G. K., Jr., . . . Carlton, B. S. (2001). Prediction of anxiety disorders using the State–Trait Anxiety Inventory for multiethnic adolescents. *Journal of Anxiety Disorders, 15,* 511–533.

Hodges, K. (1990). Depression and anxiety in children: A comparison of self-report questionnaires to clinical interview. *Psychological Assessment, 2,* 376–381.

Hofflich, S. A., Hughes, A., & Kendall, P. C. (2006). Somatic complaints and childhood anxiety disorders. *International Journal of Clinical and Health Psychology, 6,* 229–242.

Inderbitzen-Nolan, H., Davies, C. A., & McKeon, N. D. (2004). Investigating the construct validity of the SPAI-C: Comparing the sensitivity and specificity of the SPAI-C and the SAS-A. *Journal of Anxiety Disorders, 18,* 547–560.

Kagan, E. R., Frank, H. E., & Kendall, P. C. (2017). Accommodation in youth with OCD and anxiety. *Clinical Psychology: Science and Practice, 24,* 78–98.

Kazantzis, N., Deane, F. P., & Ronan, K. R. (2004). Assessing compliance with homework assignments: Review and recommendations for clinical practice. *Journal of Clinical Psychology, 60*(6), 627–641.

Kendall, P. C. (1994). Treating anxiety disorders in children: Results of a randomized clinical trial. *Journal of Consulting and Clinical Psychology, 62,* 100–110.

Kendall, P. C., Compton, S. N., Walkup, J. T., Birmaher, B., Albano, A. M., Sherrill, J., . . . Piacenti, J. (2010). Clinical characteristics of anxiety disordered youth. *Journal of Anxiety Disorders, 24,* 360–365.

Kendall, P. C., Cummings, C. M., Villabo, M. A., Narayanan, M. K., Treadwell, K., Birmaher, B., . . . Albano, A. M. (2016). Mediators of change in the child/adolescent anxiety multimodal treatment study. *Journal of Consulting and Clinical Psychology, 84*(1), 1–14.

Kendall, P. C., & Flannery-Schroeder, E. C. (1998). Methodological issues in treatment research for anxiety disorders in youth. *Journal of Abnormal Child Psychology, 26,* 27–38.

Kendall, P. C., Flannery-Schroeder, E., Panichelli-Mindel, S., Southam-Gerow, M., Henin, A., & Warman, M. (1997). Therapy for youths with anxiety disorders: A second randomized clinical trial. *Journal of Consulting and Clinical Psychology, 65,* 366–380.

Kendall, P. C., & Hedtke, K. A. (2006). *Cognitive-behavioral therapy for anxious children: Therapist manual.* Ardmore, PA: Workbook.

Kendall, P. C., & Pimentel, S. S. (2003). On the physiological symptom constellation in youth with generalized anxiety disorder (GAD). *Journal of Anxiety Disorders, 17,* 211–221.

Kerns, C. M., Maddox, B. B., Kendall, P. C., Rump, K., Berry, L., Schultz, R. T., . . . Miller, J. (2015). Brief measures of anxiety in non-treatment-seeking youth with autism spectrum disorder. *Autism, 19,* 969–979.

Kerns, K. A., & Brumariu, L. E. (2013). Is insecure parent–child attachment a risk factor for the development of anxiety in childhood or adolescence? *Child Development Perspectives, 8*(1), 12–17.

Kessler, R. C., Berglund, P., Demler, O., Jin, R., & Walters, E. E. (2005). Lifetime prevalence and age-of-onset distributions of DSM-IV disorders in the National Comorbidity Survey Replication. *Archives of General Psychiatry, 62,* 593–602.

Krain, A. L., & Kendall, P. C. (2000). The role of parental emotional distress in parent report of child anxiety. *Journal of Clinical Child Psychology, 29,* 328–335.

Kristensen, H., & Torgersen, S. (2006). Social anxiety disorder in 11–12-year-old children. *European Child and Adolescent Psychiatry, 15,* 163–171.

La Greca, A. M., Dandes, S. K., Wick, P., Shaw, K., & Stone, W. L. (1988). Development of the Social Anxiety Scale for Children: Reliability and concurrent validity. *Journal of Clinical Child Psychology, 17,* 84–91.

La Greca, A. M., & Lopez, N. (1998). Social anxiety among adolescents: Linkages with peer relations and friendships. *Journal of Abnormal Child Psychology, 26,* 83–94.

La Greca, A. M., & Stone, W. L. (1993). Social anxiety scale for children-revised: Factor structure and concurrent validity. *Journal of Clinical Child Psychology, 22*, 17–27.

Ladouceur, R., Gosselin, P., & Dugas, M. J. (2000). Experimental manipulation of intolerance of uncertainty: A study of a theoretical model of worry. *Behaviour Research and Therapy, 38*, 933–941.

Langley, A. K., Bergman, R. L., McCracken, J., & Piacentini, J. C. (2004). Impairment in childhood anxiety disorders: Preliminary examination of the Child Anxiety Impact Scale–Parent Version. *Journal of Child and Adolescent Psychopharmacology, 14*, 105–114.

Langley, A. K., Bergman, R. L., & Piacentini, J. C. (2002). Assessment of childhood anxiety. *International Review of Psychiatry, 14*, 102–113.

Larson, K., Russ, S. A., Kahn, R. S., & Halfon, N. (2011). Patterns of comorbidity, functioning, and service use for US children with ADHD, 2007. *Pediatrics, 127*, 462–470.

Lebeau, R. T., Davies, C. D., Culver, N. C., & Craske, M. G. (2013). Homework compliance counts in cognitive-behavioral therapy. *Cognitive Behavior Therapy, 42*, 171–179.

Lebowitz, E. R., Woolston, J., Bar-Haim, Y., Calvocoressi, L., Dauser, C., Warnick, E., . . . Leckman, J. F. (2013). Family accommodation in pediatric anxiety disorders. *Depression and Anxiety, 30*, 47–54.

Loeber, R., Green, S., & Lahey, B. (1990). Mental health professionals' perception of the utility of children, mothers, and teachers as informants on childhood psychopathology. *Journal of Clinical Child and Adolescent Psychology, 19*, 136–143.

Lyneham, H. J., Abbott, M. J., & Rapee, R. M. (2007). Interrater reliability of the Anxiety Disorders Interview Schedule for DSM-IV: Child and parent version. *Journal of the American Academy of Child and Adolescent Psychiatry, 46*, 731–736.

March, J. S., Parker, J. D. A., Sullivan, K., Stallings, P., & Conners, C. K. (1997). The Multidimensional Anxiety Scale for Children (MASC): Factor structure, reliability, and validity. *Journal of the American Academy of Child and Adolescent Psychiatry, 36*, 554–565.

March, J. S., Sullivan, K., & Parker, J. (1999). Test–retest reliability of the Multidimensional Anxiety Scale for Children. *Journal of Anxiety Disorders, 13*, 349–358.

Masia-Warner, C., Storch, E. A., Pincus, D. B., Klein, R. G., Heimberg, R. G., & Liebowitz, M. R. (2003). The Liebowitz Social Anxiety Scale for children and adolescents: An initial psychometric investigation. *Journal of the American Academy of Child and Adolescent Psychiatry, 42*, 1076–1084.

McClellan, J. M., & Werry, J. S. (2000). Introduction: Research psychiatric diagnostic interviews for children and adolescents. *Journal of the American Academy of Child and Adolescent Psychiatry, 39*, 19–27.

McGuire, J. F., Caporino, N. E., Palitz, S. A., Kendall, P. C., Albano, A. M., Ginsburg, G. S., . . . Piacentini, J. (2019). Integrating evidence-based assessment into clinical practice for pediatric anxiety disorders. *Depression and Anxiety, 36*(8), 744–752.

Merikangas, K. R., He, J., Burstein, M., Swanson, S. A., Avenevoli, S., Cui, L., . . . Swendsen, J. (2010). Lifetime prevalence of mental disorders in U.S. adolescents: Results from the National Comorbidity Survey Replication—Adolescent Supplement (NCS-A). *Journal of the American Academy of Child and Adolescent Psychiatry, 49*(10), 980–989.

Monga, S., Birmaher, B., Chiappetta, L., Brent, D., Kaufman, J., Bridge, J., & Cully, M. (2000). Screen for Child Anxiety-Related Emotional Disorders (SCARED): Convergent and divergent validity. *Depression and Anxiety, 12*, 85–91.

Muris, P. (2006). The pathogenesis of childhood anxiety disorders: Considerations from a developmental psychopathology perspective. *International Journal of Behavioral Development, 30*(1), 5–11.

Muris, P., Dreessen, L., Bögels, S., Weckx, M., & van Melick, M. (2004). A questionnaire for screening a broad range of DSM-defined anxiety disorder symptoms in clinically referred children and adolescents. *Journal of Child Psychology and Psychiatry, 45*, 813–820.

Muris, P., Meesters, C., & Spinder, M. (2003). Relationships between child- and parent-reported behavioural inhibition and symptoms of anxiety and depression in normal adolescents. *Personality and Individual Differences, 34*, 759–771.

Muris, P., Merckelbach, H., Ollendick, T., King, N., & Bogie, N. (2002). Three traditional and three new childhood anxiety questionnaires: Their reliability and validity in a normal adolescent sample. *Behaviour Research and Therapy, 40*, 753–772.

Muris, P., Simon, E., Lijphart, H., Bos, A., Hale, W., Schmeitz, K., & the International Child and Adolescent Anxiety Assessment Expert Group. (2016). The Youth Anxiety Measure for DSM-5 (YAM-5): Development and first psychometric evidence of a new scale for assessing anxiety disorders symptoms of children and adolescents. *Child Psychiatry and Human Development, 48*, 1–17.

Nauta, M. H., Scholing, A., Rapee, R. M., Abbott, M., Spence, S. H., & Waters, A. (2004). A parent-report measure of children's anxiety: Psychometric properties and comparison with child-report in a clinic and normal sample. *Behaviour Research and Therapy, 42*, 813–839.

Nilsen, T. S., Eisemann, M., & Kvernmo, S. (2013). Predictors and moderators of outcome in child and adolescent anxiety and depression: A systematic review of psychological treatment studies. *European Journal of Child and Adolescent Psychiatry, 22*, 69–87.

Ollendick, T. H. (1983). Reliability and validity of the revised Fear Survey Schedule for Children (FSSC-R). *Behaviour Research and Therapy, 21*, 685–692.

Ollendick, T. H., & Benoit, K. E. (2012). A parent–child interactional model of social anxiety disorder in youth. *Clinical Child and Family Psychology Review*, 15(1), 81–91.

Ollendick, T. H., Jarrett, M. A., Grills-Taquechel, A. E., Hovey, L. D., & Wolff, J. C. (2008). Comorbidity as a predictor and moderator of treatment outcomes in youth with anxiety, affective, attention deficit/hyperactivity disorder, and oppositional/conduct disorders. *Clinical Psychology Review*, 28, 1447–1471.

Pahl, K. M., Barrett, P. M., & Gullo, M. J. (2012). Examining potential risk factors for anxiety in early childhood. *Journal of Anxiety Disorders*, 26, 311–320.

Palitz, S. A., Caporino, N. E., McGuire, J., Piacentini, J., Albano, A. M., Birmaher, B., . . . Kendall, P. C. (2018). Defining treatment response and remission in youth anxiety: A signal detection analysis with the Multidimensional Anxiety Scale for Children. *Journal of the American Academy of Child and Adolescent Psychiatry*, 57, 418–427.

Pauschardt, J., Remschmidt, H., & Mattejat, F. (2010). Assessing child and adolescent anxiety in psychiatric samples with the Child Behavior Checklist. *Journal of Anxiety Disorders*, 24, 461–467.

Pilecki, B., & McKay, D. (2011). Cognitive behavioral models of phobias and pervasive anxiety. In D. McKay & E. A. Storch (Eds.), *Handbook of child and adolescent anxiety disorders* (pp. 479–503). New York: Springer.

Pina, A. A., Little, M., Wynne, H., & Beidel, D. C. (2013). Assessing social anxiety in African American youth using the Social Phobia and Anxiety Inventory for Children. *Journal of Abnormal Child Psychology*, 42, 311–320.

Pramana, G., Parmanto, B., Kendall, P. C., & Silk, J. (2014). The SmartCAT: An mHealth platform for ecological momentary intervention in child anxiety treatment. *Telemedicine and E-Health*, 20, 419–427.

Pramana, G., Parmanto, B., Lomas, J., Lindhiem, O., Kendall, P. C., & Silk, J. (2018). Using mobile health gamification to facilitate cognitive-behavioral therapy skills practice in child anxiety treatment. *JMIR Serious Games*, 6(2), e9.

Puleo, C., Conner, B., Benjamin, C., & Kendall, P. C. (2011). CBT for childhood anxiety and substance use at 7.4-year follow-up: A reassessment controlling for known predictors. *Journal of Anxiety Disorders*, 25, 690–696.

Raiker, J. S., Freeman, A. J., Perez-Algorta, G., Frazier, T. W., Findling, R. L., & Youngstrom, E. A. (2017). Accuracy of Achenbach scales in the screening of attention-deficit/hyperactivity disorder in a community mental health clinic. *Journal of the American Academy of Child and Adolescent Psychiatry*, 56, 401–409.

Rapee, R. M., Barrett, P. M., Dadds, M. R., & Evans, L. (1994). Reliability of the DSM-III-R childhood anxiety disorders using structured interview: Interrater and parent–child agreement. *Journal of the American Academy of Child and Adolescent Psychiatry*, 33, 984–992.

Rappaport, B. I., Pagliaccio, D., Pine, D. S., Klein, D. N., & Jarcho, J. M. (2017). Discriminant validity, diagnostic utility, and parent–child agreement on the Screen for Child Anxiety Related Emotional Disorders (SCARED) in treatment- and non-treatment-seeking youth. *Journal of Anxiety Disorders*, 51, 22–31.

Read, K. L., Comer, J. S., & Kendall, P. C. (2013). The Intolerance of Uncertainty Scale for Children (IUSC): Discriminating principal anxiety diagnoses and severity. *Psychological Assessment*, 25, 722–729.

Reardon, T., Spence, S. H., Hesse, J., Shakir, A., & Creswell, C. (2018). Identifying children with anxiety disorders using brief versions of the Spence Children's Anxiety Scale for children, parents and teachers. *Psychological Assessment*, 30(10), 1342–1355.

Reiss, S., Peterson, R. A., Gursky, D. M., & McNally, R. J. (1986). Anxiety sensitivity, anxiety frequency and the prediction of fearfulness. *Behaviour Research and Therapy*, 24, 1–8.

Research Units on Pediatric Psychopharmacology Anxiety Study Group. (2002). The Pediatric Anxiety Rating Scale (PARS): Development and psychometric properties. *Journal of the American Academy of Child and Adolescent Psychiatry*, 41, 1061–1069.

Reynolds, C. R., & Richmond, B. O. (1978). What I think and feel: A revised measure of children's manifest anxiety. *Journal of Abnormal Child Psychology*, 6, 271–280.

Reynolds, C. R., & Richmond, B. O. (1985). *Revised Children's Manifest Anxiety Scale: Manual*. Los Angeles: Western Psychological Services.

Roemer, L., & Orsillo, S. M. (2014). An acceptance-based behavioral therapy for generalized anxiety disorder. In D. H. Barlow (Ed.), *Clinical handbook of psychological disorders: A step-by-step treatment manual* (p. 206–236). New York: Guilford Press.

Ronan, K. R., Kendall, P. C., & Rowe, M. (1994). Negative affectivity in children: Development and validation of a self-statement questionnaire. *Cognitive Therapy and Research*, 18, 509–528.

Schleider, J., Ginsburg, G., Keeton, C., Weisz, J., Birmaher, B., Kendall, P. C., . . . Walkup, J. (2015). Parental psychopathology and treatment outcome for anxious youth: Roles of family functioning and caregiver strain. *Journal of Consulting and Clinical Psychology*, 83, 213–224.

Schniering, C. A., Hudson, J. L., & Rapee, R. M. (2000). Issues in the diagnosis and assessment of anxiety disorders in children and adolescents. *Clinical Psychology Review*, 20, 453–478.

Schreier, A., Wittchen, H. U., Höfler, M., & Lieb, R. (2008). Anxiety disorders in mothers and their children: Prospective longitudinal community study. *British Journal of Psychiatry*, 192(4), 308–309.

Scott, T. J., & Feeny, N. C. (2006). Relapse prevention techniques in the treatment of childhood anxiety disorders: A case example. *Journal of Contemporary Psychotherapy*, 36(4), 151–157.

Seligman, L. D., Ollendick, T. H., Langley, A. K., & Baldacci, H. B. (2004). The utility of measures of child and adolescent anxiety: A meta-analytic review of the Revised Children's Manifest Anxiety Scale, the State–Trait Anxiety Inventory for Children, and the Child Behavior Checklist. *Journal of Clinical Child and Adolescent Psychology, 33,* 557–565.

Shaffer, D., Gould, M. S., Brasic, J., Ambrosini, P., Fisher, P., Bird, H., & Aluwahlia, S. (1983). A Children's Global Assessment Scale (CGAS). *Archives of General Psychiatry, 40,* 1228–1231.

Shaffer, D., Schwab-Stone, M., Fisher, P., Cohen, P., Piacentini, J. C., Davies, M., . . . Regier, D. (1993). The Diagnostic Interview Schedule for Children—Revised Version (DISC-R): I. Preparation, field testing, interrater reliability, and acceptability. *Journal of the American Academy of Child and Adolescent Psychiatry, 32,* 643–650.

Shiffman, S., Stone, A. A., & Hufford, M. R. (2008). Ecological momentary assessment. *Annual Review of Clinical Psychology, 4,* 1–32.

Silverman, W. K., & Albano, A. M. (1996). *Anxiety Disorders Interview Schedule for DSM-IV: Child and Parent Versions.* Boulder, CO: Graywind.

Silverman, W. K., Fleisig, W., Rabian, B., & Peterson, R. A. (1991). Childhood Anxiety Sensitivity Index. *Journal of Clinical Child Psychology, 20,* 162–168.

Silverman, W. K., Kurtines, W. M., Ginsburg, G. S., Weems, C. F., Lumpkin, P. W., & Carmichael, D. H. (1999). Treating anxiety disorders in children with group cognitive-behavioral therapy: A randomized clinical trial. *Journal of Consulting and Clinical Psychology, 67,* 995–1003.

Silverman, W. K., & Nelles, W. B. (1988). The Anxiety Disorders Interview Schedule for Children. *Journal of the American Academy of Child and Adolescent Psychiatry, 27,* 772–778.

Silverman, W. K., & Ollendick, T. H. (2005). Evidence-based assessment of anxiety and its disorders in children and adolescents. *Journal of Clinical Child and Adolescent Psychology, 34,* 380–411.

Silverman, W. K., Saavedra, L. M., & Pina, A. A. (2001). Test–retest reliability of anxiety symptoms and diagnoses with the Anxiety Disorders Interview Schedule for DSM-IV: Child and Parent Versions. *Journal of the American Academy of Child and Adolescent Psychiatry, 40,* 937–944.

Skarphedinsson, G., Villabø, M. A., & Lauth, B. (2015). Screening efficiency of the self-report version of the Multidimensional Anxiety Scale for Children in a highly comorbid inpatient sample. *Nordic Journal of Psychiatry, 69,* 613–620.

Smokowski, P. R., Guo, S., Rose, R., Evans, C. B. R., Cotter, K. L., & Bacallao, M. (2014). Multilevel risk factors and developmental assets for internalizing symptoms and self-esteem in disadvantaged adolescents: Modeling longitudinal trajectories from the Rural Adaptation Project. *Development and Psychopathology, 26*(4, Pt. 2), 1495–1513.

Sood, E., & Kendall, P. (2007). Assessing anxious self-talk in youth: The Negative Affectivity Self-Statement Questionnaire–Anxiety Scale. *Cognitive Therapy and Research, 31,* 603–618.

Southam-Gerow, M. A., Flannery-Schroeder, E. C., & Kendall, P. C. (2003). A psychometric evaluation of the parent report form of the State–Trait Anxiety Inventory for Children—Trait Version. *Journal of Anxiety Disorders, 17,* 427–446.

Southam-Gerow, M. A., & Kendall, P. C. (2002). Emotion regulation and understanding: Implications for child psychopathology and therapy. *Clinical Psychology Review, 22,* 189–222.

Spence, S. H. (1998). A measure of anxiety symptoms among children. *Behaviour Research and Therapy, 36,* 545–566.

Spence, S. H., Barrett, P. M., & Turner, C. M. (2003). Psychometric properties of the Spence Children's Anxiety Scale with young adolescents. *Journal of Anxiety Disorders, 17,* 605–625.

Spielberger, C. D. (1973). *Manual for the State–Trait Anxiety Inventory for Children.* Palo Alto, CA: Consulting Psychologists Press.

Storch, E. A., Masia-Warner, C., Dent, H. C., Roberti, J. W., & Fisher, P. H. (2004). Psychometric evaluation of the Social Anxiety Scale for Adolescents and the Social Phobia and Anxiety Inventory for Children: Construct validity and normative data. *Journal of Anxiety Disorders, 18,* 665–679.

Strauss, C. (1987). *Modification of trait portion of State–Trait Anxiety Inventory for Children–Parent Form.* Available from author, University of Florida, Gainesville, at cstrauss@phhp.ufl.edu.

Streiner, D. L. (2003). Starting at the beginning: An introduction to coefficient alpha and internal consistency. *Journal of Personality Assessment, 80,* 99–103.

Suppiger, A., In-Albon, T., Hendriksen, S., Hermann, E., Margraf, J., & Schneider, S. (2009). Acceptance of structured diagnostic interviews for mental disorders in clinical practice and research settings. *Behavior Therapy, 40,* 272–279.

Swan, A. J., & Kendall, P. C. (2016). Fear and missing out: Youth anxiety and functional outcomes. *Clinical Psychology Science and Practice, 23*(4), 417–435.

Taylor, J. H., Jakubovski, E., & Bloch, M. H. (2015). Predictors of anxiety recurrence in the Coordinated Anxiety Learning and Management (CALM) trial. *Journal of Psychiatric Research, 65,* 154–165.

Thaler, N. S., Kazemi, E., & Wood, J. J. (2010). Measuring anxiety in youth with learning disabilities: Reliability and validity of the Multidimensional Anxiety Scale for Children (MASC). *Child Psychiatry and Human Development, 41,* 501–514.

Thayer, J. F., Åhs, F., Fredrikson, M., Sollers, J. J., III, & Wager, T. D. (2012). A meta-analysis of heart rate variability and neuroimaging studies: Implications for heart rate variability as a marker of stress and health. *Neuroscience and Biobehavioral Reviews, 36,* 747–756.

Tracey, S. A., Chorpita, B. F., Douban, J., & Barlow, D. H. (1997). Empirical evaluation of DSM-IV generalized anxiety disorder criteria in children and adolescents. *Journal of Clinical Child Psychology, 26,* 404–414.

Tracey, T. J., & Kokotovic, A. M. (1989). Factor structure of the Working Alliance Inventory. *Psychological Assessment, 1*(3), 207–210.

van Gastel, W., & Ferdinand, R. F. (2008). Screening capacity of the Multidimensional Anxiety Scale for Children (MASC) for DSM-IV anxiety disorders. *Depression and Anxiety, 25,* 1046–1052.

Van Meter, A. R., You, D. S., Halverson, T., Youngstrom, E. A., Birmaher, B., Fristad, M. A., . . . LAMS Group. (2016). Diagnostic efficiency of caregiver report on the SCARED for identifying youth anxiety disorders in outpatient settings. *Journal of Clinical Child and Adolescent Psychology, 47,* S161–S175.

Van Meter, A., Youngstrom, E., Youngstrom, J. K., Ollendick, T., Demeter, C., & Findling, R. L. (2014). Clinical decision making about child and adolescent anxiety disorders using the Achenbach System of Empirically Based Assessment. *Journal of Clinical Child and Adolescent Psychology, 43,* 552–565.

Viana, A. G., Rabian, B., & Beidel, D. C. (2008). Self-report measures in the study of comorbidity in children and adolescents with social phobia: Research and clinical utility. *Journal of Anxiety Disorders, 22,* 781–792.

Villabø, M., Gere, M., Torgersen, S., March, J. S., & Kendall, P. C. (2012). Diagnostic efficiency of the child and parent versions of the Multidimensional Anxiety Scale for Children. *Journal of Clinical Child and Adolescent Psychology, 41,* 75–85.

Walkup, J. T., Albano, A. M., Piacentini, J., Birmaher, B., Compton, S. N., Sherrill, J. T., . . . Kendall, P. C. (2008). Cognitive behavioral therapy, sertraline, or a combination in childhood anxiety. *New England Journal of Medicine, 359*(26), 2753–2766.

Wallace, M., McMakin, D., Tan, P., Rosen, D., Forbes, E., Cecile. D., . . . Silk, J. (2017). The role of day-to-day emotions, sleep, and social interactions in pediatric anxiety treatment. *Behaviour Research and Therapy, 90,* 87–95.

Weems, C. F., Taylor, L. K., Marks, A. B., & Varela, R. E. (2008). Anxiety sensitivity in childhood and adolescence: Parent reports and factors that influence associations with child reports. *Cognitive Therapy and Research, 34,* 303–315.

Weems, C. F., Zakem, A. H., Costa, N. M., Cannon, M. F., & Watts, S. E. (2005). Physiological response and childhood anxiety: Association with symptoms of anxiety disorders and cognitive bias. *Journal of Clinical Child and Adolescent Psychology, 34,* 712–723.

Wei, C., Hoff, A., Villabø, M. A., Peterman, J., Kendall, P. C., Piacentini, J., . . . March, J. (2014). Assessing anxiety in youth with the Multidimensional Anxiety Scale for Children (MASC). *Journal of Clinical Child and Adolescent Psychology, 43,* 566–578.

Weisz, J. R., Chorpita, B. F., Frye, A., Ng, M. Y., Lau, N., Bearman, S. K., . . . Hoagwood, K. E. (2011). Youth Top Problems: Using idiographic, consumer-guided assessment to identify treatment needs and to track change during psychotherapy. *Journal of Consulting and Clinical Psychology, 79*(3), 369–380.

Wilmshurst, L. (2015). *Essentials of child and adolescent psychopathology* (2nd ed.). Hoboken, NJ: Wiley.

Wolpe, J. (1958). *Psychotherapy by reciprocal inhibition.* Stanford, CA: Stanford University Press.

Wood, J. J., Piacentini, J. C., Bergman, R. L., McCracken, J., & Barrios, V. (2002). Concurrent validity of the anxiety disorders section of the Anxiety Disorders Interview Schedule for DSM-IV: Child and parent versions. *Journal of Clinical Child and Adolescent Psychology, 31,* 335–342.

Youngstrom, E. A., Choukas-Bradley, S., Calhoun, C. D., & Jensen-Doss, A. (2015). Clinical guide to the evidence-based assessment approach to diagnosis and treatment. *Cognitive and Behavioral Practice, 22,* 20–35.

Youngstrom, E. A., & Van Meter, A. (2016). Empirically supported assessment of children and adolescents. *Clinical Psychology: Science and Practice, 23,* 327–347.

Youngstrom, E. A., Van Meter, A., Frazier, T. W., Hunsley, J., Prinstein, M. J., Ong, M. L., & Youngstrom, J. K. (2017). Evidence-based assessment as an integrative model for applying psychological science to guide the voyage of treatment. *Clinical Psychology: Science and Practice, 24,* 331–363.

Zainal, H., Magiati, I., Tan, J. W.-L., Sung, M., Fung, D. S. S., & Howlin, P. (2014). A preliminary investigation of the Spence Children's Anxiety Parent Scale as a screening tool for anxiety in young people with autism spectrum disorders. *Journal of Autism and Developmental Disorders, 44,* 1982–1994.

CHAPTER 11

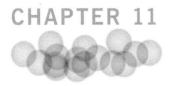

Pediatric Obsessive–Compulsive Disorder

Jonathan S. Abramowitz and Jennifer L. Buchholz

We address in this chapter the assessment and conceptualization of obsessive–compulsive disorder (OCD) in young people in order to aid the clinician in the successful evaluation and treatment of this condition. After identifying, defining, and describing the cardinal features of OCD, we address assessment for the purposes of (1) screening for OCD symptoms, (2) establishing a clinical diagnosis of OCD and ruling out alternative diagnoses, (3) measuring symptom severity and related phenomena, (4) conducting a functional analysis of OCD symptoms, and (5) assessing treatment response and guarding against relapse. Not all of the available measures for assessing OCD in children are discussed here, as some measures have either fallen out of favor, been replaced by newer versions, or have poor (or unexamined) psychometric properties.

Background and Example "Starter Kit"

Description and Diagnostic Classification

Obsessions and Compulsions

OCD is classified in the fifth edition of the *Diagnostic and Statistical Manual of Mental Disorders* (DSM-5; American Psychiatric Association, 2013) as obsessive–compulsive and related disorders characterized by *obsessions* or *compulsions*. Obsessions are persistent, intrusive thoughts, ideas, images, or doubts that are experienced as unacceptable, senseless, or bizarre. The intrusive cognitions also evoke subjective distress (e.g., anxiety, fear, doubt) and are not simply everyday worries about work, relationships, or finances. Common obsessions in children and adolescents include ideas of contamination (e.g., by floors), unwanted thoughts of harming loved ones (e.g., parents or siblings), and unwanted sexual thoughts. Although highly individualistic, obsessions typically concern the following general themes: contamination, violence, responsibility for harm, sex, exactness or completeness, and serious illnesses. Most children with OCD evidence multiple types of obsessions (James, Farrell, & Zimmer-Gembeck, 2017).

To control their obsessional anxiety, children with OCD attempt to avoid stimuli that trigger obsessions (e.g., public restrooms in the case of contamination obsessions). If such stimuli cannot be avoided, however, the child performs compulsive rituals—behavioral or mental acts that are completed according to self-generated "rules." The rituals are deliberate, yet clearly senseless or excessive in relation to the obsessional fear they are designed to neutralize (e.g., washing one's hands for 30 minutes after using the restroom). As with obsessions, compulsions are highly individualized. Common *overt* rituals include excessive decontamination (e.g., washing), checking (e.g., locks, windows), counting, and repeating routine actions (e.g., touching things a certain number of times). Examples of *covert* or *mental* rituals include using special "safe" phrases or numbers to neutralize "unsafe" thoughts or stimuli (e.g., thinking the number 2 to "undo" the number 13). Obsessions and compulsions are functionally related in that obsessions (e.g., images of germs) *increase* subjective distress and rituals (e.g., washing) *reduce* distress.

Functional Impairment

Without proper assessment and treatment, childhood OCD often exacts deleterious long-term effects, including disruptions to normative development (e.g., Piacentini, Bergman, Keller, & McCracken, 2003) and impairments in social, academic, and family functioning (Valderhaug & Ivarsson, 2005). In addition, symptoms often worsen with time, and comorbid psychological disorders (e.g., depression) may develop. This in turn leads to increased disability costs, decreased work productivity, and increased utilization of health care services (Knapp, Henderson, & Patel, 2000). Such consequences highlight the importance of careful screening and assessment for childhood OCD so as to minimize the long-term burden of the disorder.

Epidemiology

Fewer than three decades ago, OCD was thought to be a rare condition in children, with limited literature available describing childhood OCD prevalence from retrospective reviews of child psychiatric samples. The condition is now known to occur in about 1–3% of children and adolescents globally (Apter et al., 1996; Rapoport et al., 2000; Valleni-Basile, Garrison, Jackson, & Waller, 1994). The average age of onset in pediatric samples ranges from ages 7.5 to 12.5 years, with a mean of 10.3 years (Geller et al., 1998), and boys appear to outnumber girls by a 3:2 ratio. While these estimates suggest that OCD is a relatively prevalent condition, they are probably an underrepresentation of the real numbers of youth with this condition. Children and adolescents with OCD are susceptible to underdiagnosis and undertreatment due to (1) factors inherent to the disorder, such as secretiveness and lack of insight; (2) health care provider factors, such as incorrect diagnosis and either lack of familiarity with or unwillingness to use proven treatments; and (3) general factors, such as lack of access to treatment resources.

A meta-analysis of the long-term outcomes of child and adolescent OCD, based on 16 studies with a total of 521 participants, indicated that rates of persistence of OCD in childhood-onset cases are lower than previously believed (Stewart et al., 2004). Across follow-up periods ranging from 1 to 15.6 years, OCD persisted in a mean of 60% of the pooled samples, indicating an overall remission rate (not meeting criteria for full or subthreshold OCD) of 40%. This implies that the symptoms of a substantial proportion of children with OCD remit over time.

Associated Clinical Features

When establishing a diagnosis of OCD in children, clinicians should consider whether the individual's presentation warrants the assignment of a diagnostic specifier to better characterize symptoms, as subgroups can have implications for prognosis and treatment considerations. Classification to OCD subgroups can be determined during initial assessment, utilizing measures we reference later in this chapter.

Insight

Children with OCD display a range of insight into the senselessness of their obsessions and compulsions: Whereas some acknowledge the irrationality of these symptoms, others are firmly convinced that these symptoms are rational (Storch et al., 2014). Accordingly, DSM-5 (American Psychiatric Association, 2013) includes the specifier *with poor insight* to allow for a more dimensional approach to record insight: *with good or fair insight, with poor insight,* or *with absent insight/delusional beliefs.* Children tend to have less insight regarding their illness than do their adult counterparts (Foa et al., 1995); therefore, they often resist engaging in treatment or have limited motivation for change. Moreover, insight has been associated a number of clinical characteristics, including symptom severity, preponderance of compulsions, illness chronicity, limited patient resistance against and presumably control of symptoms, early symptom onset, and a family history of OCD (Storch et al., 2014).

Tics

DSM-5 also includes a specifier if the individual has a current or past history of a tic disorder. Epidemiological research has reported a high comorbidity between OCD and Tourette syndrome/tic disorders, especially among children (Eichstedt & Arnold, 2001). Tics are sudden, rapid, recurrent, nonrhythmic motor movement or vocalizations (American Psychiatric Association, 2013). Compared to children with OCD alone, those with comorbid tics usually present with an earlier age of onset and are more frequently males (Diniz et al., 2006; Leckman et al., 1994). Moreover, tic-related OCD presentations are likely to be accompanied by the presence of antecedent sensory phenomena such as localized tactile and musculoskeletal sensations; "just-right" perceptions associated with visual, tactile, or auditory stimuli; feelings of "incompleteness"; and "urges" to perform an action (Leckman et al., 2010).

Challenges in Detection and Assessment of Pediatric OCD

Children with OCD often have difficulty discussing their obsessions and compulsions. Embarrassment over the theme (e.g., sexual) and senselessness of such symptoms are primary factors. The interviewer should be sensitive to such concerns and demonstrate appropriate empathy regarding the difficulties inherent in discussing these problems with others. Often, parents end up being an important source of information about embarrassing symptoms, but parents may also be unaware of highly embarrassing obsessions and compulsions. Clearly, the clinician should avoid appearing shocked or disturbed by descriptions of obsessions and compulsions. Semistructured instruments, as we describe later in this chapter, can help the interviewer normalize such symptoms. Children may also have difficulty describing their symptoms if they are unaware that such thoughts and behaviors represent obsessions and compulsions. Thus,

including multiple informants in the interview can further help identify such symptoms.

Occasionally, features of OCD itself—such as fear, indecisiveness, rigidity, and the need for reassurance—attenuate the assessment process. Children may be afraid to verbalize obsessional thoughts for fear that doing so will cause harm to befall themselves or others (e.g., "If I mention the idea of mother dying aloud, then mother will die"). They might also be highly circumstantial in their responses because of fears that if they do not provide "all the details," they will not benefit from therapy. Such obstacles require the clinician's patience but can often be managed with gentle, yet firm, reminders of the importance of accurate reporting.

Assessment of OCD in Children: Starter Kit of Measures

There are a handful of useful measures and rating scales to detect the presence and clinical features of OCD in youth. Table 11.1 provides a list of recommended assessment tools to use when evaluating OCD as a potential diagnosis. A more complete review of OCD-specific instruments appears in the sections that follow.

Screening Tools, Different Informants, and Assessment of Risk

Children presenting with complaints of intrusive thoughts, recurrent worries, excessive reassurance seeking, and repetitive rituals or behaviors should be screened for the presence of OCD. In this section, we review several measures appropriate for this purpose. We also describe the use of multiple informants in assessment and diagnosis. Finally, we address risk factors for childhood OCD that require careful attention during assessment.

Screening Tools and Diagnostic Aids

It is useful to begin the screening and assessment for OCD in an unstructured way by asking the child (and any other available informant) to provide a general description of his or her difficulties. Reviewing a typical day can highlight, for example, the frequency and duration of possible OCD symptoms, how these symptoms are managed, and the ways in which the person is functionally impaired. Examples of initial open-ended questions to ask regarding presence of obsessions, compul-

TABLE 11.1. Empirically Supported Tools for Assessing OCD and Related Phenomena in Young People

Assessment tool	Administration	Described further
Screening measures		
Children's Florida Obsessive–Compulsive Inventory (C-FOCI; Storch et al., 2009)	Self-report	Page 311
Obsessive–Compulsive Inventory—Child Version (OCI-CV; Foa et al, 2010)	Self-report	Page 311
Children's Obsessional Compulsive Inventory (CHOCI; Shafran et al., 2003)	Self-report	Page 311
Diagnostic measures		
OCD module of the Structured Clinical Interview for DSM-5 (SCID-5; First, Williams, Karg, & Spitzer, 2015)	Clinician-rated semistructured interview	Page 313
Differential diagnoses		
Anxiety and Related Disorders Interview Schedule for DSM-5 (ADIS-5; Brown & Barlow, 2014).	Clinician-rated semistructured interview	Pages 313–314
Mini-International Neuropsychiatric Interview for Children and Adolescents (MINI-KID; Sheehan et al., 2010)	Clinician-rated structured interview	Page 314
OCD severity, insight, and related impairment		
Children's Yale–Brown Obsessive–Compulsive Symptom Checklist and Severity Scale (CY-BOCS; Scahill et al., 1997)	Clinician-rated semistructured interview	Pages 314–315
Brown Assessment of Beliefs Scale Adolescent Version (BABS; Eisen et al., 1998)	Clinician-rated semistructured interview	Page 315
Child Obsessive Compulsive Impact Scale—Revised (COIS-C/P; Piacentini et al., 2007)	Self-report and parent report	Pages 315–316
OCD-related cognitive distortions		
Obsessive Beliefs Questionnaire—Child Version (OBQ-CV; Coles et al., 2010)	Self-report	Page 318
Interpersonal factors and family functioning		
Family Accommodation Scale for OCD (FAS-OCD; Calvocoressi et al., 1995, 1999)	Semistructured interview	Page 319
Parental Attitudes and Beliefs Scale (PABS; Peris et al., 2008)	Parent report	Page 319

sions, and related signs and symptoms include the following:

- "What kinds of activities or situations trigger anxiety or fear?"
- "What kinds of upsetting or scary thoughts have you been experiencing?"
- "What places or situations have you have been avoiding?"
- "Tell me about any behaviors that you feel the urge to perform over and over."
- "What do you think might happen if you couldn't perform these behaviors?"

As indicated in Table 11.1, there are also a number of empirically supported self-report instruments available for the purpose of screening for obsessions and compulsions if one suspects the presence of such symptoms. In our clinic, we send one or more of these measures (as part of a larger battery of self-report scales) to clients and their families in advance of their initial assessment/consultation visit in order to help guide the in-person diagnostic assessment. These measures may be administered via paper and pencil or online, as research indicates no effect of administration method for self-report instruments related to OCD (Coles, Cook, & Blake, 2007). It is important, however, to interpret scores with some caution, as responses to certain questions might be unclear without further functional assessment of symptoms (as described later in this chapter). Accordingly, these measures are useful as a guide, but they should not be used alone to make a diagnosis.

Children's Florida Obsessive–Compulsive Inventory

The Children's Florida Obsessive–Compulsive Inventory (C-FOCI; Storch et al., 2009) is a brief self-report screening measure for childhood OCD with good psychometric properties. The instrument has two parts: a symptom checklist and a severity scale. The checklist includes questions about 17 obsessions and compulsions across three categories: (1) unpleasant thoughts and images, (2) worries about terrible things happening, and (3) the need to repeat certain acts. Items on the severity scale ask about the symptoms endorsed on the checklist and assess (1) the amount of time occupied by the thoughts and behaviors endorsed, (2) how much the thoughts and behaviors bother the child, (3) the amount of control over the thoughts and behaviors, and (4) the level of avoidance and interference.

Obsessive–Compulsive Inventory—Child Version

The Obsessive–Compulsive Inventory—Child Version (OCI-CV; Foa et al., 2010) is a 21-item self-report measure that assesses OCD symptom severity in children and adolescents ages 7–17 years old. Each of the 21 items is scored on a 3-point Likert-type scale (0—*never*, 1—*sometimes*, 2—*always*). According to the original study (Foa et al., 2010), its factor structure is comprises six subscales that represent different dimensions of OCD: Doubting/Checking (five items), Obsessing (four items), and Washing, Hoarding, Ordering, and Neutralizing (each with three items). Thus, an advantage of the OCI-CV is that it assesses the dimensionality of OCD symptoms. Several studies have demonstrated strong internal consistency and excellent psychometric properties for the total score and subscales in clinical and community samples, except that the Neutralizing subscale has somewhat reduced reliability (e.g., Rodriguez-Jimenez et al., 2016). Scores on the OCI-CV are correlated with other measures of OCD symptoms, and the scale is sensitive to changes with treatment (Foa et al., 2010).

Children's Obsessional Compulsive Inventory

The Children's Obsessional Compulsive Inventory (CHOCI; Shafran et al., 2003) is a self-report measure designed to assess OCD symptoms and the impairment associated with them. The symptom presence section includes 19 symptom items that are classified as obsessions or compulsions and rated on a 3-point scale, from *Not at all* to *A lot*. The impairment section includes five items for impairment related to obsessions and five related to compulsions. There are two forms of the CHOCI: a parent report and a child report. Internal consistency is good for both the total score and subscales (Shafran et al., 2003; Uher, Heyman, Turner, & Shafran, 2008). The CHOCI also shows evidence of convergent validity, with moderate to strong correlations with other measures of OCD symptoms. Uher and colleagues (2008) revised the CHOCI, deleting nine of the 19 symptom items and using a 5-point rating scale. This shortened measure has strong concurrent and discriminative validity and is able to discriminate well between children with and without OCD.

Cross-Informant Assessment

Ideally, a comprehensive assessment with multiple informants (i.e., the child, the parent(s), and possibly teachers) should be conducted to differentiate developmentally appropriate behaviors from compulsive rituals, as well as to make a distinction between OCD-related thoughts, behaviors, and other repetitive thinking and behavior patterns that are functionally distinct from OCD but often confused with symptoms of OCD.

Children and adolescents with OCD may be hesitant to disclose their obsessional thoughts and compulsive behaviors due to shame or embarrassment. Indeed, the focus of obsessions can concern personal, upsetting, or sensitive issues such as sex, morality, and religion. Compulsive behaviors may seem bizarre and senseless. Therefore, it may be helpful for clinicians to obtain information from additional informants about the child's symptoms.

Parents, as opposed to children, may be able to provide more accurate information about the amount of the child's time occupied by compulsive rituals, as well as degree to which OCD symptoms interfere with personal functioning (e.g., at school, socially) and the family's daily routine. This is especially the case if the child tends to downplay or minimize his or her difficulties with OCD. Parents may also be able to shed light on family members' accommodation of the child's OCD symptoms (e.g., helping with compulsive rituals, avoiding certain situations, allowing the child to skip activities due to distress, providing excessive reassurance related to obsessional fear). Family accommodation is usually well intentioned, with the aim of reducing the child's distress, yet it has the longer-term effect of maintaining obsessional fear.

In some instances, teachers may be able to provide helpful information about a child's OCD symptoms. Yet given the degree of embarrassment associated with obsessions and compulsions, we recommend only seeking input from teachers with the child's consent. A teacher may specifically be able to report on the extent to which the child appears distracted in class, is performing compulsive behaviors (e.g., using the bathroom throughout the day to possibly be completing compulsive hand-washing rituals), or is disengaged socially, which may capture interference due to OCD.

Risk Factors

Predictors of OCD Development

A large and consistent body of research demonstrates that certain ways of appraising one's own intrusive thoughts predict the development and persistence of OCD symptoms. More specifically, perceiving thoughts as personally significant or threatening and believing that merely *thinking about* bad behavior is morally equivalent to performing the corresponding behavior appear to be psychological risk factors (e.g., Abramowitz, Khandker, Nelson, Deacon, & Rygwall, 2006; Abramowitz, Nelson, Rygwall, & Khandker, 2007). An international group of researchers interested in the cognitive basis of OCD, the Obsessive Compulsive Cognitions Working Group (OCCWG; 2005) also identified three domains of "core beliefs" thought to underlie the development of obsessions from normal intrusive thoughts, including (1) the tendency to overestimate threat and responsibility, (2) catastrophic beliefs about the importance of and need to control thoughts, and (3) the need for certainty and perfection.

A number of researchers have also examined the possible contributions of parental rearing practices to the development of OCD, yet these have yielded largely conflicting results. For example, some researchers have found high levels of parental overprotection in people with OCD (e.g., Turgeon, O'Connor, Marchand, & Freeston, 2002), whereas others have reported more rejection and less caring as compared to nonpatients (e.g., Hoekstra, Visser, & Emmelkamp, 1989), or no significant differences between individuals with and without OCD (e.g., Alonso et al., 2004). Thus, there is no convincing evidence that certain styles of parental rearing cause OCD.

Other authors (Rachman, 1997; Salkovskis, Shafran, Rachman, & Freeston, 1999) have proposed that strict religious orthodoxy gives rise to the overvaluation of thoughts, especially if certain standards for behaving and thinking are repeatedly admonished by authority figures (e.g., learning from clergy that thinking certain thoughts amounts to sin). The influence of cultural and religious background on OCD symptoms has been examined in several studies with largely consistent results. For example, strictly religious Protestants reported more obsessionality, contamination concerns, intolerance of uncertainty, beliefs about the importance of thoughts, beliefs about the need to control thoughts, and inflated responsibility, compared to Atheists and less religious Protestants (Abramowitz, Deacon, Woods, & Tolin, 2004). A similar investigation of Catholics revealed almost identical results (Sica, Novara, & Sanavio, 2002).

Salkovskis and colleagues (1999) proposed several learning experiences that might put one at risk for OCD. For example, a childhood in which one's parents convey the message that certain situations or objects are very dangerous, or that the child is incapable of dealing with the resulting harm, could lead to obsessions regarding the specific harbinger of perceived danger. This idea is consistent with previous research in which patients with severe contamination obsessions came from families in which cleanliness and perfectionism were emphasized (Hoover & Insel, 1984). Shafran, Thordarson, and Rachman (1996) proposed that certain experiences, such as a chance pairing between a thought and a negative event, could lead to a heightened threat value for intrusive mental processes, although research has not yet addressed this possibility.

Accordingly, it is important to assess the young person's beliefs about responsibility, uncertainty, perfectionism, and the importance of thoughts (as we discuss in a later section). Although it might also be interesting to ascertain and discuss examples of experiences that might have led to such cognitive distortions (e.g., traumatic learning experiences and religious, family, or cultural perspectives), treatment focuses more on modifying the more proximal appraisals and responses to obsessional thoughts rather than the more distal experiences that may have contributed to learning to have such cognitions.

Using Assessment to Guide Diagnosis, Case Formulation, and Treatment Planning

In this section we address measures and diagnostic considerations for thorough assessment and treatment planning for youngsters with OCD. Once a diagnosis is established, OCD-specific symptoms, severity, and insight can be characterized. This section also provides information about differential diagnostic considerations, which are particularly important when evaluating symptoms of OCD that overlap with or are often confused with other psychological conditions. Last, we discuss the functional assessment of OCD, which is an important step in developing a case conceptualization and treatment plan.

Information about the onset, historical course of the problem, comorbid conditions, social and developmental history, and personal/family history of mental health treatment should also be obtained. The most common comorbid conditions in youngsters with OCD are unipolar mood disorders and other anxiety disorders (e.g., social anxiety disorder). The use of a structured diagnostic interview is suggested when it is (1) difficult to distinguish between OCD and an alternative diagnosis, and (2) necessary to determine the precise diagnosis (e.g., for research purposes or for insurance reimbursement).

Structured Diagnostic Interviews

OCD Module of the Structured Clinical Interview for DSM-5

The Structured Clinical Interview for DSM-5 (SCID-5; First, Williams, Karg, & Spitzer, 2015) is a semistructured clinical interview designed to assess DSM-5 diagnostic criteria for a range of psychiatric disorders, including OCD. It can also be used to evaluate comorbid and differential conditions. The language and diagnostic coverage make the SCID-5 most appropriate for use with adults (age 18 and over). With slight modification to the wording of the questions, the SCID-5 may be administered to adolescents. Plans are under way to develop a SCID-5 version specifically tailored for children and adolescents that will include self- and parent/guardian-reporting features. The interview begins with an open-ended assessment of demographic information and various domains of functioning. The OCD section includes probe questions about the presence of obsessions and compulsions. Next to each probe appear the corresponding DSM-5 diagnostic criteria, which are rated as absent (false), subthreshold, or present (true). Thus, ratings are of diagnostic criteria, not of interviewees' responses. Research on the reliability of the SCID scores for assessing the presence of OCD has only been conducted with adults and has provided mixed results. Whereas some studies report low kappas, others report more acceptable interrater reliability (e.g., Williams et al., 1992). We recommend that the SCID-5 be completed by an assessor who has clinical training and thorough understanding of DSM-5 diagnostic criteria. The OCD module of the SCID-5 can be completed in less than 10 minutes.

Anxiety and Related Disorders Interview Schedule for DSM-5

The Anxiety and Related Disorders Interview Schedule for DSM-5 (ADIS-5; Brown & Barlow, 2014) is a clinician-administered, semistructured diagnostic interview developed to establish the differential diagnosis among anxiety and related disorders based on DSM-5 criteria. Compared with other diagnostic interviews, it provides greater detail about OCD in particular. The ADIS-5 begins with demographic questions and items about general functioning and life stress. Sections assess an array of disorders that include anxiety as a primary symptom. The OCD section begins with a screening question, a positive answer that triggers more detailed questions about obsessions and compulsions based on DSM-5 criteria. The measure is developed for adults; therefore, administration should consider the need to modify questions to be appropriate for younger clients.

Diagnoses obtained by the ADIS-5 and its predecessor, the ADIS-IV, have very good interrater reliability, with the main sources of unreliability coming from the occasional assignment of a subclinical OCD diagnosis (as opposed to a different anxiety disorder). Other advantages of the ADIS-5 include the fact that it contains a semistructured format that allows the clinician to collect detailed information. It also includes a dimensional rating of symptom severity. One limitation of the measure, however, is that administration of the entire instrument can be time consuming, although the OCD module itself is not very long.

Mini-International Neuropsychiatric Interview for Children and Adolescents

The Mini-International Neuropsychiatric Interview for Children and Adolescents (MINI-KID; Sheehan et al., 2010) is a brief, structured diagnostic interview that assesses psychological disorders in youth ages 6–17 years. It is designed to assess current symptoms of psychopathology for 24 disorders, including OCD. Unlike the SCID-5 and the ADIS-5, the MINI-KID can be administered to the child and parent together rather than separately. The interview is organized such that the clinician only proceeds with asking additional symptom questions if screening questions are endorsed. Because child and parent are both present during the interview, the clinician addresses discrepancies as they arise, using his or her clinical judgment for final decisions. Unlike the longer SCID and ADIS, the MINI-KID only takes approximately 30 minutes to administer, which makes it a more feasible alternative to longer structured interviews. The MINI-KID has adequate reliability and validity, and is highly concordant with diagnoses found on other structured interviews.

Assessment of Symptoms, Severity, and Insight

Children's Yale–Brown Obsessive–Compulsive Symptom Checklist and Severity Scale

No assessment of pediatric OCD would be complete without the semistructured interview version of the Children's Yale–Brown Obsessive–Compulsive Symptom Checklist and Severity Scale (CY-BOCS; Scahill, Riddle, McSwiggin-Hardin, & Ort, 1997). It is a modified versions of the adult Yale–Brown Obsessive–Compulsive Scale (Y-BOCS; Goodman, Price, Rasmussen, Mazure, Delgado, et al., 1989; Goodman, Price, Rasmussen, Mazure, Fleischmann, et al., 1989). Widely considered the "gold standard" measure of OCD symptom severity, the CY-BOCS requires up to 60 minutes to administer, yet it is well worth the time investment, as it yields rich information about the content and severity of obsessions and compulsions to help with case conceptualization and treatment planning.

The first section of the CY-BOCS provides definitions of obsessions and compulsions that are read to the child (often with the parent present). Next, the clinician reviews a list of over 50 common obsessions and compulsions and asks whether each symptom is currently present or has occurred in the past. Finally, the most prominent obsessions, compulsions, and OCD-related avoidance behaviors are identified from those endorsed by the patient.

Gallant and colleagues (2008) demonstrated initial psychometric support for the checklist items, but little additional psychometric research has been conducted. Moreover, although fairly comprehensive in scope, the checklist merely assesses the *form* of obsessions and rituals, without regard for the *function* of these symptoms; that is, there are no questions relating to how rituals are used to reduce obsessional fears (we discuss this further below in describing a functional approach to assessing OCD symptoms that has incremental validity over the CY-BOCS checklist for the purpose of developing a treatment plan). Furthermore, the checklist contains some items that do not pertain to OCD per se, such as hoarding obsessions (hoarding is defined as a separate disorder in DSM-5), and hair-pulling and self-injurious compulsions. Finally, because of its emphasis on the overt characteristics of obsessions and compulsions—such as their repetitiveness and thematic content (e.g., fears of illness, repetitive counting)—the CY-BOCS checklist offers little help in differentiating OCD symptoms from other clinical phenomena that might also be repetitive or thematically similar. For example, worries might be repetitive and can focus on matters of health and illness, depressive ruminations are repetitive and involve negative thinking, and hair-pulling disorder (i.e., trichotillomania) can involve repetitive behaviors. It is therefore necessary to distinguish OCD symptoms from these other entities, as we discuss further below.

The second section of the CY-BOCS is the severity scale, which is a semistructured interview that includes 10 items that assess five parameters of obsessions (items 1–5) and compulsions (items 6–10) identified using the CY-BOCS checklist. These parameters are (1) time/frequency, (2) related interference in functioning, (3) associated distress, (4) attempts to resist, and (5) degree of control. Each item is rated from 0 (*no symptoms*) to 4 (*extreme*), and the 10 items are summed to produce a total score ranging from 0 to 40. In most instances, CY-BOCS scores of 0–7 represent subclinical OCD symptoms, scores of 8–15 represent mild symptoms, scores of 16–23 relate to moderate symptoms, scores of 24–31 suggest severe symptoms, and scores of 32–40 imply extreme symptoms. A strength of the CY-BOCS is that it measures symptom severity independent of the *number* or *types* of different obsessions and compulsions. In fact, it is the only measure of OCD that assesses symptoms in this way.

The CY-BOCS can be administered to the child and parent jointly or separately, depending on developmental considerations. Psychometric properties of the CY-BOCS severity scale are strong among school-age children and adolescents (Scahill et al., 1997; Storch et al., 2004). Preliminary studies on the reliability and validity of the CY-BOCS among younger children (ages 5–8) indicate adequate psychometric properties, with the exception that scores on the Obsessions subscale should be interpreted with some caution (Freeman, Flessner, & Garcia, 2011).

Brown Assessment of Beliefs Scale

The Brown Assessment of Beliefs Scale (BABS; Eisen et al., 1998) is a seven-item, semistructured interview that provides a continuous measure of insight into the senselessness of OCD symptoms. Although the scale was developed for use with adults, it is appropriate for older children. Younger children, however, might have difficulty with some of the questions that relate to abstract concepts regarding insight into the senselessness

of symptoms. Administration begins with interviewer and patient identifying one or two of the patient's specific obsessional fears that have been of significant concern over the past week. Next, individual items (rated from 0 = *nonexistent* to 4 = *severe*) assess the patient's (1) conviction in the validity of this fear, (2) perceptions of how others view the validity of the fear, (3) explanation for why others hold a different view, (4) willingness to challenge the fear, (5) attempts to disprove the fear, (6) insight into whether the fear is part of a psychological/psychiatric problem, and (7) ideas/delusions of reference.

Only the first six items are summed to produce a total score, which ranges from 0 to 24 and can be used to categorize individuals as having excellent (0–3), good (4–7), fair (8–12), poor (13–17), or absent (≥18) insight. The seventh item, which is not included in the total score, assesses the degree to which the individual believes that others notice him or her because of these obsessional belief. Norms for adult OCD samples have been established in several studies (e.g., Eisen, Phillips, Coles, & Rasmussen, 2004). The BABS appears to yield scores that have good internal consistency, and it discriminates patients with OCD who have good insight from those with poor insight (Eisen et al., 1998). Whereas the BABS is sensitive to treatment-related changes in OCD symptoms, there is mixed evidence regarding whether higher scores are predictive of poorer response to treatment (e.g., Ravi Kishore et al., 2004).

Child Obsessive Compulsive Impact Scale— Child and Parent Versions

The Child Obsessive Compulsive Impact Scale— Child and Parent versions (COIS-C/P; Piacentini, Peris, Bergman, Chang, & Jaffer, 2007) assesses the degree of functional impairment resulting from obsessions and compulsions across multiple domains, including academic, social and family impairment. The measure's 33 items list specific activities with which OCD symptoms may interfere (e.g., "Going to a friend's house during the day," "Doing homework"). Responses are rated on a 4-point Likert scale, with 0 indicating *Not at all* and 3 indicating *Very much*. Factor analysis of the parent-report version resulted in a four-factor solution including OCD-related impairment in Daily Living Skills, School, Social, and Family/Activities (Piacentini, Peris, et al., 2007). Findings on the youth report produced a three-factor solution, including School, Social, and Activities (Piacentini, Peris, et al., 2007). Both the parent- and child-report versions demonstrated good psychometric properties. Rather than computing total scores, however, we find the COIS most useful for ascertaining areas of functional impairment before beginning treatment, as well as identifying functional improvements and changes in impairment throughout a course of treatment.

Differential Diagnosis

A number of (often repetitive) cognitive and behavioral phenomena are routinely confused for obsessions and compulsions; thus, many children and adolescents receive a diagnosis of OCD when it is not appropriate. In this section, we review the most common complaints that are misidentified as the symptoms of OCD.

Obsessions versus Worries

Whereas obsessions and worries can both involve repetitive thinking about themes related to illness and harm, obsessions focus on doubts about unrealistic disastrous consequences (e.g., "What if I murdered the boy I was babysitting and didn't realize it?"). Worries, which are characteristic of generalized anxiety disorder (GAD), in contrast, concern real life (everyday) situations such as relationships, the future, family health and safety, and school (e.g., "What if I fail the test and don't get into college?"). In addition, compared with worries, obsessions are experienced as more unacceptable and evoke greater subjective resistance (i.e., compulsions). Worries, on the other hand, tend to elicit reassurance seeking, but less resistance to the presence of the thought itself.

Obsessions versus Depressive Ruminations

Obsessions can be differentiated from depressive ruminations in young people based on content as well as subjective experience. Depressive ruminations typically involve overly negative thoughts about oneself, the world, and the future (e.g., "No one will ever love me"). Moreover, depressive ruminations do not elicit subjective resistance or ritualistic behavior.

Obsessions versus Fantasies

Whereas obsessions are experienced as distressing, unwanted, and unacceptable, *childhood fantasies* are experienced as pleasurable and therefore should not be confused with obsessions. For example, normal erotic fantasies among adolescents may lead to sexual arousal (even if the individual wishes not to have such thoughts or feels guilty about them). Obsessions about sex in OCD (e.g., the thought to molest a younger relative), however, do not lead to sexual arousal and are met with subjective resistance in the form of rituals and avoidance.

Obsessions versus Delusions

Although extremely rare in younger children, as adolescents approach the age of 18, the risk for the development of psychotic symptoms and schizophrenia may increase in vulnerable individuals. Whereas obsessions and psychotic delusions might both have a bizarre quality, delusions do not evoke rituals, whereas these behavioral responses are a cardinal feature of OCD.

Compulsions versus Tics

Tics (as in Tourette syndrome) and compulsive rituals differ primarily in that rituals are purposeful, meaningful behaviors that are performed in response to obsessional distress and intended to reduce an obsessional fear. Tics, in contrast, are often performed in response to physical urges and sensations (i.e., premonitory urges), and are not triggered by obsessional thinking or performed to reduce fear.

Compulsions versus Other Repetitive Behaviors Often Labeled as "Compulsive"

Repetitive behaviors such as "compulsive" hair pulling, skin picking, overeating, and stealing are problems with impulse control, yet they are often mistaken for OCD rituals. These impulsive behaviors, however, are not associated with obsessions and do not serve to reduce anxiety or the probability of feared outcomes. In fact, these acts are often experienced as pleasurable (and may be positively reinforced by pleasurable consequences; e.g., as an adrenaline rush) even if the person wishes he or she did not feel compelled to do these behaviors.

OCD versus Autism

Children on the autism spectrum may be highly attentive to detail, enjoy having things arranged "just so," and prefer the structure of daily patterns. They may also have rigid thinking patterns and repetitive preoccupations about highly specific stimuli (e.g., trains, plumbing). Whereas similar patterns of behaviors and thoughts may also be observed in children with OCD, in autism they are "ego-syntonic"—that is, consistent with how the child feels. In autism, the repetitive thinking does not typically provoke fear, and the repetitive behavior is not an escape from fear. In contrast, children with OCD experience their obsessions and compulsions as "ego-dystonic" in that the obsessions are resisted because they are fear stimuli and inconsistent with the individual's self image and desires. Compulsive rituals serve to reduce the probability of a feared consequence. Accordingly, it is important to look beyond the mere form or topography of thoughts and behaviors, and focus instead on the *function* of these phenomena, as we discuss next.

Functional Assessment for Case Formulation and Treatment Planning

Cognitive-behavioral therapy (CBT) is the most efficacious intervention for OCD in children and adolescents (e.g., Abramowitz, Whiteside, & Deacon, 2005). This treatment involves a few initial sessions of information gathering and treatment planning followed by systematic exposure to feared stimuli (i.e., exposure therapy) while resisting the urge to perform compulsive rituals (i.e., response prevention), then relapse prevention (see detailed description in Piacentini, Langley, & Roblek, 2007). This approach is derived from the cognitive-behavioral model of OCD (as described earlier and discussed in detail in Piacentini, Langley, et al., 2007), which specifies the relationship between obsessional thoughts and compulsive rituals.

Accordingly, the cognitive-behavioral model provides a framework for collecting patient-specific information and generating an individualized case conceptualization and treatment plan. This framework, referred to as *functional assessment* (Abramowitz, Deacon, & Whiteside, 2019), is important over and above the diagnostic assessment because identifying the particular stimuli to be confronted during exposure therapy requires detailed knowledge of the child's idiosyncratic fear triggers and cognitions (not simply that the child meets DSM-5 criteria for OCD). Similarly, assisting youth with OCD to resist compulsive urges (i.e., response prevention) requires knowing about all ritualistic maneuvers performed in response to obsessive fear. We describe in the section below

the components of and procedures for conducting this type of assessment.

Assessing Obsessional Stimuli

Guided by information already collected, a thorough catalogue of external triggers and intrusive thoughts that evoke the child's obsessional fear is obtained (some of which may be chosen as exposure therapy tasks). Because of the idiosyncratic nature of obsessional triggers, there are no psychometrically validated instruments for this purpose. Therefore, the assessor must rely on thoughtful, open-ended questioning and his or her clinical experience with OCD.

External triggers may include specific objects, situations, places, and so on, that evoke obsessional fears and urges to ritualize. Examples include toilets, doorknobs, knives, certain people, completing homework, and feared numbers (e.g., 13 or 666). Examples of questions to help the child describe such triggers include "In what situations does OCD become a problem?"; "What do you avoid?"; and "What triggers you to do compulsive rituals?"

Intrusive thoughts include unwanted mental stimuli (e.g., upsetting images) that are experienced as unacceptable, immoral, or repulsive and evoke obsessional anxiety. Examples include images of germs, impulses to harm loved ones, and thoughts of loved ones being injured. Examples of questions to elicit this information include "What intrusive thoughts do you have that trigger anxiety?" and "What thoughts do you try to avoid, resist, or dismiss?" Some children are unwilling to describe their intrusions, fearing that the therapist will not understand that these are *unwanted* thoughts. To overcome such reluctance, the assessor can educate the child about the universality of such intrusions and even self-disclose his or her own senseless or upsetting intrusions.

Assessing Cognitive Features

Information should be obtained about the cognitive basis of obsessional fear, that is, the feared consequences associated with obsessional stimuli (e.g., "If I touch urine, I will get my whole family sick," "If I write the number 13, my mother will die"). Knowing this information helps the therapist arrange exposure tasks that will disconfirm such exaggerated expectations. Although many children can articulate such fears, some are not able to do so. When feared consequences cannot be explicitly articulated, the patient might fear that anxiety itself will persist indefinitely (or escalate to "out-of-control" levels) unless a ritual is performed. Others might be afraid merely of not knowing "for sure" whether a feared outcome (usually in the more distant future) will occur. The following open-ended questions are appropriate for assessing feared consequences: "What is the worst thing that could happen if you are exposed to (obsessional trigger)?"; "What do you think might happen if you didn't complete the ritual?"; "What would happen if you didn't do anything to reduce your high levels of anxiety?"; and "What if you don't know for certain whether _____ will happen?"

Cognitive therapy techniques (e.g., Wilhelm & Steketee, 2006), which can be used to supplement exposure therapy, require assessment of the dysfunctional beliefs that underlie obsessional fear. A single instrument is available for assessing the cognitive landscape of OCD in children and adolescents: the Obsessive Beliefs Questionnaire—Child Version (OBQ-CV; Coles et al., 2010). The OBQ-CV (which is structurally based on the adult OCD-44; Obsessive-Compulsive Cognitions Working Group, 2005) consists of 44 items grouped into three subscales: Responsibility/Threat Estimation, Perfectionism/Certainty, and Importance/Control of Thoughts. Items are rated on a 5-point scale from *Disagree very much* to *Agree very much*. The OBQ-CV has strong internal consistency and test–retest reliability. Moreover, scores tend to be associated with OCD symptom severity as measured by various self-report instruments (e.g., Coles et al., 2010). The OBQ may be useful in clinical settings, as it identifies patterns of dysfunctional thinking that can be targeted by cognitive therapy techniques (e.g., Wilhelm & Steketee, 2006).

Assessing Responses to Obsessional Distress

Avoidance and compulsive rituals performed in response to obsessional stimuli serve to reduce anxiety in the short term, but they paradoxically maintain OCD symptoms by preventing the natural extinction of fear and by interfering with the disconfirmation of fears of disastrous consequences. Accordingly, it is important to ascertain the specifics of such behaviors, so that they can be response prevention targets.

Passive avoidance of situations and stimuli associated with obsessions is part of the repertoire of most children and adolescents with OCD. Such avoidance is performed to prevent obsessional thoughts, anxiety, or feared disastrous outcomes and might be overt (e.g., evasion of certain people [e.g., those with cancer], places [e.g., public bathrooms], situations [e.g., taking out the trash], and certain words [e.g., *kill*]) or subtle actions (e.g., staying away from the most often touched part of the toilet). Examples of questions to elicit information about avoidance include "What situations do you avoid because of obsessional fear and why?" and "What would happen if you couldn't avoid this situation?"

Compulsive rituals typically amount to "active avoidance" strategies that are used when avoidance is not possible or when obsessional fear has already been triggered. Some rituals can be called "compulsive" in that they are performed repetitively and in accordance with certain self-prescribed rules (e.g., touching the table an even number of times, washing for 40 seconds). Other rituals, however, would not be classified as compulsive because they might be subtle, brief, or performed only once at a time (e.g., holding the steering wheel tightly, using a shirtsleeve to open a door).

Topographically similar rituals can serve very different functions. For example, many children engage in hand-washing rituals to decontaminate themselves. Such washing rituals are typically evoked by thoughts and images of germs, or by doubts of whether one has had contact with a feared contaminant. Some youngsters with OCD, however, engage in washing rituals in response to feelings of "mental pollution" evoked by unwanted disturbing intrusive thoughts of a sexual or otherwise immoral nature (e.g., Fairbrother, Newth, & Rachman, 2005). A functional assessment, therefore, is necessary to elucidate how rituals are linked to obsessions and feared consequences, for example, checking the doors to prevent break-ins or using a certain type of soap because it specifically targets certain sorts of germs. Examples of probes to elicit this information include "What do you do when you can't avoid _____?"; "What do you do to reduce your fears of _____"; "Why does this ritual reduce your discomfort?"; and "What could happen if you didn't engage in this ritual?"

Mental rituals are functionally similar to behavioral rituals (de Silva, Menzies, & Shafran, 2003)—both of which serve to reduce anxiety and prevent feared outcomes. Mental rituals typically take the form of silently repeating special "safe" images, words (e.g., *life*), or phrases (e.g., "God is good") in a set manner to neutralize or "deal with" unwanted obsessional thoughts. Other common presentations include thought suppression, mentally reviewing one's actions over and over (e.g., to reassure oneself that one did not do or say something terrible), and mental counting. Many children fail to recognize mental rituals as part of OCD, or they confuse such rituals for obsessions. Moreover, parents might not be aware of such rituals, since they cannot be directly observed. Although mental rituals and obsessions are both cognitive events, they can be differentiated by careful questioning and by keeping in mind that the former are unwanted, intrusive, and anxiety evoking, whereas the latter are deliberate attempts to neutralize obsessional intrusions and, as such, function to reduce anxiety. Examples of questions to elicit information about mental rituals include "Sometimes people with OCD have mental strategies that they use to manage obsessional thoughts. What kinds of mental strategies do you use to dismiss unwanted thoughts?"

Assessing Interpersonal Aspects of OCD

Family members' emotional and behavioral responses to the child's OCD symptoms should also be considered as part of the functional assessment. In some instances, for example, parents or caregivers, who wish not to see their child suffer, unwittingly contribute to the persistence of OCD symptoms by performing rituals, providing frequent reassurance, and engaging in avoidance to help the youngster "cope with anxiety." Thus, family accommodation is an important factor to target in treatment. In other cases, parents are highly critical and express hostility toward their child with OCD. When parents meddle or chronically intrude into the young person's daily activities, it can affect course and treatment response. Assessment may involve observation of parent–child interactions concerning discussion of OCD symptoms. Parents can also be asked about (1) the extent to which they participate in the child's rituals and avoidance habits, (2) how they respond when repeatedly asked questions for reassurance, (3) what consequences they fear might occur if symptoms are not accommodated, and (4) the extent to which the family's daily activities are influenced by the child's OCD symptoms.

The Family Accommodation Scale for OCD (FAS-OCD; Calvocoressi, Lewis, Harris, & Trufan, 1995; Calvocoressi et al., 1999) is also recommended to guide the assessment of accommodation behavior. The first section of this measure, a symptom checklist similar to that included in the CY-BOCS, explores symptoms of which the family member is aware. The second section is a semistructured interview with 12 items assessing different accommodation behaviors (e.g., providing objects for rituals, changing routines, helping avoiding stimuli) and the level of distress related to accommodation or resistance against the symptoms of the OCD family member. All items are rated on a 5-point scale from 0 (*Never*) to 4 (*Extreme*). The FAS-OCD's internal consistency and interrater reliability are strong, as is the evidence for convergent and discriminant validity.

The Parental Attitudes and Beliefs Scale (PABS; Peris et al., 2008) is a parent-report questionnaire in which behaviors and beliefs related to a child's OCD symptoms are rated. The measure contains 42 items and includes statements regarding accommodation, anger, or frustration due to OCD symptoms, and other attitudes or emotional reactions to one's child's OCD symptoms. These are rated on a 5-point scale, from *not at all* to *very often*. Peris and colleagues (2008) developed and analyzed the psychometric properties of the PABS with parents of children and adolescents with OCD, revealing a three-factor model (Accommodation, Empowerment, and Hostility/Blame). Internal consistency of the different subscales was strong for Accommodation and Hostility/Blame subscales, but only adequate for the Empowerment subscale. Moreover, moderately strong correlations were found between the PABS and the FAS, and between the PABS and the CY-BOCS.

Self-Monitoring

Self-monitoring, in which the child (if developmentally capable) records the occurrence of obsessive–compulsive symptoms in "real-time," provides data to complement the functional assessment. Patients can be instructed to log the following parameters of each OCD episode using a form with corresponding column headers: (1) date and time of the episode, (2) situation or thought that triggered obsessional fear, and (3) rituals and the length of time engaged. The task of self-monitoring can be introduced as a means by which child and therapist can gain an accurate picture of the situations that lead to rituals and the time they occupy. It also helps to identify symptoms that might have gone unreported in the assessment sessions. The child should be instructed that, rather than guessing, he or she should use a watch to determine the exact amount of time spent ritualizing. Moreover, to maximize accuracy, each entry should be recorded immediately after it occurs (as opposed to waiting until the end of the day).

Case Conceptualization and Treatment Planning

A full description of the treatment process is outside the scope of this chapter and covered in detail elsewhere (Piacentini, Langley, et al., 2007). The functional assessment described earlier, however, yields the information necessary to develop an individualized conceptualization of the child's OCD symptoms to serve as a "road map" for CBT. This, in turn, fosters the development of a plan for exposure therapy (e.g., the hierarchy of exposure tasks), resisting rituals (i.e., response prevention), and targeting maladaptive parental involvement (i.e., accommodation).

Practical Considerations

As with the diagnostic assessment, children and adolescents may be hesitant to self-disclose some of the details of their OCD symptoms. Explaining the purpose and importance of such an in-depth analysis of obsessions and compulsions might be helpful in this regard, as might having another informant (e.g., a parent) attend the functional assessment session. One tactic that often works well in building rapport and camaraderie (thus, more self-disclosure) is to describe the functional assessment phase as an exchange of information between two "experts." The child, who is an expert on his or her particular OCD symptoms, must help the therapist to understand these symptoms so that an effective treatment plan can be drawn up. Simultaneously, the therapist, an expert on OCD *in general*, will help the patient learn to think about this problem so that he or she can get the most out of treatment.

As alluded to earlier, children might be afraid to mention certain symptoms due to beliefs about the consequences of saying certain things. For example, one adolescent was reluctant to describe his blasphemous obsessional thoughts because he feared that discussing these ideas (i.e., thinking about them) would invite divine punishment. In such instances, gentle, but firm, encouragement to openly discuss the obsession in the spirit of reducing old avoidance habits is the recommended course of action. As mentioned previously, to avoid reinforcing patients' fears, the interviewer should be sure to react in a calm and understanding manner when even the most unpleasant obsessions are self-disclosed.

Assessing Progress, Process, and Outcomes

Continual assessment of the severity of OCD and related symptoms throughout the course of treatment assists the therapist in evaluating whether, and in what ways, the child is responding to treatment. This is consistent with the empirical demonstration of treatment effectiveness. It is not sufficient for the clinician simply to conclude that the child "seems to be less obsessed" or even for an informant to report that he or she "seems better." Instead, progress should be measured systematically by comparing current functioning against a baseline. Thus, periodic assessment using the instruments described in earlier sections of this chapter should be conducted to objectively clarify in what ways treatment has been helpful and what work remains to be done. A multimethod approach is suggested, involving the use of clinician-administered interview and self-report instruments that tap into various facets of OCD and related symptoms (i.e., insight, depression, functional impairment).

The CY-BOCS Severity scale, in particular, provides a semi-idiographic assessment of the child's main OCD symptoms, since rating the 10 severity items is based on the most prominent obsessions and compulsions. Still, we recommend an even more fine-grained assessment strategy for measuring progress with treatment. This involves identifying up to three primary (1) feared stimuli (e.g., knives), (2) avoided stimuli (e.g., the kitchen), and (3) compulsive rituals (e.g., checking for harm). Beginning at baseline (i.e., before treatment), these are rated on a scale from 0 (i.e., *no fear, no avoidance, no rituals*) to 7 (*severe fear, continuous avoidance, continuous ritualizing*). Such ratings can be provided at various points during treatment to assess progress with these specific areas of OCD symptoms. Additionally, continued self-monitoring of rituals through the course of treatment (or at various intervals) can provide a measure of changes in the frequency and time occupied by compulsive rituals.

CBT using exposure and response prevention is presumed to reduce the symptoms of OCD by modifying cognitive appraisals of obsessional stimuli (Jacoby & Abramowitz, 2016); that is, exposure therapy is presumed to foster new learning that obsessional stimuli are not as dangerous as predicted, that obsessional thoughts are manageable, and that anxiety itself is safe and tolerable. It is this new learning, and its ability to inhibit previous fear-based beliefs, that leads to extinction of fear. Whereas very young children might not be able to appreciate or grasp these somewhat abstract concepts, older children can often be helped to become aware of changes in such cognitions. Accordingly, the OBQ-CV can be administered at various points during treatment to examine shifts in dysfunctional beliefs.

It is also important to monitor family reactions to OCD symptoms in the child. Especially when treatment explicitly targets family accommodation, it is necessary to continually inquire about progress with ending this behavior. It is useful to therefore administer the FAS-OCD and PABS at various points during treatment. Importantly, we suggest administering such measures at intervals of 1 month or more given that it may take time for such changes in family functioning to take hold.

Finally, patients and their caregivers should continue to observe OCD symptoms once treatment is terminated. Obsessions and compulsions may be exacerbated during times of transition and stress (e.g., moving, attending a new school); thus, it is particularly important to monitor symptoms during these periods. We find it helpful to teach children and their parents how to use the CY-BOCS, as well as the fear, avoidance, and rituals ratings scales, to track the time, distress, and impairment associated with obsessions and compulsions, as well as any increases in avoidance behaviors and family accommodations. Family members can then review patterns over time to identify any symptom rebound.

Conclusion

OCD is among the most common psychological conditions affecting children and adolescents, yet it often goes unrecognized due to embarrassment and the failure of many teachers and clinicians to assess for its symptoms. On the other hand, many ordinary behaviors of early childhood (e.g., repeating actions, perseveration) and symptoms of other conditions (e.g., Tourette's disorder) are mislabeled as OCD. A personally distressing and highly interfering condition, OCD is often associated with depression and reductions in functioning across many life domains. Accordingly, it is important for

clinicians to effectively assess for OCD in children and adolescents.

Proper assessment of OCD in young people begins with a screen, including open-ended questions and a brief self-report screening tool such as the OCI-CV. This yields data that may or may not suggest the need for a more thorough assessment. Following a positive screen, the clinician should further evaluate whether a patient meets DSM-5 diagnostic criteria for OCD using a structured clinical interview. It is also important to carefully consider (or rule out) differential diagnoses given that a number of other psychiatric conditions involve symptoms that (at least superficially) seem similar to those of OCD, including conditions categorized as obsessive–compulsive-related disorders. Properly identifying children who have problems other than OCD is critical, since they are unlikely to benefit from treatments developed especially for OCD that are derived from an understanding of the phenomenology of obsessions and compulsions (e.g., exposure and response prevention).

Once a diagnosis of OCD has been established, the current symptom severity, degree of insight into the senselessness of the symptoms, and general distress (e.g., depression and anxiety) can be assessed. Results of such initial assessment are useful in determining a course of treatment, goal setting, and treatment planning. It may also be useful to incorporate parents or other informants into the assessment in order to corroborate self-report and interview data coming directly from the child. Moreover, parents can be helpful in the assessment of accommodation behaviors by others in the home, which is critical, as such accommodation serves to maintain OCD symptoms and can be a barrier to effective treatment. Finally, it is helpful to consider possible risk factors associated with childhood OCD, including certain learning experiences, parenting practices, and other cultural norms and beliefs that could foster the types of maladaptive cognitions (which should also be assessed; e.g., exaggerated sense of responsibility, catastrophic misinterpretations of thoughts) considered to play a role in the development of obsessional thoughts. Following this initial evaluation, the clinician will have the necessary information to discuss treatment options and propose a plan for intervention. Changes in OCD symptoms, insight, and family accommodation should be examined using multiple methods and on a routine basis during treatment in order to ensure reliable short- and long-term responses.

REFERENCES

Abramowitz, J. S., Deacon, B. J., & Whiteside, S. P. H. (2019). *Exposure therapy for anxiety: Principles and practice* (2nd ed.). New York: Guilford Press.

Abramowitz, J. S., Deacon, B. J., Woods, C. M., & Tolin, D. F. (2004). Association between protestant religiosity and obsessive–compulsive symptoms and cognitions. *Depression and Anxiety, 20*(2), 70–76.

Abramowitz, J. S., Khandker, M., Nelson, C. A., Deacon, B. J., & Rygwall, R. (2006). The role of cognitive factors in the pathogenesis of obsessive–compulsive symptoms: A prospective study. *Behaviour Research and Therapy, 44*(9), 1361–1374.

Abramowitz, J. S., Nelson, C. A., Rygwall, R., & Khandker, M. (2007). The cognitive mediation of obsessive–compulsive symptoms: A longitudinal study. *Journal of Anxiety Disorders, 21*(1), 91–104.

Abramowitz, J. S., Whiteside, S. P., & Deacon, B. J. (2005). The effectiveness of treatment for pediatric obsessive–compulsive disorder: A meta-analysis. *Behavior Therapy, 36*(1), 55–63.

Alonso, P., Menchón, J. M., Mataix-Cols, D., Pifarré, J., Urretavizcaya, M., Crespo, J. M., . . . Vallejo, J. (2004). Perceived parental rearing style in obsessive–compulsive disorder: Relation to symptom dimensions. *Psychiatry Research, 127*(3), 267–278.

American Psychiatric Association. (2013). *Diagnostic and statistical manual of mental disorders* (5th ed.). Arlington, VA: Author.

Apter, A., Fallon T. J., Jr., King, R. A., Ratzoni, G., Zohar, A. H., Binder, M., . . . Cohen, D. J. (1996). Obsessive–compulsive characteristics: From symptoms to syndrome. *Journal of the American Academy of Child and Adolescent Psychiatry, 35*(7), 907–912.

Brown, T. A., & Barlow, D. H. (2014). *Anxiety and Related Disorders Interview Schedule for DSM-5.* New York: Oxford University Press.

Calvocoressi, L., Lewis, B., Harris, M., & Trufan, S. J. (1995). Family accommodation in obsessive–compulsive disorder. *American Journal of Psychiatry, 152*(3), 441–443.

Calvocoressi, L., Mazure, C. M., Kasl, S. V., Skolnick, J., Fisk, D., Vegso, S. J., . . . Price, L. H. (1999). Family accommodation of obsessive–compulsive symptoms: Instrument development and assessment of family behavior. *Journal of Nervous and Mental Disease, 187*(10), 636–642.

Coles, M. E., Cook, L. M., & Blake, T. R. (2007). Assessing obsessive compulsive symptoms and cognitions on the internet: Evidence for the comparability of paper and Internet administration. *Behaviour Research and Therapy, 45*(9), 2232–2240.

Coles, M. E., Wolters, L. H., Sochting, I., de Haan, E., Pietrefesa, A. S., & Whiteside, S. P. (2010). Development and initial validation of the Obsessive Belief Questionnaire—Child Version (OBQ-CV). *Depression and Anxiety, 27*(10), 982–991.

de Silva, P., Menzies, R. G., & Shafran, R. (2003). Spontaneous decay of compulsive urges: The case of covert compulsions. *Behaviour Research and Therapy, 41*(2), 129–137.

Diniz, J. B., Rosario-Campos, M. C., Hounie, A. G., Curi, M., Shavitt, R. G., Lopes, A. C., & Miguel, E. C. (2006). Chronic tics and Tourette syndrome in patients with obsessive–compulsive disorder. *Journal of Psychiatric Research, 40*(6), 487–493.

Eichstedt, J. A., & Arnold, S. L. (2001). Childhood-onset obsessive–compulsive disorder: A tic-related subtype of OCD? *Clinical Psychology Review, 21*(1), 137–157.

Eisen, J. L., Phillips, K. A., Baer, L., Beer, D. A., Atala, K. D., & Rasmussen, S. A. (1998). The Brown Assessment of Beliefs Scale: Reliability and validity. *American Journal of Psychiatry, 155*, 102–108.

Eisen, J. L., Phillips, K. A., Coles, M. E., & Rasmussen, S. A. (2004). Insight in obsessive–compulsive disorder and body dysmorphic disorder. *Comprehensive Psychiatry, 45*(1), 10–15.

Fairbrother, N., Newth, S. J., & Rachman, S. (2005). Mental pollution: Feelings of dirtiness without physical contact. *Behaviour Research and Therapy, 43*(1), 121–130.

First, M. B., Williams, J., Karg, R. S., & Spitzer, R. L. (2015). *User's guide to Structured Clinical Interview for DSM-5 Disorders (SCID-5-CV) Clinical Version.* Arlington, VA: American Psychiatric Publishing.

Foa, E. B., Coles, M., Huppert, J. D., Pasupuleti, R. V., Franklin, M. E., & March, J. (2010). Development and validation of a child version of the Obsessive Compulsive Inventory. *Behavior Therapy, 41*(1), 121–132.

Foa, E. B., Kozak, M. J., Goodman, W. K., Hollander, E., Jenike, M. A., & Rasmussen, S. A. (1995). DSM-IV field trial: Obsessive–compulsive disorder. *American Journal of Psychiatry, 152*(1), 90–96.

Freeman, J., Flessner, C. A., & Garcia, A. (2011). The Children's Yale–Brown Obsessive Compulsive Scale: Reliability and validity for use among 5 to 8 year olds with obsessive–compulsive disorder. *Journal of Abnormal Child Psychology, 39*, 877–883.

Gallant, J., Storch, E. A., Merlo, L. J., Ricketts, E. D., Geffken, G. R., Goodman, W. K., & Murphy, T. K. (2008). Convergent and discriminant validity of the Children's Yale–Brown Obsessive Compulsive Scale—symptom checklist. *Journal of Anxiety Disorders, 22*(8), 1369–1376.

Geller, D. A., Biederman, J., Jones, J., Shapiro, S., Schwartz, S., & Park, K. S. (1998). Obsessive–compulsive disorder in children and adolescents: A review. *Harvard Review of Psychiatry, 5*(5), 260–273.

Goodman, W. K., Price, L. H., Rasmussen, S. A., Mazure, C., Delgado, P., Heninger, G. R., & Charney, D. S. (1989). The Yale–Brown Obsessive Compulsive Scale: II. Validity. *Archives of General Psychiatry, 46*(11), 1012–1016.

Goodman, W. K., Price, L. H., Rasmussen, S. A., Mazure, C., Fleischmann, R. L., Hill, C. L., . . . Charney,

D. S. (1989). The Yale–Brown Obsessive Compulsive Scale: I. Development, use, and reliability. *Archives of General Psychiatry, 46*(11), 1006–1011.

Hoekstra, R., Visser, S., & Emmelkamp, P. M. G. (2089). A social learning formulation of the etiology of obsessive–compulsive disorders. In P. M. G. Emmelkamp (Ed.), *Fresh perspectives on anxiety disorders* (pp. 115–123). Amsterdam: Swets & Zeitlinger.

Hoover, C. F., & Insel, T. R. (1984). Families of origin in obsessive–compulsive disorder. *Journal of Nervous and Mental Disease, 172*(4), 207–215.

Jacoby, R. J., & Abramowitz, J. S. (2016). Inhibitory learning approaches to exposure therapy: A critical review and translation to obsessive–compulsive disorder. *Clinical Psychology Review, 49*, 28–40.

James, S. C., Farrell, L. J., & Zimmer-Gembeck, M. J. (2017). Description and prevalence of OCD in children and adolescents. In J. Abramowitz, D. McKay, & E. Storch (Eds.), *The Wiley handbook of obsessive compulsive disorders* (pp. 5–23). Hoboken, NJ: Wiley.

Knapp, M., Henderson, J., & Patel, A. (2000). Costs of obsessive–compulsive disorder: A review. In M. Maj, N. Sartorius, A. Okasha, & J. Zohar (Eds.), *Obsessive–compulsive disorder* (pp. 253–299). New York: Wiley.

Leckman, J. F., Denys, D., Simpson, H. B., Mataix-Cols, D., Hollander, E., Saxena, S., . . . Stein, D. J. (2010). Obsessive–compulsive disorder: A review of the diagnostic criteria and possible subtypes and dimensional specifiers for DSM-V. *Depression and Anxiety, 27*(6), 507–527.

Leckman, J. F., Grice, D. E., Barr, L. C., de Vries, A. L., Martin, C., Cohen, D. J., . . . Rasmussen, S. A. (1994). Tic-related vs. non-tic-related obsessive compulsive disorder. *Anxiety, 1*(5), 208–215.

Obsessive Compulsive Cognitions Working Group. (2005). Psychometric validation of the Obsessive Belief Questionnaire and Interpretation of Intrusions Inventory—Part 2: Factor analyses and testing of a brief version. *Behaviour Research and Therapy, 43*(11), 1527–1542.

Peris, T. S., Bergman, R. L., Langley, A., Chang, S., McCracken, J. T., & Piacentini, J. (2008). Correlates of accommodation of pediatric obsessive–compulsive disorder: Parent, child, and family characteristics. *Journal of the American Academy of Child and Adolescent Psychiatry, 47*(10), 1173–1181.

Piacentini, J., Bergman, R. L., Keller, M., & McCracken, J. (2003). Functional impairment in children and adolescents with obsessive–compulsive disorder. *Journal of Child and Adolesc Psychopharmacology, 13*, 61–69.

Piacentini, J., Langley, A., & Roblek, T. (2007). *Cognitive behavioral treatment of childhood OCD: It's only a false alarm: Therapist guide.* New York: Oxford University Press.

Piacentini, J., Peris, T. S., Bergman, R. L., Chang, S., & Jaffer, M. (2007). Functional impairment in childhood OCD: Development and psychometrics prop-

erties of the Child Obsessive–Compulsive Impact Scale—Revised (COIS-R). *Journal of Clinical Child and Adolescent Psychology, 36*(4), 645–653.

Rachman, S. J. (1997). A cognitive theory of obsessions. *Behaviour Research and Therapy, 35*(9), 793–802.

Rapoport, J. L., Inoff-Germain, G., Weissman, M. M., Greenwald, S., Narrow, W. E., Jensen, P. S., . . . Canino, G. (2000). Childhood obsessive–compulsive disorder in the NIMH MECA study: Parent versus child identification of cases methods for the epidemiology of child and adolescent mental disorders. *Journal of Anxiety Disorders, 14*, 535–548.

Ravi Kishore, V., Samar, R., Janardhan Reddy, Y. C., Chandrasekhar, C. R., & Thennarasu, K. (2004). Clinical characteristics and treatment response in poor and good insight obsessive–compulsive disorder. *European Psychiatry, 19*(4), 202–208.

Rodriguez-Jimenez, T., Piqueras, J. A., Lázaro, L., Moreno, E., Ortiz, A. G., & Godoy, A. (2016). Metric invariance, reliability, and validity of the Child Version of the Obsessive Compulsive Inventory (OCI-CV) in community and clinical samples. *Journal of Obsessive–Compulsive and Related Disorders, 9*, 1–8.

Salkovskis, P. M., Shafran, R., Rachman, S., & Freeston, M. H. (1999). Multiple pathways to inflated responsibility beliefs in obsessional problems: Possible origins and implications for therapy and research. *Behaviour Research and Therapy, 37*(11), 1055–1072.

Scahill, L., Riddle, M. A., McSwiggin-Hardin, M., & Ort, S. I. (1997). Children's Yale–Brown Obsessive Compulsive Scale: Reliability and validity. *Journal of the American Academy of Child and Adolescent Psychiatry, 36*(6), 844–852.

Shafran, R., Frampton, I., Heyman, I., Reynolds, M., Teachman, B., & Rachman, S. (2003). The preliminary development of a new self-report measure for OCD in young people. *Journal of Adolesccence, 26*(1), 137–142.

Shafran, R., Thordarson, D. S., & Rachman, S. (1996). Thought–action fusion in obsessive compulsive disorder. *Journal of Anxiety Disorders, 10*(5), 379–391.

Sheehan, D. V., Sheehan, K. H., Shytle, R. D., Janavs, J., Bannon, Y., Rogers, J. E., . . . Wilkinson, B. (2010). Reliability and validity of the Mini International Neuropsychiatric Interview for Children and Adolescents (MINI-KID). *Journal of Clinical Psychiatry, 71*, 313.

Sica, C., Novara, C., & Sanavio, E. (2002). Religiousness and obsessive–compulsive cognitions and symptoms in an Italian population. *Behaviour Research and Therapy, 40*(7), 813–823.

Stewart, S. E., Geller, D. A., Jenike, M., Pauls, D., Shaw, D., Mullin, B., & Faraone, S. V. (2004). Long-term outcome of pediatric obsessive–compulsive disorder: A meta-analysis and qualitative review of the literature. *Acta Psychiatrica Scandinavica, 110*(1), 4–13.

Storch, E. A., De Nadai, A. S., Jacob, M. L., Lewin, A. B., Muroff, J., Eisen, J., . . . Murphy, T. K. (2014). Phenomenology and correlates of insight in pediatric obsessive–compulsive disorder. *Comprehensive Psychiatry, 55*(3), 613–620.

Storch, E. A., Khanna, M., Merlo, L. J., Loew, B. A., Franklin, M., Reid, J. M., . . . Murphy, T. K. (2009). Children's Florida Obsessive Compulsive Inventory: Psychometric properties and feasibility of a self-report measure of obsessive–compulsive symptoms in youth. *Child Psychiatry and Human Development, 40*(3), 467–483.

Storch, E. A., Murphy, T. K., Geffken, G. R., Soto, O., Sajid, M., Allen, P., . . . Goodman, W. K. (2004). Psychometric evaluation of the Children's Yale–Brown Obsessive–Compulsive Scale. *Psychiatry Research, 129*(1), 91–98.

Turgeon, L., O'Cconnor, K. P., Marchand, A., & Freeston, M. H. (2002). Recollections of parent–child relationships in patients with obsessive–compulsive disorder and panic disorder with agoraphobia. *Acta Psychiatrica Scandinavica, 105*(4), 310–316.

Uher, R., Heyman, I., Turner, C. M., & Shafran, R. (2008). Self-, parent-report and interview measures of obsessive–compulsive disorder in children and adolescents. *Journal of Anxiety Disorders, 22*(6), 979–990.

Valderhaug, R., & Ivarsson, T. (2005). Functional impairment in clinical samples of Norwegian and Swedish children and adolescents with obsessive–compulsive disorder. *European Child and Adolescent Psychiatry, 14*(3), 164–173.

Valleni-Basile, L. A., Garrison, C. Z., Jackson, K. L., & Waller, J. L. (1994). Frequency of obsessive–compulsive disorder in a community sample of young adolescents. *Journal of the American Academy of Child and Adolescent Psychiatry, 33*(6), 782–791.

Wilhelm, S., & Steketee, G. S. (2006). *Cognitive therapy for obsessive compulsive disorder: A guide for professionals.* Oakland, CA: New Harbinger.

Williams, J. B., Gibbon, M., First, M. B., Spitzer, R. L., Davies, M., Borus, J., . . . Wittchen, H. U. (1992). The structured clinical interview for DSM-III-R (SCID): II. Multisite test–retest reliability. *Archives of General Psychiatry, 49*(8), 630–636.

PART V

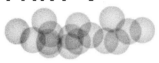

Developmental and Cognitive Disorders

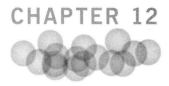

CHAPTER 12

Autism Spectrum Disorders

Elisabeth Sheridan and Catherine Lord

The assessment of children with a possible autism spectrum disorder (ASD) involves many components. This chapter provides a detailed discussion of the methods available for the assessment of core symptom areas of impairment in individuals with ASD using standardized measures of behavior, social communication, adaptive, and intellectual functioning in the context of an evaluation. We begin with a review of the diagnostic criteria and associated features of ASD, then describe components of a core assessment battery to evaluate autism symptomatology and key domains of functioning. We end with a discussion of the utility of assessment instruments in treatment planning

and evaluation, outcome assessment, and progress monitoring for youth with ASD.

Diagnostic Criteria

ASD is defined in the fifth edition of the *Diagnostic and Statistical Manual of Mental Disorders* (DSM-5; American Psychiatric Association, 2013) as persistent deficits in social communication and the presence of restricted, repetitive, and stereotyped patterns of behavior, interests, or activities across multiple contexts. Since the original description of autism by Leo Kanner in 1943, the core features of ASD have been conceptualized as social communication deficits and atypical repetitive and sensory–motor behaviors. Kanner provided detailed descriptions of 11 children seen in his psychiatric clinic who shared qualities of social aloofness, language delays or oddities, and insistence on sameness. Though it was initially believed to be a form of childhood psychosis, autism was officially recognized as a pervasive developmental disorder (PDD) in the third edition of the DSM (DSM-III; American Psychiatric Association, 1980). The term "infantile autism" was introduced to describe children with significant social impairments and unusual behaviors, and to recognize the earlier onset pattern as compared to symptoms of schizophrenia and psychoses. In response to the heterogeneous symptom presentations seen across individuals with PDD, the fourth edition of the DSM (DSM-IV; American Psychiatric Association, 1994) introduced five specific subgroups, including autistic disorder, Asperger's disorder, Rett's disorder, childhood disintegrative disorder, and pervasive developmental disorder not otherwise specified (PDD-NOS). However, given the lack of evidence to support reliable and replicable diagnostic differences among the DSM-IV-TR PDDs (Lord, Petkova, et al., 2012), the prior categorical diagnoses were subsumed under the new diagnosis of ASD in DSM-5. DSM-5 removed the PDD nomenclature and instead classifies ASD under neurodevelopmental disorders. According to DSM-5, individuals with a well-established DSM-IV diagnosis of autistic disorder, Asperger's disorder, or PDD-NOS may be assumed to meet DSM-5 criteria for ASD.

The DSM-5 revision was intended to make the diagnosis of ASD more straightforward and reliable across development using core features in two domains: social communication and interaction; and restricted, repetitive patterns of behavior, interests, or activities. Expectations are that ICD-11 will be very similar. The approach of DSM-5 ASD criteria is to describe broad mandatory and optional domains of difficulty that apply to ASD across ages and developmental levels with the expectation that a clinician, working with the referred individual and his or her caregivers, will come up with detailed examples of behaviors that fall within each domain. This places the responsibility for acquiring enough information to make an accurate diagnosis on the clinician, which means that he or she must take enough time and have sufficient sources of information to be able to apply or reasonably rule out the criteria below.

The first domain specifies persistent deficits in social communication and interaction across settings, with three criteria: (1) deficits in social emotional reciprocity; (2) deficits in nonverbal communicative behaviors used for social interaction; and (3) deficits in developing, maintaining, and understanding relationships. In the second domain of restricted, repetitive patterns of behavior, interests, or activities, there are four criteria: (1) stereotyped or repetitive motor movements, use of objects, or speech; (2) insistence on sameness, inflexible adherence to routines, or ritualized patterns of verbal or nonverbal behavior; (3) highly restricted, fixated interests that are abnormal in their intensity or focus; and (4) hyper- or hypo-reactivity to sensory input or unusual interest in sensory aspects of the environment. To have ASD,

an individual must show evidence of difficulties, either currently or by history, in each of the three social communication criteria and in at least two of the four restricted, repetitive, sensory–motor behaviors. Additionally, symptoms must be present during the early developmental period, though they may not be fully manifest until the social demands exceed limited capacities, or they may be masked by learned strategies later in life. Finally, there must currently be a clinically significant impairment in social, occupational, or other important areas of functioning even if the autism-specific features are based on history only. DSM-5 criteria specify that these deficits should not be better explained by intellectual disability or global developmental delay. Though intellectual disability and ASD may co-occur, to make a comorbid diagnosis, social communication should be below that expected for general developmental level.

The diagnosis of ASD is now made with two sets of specifiers to capture severity and specify comorbid conditions. The severity metrics for ASD are based on level of support needed for the individual and are rated separately for the social communication and the restricted, repetitive patterns of behavior domains: Level 1 (Requiring Support), Level 2 (Requiring Substantial Support), and Level 3 (Requiring Very Substantial Support), with the idea that many individuals with ASD may function well in particular contexts because of particular levels of support, and that level of severity cannot be considered without taking this support into account. DSM-5 provides examples of each severity level and suggests that the levels may change over the course of an individual's life. With the presentation of severity levels lies a concern that they will be used to exclude individuals who are either not severe enough or too severe for a particular program. In addition, to date, these levels have been shown to demonstrate limited inter-rater reliability and validity (Mazurek et al., 2018; Weitlauf, Gotham, Vehorn, & Warren, 2014).

The second set of specifiers indicates whether ASD is present with or without associated conditions: with or without accompanying intellectual impairment; with or without accompanying language impairment; associated with known medical (e.g., epilepsy) or genetic conditions (e.g., fragile X), or an environmental factor (e.g., severe deprivation); another neurodevelopmental, mental, or behavioral disorder (e.g., attention-deficit/hyperactivity disorder [ADHD]; anxiety, depressive, or bipolar disorders; feeding, elimination, or sleep disorders); or with catatonia.

Prevalence and Associated Features

A review commissioned by the World Health Organization (Elsabbagh et al., 2012) estimated the global prevalence of ASD to be approximately 1%. This estimate is consistent with a more recent review estimating the prevalence to be approximately 1.5% in developed countries (Lyall et al., 2017). The most recent prevalence estimate of ASD in the United States is 1 in 59 children (1.7%; Baio et al., 2018). It has been consistently documented that more males than females are diagnosed with ASD, with current estimates ranging from 3:1 to 4.3:1 across the spectrum (Loomes, Hull, & Mandy, 2017). The recurrence rate for ASD in families is nearly 20%, with additional risk conferred for males and in families with multiple children with ASD (Ozonoff et al., 2011). Though it is clear that prevalence rates of ASD have increased over time, upward trends in rates of prevalence cannot be directly attributed to an increase in the incidence of ASD, as changes in referral patterns and availability of services, decreasing age of diagnosis, heightened public awareness, and changes over time in diagnostic concepts and practices confound the interpretation of the data (Elsabbagh et al., 2012; Fombonne, 2005).

There is significant heterogeneity in the presentation of individuals with ASD. Specifically, individuals with ASD vary in terms of age of onset, severity of symptoms, and associated features that affect development, including intellectual functioning, language level, and comorbid psychiatric disorders (Bal, Kim, Fok, & Lord, 2019; Gotham, Risi, Pickles, & Lord, 2007; Levy et al., 2010; Salazar et al., 2015). The manifestation of social communication deficits and restricted and repetitive behaviors that define ASD are affected by these factors, which underscores the importance of considering these associated features in the context of an ASD assessment.

Chronological age has a significant effect on the way in which symptoms of ASD manifest across development. ASD emerges early in life and can be reliably diagnosed in children as young as 2 years of age (Kleinman et al., 2008). However, many children with ASD do not receive a diagnosis until older, with the average age of diagnosis in the United States occurring somewhere between ages 4 and 5 (Baio et al., 2018). Individuals with ASD also vary widely in their language abilities. Though many children with ASD were once expected to have minimal verbal abilities, this has changed greatly with the detection of milder cases of ASD and access to early intervention services.

Historically, it was thought that the majority of individuals with ASD also have an intellectual disability (ID). However, epidemiological studies have suggested that the proportion of individuals with ASD who also have an ID has decreased in recent years (Fombonne, 2005). The Autism and Developmental Disabilities Monitoring (ADDM) Network (Christensen et al., 2016) surveillance data from nine sites in the United States reported that 31.6% (range 20–50%) of 8-year-old children with ASD were classified as having IQ scores in the range of an ID. ID is characterized by cognitive and adaptive deficits, with onset in the developmental period; the level of intellectual functioning affects the presentation of core and associated features seen in ASD. Studies have shown that higher levels of intelligence are significantly associated with better clinical outcomes, while ID has been commonly associated with more severe ASD (Howlin, Moss, Savage, & Rutter, 2013). However, an increasing proportion of individuals with ASD demonstrate at least non-verbal abilities within the average range (Lord, Elsabbagh, Baird, & Veenstra-VanderWeele, 2018). Therefore, we should not make assumptions about cognitive functioning based on ASD symptoms. A cognitive assessment using standardized tools should be used to describe a child's intellectual and adaptive levels of functioning.

Contexts of ASD Assessments

Individuals are referred for diagnostic assessment of ASD for a variety of reasons. A diagnostic evaluation establishes eligibility for educational and clinical services. The assessment also provides an opportunity to identify the individual's unique profile of strengths and challenges, which can then be used to plan specific educational, therapeutic, and vocational goals. Because both outcomes and immediate goals for individuals with ASD are determined as much by factors other than autistic features, it is important to use the assessment to document functioning across a variety of domains (intellectual functioning, social communication skills, self-care, behavioral functioning). This framework and information can document baseline functioning to be used to measure progress moving forward.

The focus of the assessment of ASD and specific measures used vary depending on the age of the person being assessed. The urgency of the referral, sources of information, and differential diagnoses also often vary depending on the individual's age. It can be helpful to think about these contexts in terms of developmental stages. Language delay is often the first reason why parents of children with ASD seek help; the most common differential diagnoses in young children include language disorder and developmental delays. Parents of a young child are often seeking the assessment because they have suspected, observed, or been told by someone else that there is a concern about their child's development. Older children or adolescents referred for possible ASD often have a history of previous social or academic difficulties, but there are usually fewer concerns related to language and intellectual functioning; rather, there are likely to be concerns related to a differential or comorbid diagnosis. Individuals with ASD have higher rates of co-occurring mental health disorders than individuals with other disorders and children with other disabilities (Joshi et al., 2010; Rosen, Mazefsky, Vasa, & Lerner, 2018). While prevalence rates vary depending on both referral source and diagnostic method, an estimated 70% of youth with ASD have at least one co-occurring psychiatric disorder, most commonly ADHD, anxiety, and mood disorders (Leyfer et al., 2006; Rosen et al., 2018; Simonoff et al., 2008).

Diagnostic assessment of ASD can be performed by a variety of professionals, including developmental–behavioral pediatricians, psychiatrists, neurologists, and psychologists. Some speech–language pathologists and occupational therapists may also have significant experience with children or adolescents with ASD and can provide important input to a diagnosis. Across different disciplines or areas of expertise, it is imperative that professionals who conduct ASD assessments have appropriate clinical training and be familiar with typical development, other common diagnoses, and individuals with ASD; have clinical skill in working with people with suspected developmental delays or behavioral difficulties; and use standardized tools.

Several professional groups, including the American Academy of Child and Adolescent Psychiatry (Volkmar, Cook, Pomeroy, Realmuto, & Tanguay, 1999), the American Academy Neurology (Filipek et al., 1999), and the American Academy of Pediatrics (Johnson, Myers, & American Adacemy of Pediatrics Committee on Children with Disabilities, 2007) have issued practice parameters focused on the early identification and diagnosis of children ASD. Screening is intended to identify children who are in need of a more comprehensive diagnostic evaluation due to risk of delay in development or disability. A screening measure for ASD attempts to maintain a balance between identifying as many children with symptoms of ASD as possible and successfully excluding children without ASD symptoms, who make up by far the majority of the general population. Two widely used and well-validated screening tools for infants and toddlers are the Infant–Toddler Checklist (ITC; Wetherby, Brosnan-Maddox, Peace, & Newton, 2008) for ages 6–30 months and the Modified Checklist for Autism in Toddlers—Revised with Follow-Up (M-CHAT-R/F; Robins et al., 2014) for ages 16–24 months. Both are examples of parent/primary caregiver report measures that are freely available online and frequently administered during pediatric well-child visits. The screening measures are intended to identify risk level for ASD and refer those who screen positive for more comprehensive assessments.

Core ASD Assessment Battery

In the absence of biological markers, the best-estimate clinical diagnosis based on a constellation of behavioral features remains the "gold standard" for the diagnosis of ASD. Given the significant heterogeneity in syndrome expression, the diagnostic process involves consideration of multiple sources of information (Kim & Lord, 2012b; Risi et al., 2006), including results of ASD diagnostic tools, assessment of developmental and cognitive skills, langauge and communication, adaptive functioning, as well as information obtained in the family and medical history. There is a great deal of evidence documenting that the diagnosis of ASD can be made with excellent sensitivity (successfully identifying all people with the disorder) and specificity (identifying only the people with the disorder and not people with other disorders), with a detailed caregiver report and observation by a skilled clinician (Charman et al., 2005; Chawarska, Klin, Paul, Macari, & Volkmar, 2009; Guthrie, Swineford, Nottke, & Wetherby, 2013). Professional practice parameter guidelines emphasize the need to collect data from the parent about early development and specific symptoms of ASD, as well as to observe the child directly using standardized instruments that we review in this chapter. A summary of these measures may be found in Table 12.1.

TABLE 12.1. Descriptive Information of Selected Assessment Measures for ASD in Childhood

Measure	Age range	Format	Level of training needed	Time to administer	Cost	Where to access
Autism Diagnostic Interview—Revised (ADI-R)	>2 years mental age	Semistructured, standardized parent interview	Intensive	90–150 minutes	Yes	www.wpspublish.com/adi-r-autism-diagnostic-interview-revised
Autism Diagnostic Observation Schedule, Second Edition (ADOS-2)	12 months through adulthood	Semistructured, standardized clinician observation	Intensive	40–60 minutes	Yes	www.wpspublish.com/ados-2-autism-diagnostic-observation-schedule-second-edition
Childhood Autism Rating Scale, Second Edition (CARS2)	2 years and older	Clinician observation and parent interview	Moderate	5–10 minutes (to complete ratings)	Yes	www.wpspublish.com/cars-2-childhood-autism-rating-scale-second-edition
Developmental, Dimensional, and Diagnostic Interview (3Di)	Childhood through adulthood	Structured interview	Moderate	45–60 minutes	Yes	http://lixdx.org/3di-index.html
Diagnostic Instrument for Social Communication Disorders (DISCO-11)	Childhood through adulthood	Structured interview	Intensive	120–150 minutes	Yes	www.autism.org.uk/professionals/training-consultancy/disco.aspx
Infant–Toddler Checklist (ITC)	6–24 months	Parent questionnaire	Minimal	5–10 minutes	No	https://brookespublishing.com/product/csbs-dp-itc
Modified Checklist for Autism in Toddlers (M-CHAT)	16–30 months	Parent questionnaire with a follow-up parent interview (when indicated)	Minimal	<5 minutes for the questionnaire; 5–10 minutes for the parent interview	No	https://mchatscreen.com
Screening Tool for Autism in Toddlers (STAT)	24–36 months	Semistructured, standardized clinician observation	Intensive	20 minutes	Yes	http://stat.vueinnovations.com/about
Social Communication Questionnaire (SCQ)	Mental age >2 years	Parent questionnaire	Minimal	<10 minutes	Yes	www.wpspublish.com/scq-social-communication-questionnaire
Social Responsiveness Scale, Second Edition (SRS-2)	2 years, 5 months through adulthood	Parent/other questionnaire (preschool, school age, adults); self-report (adults)	Minimal	15–20 minutes	Yes	www.wpspublish.com/srs-2-social-responsiveness-scale-second-edition

The first step of the diagnostic assessment is to review with parents or caregivers their current concerns and the early developmental history. It is important to carefully review medical history and information regarding the physical health of the individual being evaluated because medical issues may explain some autism-like behaviors or influence an individual's performance on standardized tests. Significant visual impairments may affect eye contact, and hearing impairments may explain language difficulties and reduced responsivity (i.e., not responding when one's name is called). A review of available records from previous evaluations, school reports, and other providers should also be integrated into the background interview. This developmental history and review is then combined with both direct observation of the child, and when possible, teacher input regarding performance in the school setting.

The use of standardized assessment measures for ASD has helped to increase identification of ASD and enhance the diagnostic accuracy in both clinical and research settings (Johnson et al., 2007). However, standardized measures have strengths and limitations that should be taken into account in the context of the evaluation. Psychometrics can be affected by the setting, sample characteristics, purpose of the assessment, and presence of comorbid diagnoses (Charman & Gotham, 2013). Diagnostic scales and tools for ASD are not meant to be used in isolation but as objective and standardized measures (similar to obtaining a reading of one's temperature, white blood cell count, or heart rate in a physical exam) that can be considered by clinicians as they also gather information regarding the individual's developmental history, cognitive functioning, and language, social, and adaptive skills across a variety of contexts (Lord & Corsello, 2005).

Structured Questionnaires and Rating Scales

In the context of an assessment, structured questionnaires and rating scales offer the opportunity to collect a large amount of information from multiple informants across settings. Many scales have been developed to specifically differentiate individuals at risk for ASD from those at risk for other developmental disorders. These parent/caregiver-completed questionnaires can be used both to refer individuals in need of additional assessment for a more comprehensive evaluation, and to complement the information obtained during the clinical interview and direct observation of the child.

The Social Communication Questionnaire (SCQ; Rutter, Bailey, & Lord, 2003), formerly the Autism Screening Questionnaire (ASQ; Berument, Rutter, Lord, Pickles, & Bailey, 1999), is a widely used caregiver-completed questionnaire available from a publisher that is based on the Autism Diagnostic Interview—Revised (ADI-R; Lord, Rutter, & LeCouteur, 1994). It consists of 40 items answered yes–no that are assigned a point rating of 1 (*presence of abnormal behavior*) or 0 (*absence of abnormal behavior*). The first item is not included in scoring, as it indicates whether the child has sufficient language for the verbal items to be scored. If the child is not scored as verbal, the six language items are skipped. The SCQ was initially designed for use in children 4 years of age and older, though it can be used to screen children younger than age 4 years. There are two different versions of the SCQ: the Lifetime Form, which focuses on developmental history and behavior, and the Current Form, which focuses on the behavior during the most recent 3 months. Initial studies raised some concerns about the use of the SCQ with younger children (Baranard-Brak, Brewer, Chestnut, Richman, & Schaeffer, 2016; Corsello et al., 2007; Eaves, Wingert, Ho, & Mickelson, 2006), while other studies have used the SCQ to confirm ASD diagnoses in young children (Marvin, Marvin, & Lipkin, 2017; Moody et al., 2017). The authors suggest a cutoff score of 15 or more, though they acknowledge that other cutoffs may be desirable for general populations and other purposes. Researchers have suggested different cutoff points for different populations (i.e., younger vs. older children, clinical vs. nonclinical populations) and highlighted the importance of adjusting cutoff scores based on the research or screening goals (Corsello et al., 2007; Eaves et al., 2006).

The Social Responsiveness Scale, Second Edition (SRS-2; Constantino & Gruber, 2012) is a 65-item questionnaire that assesses communication, social interaction, and repetitive, stereotyped behaviors and interests across the lifespan, including a Preschool form (ages 2 years, 5 months to 4 years, 5 months), a School-Age form (ages 4 years, 6 months to 18 years), and the Adult Self-Report and Adult Relative/Other-Report forms (ages 19 years and older), all of which are available through a publisher. The SRS-2 is designed to measure ASD symptoms and provides *T*-scores and cutoffs for clinically significant ASD symptoms according to population-based norms by age and sex. Some studies have suggested that the SRS raw scores are influenced by non-ASD-specific child characteristics, such as internalizing and externalizing behaviors and developmental level, highlighting the need to exercise caution. The SRS-2 is not a specific measure of social deficits or ASD severity, but it can be very helpful as a continuous measure of general behavior difficulties, including social symptoms and some autism-related behaviors (Charman et al., 2007; Hus, Bishop, Gotham, Huerta, & Lord, 2013).

The Gilliam Autism Rating Scale, Third Edition (GARS-3; Gilliam, 2013) is an informant-report instrument used in schools and diagnostic clinics for rating the behavior of children and young adults ages 3–22. Ratings are made on a 4-point scale, summed, and converted to standard scores based on a reference sample across six subscales, including Restrictive/Repetitive Behaviors, Social Interaction, Social Communication, Emotional Responses, Cognitive Style, and Maladaptive Speech. The primary score of interest is the overall Autism Quotient, which has an average of 100 and a standard deviation of 15. The GARS-3 was standardized only on individuals with ASD, with the mean score of 100 indicating that a child has symptoms similar to the average child with ASD, with lower scores indicating fewer symptoms, so specificity cannot be determined. Research concerning the original GARS and GARS-2 reported both low sensitivity and specificity, which dramatically limits the usefulness of this measure for diagnostic assessment (Norris & Lecavalier, 2010; Pandolfi, Magyar, & Dill, 2010). To date, there have been no independent studies examining the sensitivity and specificity of the GARS-3.

ASD Diagnostic Interviews

Several standardized diagnostic interviews have been developed to specifically assess ASD symptomatology with parents or caregivers, including the ADI-R, the Diagnostic Instrument for Social Communication Disorders, and the Developmental, Dimensional, and Diagnostic Interview.

The ADI-R (Lord et al., 1994; Rutter, LeCouteur, & Lord, 2003), a semistructured, standardized parent interview, is administered by a trained clinician to probe for symptoms of autism. Administration and scoring of this interview takes approximately 1.5–2.5 hours in a face-to-face setting and consists of 93 questions focusing on Early Development, Language/Communication, Reciprocal Social Interactions, and Restricted Stereotyped Behaviors and Interests. The questions across these domains are meant to elicit information from the caregiver on both current behavior and developmental history, capturing codes for the behavior "currently" and whether it "ever" occurred, with the significant developmental time point being from ages 4 to 5 (referred to as "most abnormal 4 to 5") for social and communication behaviors. This examiner-based interview allows clinicians to describe in detail the individual's strengths and challenges as described in the caregiver's own words, and provides researchers the opportunity to study different behavioral differences across the domains. The ADI-R provides a way for clinicians to obtain a history, code it in a standardized way that allows comparisons with other samples, and understand a caregiver's perspective on the child's functioning and symptoms associated with ASD.

The items that distinguish between individuals with and without autism are summed into three algorithm scores, measuring abnormalities in reciprocal social interaction, communication, and repetitive behaviors. The ADI-R diagnostic algorithms, which yield classification of "autism" or "nonspectrum," is based on the "ever/most abnormal" codes in preschool years, though current scores can be used to facilitate a clinical diagnosis. Additional criteria, including using lower cutoffs with the same set of algorithm items, have been used to create an algorithm for broader classification of ASD in several collaborative research studies (Collaborative Programs of Excellence in Autism and Studies to Advance Autism Research and Treatment [CPEA–STAART] criteria; Dawson, Webb, Carver, Panagiotides, & McPartland, 2004; Lainhart et al., 2006; Risi et al., 2006). When interpreting results of the ADI-R, reference to developmental level is imperative because children with nonverbal mental ages below 18 months or individuals with profound to severe ID very often fall within the cutoff threshold of ASD, regardless of their clinical diagnosis (Cox et al., 1999; Risi et al., 2006). Therefore, though the ADI-R may provide important information regarding the behaviors of individual with severe ID, the inferred diagnostic classifications should be interpreted with caution. Revised ADI-R algorithms for toddlers and young preschoolers (Kim & Lord, 2012a, 2012b) have shown improved predictive validity for young children ages 12–47 months compared to the original ADI-R algorithm forms (de Bildt et al., 2015). The toddler algorithms expand the lowest age of application to 12 months, with a lowest nonverbal developmental level of 10 months.

While the ADI-R provides information from broad contexts, including a history and a description of the individual's functioning, the ADI-R alone cannot be used to make a clinical diagnosis. It is important to recognize that results from the diagnostic algorithm and a true clinical diagnosis are not the same thing. The clinical diagnosis should be based on multiple sources of information, including direct observation of the individual and parent report (Kim & Lord, 2012a, 2012b; Risi et al., 2006). Additionally, appropriate use of the ADI-R, which is dependent on accurate administration and interpretation of the informant's responses, requires specialized training and substantial practice (Lord et al., 1994) that is available through courses or as part of graduate or clinical training. Training workshops and videos for practice are available to help clinicians and researchers understand the scoring and administration of the ADI-R (see *www.wpspublish.com*).

The Diagnostic Instrument for Social Communication Disorders (DISCO; Wing, Leekam, Libby, Gould, & Larcombe, 2002), currently in its 11th version, is a semistructured standardized interview with more than 300 questions. It takes a dimensional approach to obtain a profile of behavior, while also assessing for specific features associated with ASD. This measure is used primarily in the United Kingdom and Europe. The DISCO can be used at any age and has a strong developmental focus, including a detailed assessment of current developmental level and developmental delay. It is administered face-to-face by a trained examiner interviewing a parent or caregiver of the individual suspected of having ASD and takes approximately 3 hours to complete. The DISCO is organized into eight parts, covering the following topics: (1) factual record of family, medical, and identifying information; (2) infancy; (3) developmental skills; (4) repetitive activities; (5) emotions; (6) maladaptive behavior; (7) clinical judgment independent of quantitative results; and (8) psychiatric conditions and forensic problems. The majority of the items are scored in three levels of severity: *marked problem*, *minor problem*, or *no problem*. Additionally, the DISCO distinguishes both "ever" and "current" ratings of behavior and has diagnostic algorithms.

The computer-generated Developmental, Dimensional, and Diagnostic Interview (3Di; Skuse et al., 2004), a computerized interview adminstered face-to-face by a trained examiner, is designed to assess symptoms of ASD from a dimensional perspective. It includes both mandatory and optional modules, including the Pervasive Developmental Disorder (PDD) Module, which specifically assesses ASD symptoms. Prior to the interview, parents complete questionaires that are entered into the software and used to tailor the wording and order of questions asked during the in-person interview. In contrast to other semistructured diagnostic interviews (e.g., ADI-R, DISCO), the 3Di requires minimal training to administer. During the 90-minute interview, the parents' responses are entered into the computer in real time. Upon completion of the interview, computer-generated reports are provided to inform diagnosis (Skuse et al., 2004).

Observational Assessment of ASD Symptoms

The direct observation by a trained clinician is a core component of any ASD diagnostic assessment. A diagnosis should not be made without the clinician interacting with the referred individual. For young children, a diagnosis can be made by a number of professionals (e.g., psychologist, physician, social worker) and should involve assessment using one of the well-researched, standardized instruments of ASD symptoms. A substantial amount of experience, skill, and practice in working with children and/or adolescents with ASD, developmental disabilities, and other neurodevelopmental disorders is necessary to use these instruments effectively.

The Autism Diagnostic Observation Schedule, Second Edition (ADOS-2; Lord, Rutter, et al., 2012) is a semistructured, standardized, interactive assessment of communication, social interaction, and restricted and repetitive behaviors in children, adolescents, and adults suspected of having ASD. Clinicians across disciplines, including physicians, psychologists, social workers, and speech pathologists, can participate in training to master reliability in both administration and coding of the ADOS-2. It consists of five different published modules, as well as two modules adapted for older children and adults with minimal verbal skills, that are currently available for research (Hus, Jackson, Guthrie, Liang, & Lord, 2011). The modules are graded according to language and developmental levels, making possible its use with a range of ages, from very young children with no language to verbally fluent adults. Each module can be completed in approximately 40–60 minutes and consists of a variety of standard activities and multiple opportunities for social interaction and communication by creating "presses" that elicit spontaneous behaviors in a standardized manner. Item scores of 0–3 are assigned to codes immediately after completing the administration.

Due to its strong predictive and discriminant validity, the ADOS-2 is widely used in international clinical and research efforts, and has been translated to more than 20 languages. Both the original ADOS and revised ADOS-2 diagnostic algorithms show strong predictive validity against best-estimate clinical diagnoses, with the revised ADOS-2 algorithms showing generally decreased association between ADOS-2 total scores and verbal IQ compared to the original algorithms, minimal association between ADOS-2 totals and chronological age, and improved sensitivity for individuals with lower cognitive skills (Gotham et al., 2007; Oosterling et al., 2010). The total scores from the ADOS-2 algorithms have been standardized to provide Calibrated Severity Scores (CSS) that provide a continuous measure of symptom severity and are less strongly associated with language and age compared to the raw ADOS-2 algorithm total scores (de Bildt et al., 2011; Gotham, Pickles, & Lord, 2009). These scores are intended to recognize that ASD is characterized by social communication and behavioral dimensions in children that can range from mildly to severely affected, in ways that also affect individuals with other disorders. The CSS can be used to compare individuals of different developmental levels and also to track symptoms within the same individual over time across both the social-affective and repetitive behavior domains (Esler et al., 2015; Hus, Gotham, & Lord, 2014); CSS scores are available in research reports and have been replicated across large independent samples (Bieleninik et al., 2017). The CSS can also be used to describe the severity of a person's core symptoms relative to his or her language level (i.e., the ADOS module), providing a way to document cases when there is clear clinical abnormality even though the child may not meet formal criteria for ASD. However, in itself, the ADOS is not sufficient for a diagnosis. The CSS should be used together with additional information regarding the child's cognitive abilities and adaptive functioning to adequately describe overall functioning.

The Screening Tool for Autism in Toddlers (STAT; Stone, Coonrod, & Ousley, 2000), an interactive observation measure for children between ages 24 and 35 months, consists of a 20-minute play session during which several different activities are presented to the child to assess communication, reciprocal social behavior, imitation, joint atten-

tion, and symbolic play. The STAT was designed to differentiate children at risk for ASD from those at risk for other developmental problems. The 12 empirically derived items administered within the play-based context assess behaviors in four social-communicative domains: Play, Requesting, Directing Attention, and Motor Imitation. The psychometric properties of the STAT suggested high sensitivity, specificity, and predictive values, as well as concurrent reliability with the ADOS, suggesting promising utility as a screening measure for ASD (Stone, Coonrod, Turner, & Pozdol, 2004; Stone, McMahon, & Henderson, 2008).

The Childhood Autism Rating Scales, Second Edition (CARS2; Schopler, Van Bourgondien, Wellman, & Love, 2010), an autism diagnostic scale, is scored using both the examiner's direct observations and other information that may be available, including parent report. The CARS-2 has two versions: the Standard form (CARS2-ST) and the High Functioning form (CARS2-HF). The CARS2-ST is for children age 6 and younger, or over age 6, with an estimated IQ of 79 or lower, or with notably impaired communication; the CARS2-HF is intended for individuals age 6 and older, with an estimated IQ of 80 or higher, with fluent communication. Each scale has 15 items focused on behaviors that are described in one to two sentences and rated on a 7-point scale (with a range of 1–4), with higher scores indicating greater severity. Additionally, the Questionnaire for Parents or Caregivers (CARS2-QPC) form is designed to gather information from parents or caregivers to help inform the scoring of the CARS2-ST and CARS2-HF (Schopler et al., 2010). The CARS2 is a well-validated measure that can be used as part of the diagnostic assessment process for individuals with ASD and emcompasses multiple sources of information (Dawkins, Meyer, & Van Bourgondien, 2016). While the CARS2 is a frequently used tool, it is based on pre-DSM conceptualizations of ASD (Van Bourgondien, Marcus, & Schopler, 1992) and does not fully capture some constructs considered to be important in the ASD diagnosis (e.g., joint attention).

Utility of Combining ASD Diagnostic Tools

Diagnoses based on combined clinician observation and caregiver reports are more reliable than those based on either observation or reports alone, emphasizing the utility of combining sources of information and diagnostic tools during an evaluation. For example, the SRS-2 resulted in higher diagnostic specificity for children with ASD when information from both teacher and parent reports were combined (Constantino et al., 2007). Risi and colleagues (2006) found a better balance of sensitivity and specificity when the ADI-R and the ADOS were used in combination than when each instrument was used alone. LeCouteur, Haden, Hammal, and McConachie (2008) also examined the combined use of the ADOS and ADI-R for preschoolers with ASD using revised ADOS algorithms (Gotham et al., 2007). For these children, consistent with the study by Risi and colleagues (2006), combining information from both ADOS and ADI-R provided improved diagnostic accuracy compared to that of either instrument in isolation. Similarly, Kim and Lord (2012a, 2012b) demonstrated that the ADI-R and ADOS made independent, additive contributions to more accurate diagnostic decisions for clinicians evaluating toddlers and young preschoolers with ASD. Overall, these studies illustrate the value added by both a skilled clinician directly working with the child and the caregiver account, especially for more complex cases.

Cognitive Assessment

Intellectual testing is a key component of an ASD diagnostic evaluation, as information about developmental level and cognitive functioning helps frame the observed social-communication difficulties relative to overall development (Johnson et al., 2007). Results of the intellectual assessment should be used to determine whether there is a comorbid developmental delay or an ID (Kamphaus & Walden, Chapter 13, this volume), and to clarify specific strengths and challenges for the given individuals who may be targets for interventions. It is important for an examiner to carefully consider the individual's chronological and mental ages when selecting and administering measures of intellectual functioning. Additionally, the measure should provide a full range of standard scores and measure verbal and nonverbal skills independently.

There are a variety of measures available to assess developmental level and intellectual functioning of individuals with ASD. For younger children or those with lower mental ages, the most commonly used measures include the Mullen Scales of Early Learning (MSEL; Mullen, 1995), the Bayley Scales of Infant and Toddler Development, Third Edition (Bayley-III; Bayley, 2016), the Develop-

mental Assessment of Young Children, Second Edition (DAYC-2, Voress & Madoxx, 2013), and the Battelle Developmental Inventory, Second Edition (BDI-2; Newborg, 2005). While these measures vary in terms of the specific dimensions and administration (e.g., the use of parent report to score specific items vs. direct observation), each measure is developed across domains of functioning, including verbal, nonverbal, fine-motor, and gross-motor abilities. Additionally, they provide standard scores and developmental age equivalents. Access to developmental age estimates can be important when a measure is needed to estimate a child's developmental level when his or her skills are not high enough to administer the more age-appropriate instruments or to use standard scores. The MSEL has been used extensively in research with children with ASD and has demonstrated good convergent and divergent validity in measuring developmental skills (Swineford, Guthrie, & Thurm, 2015). Children with ASD have demonstrated profiles on the MSEL of strengths in nonverbal reasoning skills and weaknesses in verbal skills (Barbaro & Dissanayake, 2012; Munson et al., 2008). The Leiter International Performance Scales—Third Edition (Leiter-3; Roid, Miller, Pomplum, & Koch, 2013) requires no expressive language skills and is appropriate for children, adolescents, and adults between ages 3 and 75 years. The adminstration requires no verbal instructions from the examiner or verbal responses from the individual. The Stanford–Binet Intelligence Scales, Fifth Edition (SB5; Roid, 2003) is appropriate for individuals ranging in age from 2 to 85 and contains separate sections for Nonverbal IQ and Verbal IQ, which can be helpful when testing individuals with ASD who have limited language abilities or are nonverbal.

The Differential Ability Scales, Second Edition (DAS-II; Elliot, 2007) may be administered across a wide chronological and mental age range (ages 2.5–17 years). It is commonly used to assess individuals with ASD because it is ideal for repeat administrations that allow for tracking of progress over time and for research projects in which the developmental levels of the participants may vary widely. The DAS-II also provides the option for out-of-range testing, which facilitates the use of the test with an older child who has significant intellectual limitations (i.e., norms available for a school-age child in the preschool battery). For individuals capable of spoken language, the Wechsler Scales are often used, including the Wechsler Preschool and Primary Scale of Intelligence—Fourth Edition (WPPSI-IV; Wechsler, 2012) and the Wechsler Intelligence Scale for Children—Fifth Edition (WISC-V; Wechsler, 2014). The WPPSI-IV assesses cognitive functioning from ages 2 years, 6 months to 7 years, 7 months, and the WISC-V assesses from ages 6 years, 0 months to 16 years, 11 months.

Brief IQ or short forms of intelligence tests may also be appropriate for educational reassessment, research, or when time constraints do not allow for the administration of an entire battery. Both the Leiter-3 and the SB5 have brief IQ scales that only involve select subtests from the measure; a stand-alone Brief IQ measure may also be preferred. These include the Wechsler Abbreviated Scale of Intelligence—Second Edition (WASI-II; Wechsler, 2011) and the Kaufman Brief Intelligence Test, Second Edition (KBIT-2; Kaufman & Kaufman, 2004). For the initial assessment, the administration of full intelligence scales is recommended to help inform educational placement decisions and treatment plans.

Assessment of Adaptive Behavior

Obtaining information about an individual's adaptive behavior is important because it provides an objective index of actual day-to-day functioning. The most widely used measures of adaptive behavior include the Vineland Adaptive Behavior Scales, Third Edition (Vineland–3; Sparrow, Cicchetti, & Saulnier, 2016) and the Adaptive Behavior Assessment System—Third Edition (ABAS-3; Harrison & Oakland, 2015). Both of these measures are reviewed in more detail by Kamphaus and Walden (Chapter 13, this volume). The use of these standardized measures of adaptive behavior provides valuable information about the individual's communication, socialization, daily living skills, and other behavior relative to expectations of their age. Adaptive behavior has been found to be a strong predictor of outcome in children with ASD (Bal, Kim, Cheong, & Lord, 2015; Gillham, Carter, Volkmar, & Sparrow, 2000). The measurement of adaptive behavior is particularly important in individuals with ASD because adaptive skills contribute most to the individual's ability to function successfully and independently in the world (Liss et al., 2001). Additionally, measures of adaptive functioning inform diagnostic decisions (i.e., if the individual also meets the diagnostic threshold for a dual diagnosis of ID) and help identify areas of strengths and weaknesses, beyond cognitive ability, for the individual with ASD. Significant impairments in daily living skills have been consistently documented for individuals with ASD. This information is useful in identifying functional adaptive skills to target in intervention programs (Anderson, Liang, & Lord, 2014; Bal et al., 2015; Dawson et al., 2010).

Using Assessment to Guide Diagnosis, Case Formulation, and Treatment Planning

Value of a Diagnostic Evaluation

In training, there is often great emphasis on the processes involved in making diagnoses and carrying out careful assessments; the value of these efforts is often assumed. Yet considering the question of what can be accomplished by the diagnosis and assessment of a child or an adult with possible autism may make the difference between a minimally useful or useless evaluation that is frustrating for the family and the individual, and an evaluation that can make a difference in several people's lives.

Autism overlaps with other neurodevelopmental disorders and psychological difficulties experienced at different ages but is unique in certain ways because of the very basic social communication deficits that occur from early on, the complexity of the diagnosis based on the two quite different domains, and its frequent, but not consistent, association with ID and language delay, as well as other common psychological difficulties (Jones & Lord, 2013; Simonoff et al., 2008). Each of these factors contributes to developmental trajectories, rate of progress, and outcome (Lord, Bishop, & Anderson, 2015). Treatment responses are variable in autism, often more variable than in other disorders (e.g., MTA Cooperative Group, 1999), likely because of both neurobiological differences among individuals with the syndrome and the contribution of these factors (Masi, DeMayo, Glozier, & Guastella, 2017). Thus, an initial diagnosis of autism, without additional information, is rarely sufficient to accomplish very much.

A first step is to consider the individual's and the family's goals for an evaluation. How does the clinician expect that the individual and family will use the information he or she is providing? In many cases, a diagnosis of autism is perceived as a ticket to services; in a number of regions, and with some insurance companies, an autism diagnosis can result in increased services such as applied behavior analysis (ABA), speech therapy, or occupational therapy. For an adult, it can lead to eligibility for Social Security benefits. This is not a negligible aspect of the diagnosis, but it just scratches the surface of what a well-organized, thoughtful assessment can provide an individual or family.

Second, a diagnostic label can provide access to information through the identification of relevant parents' groups, the Internet, and other media. For many families, groups can be valuable sources of support, and the Internet can be a mainstay of contact and information—but both also may be overwhelming. The sheer amount of information and the variability in quality available over the Internet about autism is astounding. For example, searching "autism" on Google in September 2019 resulted in 249 million results, over three times the number of hits from September 2015, at which time there were 68.6 million results. There are many good sources but probably even more questionable ones. Parents' groups and advocacy groups can make a difference for families, but they also can have adverse effects if the needs of the group members are greater or different than those of the family seeking to join.

Theoretically, a third benefit of a diagnosis is clarity about the cause of a disorder. In autism, this means that parents can be assured that they did not cause their child's behaviors. For an adult or adolescent receiving a first diagnosis, it means that there is a neurobiological cause to their difficulties and, again, that this is no one's fault. Over the last 20 years, it has been established that autism is associated with changes in brain development that are likely present by the second trimester of fetal development (Alarcón et al., 2008; Baron-Cohen et al., 2015; Voineagu et al., 2011; Wang et al., 2009). Autism is strongly linked to a host of different genetic patterns—some are rare; others are common, and many are not inherited but rather are changes that occur early in embryonic development for no reason that has been determined. Consequently, though a specific genetic cause to date can only be identified in a minority of cases, the general pattern of neurobiological differences may free families from guilt about how they have contributed. These findings may also provide some solace to adolescents and adults who have been told or have wondered whether they are deliberately uncooperative or difficult. On the other hand, some children or adults with autism are uncomfortable feeling that something is "different about how their brains are wired," so this information needs to be presented thoughtfully in context.

A fourth benefit of a diagnosis should be information about prognosis and what to expect in the future. We discuss this in more detail below, but because autism is so heterogeneous, long-term predictions solely on the basis of an early diagnosis are not possible, though the diagnosis itself is often stable (Kleinman et al., 2008; Lord et al., 2006; Woolfenden, Sarkozy, Ridley, & Williams, 2012). Many writers have stressed how much uncertainty comes with a diagnosis of autism, particularly for preschool children, because the behavior patterns and outcomes differ so greatly (Eaves & Ho, 2008). Parents wonder whether their child will ever talk, have a friend, or go to a regular school. For school-age children and adults receiving a first diagnosis, how the concept of autism and behaviors and issues specific to autism interact with other aspects of the person's life can vary. Autism is usually a lifelong disorder, but a small minority of people move out of it, and sometimes people move into an autism diagnosis later on (having had other diagnoses earlier), in part depending on other difficulties and the context in which the diagnosis is made (Anderson et al., 2014). An evaluation can reduce this uncertainty to some degree, but clinicians must be careful.

Finally, an evaluation, including a diagnosis, should help families understand a child's current behavior and, ideally, help an adult understand some of his or her own difficulties. We hope this understanding can lead to a reduction in stress and to better treatment and education planning. The best way to approach this through an evidence-based diagnostic formulation is the main topic of our next section.

Important Underlying Issues

The first premise, which is easy to forget, is that for autism, parent participation and involvement is likely to make more difference than any specific treatment or recommendation that we, as clinicians, make. While there is solid evidence supporting the positive effects of a number of behavioral treatments and a few medications on various aspects of development and functioning in children and adults with autism, in the long run, families are with their children for far longer and far more time than any specific treatment. Thus, although practical recommendations and goals and plans are important, a clinician always needs to consider how these fit into what a family is likely to do and the family members' understanding of how they can help. Over and over, parent-mediated interventions (Green et al., 2010; Kasari, Gulsrud, Wong, Kwon, & Locke, 2010; Kasari et al., 2014), caregiver participation in specific treatments, and parent engagement in early intervention (Anderson, Avery, DiPietro, Edwards, & Christian, 1987) have been found to make a difference. However, often, because the process of an evaluation takes on a life of its own, the unique needs, strengths, and resources available to a family are not considered as much as test scores and diagnostic formulations. Somehow, we need to build components into an assessment, so that this does not happen.

A second important issue in the use of classification systems in autism, as well as other neurodevelopmental disorders and child mental health conditions, is the question of impairment. The diagnosis of autism can technically be made on the basis of history of symptoms if there is some sort of current impairment. In medicine, quantification of impairment (how much functioning level is decreased from what is expected) is typically separate from diagnosis—in the sense that a diagnosis may be made by neurobiological markers (e.g., X-ray, blood tests, electroencephalography [EEG]) associated with known etiologies or specific diseases, while impairment is determined by behavior and skills. However, autism is not a disease and likely has varied etiologies that, at this point, have mostly (though not always) failed to be linked in a specific way to symptoms (Geschwind, 2011; Happé, Ronald, & Plomin, 2006). To make the situation more complex, various factors, particularly ID in later years, and language delay in early years, may be more associated with restrictions in functioning than are autism symptoms in many cases (Charman et al., 2011).

As we discussed earlier, DSM-5 provides a framework for level of severity in ASD, but to date, this model has not been empirically supported (Weitlauf et al., 2014). In most of medicine, severity of symptoms is not the same as severity of impairment. However, in autism, the overlap between severity of symptoms and degree of impairment is more complicated. This is because the behavioral symptoms we use to define autism are present in typical development to some degree. Use of eye contact, facial expressions, gestures, imagination, flexibility, social reciprocity—all vary within a normal population and across contexts. A person in distress may show fewer nonverbal forms of communication than a person who is very relaxed. A young child may be less flexible than an older child who understands more language or may be more flexible when his mother or father is present. To discriminate among these variations in typical behavior from autism, we rely on whether the diminution of these behaviors consistently interferes with functioning, which is essentially a measure of impairment, to determine whether this is a symptom of autism (e.g., whether a child fails to compensate for lack of language by using alternative methods of communication, such as gesture or facial expressions).

In addition, individuals with ID and autism in many cases have fewer life skills than those without ID and autism and may, in some senses, be considered more impaired and more severely. However, a person without ID can also be relatively impaired by symptoms of autism, in the sense of the degree to which autism prevents him or her from carrying out activities that in other circumstances he or she could do. To address this issue, we have tried to develop ways of quantifying autism severity that are as independent as possible from intelligence or language level; this is the purpose of the calibrated severity scores of the ADOS-2. The SRS-2 also offers a continuous distribution of T-scores that reflect social and behavioral difficulties that are minimally affected by differences in intelligence within the average range or higher (Constantino et al., 2003), though they are affected by greater differences in ID or language level (Hus et al., 2013). These distinctions have value in terms of predicting progress (Anderson et al., 1987). Thus, it is important that clinicians have separate measures of ID, language level, autism severity, and adaptive skills and levels of functioning in daily life.

Case Formulation and Preparation for Feedback

As shown in Figure 12.1, the case formulation should begin with the reasons that brought the family or the individual to the clinic for an assessment. A quick sense of how much the family or the individual already knows about autism and about the identified patient's diagnostic history can be very helpful because there is so much variability in experiences, from very first diagnoses, when families might not understand why they have been sent to a clinician, to individuals or families seeking a

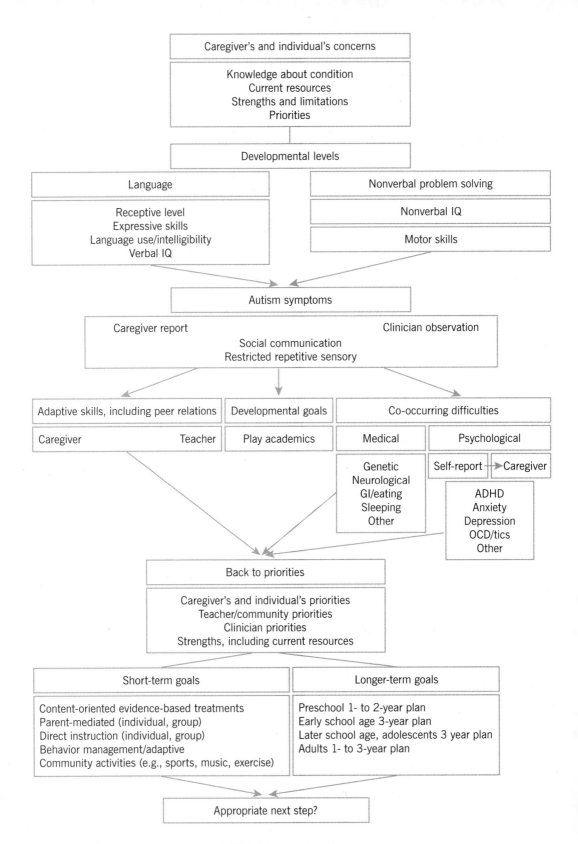

FIGURE 12.1. Case formulation.

second opinion, to families that have already seen five or more clinicians. Documentation of current resources, as much as possible, can also be worth the time it takes because often the clinician's impulse is to recommend what he or she knows rather than to start with what is most accessible to the family. Ideally, information from community providers (teachers, preschool teachers, therapists) is sought before an assessment or at least before feedback.

In some clinics, a first step is a meeting with the caregivers or parents and the clinician to get initial information about diagnostic symptoms, history, and priorities, as well as to convey to the family what will happen during the diagnostic evaluation. For example, in several clinics, the ADI-R and Vineland–3 are administered during this time. At other clinics, a developmental– behavioral pediatrician may carry out a general medical history and developmental screening before more standardized assessments. In both models, a clinician can use the initial time to acquaint parents with possible differential diagnoses (e.g., make them aware that a proportion of children with autism also have ID and/or language delays). Many parents are not aware of these possibilities, so giving them a little warning phrased in a general way can make later discussions easier if, for example, ID or other disabilities, are identified.

If the parents have an opportunity to describe their child and their concerns (particularly without the child underfoot), then the clinician may get unique insights into ways to interact with the family and provide a base for a relationship that later makes communication about diagnosis easier. This first step is appropriate for families who are seeking help for their children; it does not necessarily make sense for adults (unless the family is bringing an adult who cannot speak for him- or herself to an evaluation) or for families who have sought the evaluation because of a referral that they may not understand. In these cases, directly working with the identified patient first may make more sense.

Ideally, caregivers should always be able to observe their child's full assessment, unless the child (particularly an adult or sometimes an adolescent) requests otherwise. Because of time constraints and travel for families who come to centers from far away, sometimes parent interviews and child testing occur concurrently. Particularly for very young children, it is critical that at least one parent is present during social communication testing, both to participate and to inform the clinician

how typical the child's behavior is of how he or she usually behaves. For older children and adolescents, often it is better that parents not be in the testing room but are able to watch the assessment through a one-way mirror or video link, so that they see for themselves how the child behaves and on what the clinician is basing his or her impression. Both the information that families provide about symptoms and history and their reactions to what they observe during testing should be part of a case formulation.

As shown next in Figure 12.1, before symptoms of autism can be considered, a developmental level for language (receptive and expressive) and nonverbal problem solving must be determined. Some older children may have had previous neuropsychological or cognitive testing, and this information can be used, but it is worth being careful because, in many cases, initial impressions of cognitive levels in autism are not accurate. Thus, standardized intelligence testing (and language testing, if there are any doubts about deficits), by an examiner experienced in working with children or adults with autism using an appropriate test is necessary. If these tests are administered early in an evaluation, often the child or adult responds to their inherent structure and begins to relax, making subsequent direct assessment of autism symptoms less anxiety provoking. This information also allows the clinician to decide whether additional testing, with a particular focus, on executive functioning or attention or motor skills, for example, would be helpful.

In case formulation, the role of cognitive and language testing changes with development. For very small children with autism (under age 3 years), developmental levels (e.g., developmental quotients or early IQs), are often below average (Mayes & Calhoun, 2003). These scores are not very stable, except that children who receive standard scores below 50 (in IQ terms) or below 20 (in T-score terms) on nonverbal tests even at age 2 years, when given by experienced and competent assessors, generally continue to have scores in the range of ID as they grow older (Bishop, Farmer, & Thurm, 2015). Most children who receive nonverbal standard scores above 70 at age 2 continue to score above 70 as they grow older, but there are some who do not, particularly children who do not go on to develop fluent language. For children who score between 50 and 70, there is enormous variation.

By age 3 years, developmental quotients and IQ scores are much more predictive of later intelligence in autism (though not necessarily in typical populations) than at age 2. What is most striking is that verbal scores in children with autism are often very low at age 2; by age 3, most children who will eventually speak fluently have improved; they still remain significantly delayed but with an upward trajectory that continues into later school age. Thus, the interpretation of these scores is complex and needs to take into account their reliability and validity at different ages.

In later elementary school years, scores on intelligence tests are more stable when similar tests are used (e.g., the Wechsler scales, Stanford–Binet, or DAS-II). Yet a substantial number of people with autism do not receive basal scores on these instruments. For these individuals, estimating an IQ using tests for younger children or nonverbal tests such as the Leiter-3 may be worthwhile in a few situations (e.g., proving disability for administrative purposes or providing an opportunity to make sure the person does not have more skills than expected when he or she cannot speak for him- or herself), but specific scores below 30 are not very useful. Probably because of the complexity of measurement, IQs often decrease from elementary school years to adulthood for individuals with autism whose scores fall below 50, something probably not specific to autism (Bishop et al., 2015).

For a diagnostic formulation, clinicians put together information from their own observations and caregiver and community reports, as well as from parent or caregiver comments throughout the assessment. There are no standard ways to do this. One of the most obvious ways to start is to recommend that clinicians follow standard cutoffs on instruments such as the ADOS-2, ADI-R, SRS-2, or CARS2. One strategy is that clinicians use diagnoses provided by standard assessments unless they can specify why they feel the instruments are incorrect. However, the instruments may not yield identical results in terms of diagnostic classifications (Bishop & Norbury, 2002), and none of them are perfect. They are intended as tools, similar to blood tests, which a clinician should take into account but not accept as a simple answer. In studies, when diagnoses automatically have been made if a child meets autism criteria on only one out of several instruments administered, specificity is poor (many children whom clinicians don't believe have autism are found to have autism, and about 20% of children who later receive clinical diagnoses of autism without ID are missed) (Corsello, Akshoomoff, & Stahmer, 2013; Risi et al., 2006).

Another approach that has been suggested is to consider how high scores are on one instrument (e.g., calibrated severity score on the ADOS-2 of 7 or higher) and, taking that into account, allow for a more borderline score on another instrument (Kim & Lord, 2012a). When more than one instrument indicates a borderline score, the clinician should acknowledge this, no matter what the diagnostic decision is, and recognize that there is no true, single cutoff for autism; there will always be children and adults who fall on the crux. Rereading criteria from DSM-5 may also be helpful. Particularly with younger children, repeating the assessment in 6 months, while moving ahead with treatment as if the diagnosis is possibly autism is appropriate (Fein, Helt, Brennan, & Barton, 2016). In addition, observing a child at school or at home, getting home videos, or acquiring more information from teachers and current therapists may also be helpful.

In several earlier chapters in this volume (Fleischer, Crane, & Kendall, Chapter 10; Hankin & Cohen, Chapter 7; Van Meter, Chapter 2), more formal methods of determining diagnostic likelihoods, using diagnostic likelihood ratios (DLRs) to propose evidence-based medicine (EBM)–informed decisions, are proposed. These strategies depend on data provided from relatively large samples that are either stratified, so that the clinician can identify classes within the samples relevant for a particular child and family, or are assumed to be sufficiently homogeneous and similar to the relevant child and family that they are a good source of information. Within ASD, such data are not generally available, in part because children and adults with ASD are so heterogeneous and likely to have multiple comorbidities. However, the process that we recommend is actually very similar to the steps suggested for use of EBM and DLR approaches to assessment, but it relies less on specific likelihoods that, at least at this point, would be very difficult to accurately compute for children and adolescents of different ages, intellectual levels, language levels, and comorbidities. For example, Kim and Lord (2012a) proposed a strategy for reducing the need for both an ADOS-2 and an ADI-R on the basis of the likelihood of clinical diagnoses in young toddlers. However, the reality in ASD is also that each of the measures described earlier is not a "pure" measure of behavior but a reflection of the culture, concerns, and goals of the family and the child or adolescent, as well as their language levels, experience, and other behavioral problems. Even when we have very large samples, they are often dependent on the simplest data (e.g., brief questionnaires). Right now, the most sophisticated statistics or machine learning approaches cannot yet improve the quality of such data, at least in ASD, to match the usefulness of observations and reliable, valid, real-life descriptions, ideally from multiple sources, considered by an experienced clinician.

Thus, as part of the diagnostic formulation, it is also worth considering the severity of a child's symptoms in each of the two main domains of autism: (1) social communication and (2) restricted, repetitive, and sensory behaviors. It is possible to do this in a standard fashion with the CSSs from the ADOS-2 in a way that controls for language level (and to some extent, IQ) (Gotham et al., 2007). Using the ADI-R, it is possible at least to observe the differences between a child's earlier and current functioning across subdomains that are similar to DSM-5 subdomains, so this can also be helpful sometimes in considering areas of strength or improvement, as well as areas to target for intervention (Pickles, McCauley, Pepa, Huerta, & Lord, in press).

Beyond considering intelligence, language function, and diagnostic symptoms, a comprehensive assessment should include an estimate of adaptive functioning. Research has shown that adaptive functioning predicts adult outcome; often the everyday living skills of children and adults with autism are quite far below their intellectual levels, which also have immediate practical relevance. For younger children, "play" is the primary activity, and observation of play skills, at some level, is appropriate. For older children, we also know that academic achievement (measured through standard tests, not grades) also predicts adult independence in autism. If not available through the school, it may be worth testing reading comprehension and math problem solving, at a minimum, because these are the usual areas of greatest weakness in ASD. In a recent study, a relatively high proportion of children with ASD without ID met various standards for specific learning disabilities either in math or reading comprehension (Lord, McCauley, Huerta, & Pickles, in press). Often these discrepancies are not taken as seriously in educational planning as they should be.

Ensuring that children and, often of more concern, adults, receive regular, appropriate medical care is important. Genetics, particularly for children with more severe ID or dysmorphic features, or other physical abnormalities may be useful and is considered by the American Academies of Pe-

diatrics and Neurology to be a critical part of an autism evaluation, though this is less the case in other countries. Knowing that a child has a particular genetic syndrome may not change specific behavioral recommendations, but it may put some behaviors in a clearer context.

Recognition of the impact of common but distressing difficulties in eating, sleeping, and gastrointestinal function is also important in terms of recommendations and addressing parent priorities. It may be more important to take 15 minutes to observe and discuss how a child will only eat with an iPad on or only sleep with shoes on, than to do another subtest of a cognitive test. Finally, considering co-occurring difficulties, including ADHD symptoms and anxiety, which occur in more than half of children with autism in some samples (Di Martino et al., 2013; Simonoff et al., 2008; van Steensel, Bögels, & Perrin, 2011), as well as depression, tics, and obsessive–compulsive behaviors beyond the defining rituals and repetitive behaviors of autism, are also part of a diagnostic formulation. In the end, returning to the parents' initial reason for coming and perhaps new priorities that emerged during the assessment, combined with priorities from community sources (e.g., a teacher who requests help with engaging the child with peers) and the clinician's own ideas of both short-term and long-term goals, is the beginning of recommendations.

Having considered all this information, the ultimate endpoint is a formal diagnosis of ASD, with or without ID or language delay, with or without identifiable etiologies or neurobiological factors, then with or without various potential co-occurring mental health problems. This is quite complex information to convey to a family, so, separate from the formal diagnostic formulation, the clinician must consider how to relay this information to the family and how to link it with treatment recommendations. An example is presented in Table 12.2.

Finally, the clinician needs to consider what and how to recommend going forward. There are typically three types of recommendations: (1) recommendations of evidence-based treatment approaches found to be beneficial for children or adults of similar age and sometimes similar needs, such as early interventions (parent-mediated and direct instruction, which the literature suggest have somewhat different effects; Lord et al., 2018), groups for parents and children, such as the Program for the Education and Enrichment of Relational Skills (PEERS; Laugeson & Frankel, 2010), or individualized therapies such as cognitive-be-

TABLE 12.2. Example of a Case Formulation for 3-Year-Old "Joey"

	Evidence
Diagnosis	
Autism spectrum disorder	ADOS-2 and ADI-R
Moderate social communication deficits	ADOS-2 CCS = 7; ADI-R Social = 12; ADI-R Communication = 10
Mild sensory, restricted, and repetitive behaviors	ADOS-2 CCS = 5; ADI-R RRB = 4
Specifiers	
With significant receptive and expressive language delay	DAS-II VIQ = 62
With delayed fine-motor and nonverbal problem solving/monitor for developmental delay (intellectual disability)	DAS-II NVIQ = 75; Vineland–3; ABC = 72
Supportive family environment; inadequate services for now	Parent report
No genetic findings; no sign of epilepsy; no regression	Full microarray

Note. CCS, Communication Complexity Scale; RRB, restricted and repetitive behaviors; ABC, adaptive behavior composite; VIQ, Verbal IQ; NVIQ, Nonverbal IQ.

havioral therapy; (2) specific "content" goals that may be based on gaps in the child's knowledge or behavior that arise from observations, such as working on joint attention, self-regulation, task completion, or behavior management; and (3) general recommendations for placements or hours of therapies in school (e.g., speech therapy, occupational therapy, ABA therapy), moving into or out of a specialized program or simply sitting near the front of the class. Often parents are encouraged to value their relationship with each other and not forget their other children. Another approach is the Hudziak model (Hudziak & Ivanova, 2016), which emphasizes balance in life and basic activities such as sleep and exercise, pleasure in being outdoors, sports, music and crafts or art.

Monitoring Progress

In this section, we talk about outcomes and monitoring progress, but given how complex decisions are about recommendations for individuals, it is helpful to have a place to start. Clinicians may respond to this challenge by having lists of typical recommendations from which they choose. Table 12.3 presents an outline of one way to organize recommendations, following the previous discussion, and Table 12.4 provides an example of recommendations for one specific child. The following clinical case example is provided to illustrate the profile of a child, "Joey," whose clinical profile follows.

TABLE 12.3. Outline of Case Formulation and Recommendations

	Treatment approaches	Site/who?	How to measure progress?
Moderate to short term goals			
1. Start with family or individual priorities			
2.			
3.			
4. Then community-initiated goals			
5.			
6. Then clinician goals			
7.			
Longer-term goals			
1. Moving toward independence			
2. Moving toward community participation			
3. Happiness			
4. Other			

TABLE 12.4. Example Recommendations for 3-Year-Old "Joey"

	Treatment approaches	Site/who?	How to measure progress?
Short-term goals (3 months)			
Family/self priorities			
1. Improve expressive language			
a. Increase vocabulary *used*	1:1 speech therapy 3× a week	Preschool, clinic/ therapist	Language sample; VB-MAPP
b. Target word of the week	Repeated demonstration	School/family	Parent diary
c. Family training for communication	JASPER-EMT; ESI/ PACT	Clinic or home/family	BOSCC; parent ratings
2. Decrease tantrums			
a. Family members understand sequence of events and alternatives	Behavioral parent coaching or predictive parenting	Clinic, home/family	Youth Top Problems
b. Functional analysis	ABA	Home/BCBA	Behavioral records
Community priorities			
3. Participate in more preschool activities and play			
a. Functional analysis	Consultation; TEACCH training	School/psychologist, BCBA	Teacher diary/ observation
Clinician priorities			
4. Support for parents and sibling	Group or individual	Clinic/community	Family support questionnaire
5. Develop positive play activities with family/positive moments	JASPER/EMT; Floortime	Clinic, home/ psychologist	Parent diary
Longer-term goals (1–2 years)			
Independence			
1. Increase spontaneous use of words	See above	Preschool/family, therapist	Language sample
2. Support development of phrases	See above	Speech therapist	Language sample
3. Improve receptive understanding	Parent training or consultant?	All of the above	DAS-II; VB-MAPP
4. Address issues related to sleep and eating	Sleep training/feeding sessions	Clinic/occupational therapist, speech therapist, developmental pediatrician	Parent report

Note. VB-MAPP, Verbal Behavior Milestones Assessment and Placement Program; BOSCC, Brief Observation of Social Communication; ABA, applied behavior analysis; BCBA, board certified behavior analyst; JASPER–EMT, Joint Attention, Symbolic Play, Engagement, and Regulation and enhanced milieu teaching; ESI, Early Social Interaction; PACT, Pre-school Autism Communication Therapy; TEACCH, Treatment and Education of Autistic and Related Communication-Handicapped Children; DAS-II, Differential Ability Scales, Second Edition.

Clinical Case Example

Joey, a 3-year-old boy, was referred by his pediatrician to a university-based child assessment outpatient clinic due to concerns regarding his delayed language development and repetitive behaviors. In terms of early developmental history, Joey was born at 38 weeks' gestation, and no complications were noted at birth. Joey was recently evaluated by an audiologist, and results suggest his hearing is within normal limits. In terms of developmental milestones, Joey first walked at age 16 months, used spontaneous, single words around 26 months, and used phrase speech when he was 34 months old, including "go outside" and "another show." In the area of communication, Joey currently speaks in short phrases. Since Joey began to speak, he has often lifted lines from movies or shows and uses them repeatedly with mimicked affect and intonation regardless of the context. Joey does not typically use his language for social purposes, such as making comments or small talk with other people. He occasionally answers questions, but then has difficulty with conversation because he rarely picks up the thread to keep it going. He is most likely to talk about things that he finds very interesting (e.g., shows, movies). He sometimes uses some gestures to communicate with others, including nodding and shaking his head, waving good-bye, and using a communicative reach. In the area of reciprocal social interactions, Joey's parents indicate that he has a great deal of difficulty navigating social relationships with others. He demonstrates limited interest in other children, though he will sometimes watch from afar. Joey is sometimes responsive to the approach of other children, but then he has difficulty maintaining the interaction. Joey often plays alone for long periods of time and sometimes joins in with other children when they are doing activities he is interested in, such as playing chase. He sometimes shares with others, but usually needs to be prompted. Joey occasionally looks people in the eye when he wants something, but his use of eye contact is inconsistent, and he often looks away when he is talking to someone. His parents note that Joey has a somewhat limited range of facial expressions, but he does direct happy/amused and sad/upset facial expressions consistently. In the area of restricted and repetitive behaviors, Joey's play is described as repetitive; he often lines up figurines and toys, and becomes very upset if the line is changed or moved. Joey also demonstrates several rituals that

he wants to perform the same way each time and reportedly becomes very upset if these routines are interrupted. Joey has always had an undue sensitivity to noise (e.g., vacuum cleaners, blenders, and automatic hand dryers); Joey covers his ears with his hands when he hears these sounds. When Joey is excited or upset, he sometimes flaps and moves his hands repetitively.

Assessment over the Course of Treatment

Directly addressing family concerns (or the concerns that an older child or adult expresses about his or her own life) is critical, as well as addressing issues raised by community providers, but the clinician can also add his or her own perspective. Usually, having very long lists of recommendations based on a single feedback session and one, even long evaluation, is less appropriate than limiting the recommendations to the highest priorities for the next 3 months, then scheduling further contacts to expand on these if families want more details. Sometimes families come from far away and visits are limited, so there is a temptation to provide many, many ideas, but the frequency with which these ideas are used is questionable. If there are many, many recommendations, time may be better spent identifying a provider who can do follow-up or even referring the family to well-documented sources of goals, such as the Social Communication, Emotion Regulation, Transactional Support model (SCERTS; Prizant, Wetherby, Rubin, Rydell, & Laurent, 2003), the Early Start Denver Model checklist (ESDM; Rogers & Dawson, 2010), or the Verbal Behavior Milestones Assessment and Placement Program (VB-MAPP; Sundberg, 2008).

Initial recommendations should be for changes that can occur within 3 months; longer-term goals can be listed as well, but it should be clear that these are achievable more gradually (National Research Council, 2001). Longer-term goals can be ways of reminding parents (and school and clinicians) about issues that may not be appropriate for school or individualized educational plans (IEP) or individual family service plans (IFSP), as well as the eventual objectives. It may also be a way to keep track of goals that are not appropriate to take on immediately after a first diagnosis (e.g., sleep training, feeding, addressing a parent's possible mood disorder) but are important. These can be raised as issues to address in time.

Process Measurement

Following directly on the framework we described earlier for creating goals, measurement of objectives should be specified along with recommendations. Ideally, such a list would be generated together with the family or the community providers who would do most of the measurement, but sometimes this is not possible. A clinician needs to remember that others will likely be the people who directly attempt to reach these goals, so that the objectives need to be framed in a way that is meaningful and useful to them. This is different than a clinician who is using CBT to treat depressive symptoms in his or her own patient. Here, coming up with a few high-priority, well-thought-out goals and feasible ways to measure them can be extremely helpful to a family. Providing general lists of many goals with little clarification of how to measure them is seldom useful and may be overwhelming to families and to other providers.

Another important factor to consider is how context-specific the goals are. In autism, one of the biggest concerns is that children and adults may not generalize behaviors or skills across contexts (Schreibman, 2000). It is appropriate that goals would first be met in the context in which they are taught, but at some point, it is also necessary to test the degree to which goals are generalized. This practice does not often occur in the IEP or the IFSP and is not part of most educational plans, except when standardized achievement tests are carried out with older students. Even in this case, standardized educational testing does not usually cover many of the goals for children with autism. Psychologists, more than the immediate provider, can help families, community providers, and even medication prescribers realize the need for awareness of generalization, as well as measure more general changes. For example, in one study in which children at risk for possible autism were followed on approximately a monthly basis during late infancy and toddler years, the judgments of change made by the clinicians who saw the children regularly were less sensitive to change than scores on the Toddler ADOS-2, suggesting that providers' informal opinions over a short term may not be the best measure of general changes without more empirical support (Lord, Luyster, Guthrie, & Pickles, 2012).

The first step in this process is defining what the goal actually is. Again, ideally there is a process of negotiation and consensus with the family and other providers in setting a goal, but this cannot always happen. The Youth Top Problems (Weisz et al., 2011) approach documents this strategy. For example, in Table 12.3, a goal to increase the child's vocabulary actually entails two parts: increasing the number of different words a child says spontaneously and the frequency with which the child says the words. How big these increases might be depends on the age of the child and his or her current level; how often we would expect the child to speak also depends on the context in which this is measured and his or her existing frequency of speech production. It may be that a psychologist can estimate this from information obtained during the evaluation, but it may not, in which case he or she needs to encourage the family to seek help from someone who can. In the meantime, the psychologist can specify how progress can be measured, for example, through language samples in a standardized context (15 minutes during play with a standard set of toys with a speech therapist or the mother) or through family and teacher diaries of new words or reports on the Communication Development Inventory (Fenson et al., 2006; Kasari, Brady, Lord, & Tager-Flusberg, 2013).

In our longitudinal studies of children who were referred for autism at age 2 and are now adults, we have been able to identify a number of milestones, often either proposed or confirmed by other investigators, that predict adult outcomes of independence and increased well-being (Anderson et al., 2014; Bal et al., 2015; Kim, Bal, & Lord, 2018). Figure 12.2 shows some of these milestones that we have documented as predicting later independence and reduced symptoms of autism in adulthood. These may be helpful in terms of longer-term goals, as described earlier, as well as helping the clinician attend to the relevant milestones at a given age that are most important.

In the United States, IFSP and IEP goals are required to be written, so that outcomes can be measured. Sometimes this is useful, and sometimes it is not (e.g., one goal stated that a child will make eye contact for 15 minutes—a statement that is not specific enough to be sure what is meant by that goal). Because so many of the goals for children and adults with autism have to do with social communication and play or self-regulation, it is absolutely critical to specify the context in which changes are expected. Many of the standardized measures identify contexts in which behaviors are to occur. For example, teacher coding of peer

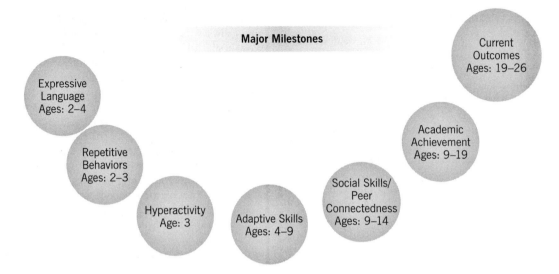

FIGURE 12.2. Milestones predicting later independence and reduced symptoms of ASD in adulthood.

relationships may specify whether the child interacts with other children on the playground or in activity-based groups formed by the teacher. On the Early Social Communication Scales, eye contact or gestures during requests versus those that are purely social initiations are counted (Mundy et al., 2003). Identifying contexts can be difficult because self-reports from children with autism, and even adults with autism, are not as valid as self-reports from other populations (Mazefsky, Kao, & Oswald, 2011). Reduced insight, which is associated with autism, may affect the ways even highly verbal adults with autism describe their emotions and skills (Hill, Berthoz, & Frith, 2004; Rieffe, Meerum Terwogt, & Kotronopoulou, 2007; Silani et al., 2008). Yet we now have a growing literature examining factors that mark transitions and predictors of positive outcomes that can be helpful. The problem is that many of these factors, such as IQ and the development of phrase speech, are not the most malleable characteristics, but we can try. Early interventions have been associated with some improvements in IQ and language, though typically ranging from about 5 to 15 points (Dawson et al., 2010; Smith, Groen, & Wynn, 2000; Wetherby et al., 2014).

Two opposite issues are also important to recognize relative to autism treatments. One issue is that autism is a developmental disorder that affects and is affected by development. Most children with autism improve gradually, in different domains, over time. The role of treatment is often

to accelerate these improvements or perhaps to "trigger" changes in behavior that might not have happened or might not have happened for a very long time, which in turn produces changes in the environment that make a difference in long-term outcome. However, even without specialized treatments, most children with autism eventually become toilet trained, learn to read at some level, and speak in some way. Thus, a finding that a child has changed cannot necessarily be attributed to a particular treatment unless there is a clear and unique relationship between the treatment and the behavior beyond what is accounted for by general development. This can be very difficult to determine without a control group. Second, it is sometimes possible, not so much with developmental goals, but with pragmatics, stress and, mood, that treatments could conceivably make children worse. Consequently, there has to be a way to monitor the direction of change and to ensure that nothing negative is happening. Studies indicate that groups, including group treatments such as that of Hanen (Carter et al., 2011), sometimes have negative effects that are not expected.

Milestones and outcomes that are appropriate as the endpoints of goals may be identified in a variety of ways. One approach is to simply describe the frequency or breadth of the behavior identified as a goal (e.g., learn five new words and use each word spontaneously at least twice a day; have at least two playdates a month and spend at least half the time in each playdate interacting with the peer).

This long-standing practice arising from the behavioral literature has substantial evidence behind it in terms of showing that goals are more likely to be met when specified in a measureable way (National Research Council, 2001). It could be fixed numbers that predict or continuous numbers that might be interpreted statistically for a group, such as the Jacobson–Truax Reliable Change Index or variations of this approach (de Beurs et al., 2018).

Another is to use standardized measures that may be more generic but provide built-in contexts and norms. One study indicated that more specific measures were more likely to show change (in adults being treated with outpatient psychotherapy) (Nugter et al., 2019); however, several treatment studies have been able to show changes on the Vineland–3 (Sparrow et al., 2016) or the SRS-2 (Constantino & Gruber, 2012), both general measures of adaptive function and behavior. In a recent presentation, Fok, Rosenberg, and Bal (2017), using the Aberrant Behavior Checklist (Aman, Singh, Stewart, & Field, 1985), showed that emotion and behavior problems were more widely distributed in children and adults with autism who were minimally verbal, and using the Child Behavior Checklist and Adult Behavior Checklist (Achenbach, Dumenci, & Rescorla, 2003; Achenbach & Rescorla, 2000) with children and adults who could speak fluently. In another study about changes in youth involved in psychotherapy (not with autism), no reliable change was seen for most children or adolescents, and the factors that predicted change were complex and somewhat contradictory (Smith & Jensen-Doss, 2017). It is important to match the skills of the child or adult with the instrument selected to measure outcome or progress.

Progress Measurement

We often assume that progressive feedback will be helpful in treatments, yet this may depend on the how the therapist uses it and how much he or she believes in it (de Jong, van Sluis, Nugter, Heiser, & Spinhoven, 2012), as well as whether the goal is greater change or faster change (Koementas-de Vos, Nugter, Engelsbel, & De Jong, 2018). The clinician should make an educated estimate of the time period in which visible change would be expected in deciding how often to measure progress.

Behaviorism is built on the assumption that more data are better, and that continuous data collection is inherently valuable, but it is not clear how continuous the data collection really needs to be, particularly if goals have to do with generalization rather than gradually improving performance in a highly structured situation (e.g., a discrete trial in ABA). There can be a trade-off between taking continual data (thus having lots of it) versus taking intermittent data (thus missing some information) and the degree to which the provider can attend to the actual treatment. The supervising or treating clinician needs to consider whether having data about the exact number of trials and responses provides important information (sometimes it does) versus more episodic information (e.g., general ratings of how a session went or more specific counts of behaviors in specific contexts—how did the child respond to losing a game?). Sometimes records of progress are important as records of process, as discussed below.

A number of standardized checklists can be used to monitor progress. These are typically lists of behaviors in approximate developmental order that were created as guides for program planning more than as outcome measures. They include the ESDM Checklist, SCERTS, and the VB-MAPP. Each lists specific behaviors in different domains that follow a general developmental pathway. They can be very helpful in identifying new goals, maintenance goals, and aspiration goals because they lay out tasks developmentally (Koegel & Koegel, 2006; Rogers & Dawson, 2010). The Vineland in its various forms (Vineland–2 and –3) is similar; it comes as an interview and a survey form, and most researchers use the interview form because of its greater validity (Sparrow, Cicchetti, & Balla, 2005; Sparrow, Cicchetti, & Saulnier, 2016). The Vineland can be used every 3–6 months but is unlikely to show much change in a short time. The Autism Impact Measure (AIM; Mazurek et al., 2018) and the Pervasive Developmental Disorder Behavior Inventory (PDD-BI; Cohen, Schmidt-Lackner, Romanczyk, & Sudhalter, 2003) both have been found to document general changes in communication, social reciprocity, and other domains over periods of several months or longer, and so can be used as both outcome and progress measures. There are also statistical methods, such as the Jacobson–Truax Reliable Change Index (Jacobson & Truax, 1991) that allow comparison of an individual to estimated rates of change in other populations that could be used with scores such as Vineland–3 or achievement tests when there are well-documented expectations for progress across development.

Finally, our research group (Catherine Lord) has been working on the development of an observational measure that provides codes of social-communicative behaviors and repetitive behaviors that we hope will be sensitive to changes in response to treatment within 12–16 weeks or longer. It is called the Brief Observation of Social Communication (BOSCC) and takes about 12–16 minutes to administer. The child interacts with an adult—which can be a caregiver, a therapist, or a teacher, or a "blinded" research assistant—for two interactions that consist of 4–6 minutes of play with a defined set of toys or materials, then, depending on the age of the child, either 2 minutes of bubble blowing, playing together with a house that has doors and locks or engaging in conversation with no materials. Videos are coded by "blinded" research assistants either locally or submitted to the publisher, who will provide coding. Naive interactors do not need much training other than not to teach or prompt the child during the session; coders require some training, but not to the degree that the ADOS-2 or ADI-R would entail. Several studies have shown significant changes in minimally verbal children receiving early intervention (Grzadzinski et al., 2016; Kitzerow, Teufel, Wilker, & Freitag, 2016; Pijl et al., 2018), though other studies have not (Fletcher-Watson et al., 2016; Nordahl-Hansen, Fletcher-Watson, McConachie, & Kaale, 2016), which is what we would expect. These codes can also be used to measure change in ADOS-2 videos and seem to be more sensitive than the ADOS-2 diagnostic items (Kim, Grzadzinski, Martinez, & Lord, 2018). Versions for minimally verbal children from ages 2 to 12 years are available, and administration instructions are available for older and more verbal children and adolescents while we finalize the codes and psychometrics. We hope this will provide an additional way to measure progress, particularly for children who are receiving ABA, for whom there is very good documentation of change within treatment but often little information about generalization. The BOSCC also may be useful in clinical trials of other interventions and medications.

Process Changes

Process can be documented in a number of ways. Because many children and adults with autism are much more comfortable when they can predict what happens, use of schedules and agendas within treatment is very common. Saving these agendas as records of process, with very brief notes (of what did or did not happen, or any unusually positive or negative reactions) is an easy way to keep records of the process of treatment, particularly if this can be done online or using templates that make collapsing data easier. Many older children and adults with autism enjoy sending online updates or homework in advance of sessions, which can be helpful in monitoring what they are doing or feeling outside of sessions.

Using the Top Problems approach (Weisz et al., 2011), sharing a form with families or children that summarizes behaviors related to each goal or factors that may mediate progress within treatment sessions (e.g., relaxed, irritable, anxious, motivated) may be helpful to denote progress. Other factors that may mediate or moderate progress, such as attendance, family and teacher involvement, adverse events and medication, can also be recorded as part of process notes.

Many of the ASD early intervention approaches have fidelity measures for parents that can be used to note their changes in parent-mediated treatments (including Pivotal Response Treatment [PRT], ESDM, Early Social Interaction [ESI], and Joint Attention Symbolic Play and Engagement Regulation [JASPER]). Recently, Vibert and colleagues (2020) combined several approaches to create an integrated coding scheme of caregiver (or any interactor) behavior that can be used to describe behavior during the BOSCC. This would provide an important measure of what we believe is the most significant mediator of child improvement, changes in caregiver behaviors, which could eventually be a step in process measurement.

Conclusion

The assessment of ASD is complex and requires an appreciation and understanding of the diagnostic criteria and assessment tools that have been developed to standardize diagnostic practices. As we have already discussed, assessment of ASD is not a one-time, single event. For young children, under age 5, yearly reevaluations are critical to monitor progress and make recommendations. Trajectories at these ages are more important than absolute levels. For older children, adolescents and adults, because ASD is so heterogeneous, evaluations that precede transitions can be extremely helpful for families making decisions about school placements, amount of therapy, and expectations for their children. These evaluations can be briefer than a first, comprehensive evaluation and should focus on issues most important to the family, as well as short and long-term planning. Follow-up visits after briefer periods of time may be warranted for very young children or when situations change (e.g., a child begins an intensive program or for the first time, or attends a less structured, more integrated school). Because we cannot predict outcome in very young preschoolers, and because trajectories vary so greatly, it is important to keep adequate records that can be shared with other providers, and monitor change (or lack of change) over time and be sure that families are involved in this process.

Across the last two decades, both research and clinical practice have seen tremendous growth in the development, refinement, and application of standardized diagnostic tools in ASD. While these tools provide valuable sources of information to help clinicians make more informed diagnostic decisions, there is no single tool that equates to a diagnosis in isolation. There is a need for continued research and multimodal validation of assessment tools. Despite the heterogeneity of symptom expression observed in ASD, comprehensive evaluations using evidence-based tools can lead to a reliable diagnosis that can improve the prospect for enhanced quality of life for individuals with ASD and their families.

REFERENCES

Achenbach, T. M., Dumenci, L., & Rescorla, L. A. (2003). Are American children's problems still getting worse?: A 23-year comparison. *Journal of Abnormal Child Psychology, 31*(1), 1–11.

Achenbach, T. M., & Rescorla, L. A. (2000). Validity of ASEBA preschool scales. *Manual for the ASEBA Preschool Forms and Profiles*. Burlington: University of Vermont, Research Center for Children, Youth, and Families.

Alarcón, M., Abrahams, B. S., Stone, J. L., Duvall, J. A., Perederiy, J. V., Bomar, J. M., & Geschwind, D. H. (2008). Linkage, association, and gene-expression analyses identify CNTNAP2 as an autism-susceptibility gene. *American Journal of Human Genetics, 82*(1), 150–159.

Aman, M. G., Singh, N. N., Stewart, A. W., & Field, C. J. (1985). The Aberrant Behavior Checklist: A behavior rating scale for the assessment of treatment effects. *American Journal of Mental Deficiency, 89,* 485–491.

American Psychiatric Association. (1980). *Diagnostic and statistical manual of mental disorders* (3rd ed.). Washington, DC: Author.

American Psychiatric Association. (1994). *Diagnostic and statistical manual of mental disorders* (4th ed.). Washington, DC: Author.

American Psychiatric Association. (2013). *Diagnostic and statistical manual of mental disorders* (5th ed.). Arlington, VA: Author.

Anderson, D. K., Liang, J. W., & Lord, C. (2014). Predicting young adult outcome among more and less cognitively able individuals with autism spectrum disorders. *Journal of Child Psychology and Psychiatry, 55*(5), 485–494.

Anderson, S. R., Avery, D. L., DiPietro, E. K., Edwards, G. L., & Christian, W. P. (1987). Intensive home-based early intervention with autistic children. *Education and Treatment of Children, 10,* 353–366.

Baio, J., Wiggins, L., Christensen, D. L., Maenner, M. J., Daniels, J., Warren, Z., . . . Dowling, N. F. (2018). Prevalence of autism spectrum disorder among children aged 8 years—Autism and Developmental Disabilities Monitoring Network, 11 sites, United States, 2014. *MMWR Surveillance Summary, 67*(6), 1–23.

Bal, V. H., Kim, S.-H., Cheong, D., & Lord, C. (2015). Daily living skills in individuals with autism spectrum disorder from 2 to 21-years of age. *Autism, 19*(7), 774–784.

Bal, V. H., Kim, S., Fok, M., & Lord, C. (2019). Autism spectrum disorder symptoms from ages 2 to 19 years: Implications for diagnosing adolescents and young adults. *Autism Research, 12,* 89–99.

Baranard-Brak, L., Brewer, A., Chestnut, S., Richman, D., & Schaeffer, A. M. (2016). The sensitivity and specificity of the Social Communication Questionnaire (SCQ) for autism spectrum with respect to age. *Autism Research, 9,* 838–845.

Barbaro, J., & Dissanayake, C. J. (2012). Developmental profiles of infants and toddlers with autism spectrum disorders identified prospectively in a community-based setting. *Journal of Autism and Developmental Disorders, 42*(9), 1939–1948.

Baron-Cohen, S., Auyeung, B., Nørgaard-Pedersen, B., Hougaard, D. M., Abdallah, M. W., Melgaard, L., & Lombardo, M. V. (2015). Elevated fetal steroidogenic activity in autism. *Molecular Psychiatry, 20*(3), 369–376.

Bayley, N. (2016). *Bayley Scales of Infant and Toddler Development* (3rd ed.). San Antonio, TX: Harcourt Assessment.

Berument, S. K., Rutter, M., Lord, C., Pickles, A., & Bailey, A. (1999). Autism Screening Questionnaire: Diagnostic validity. *British Journal of Psychiatry, 175*(5), 444–451.

Bieleninik, L., Geretsegger, M., Mössler, K., Assmus, J., Thompson, G., Gattino, G., . . . TIME-A Study Team. (2017). Effects of improvisational music therapy vs. enhanced standard care on symptom severity among children with austism spectrum disorder: The TIME-A randomized clinical trial. *Journal of the American Medical Association, 318*(6), 525–535.

Bishop, D. V. M., & Norbury, C. F. (2002). Exploring the borderlands of autistic disorder and specific language impairment: A study using standardised diagnostic instruments. *Journal of Child Psychology and Psychiatry, 43*(7), 917–929.

Bishop, S., Farmer, C., & Thurm, A. (2015). Measurement of nonverbal IQ in autism spectrum disorder: Scores in young adulthood compared to early childhood. *Journal of Autism and Developmental Disorders, 45*(4), 966–974.

Carter, A. S., Messinger, D. S., Stone, W. L., Celimli, S., Nahmias, A. S., & Yoder, P. (2011). A randomized controlled trial of Hanen's "More Than Words" in toddlers with early autism symptoms. *Journal of Child Psychology and Psychiatry, 52*(7), 741–752.

Charman, T., Baird, G., Simonoff, E., Loucas, T., Chandler, S., Meldrum, D., & Pickles, A. (2007). Efficacy of three screening instruments in the identification of autism spectrum disorder. *British Journal of Psychiatry, 191,* 554–559.

Charman, T., & Gotham, K. (2013). Measurement issues: Screening and diagnostic instruments for autism spectrum disorders—lessons from research and practice. *Child and Adolescent Mental Health, 18,* 52–63.

Charman, T., Pickles, A., Simonoff, E., Chandler, S., Loucas, T., & Baird, G. (2011). IQ in children with autism spectrum disorders: Data from the Special Needs and Autism Project (SNAP). *Psychological Medicine, 41*(3), 619–627.

Charman, T., Taylor, E., Drew, A., Cockerill, H., Brown, J.-A., & Baird, G. (2005). Outcome at 7 years of children diagnosed with autism at age 2: Predictive validity of assessments conducted at 2 and 3 years of age and pattern of symptom change over time. *Journal of Child Psychology and Psychiatry, 46*(5), 500–513.

Chawarska, K., Klin, A., Paul, R., Macari, S., & Volkmar, F. (2009). A prospective study of toddlers with ASD: Short-term diagnostic and cognitive outcomes. *Journal of Child Psychology and Psychiatry, 50*(10), 1235–1245.

Christensen, D. L., Bilder, D. A., Zahorodny, W., Pettygrove, S. D., Durkin, M. S., Fitzgerald, R. T., . . . Yeargin-Allsopp, M. (2016). Prevalence and characteristics of autism spectrum disorder among 4-year-old children in the autism and developmental disabilities monitoring network. *Journal of Developmental and Behavioral Pediatrics, 37*(1), 1–8.

Cohen, I. L., Schmidt-Lackner, S., Romanczyk, R., & Sudhalter, V. (2003). The PDD Behavior Inventory: A rating scale for assessing response to intervention in children with pervasive developmental disorder. *Journal of Autism and Developmental Disorders, 33*(1), 31–45.

Constantino, J. N., Davis, S. A., Todd, R. D., Schindler, M. K., Gross, M. M., Brophy, S. L., & Reich, W. (2003). Validation of a brief quantitative measure of autistic traits: Comparison of the Social Responsiveness Scale with the Autism Diagnostic Interview—Revised. *Journal of Autism and Developmental Disorders, 33*(4), 427–433.

Constantino, J. N., & Gruber, C. P. (2012). *Social Responsive Scale–Second Edition (SRS-2) manual.* Los Angeles: Western Psychological Services.

Constantino, J. N., LaVesser, P. D., Zhang, Y., Abbacchi, A. M., Gray, T., & Todd, R. D. (2007). Rapid quantitative assessment of autistic social impairment by classroom teachers. *Journal of the American Academy of Child and Adolescent Psychiatry, 46,* 1668–1676.

Corsello, C. M., Akshoomoff, N., & Stahmer, A. C. (2013). Diagnosis of autism spectrum disorders in 2-year-olds: A study of community practice. *Journal of Child Psychology and Psychiatry, 54*(2), 178–185.

Corsello, C., Hus, V., Pickles, A., Risi, S., Cook, E. H., Leventhal, B. L., & Lord, C. (2007). Between a ROC and a hard place: Decision making and making decisions about using the SCQ. *Journal of Child Psychology and Psychiatry, 48*(9), 932–940.

Cox, A., Klein, K., Charman, T., Baird, G., Baron-Cohen, S., Swettenham, J., . . . Wheelwright, S. (1999). Autism spectrum disorders at 20 and 42 months of age: Stability of clinical and ADI-R diagnosis. *Journal of Child Psychology and Psychiatry, 40*(5), 719–732.

Dawkins, T., Meyer, A. T., & Van Bourgondien, M. E. (2016). The relationship between the childhood autism rating scale: Second edition and clinical diagnosis utilizing the DSM-IV-TR and the DSM-5. *Journal of Autism and Developmental Disorders, 46*(10), 3361–3368.

Dawson, G., Rogers, S., Munson, J., Smith, M., Winter, J., Greenson, J., & Varley, J. (2010). Randomized, controlled trial of an intervention for toddlers with autism: The Early Start Denver Model. *Pediatrics, 125*(1), e17–e23.

Dawson, G., Webb, S., Carver, L., Panagiotides, H., & McPartland, J. (2004). Young children with autism show atypical brain responses to fearful versus neutral facial expressions of emotion. *Developmental Science, 7*(3), 340–359.

de Beurs, E., Blankers, M., Delespaul, P., van Duijn, E., Mulder, N., Nugter, A., & van Weeghel, J. (2018). Treatment results for severe psychiatric illness: Which method is best suited to denote the outcome of mental health care? *BMC Psychiatry, 18*(1), 225.

de Bildt, A., Oosterling, I. J., van Lang, N. D., Sytema, S., Minderaa, R. B., van Engeland, H., . . . de Jonge, M. V. (2011). Standardized ADOS scores: Measuring severity of autism spectrum disorders in a Dutch sample. *Journal of Autism and Developmental Disorders, 41*(3), 311–319.

de Bildt, A., Sytema, S., Zander, E., Bölte, S., Sturm, H., Yirmiya, N., . . . Oosterling, I. J. (2015). Autism Diagnostic Interview—Revised (ADI-R) algorithms for toddlers and young preschoolers: Application in a non-US sample of 1,104 children. *Journal of Autism and Developmental Disorders, 45*(7), 2076–2091.

de Jong, K., van Sluis, P., Nugter, M. A., Heiser, W. J., & Spinhoven, P. (2012). Understanding the differential impact of outcome monitoring: Therapist variables that moderate feedback effects in a randomized clinical trial. *Psychotherapy Research, 22*(4), 464–474.

Di Martino, A., Zuo, X.-N., Kelly, C., Grzadzinski, R., Mennes, M., Schvarcz, A., & Milham, M. P. (2013).

Shared and distinct intrinsic functional network centrality in autism and attention-deficit/hyperactivity disorder. *Biological Psychiatry, 74*(8), 623–632.

Eaves, L. C., & Ho, H. H. (2008). Young adult outcome of autism spectrum disorders. *Journal of Autism and Developmental Disorders, 38*(4), 739–747.

Eaves, L. C., Wingert, H. D., Ho, H. H., & Mickelson, E. C. (2006). Screening for autism spectrum disorders with the Social Communication Questionnaire. *Journal of Developmental and Behavioral Pediatrics, 27,* S95–S103.

Elliott, C. (2007). *Differential Ability Scales* (2nd ed.). San Antonio, TX: Harcourt Assessment.

Elsabbagh, M., Divan, G., Koh, Y. J., Kim, Y. S., Kauchali, S., Marcín, C., & Yasamy, M. T. (2012). Global prevalence of autism and other pervasive developmental disorders. *Autism Research, 5*(3), 160–179.

Esler, A. N., Bal, V. H., Guthrie, W., Wetherby, A., Weismer, S. E., & Lord, C. (2015). The Autism Diagnostic Observation Schedule, Toddler Module: Standardized severity scores. *Journal of Autism and Developmental Disorders, 45*(9), 2704–2720.

Fein, D., Helt, M., Brennan, L., & Barton, M. (2016). *The Activity Kit for Babies and Toddlers at Risk: How to use everyday routines to build social and communication skills.* New York: Guilford Press.

Fenson, L., Marchman, V. A., Thai, D. J., Dale, P. S., Reznick, J. S., & Bates, E. (2006). *The MacArthur–Bates Communicative Development Inventories user's guide and technical manual* (2nd ed.). Baltimore: Brookes.

Filipek, P. A., Accardo, P. J., Baranek, G. T., Cook, E. H., Jr., Dawson, G., Gordon, B., . . . Volkmar, F. R. (1999). The screening and diagnosis of autistic spectrum disorders. *Journal of Autism and Developmental Disorders, 29*(6), 439–484.

Fletcher-Watson, S., Petrou, A., Scott-Barrett, J., Dicks, P., Graham, C., O'Hare, A., & McConachie, H. (2016). A trial of an iPad™ intervention targeting social communication skills in children with autism. *Autism, 20*(7), 771–782.

Fok, M., Rosenberg, E., & Bal, V. H. (2017, May). Assessing emotional/behavior problems in children with ASD: Differences in ABC and CBCL profiles by language level. In C. DiStefano (Chair), *Variability at the minimally verbal end of the spectrum: Evidence from biology and behavior.* Paper presented at the International Meeting for Autism Research, San Francisco, CA.

Fombonne, E. (2005). The changing epidemiology of autism. *Journal of Applied Research in Intellectual Disabilities, 18,* 281–294.

Geschwind, D. H. (2011). Genetics of autism spectrum disorders. *Trends in Cognitive Sciences, 15*(9), 409–416.

Gillham, J. E., Carter, A. S., Volkmar, F. R., & Sparrow, S. S. (2000). Towards a developmental operational definition of autism. *Journal of Autism and Developmental Disorders, 30*(4), 269–278.

Gilliam, J. E. (2013). *Gilliam Autism Rating Scale–Third Edition* (GARS-3). Austin, TX: PRO-ED.

Gotham, K., Pickles, A., & Lord, C. (2009). Standardizing ADOS scores for a measure of severity in autism spectrum disorders. *Journal of Autism and Developmental Disorders, 39*(5), 693–705.

Gotham, K., Risi, S., Pickles, A., & Lord, C. (2007). The Autism Diagnostic Observation Schedule (ADOS): Revised algorithms for improved diagnostic validity. *Journal of Autism and Developmental Disorders, 37*(4), 613–627.

Green, J., Charman, T., McConachie, H., Aldred, C., Slonims, V., Howlin, P., & Pickles, A. (2010). Parent-mediated communication-focused treatment in children with autism (PACT): A randomised controlled trial. *Lancet, 375*(9732), 2152–2160.

Grzadzinski, R., Carr, T., Colombi, C., McGuire, K., Dufek, S., Pickles, A., & Lord, C. (2016). Measuring changes in social communication behaviors: Preliminary development of the Brief Observation of Social Communication Change (BOSCC). *Journal of Autism and Developmental Disorders, 46*(7), 2464–2479.

Guthrie, W., Swineford, L. B., Nottke, C., & Wetherby, A. M. (2013). Early diagnosis of autism spectrum disorder: Stability and change in clinical diagnosis and symptom presentation. *Journal of Child Psychology and Psychiatry, 54*(5), 582–590.

Happé, F., Ronald, A., & Plomin, R. (2006). Time to give up on a single explanation for autism. *Nature Neuroscience, 9*(10), 1218–1220.

Harrison, P., & Oakland, T. (2015). *Adaptive Behavior Assessment Systems* (3rd ed.). Torrance, CA: Western Psychological Services.

Hill, E., Berthoz, S., & Frith, U. (2004). Brief report: Cognitive processing of own emotions in individuals with autistic spectrum disorder and in their relatives. *Journal of Autism and Developmental Disorders, 34*(2), 229–235.

Howlin, P., Moss, P., Savage, S., & Rutter, M. (2013). Social outcomes in mid- to later adulthood among individuals diagnosed with autism and average nonverbal IQ as children. *Journal of the American Academy of Child and Adolescent Psychiatry, 52*(6), 572–581.

Hudziak, J., & Ivanova, M. Y. (2016). The Vermont family based approach: Family based health promotion, illness prevention, and intervention. *Child and Adolescent Psychiatric Clinics of North America, 25*(2), 167–178.

Hus, V., Bishop, S., Gotham, K., Huerta, M., & Lord, C. (2013). Factors influencing scores on the Social Responsiveness Scale. *Journal of Child Psychology and Psychiatry, 54*(2), 216–224.

Hus, V., Gotham, K., & Lord, C. (2014). Standardizing ADOS Domain Scores: Separating severity of social affect and restricted and repetitive behaviors. *Journal of Autism and Developmental Disorders, 44*(10), 2400–2412.

Hus, V., Jackson, L., Guthrie, W., Liang, J., & Lord, C. (2011, May). *The Adapted ADOS—Preliminary find-*

ings using a modified version of the ADOS for adults who are nonverbal or have limited language. Paper presented at the International Meeting for Autism Research, San Diego, CA.

Jacobson, N. S., & Truax, P. (1991). Clinical significance: A statistical approach to denning meaningful change in psychotherapy research. Journal of Consulting and Clinical Psychology, 59(1), 9–12.

Johnson, C. P., Myers, S. M., & American Academy of Pediatrics Council on Children with Disabilities. (2007). Identification and evaluation of children with autism spectrum disorders. Pediatrics, 120(5), 1183–1215.

Jones, R. M., & Lord, C. (2013). Diagnosing autism in neurobiological research studies. Behavioural Brain Research, 251, 113–124.

Joshi, G., Petty, C., Wozniak, J., Henin, A., Fried, R., Galdo, M., . . . Biederman, J. (2010). The heavy burden of psychiatric comorbidity in youth with autism spectrum disorders: A large comparative study of a psychiatrically referred population. Journal of Autism and Developmental Disorders, 40, 1361–1370.

Kanner, L. (1943). Autistic disturbances of affective contact. Nervous Child, 2, 217–250.

Kasari, C., Brady, N., Lord, C., & Tager-Flusberg, H. (2013). Assessing the minimally verbal school-aged child with autism spectrum disorder. Autism Research, 6(6), 479–493.

Kasari, C., Gulsrud, A. C., Wong, C., Kwon, S., & Locke, J. (2010). Randomized controlled caregiver mediated joint engagement intervention for toddlers with autism. Journal of Autism and Developmental Disorders, 40(9), 1045–1056.

Kasari, C., Lawton, K., Shih, W., Barker, T. V., Landa, R., Lord, C., & Senturk, D. (2014). Caregiver-mediated intervention for low-resourced preschoolers with autism: An RCT. Pediatrics, 134(1), e72–e79.

Kaufman, A. S., & Kaufman, N. L. (2004). Kaufman Brief Intelligence Test, Second Edition (KBIT-2). Circle Pines, MN: American Guidance Service.

Kim, S. H., Bal, V. H., & Lord, C. (2018). Longitudinal follow-up of academic achievement in children with autism from age 2 to 18. Journal of Child Psychology and Psychiatry, 59(3), 258–267.

Kim, S. H., Grzadzinski, R., Martinez, K., & Lord, C. (2019). Measuring treatment response in children with autism spectrum disorder: Applications of the Brief Observation of Social Communication Change to the Autism Diagnostic Observation Schedule. Autism?: The International Journal of Research and Practice, 23(5), 1176–1185.

Kim, S. H., & Lord, C. (2012a). Combining information from multiple sources for the diagnosis of autism spectrum disorders for toddlers and young preschoolers from 12 to 47 months of age. Journal of Child Psychology and Psychiatry, 53(2), 143–151.

Kim, S. H., & Lord, C. (2012b). New Autism Diagnostic Interview—Revised algorithms for toddlers and young preschoolers from 12 to 47 months of age.

Journal of Autism and Developmental Disorders, 42(1), 82–93.

Kitzerow, J., Teufel, K., Wilker, C., & Freitag, C. M. (2016). Using the Brief Observation of Social Communication Change (BOSCC) to measure autism-specific development. Autism Research, 9(9), 940–950.

Kleinman, J. M., Ventola, P. E., Pandey, J., Verbalis, A. D., Barton, M., Hodgson, S., . . . Fein, D. (2008). Diagnostic stability in very young children with autism spectrum disorders. Journal of Autism and Developmental Disorders, 38(4), 606–615.

Koegel, R. L., & Koegel, L. K. (2006). Pivotal response treatment for autism: Communication, social, and academic development. Baltimore: Brookes.

Koementas-de Vos, M. M. W., Nugter, M. A., Engelsbel, F., & De Jong, K. (2018). Does progress feedback enhance the outcome of group psychotherapy? Psychotherapy, 55(2), 151–163.

Lainhart, J., Bigler, E., Bocain, M., Coon, H., Dinh, E., Dawson, G., . . . Volkmar, F. R. (2006). Head circumference and height in autism: A study by the collaborative program of excellence in autism. American Journal of Medical Genetics A, 140(21), 2256–2274.

Laugeson, E. A., & Frankel, F. (2010). Social skills for teenagers with developmental and autism spectrum disorders: The PEERS treatment manual. New York: Routledge.

LeCouteur, A., Haden, G., Hammal, D., & McConachie, H. (2008). Diagnosing autism spectrum disorder in pre-school children using two standardised assessment instruments: The ADI-R and the ADOS. Journal of Autism and Developmental Disorders, 38(2), 362–372.

Levy, S. E., Giarelli, E., Lee, L. C., Schieve, L. A., Kirby, R. S., Cunniff, . . . Rice, C. E. (2010). Autism spectrum disorder and co-occurring developmental, psychiatric, and medical conditions among children in multiple populations of the United States. Journal of Developmental and Behavioral Pediatrics, 31, 267–275.

Leyfer, O. T., Folstein, S. E., Bacalman, S., Davis, N. O., Dinh, E., Morgan, J., . . . Lainhart, J. E. (2006). Comorbid psychiatric disorders in children with autism: Interview development and rates of disorders. Journal of Autism and Developmental Disorders, 36, 849–861.

Liss, M., Harel, B., Fein, D., Allen, D., Dunn, M., Feinstein, C., . . . Rapin, I. (2001). Predictors and correlates of adaptive functioning in children with developmental disorders. Journal of Autism and Developmental Disorders, 31(2), 219–230.

Loomes, R., Hull, L., & Mandy, W. P. (2017). What is the male-to-female ratio in autism spectrum disorder?: A systematic review and meta-analysis. Journal of the American Academy of Child and Adolescent Psychiatry, 56(6), 466–474.

Lord, C., Bishop, S., & Anderson, D. (2015). Developmental trajectories as autism phenotypes. American Journal of Medical Genetics C: Seminars in Medical Genetics, 169(2), 198–208.

Lord, C., & Corsello, C. (2005). Diagnostic instruments in autism spectrum disorders. In F. R. Volkmar, R. Paul, A. Klin, & D. J. Cohen (Eds.), *Handbook of autism and pervasive developmental disorders* (3rd ed., pp. 730–771). New York: Wiley.

Lord, C., Elsabbagh, M., Baird, G., & Veenstra-Vander-Weele, J. (2018). Autism spectrum disorder. *Lancet, 392*, 508–520.

Lord, C., Luyster, R., Guthrie, W., & Pickles, A. (2012). Patterns of developmental trajectories in toddlers with autism spectrum disorder. *Journal of Consulting and Clinical Psychology, 80*(3), 477–489.

Lord, C., McCauley, J., Huerta, M., & Pickles, A. (in press). Work, living, and the pursuit of happiness: Vocational and psychosocial outcomes for young adults with autism. *Autism.*

Lord, C., Petkova, E., Hus, V., Gan, W., Lu, F., Martin, D. M., . . . Risi, S. (2012). A multisite study of the clinical diagnosis of different autism spectrum disorders. *Archives of General Psychiatry, 69*(3), 306–313.

Lord, C., Risi, S., DiLavore, P. S., Shulman, C., Thurm, A., & Pickles, A. (2006). Autism from 2 to 9 years of age. *Archives of General Psychiatry, 63*(6), 694–701.

Lord, C., Rutter, M., DiLavore, P. C., Risi, S., Gotham, K., & Bishop, S. L. (2012). *Autism Diagnostic Observation Schedule, Second Edition (ADOS-2) Modules 1–4.* Los Angeles: Western Psychological Services.

Lord, C., Rutter, M., & LeCouteur, A. (1994). *Autism Diagnostic Interview—Revised.* Los Angeles: Western Psychological Services.

Lyall, K., Croen, L., Daniels, J., Fallin, M. D., Ladd-Acosta, C., Lee, B. K., . . . Volk, H. E. (2017). The changing epidemiology of autism spectrum disorders. *Annual Review of Public Health, 38*, 81–102.

Marvin, A. R., Marvin, D. J., & Lipkin, P. H. (2017). Analysis of Social Communication Questionnaire (SCQ) screening for children less than age 4. *Current Developmental Disorders Reports, 4*(4), 137–144.

Masi, A., DeMayo, M. M., Glozier, N., & Guastella, A. J. (2017). An overview of autism spectrum disorder, heterogeneity and treatment options. *Neuroscience Bulletin, 33*(2), 183–193.

Mayes, S. D., & Calhoun, S. L. (2003). Analysis of WISC-III, Stanford–Binet: IV, and academic achievement test scores in children with autism. *Journal of Autism and Developmental Disorders, 33*(3), 329–341.

Mazefsky, C. A., Kao, J., & Oswald, D. P. (2011). Preliminary evidence suggesting caution in the use of psychiatric self-report measures with adolescents with high-functioning autism spectrum disorders. *Research in Autism Spectrum Disorders, 5*(1), 164–174.

Mazurek, M. O., Carlson, C., Baker-Ericzén, M., Butter, E., Norris, M., & Kanne, S. (2018). Construct validity of the Autism Impact Measure (AIM). *Journal of Autism and Developmental Disorders.* [Epub ahead of print]

Moody, E. J., Reyes, N., Ledbetter, C., Wiggins, L., DiGi-useppi, C., Alexander, A., . . . Rosenberg, S. A. (2017). Screening for autism with SRS and SCQ: Variations across demographic, developmental and behavioral factors in preschool children. *Journal of Autism and Developmental Disorders, 47*(11), 3550–3561.

MTA Cooperative Group. (1999). A 14-month randomized clinical trial of treatment strategies for attention-deficit/hyperactivity disorder: The MTA Cooperative Group Multimodal Treatment Study of Children with ADHD. *Archives of General Psychiatry, 56*(12), 1073–1086.

Mullen, E. M. (1995). *Mullen Scales of Early Learning.* Circle Pines, MN: American Guidance Service.

Mundy, P., Delgado, C., Block, J., Venezia, M., Hogan, A., & Seibert, J. (2003). *A manual for the abridged early social communication scales.* Coral Gables, FL: University of Miami.

Munson, J., Dawson, G., Sterling, L., Beauchaine, T., Zhou, A., Elizabeth, K., . . . Abbott, R. (2008). Evidence for latent classes of IQ in young children with autism spectrum disorder. *American Journal of Mental Retardation, 113*(6), 439–452.

National Research Council. (2001). *Educating children with autism.* Washington, DC: National Academy Press.

Newborg, J. (2005). *Battelle Developmental Inventory* (2nd ed.). Itasca, IL: Riverside.

Nordahl-Hansen, A., Fletcher-Watson, S., McConachie, H., & Kaale, A. (2016). Relations between specific and global outcome measures in a social-communication intervention for children with autism spectrum disorder. *Research in Autism Spectrum Disorders, 29–30*, 19–29.

Norris, M., & Lecavalier, L. (2010). Screening accuracy of Level 2 autism spectrum disorder rating scales: A review of selected instruments. *Autism, 14*(4), 263–284.

Nugter, M. A., Hermens, M. L. M., Robbers, S., Van Son, G., Theunissen, J., & Engelsbel, F. (2019). Use of outcome measurements in clinical practice: How specific should one be? *Psychotherapy Research, 29*(4), 432–444.

Oosterling, I. J., Roos, S., de Bildt, A., Rommelse, N., de Jonge, M., Visser, J., . . . Buitelaar, J. (2010). Improved diagnostic validity of the ADOS revised algorithms: A replication study in an independent sample. *Journal of Autism and Developmental Disorders, 40*(6), 689–703.

Ozonoff, S. J., Young, G. S., Carter, A., Messinger, D., Yirmiya, N., Zwaigenbaum, L., . . . Stone, W. L. (2011). Recurrence risk for autism spectrum disorders: A baby siblings research consortium study. *Pediatrics, 128*(3), e488–e495.

Pandolfi, V., Magyar, C. I., & Dill, C. A. (2010). Constructs Assessed by the GARS-2: Factor analysis of data from the standardization sample. *Journal of Autism and Developmental Disorders, 40*, 1118–1130.

Pickles, A., McCauley, J. B., Pepa, L. A., Huerta, M., & Lord, C. (in press). The adult outcome of children referred for autism: Typology and prediction from childhood. *Journal of Child Psychology and Psychiatry.*

Pijl, M. K., Rommelse, N. N., Hendriks, M., De Korte, M. W., Buitelaar, J. K., & Oosterling, I. J. (2018). Does the Brief Observation of Social Communication Change help moving forward in measuring change in early autism intervention studies? *Autism, 22*(2), 216–226.

Prizant, B. M., Wetherby, A., Rubin, E., Rydell, P., & Laurent, A. (2003). THE SCERTS model: A family-centered, transactional approach to enhancing communication and socioemotional abilities of young children with ASD. *Infants and Young Children, 16,* 296–316.

Rieffe, C., Meerum Terwogt, M., & Kotronopoulou, K. (2007). Awareness of single and multiple emotions in high-functioning children with autism. *Journal of Autism and Developmental Disorders, 37*(3), 455–465.

Risi, S., Lord, C., Gotham, K., Corsello, C., Chrysler, C., Szatmari, P., & Pickles, A. (2006). Combining information from multiple sources in the diagnosis of autism spectrum disorders. *Journal of the American Academy of Child and Adolescent Psychiatry, 45*(9), 1094–1103.

Robins, D. L., Casagrande, K., Barton, M., Chen, C-M. A., Dumont-Mathieu, T., & Fein, D. (2014). Validation of the Modified Checklist for Autism in Toddlers, revised with follow-up (MCHAT-R/F). *Pediatrics, 133*(1), 37–45.

Rogers, S. J., & Dawson, G. (2010). *Early Start Denver Model for young children with autism: Promoting language, learning, and engagement.* New York: Guilford Press.

Roid, G. H. (2003). *Stanford–Binet Intelligence Scales, Fifth Edition.* Ithasca, IL: Riverside.

Roid, G. H., Miller, L. J., Pomplun, M., & Koch, C. (2013). *Leiter International Performance Scale—Third Edition (Leiter-3).* Wood Dale, IL: Stoelting.

Rosen, T. E., Mazefsky, C. A., Vasa, R. A., & Lerner, M. D. (2018). Co-occurring psychiatric conditions in autism spectrum disorder. *International Review of Psychiatry, 30*(1), 40–61.

Rutter, M., Bailey, A., & Lord, C. (2003). *Social Communication Questionnaire: Manual.* Los Angeles: Western Psychological Services.

Rutter, M., LeCouteur, A., & Lord, C. (2003). *ADI-R: Autism Diagnostic Interview—Revised (ADI-R).* Los Angeles: Western Psychological Services.

Salazar, F., Baird, G., Chandler, S., Tseng, E., O'Sullivan, T., Howlin, P., . . . Simonoff, E. (2015). Co-occurring psychiatric disorders in preschool and elementary school-aged children with autism spectrum disorder. *Journal of Autism and Developmental Disorders, 45*(8), 2283–2294.

Schopler, E., Van Bourgondien, M. E., Wellman, G. J., & Love, S. R. (2010). *Childhood Autism Rating Scale—Second Edition.* Los Angeles: Western Psychological Services.

Schreibman, L. (2000). Intensive behavioral/psychoed-ucational treatments for autism: Research needs and future directions. *Journal of Autism and Developmental Disorders, 30*(5), 373–378.

Silani, G., Bird, G., Brindley, R., Singer, T., Frith, C., & Frith, U. (2008). Levels of emotional awareness and autism: An fMRI study. *Social Neuroscience, 3*(2), 97–112.

Simonoff, E., Pickles, A., Charman, T., Chandler, S., Loucas, T., & Baird, G. (2008). Psychiatric disorders in children with autism spectrum disorders: Prevalence, comorbidity, and associated factors in a population-derived sample. *Journal of the American Academy of Child and Adolescent Psychiatry, 47*(8), 921–929.

Skuse, D., Warrington, R., Bishop, D., Chowdhury, U., Lau, J. Y., Mandy, W., & Place, M. (2004). The developmental, dimensional and diagnostic interview (3di): A novel computerized assessment for autism spectrum disorders. *Journal of the American Academy of Child and Adolescent Psychiatry, 43*(5), 548–558.

Smith, A. M., & Jensen-Doss, A. (2017). Youth psychotherapy outcomes in usual care and predictors of outcome group membership. *Psychological Services, 14*(1), 66–76.

Smith, T., Groen, A. D., & Wynn, J. W. (2000). Randomized trial of intensive early intervention for children with pervasive developmental disorder. *American Journal on Mental Retardation, 105*(4), 269–285.

Sparrow, S. S., & Cicchetti, D. V. (1985). Diagnostic uses of the Vineland Adaptive Behavior Scales. *Journal of Pediatric Psychology, 10*(2), 215–225.

Sparrow, S., Cicchetti, D., & Balla, D. (2005). *Vineland Adaptive Behavior Scales* (2nd ed.). Minneapolis, MN: Pearson Assessments.

Sparrow, S. S., Cicchetti, D. V., & Saulnier, C. A. (2016). *The Vineland Adaptive Behavior Scales* (3rd ed). Minneapolis, MN: Pearson Assessments.

Stone, W. L., Coonrod, E. E., & Ousley, O. Y. (2000). Screening tool for autism two-year-olds (STAT): Development and preliminary data. *Journal of Autism and Developmental Disorders, 30,* 607–612.

Stone, W. L., Coonrod, E. E., Turner, L. M., & Pozdol, S. L. (2004). Psychometric properties of the STAT for early autism screening. *Journal of Autism and Developmental Disorders, 34*(6), 691–701.

Stone, W. L., McMahon, C. R., & Hederson, L. M. (2008). Use of screening tool for autism in two-year-olds (STAT) for children under 24 months. *Autism, 12*(5), 557–573.

Sundberg, M. L. (2008). *VB-MAPP Verbal Behavior Milestones Assessment and Placement Program: A language and social skills assessment program for children with autism or other developmental disabilities.* Concord, CA: AVB Press.

Swineford, L. B., Guthrie, W., & Thurm, A. (2015). Convergent and divergent validity of the Mullen Scales of Early Learning in young children with and without autism spectrum disorder. *Psychological Assessment, 27*(4), 1364–1378.

Van Bourgondien, M. E., Marcus, L. M., & Schopler, E. (1992). Comparison of DSM-III-R and Childhood Autism Rating Scale diagnoses of autism. *Journal of Autism and Developmental Disorders, 22,* 493–506.

van Steensel, F. J., Bögels, S. M., & Perrin, S. (2011). Anxiety disorders in children and adolescents with autistic spectrum disorders: A meta-analysis. *Clinical Child and Family Psychology Review, 14*(3), 302–317.

Vibert, B., Dufek, S., Klein, C., Choi, Y. B., Winter, J., Lord, C., & Kim, S. H. (2020). Quantifying caregiver change across early autism interventions using the Measure of NDBI Strategy Implementation–Caregiver Change (MONSI-CC). *Journal of Autism and Developmental Disorders, 50,* 1364–1379.

Voineagu, I., Wang, X., Johnston, P., Lowe, J. K., Tian, Y., Horvath, S., & Geschwind, D. H. (2011). Transcriptomic analysis of autistic brain reveals convergent molecular pathology. *Nature, 474*(7351), 380–384.

Volkmar, F. R., Cook, E. H. J., Pomeroy, J., Realmuto, G., & Tanguay, P. (1999). Practice parameters for autism and pervasive developmental disorders. *Journal of the American Academy of Child and Adolescent Psychiatry, 38,* 32s–54s.

Voress, J. K., & Maddox, T. (2013). *Developmental assessment of young children* (2nd ed.). Austin, TX: PRO-ED.

Wang, K., Zhang, H., Ma, D., Bucan, M., Glessner, J. T., Abrahams, B. S., . . . Hakonarson, H. (2009). Common genetic variants on 5p14.1 associate with autism spectrum disorders. *Nature, 459*(7246), 528–533.

Wechsler, D. (2011). *Wechsler Abbreviated Scale of Intelligence–Second Edition.* San Antonio, TX: NCS Pearson.

Wechsler, D. (2012). *Wechsler Preschool and Primary Scale of Intelligence–Fouth Edition.* San Antonio, TX: NCS Pearson.

Wechsler, D. (2014). *Wechsler Intelligence Scale for Children* (5th ed.). San Antonio, TX: Pearson.

Weisz, J. R., Chorpita, B. F., Frye, A., Ng, M. Y., Lau, N., Bearman, S. K., . . . Hoagwood, K. E. (2011). Youth top problems: Using idiographic, consumer-guided assessment to identify treatment needs and to track change during psychotherapy. *Journal of Consulting and Clinical Psychology, 79*(3), 369–380.

Weitlauf, A. S., Gotham, K. O., Vehorn, A. C., & Warren, Z. E. (2014). Brief report: DSM-5 "levels of support": A comment on discrepant conceptualizations of severity in ASD. *Journal of Autism and Developmental Disorders, 44*(2), 471–476.

Wetherby, A. M., Brosnan-Maddox, S., Peace, V., & Newton, L. (2008). Validation of the Infant–Toddler Checklist as a broadband screener for autism spectrum disorders from 9 to 24 months of age. *Autism, 12*(5), 487–511.

Wetherby, A. M., Guthrie, W., Woods, J., Schatschneider, C., Holland, R. D., Morgan, L., & Lord, C. (2014). Parent-implemented social intervention for toddlers with autism: An RCT. *Pediatrics, 134*(6), 1084–1093.

Wing, L., Leekam, S., Libby, S., Gould, J., & Larcombe, M. (2002). Diagnostic Interview for Social and Communication Disorders: Background, inter-rater reliability and clinical use. *Journal of Child Psychology and Psychiatry, 43,* 307–325.

Woolfenden, S., Sarkozy, V., Ridley, G., & Williams, K. (2012). A systematic review of the diagnostic stability of autism spectrum disorder. *Research in Autism Spectrum Disorders, 6*(1), 345–354.

CHAPTER 13

Intellectual Disability

Randy W. Kamphaus and Emily Walden

Intellectual disability (ID) has been recognized by societies since at least the time of the Roman Empire; the Romans were reported to have discarded children with ID, and Spartans treated offspring with ID similarly. The education and care of these children came about in the 1800s as a result of the emergence of definitions of the disability and development of measures to assess intelligence. While intelligence assessment remains a core component of the diagnosis, the assessment of adaptive behavior and other definitional and diagnostic considerations remain in a state of change.

Prevalence of ID

The Centers for Disease Control and Prevention reported that in 2016, 1.14% of U.S. children ages 13–17 years-old had a diagnosed ID, which was not a significant change from the prior 2 years (Zablotsky, Black, & Blumberg, 2017). Prevalence rates show that boys and children ages 8–12 years especially had higher rates, but there were no differences in rates by race or Hispanic ethnicity (Zablotsky et al., 2017). Of the 6.7 million U.S. students ages 3–21 years who qualify for special education under the Individuals with Disabilities Education Act, 6% were served under the eligibility of ID (National Center for Education Statistics, Institute of Education Sciences, & U.S. Department of Education, 2018). In a meta-analysis published during 2010–2015, McKenzie, Milton, Smith, and Oullette-Kuntz (2016) examined prevalence rates of children and adults with ID in 17 studies across the United States, Canada, Australia, India, Taiwan, Norway, and Denmark. Prevalence in children/adolescents ranged from 0.22 to 1.55% (both estimates were recorded in the United States), while prevalence in adults was reported to range from 0.05% (in Australia) to 0.8% (in Canada). ID prevalence rates differ globally by a small margin, which may be dependent on different assessment and sampling methods (McKenzie et al., 2016).

Risk Factors and Causes

Biological and environmental risk factors and causes are associated with the development of ID. The fifth edition of the *Diagnostic and Statistical Manual of Mental Disorders* (DSM-5; American Psychiatric Association, 2013) describes several risk factors at different developmental levels, including prenatal, perinatal, and postnatal events. During the prenatal stage, children are at risk for ID from biological causes due to genetics or chromosome disorders, maladaptive brain development, placental disease of the mother, or a metabolism disorder; exposure to toxins prenatally can also cause ID, including alcohol and drugs (American Psychiatric Association, 2013). In a review of genetic causes of ID, Vissers, Gilissen, and Veltman (2016) discussed how fragile X and Down syndrome are specific genetic disorders that are often risk factors for inherited ID, with Down syndrome in particular accounting for 6–8% of the causes of ID in general; however, even rarer genetic disorders such as Kabuki syndrome and Schinzel–Giedion syndrome also result in ID. Even in individuals with ID who predominately were diagnosed due to a genetic disorder there may be many different root causes, as each genetic disorder is different, along with differing co-occurring symptoms.

Children are also at-risk for ID due to events during labor and birth, including complications during delivery, especially those that result in a traumatic birth and lack of oxygen for the child (American Psychiatric Association, 2013). As reviewed by Modabbernia, Mollon, Boffeta, and Reichenberg (2016), neonatal hypoxia is especially detrimental to oxygen levels at birth, which can result in brain damage and ID. Families may have no genetic risk factors for the development of ID, but traumatic birth can put children at risk, though neither will absolutely result in the development of ID, as this is dependent upon multiple factors.

Environmental causes after birth can further put children at risk for ID. These can include exposure to toxins or infectious diseases, seizures, experiencing head injuries that result in traumatic brain injury, and severe social isolation (American Psychiatric Association, 2013). Severe neglect in early childhood can also result in poor cognitive development by adolescence (Hanson et al., 2013). Therefore, children who experience early environmental trauma may be especially at risk for development of ID, though impacts can differ depending on other risk factors and developmental timing. It may be helpful for practitioners to be aware of the causes of a particular child's ID if relevant for providing individualized services to that child, depending on that child's needs.

Comorbidity

The comorbidity of ID and other disorders is important to consider for assessment of children. ID can potentially influence or be influenced by other disorders; symptoms of each disorder may co-occur.

Prevalence of comorbid disorders with ID is necessary to understand given that comorbidity with other disorders is high in this population. To better understand the prevalence of comorbid ID and other disorders, Platt, Keyes, McLaughlin, and Kaufman (2018) conducted a study with 6,000 adolescents ages 13–18 years in a nonclinical sample that was representative of the U.S. population and found a 3.2% prevalence of ID within this sample. Of adolescents who could be diagnosed with ID, 65.1% had symptoms suggestive of a comorbid mental illness. When controlling for socioeconomic-related factors that were more often associated with ID, including low income, low parent education, and fewer biological caregivers, ID was comorbid with only bipolar disorder, specific phobia, and agoraphobia. They also examined severity of symptoms, comparing adolescents with and without ID, and found that students with ID had significantly more severe symptoms across many disorders, from anxiety disorders to attention-deficit/hyperactivity disorder (ADHD), from bipolar disorder to different phobias, as well as substance disorders. Adolescents with ID especially had significantly more severe symptoms of generalized anxiety disorder, oppositional defiant disorder, and drug abuse compared to adolescents without ID with any of these disorders. This study highlights not only the prevalence of ID with comorbid disorders but the importance of family context and symptom differences when considering assessment and recommendations.

The following explores specific disorders that often are comorbid with ID. Autism spectrum disorder (ASD) is especially salient because of comorbidity rates of ID and ASD among 8-year-old children in the most recent findings to date by the Centers for Disease Control and Prevention (Zablotsky et al., 2017). Prevalence of ASD varied across study sites from 13.1 to 29.3 for every 1,000 children, and of the children who had ASD, 31% had an IQ score of 70 or lower, indicating possible ID, and one-fourth of children with ASD had IQ scores between 71 and 85 that were marginal for ID diagnosis (Zablotsky et al., 2017). In a sample of over 2,000 children with ASD, over 18% also had ID (Levy et al., 2010; Tonnsen et al., 2016), further indicating the need to consider evaluation for ID when assessing for ASD. Differentiating between ID and ASD when diagnosing or working with individuals can be challenging given some overlapping symptoms (Tonnsen et al., 2016), so a practitioner needs to be aware of both sets of symptoms to provide an accurate diagnosis, recognize when comorbidity exists, and provide the best recommendations for the individual child's treatment plan.

ADHD is another disorder that often is comorbid with ID (Neece, Baker, Blacher, & Crnic, 2011), with 3.5% of children and adolescents with ID also having ADHD, similar to the 3.9% of children and adolescents without ADHD (Platt et al., 2018). In a study by Ahuja, Martin, Langley, and Thapar (2013), children with ADHD and children with ADHD and mild ID were compared on several factors related to ADHD or ID. This study found that children with ADHD and ID had significantly lower intelligence test scores than children with only ID. Children with comorbid ADHD and ID also were more likely to experience symptoms related to oppositional defiant disorder and conduct disorder compared to children with only ID. The researchers also examined ADHD symptoms within both groups, noting that both groups had similar numbers and types of ADHD symptoms. Neece and colleagues (2011) also found that young children ages 5–8 years assessed annually often received a diagnosis of ADHD earlier if they had a diagnosis of ID than did children who did not have ID, which means that ADHD symptoms developed or were noted sooner in children with ID. However, Neece and colleagues determined that symptoms of ADHD were similar for children with and without ID across the 3-year study, though children with ID were three more times likely to also receive an ADHD diagnosis than typically developing children. For children with comorbid ID and other disorders, more intensive treatment may be needed, considering that children with ID are more likely to have ADHD than typically developing children, and considering the earlier development of ADHD.

Internalizing disorders, such as anxiety and depression, also may be comorbid with ID. Rodas, Chavira, and Baker (2017) found that across mother and father reports of internalizing behaviors of their children ages 4–8 years with ID, 10% had a high degree of internalizing symptoms and 5% had a clinically significant rating of symptoms. In the Platt and colleagues (2018) study of children with ID, 13.2% had a major depressive episode or dysthymia and 6.0% had generalized anxiety disorder, compared to 12.7 and 3.2% of children without ID, respectively. High rates of anxiety were also found in children with ID. In a systematic review of the literature, Reardon, Gray, and Melvin (2015) found that anxiety disorders were prevalent in 3–22% of children with ID, but they caution practitioners that measures of internalizing symptoms validated for children with ID are limited. Yet being aware of the impact of internalizing behaviors on children with ID during assessment may help to inform recommendations and diagnostic decisions, so practitioners are urged to consider these disorder types when assessing children with ID and when providing recommendations for treatment.

Contextual Considerations

Several contextual considerations exist regarding assessment of children with ID in determining comorbid disorders. While rates of comorbidity are high for children with ID, especially for anxiety, ADHD, ASD, and other disorders, recognizing how the environment informs these comorbidities is critical. The environment may exacerbate or mask symptoms, so being aware of how the environment shapes behavior is crucial for providing the best support to students. While many types of settings can contribute to differences in recognizing comorbidities, the following describes a few key factors that practitioners should consider.

Exposure to traumatic experience is an important consideration when assessing for ID, in considering comorbidity relative to other trauma-related disorders, and in better recognizing whether behaviors are characteristic of ID or related to trauma. McDonnell and colleagues (2019) found that children who had either ASD, ID, or both ASD and ID were much more likely to have experienced maltreatment compared to children who had neither disorder. In a review, Byrne (2018) determined that children with ID are at an increased risk especially for sexual abuse, and across studies, risk factors tended to include difficulty with adaptive skills related to daily living, female gender, and lack of education regarding prevention of sexual abuse. When assessing for comorbidity, clinicians should consider any traumatic experiences and be aware of how symptoms may be recognized within an individual with ID and/or how the symptoms related to ID may interact with behaviors related to trauma. Practitioners can utilize trauma screening tools, such as the Trauma Symptom Checklist for Children (Briere, 1996), the UCLA Posttraumatic Stress Disorder Reaction Index (Steinberg, Brymer, Decker, & Pynoos, 2004), or the Social Behavior Inventory (Gully, 2003) to better understand the extent of traumatic experiences in children with ID.

Comorbidity may be present but undiagnosed. In a study of adults with ID, Peña-Salazar and colleagues (2018) determined that 29.6% of the adults in the study could be diagnosed with a mental illness (which had not previously been documented). This indicates that this population may be at risk for experiencing undiagnosed disorders that may have an impact on appropriate intervention options. While these disorders may have been present in childhood, they may have been missed, thus indicating further need for rigorous assessment in childhood so as to best support children who are experiencing comorbid disorders.

Assessment, Diagnosis, and Classification

Most modern diagnostic systems are based on criteria set by the American Association on Intellectual and Developmental Disabilities (AAIDD). According to the AAIDD, intellectual disability is characterized by significant limitations in both *intellectual functioning* and *adaptive behavior*, which covers many everyday social and practical skills. This disability originates *before the age of 18* (Schalock et al., 2010).

All of the major diagnostic systems have adopted the view that an intelligence deficit is, at best, only one of the core deficits of ID. Most diagnostic systems also mimic DSM-5 (American Psychiatric Association, 2013) by defining significantly below-average intelligence as a standard score (M = 100,

SD = 15 or 16) of about 70 or below. Often individual state departments of education also stipulate, in their Individuals with Disabilities Education Improvement Act (IDEIA) implementation regulations, that the standard error of measurement may be taken into account. Specifically, scores of about 67–73 may be considered as either qualifying or disqualifying a child for the diagnosis of ID when other variables, such as adaptive behavior and age of onset, are taken into account.

The core logic of the criteria for the diagnosis of ID can be simplistically applied to the examples shown in Table 13.1.

These sample cases, while oversimplifications of the diagnostic principles involved in ID diagnosis, do give some indication of the general parameters that are considered in making the diagnosis. Case 1 is probably the trickiest because the sole reason that the diagnosis cannot be made is because the age of onset is outside that which is typically considered to be the developmental period.

With regard to intellectual assessment, the AAIDD (Schalock et al., 2010, p. 1) provides the following guidelines:

- Determination of subaverage intellectual functioning requires the use of global measures that include different types of items and different factors of intelligence. The instruments more commonly used include the Wechsler Intelligence Scale for Children—Fifth Edition (WISC-V), the Woodcock–Johnson Tests of Cognitive Ability—Fourth Edition, or the newer Reynolds Intellectual Assessment Scales—Second Edition (RIAS-2).
- If a valid IQ is not possible, significantly subaverage intellectual capabilities means a level of performance that is less than that observed in the vast majority (approximately 97%) of persons of comparable background.
- In order to be valid, the assessment of cognitive performance must be free from errors caused by motor, sensory, emotional, or cultural factors.

TABLE 13.1. Examples of ID Diagnoses

Case no.	Intelligence test composite score	Adaptive behavior composite score	Age (in years) of onset	ID diagnosis (yes or no)
1	55	62	27	No
2	60	81	2	No
3	84	63	7	No
4	58	59	2	Yes

These guidelines have several sensible implications for assessment practice. First, screening measures are discouraged. Second, it is recognized that a standardized assessment of IQ is not always possible. Later, we suggest that an adaptive measure be used for the intelligence tests in these extreme cases. Third, psychologists must use good common sense and rule out nonintellective causes for low intelligence test scores.

Elements of a Comprehensive Assessment of Intelligence

History Taking

Although often not emphasized, qualitative assessment of the onset of ID is crucial for making the diagnosis. Intelligence tests, adaptive behavior scales, and other formal "tests" are of no value for documenting the presence of disability prior to age 18. As such, a thorough assessment of history via parent or other caretaker interviews is required, as is careful collection of quantitative assessment results prior to age 18. This information is all the more important when the diagnosis of ID is made in adulthood—after age 18—for the first time. With a thorough history in place, intellectual and adaptive behavior assessment is necessary to document the two core deficits associated with the ID diagnosis. An overview of some of the more widely used measures follows.

Individually Administered Assessment of Intelligence

Although intelligence tests and intelligence testing has been criticized on many fronts for many decades, for many reasons, the practice of assessing intelligence, intellectual development, or developed cognitive abilities remains central to the diagnosis of ID. In fact, it is helpful to remind ourselves that intelligence tests were developed for just this purpose—to differentiate ID disability from psychiatric disorders such as schizophrenia (Kamphaus, 2001). Furthermore, the construct of general intelligence has stood the test of time. Reviewers of almost two centuries of research have concluded that the concept of general intelligence is one of the most robust findings in all of psychology and the social sciences (Lubinski, 2004). For these reasons, modern diagnostic systems and standards continue to depend on the use of an intellectual assessment to document the presence of an ID. Despite recognition of imperfections and

a history of misuse, an individually administered assessment, with a modern and well-researched test of general intelligence by an individual with proper training in standardized test administration procedures provides valuable information for ruling in, or ruling out, the presence of ID. In the section that follows we provide some exemplars of such tests. The universe of possible measures is quite large and beyond the scope of this chapter. Thus, the reader is advised to read comprehensive compendia of intelligence measures. The measures included herein, however, are relatively modern, researched, and widely used internationally.

Wechsler Intelligence Scale for Children—Fifth Edition

The Wechsler Intelligence Scale for Children—Fifth Edition (WISC-V; Wechsler, 2014) is an individually administered test of intelligence for individuals ages 6–16 years; examiners assess individuals through 21 subtests, with 10 primary subtests, that fall within five domains: Fluid Reasoning, Verbal Comprehension, Processing Speed, Visual Spatial, and Working Memory. For example, examinees are asked to repeat sequences of numbers, copy block patterns, and explain vocabulary words, among other tasks. Administration takes approximately 60–90 minutes, completed by an assessor who is competent and qualified to give the test. In addition to the paper-based test, there is an iPad version using linked examiner–examinee iPads. Test materials are provided by Pearson.

Wechsler Abbreviated Scale of Intelligence— Second Edition

The Wechsler Abbreviated Scale of Intelligence—Second Edition (WASI-II; Wechsler, 2011) is an individually administered screening test of intelligence for individuals ages 6–90 years; examiners assess individuals by selecting the four- or two-subtest form, allowing for flexibility in time and comprehensiveness. The four-subtest form provides three scores: Overall Cognitive Ability, Crystallized Abilities, and Nonverbal Fluid Abilities and Visual–Motor/Coordination Skills; the two-subtest form provides only the Overall Cognitive Ability score. This assessment offers clinicians a method of assessing cognitive abilities in a briefer time frame, typically 15–30 minutes, depending on whether the two- or four-subtest form is used. An individual must be qualified to administer the WASI-II. The WASI-II provides a method of screening for clinicians to understand, through a shorter measure, whether an individual is experiencing any cognitive issues, for which longer intellectual assessments may be useful to provide a deeper understanding of the individual's cognitive abilities. In effect, the WASI-II may serve as a "rule out" for ID if it provides scores in the average range or above. In addition, this measure may be used for periodic reassessment of intellectual status. For example, an individual recovering from head injury could be reassessed more practically and frequently with a screening form such as the WASI-II in order to track cognitive recovery.

Woodcock–Johnson Tests of Cognitive Abilities—Fourth Edition

The Woodcock–Johnson Tests of Cognitive Abilities—Fourth Edition (WJ-IV-COG; Schrank, McGrew, & Mather, 2014) is an individually administered test of intelligence for individuals ages 2–over 90 years. A qualified clinician administers 10 primary subtests, with an option for eight extended battery tests; subtests measure specific aspects of intelligence, such as fluid reasoning or working memory. For example, individuals must think through visual patterns, solve problems, and remember and repeat auditory information, among other tasks. The WJ-IV-COG takes approximately 60–90 minutes to complete and is part of a battery of tests, which also includes the WJ-IV Tests of Achievement and the WJ-IV Tests of Oral Language. For a full review of the WJ-IV-COG, see the review by Canivez (2017). Test materials are provided by Houghton Mifflin Harcourt.

Reynolds Intellectual Assessment Scales—Second Edition and Reynolds Intellectual Screening Test—Second Edition

The Reynolds Intellectual Assessment Scales—Second Edition (RIAS-2; Reynolds & Kamphaus, 2015b) is an individually administered test of intelligence for individuals ages 3–94 years. Test administration takes approximately 45 minutes and covers four primary tests that measure Verbal Intelligence (both crystallized and reasoning) and Nonverbal Intelligence (both fluid and overall nonverbal). Additional subtests may be completed to understand more about an individual's processing speed and memory. The primary purpose of the RIAS-2 is to provide information on an individual's intellectual functioning to determine whether that individual is at risk for ID; in addition, this assessment was especially developed for individuals with mental illness to better understand their intellectual functioning. For additional information, see a review by Ward (in press). Test materials are available through Psychological Assessment Resources, Inc.

Universal Nonverbal Intelligence Test—Second Edition

The Universal Nonverbal Intelligence Test—Second Edition (UNIT2; Bracken & McCallum, 2016) continues to improve on the foundation of the first edition. The UNIT2 has distinguished itself as a nonverbal measure that better approximates a comprehensive measure of general intelligence using an entirely nonverbal format for examinees. Evidence that it provides a more comprehensive assessment of intelligence is provided by the composite scores available, including Memory, Reasoning, Quantitative, Abbreviated Battery, Standard Battery with Memory, Standard Battery without Memory, and Full-Scale Battery. The UNIT2 may be used in specialized circumstances to estimate general intelligence in cases of verbal impairment due to brain injury, disorders such as cerebral palsy, or higher-frequency disorders of verbal fluency, such as some cases of autism. It may also be valuable for estimating intelligence in cases of limited English speakers.

Adaptive Behavior Assessment

Adaptive behavior scales assess the degree to which an individual meets the standards of personal independence and social responsibility expected for a child's age or cultural group (Grossman, 1983). This construct is more variable than intelligence, since the standards of behavior and achievement are determined by an individual's society. For example, adult expectations to vote may be relevant in some societies and not others. Cooking skills may be deemed necessary for some cultural groups and not for others. As it turns out, however, some standards of adaptive behavior are relatively universal, such as toilet training, control of aggression, and respect for authority figures. These skills are the ones typically assessed by adaptive behavior scales.

Vineland–3

One of the oldest and premier measures of adaptive behavior is the Vineland Adaptive Behavior Scales, Third Edition (Vineland–3; Sparrow, Cicchetti, & Saulnier, 2016). The latest Vineland is a revision of the Vineland Social Maturity Scale, developed by Edgar Doll in the 1930s. Doll essentially founded the field of adaptive behavior assessment by noting that although all of his patients at the Vineland (New Jersey) State Training School suffered from intellectual problems, there were vast differences in their day-to-day lives and coping skills. If, for example, two children have intelligence test composite scores of 60, and one is toilet trained and the other is frequently incontinent, these children would place considerably different demands on an adult's time. The toilet-trained child is more mobile and can be involved in many more activities than the incontinent child, who requires considerably more attention and care.

Clinicians may use the Vineland–3 to assess adaptive behavior, as reported by parents/caregivers through a structured interview and/or rating scale and teachers (if applicable) through a rating scale; online formats also exist for both the structured interview and rating forms. The purpose of this measure is to understand adaptive behavior in individuals from birth through age 90 years, specific to each of five domains, including Daily Living Skills, Socialization, and Communication, as well as Optional Motor Skills and Maladaptive Behavior. In each measure, behaviors are rated on a Likert scale for the individual's independence level (i.e., *never, sometimes, usually/often*) in performing an action (e.g., bathing, writing, or spending time with peers). Administration takes approximately 40 minutes for the structured interview, while rating forms take about 10 minutes to complete. Examiners should possess a master's degree or higher in a field relevant to work with those with ID. For further information, see Pepperdine and McCrimmon's (2018) test review. Test materials are provided by Pearson.

Adaptive Behavior Assessment System—Third Edition

The Adaptive Behavior Assessment System—Third Edition (ABAS-3; Harrison & Oakland, 2015) measures adaptive behavior in individuals from birth through age 89 years across three domains (i.e., Social, Practical, Conceptual). Parents/caregivers complete separate forms for individuals from birth to age 5 years and from ages 5 to 21 years; teachers (or day care providers for young children) complete separate forms for individuals ages 2–5 years and 5–21 years; individuals ages 16–89 years may complete a self-assessment. Rating forms take approximately 15–20 minutes to complete, with raters choosing on a Likert scale how often the individual does a specific action,

such as saying a known person's name or using gestures to convey ideas. In addition, planning tools with progress monitoring for interventions are also included in the test kit. An online format for completing rating forms also exists. Test materials may be found through Western Psychological Services.

Anecdotally, I (Randy W. Kamphaus) learned to appreciate the difference between intelligence and adaptive behavior early in my career. My third job after completing college (yes, I had trouble finding a job I liked with a bachelor's degree in psychology) was a temporary position as Rehabilitation Workshop Supervisor in a modern version of a state mental hospital. I helped patients build birdhouses and stools, and I served as the favorite target for adolescents who felt the need to throw paint at someone—but that is another story. I vividly recall an experience with a young man, about age 30, who was in the hospital for alcoholism treatment. I remember this man so well because he was well groomed, mannered, and pleasant. We had many enjoyable conversations about his family and his work, and I looked forward to his visits to the workshop. I also remember being stunned when one of the staff members from the alcoholism treatment unit told me that the young man was diagnosed with mild ID. I remember feeling a sense of empathy and also wishing that all of the clients who did not have cognitive deficits would be as polite and enjoyable to work with as this man.

Levels of ID

A standard score of less than 70 has long been accepted as a criterion of ID (Flynn, 1985). To date, very few have questioned the ability of the Wechsler Scales or other major intelligence tests to provide a meaningful criterion of ID. This acceptance exists, although Flynn (1985), in an interesting investigation, showed how sampling problems and changes in norms over time have served to effectively change the numbers of individuals (the percentage of the population) who are identified by the standard score = 70 criterion. He found the criterion of ID (standard score = 70) to vary as much as a full standard deviation on the particular Wechsler scale selected. Among other results, Flynn concluded that in order to have a coherent and consistent cutoff score for ID, the Psychological Corporation would have to re-norm the Wechsler Scales every 7 years. Despite such contrary findings, an intelligence test overall composite standard score of about 70 or lower will likely be used as a cutoff for some time.

It is in the differentiation of levels of ID that psychologists have come face-to-face with the limitations of intelligence tests. The scholastic nature of many of the items does not provide easy enough items for children with severe impairments. Infant and some preschool tests do have enough easy items because intelligence is defined differently, more globally, for these ages. Motor scales, for example, are common and contribute to developmental indices. Some individuals have advised using infant scales such as the Bayley Scales with children who are beyond the test's age range, yet have mental ages that are within the age range (Sullivan & Burley, 1990). Differentiating between severe and profound levels of disability remains a murky area in which the intelligence testing technology usually fails. In fact, the AAIDD approach, which places less emphasis on the differentiation of levels, may be of greater value for clinical assessment purposes with severely disabled populations.

Different levels of ID used to be recognized by most diagnostic systems. The newest version of the AAIDD diagnostic manual has eschewed this practice by emphasizing the assessment of patient needs in a variety of domains. DSM-5, however, has retained the practice by defining three levels of disability—mild, moderate, severe and profound. DSM-5 has recognized that adaptive behavior test results are best suited for determining these levels than intelligence tests.

Selecting a Score for ID Diagnosis

An important issue regarding the use of intelligence tests for the purposes of ID diagnosis is the decision about which composite score to use in making a diagnosis when there is a composite score (e.g., Verbal Comprehension [VC] vs. Visual/ Spatial [V/P]) difference and one of these scores is outside that which is typically considered to be the ID range. A child, for example, could obtain a Wechsler Verbal Comprehension score of 78 and a Visual Spatial score of 65. In this scenario, the Full Scale score of 70 is not too problematic. If the child's Adaptive Behavior Composite score is also about 70 or less, the diagnosis of ID becomes more likely as dual deficits in intelligence and adaptive behavior are clearly documented.

There are, however, more difficult cases where a large V/P discrepancy is evident. A good example of this latter situation would be a child who obtains a Visual Spatial score of 88, Verbal Comprehension score of 60, Full Scale score of 72, and Adaptive Behavior Composite score of 71. This case

is more difficult to decide based on scores alone, forcing logic and prior research to come into play. This case is also a good example of why rigid cutoff scores should not be used when making diagnoses based on intelligence test results (Kaufman, 1990). One may make quite different diagnostic decisions with this same set of scores, depending on other information about the child. This child may be diagnosed with ID given information that he or she

- Is 9 years old and has failed most academic subjects every school year despite the fact that his or her parents have hired tutors and he or she seems to be putting forth great effort in school;
- Was born in the United States and speaks English as his or her native language; and
- Has a developmental history indicating that he or she achieved major language and motor milestones considerably later than normal.

A child with these scores may just as well not be diagnosed with ID if he or she

- Is 7 years old, has lived in the United States for only 1 year, and Spanish was his or her first language acquired;
- Has failed only language arts subjects; and
- Was reared in a high-socioeconomic-status (SES) family environment in which his or her needs were met by others, and the acquisition of adaptive life skills was not emphasized or deemed necessary (e.g., the household employed both a maid and a cook). This privileged environment resulted in a very low score on the Daily Living Skills domain of the Vineland, with other domain scores being considerably higher.

Since background information, other test scores, developmental history, and other factors are so important in making diagnostic decisions with intelligence tests, perhaps the most reasonable approach is to consider developmental history, other test scores, and related information as central to the ID diagnostic process. In cases where there are composite score differences, with some scores within the ID range and others outside this range, the examiner should explain why the diagnostic decision was made, whatever that decision may be. This practice at least allows for peer review and collaboration. If the reason is defensible to other professionals who know the child's circumstances, then the clinician can feel more comfortable with the decision made. Writing the rationale for the diagnosis has an additional benefit in that it may also help the clinician clarify his or her thought processes regarding the diagnostic decision.

Unfortunately, the use of intelligence tests in isolation has been reinforced by statutory guidelines, such as those offered by some state departments of education and U.S. federal agencies (e.g., the Social Security Administration). A cutoff score of 70 has been identified by various agencies to decide everything from special education class placement to eligibility for monetary benefits. One can imagine the ire of physicians if the use of medical diagnostic tests was similarly regulated. What if, for example, some governmental body decided that a person had to have a cholesterol level of 200 (low-density lipoproteins [LDL]) to be eligible to receive medicine to reduce serum cholesterol (a practice that is now more likely due to the ubiquitous nature of managed care)? Patients with levels of 195 would likely be very angry at being denied treatment, and those patients with levels of 205 who wanted to treat themselves with diet modifications would be similarly angry. This situation is not far removed from current ID diagnostic practice that occurs with school-age children under the aegis of various governmental regulatory bodies. If intelligence tests are going to be used in a larger context for decision making, then clinicians have to use discretion as opposed to rigid cutoff scores or diagnostic formulas. To do otherwise is to promote the simplistic and inappropriate use of intelligence tests, which serves no one.

Intelligence and Adaptive Behavior Revisited

The relationship between adaptive behavior scales and intelligence scales should also be kept in mind for appropriate use of intelligence tests in diagnosing ID (Kamphaus, 1987). I (Randy W. Kamphaus) found that the correlation between the WISC-R and the Kaufman Assessment Battery for Children (KABC) and adaptive behavior scales such as the Vineland–3, where parents serve as the informant, is moderate to low in most studies (i.e., correlations in the .20 to .60 range). This finding has several practical implications for the use of an intelligence test along with an adaptive behavior scale in the diagnosis of ID. These implications include:

- Psychologists should not expect intelligence and parent-reported adaptive behavior scores to show a great deal of agreement, especially when the child is outside the ID range.
- The limited correlation of these measures with intelligence tests suggests that adaptive behav-

ior scales are adding information to the diagnostic process that is different from that of intelligence tests (Kamphaus, 1987).
- The correlation between intelligence tests and adaptive behavior scores as rated by teachers may be somewhat higher (Kamphaus, 1987). Teacher-rated adaptive behavior, therefore, may not be considered as a substitute for parent-reported adaptive behavior, and vice versa.

All of these findings also support the notion that adaptive behavior is likely to become more central to the diagnosis of ID and to treatment plan design (DeStefano & Thompson, 1990). In fact, the latest AAIDD (Schalock et al., 2010) criteria emphasize the assessment of adaptive behavior in three domains in order to establish need for services—Conceptual, Social, and Practical Skills. These same AAIDD criteria have expanded the advised diagnostic procedures to include two new assessment domains.

First, clinicians are admonished to systematically assess the "individual's health and physical well-being." Second, the "elements of an individual's current environment" are to be assessed to determine any factors that restrict or assist an individual's current level of daily functioning. Consideration of these new domains should aid further in the rehabilitation process.

Regression Effects

Yet another issue to consider in the diagnosis of ID is the likelihood of regression effects. Since intelligence tests are not perfectly reliable, one can expect the composite score means for samples of children with ID to move toward the normative mean. A good example of this is a study by Spitz (1983) in which the original mean for the ID group was 55 (54.96) at age 13 and 58 (58.33) at age 15. This fact can make diagnosis very difficult, especially if a child moves from a score of 68 to 74. Is this child still appropriately diagnosed as ID? At least a few of the possibilities to consider include the following:

- The child's first evaluation was conducted under less than ideal circumstances, and the first test results were inordinately low.
- The second score is higher primarily due to regression effects. This hypothesis is especially plausible when the difference between the first and second scores is rather small (e.g., less than 10 points or so).

- Practice effects could play a role in the second score being higher. This result could also be obtained when the difference between tests is very small—about 6 points or less—and there is greater gain on nonverbal–spatial–simultaneous tests that are more prone to practice effects.
- The second score could reflect gains in cognitive development. This explanation is more likely when the first evaluation was conducted when the child was very young—in the preschool years. The child's intellectual skills could have simply unfolded during the early school years, when cognitive development is fairly rapid. Another possibility is that the child has been the beneficiary of an effective intervention program.

These possibilities and others should be considered when evaluating a child's gain on retest. However, equally important are the child's scores on measures of other traits. If a child's overall composite is 74 on retest and his or her achievement and adaptive behavior test scores are both 69 and below, then it is more difficult to argue that there has been a substantial and important cognitive change for the better that is not due to regression and practice effects. On the other hand, if a child with this same composite on retest has achievement test and adaptive behavior scores that have also moved above 70, then retaining the diagnosis of ID becomes questionable.

Another finding that could mitigate against regression effects is the "cumulative deficit phenomenon." If a child scores lower on retesting and is the product of an impoverished environment, then the effects of the impoverishment may accumulate over ontogeny (Haywood [1987] refers to this as the "mental age [MA] deficit"), resulting in a child achieving increasingly lower standard scores with increasing age in comparison to chronological age peers. The child's raw scores may be increasing over the course of development, but a relatively flat developmental trajectory makes the child look like he or she is losing ground when standard scores are computed. It may be that children without early cognitive delay are developing at a faster rate, which serves to make the norm-referenced standard scores look like no growth or reversal of cognitive growth is occurring for the child who experiences developmental delay.

The Range of Scores Issue

A common complaint about intelligence tests is their inability to differentiate between the various levels of ID. Few intelligence tests offer standard scores that go so low as to be able to differentiate among moderate, severe, and profound levels of disability. Many popular scales only produce standard scores as low as 45 or 50. The DAS (Differential Ability Scales) is a notable exception in this regard.

It is first important to consider the psychometric limitations inherent in this situation. One limitation is the availability of data for calculating norms for these groups. If, for example, a test has collected only 200 cases at age 7 for norming purposes, then there are only going to be about four cases, or data points, below a standard score of 70 (the second percentile). Consequently, the calculation of norms below the second percentile may be based more on the computer algorithms used for calculating the norms than actual data for children with disabilities.

Even if this psychometric limitation is conquered with statistical or sampling procedures, the practice may still be questionable. At the very low levels of functioning, the type of scholastic intelligence assessed by most intelligence tests is less relevant. Adaptive behavior issues such as ambulation, speech, toileting, and eating skills are more important at these low levels of functioning. Reschly (1980) recognized this difference between mild and other levels of ID by pointing out that mild ID is not characterized by physical abnormalities, it is usually only apparent in school settings, and it may not be permanent. It may well be that not only does the nature of ID differ across levels but also the relative importance of adaptive behavior and intelligence tests changes across the levels of ID. Intelligence tests may be important for differentiating between mild and moderate levels of ID. Adaptive behavior scales, however, such as the Vineland do produce standard scores as low as 20.

Adaptive behavior scales are also more likely to produce much more important information for intervention design than intelligence scales. It is also theoretically defensible to use adaptive behavior scales as measures of intelligence with those who have severe disabilities because the content domain at low levels of adaptive behavior scales is strikingly similar to that of infant intelligence tests, such as the Bayley scales. Motor skills are part of intelligence scales for preschoolers; why can't they be part of a developmental assessment for the older child or adolescent who has a significant cognitive impairment? Our opinion is that adaptive behavior scales are the tests of choice for differentiating among moderate, severe, and profound levels of ID or developmental disability.

Unfortunately, some regulatory agencies still insist that every child diagnosed with ID have a recent intelligence test score on record. This requirement results in psychologists engaging in questionable practices, such as using preschool tests to obtain a mental age for adolescents with ID, and using the old ratio IQ formula (MA/CA × 100 = IQ) to produce an IQ score. An intelligence test should never be used outside its age range to produce a norm-referenced score to be used in making diagnostic decisions. If an intelligence test is used in this manner, it is likely no better, and it may be worse, than an educated guess by a skilled professional. The sample case for Kent (in this chapter) shows how a credible evaluation of a child with a severe disability may be completed without using an intelligence test.

Other Diagnostic Issues

With problems and limitations duly recognized (Spitz, 1983, 1986, 1988), intelligence tests will likely continue to play an important role in the diagnosis of ID. The potential for misuse of intelligence tests in making the ID diagnosis, however, looms large, especially when intelligence test scores are interpreted in isolation, without giving due consideration to adaptive behavior evaluations and background information. A good example is the case of Daniel Hoffman, who was diagnosed by a school board psychologist as having an ID (Payne & Patton, 1981). He spent 12 years in a class for students with ID before it was discovered that the initial diagnosis was incorrect. He, in fact, was above average intellectually, but he had a severe speech defect. Remarkably, he had even accepted the fact that he was intellectually disabled.

The reasons for making the diagnosis of ID, since it does depend so heavily on the use of intelligence test results, should be explained in writing. Simply reporting scores that are 70 or below and concluding that a child has ID is not adequate for modern assessment practice. Above all, intelligence test results should not be used rigidly in making ID diagnoses. The use of strict cutoff scores serves to place too much emphasis on those very scores and causes evaluators to lose sight of the child's full spectrum of strengths and weaknesses. Gone are the days when the diagnosis of ID is based solely on one-measure intelligence tests. The practice of using intelligence tests in

isolation is analogous to using only the LDL serum cholesterol level to diagnose risk for heart disease. It is now clear that other factors (e.g., high-density lipoproteins [HDL]) must be considered. The AAIDD (Schalock et al., 2010) diagnostic manual has provided compelling empirical evidence and logical arguments to support the identification of adaptive behavior, emotional functioning, health, and intellectual abilities as part of ID diagnosis and treatment planning.

Assessment during Treatment

As prevalence data show, comorbid psychological disorders can exist in children with ID, making it critical that practitioners assess for symptoms and disorders, so that children may best be supported. Reliable and valid assessment of comorbidities is then needed, which incorporates recognizing symptoms early through screening, tracking symptoms across time through progress monitoring, and being aware of how to effectively use functional behavioral assessment (FBA) when focusing on specific behavioral problems. In any individual case, practitioners should be aware of individual differences that also can inform their screening and progress monitoring practices, especially given contextual considerations for comorbid symptoms and which measures would best be suited for the given situation.

Screening

Screening for comorbidity is essential for supporting students with ID. The screening process allows for examination of comorbid psychological disorders in children who have ID, often through rating scales, interviews, or observations. For example, the Behavior Assessment System for Children, Third Edition (BASC-3) is a rating form used by teachers, caregivers, and children to rate a child's behavior across several domains, including internalizing, externalizing, anxiety, attention, depression, daily living skills, communication, among others (Reynolds & Kamphaus, 2015a). The rating scale takes approximately 10–30 minutes to complete and provides essential information that can inform intervention, such as supplying teachers and caregivers with severity ratings of behaviors by behavior type. The Child Behavior Checklist (CBCL; Achenbach, 2009) is another rating scale that provides crucial information on potential psychological symptoms of a child, including internalizing and externalizing characteristics, aggression, withdrawal, and others. While the BASC-3 and CBCL both provide information important for screening, neither rating scale alone can be used for diagnosis. However, these rating scales can be used to assess symptoms that may provide information on problem behaviors that can inform practitioners of relevant interventions, and these rating scales and others can be used to inform potential diagnoses of comorbid disorders.

Rating scales provide efficient and reliable methods of tracking comorbid symptoms of psychological disorders in children with ID; however, it is necessary to consider whether rating scales have included children in special education in the norming sample when using the scale. While the BASC-3 did include children with special education diagnoses in the norming sample, this may not always be true of other rating scales. Therefore, practitioners are cautioned to consider the validity and reliability of assessing children with ID before using a rating scale or other form of measurement of psychological disorder symptoms. Other disorders in children with ID, such as those related to attachment, can be screened using parent interviews and questionnaires (Giltaij, Sterkenburg, & Schuengel, 2015). Practitioners can utilize multiple methods to inform symptoms, as some symptoms may be captured in home versus school environments or other settings, so it is important to use a multimethod approach.

Type of method used is important to consider, as measures may differ even when they are attempting to measure similar constructs, as is the case with measurement of anxiety in children with ID. Reardon and colleagues (2015) conducted a systematic review of anxiety screening measures for children and adolescents with ID, identifying 13 measures in the literature. Some measures were broad in assessing many different areas in addition to anxiety, such as the CBCL; others involved self-report, with some including accommodations or modifications for students with ID, yet studies differed regarding the severity of ID reported, so not all samples were necessarily the same. Reardon and colleagues also point out that across the literature, only few studies really specifically examined students with ID in relation to anxiety screening, and further research is needed. Differences also may be found in other comorbid psychological disorder symptoms with ID depending on screening measure. Prevalence across comorbidities can differ in children with ID, especially depending on screening measure, so it is important for practitio-

ners to be aware of the pros and cons of measures they are using with this population and to make sure that these measures are valid. When using screening measures, whether for anxiety or other psychological disorder symptoms, it is important to remember that the type of measure used may or may not be as valid for individuals with ID, so interpreting and reporting results with more caution is needed.

Progress Monitoring

While screening can help capture comorbidity of mental health concerns and behaviors, progress monitoring is critical for tracking these symptoms over time to ensure that intervention is effective and symptoms are decreasing, or whether more intense or alternative interventions are needed. The literature regarding progress monitoring of mental health concerns in the context of ID is sparse, but practitioners can still utilize current literature and best practices generally for progress monitoring of mental health concerns. Any measure chosen for progress monitoring should be sensitive to change and capture the specific behaviors that intervention is targeting. Measures that are too broad or not sensitive to change risk showing a lack of progress, when progress may have been made from intervention.

Rating scales are a method that can be used for progress monitoring. Yet understanding the validity of rating scales in close time succession should be noted. Rating scales may only be valid if administered every 3 or 6 months, or perhaps a longer time frame, depending on the measure. Typically, traditional rating scales are not administered daily or weekly, though these shorter time frames may be best practice for progress monitoring. First, for many measures, this would be too much to expect of a teacher or parent given time constraints, and second, sensitivity to change may be problematic in too short of a time. However, other methods also exist to progress-monitor behaviors related to mental health concerns, such as through shorter, progress monitoring report forms and direct observation. For example, the BASC-3 provides a progress monitoring system called the BASC-3 Flex Monitor, in which teachers and parents can fill out forms that capture behaviors, such as those related to internalizing and externalizing concerns, disruption, hyperactivity, and other social behaviors related to development, all of which can inform current mental health concerns; there is also a self-report form for students, which should be used depending on assessment of the student's individual skills levels, and whether this would be appropriate for a student with ID. This system can be used much more frequently than traditional rating scales, so it allows for easier and more reliable progress monitoring.

Behavioral Observations

Behavioral observations are critical for assessment of disability, as they allow a direct method of assessing for difficulties that may be the result of symptoms of a disability. In addition, behavioral observations offer a more natural account of how a student's disability may be impacting his or her behavior in different settings, so understanding behavior through observation can give a more nuanced guide for recommendations during screening, progress monitoring, and the FBA process.

Comorbidity should also be considered when conducting behavioral observations, as these types of observations can give a better understanding of how individuals may be impacted by co-occurring disorders. Anderson and colleagues (2015) reported that in a study of children and adolescents, similar behavior problems were found between individuals with ID or ASD, and that these behaviors differed significantly from what was reported for students with neither disorder. FBAs were conducted with each of these students. For students with ID or ASD, self-injury, eloping from an area, having aggressive behaviors, inappropriate verbalizations, tantrums, and stereotyped behavior were often reported. However, for students without ID or ASD, behaviors reported to be problematic were different; often behaviors including verbal aggression, defiance, not being on task, talking when not supposed to, or being out of one's seat were reported as problematic.

Therefore, considering these differences in behaviors, it is important to look for behaviors that might be more common for a child with ID, and to be aware of these behaviors; however, as Anderson, Rodriguez, and Campbell (2015) also note, each of the behaviors listed for each group were experienced by the other group as well. While far fewer children with ID were reported to be out of their seats, as exhibiting the problem behavior, there were still some students with ID or autism who were reported to have this issue. Knowing how to talk with teachers or parents when conducting an FBA to fully understand the function of behavior may require being aware of a range of potential behaviors.

Tools for direct observation of mental health concerns exist. The BASC-3 provides a tool for direct observations of a child's behavior by a qualified professional, called the BASC-3 Student Observation System (Reynolds & Kamphaus, 2015a), which can provide crucial information on symptoms of psychological disorders that are present under direct observation. Yet, with any direct observation, it is important to consider how measurement is being used for children with ID to ensure appropriate capture of symptoms, interpret results with caution, and use multiple methods to inform comorbidity.

Functional Behavioral Assessment

An FBA is a type of analysis conducted typically in clinical or school-based settings to determine the function of a challenging behavior experienced by an individual and usually involves gathering data through observations and interviews to define and understand a problem behavior (Anderson et al., 2015). As Anderson and colleagues (2015) reported in a systematic literature review of FBAs, individuals with ID in particular are most likely to be assessed through the FBA process. While screening and progress monitoring can provide information on comorbid psychological symptoms, the FBA process may especially be useful for a single, focused problem. The FBA process is more intensive and longer, often requiring more detailed measures and interviews for teachers and caregivers, and more time and resources from practitioners. Direct observation is also included in the FBA process, in which practitioners record antecedents, behaviors, and consequences of a student's behavior, often in the classroom, to better understand the function of problem behavior and learn what is maintaining that behavior, which then informs intervention targets (Sugai et al., 2000).

Before engaging in the FBA process, it may be useful to also conduct screening of psychological symptoms, which could then inform the FBA process. If psychological symptoms of comorbid disorders exist, then other treatment options may be necessary; if the FBA process is still viewed as the logical next step, though, at least knowledge of comorbid symptoms from the screening process can inform the FBA process and possible interventions.

Researchers have documented success of the FBA process with elementary school children with ID often through single-subject research, as is the case in the Wadsworth, Hansen, and Wills (2015) study documenting how FBAs supported children with ID regarding noncompliance. Other studies have also determined that severe problem behaviors of children with ID, such as harming of self, others, or property, can also be reduced through the use of FBA (Doehring, Reichow, Palka, Phillips, & Hagopian, 2014).

When conducting an FBA with individuals with ID, it is also important to consider the context when determining the function of behavior. Platt and colleagues (2018) found that children with ID are much more likely to be living in lower SES families, have parents with less education, and have fewer biological caregivers living with them. Being aware of this context can be critical when assessing behavior and learning more about whether the behavior is due to ID, the context, or a combination of both. This can help to inform both the function of that problem behavior and possible comorbid psychological disorders. For example, the FBA process may also reveal more details about a child's other psychological symptoms that have not been captured previously, even if screening was performed. Therefore, it is an ongoing cycle of conducting interventions and receiving new information that may prove vital for understanding problem behaviors, especially if a child is experiencing comorbid psychological disorders with ID.

Performance-Based Assessment

Assessing a child's performance of skills can inform not only the severity of ID but also comorbid psychological symptoms. Individuals who experience cognitive disorders often lack daily living skills, such as care of personal hygiene, getting dressed, and eating (Mlinac & Feng, 2016). When assessing children with ID, daily living skills can be observed or reported by caregivers or teachers as part of the assessment process to determine disability, as well as to inform recommendations for intervention. Sparrow and colleagues (2016) developed a tool for measuring adaptive behavior that includes daily living skills, called the Vineland–3. This assessment incorporates detailed interviews of caregivers and teachers and rating forms to get a full understanding of the student in multiple settings to best understand his or her level of daily living skills.

Performance-based assessment can be measured through specific tasks, which can be especially useful in the context of intervention, as this can inform interventionists as to the current skill levels of students in a task as they attempt to increase performance (Shepley, Spriggs, Samudre, & Elliott, 2018). Tasks could include knowing and following the steps for getting a book in the library, making a meal at home, or getting dressed in the morning. When observing how children complete these steps, assessment of this performance can lead to better understanding of specific areas in which the child may struggle and need further instruction. To measure daily living skills in this manner, often observation protocols need to be developed, with specific steps that are expected for a task so as to provide an unbiased account of that student's performance on a task, as has been documented in prior research with children (Shepley et al., 2018; Wynkoop, Robertson, & Schwartz, 2018).

Conclusion

Intellectual disability and its prevalence, comorbidity, and treatment outcomes remain challenging for families, educational institutions, other institutions (e.g., correctional), and society. The need for continuing research, identifying better treatments and prevention methods, and accurate diagnosis is as great today as ever. Many gains have been made. The longevity of some affected individuals and their potential for independent living (e.g., Down syndrome) has improved significantly due to advances in medicine, vocational training, and general acceptability in society and the workplace. Advances in research and practice remain the focus of many of us academics, and we have to remain confident that progress will not only continue but also be accelerated.

For today, however, accurate diagnosis can and should be the focus of our efforts to help individuals with ID live better lives. Failure to detect ID, for example, can deprive individuals of needed services that are known to lead to better life outcomes. And, detecting ID can still be difficult due to the complexities of comorbidity and the unavailability of service providers or systems, particularly in societies with fewer financial resources. Limited service provision is probably the major detriment to early identification of ID and initiation of intervention/treatment. For the time being, increasing access to diagnostic, prevention, and early intervention services should be the focus of our efforts as we wait for the scientific breakthroughs that surely lie ahead.

REFERENCES

Achenbach, T. M. (2009). *The Achenbach System of Empirically Based Assessment (ASEBA): Development, findings, theory, and applications.* Burlington: University of Vermont Research Center for Children, Youth, and Families.

Ahuja, A., Martin, J., Langley, K., & Thapar, A. (2013). Intellectual disability in children with attention deficit hyperactivity disorder. *Journal of Pediatrics, 163*(3), 890–895.

American Psychiatric Association. (2013). *Diagnostic and statistical manual of mental disorders* (5th ed.). Arlington, VA: Author.

Anderson, C. M., Rodriguez, B. J., & Campbell, A. (2015). Functional behavior assessment in schools: Current status and future directions. *Journal of Behavioral Education, 24*(3), 338–371.

Bracken, B. A., & McCallum, R. S. (2016). *Universal Nonverbal Intelligence Test™ 2.* Torrance, CA: Western Psychological Services.

Briere, J. (1996). *Trauma Symptom Checklist for Children (TSCC), professional manual.* Odessa, FL: Psychological Assessment Resources.

Byrne, G. (2018). Prevalence and psychological sequelae of sexual abuse among individuals with an intellectual disability: A review of the recent literature. *Journal of Intellectual Disabilities, 22*(3), 294–310.

Canivez, G. L. (2017). Test review of Woodcock–Johnson IV. In J. F. Carlson, K. F. Geisinger, & J. L. Jonson (Eds.), *The twentieth mental measurements yearbook* (pp. 2–27). Lincoln, NE: Buros Center for Testing.

DeStefano, L., & Thompson, D. S. (1990). Adaptive behavior: The construct and its measurement. In C. R. Reynolds & R. W. Kamphaus (Eds.), *Handbook of psychological and educational assessment of children: Personality, behavior, and context* (pp. 445–469). New York: Guilford Press.

Doehring, P., Reichow, B., Palka, T., Phillips, C., & Hagopian, L. (2014). Behavioral approaches to managing severe problem behaviors in children with autism spectrum disorder and related developmental disorders: A descriptive analysis. *Child and Adolescent Psychiatric Clinics of North America, 23*(1), 25–40.

Doll, E. (1936). *The Vineland Social Maturity Scale: Revised condensed manual of directions.* Vineland, NJ: Training School at Vineland.

Flynn, J. R. (1985). Wechsler intelligence tests: Do we really have a criterion of mental retardation? *American Journal of Mental Deficiency, 90,* 236–244.

Giltaij, H. P., Sterkenburg, P. S., & Schuengel, C. (2015). Psychiatric diagnostic screening of social maladaptive behaviour in children with mild intellectual disability: Differentiating disordered attachment and pervasive developmental disorder behaviour. *Journal of Intellectual Disability Research, 59*(2), 138–149.

Grossman, H. J. (1983). *Classification in mental retardation.* Washington, DC: American Association on Mental Deficiency.

Gully, K. J. (2003). *Social Behavior Inventory: Professional manual.* Salt Lake City, UT: PEAK Ascent.

Hanson, J. L., Adluru, N., Chung, M. K., Alexander, A. L., Davidson, R. J., & Pollak, S. D. (2013). Early neglect is associated with alterations in white matter integrity and cognitive functioning. *Child Development, 84*(5), 1566–1578.

Harrison, P., & Oakland, T. (2015). *Adaptive Behavior Assessment System, Third Edition (ABAS-3).* San Antonio, TX: Pearson Education.

Haywood, H. C. (1987). The mental age deficit: Explanation and treatment. *Uppsala Journal of Medical Science Supplement, 44,* 191–203.

Kamphaus, R. W. (1987). Defining the construct of adaptive behavior by the Vineland Adaptive Behavior Scales. *Journal of School Psychology, 25*(1), 97–100.

Kamphaus, R. W. (2001). *Clinical assessment of child and adolescent intelligence* (2nd ed.). New York: Springer.

Kaufman, A. S. (1990). *Assessing adolescent and adult intelligence.* Boston: Allyn & Bacon.

Levy, S. E., Giarelli, E., Li-Ching, L., Schieve, L. A., Kirby, R. S., Cunniff, C., . . . Rice, C. E. (2010). Autism spectrum disorder and co-occurring developmental, psychiatric, and medical conditions among children in multiple populations of the United States. *Journal of Developmental and Behavioral Pediatrics, 31*(4), 267–275.

Lubinski, D. (2004). Introduction to the special section on cognitive abilities: 100 years after Spearman's (1904) "'General Intelligence,' Objectively Determined and Measured." *Journal of Personality and Social Psychology, 86*(1), 96–99.

McDonnell, C. G., Boan, A. D., Bradley, C. C., Seay, K. D., Charles, J. M., & Carpenter, L. A. (2019). Child maltreatment in autism spectrum disorder and intellectual disability: Results from a population-based sample. *Journal of Child Psychology and Psychiatry, 60*(5), 576–584.

McKenzie, K., Milton, M., Smith, G., & Oullette-Kuntz, H. (2016). Systematic review of the prevalence and incidence of intellectual disabilities: Current trends and issues. *Current Developmental Disorders Reports, 3*(2), 104–115.

Mlinac, M. E., & Feng, M. C. (2016). Assessment of activities of daily living, self-care, and independence. *Archives of Clinical Neuropsychology, 31,* 506–516.

Modabbernia, A., Mollon, J., Boffetta, P., & Reichenberg, A. (2016). Impaired gas exchange at birth and risk of intellectual disability and autism: A meta-analysis. *Journal of Autism and Developmental Disorders, 46,* 1847–1859.

National Center for Education Statistics, Institute of Education Sciences, U.S. Department of Education. (2018). *The Condition of Education 2018.* Washington, DC: Authors.

Neece, C. L., Baker, B. L., Blacher, J., & Crnic, K. A. (2011). Attention-deficit/hyperactivity disorder among children with and without intellectual disability: An examination across time. *Journal of Intellectual Disability Research, 55*(7), 623–635.

Payne, J. S., & Patton, J. R. (1981). *Mental retardation.* Columbus, OH: Merrill.

Peña-Salazar, C., Arrufat, F., Santos, J. M., Fontanet, A., González-Castro, G., Más, S., . . . Valdés-Stauber, J. (2018). Underdiagnosis of psychiatric disorders in people with intellectual disabilities: Differences between psychiatric disorders and challenging behaviour. *Journal of Intellectual Disabilities.* [Epub ahead of print]

Pepperdine, C. R., & McCrimmon, A. W. (2018). Test review: Vineland Adaptive Behavior Scales, Third Edition (Vineland-3) by Sparrow, S. S., Cicchetti, D. V., & Saulnier, C. A. *Canadian Journal of School Psychology, 33*(2), 157–163.

Platt, J. M., Keyes, K. M., McLaughlin, K. A., & Kaufman, A. S. (2018). Intellectual disability and mental disorders in a U.S. population representative sample of adolescents. *Psychological Medicine, 49*(6), 952–961.

Reardon, T. C., Gray, K. M., & Melvin, G. A. (2015). Anxiety disorders in children and adolescents with intellectual disability: Prevalence and assessment. *Research in Developmental Disabilities, 36,* 175–190.

Reschly, D. J. (1980). Psychological evidence in the Larry P. opinion: A case of right problem–wrong solution? *School Psychology Review, 9*(2), 123–135.

Reynolds, C. R., & Kamphaus, R. W. (2015a). *Behavior Assessment System for Children, Third Edition (BASC-3).* San Antonio, TX: Pearson Education.

Reynolds, C. R., & Kamphaus, R. W. (2015b). *Reynolds Intellectual Assessment Scale, Second Edition (RIAS-2).* Lutz, FL: Psychological Assessment Resources.

Rodas, N. V., Chavira, D. A., & Baker, B. L. (2017). Emotion socialization and internalizing behavior problems in diverse youth: A bidirectional relationship across childhood. *Research in Developmental Disabilities, 62,* 15–25.

Schalock, R., Borthwick-Duffy, S. A., Bradley, V. J., Buntinx, W. H. E., Coulter, D. L., Craig, E. M., . . . Yeager, M. H. (2010). *Intellectual disability: Definition, classification, and systems of supports* (11th ed.). Silver Spring, MD: American Association on Intellectual and Developmental Disabilities.

Schrank, F. A., McGrew, K. S., & Mather, N. (2014). *Woodcock–Johnson IV Tests of Cognitive Abilities, Fourth Edition (WJ-IV-COG).* Rolling Meadows, IL: Riverside.

Shepley, S. B., Spriggs, A. D., Samudre, M., & Elliott, M. (2018). Increasing daily living independence using video activity schedules in middle school students with intellectual disability. *Journal of Special Education Technology, 33*(2), 71–82.

Sparrow, S. S., Cicchetti, D. V., & Saulnier, C. A. (2016). *Vineland Adaptive Behavior Scales, Third Edition (Vineland-3).* San Antonio, TX: Pearson.

Spitz, H. H. (1983). Intratest and intertest reliability and stability of the WISC, WISC-R, and WAIS full scale IQs in a mentally retarded population. *Journal of Special Education, 17*(1), 69–80.

Spitz, H. H. (1986). *The raising of intelligence: A selected history of attempts to raise retarded intelligence.* Hillsdale, NJ: Erlbaum.

Spitz, H. H. (1988). Mental retardation as a thinking disorder: The rationalist alternative to empiricism. In N. W. Bray (Eds.), *International review of research in mental retardation* (Vol. 15, pp. 1–32). New York: Academic Press.

Steinberg, A. M., Brymer, M., Decker, K., & Pynoos, R. S. (2004). The University of California at Los Angeles Post-Traumatic Stress Disorder Reaction Index. *Current Psychiatry Reports, 6,* 96–100.

Sugai, G., Horner, R. H., Dunlap, G., Hieneman, M., Nelson, C. M., Scott, T., . . . Ruef, M. (2000). Applying positive behavior support and functional behavioral assessment in schools. *Journal of Positive Behavior Interventions, 2*(3), 131–143.

Sullivan, P. M., & Burley, S. K. (1990). Mental testing of the deaf child. In C. R. Reynolds & R. W. Kamphaus (Eds.), *Handbook of psychological and educational assessment of children* (pp. 761–788). New York: Guilford Press.

Tonnsen, B. L., Boan, A. D., Bradley, C. C., Charles, J., Cohen, A., & Carpenter, L. A. (2016). Prevalence of autism spectrum disorders among children with intellectual disability. *American Journal of Intellectual and Developmental Disabilities, 121*(6), 487–500.

Vissers, L. E., Gilissen, C., & Veltman, J. A. (2016). Genetic studies in intellectual disability and related disorders. *Nature Reviews Genetics, 17,* 9–18.

Wadsworth, J. P., Hansen, B. D., & Wills, S. B. (2015). Increasing compliance in children with intellectual disabilities using functional behavioral assessment and self-monitoring. *Remedial and Special Education, 36*(4), 195–207.

Ward, S. (in press). Test review of Reynolds Intellectual Assessment Scales, Second Edition and Reynolds Intellectual Screening Test, Second Edition. In J. F. Carlson, K. F. Geisinger, & J. L. Jonson (Eds.), *The twenty-first mental measurements yearbook.* Lincoln, NE: Buros Center for Testing.

Wechsler, D. (2011). *Wechsler Abbreviated Scale of Intelligence, Second Edition (WASI-II).* San Antonio, TX: NCS Pearson.

Wechsler, D. (2014). *Wechsler Intelligence Scale for Children, Fifth Edition (WISC-V).* Bloomington, MN: Pearson.

Wynkoop, K. S., Robertson, R. E., & Schwartz, R. (2018). The effects of two video modeling interventions on the independent living skills of students with autism spectrum disorder and intellectual disability. *Journal of Special Education Technology, 33*(3), 145–158.

Zablotsky, B., Black, L. I., & Blumberg, S. (2017). Estimated prevalence of children with diagnosed developmental disabilities in the United States, 2014–2016 (NSCHS Data Brief, No. 291). Washington, DC: U.S. Department of Health and Human Services, Centers for Disease Control and Prevention.

CHAPTER 14

Learning Disabilities

Ryan J. McGill, Kara M. Styck, and Stefan C. Dombrowski

Learning disability (LD [a.k.a. specific learning disorder, or SLD]) is an umbrella term that describes a condition in which individuals present with low achievement that cannot be explained by other psychological disorders or environmental factors. Despite much persistence and effort, LD remains difficult to demarcate, and considerable controversy has been associated with each attempt to operationally define the construct over the last 50 years. As a result, clinicians are forced to navigate an array of complex, and in some cases, conflicting statutes, regulations, and classification criteria when attempting to identify LD in children and adolescents. As an example, a client may meet the all of the diagnostic criteria for SLD in the fifth

edition of the *Diagnostic and Statistical Manual of Mental Disorders* (DSM-5; American Psychiatric Association, 2013) yet be denied special education and related services in that same category under local educational regulations. Further complicating the matter are the numerous classification approaches that pervade professional practice. While scholars continue to debate the merits of LD assessment methods and what new approaches may portend for the field, practitioners must adhere to state and federal guidelines, and, in some cases, implement new approaches that have yet to be empirically validated (Kavale, Kauffman, Bachmeier, & LeFever, 2008; McGill, Styck, Palomares, & Hass, 2016). Apropos of this dilemma, we begin this chapter by outlining the salient diagnostic features of LD and describe the history of approaches to LD assessment and identification before proceeding to elaborate on contemporary assessment methods and classification approaches.

Diagnostic Features

Within DSM-5, LDs fall under the broader category of neurodevelopmental disorders and are characterized by focal impairments in academic learning that limit the acquisition and performance of academic skills. Epidemiological surveys indicate that approximately 5–15% of school-age children present with a LD (Moll, Kunze, Neuhoff,

Bruder, & Schulte-Korne, 2014). Reading disorder is the most researched and most common variant of LD, and the vast majority of assessment and intervention research has been focused in this area. Evidence suggests that approximately 70–80% of individuals with LDs have primary deficits in reading (Ferrer, Shaywitz, Holahan, Murchione, & Shaywitz, 2010).

Although conceptualizations of LD may differ across clinical settings, all operational LD definitions share the same fundamental assumption that LDs reflect *unexpected* underachievement (Beaujean, Benson, McGill, & Dombrowski, 2018). Unlike other psychological disorders, LD represents both a clinical condition and an educational policy category. As a result, the makeup of the population of individuals diagnosed with LD may vary considerably when applicable laws and regulations change (Lewandowski & Lovett, 2014). As an example, if a school district uses one assessment method for classification and a neighboring school district uses another, an individual may be classified as having LD in the former district but upon moving to the later district, their eligibility for services may be removed for failure to meet the different criteria that is employed in that particular jurisdiction (Miciak, Fletcher, Stuebing, Vaughn, & Tolar, 2014). As we discuss later, even when different jurisdictions employ the same assessment method or model, identification practices may still fluctuate because of nontrivial differences in how various features of that model are operationalized. It is important to note that these issues are not limited to educational settings, as clinicians in private practice may employ different assessment and identification methods due to the opaque diagnostic criteria presently contained in DSM-5.

Changes in DSM-5

Numerous terms have been used to describe LD in previous DSM editions, including "learning disturbance" and "academic skills disorders." The current version of DSM-5 uses the term "specific learning disorder," which it operationally defined as "difficulties learning and using academic skills . . . that have persisted for at least 6 months, despite the provision of interventions that target those difficulties" (American Psychiatric Association, 2013, p. 66). Subtypes demarcate impairment in three academic domains: reading (marked by deficits in word-reading accuracy, reading fluency, and reading comprehension), written expression (marked by deficits in spelling, grammar, and clar-

ity and organization of writing), and mathematics (marked by deficits in number sense, memorization of math facts, calculation, and math reasoning). Whereas DSM-IV listed a nonspecified subtype of SLD (LD not otherwise specified [LD NOS]), this subtype has been omitted from the current DSM edition. As with other psychological disorders, clinicians are also required to grade the severity of symptom presentation (i.e., mild, moderate, or severe).

Despite the fact that assessment of intellectual functioning has historically played a prominent role in many of the LD identification assessment models developed since the 1960s, the potential value of cognitive assessment for diagnosis is downplayed in DSM-5. It is noted that "individuals with specific learning disorder typically (but not invariably) exhibit poor performance on psychological tests of cognitive processing. However, it remains unclear whether these cognitive abnormalities are the cause, correlate, or consequence of the learning difficulties" (American Psychiatric Association, 2013, p. 70). Consequently, evidence for the presence of a cognitive processing disorder or a significant discrepancy between measured IQ and achievement are no longer required for diagnosis. Instead, the core diagnostic feature in DSM-5 is the presence of academic dysfunction that is resistant to remediation. This change has been a source of significant criticism within the professional literature, as it seemingly moves the diagnostic criteria from what was previously an ability–achievement discrepancy model to one that is largely based on low achievement and/or response to intervention (RTI),[1] a move that is consistent with current professional practice trends (Cavendish, 2013).

In spite of these developments, cognitive discrepancy methods are still widely utilized in school-based settings, and nothing explicitly prohibits their use in DSM or in federal regulations (Maki, Floyd, & Roberson, 2015). Given the current absence of a consistent diagnostic approach, Schroeder, Drefs, and Cormier (2017) note that it is not uncommon for clinicians to rely on clinical judgment and elect to disregard or be lenient in their application of a particular assessment approach. As should be evident, it is imperative for practitioners, regardless of the setting in which they are working, to be cognizant of the regulations (i.e., state and federal educational codes)

---

[1]DSM-5 and ICD-10 (World Health Organization, 1992) do not presently endorse any particular assessment method for LD identification.

and assessment practices that are prevalent in their particular jurisdiction, in order for their assessment results and diagnostic recommendations to have ecological validity across various clinical settings.

Assessment and Identification: Historical Context

Many authorities credit Samuel Kirk for originating the term "learning disability." In the original edition of *Educating Exceptional Children*, Kirk (1962) provided one of the first operational definitions of LD, on which he explicated a year later in a speech delivered at the annual meeting of the organization that eventually became the Learning Disabilities Association of America. According to Hallahan and Mercer (2002), this was the first time that the term was used at an educational conference. The importance of these events cannot be overstated, as they gave rise to a decade-long series of events that led to federal involvement in LD and the eventual passage of the Education for All Handicapped Act (Public Law 94-142) in 1975. This act contained a federal operational definition for LD that continues to be used to this day. The pace of adoption in clinical practice was much faster, as the original DSM published in 1968 contained a preliminary category (learning disturbance) that eventually morphed into SLD.

Although federal involvement in LD has only been evident since the 1960s, scholars have traced the roots of LD all the way back to the early 1800s, and much of the assessment logic that clinicians employ today can be sourced to this "prefoundational" period; that is, many assessment and identification approaches were conceived of prior to the development and eventual acceptance of formal operational definitions of the construct. As a result, typical LD assessment practices have not kept pace with advances in evidence-based practices (Fletcher, Stuebing, Morris, & Lyon, 2013).

Prefoundational Period

The origins of the LD field can be traced to a series of case study publications by prominent physicians and researchers in early 19th-century Europe. Most of these investigations were conducted with adult patients who had sustained traumatic brain injury resulting in peculiar language deficits. Although limited by the technology of the time, seminal discoveries during this era continue to serve as points of reference for the field. For example, Joseph Gall was one of the first individuals to explore relationships between brain injury and impairment. Based on these observations, Head (1926) concluded that each of the "intellectual qualities of the mind" (p. 4) was localized in a different portion of the brain. These findings gave rise to the practice of phrenology—an approach in which the shape and size of an individual's cranium were evaluated in order to make inferences about his or her character and mental abilities. Although phrenology was soon disavowed by the medical and psychological communities, the localization of function idea (i.e., that specific cognitive tests can be used to make inferences about potential deficits in focal areas of the brain) continues to undergird many LD assessment methods (McGill & Busse, 2017).

It is interesting to note that early assessment approaches focused mostly on using assessment to inform intervention by administering rudimentary reading and language tasks to individuals with reading difficulties (i.e., direct measures of academic skills). Clinical evaluations focused mostly on academic strengths and weaknesses and identifying the component skills that were in need of remediation. For example, Monroe (1932) developed a "reading index" that calculated the discrepancy between actual and expected reading achievement for a student, and it was thought that this index could be used to identify students in need of special assistance. Additionally, she was an early proponent of using error analysis to help guide treatment selection, and she encouraged practitioners to give equal consideration to a child's quantitative and qualitative performance on academic achievement tasks. With the advent of IQ tests, the administration of these measures soon became routine in case studies that emerged in the early 20th century. Initially, the relative value of IQ tests for the diagnosis or remediation or reading disability was called into question. Orton (1925) noted that "the test [IQ test] is inadequate to gage the equipment in a case of such a special disability" (p. 584).

Developments in psychological assessment and individual-differences research led to a paradigm shift in LD assessment in the mid-20th century. Principle among these were Samuel Kirk's research program, which stressed the importance of intraindividual differences and assessment-based instruction, and the rise of commercial IQ tests measuring multiple factors that were thought to reflect different cognitive attributes. Whereas IQ tests were given modest consideration by early LD practitioners, they soon became prominent features of emerging LD classification models.

After obtaining his doctorate from the University of Michigan, Kirk obtained a faculty position at the University of Illinois and established an experimental preschool for children with intellectual disabilities. In order to better educate these children, Kirk believed that he needed assessments that could amplify relevant psychoeducational strengths and weaknesses. Put simply, the goal was to develop a series of diagnostic tests that would be useful for instruction. This experimental research culminated in the development of the Illinois Test of Psycholinguistic Abilities (ITPA; Kirk, McCarthy, & Kirk, 1961). The ITPA contained 12 subtests measuring perceptual, linguistic, and memory abilities, and it was believed that particular ITPA profiles could be matched to training activities that were developed in conjunction with the instrument. A critical goal of the ITPA research program was to identify relevant aptitude-by-treatment interactions (ATIs), the notion that some instructional strategies are more or less effective for particular individuals depending on their abilities.

Although use of the ITPA was widespread in the 1960s and 1970s, numerous critiques of the instrument's psychometric properties and efficacy of its training procedures emerged (e.g., Hammill & Larsen, 1974; Mann, 1979) and it soon fell out of favor. On the basis of 18 years of largely unsuccessful research, Cronbach (1975) concluded that the search for ATIs was plagued by the fact that "once we attend to interactions, we enter into a hall of mirrors that extends to infinity" (p. 119) and that scientific psychology would be better served by eschewing the correlational approach in favor of short-run empiricism. Nevertheless, Hallahan, Pullen, and Ward (2013) argue that the development of the ITPA remains historically important because it reinforced the notion that children with LDs have important individual differences and that psychoeducational assessment may be used to guide instruction. Despite their intuitive appeal, few ATIs have been empirically validated for children with LD since Cronbach's seminal critique, and the ATI validation remains a topic of controversy within the field (see Burns et al., 2016).

Origins of the Ability–Achievement Discrepancy Model

Although the term "learning disability" was introduced in the early 1960s, existing operational definitions are relatively opaque and shed little insight on how LD should be assessed or identified. This began to change when Barbara Bateman (1965) expanded on Kirk's definition and offered the following definition for LD:

> Children who have learning disorders are those who manifest an educationally significant discrepancy between their estimated potential and actual level of performance related to basic disorders in the learning process, which may or may not be accompanied by demonstrable central nervous system dysfunction. (p. 220)

Bateman's definition served as a critical inflection point in the field, as it reinforced Monroe's (1932) earlier notion that a discrepancy between achievement and potential may be used to formally diagnose students with LD and, more importantly, that cognitive tests are vital for assessment and identification. As a result of this development, discrepancy soon became linked with the identification of LDs and a focal point of subsequent modifications to the operational definitions and regulations produced by federal task forces.

As previously mentioned, with the passing of Public Law 94-142 in 1975, the federal government produced an operational definition for SLD that has subsequently undergone only slight modifications and has additional implications for LD classification in school-based settings. That definition, as quoted in the final regulations adopted by the U.S. Office of Education (USOE) in 1977 is as follows:

> The term "specific learning disability" means a disorder in one or more of the basic psychological processes involved in understanding or in using language, spoken, or written, which may manifest itself in an imperfect ability to listen, speak, read, write, spell, or do mathematical calculations (p. 65083).

Given the integral role of "psychological processes" in the federal definition, it is frequently asserted that LD assessment methods should focus on identifying relevant processing strengths and weaknesses (PSWs; Hale et al., 2010). However, in an interesting paradox, more recent federal regulations seem to deemphasize processing assessment entirely (Lichtenstein, 2014). Nevertheless, as this definition implies that a disorder in cognitive processing is the putative cause of LD, many assessment methods (e.g., PSW approaches) focus exclusively on documenting the presence of a processing deficit, and practitioners have long been encouraged to evaluate ability profiles for unique patterns and signs that portend to have implications for the presence of LD (Fletcher et al., 2013).

Prior to Public Law 94-142 implementation in 1977, the USOE (1976) furnished additional regulations pertaining to the identification of individuals with LD and proposed a formula that defined a severe discrepancy as "when achievement in one or more of the areas falls at or below 50% of the child's expected achievement level" (p. 52405). Public response to the formula was overwhelmingly negative (Hallahan & Mercer, 2002). Although the USOE continued to endorse the idea of an ability–achievement discrepancy in the regulations, no formula was included, giving each state the power to determine how the discrepancy model would be operationalized within its borders. The discrepancy model soon became the dominant method for conferring an educational classification of SLD in a most states, as well as a prominent element in the diagnostic criteria outlined in the DSM.

What is particularly striking about the process that led to the reification of the discrepancy model is the limited empirical evidence available at that time to support use of the method. The only compelling evidence validating the IQ discrepancy hypothesis that could be located came from the Isle of Wight epidemiological studies conducted by Rutter and Yule (1975), who administered the Performance IQ scale from the Wechsler Intelligence Scale for Children (WISC) and additional reading measures to a large sample of children. Using a regression-based definition, they found that they were able to distinguish between "specific reading retardation [sic]" and "general reading backwardness," with the bulk of the children in the former group producing reading scores that were two standard deviations or more below their IQ scores. This resulting "hump" was interpreted as a useful cutoff point for distinguishing between children with LDs and "garden variety" poor learners. However, subsequent attempts to replicate these findings have been unsuccessful (e.g., Shaywitz, Escobar, Shaywitz, Fletcher, & Makuch, 1992) and the discrepancy model has been maligned since its inception (Aaron, 1997).

Given the widespread dissatisfaction with the discrepancy model and additional concerns by some researchers with the field's perceived devotion to processing assessment and cognitive process training (see Mann, 1979), the USOE funded five LD research institutes to identify and advance research-based assessment and intervention practices. The institutes were housed at the University of Illinois at Chicago, the University of Kansas, the University of Minnesota, the University of Virginia, and Columbia University. In spite of making substantive advances in the development of curriculum-based assessment procedures and the identification of numerous empirically supported treatments, researchers were unable to come to a consensus on an alternative assessment method to replace the discrepancy model. In summarizing the results of 5 years of research findings produced by the institute at the University of Minnesota, Ysseldyke and colleagues (1983) noted, "After five years of trying, we cannot describe, except with considerable lack of precision, students called LD. We think that LD can best be defined as 'whatever society wants it to be, needs it to be, or will let it be' at any point in time" (p. 89). Whereas this may be viewed by some as an overly draconian account of the state of affairs at that time, we suspect that there are likely many clinicians who believe this quote is as accurate today as it was 25 years ago.

The Search for Diagnostic Signs and Unique PSWs

Although dissemination of the discrepancy method was instrumental in popularizing the use of IQ tests for LD assessment and identification, this was not the first attempt to utilize cognitive tests in this capacity. It has long been speculated that cognitive test scatter and variability could serve as a potential pathognomonic sign for a host of psychological disorders, including LD. Early researchers hypothesized that subtest scatter would predict scholastic potential and membership in exceptional groups (Harris & Shakow, 1937), and formal methods for these types of analyses have been proposed in the literature for well over 70 years. Rapaport, Gil, and Schafer (1945) developed a formal process for evaluating cognitive scatter in a two-volume series devoted to diagnostic testing. Their system involved graphically plotting subtest profiles, then visually inspecting the peaks and valleys in an examinee's scores and generating pathognomonic inferences from these observations. Given the intuitive nature of these procedures, they soon became a staple of clinical tradition. As tests expanded, clinicians were provided with more scores and score comparisons to interpret, and questionable interpretive practices emerged and remained popular through the 1970s (Kaufman, Raiford, & Coalson, 2016).

As a remedy, Kaufman (1979) proposed a step-by-step profile analysis interpretive approach for the WISC-R[2] that he termed "intelligent testing." According to Kaufman, Raiford, and Coalson (2016), Kaufman was motivated by a need to "impose some empirical order on profile interpretation; to make sensible inferences from the data with full awareness of errors of measurement and to steer the field away from the psychiatric coach" (p. 7). In the intelligent testing approach, practitioners are encouraged to interpret test scores in a systematic fashion, beginning with the full scale intelligence quotient (FSIQ) and culminating at the subtest level. However, users are encouraged to focus most of their interpretive weight on the scatter and elevation (i.e., strengths and weaknesses) that are observed in lower-order scores (e.g., subtest and broad ability composite and index scores), and interpretation of the FSIQ is deemphasized. Inferential hypotheses are then generated from these observations, as well as the qualitative behaviors observed during the test administration.

Consonant with the publication of the WISC-III, Kaufman (1994) produced a revision of the so-called "Kaufman method," outlining several schemes based on different configurations of Wechsler subtests that were thought to be useful for the diagnosis of LD. For instance, Kaufman noted that individuals with disabilities tended to score lower on the subtests comprising the SCAD profile (Symbol Search [S], Coding [C], Arithmetic [A], and Digit Span [D]). Additional profiles included the ACID profile, Bannatyne (1968) pattern, and the Learning Disability Index (LDI). Although it is common to find abnormal scatter and patterns of PSWs within clinical groups, the uniqueness of these differences tends to evaporate whenever normal controls are included in the samples due to the large amount variability that is endemic in the population (Zimmerman & Woo-Sam, 1985). Empirical research studies have consistently indicated that the diagnostic accuracy of these profiles rarely exceeds chance levels, rendering them ineffectual for LD classification (e.g., Smith & Watkins, 2004; Watkins, Kush, & Glutting, 1997a, 1997b; Watkins, Kush, & Schaefer, 2002).

Another popular heuristic emerging out of the Kaufman tradition is the hypothesis that children with LD are characterized by significant Verbal IQ–Performance IQ (VIQ–PIQ) discrepancies, and these types of composite score pairwise comparisons have long been a core feature of the Kaufman interpretive approach. This notion stems from belief that such discrepancies reflect underdevelopment in focal areas of the brain or neural circuits that may have implications for matching instruction to a client's learning style (Elliott & Resing, 2015). Beyond the fact that the learning styles concept has been the subject of significant research criticism, the evidence base for matching students with learning difficulties to effective instruction based on the information furnished by cognitive tests is less than compelling (Burns et al., 2016; Cronbach & Snow, 1977; Fletcher & Miciak, 2017; Pashler, McDaniel, Rohrer, & Bjork, 2008). Furthermore, in a comprehensive meta-analysis of 94 studies, Kavale and Forness (1984) found that the mean VIQ–PIQ difference in individuals that were diagnosed with LDs was only 3.46 points. Based on this finding they concluded that 79% of the population was likely to exhibit the same or greater discrepancy between those scores. As a result, they concluded, "V-P differences appear to be of little value in LD diagnosis" (p. 139).

Additional studies have illuminated psychometric limitations of profile analysis that may have implications for the application of these procedures for the diagnosis of LD. McDermott, Fantuzzo, and Glutting (1990) surveyed the extant literature on intraindividual and interindividual subtest analysis and concluded that there was little empirical support for interpretation of these metrics. These findings have since been replicated (McDermott, Fantuzzo, Glutting, Watkins, & Baggaley, 1992; Watkins, 2005). As an example, Watkins tested the diagnostic validity of four different configurations of WISC-III subtest scatter, and receiver operating characteristic curve (ROC) analyses revealed that the scatter indices correctly diagnosed preidentified LD only 50–55% of the time. The results produced by Macmann and Barnett (1997) may be instructive for understanding why psychometric researchers investigating the diagnostic utility of profile analysis methods have consistently obtained negative research results. Macmann and Barnett used computer simulations to measure the impact of measurement error on the reliability of cognitive profile analysis interpretations (e.g., pairwise comparisons, PSWs, and scatter) and

---

[2]The intelligent testing approach can be used with other measures, and the levels-of-analysis approach to test interpretation is featured in virtually every test technical manual and clinical guidebook.

found that 62.4% of the sample presented with at least one significant composite score strength or weakness, and the base rate was even higher at the subtest level. As a result, they concluded that there was strong potential for clinical error and confirmation bias when attempting to ascribe *meaning* to these observations. Relatedly, Watkins and Canivez (2004) examined the temporal stability of PSWs and found low longitudinal agreement. As a consequence, they suggested that the inferences generated from these patterns of scores are likely to be unreliable.

More recently, McGill (2018) utilized the evidence-based assessment framework outlined by Youngstrom and Van Meter (2016) to evaluate whether cognitive scatter accurately discriminated between individuals predetermined to have LD and non-LD controls in a nationally representative normative sample ($N = 2,025$). Diagnostic efficiency statistics revealed that increasing levels of scatter did not function as a useful diagnostic sign. Area under the curve (AUC) values ranged from .46 to .51, indicating that cognitive scatter, at best, functioned as the diagnostic equivalent of flipping a coin, and positive predictive values (.04 to .05) were even more dismal. As a result, probability nomograms for each level of scatter indicated that scatter assessment did not improve the posterior odds of correct diagnosis from prior base rates. Based on these results, it appears that practitioners who engage in scatter and other, related PSW analyses may be spending a significant amount of time and resources to obtain information that may not be clinically useful.

Nevertheless, Kaufman (1994) has long argued that these limitations are managed by clinical acumen. For example, Kaufman and Lichtenberger (2006) argue that validity studies using group data (e.g., Macmann & Barnett, 1997) may obscure important individual differences; thus, clinicians should use their professional judgment to discern when these results are applicable when interpreting the assessment data obtained from individuals; that is, it is possible for a child to have a LD even when a specific pattern or sign hypothesized to reflect that disorder is not present and clinicians may be able to discern when this phenomenon may occur at the level of the individual through skilled detective work. In spite of a long-standing body of literature recommending that these practices be eschewed (e.g., Bray, Kehle, & Hintze, 1998; Canivez, 2013; Glutting, Watkins, & Youngstrom, 2003; Kranzler et al., 2016a; Watkins, 2000, 2003), surveys reveal that these procedures remain a core staple of LD assessment training and practice (Benson, Floyd, Kranzler, Eckert, & Fefer, 2018; Sotelo-Dynega & Dixon, 2014).

Decline of the Discrepancy Model and the Rise of RTI

By the 1990s, the majority of states had adopted some variant of the discrepancy method as part of their identification procedures (Hallahan & Mercer, 2002). However, empirical investigations began to identify considerable conceptual and psychometric problems with the method. For example, in a meta-analysis, Stuebing and colleagues (2002) evaluated the cognitive correlates of poor reading groups containing individuals with significant discrepancies and those that were not discrepant. Results indicated that there was significant overlap between the two groups on the core cognitive skills that were most associated with reading, indicating that those dimensions did not discriminate between children with and without discrepancies.

The discrepancy model has also been criticized as a "wait to fail" approach due to the fact that younger children, who are referred for an evaluation, often do not present with a discrepancy that is large enough to meet diagnostic criteria for LD (Restori, Gresham, & Cook, 2008). Accordingly, these students must continue to fail until their achievement is sufficiently low compared to their IQ. To buttress this claim, critics point to surveys indicating that identification rates tend to peak between third and fourth grade, even though the manifest symptoms of academic dysfunction are often apparent much earlier (Lyon, Fletcher, Fuchs, & Chhabra, 2006). Of concern, some "gold standard" treatments may begin to lose their effectiveness by the time these children are identified (Wanzek et al., 2013). This limitation also appears to have impacted the integrity of identification practices in some jurisdictions. MacMillan, Gresham, and Bocian (1998) conducted an audit of students who were identified as LD in a California school district employing the discrepancy model and found that less than half of students identified as LD met the regulatory criteria for eligibility. These findings are not intrinsic to California, and similar results have been obtained in numerous jurisdictions since the imposition of the discrepancy model in the 1970s. As noted by Peterson and Shinn (2002), school personnel tend to base eligibility decision on an "absolute low achievement" criterion, even at the expense of the law.

By the turn of the century, resistance to the discrepancy model reached a crescendo, culminating in a Learning Disabilities Summit of leading researchers in 2001. A majority of the white papers that were presented argued for an alternative (RTI) to the discrepancy model that focused on providing targeted interventions to children with academic difficulties and using low-inference progress monitoring assessments to evaluate treatment outcomes (Al Otaiba, Wagner, & Miller, 2014). It is interesting to note that much of this effort grew out of the assessment and intervention research that begun at the federal LD institutes in the 1970s. By the turn of the century, there was abundant evidence to indicate that the discrepancy model did not predict treatment response between difficult-to-remediate and readily remediated children (e.g., Vellutino et al., 1996) and that children with reading difficulties were able to benefit from targeted reading interventions, in particular, remedial phonics-based instruction.

In 2004, the Individuals with Disabilities Education Act (IDEA) was reauthorized, and the regulations pertaining to the identification of SLDs were modified, based largely on the findings and recommendations produced from the 2001 Summit. The final regulations authored by the Office of Special Education and Rehabilitation Services (OSERS) specify that use of the discrepancy method is no longer required (but is not prohibited), that states must allow for the use of RTI procedures for identification, and that states are free to adopt a *research-based* alternative to discrepancy and/or RTI. Over the course of the last decade, numerous states and jurisdictions (some states permit local educational agencies to adopt their own local LD identification criteria) have implemented RTI models and procedures, and the dissemination of these methods has been a prominent topic within the professional literature.

The debate that produced the RTI "consensus" was not without controversy. Several rival models that emphasized the importance of a processing-based approach for diagnosis were presented and considered at the Summit. Critics argue that the RTI model is not consistent with the federal operational definition of LD, as its assessment procedures do not yield information that is useful for identifying a deficit in cognitive processing (e.g., Hale, Kaufman, Naglieri, & Kavale, 2006). Emerging out of the radical behavior tradition, RTI represents a profound paradigm shift in which assessment is focused exclusively on treatment utility, and cognitive testing is given little, if any, consid-

eration in the diagnostic process outside of ruling out the presence of intellectual disability. Scruggs and Mastropieri (2002) suggest that such radical alterations to identification criteria are akin to "throwing the baby out with the bath water" (p. 155). Since 2000, a number of rival processing-based approaches for assessment and identification (e.g., PSW) have been proposed in the literature.

In general, the PSW approach is essentially a cognitive discrepancy method. According to McGrady (2002), "The discrepancy comparisons are made *among* apparently discrete skills and abilities, not as a comparison of such skills with performance on a general estimate of intellectual potential—the traditional discrepancy formula approach" (p. 628, original emphasis). Although these models were debated and ultimately found wanting at the Learning Disabilities Summit, enthusiasm for their implementation by practitioners and scholars has increased over the last 5 years. As a result, LD identification practices vary considerably across states. In a survey, Maki and colleagues (2015) found that 67% of states continue use the discrepancy method, 16% require the use of RTI procedures as a primary method of LD identification, and 28% now permit use of a PSW approach.

Summary

Although there is considerable agreement about the definition of LD as a construct, a consensus method for identifying LD has been elusive. As a result, it is important for practitioners to understand the history and context that has led to the development of various classification models and the perceived weaknesses for each of these approaches. Ironically, the very method that has long dominated the field (discrepancy) was adopted by default when researchers and practitioners were unable to agree on a suitable alternative (Dombrowski & Gischlar, 2014). The field has essentially been on a path of course correction ever since. Presently, these debates largely focus on the role of cognitive testing in assessment and diagnosis and whether any approach can *validly* and *reliably* distinguish between individuals with LD and those with broader academic dysfunction (i.e., "garden variety" poor learners). As should be evident in this review, these issues are not new and have plagued the field since its inception. In the following sections of this chapter, we outline and describe commonly used assessment tools and contemporary classification schemes in more detail.

Assessments Commonly Used in LD Classification

Contemporary surveys (e.g., Sotelo-Dynega & Dixon, 2014) reveal that norm-referenced tests of intelligence and achievement, and curriculum-based measurement are the most commonly used measures across settings for the assessment of LD. In this section we provide examples and describe each of these assessment types in more detail. It should be noted that even in classification models that employ a cognitive discrepancy approach, a comprehensive evaluation should include additional elements that are common to other areas of psychopathology (e.g., review of records, diagnostic interview, direct behavioral observations) to rule out relevant exclusionary factors or to examine other areas of psychological functioning that may contribute to a child's learning problems. For example, behavioral rating scales may be used to screen for social–emotional dysfunction or conduct differential diagnosis for relevant comorbid disorders such as ADHD. As these applications are described in more detail in other areas of this text, we defer elaborating on them further here.

Wechsler Intelligence Scale for Children— Fifth Edition

The Wechsler Intelligence Scale for Children— Fifth Edition (WISC-V; Wechsler, 2014) is the latest version of one of the most frequently used intelligence tests for children. It includes 16 subtests; five factor index scores (Verbal Comprehension, Visual–Spatial, Fluid Reasoning, Working Memory, and Processing Speed); and a hierarchically ordered FSIQ score. Users can also use various combinations of secondary and complimentary subtests to produce a series of ancillary index scores (General Ability, Cognitive Proficiency, Quantitative Reasoning, Nonverbal, and Auditory Working Memory). However, these scores are not derived from factor analysis; instead, they are logically or theoretically constructed and should be interpreted with caution.

The WISC-V is a substantial revision of the previous version of the instrument. The Word Reasoning and Picture Completion subtests were eliminated, and several new subtests were added. The Picture Span subtest (adapted from the Wechsler Preschool and Primary Scale of Intelligence— Fourth Edition [WPPSI-IV]) was added to measure visual working memory, and the Visual Puzzles and Figure Weights subtests (adapted from the

Wechsler Adult Intelligence Scale, Fourth Edition [WAIS-IV]) were added to measure visual–spatial and fluid reasoning, respectively. A major goal of the WISC-V revision was to split the former Perceptual Reasoning Index (PRI) into separate Visual–Spatial and Fluid Reasoning indices.

The technical manual suggests that primary index scores should be the main focus of clinical interpretation and that the patterns observed in these scores may be used to make logical inferences about PSWs that may have implications for LD assessment. In the descriptions of the subtests in the manual, there are descriptions of relations to cognitive and neuropsychological theories to facilitate inferences onto which narrow abilities these measures may map. As a result, the FSIQ (or a substitute ancillary index) may be used to identify children with a severe discrepancy, and the lower-order scores may be used to generate unique PSW profiles.

Kaufman Assessment Battery for Children— Second Edition

The Kaufman Assessment Battery for Children— Second Edition (KABC-II; Kaufman & Kaufman, 2004) measures the processing and cognitive abilities of children and adolescents between ages 3 and 18 years. According to the test authors, KABC-II underwent a major structural and conceptual revision. Eight subtests were eliminated from the original K-ABC, 10 measures were created and added to the current battery, and the KABC-II theoretical foundation was updated. The KABC-II utilizes a dual-theoretical foundation: Cattell–Horn–Carroll theory (CHC; Schneider & McGrew, 2018) and Luria's neuropsychological theory of cognitive processing (Luria, 1966). One of the features of the KABC-II is the flexibility that it affords the examiner in determining the theoretical model to administer to the examinee. Although examiners may select either the Luria or CHC interpretive models, users are advised to interpret the KABC-II primarily from the CHC perspective.

The CHC model for school ages features 16 subtests (10 core and six supplemental), which combine to yield five first-order factor scale scores (Short-Term Memory [Gsm], Long-Term Storage and Retrieval [Glr], Visual Processing [Gv], Fluid Reasoning [Gf], and Crystallized Ability [Gc]), and a second-order full scale Fluid Crystallized Index (FCI) that is thought to represent psychometric g (general intelligence). Each CHC factor scale comprises two subtest measures, and the FCI is derived from a linear combination of the 10 core subtests that comprise the constituent factor scores. Although the KABC-II manual encourages a stepwise progression of interpretation from the FCI to the factor scores (consistent with the Kaufman method), clinicians are encouraged to use the CHC factor scores as the primary point of interpretation for the instrument. The Luria model omits measures of Crystallized Ability and thus features eight core subtests that combine to form an alternative full scale Mental Processing Index (MPI). If interpreting from the Luria perspective, the factor scores also employ a different nomenclature (Sequential [Gsm], Learning [Glr], Simultaneous [Gv], and Planning [Gf]). Given its versatility, it is suggested that it may be a particularly useful measure for examinee's who are culturally and linguistically diverse. However, an independent review by Braden and Ouzts (2005) suggests caution in employing the verbiage associated with the Luria model to interpret KABC-II scores, as it is psychometrically implausible for subtests to measure two distinct and theoretically divergent constructs simultaneously.

Kaufman Test of Educational Achievement— Third Edition

The Kaufman Test of Educational Achievement— Third Edition (KTEA-3; Kaufman & Kaufman, 2014) is an individually administered, norm-referenced test of achievement for individuals ages 4–25. It features 19 subtests (six core, 13 supplemental) that combine to form three subscale scores (Reading, Math, Writing), as well as an omnibus full scale score of overall academic achievement (Academic Skills Battery [ASB]). Various combinations of the core and supplemental tests can also be combined to form four reading-related composite scores (Sound–Symbol, Decoding, Reading Fluency, and Reading Understanding), two oral language composites (Oral Language and Oral Fluency), and four cross-domain composites (Comprehension, Expression, Orthographic Processing, and Academic Fluency). The measure provides both age- and grade-based normative scores which is a useful feature when assessing clients who may have been retained.

Another useful feature that is unique to the KTEA-3 is the incorporation of error analysis procedures for 10 of the 19 subtests. For example, when administering the Math Computation subtest, examiners can inspect the completed worksheet and complete a supplemental standardized protocol,

highlighting specific reasons for a student's incorrect responses to individual items. In contrast to previous editions, base rates for these observations are now provided by the test publisher. Error analysis on the KTEA-3 was the subject of a special issue of the *Journal of Psychoeducational Assessment* in 2017 (Breaux, Bray, Root, & Kaufman, 2017). In that issue, containing 13 articles and commentaries, preliminary evidence was presented, using the normative sample data for the KTEA-3, that error analysis patterns may be useful for discriminating among various LD subtypes.

Woodcock–Johnson IV

The Woodcock–Johnson IV (WJ-IV; Schrank, McGrew, & Mather, 2014) is a comprehensive battery of psychoeducational abilities for individuals ages 2–90 years. The measure contains 47 subtests allocated to three different batteries that allow for a comprehensive assessment of cognitive ability, achievement, and oral language. The battery was principally designed, and is the only commercial ability test to measure, all of the consensus factors posited by CHC theory (see Table 14.1). The WJ-IV presently serves as the preeminent reference instrument for making refinements to CHC and the understanding of cognitive–achievement relations in the psychological sciences. Each of the batteries is designed to be administered in isolation, although an examiner may elect to administer selected subtests from each battery utilizing a cross-battery assessment (XBA) framework. Interested readers are encouraged to consult Schrank and Wendling (2018) for an in-depth description of the panoply of scores afforded by the instrument. In addition to CHC-based factor scores, there are well over 20 broad and narrow cognitive–achievement clusters that can be calculated from different configurations of WJ-IV subtests. Whereas all of the tests that have been previously reviewed in this section can be hand-scored, standardized scores for the WJ-IV can only be obtained from an online scoring platform that charges a per-use fee.

Given its relation to CHC theory, the WJ-IV features prominently in several interpretive approaches based on that theory that may be used as part of LD diagnosis. For example, McGrew and Wendling (2010) provide a summary of relations between CHC abilities and specific areas of achievement which, when combined with the WJ-IV CHC subtest classifications reported in the most recent XBA handbook (Flanagan, Ortiz, & Alfonso, 2013), may be used to guide selective assessment. In fact, an emerging PSW method, the Core-Selective Evaluation Process (C-SEP; Schultz & Stephens-Pisecco, 2015) seemingly was designed to align with core sets of tests from the WJ-IV. There are two sources that describe how to utilize the WJ-IV within that model (Schrank, Stephens-Pisecco, & Schultz, 2017; Schultz & Stephens-Pisecco, 2015), and the C-SEP was outlined in an advertorial by the publisher in the *Communique*, a practitioner newsletter published each month by the National Association of School Psychologists.

TABLE 14.1. Consensus Cattell–Horn–Carroll (CHC) Broad Cognitive Abilities (Schneider & McGrew, 2018)

CHC dimension	Description
Comprehension–Knowledge (Gc)	Depth and breadth of knowledge and skills that are valued by one's culture.
Fluid Reasoning (Gf)	The deliberate but flexible control of attention to solve novel "on the spot" problems that cannot be performed by relying exclusively on previously learned habits, schemas, and scripts.
Short-Term Memory (Gsm)	The ability to encode, maintain, and manipulate information in one's immediate awareness.
Long-Term Storage and Retrieval (Glr)	The ability to store, consolidate, and retrieve information over periods of time measured in minutes, hours, days, and years.
Visual Processing (Gv)	The ability to make use of simulated mental imagery (often in conjunction with currently perceived images) to solve problems.
Auditory Processing (Ga)	The ability to detect and process meaningful nonverbal information in sound.
Processing Speed (Gs)	The ability to perform simple, repetitive cognitive tasks quickly and fluently.
Reading and Writing (Grw)	Depth and breadth of knowledge and skills related to written language.
Quantitative Reasoning (Gq)	Depth and breadth of knowledge related to mathematics.

Curriculum-Based Measurement

Although curriculum-based measurement (CBM) is frequently used to document treatment response within an RTI intervention framework, it can also be used to conduct a diagnostic assessment of academic skills. CBM represents a series of alternative probes of core academic skills (e.g., Oral Reading Fluency, Phonemic Awareness, Math Computation, Writing Fluency, Spelling, Maze [as a proxy for reading comprehension]). The measures are timed (e.g., 1–3 minutes' duration) and yield measurements of both accuracy and response rate. Probes are designed to be brief, repeatable, and sensitive to small increments in change. As a result of these properties, CBM is a useful technology for screening, as well as progress monitoring, children with academic difficulties (Deno, 2003). CBM probes are considered to be general outcome measures (GOMs); that is, they provide a consistent scale for decision making across subskills that serve as the focal target for intensive interventions. CBM works much like GOMs in other disciplines (e.g., thermometer in medicine, stock market index in economics). For example, even though a reading intervention may target a specific subskill of reading (e.g., sound blending), the effects of that intervention will be captured by corresponding changes in a person's reading fluency rate over time. In a comparison of progress monitoring data from reading fluency probes and specific subskill mastery measures of reading (SSMM) that more closely matched intervention targets, Van Norman, Maki, Burns, McComas, and Helman (2018) found that while some SSMM's provided an incremental benefit beyond GOM's for early struggling readers, this distinction became less meaningful as readers were exposed to more complex phonetic patters as they got older.

A number of studies have validated the use of CBM with children suffering from academic dysfunction, and grade norms and expected growth rates have been established for every major type of CBM (e.g., Deno, Fuchs, Marston, & Shin, 2001). Thus, if a child's CBM level (absolute difference) or slope (growth) of learning deviates significantly from expected levels of performance, this may indicate the presence of LD. More importantly, CBM data directly inform academic intervention and instructional planning and have been shown to predict year-end high-stakes test outcomes. Several resources for CBM assessment and interpretation are provided in Appendix 14.1.

Contemporary Classification Approaches

LD assessment methods have been influenced by changes and modifications to federal regulations over the course of the last 40 years. The final regulations adopted by the USOE (1977) focused on a severe discrepancy resulting in a conceptual shift away from a deficit in processing to explain underachievement. According to Fletcher and colleagues (2013), this shift was a response to concerns about the validity of processing-based approaches to identification and the perceived lack of efficacy of related process training (e.g., Mann, 1979). Ironically, the field is presently experiencing a "back to the future"-type moment as enthusiasm for new processing-based approaches (i.e., PSW) has increased. Nevertheless, existing federal regulations and diagnostic criteria permit the use of multiple assessment methods for LD identification, and these methods have different assumptions regarding LD as a construct. What follows is a review of the three classification methods that have been featured prominently in the professional literature. We should note that even though our discussion focuses on the salient inclusionary criteria in each of the models, all identification models stipulate that LD classification should be based on a comprehensive evaluation of other relevant factors beyond these inclusionary criteria (i.e., exclusionary factors). We point this out because proponents (e.g., Hale et al., 2010) of various methods frequently invoke the term *comprehensive assessment* to suggest that the use of particular types of assessments (i.e., neuropsychological measures) may be required by existing codes and guidelines, even though this may not actually be the case (Zirkel, 2013). When considering whether to add a new test to a preferred battery, it is important for practitioners to consider the incremental validity associated with the use of that instrument in clinical practice. More testing does not always result in improved decision making and may in some circumstances actually create a dilution effect in which aggregate validity is lowered (Kraemer, 1992).

Ability–Achievement Discrepancy

The discrepancy method is based on the logic of cognitive referencing, in which a child's IQ is used as a benchmark for achievement. When measured achievement deviates significantly from measured IQ, this underachievement is thought to be unexpected. As the federal regulations do not specify a preferred discrepancy formula, numerous variations of this model have been employed. Most jurisdictions employ a "simple-difference" standard score comparison, in which a discrepancy is considered severe only if the difference between IQ and achievement meets or exceeds an a priori cutoff point or threshold. Most existing simple-difference thresholds range from one to two standard deviations (15–30 standard score points). For example, in a state that utilizes a 1.5 standard deviation cutoff point (22.5 points), a child with an IQ score of 100 would have to obtain an achievement score ≤ 77 in order to have a severe discrepancy.

Other methods that have been employed include expectancy formulas (based on chronological age) and regression-based formulas that seek to control for regression to the mean. Using the regression method, a critical value is established between two scores, and the observed discrepancy must be greater than this value in order to be considered severe. According to Reynolds (1984–1985), the latter is the most psychometrically defensible method, but it is not commonly utilized by practitioners due to its computational complexity. Whereas in the majority of states employing the discrepancy model, a severe discrepancy alone represents the de facto inclusionary criteria for LD eligibility, a handful of states also require examiners to furnish evidence of a concomitant deficit in cognitive processing.

Strengths of the Discrepancy Model

The discrepancy model has several strengths. Most notably, it is the easiest of the three methods to implement, and it aligns well with the idea that LD is marked by unexpected underachievement. Among existing models, it most closely approximates an actuarial model in which the effects of clinical judgment are minimized and decision making *should be* relatively consistent across practitioners and jurisdictions in which the same formula is employed (Canivez, 2013).

Weaknesses of the Discrepancy Model

In addition to the issues that were raised previously, additional measurement issues have been raised about the method. Before proceeding, it is important to point out that all of the cognitive and achievement attributes that are commonly assessed as part of a comprehensive evaluation appear normally distributed, representing continua with no natural demarcations. In the discrepancy model, these attributes are reduced to categorical (yes–no) classifications. The problems with artificially dichotomizing continuous data have long been known (MacCallum, Zang, Preacher, & Rucker, 2002). In particular, decision error (i.e., diagnostic misses) will likely be exacerbated around the cutoff point due to the fact that we are unable to measure these attributes without error. Even though discrepancy models require practitioners to interpret observed differences as "point" estimates, traditional norm-referenced tests may not be capable of measuring attributes with that level of precision (Beaujean et al., 2018).

Whenever scores are positively correlated (which is almost always the case with IQ and achievement), the discrepancy between those scores will always be *less* reliable than its reference scores. If the confidence band associated with a discrepancy score straddles a diagnostic threshold, the likelihood of *actually* meeting or not meeting discrepancy criteria is relatively equivalent. Not surprisingly, in a longitudinal study of the reliability of LD classification using the discrepancy method, Francis and colleagues (2005) found that 30% of the children in the LD and non-LD groups changed group membership between grades 3 and 5 as a function of being reassessed. Put simply, many examinees who present with a severe discrepancy at Time 1 may not maintain the discrepancy when assessed again at Time 2 due to factors (e.g., measurement error, test selection[3]) not having to do with actual individual differences.

Furthermore, studies indicate that a severe discrepancy only accounts for approximately 1–2% of the variance in treatment response (e.g., Stuebing, Barth, Molfese, Weiss, & Fletcher, 2009) and that it disproportionally favors individuals with higher IQs as an artifact of regression to the mean. There has also been significant concern about the lack of decision-making consistency within and between jurisdictions (Peterson & Shinn, 2002). As a consequence, Wilson (1987) concludes that the discrepancy model represents an "atheoreti-

cal, psychologically uninformed solution to the problem of LD classification" (p. 28). Even so, the method continues to be widely used in clinical and educational settings, and epidemiological studies indicate that the vast majority of individuals diagnosed with LD are likely identified using some variation of this method (McDermott, Goldberg, Watkins, Stanley, & Glutting, 2006).

Processing Strengths and Weaknesses

In contrast to the IQ–achievement discrepancy model, which places greater importance on the interpretation of an individual's FSIQ score, an emerging class of LD identification models focuses more on inspecting the variability and scatter among cognitive scores in order to make inferences about the PSWs that are thought to underlie LD, and it is thought that LD subtypes can be distinguished by these unique score patterns. This approach to LD identification is broadly referred to as patterns of PSWs.

To date, several models have been proposed that attempt to operationalize PSW, including (1) the concordance/discordance model (C/DM; Hale & Fiorello, 2004), (2) the dual-discrepancy/consistency model (DD/C; Flanagan et al., 2018), and (3) the discrepancy/consistency model (D/CM; Naglieri, 2011). Although they have different theoretical orientations and employ different criteria to identify PSWs, all three models apply the same fundamental logic for identifying a confirmatory PSW pattern in assessment data; that is, in order to confirm LD, there must be evidence of cognitive and academic weaknesses in the presence of otherwise spared abilities, and the cognitive weakness should be linked theoretically[4] to the area of academic concern.

Concordance/Discordance Model

The C/DM approach suggests that LD is demonstrated by an exclusive pattern of concordant (consistent performance with a reference variable) and discordant (inconsistent performance with a reference variable) in an ability profile. Potential concordances and discordances are determined to be statistically significant if they exceed critical

---

[3]In our experience, it does not take long for skilled practitioners to become adept at selecting instruments and/or scores as the focal point of discrepancy analyses that are more likely or not to yield a severe discrepancy depending on which outcome is preferred. For example, practitioners are frequently taught to "invalidate" the FSIQ score when an examinee presents with significant variability in his or her cognitive profile. Although this practice is popular, its validity has been questioned (see McGill, 2016).

---

[4]The decision about whether a particular cognitive weakness meets this standard is based largely on the clinical judgment of the assessor. Recent attempts to operationalize these procedures are based largely on qualitative interpretations of the professional literature.

values obtained using the standard error of the difference (SE_d) formula (see Hale, Wycoff, & Fiorello, 2011, for a demonstration). The C/DM is one of the few PSW models that explicitly endorses use of a statistical approach for evaluating pairwise discrepancies. To facilitate these comparisons, users are encouraged to select subtests and/or composite scores from different batteries that are most likely to yield beneficial information based on the referral concern. When a confirmatory PSW pattern is observed in these data, examiners must cross-validate that finding with additional sources of information (i.e., records reviews, observations) to ensure that the assessment has ecological validity. This notion is stressed in every approach to PSW assessment. Although these types of default statements imply that a confirmatory PSW pattern, in and of itself, is not diagnostic, it is important to note that the presence of a unique PSW represents the de facto inclusionary criteria for the method.

Discrepancy/Consistency Model

It can be argued that the D/CM model, first described by Naglieri (1999), was the first systematic PSW model to be proposed in the professional literature. The D/CM utilizes the same conceptual approach as C/DM to examine profile variability for the presence of LD; however, it employs different criteria to identify a cognitive weakness. According to Naglieri (2011), dual criteria are applied to determine whether the score reflects a legitimate cognitive weakness: The score must be both a relative weakness (via ipsative analysis) and a normative weakness (e.g., standard score < 90). If a child presents with a cognitive weakness that is related to an achievement weakness in the presence of otherwise spared abilities, this may be regarded as a confirmatory PSW pattern. Although most descriptions of the D/CM have illustrated its application using various iterations of the cognitive assessment system, the method can be applied to any cognitive tests. In contrast to other methods, the D/CM is designed primarily to be applied to scores obtained from the same test battery.

Dual-Discrepancy Consistency Model

The DD/C (Flanagan et al., 2018) was originally proposed in the XBA literature but is conceptually different from that approach. The DD/C uses the CHC model as a theoretical foundation for creating an operational definition for LD. Clinicians are encouraged to administer cognitive measures that correspond with the broad abilities posited in the CHC model, then compare those scores to scores obtained from a norm-referenced test of achievement. SLD identification using the DD/C requires users to (1) identify an academic weakness, (2) determine that the academic weakness is not primarily due to exclusionary factors, (3) identify a cognitive weakness, and (4) determine whether a student displays a confirmatory PSW consistent with several criteria specific to the DD/C model (see Flanagan et al., 2018, for an in-depth description of these criteria). Although normative cutoffs (e.g., standard score < 90) have been provided in the DD/C literature, clinicians may use professional judgment in determining whether a child manifests a relevant weakness in cognition or achievement.

To aid decision making, Flanagan, Ortiz, and Alfonso (2017) have developed a cross-battery assessment software system (X-BASS) that contains a PSW score analyzer inspired by XBA/CHC theory. It should be noted that the software requires that users input scores for all of the consensus broad ability factors in CHC theory. As a result, clinicians favoring a test other than the WJ will likely have to administer measures from other tests in order to utilize the program. Whereas the DD/C approach is presently the most commonly referenced PSW method in the professional literature, it remains unclear to what degree users *actually* adhere to the operational procedures described in DD/C materials (Beaujean et al., 2018).

Strengths of the PSW Model

Before proceeding, we must acknowledge that any discussion regarding PSWs associated with the PSW model should be interpreted as speculative, as this is a relatively new method of LD identification, and empirical data for its potential efficacy have only recently began to accumulate. Proponents of these methods point to studies showing the differential predictive effects of cognitive abilities for achievement across the lifespan (e.g., Cormier, Bulut, McGrew, & Singh, 2017; McGrew & Wendling, 2010) and that groups formed using PSW approaches have statistically significant means differences on scores (e.g., Feifer, Nader, Flanagan, Fitzer, & Hicks, 2014). The latter form of evidence has been interpreted as indicating that PSW may be useful in isolating and amplifying various LD subtypes. However, Miciak and colleagues (2014) note that "evidence for the existence of distinct disability subtypes is not *ipso facto* evidence for the reliability, validity, or utility of PSW methods for LD identification" (p. 23).

Additionally, as compared to the traditional discrepancy model, there is a greater focus on prevention and using assessment data for intervention. As an example, all of the PSW models that we have described assume that each child has been the recipient of preventive interventions (i.e., RTI) prior to being referred for a comprehensive evaluation. In this way, these models may be regarded as *hybrid* or "third-method" approaches, as they seek to marry elements of RTI and PSW, and it is suggested that assessment data generated from both approaches can be used as part of a comprehensive assessment to determine whether a child has LD (Flanagan, Fiorello, & Ortiz, 2010).

Potential Weaknesses of the PSW Model

At face value, it may appear that these models provide users with the best of both worlds; however, they have been the subject of considerable research criticism. In a review, McGill and colleagues (2016) identified several concerns with the PSW method. Specifically, (1) cognitive weaknesses are ill-defined, and their identification is not consistent across the models; (2) there is presently limited evidence for PSW diagnostic utility; (3) scores that are the focal point of PSW analyses may not be suitable for individual decision making; and (4) it remains unclear whether psychologists have adequate training to implement these assessment procedures with integrity given prior integrity concerns with less complex approaches such as the discrepancy model. Available research has largely supported these concerns.

In a simulation study, Stuebing, Fletcher, Branum-Martin, and Francis (2012) evaluated the technical adequacy of three PSW methods and found that all three methods were very good at identifying "not-LD" but had low to moderate sensitivity and very low positive predictive values indicating that the methods were not very good at identifying LD as defined in the simulations. These findings were replicated in a more recent investigation by Kranzler and colleagues (2016a), who reported diagnostic efficiency statistics associated with the application of DD/C procedures to assessment data for 900 participants in the WJ-III normative sample. Consistent with DD/C parameters, a true positive was indicated when participants had an academic weakness, and a predicted cognitive weakness also occurred in the presence of average or better general ability. Prevalence

rates for SLD, as defined in the study, ranged from 0 to 7% depending on the target area of cognitive weakness. Mean specificity and negative predictive values were 92 and 89% across CHC cognitive abilities and achievement domains, indicating that the absence of a cognitive weakness was very accurate in detecting what they deemed to be "true negatives" (individuals without an achievement weakness). On the other hand, sensitivity and positive predictive value (PPV) estimates (21 and 34%, respectively) were quite low, indicating that the presence of a cognitive weakness may not be very useful at accurately identifying what they classified as "true positives."

Of additional concern, diagnostic decisions based on PSW assessment appear to be highly unstable, and the reliability of decisions appears to worsen as more assessment data are gathered (Taylor, Miciak, Fletcher, & Francis, 2017). These findings seem to counter one of the core axioms of psychological assessment that additional information about a client helps to reduce uncertainty. As we mentioned previously, additional information is only useful when it is not redundant. Furthermore, overlap between the methods has been found to be low, and classification agreement may be impacted by nontrivial factors such as test selection (Miciak, Taylor, Denton, & Fletcher, 2015), model choice (Miciak et al., 2014), and the arbitrary use of cutoff points (McGill et al., 2016). Even so, proponents of these methods suggest that these studies merely illustrate a mechanistic approach to decision making and fail to take into account that "other data gathered through multiple methods and multiple sources need to be considered and must corroborate any conclusions that are drawn from the PSW analyses" (Flanagan & Alfonso, 2017, p. 488). Despite the intuitive appeal of such declarative statements, it remains unclear what these *other* data sources are or how practitioners should weight various pieces of information they encounter in the data gathering process. Although clinicians often claim to base conclusions on the complex integration of most or all of available data, studies emanating out of the decision science literature have consistently indicated that individuals often overweigh nondiagnostic information and have difficulty accounting for interactions in as little as two or three pieces of information during the decision-making process (e.g., Faust, 1989; Nisbett, Zukier, & Lemley, 1981). As a consequence, it is difficult to envision the psychometric shortcomings of PSW analyses being overcome by additional data collection alone.

As we mentioned previously, it is important to realize that, at its heart, the PSW method may very well be a reparameterization of the discrepancy model; that is, a confirmatory pattern in many of the models requires users to identify whether there are significant differences (i.e., discrepancies) between cognitive–achievement scores. Except, instead of evaluating one pairwise comparison (IQ–achievement), users are required to appraise multiple pairwise comparisons simultaneously, which may result in inflated Type I decision error. Thus, the measurement issues associated with the discrepancy model are likely to be exacerbated. Whereas PSW proponents (e.g., Hale et al., 2011) raise these concerns when discussing rival models, their potential implications for PSW decision making are rarely discussed.

To be fair, some PSW models do not employ traditional discrepancy procedures and instead adopt ad hoc cutoff points for determining what constitutes a cognitive–achievement weakness. Typically, suggested thresholds are derived on a normative basis wherein a standard score ≤ 85 or 90 indicates the presence of a cognitive or achievement weakness. According to Streiner (2002), dichotomizing a continuous variable results in lost information

and increased probability of decision error regardless of where the cutoff point is imposed. Figure 14.1 illustrates the logic of cutoff point analyses in the PSW model using simulated test scores for a hypothetical cognitive and achievement score. As can be seen in the figure, many hundreds of cases cluster together right at the intersection of the cutoff point threshold (< 85) for both tests. Similar to the issues we discussed when describing the issues with cutoff points associated with the discrepancy model, the corresponding confidence intervals associated with scores that reside right around a cutoff point are likely to contain values that fall above and below the threshold. In this scenario, it is incredibly difficult for a practitioner to validly determine whether a patient is a true positive (lower left-hand quadrant) or a true negative case (all other quadrants) as posited by the PSW model.

Although it is often suggested that PSW assessment may be useful for treatment planning, these claims run counter to a long-standing body of empirical evidence that calls into question the utility of ATI prescriptions (Fletcher & Miciak, 2017). For example, in a meta-analysis, Burns and colleagues (2016) found that the effect sizes associated with

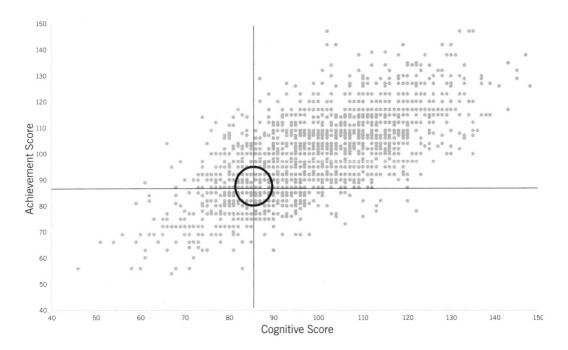

FIGURE 14.1. Probability nomogram used to combine prior probability (i.e., base rate [15%]) with the likelihood ratio (+3.13) to estimate revised posterior probability (37%). Using the clinical decision-making guidelines outline in Youngstrom and Van Meter (2013), additional assessment is needed to provide focused targets for LD.

academic interventions guided by cognitive data were mostly small, with only the effects associated with interventions informed by phonological awareness providing moderate treatment effects. As a result, they concluded that "the current and previous data indicate that measures of cognitive abilities have little to no utility in screening or planning interventions for reading and mathematics" (p. 37). It should be noted that even those who support the use of these methods have begun to acknowledge discrepancies between the laudatory ATI rhetoric and available research evidence. To wit, Schneider and Kaufman (2017, p. 8) asserted, "After rereading dozens of papers defending such assertions, including our own, we can say that this position is mostly backed by rhetoric in which assertions are backed by citations of other scholars making assertions backed by citations of still other scholars making assertions."

In summation, it remains to be seen whether PSW implementation represents a legitimate step forward for identification and treatment. Although billed as new and revolutionary, these models rely on the use of profile analytic logic that has considerable psychometric limitations. According to Fletcher and colleagues (2013) "It is ironic that methods of this sort continue to be proposed when the basic psychometric issues are well understood and have been documented for many years" (p. 40). Unfortunately, this body of literature is *rarely* cited by proponents of these methods, a practice that should cause concern in an era of psychological science that stresses evidence-based practice. As a result, practitioners are encouraged to carefully consider the value of the information yielded by these assessment practices relative to the costs in time and resources associated with their adoption costs (Williams & Miciak, 2018). Although PSW is described as a "research-based" method, compelling evidence that a confirmatory PSW pattern is necessary for the diagnosis or treatment of LD is presently lacking (Kranzler et al., 2016b; Miciak, Taylor, Stuebing, & Fletcher, 2018).

Response to Intervention

It is somewhat difficult to define RTI as a method for LD identification, as RTI represents a prevention and intervention framework and not an assessment model per se. However, due to revisions in the federal regulations in 2006, RTI has become synonymous with LD identification in the professional literature (Burns, Jacob, & Wagner, 2008).

RTI is an umbrella term that generally refers to three tiers of increasingly intense instruction, using ongoing progress monitoring to evaluate treatment response and movement between the tiers. Tier 1 represents instruction in the general education classroom. It is assumed that if instruction is effective, then this will benefit the overwhelming majority of children. Tier 2 involves providing supplemental instruction to children who do not benefit from the general education curriculum at Tier 1. This represents the first attempt to remediate academic dysfunction and usually involves some type of evidence-based group or individualized treatment. Tier 3 can differ significantly across models and may represent providing a child with a more intensive intervention in comparison to that provided at Tier 2 (i.e., higher dose, targeted individualized treatment based on further assessment) or a referral for a comprehensive evaluation. The core tenets of RTI are providing evidence-based instruction with fidelity and monitoring treatment progress frequently using low-inference assessment tools such as CBM. As such, even though classification may be a terminal outcome of an RTI model, it is not an explicit goal of the framework.

Whether implicated once a child reaches Tier 3, or after he or she has not benefited from the intervention(s) employed at that tier, a comprehensive evaluation typically includes multiple measures to supplement available RTI intervention data (i.e., CBM). These assessments may include a norm-referenced test of achievement to further validate the presence of low achievement, behavioral rating scales, direct behavioral observations, and/or a diagnostic interview to rule out exclusionary factors or provide information that is relevant for differential diagnosis. Thus, classification in the RTI model is not based solely on treatment outcome data. However, this information can be important for establishing that a child's rate and level of learning falls below expected level of performance.

Fuchs and Fuchs (1998) describe what is referred to as a dual-discrepancy identification model in which LD is characterized by concomitant deficits in learning rate (i.e., slope) and level (i.e., below average performance on a norm-referenced test of achievement). "Low achievement" models (e.g., Dombrowksi, Kamphaus, & Reynolds, 2004), in which LD is marked by deficient achievement across multiple measures, may also be applied within the context of an RTI classification model.

In contrast to cognitive discrepancy models, unexpected underachievement is documented by the presence of spared achievement indicating that the area(s) of deficit are focal in nature. Cognitive testing is typically deemphasized in RTI, although it may be used to rule out intellectual disability or to assess areas of cognitive processing that have been linked to beneficial treatment outcomes (i.e., phonological awareness).

Strengths of the RTI Model

As we discussed previously, the RTI model is a direct response to the perceived shortcomings of the traditional discrepancy method. In particular, the explicit focus on prevention illustrates well that a child no longer has to "wait to fail" in order to receive intervention. Although RTI methods may require a profound shift in how psychologists conceptualize and assess LD, surveys indicate that clinicians prefer it to the discrepancy method (O'Donnell & Miller, 2011). Thus, there is evidence of social validity among practitioners in areas in which it has been implemented.

Although "true LD" is a somewhat amorphous construct in RTI because eligibility is not based on previously accepted inclusionary criteria (i.e., discrepancy, processing deficit), prevalence studies suggest that the model may be useful in identifying a subset of children that are likely to be LD. Speece and Case (2001) evaluated the technical adequacy of several LD identification methods and found that use of a dual-discrepancy CBM approach identified 8% of the population before Tier 2 intervention, which is close to the ~5–10% estimated rate of LD. The results have been replicated by Fuchs and colleagues (2005), who found similar estimates in a rare RTI model for math intervention. Relatedly, Fuchs, Compton, Fuchs, and Bryant (2008) found that the CBM assessments commonly used in RTI had adequate sensitivity and specificity for determining future disability status in 252 children evaluated in first grade. Additionally, there is also some evidence to indicate that RTI may be useful at reducing disproportionality in LD classification (VanDerHeyden, Witt, & Gilbertson, 2007), a major concern that was expressed in the 2001 LD Summit.

Weaknesses of the RTI Model

In spite of the many positives associated with the model, Kavale and colleagues (2008) warn that there may be a rhetoric of self-congratulation in the RTI literature regarding its use as a classification method. One of the major factors complicating its use in this context is the fact that classification is essentially conferred by default as a result of poor treatment outcomes, and little consideration is given to the underlying etiology of the disorder. Group studies indicate that individuals with LDs have large cognitive processing deficits compared to normal controls (Johnson, Humphrey, Mellard, Woods, & Swanson, 2010). Although, the implications of these findings have been difficult to translate into practice, Fuchs, Hale, and Kearns (2011) suggest that even if one supports the preventive mission of RTI, it is difficult to argue against the notion that it may be necessary for practitioners to go beyond RTI data, including the careful use of cognitive measures.

Additionally, Reynolds and Shaywitz (2009) suggest that a rigid application of RTI, in which children at-risk for LD are required to progress linearly through various tiers of instruction that may be of dubious quality, seemingly shifts the process of LD identification from a "wait to fail" to a "watch them fail" approach. Emerging research on the efficacy of RTI assessment and intervention methods seems to support this notion. In an RTI efficacy study, Compton and colleagues (2012) found that, among 129 first grade children who were unresponsive to Tier 1 instruction, chronic nonresponders (i.e., children who failed to respond to instruction at Tiers 1 and 2) could be identified from Tier 1 data alone. These results suggest that a different approach to RTI assessment may be necessary to avoid prolonged periods of failure.

Burns and colleagues (2008) have identified a series of threats to valid RTI practice, including but not limited to (1) the lack of established research-based interventions for diverse groups and academic domains; (2) uncertainty about when a comprehensive assessment is warranted; (3) difficulty translating implementation science to conventional school settings; and (4) inadequate training and fidelity. As a result of these threats, it is not surprising that a recent large-scale Institute of Educational Sciences (IES) outcome study (Balu et al., 2015), purporting to evaluate the effectiveness of RTI models, found that assignment to a targeted intervention in Tiers 2 or 3 had little effect on reading performance in elementary schools nationwide and, in some cases, the intervention outcomes were contraindicated (i.e., students' performance worsened in response to treatment).

Summary

Prominent LD identification methods (discrepancy, PSW, RTI) provide different conceptualizations of LD, employ different assessment procedures, and possess different strengths as well as limitations relative to rival methods. As should be evident, model selection is not arbitrary, as different models will likely identify different subsets of children who present with academic difficulties. Similar to the previous edition of this chapter, LD assessment remains a subjective exercise in clinical judgment; regardless of the method used, clinicians do not appear to consistently employ or adhere to extant identification criteria.

In a relatively recent study, Maki, Burns, and Sullivan (2017) evaluated the consistency of practitioners in rendering LD classifications using a series of vignettes representing the three major classification approaches. No differences between the methods were found, but overall consistency was low. In an interesting follow-up to that study, Maki and colleagues (2018) found that diagnostic (over)confidence may be an important moderator variable within these results. In a survey of 376 school psychologists, practitioners who reported moderate levels of confidence produced less consistent decisions with ambiguous assessment data than clinicians who reported being "not very confident" in their appraisals. We would argue that part of the problem is that the data (i.e., cognitive test scores) used to render these types of judgments contain measurement error that will likely degrade any decisions-making model in which these data are the primary focus of clinical interpretation. In confronting this reality, it is important for practitioners not to fall prey to what Lilienfeld, Wood, and Garb (2006) term the *alchemist's fantasy*— the belief that powers of intuition enable them to transform questionable test scores into clinical gold.

As a result of these limitations, the search for a "gold standard" method for LD identification remains elusive. Even so, we are mindful that many clinicians practice in jurisdictions where they may be compelled to engage in one particular method or another. Thus, "saying no" to methods that have been shown to be problematic (e.g., cognitive discrepancy methods) simply is not an option. In these circumstances, we gently remind practitioners of their responsibility to fully disclose the potential limitations of various assessment methods as part of their informed consent mandate.

Current Issues with LD Assessment

Other difficulties for assessment are the lack of a diagnostic "gold standard" for LD, which complicates any attempt to validate proposed identification frameworks. Additional psychometric and conceptual concerns include issues that have been raised about some of the scores that are the focal point of clinical interpretation in many diagnostic schemes, as well as potential conflicts of interest that pervade the field. We next provide a brief overview of these factors.

Lack of a Diagnostic "Gold Standard"

Presently, there is no diagnostic "gold standard" for LD, which makes translating LD assessment research to clinical settings difficult. As an example, although diagnostic validity studies of various PSW permutations have consistently furnished negative results, the lack of a "gold standard" means that there is no way to truly know the rate at which the method may or may not accurately identify true LD. Thus, at best, these studies should only be regarded as a sort of "best guess" for the potential utility of the method.

In a review of LD research published from 2001 to 2013, Williams, Miciak, McFarland, and Wexler (2016) found that identification varied widely and nearly one-third of all studies investigating LD failed to describe how the participants were identified, illustrating well that LD identification remains ill-defined. According to Meehl (1978), substantive theory building from an open concept is conceptually difficult because, by definition, the boundary conditions for the construct have not been established; thus, it is difficult to articulate the conditions necessary for knowledge claims about it to be falsified. Apropos, Kranzler and colleagues (2016b) raise this very concern with respect to the DD/C model and encourage practitioners to view these methods with skepticism until additional empirical evidence is furnished to support its use.

Validity of Scores from Commercial Ability Tests

Validation of commercial ability measures involves consideration of evidence on test content, internal structure (i.e., structural validity), and relations with other measures. Whereas each of these elements is important in its own right, structural validity is especially important because it provides the theoretical and statistical rational for the scores that are provided to users. For example, if a factor that is thought to measure a particular cognitive ability (e.g., long-term memory) is not located by a factor analysis, the score representing that construct may be illusory. Factor validity is a foundational validity measure and supports all other attempts at establishing construct validity.

Since 2000, a body of independent factor analytic research has emerged raising concerns about the integrity of many of the structures and interpretive models promoted by the publishers of commonly used intelligence tests (Canivez, 2013). In some cases, these discrepancies are small and involve only one or two factors (e.g., Canivez, Watkins, & Dombrowski, 2017; McGill & Dombrowksi, 2018); in other cases, whole aspects of the posited structure cannot be replicated (e.g., Canivez, 2008; Dombrowski, McGill, & Canivez, 2018).

Even when posited dimensions can be located, these indices often contain insufficient unique variance for confidant clinical interpretation and mostly reflect systematic variance that is attributable to g. As a result, many broad ability scores and composites may lack the requisite incremental validity to predict meaningful achievement outcomes beyond g (Canivez, 2013). These results are not unique to any particular instrument, and virtually every current ability measure has been implicated by these analyses. As structural and incremental validity have important implications for the potential clinical utility of scores, these results challenge the interpretive foundations of identification models that rely predominantly on the clinical interpretation of subscale scores (i.e., PSW). To date, proponents of these methods (e.g., Decker, Hale, & Flanagan, 2013) have yet to demonstrate a method by which these potential psychometric limitations may be overcome when using these scores to make decisions about individuals.

Processing Assessment: Just Say "Maybe"?

The assumption that a deficit in cognitive processing underlies a LD is an idea that predates the advent of PSW and can be traced to the initial conceptualization of the current federal definition of SLD. Nevertheless, many PSW guidebooks and interpretive manuals encourage practitioners to engage in elaborate processing assessment procedures and speculate about the potential linkages between cognitive processing and achievement. For example, in the Ventura County PSW manual (Ventura County SELPA, 2017), users are provided a matrix of cognitive–achievement relationships to help facilitate the identification of confirmatory PSW patterns in assessment data. The strength of these relationships are evaluated on a 5-point scale after appraising the "research base of processing-achievement relations" (p. B8). In that document, it is suggested that long-term storage and retrieval (Glr) is one of the strongest predictors (4; highest rating) for mathematics achievement. However, the results furnished in a recent study did not support this claim; McGill, Conoyer, and Fefer (2018) employed elements of the evidence-based assessment framework to shed insight on how well a processing weakness (< 85) in Glr discriminated between individuals with and without achievement weaknesses in mathematics using data from the KABC-II normative sample.

Results indicate that individual decisions based on the Glr and mathematics linkage posited in the Ventura County PSW manual are likely specious. The true positive rate (sensitivity) was .381 and the true negative rate (specificity) was .888. Positive predictive power was .394 and negative predictive power was .882, indicating that the presence of a processing weakness in Glr functions below chance as a potential rule-in test of an achievement weakness in math. Accordingly, the diagnostic odds ratio for a positive test (+3.40) falls well below recommended guidelines for a quality diagnostic indicator (Streiner, 2003). An AUC value of .634 was found, indicating that this particular PSW pattern has relatively low classification accuracy overall (Youngstrom, 2014). To better understand the utility afforded by assessment procedures, Meehl (1954) encouraged clinicians to "bet the base rate" to determine whether assessment information meaningfully improves our understanding of a clinical phenomenon in comparison to conducting no assessment at all. Probability theory dictates that ~15% of the population has an academic weakness in any given area (i.e., < 85). So how much does the presence of a cognitive weakness in Glr increase the posterior probability of having an academic weakness in mathematics? The probability nomogram in Figure 14.2, produced from these data, results in a posterior probability of only 37%. This means that out of 100 cases presenting in a clinical setting with similar assessment results (evidence of processing weakness), only 37 would be expected to have an

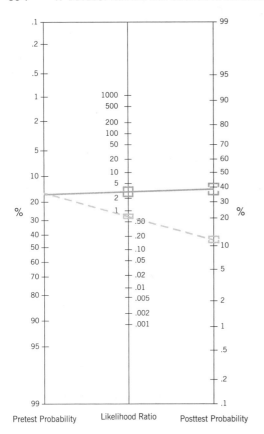

Pretest Probability   Likelihood Ratio   Posttest Probability

FIGURE 14.2. Probability nomogram used to combine prior probability (i.e., base rate [15%] of individuals assumed to have a normative weakness in achievement) with the likelihood ratio (+3.40) to estimate revised posterior probability (37%). Using the clinical decision-making guidelines outlined in Youngstrom and Van Meter (2013), additional assessment is needed to provide a focused target for LD.

academic disorder in mathematics. Whereas this is an improvement from the base rate, clearly, additional assessment data are needed in order for us to feel confident in treating this individual as having LD.

However, establishing linkages between cognitive–achievement weaknesses represents only one step in the broader PSW process. Flanagan and Schneider (2016) note that there are many *potential* reasons why cognitive deficits may not lead to academic deficits for some individuals, as "cognitive abilities are causally related to academic abilities, but the causal relationship is of moderate size, and only probabilistic, not deterministic" (p. 141).

Even so, it is difficult to regard an assessment variable as important when it predicts a relevant diagnostic outcome at lower than chance levels. Proponents of these methods must also come to terms with the fact that a specific pattern, ruling in or ruling out LD has yet to be established (Mather & Schneider, 2015). To be clear, we are not suggesting that practitioners should "just say no" to cognitive testing as a matter of course. Although we are sympathetic to the position expressed by Fuchs and colleagues (2011), we believe that available empirical evidence indicates that the use of IQ tests should be limited to ruling out exclusionary factors (i.e., intellectual disability), with additional applications related to the assessment of cognitive processing employed cautiously, if at all.

Potential Conflicts of Interest in the Assessment Literature

Over the course of the last 20 years, proponents of various methods have tended to marginalize competing frameworks, while magnifying the strengths and minimizing the weaknesses of a favored assessment approach (Dombrowski, Ambrose, & Clinton, 2007). The potential contraindicated effects of this insularity should be considered given the potential conflicts of interest that pervade assessment training and practice. For example, a nontrivial proportion of workshops where LD assessment methods are disseminated to practitioners feature authors who receive royalties from books, chapters, and commercial tests featuring the use of these methods, and the use of disclosures of conflict of interest has historically been inconsistent in clinical science (Truscott, Baumgart, & Rogers, 2004). There have been marked changes in the standards of practice in terms of disclosing conflicts of interest in medical research, publishing, and continuing medical education, and a similar move toward increased reporting and transparency is happening in other areas of psychology. Still, given these complexities, it is imperative that practitioners develop a skills set that helps them to discern between evidence-based and non-evidence-based practices.

Conclusion

As a result of the numerous psychometric and conceptual limitations that continue to plague LD identification and assessment, it is relevant to ask, "What should practitioners do?" Admittedly, this is a difficult question to answer, as there is limited empirical evidence to indicate that any of the prevailing approaches can be used to reliably and validly identify LD, and endorsing any particular approach at the expense of the anther will no doubt engender significant controversy. Accordingly, we believe that the most defensible position at the present time is to encourage practitioners and scholars to consider adopting more parsimonious assessment methods that align with DSM-5. The dual-deficit functional academic impairment (DDFAI) model described by Dombrowski and colleagues (2004) and the "hybrid" approach articu-lated by Fletcher and colleagues (2013) are model frameworks that bear further consideration. As can be seen in Table 14.2, both approaches emphasize that an academic deficit must be established using dual-deficit criteria. Whereas both approaches require that a deficit be established using conventional norm-referenced achievement tests as part of the first criterion, they differ on the process used to indicate the secondary criterion. Dombrowski and colleagues suggest that, beyond low achievement, a child must also have a *functional* impairment in academics, which can be established through measures of performance in the child's

TABLE 14.2. Classification Criteria for Alternative Hybrid Models for LD Identification

Dual-deficit functional academic impairment model (Dombrowski et al., 2004)	"Hybrid" approach (Fletcher et al., 2013)
Normative deficit: Norm-referenced academic achievement test score more than one standard deviation below the mean (below standard score of about 85 on most tests, in order to incorporate standard error of measurement).	*Low achievement:* Establish that a child has a normative deficit in achievement using a comprehensive norm-referenced achievement battery of a narrow-band measure of focal academic skills.
Functional deficit: Evidence of impairment in educational performance. Normative deficit must be corroborated by measures of performance in the academic setting, such as CBM (below the 17th percentile in child's local cohort), teacher ratings of academic performance, grades, high-stakes test scores.	*Inadequate response to instruction:* Having low achievement is singularly insufficient for determining whether a child has an LD. Low achievement merely informs us where the child is presently performing (level) but does not inform learning rate. In order to be classified as having an LD, a child must have a deficit in both level and learning rate, as evidenced through inadequate response to quality targeted instruction.
Exclusionary factors: The academic dysfunction is not primarily attributable to another DSM-5 condition that would preclude the diagnosis of LD (e.g., ADHD, intellectual disability [ID], emotional or behavioral disturbance).	*Exclusionary criteria:* Low achievement is not primarily attributable to exclusionary factors such as ID, sensory deficits, emotional disturbance, cultural and linguistic diversity, and/or lack of opportunity to learn. A comprehensive assessment must include consideration of other disabilities or environmental circumstances.
Alternative explanatory factors: According to DSM-5 and the IDEA, a number of factors could potentially exclude individuals from an LD diagnosis. However, these factors are considered to be explanatory rather than exclusionary and include, but are not limited to, cultural and linguistic diversity, lack of educational opportunity, and lack of access to quality instruction.	*Note:* The presence of a processing deficit in not required for the diagnosis of LD; however, intelligence tests may be administered to rule out ID as an exclusionary factor.
Diagnosis by age 18: LD is a developmental phenomenon that is typically diagnosed before age 18. However, an adult may be classified as having an LD if there is evidence to indicate that academic dysfunction occurred during the developmental period.	
Note: The presence of a processing deficit is not a required element for the diagnosis of LD; however, intelligence tests may be administered to rule out ID as an exclusionary factor.	

Note. In both approaches, nothing precludes a clinician from conducting additional assessment to rule out rival hypotheses about why a child's learning is not adequate. For example, if ADHD is expected, a comprehensive assessment may include broad- and narrow-band rating scales or direct assessments of behaviors of interest.

academic setting (i.e., grades, test scores). Alternatively, the hybrid approach suggested by Fletcher and colleagues requires evidence specifically of inadequate response to instruction. Whereas RTI could be used to establish a functional impairment in the DDFAI approach, it is not required. Aside from this difference, both approaches are similar in that once the dual criteria for academic impairment have been met, the goal of the comprehensive assessment is to rule out rival hypotheses that might better explain why a child is not performing well academically. In this way, assessments are administered to answer specific clinical questions. For example, although cognitive testing is not required in both of these approaches, a clinician may administer an intelligence test to rule out the presence of intellectual disability when that condition is suspected. Appendix 14.2 contains a case study and sample assessment illustrating the application of the DDFAI model.

Whereas both hybrid models meet the IDEA statutory requirements for a comprehensive assessment and are consistent with the diagnostic criteria for LD in DSM-V, we realize that some clinicians may be wary of adopting these models in clinical practice because of the deemphasis on cognitive testing and the perceived value afforded by these practices. However, if the implicit goal of clinical assessment is *actually* to remedy the presenting problem, clinicians continuing to endorse classification approaches centered around cognitive testing will have to consider the present evidentiary status for these assessment practices (McGill, Dombrowski, & Canivez, 2018). As noted by Schneider and Kaufman (2017, p. 18), "It is not irrational to believe that comprehensive cognitive assessment is more beneficial than can be supported by current evidence. It is irrational to pretend that the evidence is not needed and that all is well in our field."

REFERENCES

Aaron, P. G. (1997). The impending demise of the discrepancy model. *Review of Educational Research, 67,* 461–502.

Al Otaiba, S., Wagner, R. K., & Miller, B. (2014). "Waiting to fail" redux: Understanding inadequate response to intervention. *Learning Disability Quarterly, 37,* 129–133.

Alfonso, V. C., & Flanagan, D. P. (Eds.). (2018). *Essentials of specific learning disability identification* (2nd ed.). Hoboken, NJ: Wiley.

American Psychiatric Association. (2013). *Diagnostic and statistical manual of mental disorders* (5th ed.). Arlington, VA: Author.

Balu, R., Zhu, P., Doolittle, F., Schiller, E., Jenkins, J., & Gersten, R. (2015). *Evaluation of response to intervention practices for elementary school reading.* Washington, DC: Institute of Education Sciences.

Bannatyne, A. (1968). Diagnosing learning disabilities and writing remedial prescriptions. *Journal of Learning Disabilities, 1,* 242–249.

Bateman, B. B. (1965). An educational view of a diagnostic approach to learning disorders. In J. Hellmuth (Ed.), *Learning disorders* (Vol. 1., pp. 219–239). Seattle, WA: Special Child.

Beaujean, A. A., Benson, N. F., McGill, R. J., & Dombrowski, S. C. (2018). A misuse of IQ scores: Using the dual discrepancy/consistency model for identifying specific learning disabilities. *Journal of Intelligence, 6*(3). [Epub ahead of print]

Benson, N., Floyd, R. G., Kranzler, J. H., Eckert, T. L., & Fefer, S. (2018, February). *Contemporary assessment practices in school psychology: National survey results.* Paper presented at the meeting of the National Association of School Psychologists, Chicago, IL.

Braden, J. P., & Ouzts, S. M. (2005). Review of Kaufman assessment battery for children. In R. A. Spies & B. S. Plake (Eds.), *The sixteenth mental measurements yearbook* (2nd ed., pp. 517–520). Lincoln, NE: Buros Center for Testing.

Bray, M. A., Kehle, T. J., & Hintze, J. M. (1998). Profile analysis with the Wechsler Scales: Why does it persist? *School Psychology International, 19,* 209–220.

Breaux, K. C., Bray, M. A., Root, M. M., & Kaufman, A. S. (2017). Introduction to the special issue and to KTEA-3 error analysis. *Journal of Psychoeducational Assessment, 35,* 4–6.

Burns, M. K., Jacob, S., & Wagner, A. R. (2008). Ethical and legal issues associated with using response-to-intervention to assess learning disabilities. *Journal of School Psychology, 46,* 263–279.

Burns, M. K., Peterson-Brown, S., Haegele, K., Rodriguez, M., Schmitt, B., . . . VanDerHeyden, A. M. (2016). Meta-analysis of academic interventions derived from neuropsychological data. *School Psychology Quarterly, 31,* 28–42.

Canivez, G. L. (2008). Orthogonal higher order factor structure of the Stanford–Binet Intelligence Scales—Fifth Edition for children and adolescents. *School Psychology Quarterly, 23,* 533–541.

Canivez, G. L. (2013). Psychometric versus actuarial interpretation of intelligence and related aptitude batteries. In D. H. Saklofske, C. R. Reynolds, & V. L. Schwean (Eds.), *The Oxford handbook of child psychological assessment* (pp. 84–112). New York: Oxford University Press.

Canivez, G. L., Watkins, M. W., & Dombrowski, S. C. (2017). Structural validity of the Wechsler Intelligence Scale for Children—Fifth Edition: Confirmatory factor analyses with the 16 primary and secondary subtests. *Psychological Assessment, 29,* 458–472.

Cavendish, W. (2013). Identification of learning disabilities: Implications of proposed DSM-5 criteria for school-based assessment. *Journal of Learning Disabilities, 46,* 52–57.

Compton, D. L., Gilbert, J. K., Jenkins, J. R., Fuchs, D., Fuchs, L. S., Cho, E., . . . Bouton, B. (2012). Accelerating chronically unresponsive children to tier 3 instruction: What level of data is necessary to ensure selection accuracy? *Journal of Learning Disabilities, 45,* 204–216.

Cormier, D. C., Bulut, O., McGrew, K. S., & Sing, D. (2017). Exploring the relations between Cattell–Horn–Carroll (CHC) cognitive abilities and mathematics achievement. *Applied Cognitive Psychology, 31,* 530–538.

Cronbach, L. J. (1975). Beyond the two disciplines of scientific psychology. *American Psychologist, 30,* 116–127.

Cronbach, L. J., & Snow, R. E. (1977). *Aptitudes and instructional methods: A handbook for research on interactions.* New York: Irvington.

Decker, S. L., Hale, J. B., & Flanagan, D. P. (2013). Professional practice issues in the assessment of cognitive functioning for educational applications. *Psychology in the Schools, 50,* 300–313.

Deno, S. L. (2003). Developments on curriculum-based measurement. *Journal of Special Education, 37,* 184–192.

Deno, S. L., Fuchs, L. S., Marston, D., & Shin, J. (2001). Using curriculum-based measurement to establish growth standards for students with learning disabilities. *School Psychology Review, 30,* 507–524.

Dombrowski, S. C., Ambrose, D., & Clinton, A. (2007). Dogmatic insularity in learning disabilities identification classification and the critical need for a philosophical analysis. *International Journal of Special Education, 22,* 2–10.

Dombrowski, S. C., & Gischlar, K. L. (2014). Ethical and empirical considerations in the identification of learning disabilities. *Journal of Applied School Psychology, 30,* 68–82.

Dombrowski, S. C., Kamphaus, R. W., & Reynolds, C. R. (2004). After the demise of the discrepancy: Proposed learning disabilities diagnostic criteria. *Professional Psychology: Research and Practice, 35,* 364–372.

Dombrowski, S. C., McGill, R. J., & Canivez, G. L. (2018). An alternative conceptualization of the theoretical structure of the WJ IV Cognitive at school age: A confirmatory factor analytic investigation. *Archives of Scientific Psychology, 6,* 1–13.

Elliott, J. G., & Resing, W. C. M. (2015). Can intelligence testing inform educational intervention for children with reading disability? *Journal of Intelligence, 3,* 137–157.

Faust, D. (1989). Data integration in legal evaluations:

Can clinicians deliver on their premises? *Behavioral Sciences and the Law, 7,* 469–483.

Feifer, S. G., Nader, R. G., Flanagan, D. P., Fitzer, K. R., & Hicks, K. (2014). Identifying specific reading subtypes for effective educational remediation. *Learning Disabilities: A Multidisciplinary Journal, 20,* 18–30.

Ferrer, E., Shaywitz, B. A., Holahan, J. M., Marchione, K., & Shaywitz, S. E. (2010). Uncoupling of reading and IQ over time: Empirical evidence for a definition of dyslexia. *Psychological Science, 21,* 93–101.

Flanagan, D. P., & Alfonso, V. C. (2017). *Essentials of WISC-V assessment.* Hoboken, NJ: Wiley.

Flanagan, D. P., Alfonso, V. C., Sy, M. C., Mascolo, J. T., McDonough, E. M., & Ortiz, S. O. (2018). Dual discrepancy/consistency operational definition of SLD: Integrating multiple data sources and multiple data gathering methods. In V. C. Alfonso & D. P. Flanagan (Eds.), *Essentials of specific learning disability identification* (2nd ed., pp. 431–476). Hoboken, NJ: Wiley.

Flanagan, D. P., Fiorello, C. A., & Ortiz, S. O. (2010). Enhancing practice through application of Cattell–Horn–Carroll theory and research: A "third-method" approach to specific learning disability identification. *Psychology in the Schools, 47,* 739–760.

Flanagan, D. P., Ortiz, S. O., & Alfonso, V. C. (2013). *Essentials of cross-battery assessment* (3rd ed.). Hoboken, NJ: Wiley.

Flanagan, D. P., Ortiz, S. O., & Alfonso, V. C. (2017). *Cross-Battery Assessment Software System 2.0 (X-BASS).* Hoboken, NJ: Wiley.

Flanagan, D. P., & Schneider, W. J. (2016). Cross-battery assessment? XBA PSW? A case of mistaken identity: A commentary on Kranzler and colleagues' "Classification agreement analysis of cross-battery assessment in the identification of specific learning disorders in children and youth." *International Journal of School and Educational Psychology, 4,* 137–145.

Fletcher, J. M., Lyon, G. R., Fuchs, L. S., & Barnes, M. A. (2019). *Learning disabilities: From identification to intervention* (2nd ed.). New York: Guilford Press.

Fletcher, J. M., & Miciak, J. (2017). Comprehensive cognitive assessments are not necessary for the identification and treatment of learning disabilities. *Archives of Clinical Neuropsychology, 32,* 2–7.

Fletcher, J. M., Stuebing, K. K., Morris, R. D., & Lyon, G. R. (2013). Classification and definition of learning disabilities: A hybrid model. In H. L. Swanson, K. R. Harris, & S. Graham (Eds.), *Handbook of learning disabilities* (2nd ed., pp. 33–50). New York: Guilford Press.

Francis, D. J., Fletcher, J. M., Stuebing, K. K., Lyon, G. R., Shaywitz, B. A., & Shaywitz, S. E. (2005). Psychometric approaches to the identification of LD: IQ and achievement scores are not sufficient. *Journal of Learning Disabilities, 38,* 98–108.

Fuchs, D., Compton, D. L., Fuchs, L. S., & Bryant, J. (2008). Making "secondary intervention" work in a three-tier responsiveness-to-intervention model:

Findings from the first-grade longitudinal reading study at the National Research Center on Learning Disabilities. *Reading and Writing: An Interdisciplinary Journal, 21,* 413–436.

Fuchs, D., Hale, J. B., & Kearns, D. M. (2011). On the importance of a cognitive processing perspective: An introduction. *Journal of Learning Disabilities, 44,* 99–104.

Fuchs, L. S., Compton, D. L., Fuchs, D., Paulsen, K., Bryant, J. D., & Hamlett, C. L. (2005). The prevention, identification, and cognitive determinants of math difficulty. *Journal of Educational Psychology, 97,* 493–513.

Fuchs, L. S., & Fuchs, D. (1998). Treatment validity: A unifying concept for reconceptualizing the identification of learning disabilities. *Learning Disabilities Research and Practice, 13,* 204–219.

Glutting, J. J., Watkins, M. W., & Youngstrom, E. A. (2003). Multifactored and cross-battery assessments: Are they worth the effort? In C. R. Reynolds & R. W. Kamphaus (Eds.), *Handbook of psychological and educational assessment of children: Intelligence aptitude, and achievement* (2nd ed., pp. 343–374). New York: Guilford Press.

Hale, J., Alfonso, V., Berninger, V., Bracken, B., Christo, C., Clark, E., . . . Yalof, J. (2010). Critical issues in response-to-intervention, comprehensive evaluation, and specific learning disabilities identification and intervention: An expert white paper consensus. *Learning Disabilities Quarterly, 33,* 223–236.

Hale, J. B., & Fiorello, C. A. (2004). *School neuropsychology: A practitioner's handbook.* New York: Guilford Press.

Hale, J. B., Kaufman, A., Naglieri, J. A., & Kavale, K. A. (2006). Implementation of IDEA: Integrating response to intervention and cognitive assessment methods. *Psychology in the Schools, 43,* 753–770.

Hale, J. B., Wycoff, K. L., & Fiorello, C. A. (2011). RTI and cognitive hypothesis testing for identification and intervention of specific learning disabilities: The best of both worlds. In D. P. Flanagan & V. C. Alfonso (Eds.), *Essentials of specific learning disability identification* (pp. 173–201). Hoboken, NJ: Wiley.

Hallahan, D. P., & Mercer, C. D. (2002). Learning disabilities: Historical perspectives. In R. Bradley, L. Danielson, & D. P. Hallahan (Eds.), *Identification of learning disabilities: Research to practice* (pp. 1–67). Mahwah, NJ: Erlbaum.

Hallahan, D. P., Pullen, P. C., & Ward, D. (2013). Brief history of the field of learning disabilities. In H. L. Swanson, K. R. Harris, & S. Graham (Eds.), *Handbook of learning disabilities* (2nd ed., pp. 15–32). New York: Guilford Press.

Hammill, D. D., & Larsen, S. C. (1974). The effectiveness of psycholinguistic training. *Exceptional Children, 41,* 429–436.

Harris, A. J., & Shakow, D. (1937). The clinical significance of numerical measures of scatter on the Stanford–Binet. *Psychological Bulletin, 34,* 134–150.

Head, H. (1926). *Aphasia and kindred disorders of speech.* London: Cambridge University Press.

Hosp, M. K., Hosp, J. L., & Howell, K. W. (2016). *The ABCs of CBM* (2nd ed.). New York: Guilford Press.

Johnson, E. S., Humphrey, M., Mellard, D. F., Woods, K., & Swanson, H. L. (2010). Cognitive processing deficits and students with specific learning disabilities: A selective meta-analysis of the literature. *Learning Disability Quarterly, 33,* 3–18.

Kaufman, A. S. (1979). *Intelligent testing with the WISC-R.* New York: Wiley.

Kaufman, A. S. (1994). *Intelligent testing with the WISC-III.* New York: Wiley.

Kaufman, A. S., & Kaufman, N. L. (2004). *Kaufman Assessment Battery for Children—Second Edition.* Circle Pines, MN: American Guidance Service.

Kaufman, A. S., & Kaufman, N. L. (2014). *Kaufman Test of Educational Achievement* (3rd ed.). San Antonio, TX: NCS Pearson.

Kaufman, A. S., & Lichtenberger, E. O. (2006). *Assessing adolescent and adult intelligence* (3rd ed.). Hoboken, NJ: Wiley.

Kaufman, A. S., Raiford, S. E., & Coalson, D. L. (2016). *Intelligent testing with the WISC-V.* Hoboken, NJ: Wiley.

Kavale, K. A., & Forness, S. R. (1984). A meta-analysis of the validity of Wechsler scale profiles and recategorizations: Patterns or parodies? *Learning Disability Quarterly, 7,* 136–156.

Kavale, K. A., Kauffman, J. M., Bachmeier, R. J., & LeFever, G. B. (2008). Response-to-intervention: Separating the rhetoric of self-congratulation from the reality of specific learning disability identification. *Learning Disability Quarterly, 31,* 135–150.

Kraemer, H. C. (1992). *Evaluating medical tests: Objective and quantitative guidelines.* Thousand Oaks, CA: SAGE.

Kranzler, J. H., Floyd, R. G., Benson, N., Zaboski, B., & Thibodaux, L. (2016a). Classification agreement analysis of cross-battery assessment in the identification of specific learning disorders in children and youth. *International Journal of School and Educational Psychology, 4,* 124–136.

Kranzler, J. H., Floyd, R. G., Benson, N., Zaboski, B., & Thibodaux, L. (2016b). Cross-battery assessment pattern of strengths and weaknesses approach to the identification of specific learning disorders: Evidence-based practice or pseudoscience? *International Journal of School and Educational Psychology, 4,* 146–157.

Kirk, S. A. (1962). *Educating exceptional children.* Boston: Houghton Mifflin.

Kirk, S. A., McCarthy, J. J., & Kirk, W. D. (1961). *Illinois Test of Psycholinguistic Abilities.* Urbana: University of Illinois Press.

Lewandowski, L. J., & Lovett, B. J. (2014). Learning disabilities. In E. J. Mash & R. A. Barkley (Eds.), *Child psychopathology* (3rd ed., pp. 625–669). New York: Guilford Press.

Lichtenstein, R. (2014). Best practices in identifying learning disabilities. In P. L. Harrison & A. Thomas (Eds.), *Best practices in school psychology: Data-based and collaborative decision making* (pp. 331–354). Bethesda, MD: National Association of School Psychologists.

Lilienfeld, S. O., Wood, J. M., & Garb, H. N. (2006). Why questionable psychological tests remain popular. *Scientific Review of Alternative Medicine, 10*, 6–15.

Luria, A. R. (1966). *Human brain and psychological processes.* New York: Harper & Row.

Lyon, G. R., Fletcher, J. M., Fuchs, L. S., & Chhabra, V. (2006). Learning disabilities. In E. J. Mash & R. A. Barkley (Eds.), *Treatment of childhood disorders* (3rd ed., pp. 512–591). New York: Guilford Press.

MacCallum, R. C., Zhang, S., Preacher, K. J., & Rucker, D. D. (2002). On the practice of dichotomization of quantitative variables. *Psychological Methods, 7,* 19–40.

Macmann, G. M., & Barnett, D. W. (1997). Myth of the master detective: Reliability of Interpretations for Kaufman's "intelligent testing" approach to the WISC-III. *School Psychology Quarterly, 12,* 197–234.

MacMillan, D. L., Gresham, F. M., & Bocian, K. M. (1998). Discrepancy between definitions of learning disabilities and school practices: An empirical investigation. *Journal of Learning Disabilities, 31,* 314–326.

Maki, K. M., Burns, M. K., & Sullivan, A. (2017). Learning disability identification consistency: The impact of methodology and student evaluation data. *School Psychology Quarterly, 32,* 254–267.

Maki, K. M., Burns, M. K., & Sullivan, A. L. (2018). School psychologists' confidence in learning disability identification decisions. *Learning Disability Quarterly, 41,* 243–256.

Maki, K. M., Floyd, R. G., & Roberson, T. (2015). State learning disability eligibility criteria: A comprehensive review. *School Psychology Quarterly, 30,* 457–469.

Mann, L. (1979). *On the trail of process.* New York: Grune & Stratton.

Mather, N., & Schneider, D. (2015). The use of intelligence tests in the diagnosis of specific reading disability. In S. Goldstein, D. Princiotta, & J. A. Naglieri (Eds.), *Handbook of intelligence: Evolutionary theory, historical perspective, and current concepts* (pp. 415–434). New York: Springer.

McDermott, P. A., Fantuzzo, J. W., & Glutting, J. J. (1990). Just say no to subtest analysis: A critique on Wechsler theory and practice. *Journal of Psychoeducational Assessment, 8,* 290–302.

McDermott, P. A., Fantuzzo, J. W., Glutting. J. J., Watkins, M. W., & Baggaley, A. R. (1992). Illusions of meaning in the ipsative assessment of children's ability. *Journal of Special Education, 25,* 504–526.

McDermott, P. A., Goldberg, M. M., Watkins, M. W., Stanley, J. L., & Glutting, J. J. (2006). A nationwide epidemiologic modeling study of LD: Risk, protection, and unintended impact. *Journal of Learning Disabilities, 39,* 230–251.

McGill, R. J. (2016). Invalidating the full scale IQ score in the presence of significant factor score variability: Clinical acumen or clinical illusion? *Archives of Assessment Psychology, 6*(1), 49–79.

McGill, R. J. (2018). Confronting the base rate problem: More ups and downs for cognitive scatter analysis. *Contemporary School Psychology, 22,* 384–393.

McGill, R. J., & Busse, R. T. (2017). When theory trumps science: A critique of the PSW model for SLD identification. *Contemporary School Psychology, 21,* 10–18.

McGill, R. J., Conoyer, S. J., & Fefer, S. (2018). Elaborating on the linkage between cognitive and academic weaknesses: Using diagnostic efficiency statistics to inform PSW assessment. *School Psychology Forum, 12,* 118–132.

McGill, R. J., & Dombrowski, S. C. (2018). Factor structure of the CHC model for the KABC-II: Exploratory factor analyses with the 16 core and supplemental subtests. *Contemporary School Psychology, 22,* 279–293.

McGill, R. J., Dombrowski, S. C., & Canivez, G. L. (2018). Cognitive profile analysis in school psychology: History, issues, and continued concerns. *Journal of School Psychology, 71,* 108–121.

McGill, R. J., Styck, K. S., Palomares, R. S., & Hass, M. R. (2016). Critical issues in specific learning disability identification: What we need to know about the PSW model. *Learning Disability Quarterly, 39,* 159–170.

McGrady, H. J. (2002). A commentary on "Empirical and Theoretical Support for Direct Diagnosis of Learning Disabilities by Assessment of Intrinsic Processing Weaknesses." In R. Bradley, L. Danielson, & D. P. Hallahan (Eds.), *Identification of learning disabilities: Research to practice* (pp. 623–651). Mahwah, NJ: Erlbaum.

McGrew, K. S., & Wendling, B. J. (2010). Cattell–Horn–Carroll cognitive–achievement relations: What we have learned from the past 20 years of research. *Psychology in the Schools, 47,* 651–675.

Meehl, P. E. (1954). *Clinical versus statistical prediction: A theoretical analysis and a review of the evidence.* Minneapolis: University of Minnesota Press.

Meehl, P. E. (1978). Theoretical risks and tabular asterisks: Sir Karl, Sir Ronald, and the slow progress of soft psychology. *Journal of Consulting and Clinical Psychology, 46,* 806–834.

Miciak, J., Fletcher, J. M., Stuebing, K. K., Vaughn, S., & Tolar, T. D. (2014). Patterns of cognitive strengths and weaknesses: Identification rates, agreement, and validity for learning disabilities identification. *School Psychology Quarterly, 29,* 21–37.

Miciak, J., Taylor, W. P., Denton, C. A., & Fletcher, J. M. (2015). The effect of achievement test selection on identification of learning disabilities within a patterns of strengths and weaknesses framework. *School Psychology Quarterly, 30,* 321–334.

Miciak, J., Taylor, W. P., Stuebing, K. K., & Fletcher, J.

M. (2018). Simulation of LD identification accuracy using a patterns of processing strengths and weaknesses method with multiple measures. *Journal of Psychoeducational Assessment, 36,* 21–33.

Moll, K., Kunze, S., Neuhoff, N., Bruder, J., & Schulte-Korne, G. (2014). Specific learning disorder: Prevalence and gender differences. *PLOS ONE, 9*(7), 1–8.

Monroe, M. (1932). *Children who cannot read.* Chicago: University of Chicago Press.

Naglieri, J. A. (1999). *Essentials of CAS assessment.* New York: Wiley.

Naglieri, J. A. (2011). The discrepancy/consistency approach to SLD identification using the PASS theory. In D. P. Flanagan & V. C. Alfonso (Eds.), *Essentials of specific learning disability identification* (pp. 145–172). Hoboken, NJ: Wiley.

Nisbett, R. E., Zukier, H., & Lemley, R. E. (1981). The dilution effect: Nondiagnostic information weakens the implications of diagnostic information. *Cognitive Psychology, 13,* 248–277.

O'Donnell, P. S., & Miller, D. N. (2011). Identifying students with specific learning disabilities: School psychologists' acceptability of the discrepancy model versus response to intervention. *Journal of Disability Policy Studies, 22,* 83–94.

Orton, S. T. (1925). "Word-blindness" in school children. *Archives of Neurology and Psychiatry, 14,* 581–615.

Pashler, H., McDaniel, M., Rohrer, D., & Bjork, R. (2008). Learning styles: Concepts and evidence. *Psychological Science in the Public Interest, 9,* 105–119.

Peterson, K. M. H., & Shinn, M. H. (2002). Severe discrepancy models: Which best explains school identification practices for learning disabilities? *School Psychology Review, 31,* 459–476.

Rapaport, D., Gil, M., & Schafer, R. (1945). *Diagnostic psychological testing: The theory, statistical evaluation, and diagnostic application of a battery of tests* (Vol. 1). Chicago: Yearbook Medical.

Restori, A. F., Gresham, F. M., & Cook, C. R. (2008). "Old habits die hard": Past and current issues pertaining to response-to-intervention. *California School Psychologist, 13,* 67–78.

Reynolds, C. R. (1984–1985). Critical measurement issues in learning disabilities. *Journal of Special Education, 18,* 451–476.

Reynolds, C. R., & Shaywitz, S. E. (2009). Response to intervention: Ready or not? Or, from wait-fail to watch-them fail. *School Psychology Quarterly, 24,* 130–145.

Riley-Tillman, T. C., & Burns, M. K. (2009). *Evaluating educational interventions: Single-case design for measuring response to intervention.* New York: Guilford Press.

Rutter, M., & Yule, W. (1975). The concept of specific reading retardation. *Journal of Child Psychology and Psychiatry, 16,* 181–197.

Schneider, W. J., & Kaufman, A. S. (2017). Let's not do away with comprehensive cognitive assessments just yet. *Archives of Clinical Neuropsychology, 32,* 8–20.

Schneider, W. J., & McGrew, K. S. (2018). The Cattell–Horn–Carroll theory of cognitive abilities. In D. P. Flanagan & E. M. McDonough (Eds.), *Contemporary intellectual assessment: Theories, tests, and issues* (4th ed., pp. 73–163). New York: Guilford Press.

Schrank, F. A., McGrew, K. S., & Mather, N. (2014). *Woodcock–Johnson IV.* Rolling Meadows, IL: Riverside.

Schrank, F. A., Stephens-Pisecco, T. L., & Schultz, E. K. (2017). *The WJ IV core-selective evaluation process applied to identification of a specific learning disability* (Woodcock–Johnson IV Assessment Service Bulletin No. 8). Itasca, IL: Houghton Mifflin/Harcourt.

Schrank, F. A., & Wendling, B. J. (2018). The Woodcock–Johnson IV: Tests of cognitive abilities, tests of oral language, tests of achievement. In D. P. Flanagan & E. M. McDonough (Eds.), *Contemporary intellectual assessment: Theories, tests, and issues* (4th ed., pp. 383–451). New York: Guilford Press.

Schroeder, M., Drefs, M. A., & Cormier, D. C. (2017). The messiness of LD identification: Contributions of diagnostic criteria and clinical judgment. *Canadian Psychology, 58,* 218–227.

Schultz, E. K., & Stephens-Pisecco, T. L. (2015). Core-Selective Evaluation Process: An efficient and comprehensive approach to identify students with SLD using the WJ IV. *The Dialog, 44*(2), 5–12.

Scruggs, T. E., & Mastropieri, M. A. (2002). On babies and bathwater: Addressing the problems of identification of learning disabilities. *Learning Disability Quarterly, 25,* 155–168.

Shaywitz, S. E., Escobar, M. D., Shaywitz, B. A., Fletcher, J. M., & Makuch, R. (1992). Evidence that dyslexia may represent the lower tail of a normal distribution of reading ability. *New England Journal of Medicine, 326,* 145–150.

Smith, C. B., & Watkins, M. W. (2004). Diagnostic utility of the Bannatyne WISC-III pattern. *Learning Disabilities Research and Practice, 19,* 49–56.

Sotelo-Dynega, M., & Dixon, S. G. (2014). Cognitive assessment practices: A survey of school psychologists. *Psychology in the Schools, 51,* 1031–1045.

Speece, D. L., & Case, L. P. (2001). Classification in context: An alternative approach to identifying early reading disability. *Journal of Educational Psychology, 93,* 735–749.

Stephens-Pisecco, T. L., & Schultz, E. K. (2019). *Core-Selective Evaluation Process (C-SEP): Overview and procedures.* Unpublished manuscript.

Streiner, D. L. (2002). Breaking up is hard to do: The heartbreak of dichotomizing continuous data. *Canadian Journal of Psychiatry, 47,* 262–266.

Streiner, D. L. (2003). Diagnosing tests: Using and misusing diagnostic and screening tests. *Journal of Personality Assessment, 81,* 209–219.

Stuebing, K. K., Barth, A. E., Molfese, P. J., Weiss, B., & Fletcher, J. M. (2009). IQ is not strongly related to response to reading instruction: A meta-analytic interpretation. *Exceptional Children, 76*, 31–51.

Stuebing, K. K., Fletcher, J. M., Branum-Martin, L., & Francis, D. J. (2012). Evaluation of the technical adequacy of three methods for identifying specific learning disabilities based on cognitive discrepancies. *School Psychology Review, 41*, 3–22.

Stuebing, K. K., Fletcher, J. M., LeDoux, J. M., Lyon, G. R., Shaywitz, S. E., & Shaywitz, B. A. (2002). Validity of IQ-discrepancy classifications of reading disabilities: A meta-analysis. *American Educational Research Journal, 39*, 469–518.

Taylor, W. P., Miciak, J., Fletcher, J. M., & Francis, D. J. (2017). Cognitive discrepancy models for specific learning disabilities identification: Simulations of psychometric limitations. *Psychological Assessment, 29*, 446–457.

Truscott, S. D., Baumgart, M. B., & Rogers, K. M. (2004). Financial conflicts of interest in the school psychology assessment literature. *School Psychology Quarterly, 19*, 166–178.

U.S. Office of Education. (1976). Proposed rulemaking. *Federal Register, 41*(230), 52404–52407.

U.S. Office of Education. (1977). Assistance to the states for education of handicapped children: Procedures for evaluating specific learning disabilities. *Federal Register, 42*(250), 65082–65085.

Van Norman, E. R., Maki, K. E., Burns, M. K., McComas, J. J., & Helman, L. (2018). Comparison of progress monitoring data from general outcome measures and specific subskill mastery measures for reading. *Journal of School Psychology, 67*, 178–189.

VanDerHeyden, A. M., Witt, J. C., & Gilbertson, D. (2007). A multi-year evaluation of the effects of a response to intervention (RTI) model on identification of children for special education. *Journal of School Psychology, 45*, 225–256.

Vellutino, F. R., Scanlon, D. M., Sipay, E. R., Small, S. G., Pratt, A., Chen, R., & Denckla, M. B. (1996). Cognitive profiles of difficult-to-remediate and readily remediated poor readers: Early intervention as a vehicle for distinguishing between cognitive and experiential deficits as basic causes of specific reading disability. *Journal of Educational Psychology, 88*, 601–638.

Ventura County SELPA. (2017). The Ventura County SELPA pattern of strengths and weaknesses model for specific learning disability eligibility procedural manual. Retrieved from *www.venturacountyselpa.com*.

Wanzek, J., Vaughn, S., Scammacca, N. K., Metz, K., Murray, C. S., Roberts, G., & Danielson, L. (2013). Extensive reading interventions for students with reading difficulties after grade 3. *Review of Education Research, 83*, 163–195.

Watkins, M. W. (2000). Cognitive profile analysis: A shared professional myth. *School Psychology Quarterly, 15*, 465–479.

Watkins, M. W. (2003). IQ subtest analysis: Clinical acumen or clinical illusion? *Scientific Review of Mental Health Practice, 2*, 118–141.

Watkins, M. W. (2005). Diagnostic validity of Wechsler subtest scatter. *Learning Disabilities: A Contemporary Journal, 3*, 20–29.

Watkins, M. W., & Canivez, G. L. (2004). Temporal stability of WISC-III subtest composite: Strengths and weaknesses. *Psychological Assessment, 16*, 133–138.

Watkins, M. W., Kush, J. C., & Glutting, J. J. (1997a). Discriminant and predictive validity of the WISC-III ACID profile among children with learning disabilities. *Psychology in the Schools, 34*, 309–319.

Watkins, M. W., Kush, J. C., & Glutting, J. J. (1997b). Prevalence and diagnostic utility of the WISC-III SCAD profile among children with disabilities. *School Psychology Quarterly, 12*, 235–248.

Watkins, M. W., Kush, J. C., & Schaefer, B. A. (2002). Diagnostic utility of the WISC-III learning disability index. *Journal of Learning Disabilities, 35*, 98–103.

Wechsler, D. (2014). *Wechsler Intelligence Scale for Children* (5th ed.). San Antonio, TX: NCS Pearson.

Williams, J., & Miciak, J. (2018). Adoption costs associated with processing strengths and weaknesses methods for learning disabilities identification. *School Psychology Forum, 12*, 17–29.

Williams, J. L., Miciak, J., McFarland, L., & Wexler, J. (2016). Learning disability identification criteria and reporting in empirical research: A review of 2001–2013. *Learning Disabilities Research and Practice, 31*, 221–229.

Wilson, V. L. (1987). Statistical and psychometric issues surrounding severe discrepancy. *Learning Disabilities Research, 3*, 24–28.

World Health Organization. (1992). *The ICD-10 classification of mental and behavioural disorders: Clinical descriptions and diagnostic guidelines.* Geneva: Author.

Youngstrom, E. A. (2014). A primer on receiver operating characteristic analysis and diagnostic efficiency statistics for pediatric psychology: We are ready to ROC. *Journal of Pediatric Psychology, 39*, 204–221.

Youngstrom, E. A., & Van Meter, A. (2016). Empirically supported assessments of children and adolescents. *Clinical Psychology: Science and Practice, 23*, 327–347.

Ysseldyke, J. E., Thurlow, M., Graden, J., Wesson, C., Algozzine, B., & Deno, S. L. (1983). Generalizations from five years of research on assessment and decision making: The University of Minnesota Institute. *Exceptional Education Quarterly, 4*(1), 75–93.

Zimmerman, I. L., & Woo-Sam, J. M. (1985). Clinical applications. In B. B. Wolman (Ed.), *Handbook of intelligence: Theories, measurements, and applications* (pp. 873–898). New York: Wiley.

Zirkel, P. A. (2013). A comprehensive evaluation of the Supreme Court's Forest Grove decision? *Journal of Psychoeducational Assessment, 31*, 313–317.

APPENDIX 14.1. Clinical Resources for Practitioners

LD Assessment and Identification Resources

National Center for Learning Disabilities (*www.ncld. org*)

Texas Center for Learning Disabilities (*www. texasldcenter.org*)

Essentials of Specific Learning Disability Identification (Alfonso & Flanagan, 2018)

Learning Disabilities: From Identification to Intervention (Fletcher, Lyon, Fuchs, & Barnes, 2019)

CBM (RTI) Assessment

Evaluating Educational Interventions: Single-Case Design for Measuring RTI (Riley-Tillman & Burns, 2009)

Dynamic Indicators of Basic Early Literacy Skills (*https://dibels.uoregon.edu*)

easyCBM (*www.easycbm.com*)

The ABCs of CBM: A Practical Guide to Curriculum-Based Measurement (Hosp, Hosp, & Howell, 2016)

APPENDIX 14.2. LD Identification Assessment Case Study

Background

Matthew Smith, an 8-year-old second-grade student, is experiencing significant reading and behavioral difficulties at school. Mathew was born prematurely at 34 weeks gestation. Background information did not reveal any immediate adverse development delays other than skipping the babbling stage preceding talking. Matthew attended a Montessori preschool, and reports from the school did not reveal academic or behavioral struggles at that time. Upon primary school entry in kindergarten, Matthew was observed to struggle with basic reading skills during early literacy development and task persistence when assigned independent work. These difficulties have persisted to the present time period. Matthew's pediatrician referred Matthew to a child psychiatrist for his struggles with attention-deficit/hyperactivity disorder (ADHD). Ms. Smith thought it was a good idea to obtain a non-school-based evaluation to address the reading difficulties prior to the meeting with the psychiatrist.

Psychological Report—Confidential

Reason for Referral

Matthew was referred for a comprehensive evaluation (1) to gain insight into his present level of functioning, (2) to ascertain diagnostic impressions, and (3) to determine treatment recommendations and accommodations that might be appropriate for him. Background information and teacher reports reveal that Matthew struggles with all aspects of reading. Specifically, Matthew experiences difficulty with word decoding, oral reading fluency, and reading comprehension. Additionally, Matthew's faces difficulties with attention, hyperactivity, and distractibility.

Assessment Methods and Sources of Data

Reynolds Intellectual Assessment Scale—Second Edition (RIAS-2)

Woodcock–Johnson Tests of Achievement—Fourth Edition (WJ-IV)

Comprehensive Test of Phonological Processing, Second Edition (CTOPP-2)

Behavior Assessment System for Children, Third Edition (BASC-3)

Child Development Questionnaire (CDQ)

ADHD Rating Scale, Fifth Edition

Teacher Interview

Parent Interview

Child Interview

Classroom Observations

Review of Academic Records

Review of School Records

Review of Pediatrician's Records

Comment: Background information reveals that there additional concerns related to attention and suspicion that Matthew may have ADHD. Therefore, additional attention rating scales have been added to the assessment battery to shed insight on potential comorbidity with LD.

Background Information and Developmental History

Matthew Smith is an 8-year-old child in the second grade at the Cherry Hill Public School District (CHPS). Matthew faces difficulty with paying attention, organization, and remaining on task. Background information also revealed difficulty with reading comprehension. Ms. Smith, Matthew's mother, indicates that Matthew has been diagnosed by his pediatrician with ADHD. Ms. Smith noted that Matthew's pediatrician offered the diagnosis based on his observation and a computerized test on which Matthew scored poorly on a measure of attention. Matthew is not presently taking any medication for the management of his symptoms, but Ms. Smith reports that he is scheduled for a psychiatric evaluation in mid-July at the ADHD Clinic within the Children's Hospital of Philadelphia. She explained that she sought this psychological evaluation to gain a better sense of Matthew's overall functioning prior to the psychiatric evaluation.

Prenatal, Perinatal, and Early Developmental History

Ms. Smith experienced gestational diabetes during her pregnancy with Matthew. Matthew was born at 34 weeks weighing 6 pounds, 5 ounces. He had a 2-week stay in the neonatal intensive care unit (NICU) for jaundice. Matthew's early developmental milestones were generally attained within normal limits, with the exception of skipping the babbling stage that precedes learning to talk. Matthew attended a Montessori school and was determined to be developing at an age-expected level with no behavioral, social, or academic concerns noted.

Medical

Ms. Smith indicated that Matthew is not currently taking any medications but suffers from occasional migraines (averaging six times per month). Matthew will be evaluated by a child psychiatrist in mid-July. Matthew's hearing and vision are intact. Ms. Smith reported no prior incidence of head injury, accident, or major infection.

Cognitive, Academic, and Language Functioning

Background information and teacher reports indicate that Matthew struggles with all aspects of reading. Ms. Smith commented that Matthew's reading is below grade level, noting that he rarely stays focused on the lesson or during independent reading time. Teacher reports confirmed difficulties with these academic areas. Background information suggests that Matthew's guided reading level is approximately two grades below where he is expected to be at this point in the school year. Background reports indicated that Matthew's mathematics progress is at grade level. Results of Matthew's state benchmark testing for last spring were as follows: reading (5th percentile), written expression (8th percentile) and mathematics (25th percentile). Ms. Jones indicated that Matthew has a good understanding of basic mathematics skills but struggles when required to sustain attention in multistep math problems. She noted that his writing progress is slightly below that of other students his age.

Comment: Teacher reports and review of academic records indicate that Matthew is presently functionally impaired in reading and that his performance in mathematics is at expected levels, indicating these deficits are specific in nature. These deficits began to occur almost immediately at the onset of early literacy instruction during kindergarten, persisted since that time during the developmental period, and have persisted for longer than 6 months (DSM-5 criteria).

Social–Emotional and Behavioral Functioning

Ms. Jones indicated that Matthew is a pleasant but active and impulsive child. Every once in a while, he becomes upset and stomps the ground, throws his pencil, or slams his book on the table. Ms. Jones explained that

he usually calms down after being redirected, but he can sulk for a long time. She noted that Matthew needs to pay attention to whole-class instruction, stay focused on independent work, keep his body under control by not bothering those around him, and listen to and follow the teacher's instructions. Ms. Jones noted that Matthew has been sent to the ReSet room numerous times, and this sometimes seems to help his behavior. Both Ms. Jones and Ms. Smith report that Matthew has many friends, but they are sometimes annoyed by his tendency to intrude into their activities, interrupt what they are saying, and avoid waiting for his turn. Both Ms. Smith and Ms. Jones are concerned that Matthew may become alienated from his peers at school.

Comment: Although there are clearly concerns with reading, it is presently unclear whether these deficits are due to LD or are a collateral deficit of Matthew's attention difficulties; it is common for children with ADHD to also present with academic deficits consistent with LD.

Strengths

Matthew's strengths include helping out around the classroom when asked by a teacher. He has also been described as a child with good artistic ability, a good sense of humor, and one who enjoys life. Matthew enjoys playing video games, soccer, and basketball.

Summary

Matthew struggles with symptoms of inattentiveness, hyperactivity, and impulsivity. He also struggles with all aspects of reading. Matthew enjoys helping in the classroom and is motivated to do well at school. He struggles with both academic and behavioral functioning at school.

Interview Results

Parent Interview

Ms. Smith was contacted to ascertain impressions of Matthew's academic, behavioral and social–emotional functioning at school. Ms. Smith commented first regarding Matthew's behavioral issues. She noted that he has been diagnosed with ADHD by his pediatrician, who suggested both psychological and psychiatric evaluations. Ms. Smith explained that the wait for the psychological evaluation at CHOP was over a year, so she sought out services for that elsewhere. Ms. Smith indicated that her concerns are "more behavioral than academic." Ms. Smith indicated that Matthew has a few instances of not listening, not controlling his body, and being put in time out from recess. She explained that Matthew is a generally kind child but struggles to control his activity level and exuberance for life. Commenting next on his social progress, Ms. Smith indicated that socially Matthew is OK but she has noticed that his friends are beginning to become frustrated by his tendency to jump into and intrude in their activities at inappropriate times. Commenting next on Matthew's academic progress, Ms. Smith noted that Matthew struggles with reading, and his handwriting can be sloppy. She discussed Matthew's areas of strengths and needs, noting that he can focus for long periods if he is interested in a topic or activity. For instance, Ms. Smith explained that Matthew can play video games for hours on end. She also indicted that Matthew likes to draw and play outside. She noted that math is one of his strengths. She also mentioned that Matthew is very athletic and loves to play all types of sports.

Child Interview

Matthew was interviewed to ascertain impressions of his overall social, emotional, and behavioral progress. Matthew stated that he enjoys school, especially science, art, and recess. When asked about his academic progress, Matthew explained that reading is sometimes difficult for him, but mathematics and writing are good. Matthew next discussed his behavior at school. He explained that he sometimes gets into trouble for "doing something bad." When asked to elaborate, Matthew indicated that he once went to the principal's office for making noises with his throat. He did not discuss any additional behavioral incidents. When asked about his mood or feelings, Matthew noted that he is generally a happy child who enjoys going outside and playing sports.

Teacher Interview

Ms. Jones, Matthew's second-grade teacher, was interviewed regarding Matthew's academic, behavioral, emotional, and social functioning. She explained that Matthew struggles with reading, and she is really concerned about this. Ms. Jones indicated that any language-based topic is difficult for Matthew. She explained that Matthew had regressed in reading this past summer and had forgotten many basic reading skills from the prior year. Ms. Jones noted that phonological skills are a problem for Matthew. She also mentioned that Matthew has low sight-word knowledge and places at the primer level. Ms. Jones explained that Matthew's writing skills are below those of his peers, but not as low as his reading abilities. She explained that Matthew can demonstrate some level of competence if a teacher is able to sit with him and coach him. Commenting on Matthew's behavioral progress, Ms. Jones noted that Matthew struggles with distractibility, remaining on task, loss of focus, and a high activity level. She explained that Matthew generally gets along with other children in the classroom, but other children have recently become frustrated by his tendency to interrupt them, to avoid waiting his turn, and to intrude into their activities. Ms. Jones noted that

Matthew is an athletic child, and this supports his social development at school. However, Ms. Jones explained that Matthew sulks when denied his own way but eventually comes around and regains his focus. She indicated that Matthew is motivated to do well in school despite his academic difficulties.

Comment: Additional corroborating information through teacher report indicates that Matthew is functionally impaired in reading.

Teacher Interview

Ms. Mia Riley, reading specialist, was asked to furnish her impressions of Matthew's progress in school. Matthew sees the reading specialist three times per week for 30 minutes. Ms. Riley indicated that Matthew is eager to learn and willing to try whatever is put in front of him; however, Matthew struggles with phonological awareness and with sight-word decoding. Ms. Riley comments that this impacts his comprehension of written text. Additionally, she stated that Matthew struggles with spelling and writing at an expected grade level, but this is not as much a concern as his reading capabilities. Ms. Riley explained that she has been working on fostering Matthew's basic understanding of phonemic awareness skills.

Comment: Clinicians in private practice settings may not have the resources to facilitate targeted interventions for children who are referred for LD evaluations and explicitly evaluate a student's response to instruction. However, many students who experience academic difficulties (especially in reading) are provided with some form of targeted assistance beyond the general education classroom, thus permitting inferences pertaining to RTI. Here we have evidence that Matthew has been provided with supplemental interventions through the reading specialist three times a week, which is roughly equivalent to a Tier 2 RTI intervention. Given the persistence of Matthew's difficulties, it is clear that this intervention has not been successful at remediating his reading problems (DSM-5 criteria).

Observations

Classroom Observation

Matthew was observed for 15 minutes in Ms. Jones's classroom. The observation occurred during a reading activity in which students were instructed on how to make connections between books with a partner. During this whole-group instruction, Matthew was observed to sit attentively and listen to Ms. Jones. When the activity shifted and students were asked to partner with another student to share their connections, Matthew again complied with this request. Impressions of the observation were that Matthew was on task and compliant with teacher requests.

Observation during Assessment

Matthew was very compliant during the beginning of assessment, though he struggled in both cognitive and achievement tests. Matthew grew frustrated during the Passage Comprehension subtest of the WJ-IV and received encouragement for his efforts on this subtest. Matthew responded well to encouragement and was engaged in the subtest. He needed two breaks during the assessment session. Matthew was oriented to person, place, and time. He denied any feeling of suicidal or homicidal ideation. Test results are considered a valid representation of Matthew's abilities.

Cognitive and Academic Functioning

Reynolds Intellectual Assessment Scale— Second Edition (RIAS-2)

Matthew was administered the RIAS-2, which is an individually administered measure of intellectual functioning, normed for individuals between ages 3 and 94 years. The RIAS-2 contains several individual tests of intellectual problem solving and reasoning ability that are combined to form a Verbal Intelligence Index (VIX) and a Nonverbal Intelligence Index (NIX). The subtests that comprise the VIX assess verbal reasoning ability, along with the ability to access and apply prior learning in solving language-related tasks. Although labeled the VIX, it is also a reasonable approximation of crystallized intelligence. The NIX comprises subtests that assess nonverbal reasoning and spatial ability. Although labeled the NIX, it also provides a reasonable approximation of fluid intelligence and spatial ability. These two indices of intellectual functioning are then combined to form an overall Composite Intelligence Index (CIX). By combining the VIX and the NIX into the CIX, a strong, reliable assessment of general intelligence (g) is obtained. The CIX measures the two most important aspects of g according to recent theories and research findings: reasoning or fluid abilities and verbal or crystallized abilities.

The RIAS-2 also contains subtests designed to assess verbal memory and nonverbal memory. Depending on the age of the individual being evaluated, the Verbal Memory subtest comprises a series of sentences, age-appropriate stories, or both, read aloud to the examinee. The examinee is then asked to recall these sentences or stories as precisely as possible. The Nonverbal Memory subtest comprises the presentation of pictures of various objects or abstract designs for a period of 5 seconds. The examinee is then shown a page containing six similar objects or figures and must discern which object or figure was previously shown. The scores from these subtests are combined to form a Composite Memory Index (CMX), which provides a strong, reliable assessment of working memory and may also provide indications as to whether a more detailed assessment of memory functions may be required. In addition, the high reliability of the Verbal and Nonverbal Memory subtests allows direct comparison of them to each other.

Each of these indices is expressed as an age-corrected standard score that is scaled to a mean of 100 and a standard deviation of 15. These scores are normally distributed and can be converted to a variety of other metrics if desired.

Following are the results of Matthew's performance on the RIAS-2.

	Composite IQ	Verbal IQ	Nonverbal IQ	Memory Index
RIAS-2 Index	84	79	100	97
Percentile	14	8	50	42
Confidence interval (95%)	79–90	73–87	45–57	91–103

On testing with the RIAS-2, Matthew attained a CIX of 84. On the RIAS-2, this level of performance falls within the range of scores designated as low average and exceeded the performance of 14% of individuals who were Matthew's age. His Verbal IQ (Standard Score = 79; 8th %ile) was in the below-average range and exceeded 8% of individuals who were Matthew's age. Matthew's Nonverbal IQ (Standard Score = 93; 32nd %ile) was in the average range, exceeding 32% of individuals Matthew's age. Matthew earned a CMX of 97, which falls within the average range of working memory skills and exceeds the performance of 42 out of 100 individuals Matthew's age.

Comment: The RIAS-2 was administered to rule out intellectual deficiency (ID) as a potential explanation for Matthew's reading difficulties. Interpretation is focused mostly on the CIX, as that is the most reliable and valid score on the RIAS-2, and little, if any, consideration is given to the interpretation of subscale scores, although they are reported to comport with ethical test standards. These results indicate that Matthew has enough ability to benefit from the instructional environment; thus, cognitive ability is not considered to be the reason he is struggling to learn how to read.

Woodcock–Johnson Tests of Achievement IV (WJ-IV)

The WJ-IV is an achievement test used to measure reading, writing, and mathematics skills. The Reading Index includes letter and word identification, vocabulary, and comprehension skills. The Writing Index includes spelling, writing fluency, and simple sentence writing. The Mathematics Index includes calculation, practical problems, and knowledge of mathematical concepts and vocabulary.

Matthew obtained the scores illustrated in the table at below in each of the areas of measurement.

Comment: The RIAS-2 was administered to rule out intellectual deficiency (ID) as a potential explanation for Matthew's reading difficulties. Interpretation is focused mostly on the CIX, as that is the most reliable and valid score on the RIAS-2, and little, if any, consideration is given to the interpretation of subscale scores, although they are reported to comport with ethical test standards. These results indicate that Matthew has enough ability to benefit from the instructional environment; thus, cognitive ability is not considered to be the reason he is struggling to learn how to read.

Standardized achievement test results revealed below-average performance across the broad reading composite, with low average performance on the broad written language performance. Matthew scored in the average range on the broad mathematics composite.

Comment: The below-average reading scores on the WJ-IV provide evidence of low achievement and that Matthew's reading difficulties are also a normative deficit. At this point, both of the dual-deficit criteria are satisfied.

Comprehensive Test of Phonological Processing, Second Edition (CTOPP-2)

The CTOPP-2 is a standardized test of phonological processing that yield three composite scores: (1) Phonological Awareness, (2) Phonological Memory, and (3) Rapid Naming. The Phonological Awareness composite measures a student's ability to access the phonological structure of oral language. The Phonological Memory composite measures the ability to code information phonologically for temporary storage in working or short-term memory. The Rapid Naming Composite measures a student's ability to retrieve phonological information from memory and to complete a sequence of operations quickly and repeatedly. Matthew's performance across the three index composite areas was as follows:

	Scaled score	%ile	Description
Phonological Awareness	79	7	Below average
Phonological Memory	100	50	Average
Rapid Naming	78	8	Below average

Matthew's profile on the CTOPP-2 revealed a child who falls within the below-average range on the Phonological Awareness and Rapid Naming subtests, and in the average range on the Phonological Memory subtest. The current test administration appears to provide an accurate estimate of Matthew's present phonological processing.

Comment: The CTOPP-2 provides direct assessment of one of the most important early literacy subskills: phonological awareness. These results indicate that Matthew has a normative deficit in this skill. This deficit is likely the reason for his reading difficulties. Intervention efforts should target phonics development to remediate this skill area.

	Standard score	Percentile	95% CI interval	Descriptive classification
Broad Reading Composite	**79**	**8**	**<1–6**	**Below average**
Letter–word ID	89	23	2–8	Low average
Passage comprehension	79	8	2–11	Below average
Word attack	79	8	1–31	Below average
Oral reading	87	20	<1–4	Low average
Sentence reading fluency	77	7	<1–20	Below average
Broad Written Language Composite	**87**	**17**	**9–22**	**Low average**
Sentence writing fluency	83	12	5–40	Low average
Writing samples	82	11	5–45	Low average
Spelling	92	30	2–19	Average
Broad Mathematics Composite	**93**	**32**	**9–31**	**Average**
Math facts fluency	95	38	3–38	Average
Applied problems	99	48	4–33	Average
Calculation	90	25	23–53	Average

Social–Emotional and Behavioral Functioning

Behavior Assessment System for Children, Third Edition (BASC-3)

The BASC-3 is an integrated system, designed to facilitate the differential diagnosis and classification of a variety of emotional and behavioral conditions in children. It possesses validity scales and several clinical scales that reflect different dimensions of a child's personality. T-scores between 40 and 60 are considered average. Scores greater than 70 ($T > 70$) are in the clinically significant range and suggest a high level of difficulty. Scores in the at-risk range (T-score 60–69) identify either a significant problem that may not be severe enough to require formal treatment or the potential to develop a problem that needs careful monitoring. On the Adaptive Scales, scores below 30 are considered clinically significant, while scores between 31 and 39 mean that the child is at risk. See the table below.

These results indicate at-risk elevations on Externalizing Problems, Adaptive Skills, and the School Problems composite, and clinically significant elevations on the Hyperactivity and Attention Problems clinical scales, with an at-risk rating on the Adaptive Skills and Study Skills clinical scales.

ADHD Rating Scale–5

The ADHD Rating Scale–5 comprises ADHD symptoms based on DSM-5 diagnostic criteria. In general, scores between the 85th and 93rd percentiles are considered above average or "at-risk" for symptom cluster compared to the normative sample. Scores above the 93rd percentile are generally considered clinically significant. Matthew received the following scores:

Scale	Teacher percentile	Parent percentile
Hyperactivity–Impulsivity	95th (clinically significant)	95th (clinically significant)
Inattention	94th (clinically significant)	95th (clinically significant)
Combined	97th (clinically significant)	97th (clinically significant)

	Ms. Jones		Ms. Smith	
Clinical scales	T-score	Percentile	T-score	Percentile
Hyperactivity	85**	99	72**	95
Aggression	59	82	58	80
Conduct Problems	55	74	51	55
Anxiety	43	26	54	67
Depression	47	51	59	85
Somatization	46	46	45	44
Attention Problems	73**	99	75**	96
Learning Problems	73**	99	73**	98
Atypicality	43	19	45	23
Withdrawal	55	74	53	70
Adaptability	33*	3	32*	5
Social Skills	40	20	40	22
Leadership	47	43	45	40
Study Skills	38*	15	—	—
Functional Communication	43	25	44	2
Composite scores				
Externalizing Problems	63*	88	54	67
Internalizing Problems	44	30	45	32
School Problems	67*	94	—	—
Behavioral Symptoms Index	56	75	54	66
Adaptive Skills	38*	12	40	14

Note. For clinical scales, *at-risk rating ($T = 60$–69); **clinically significant rating ($T = 70+$). For composite scores, *at-risk rating ($T = 30$–39); **clinically significant rating ($T <30$). —Not applicable/assessed on Parent Rating Scale.

The ratings on the ADHD Rating Scale–5, across both parent and teacher versions, converged to suggest clinically significant elevations across all scales.

Diagnostic Impressions

Multiple data sources and methods of assessment inform the conceptualization of Matthew's cognitive, academic, social–emotional, and behavioral functioning, including whether he meets criteria for any diagnostic category. Details in support of these findings are offered below.

Cognitive and Academic Functioning

Matthew's on measures of cognitive ability was low average (Composite IQ = 84, 14th %ile; VIQ = 79, 8th %ile; NIQ = 100, 50th %ile). Matthew's performance on the WJ-IV Achievement was below average in reading, low average in writing, and average in mathematics. Matthew's performance on the CTOPP-2 was below average on a measure of phonological processing and rapid naming. Matthew's performance on standardized measures of academic achievement is consistent with teacher reports in which Matthew was noted to struggle with reading. Matthew is performing at grade level in mathematics on both measures of academic achievement and classroom progress.

Social and Emotional Functioning

Matthew is described as a child who struggles with attention, loss of focus, distractibility, impulsivity, and hyperactivity. His has a classification of ADHD, combined type (314.01). This is consistent with BASC-3 results in which he scored in the clinically significant range on the Inattention and Hyperactivity clinical scales. It is also consistent with scores on the ADHD rating scales. Background information and standardized behavior rating scales revealed that Matthew sometimes disregards classroom rules and teacher requests, and needs structure and support for these difficulties. He sometimes sulks when he does not get his own way. His peers are becoming frustrated by his tendency to intrude at inappropriate times and in inappropriate ways into their activities. Matthew can be a helpful child when a teacher requests his assistance.

Diagnostic Impression Summary

Multiple methods and sources of evaluation including the dual-deficit academic model of LD supported by clinical judgment suggest Matthew has a classification of specific learning disorder (SLD; 315.0) with impairment in reading. Matthew also meets criteria for a diagnosis of ADHD, combined presentation (314.01). It is recommended that Ms. Smith present this report to Matthew's school district, as he will likely qualify for special education support and receive an individualized education plan (IEP) and a Section 504 plan for his difficulties with ADHD.

Comment: Matthew currently meets all of the criteria for LD classification in both "hybrid" approaches and DSM-V. There is information to indicate that he has been provided access to appropriate instruction and intervention supports, and although he has been diagnosed with ADHD, there is evidence to indicate that a separate LD diagnosis is warranted. The most compelling factor is the specific nature of his deficits in reading, with no concomitant weaknesses in mathematics or writing. If his deficits were predominately due to attention, we would expect to see those deficits also manifest in other academic area. Additionally, the results from the CTOPP-2 indicate that Matthew is currently deficient in an important subskill associated with early literacy development.

Summary and Recommendations

Matthew's overall cognitive ability falls within the low-average range. Matthew's performance on measures of academic achievement (WJ-IV) was in the below-average to average range. He qualifies for a diagnosis of SLD (315.0) with impairment in reading. Matthew also experiences a high level of activity, distractibility, impulsivity, and inattention. He qualifies for a diagnosis of ADHD, combined presentation (314.01). The following home- and school-based recommendations will benefit Matthew. Matthew's school district should consider the diagnostic impressions included in this report and consider offering him special education support for his learning and behavioral difficulties, both of which are adversely impacting his educational performance.

Strategies for Difficulties with Attention, Distractibility, Overactivity, Impulsivity, and Loss of Focus

The following recommendations might be beneficial for Matthew:

1. *Direct contingency management at home and school and clinical cognitive-behavioral therapy to help supplement these efforts.* Both caregivers and teachers should implement home- or school-based contingencies incorporating (a) positive incentives such as praise or individualized reward programs for targeted behavior; (b) negative consequences such as reprimands, response cost, or time out; or (c) combinations of positive and negative contingencies. This approach has been found to be effective in home and school settings. Caregivers specifically may benefit from parent behavioral management training to better understand how to properly implement a direct contingency management program in the home. Experienced teachers generally have the tools to implement, but consultation with the teacher may be warranted.

2. *Additional school-based strategies for ADHD*

- *Seating.* Matthew should continue to sit in a location where there are minimal distractions.
- *Provision of directions by teachers.* When Matthew's teachers interact with him, he should be encouraged to repeat and explain instructions to ensure understanding. The provision of directions to Matthew will be most effective when the teacher makes eye contact, avoids multiple commands, is clear and to the point, and permits repetition of directions when asked for or needed.
- *Positive reinforcement and praise for successful task completion.* Matthew's teachers should provide positive reinforcement and immediate feedback for completion of desired behaviors or tasks. Initially, praise and reinforcement should be offered for successful effort on a task or behavior, regardless of quality of performance.
- *Time on task.* Communicate to Matthew how long he will need to engage in or pay attention on a particular task. Open-ended expectations can be distressing to any child, let alone one with attentional difficulties.
- *Prepare student discreetly for transitions.* Furnish Matthew with verbal prompts and visual cues that a new activity or task is about to start. This should be accomplished discreetly so as to avoid student embarrassment.
- *Recess time.* Matthew should be permitted to participate in recess. Recess should not be a time to complete unfinished classwork or homework.
- *Extended time, teacher check-ins, and frequent breaks.* Matthew should be permitted additional time to complete academic tasks and projects. Matthew's teachers should also consider review of classwork as Matthew progresses on an assignment or project to assist Matthew in avoiding careless mistakes. More frequent breaks than what is typical may also reduce careless mistakes and help to maintain focus.
- *Daily behavior report card.* Key targeted behavior is monitored by the teacher, with home reinforcement contingent on positive teacher report.

3. *Behaviorally oriented social skills training.* This approach has received preliminary empirical support for social skills difficulties in children with ADHD, but not in all studies. Specific behavioral deficits such as intruding in an activity without asking, interrupting other children, and difficulty waiting one's turn in social exchange should be the initial targets for intervention. The goals of therapy should be conveyed to Matthew's teacher, so that she may reinforce prosocial behaviors or correct behaviors that are targets of intervention.

4. *Child psychiatric evaluation.* Matthew will benefit from the forthcoming child psychiatric evaluation at the Children's Hospital of Philadelphia to determine whether he would benefit from psychotropic medication as an adjunct to his behavioral intervention at school and home.

5. *Support for difficulties with reading comprehension, phonological awareness, sight-word recognition, word decoding, and reading fluency.* Matthew struggles with all aspects of reading, including word decoding, phonological/phonemic awareness, reading fluency, and reading comprehension. Matthew requires special education support for his reading difficulties, as noted below.

- *Phonological awareness and sight-word knowledge skills.* Matthew will benefit from continued intervention with basic phonemic awareness skills, such as emphasizing instruction on basic rimes (*ack, ame, all, ake*). Matthew would be well served to increase his familiarity with reading fundamentals through a focus on words via alliteration lessons (e.g., tongue twisters), a personal dictionary of sight words (i.e., most frequently used words), and word family study (e.g., *neat, beat, heat; noise, poise, choice*).
- *Reading fluency.* Matthew should practice oral reading fluency. Accordingly, Matthew will benefit from repeated reading of the passage until an appropriate grade-level fluency rate is attained. The research literature suggests that improvements in oral reading fluency via repeated passage reading generalizes to improvements in overall reading ability.
- *Reading comprehension.* Matthew struggles with the comprehension of written text and will benefit from prereading and organizational strategies that attempt to improve this skill area. Following are a few suggestions that will likely benefit Matthew:
  - Before reading, preview the text by looking at the title and illustrations.
  - Encourage the creation of a possible story from the illustrations.
  - Make predictions about the story based on story features prior to reading the story.
  - During reading, generate questions about the story that are directly related to the text and that require thinking beyond the text.
  - After reading, spend time reflecting on the material and relating it to experiences and events the child has encountered.
  - After reading, have Matthew engage in the reading material using text summarizing.

PART VI

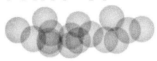

Stressful Events, Maltreatment, Trauma, and Loss

CHAPTER 15

Posttraumatic Stress Disorder

Annette M. La Greca and BreAnne A. Danzi

Preparation: Organizing Materials Relevant to Assessing Posttraumatic Stress Disorder in Youth

Recent years have witnessed a growing concern about the exposure of youth to large-scale, potentially traumatic or life-threatening events, such as mass shootings, terrorist attacks, and climate-related natural disasters (La Greca & Danzi, 2019). On an individual level, many youth are affected by other traumatic events, such as injuries or medically related trauma. For example, over 9.2 million youth are treated annually in emergency departments for potentially life-threatening injuries (e.g., due to burns, falls, motor vehicle accidents), which are the leading cause of morbidity and mor-

tality among youth ages 0–19 years (Centers for Disease Control and Prevention, 2008). Medical illness, such as cancer, also affect many youth (Price, Kassam-Adams, Alderfer, Christofferson, & Kazak, 2016).

Fortunately, most youth are resilient, even in the face of potentially traumatic events (PTEs) such as those we noted earlier. At the same time, PTEs clearly contribute to the development and maintenance of posttraumatic stress disorder (PTSD) or significant posttraumatic stress symptoms (PTSS), at least for a substantial minority of exposed youth (Bonanno, Brewin, Kaniasty, & La Greca, 2010; Furr, Comer, Edmunds, & Kendall, 2010; La Greca et al., 2013; Price et al., 2016).

Our purpose in this chapter is to provide a framework for assessing PTSD and PTSS in youth. This area of psychological assessment typically involves multiple aspects, such as identifying the target PTE to which a child or adolescent was exposed; assessing the frequency and severity of PTSD symptoms and any associated functional impairment; evaluating other psychological symptomatologies (e.g., anxiety or depression) that commonly co-occur with PTSD; and assessing risk and protective factors that may affect treatment planning or moderate treatment outcome. These are among the key assessment issues we discuss in this chapter.

In this opening section, we briefly describe studies of PTSD prevalence, then provide background information on the diagnosis of PTSD in youth, noting marked differences in the diagnostic approaches taken by the 11th edition of the *International Classification of Diseases* (ICD-11; Brewin et al., 2017) and the fifth edition of the *Diagnostic and Statistical Manual of Mental Disorders* (DSM-5; American Psychiatric Association, 2013). We also suggest a "starter kit" of assessments that might be useful for evaluating youth in clinical settings and schools—two of the most common settings for initial screening or evaluation of PTSD in youth.

In the second section, we focus in greater depth on assessment measures pertinent to screening youth exposed to PTEs, informant issues, and assessment of co-occurring conditions. We focus in the third section on diagnosis and treatment planning, including the use of structured or semi-structured interviews, considerations for case formulation, and factors that might mitigate or enhance treatment outcome and planning. In the fourth section, we discuss ways to monitor treatment progress and outcome; here, the reader is referred to La Greca and Danzi (2019) for descriptions of evidence-based treatments for PTSD in youth. Finally, we end the chapter with some overall conclusions and recommendations for the future.

Prevalence of PTSD in Youth

U.S. population-based studies suggest that PTSD develops during childhood or adolescence in about 3–4% of boys and 7% of girls (Kilpatrick et al., 2003; McLaughlin et al., 2013), and subclinical levels of PTSD occur at substantially higher rates (Bonanno et al., 2010; Copeland, Keeler, Angold, & Costello, 2007; Price et al., 2016). Even subclinical levels of PTSD interfere with academic, cognitive, social, and emotional functioning in youth and are reasons for concern (e.g., La Greca, Silverman, Lai, & Jaccard, 2010; Lai, La Greca, Auslander, & Short, 2013; Price et al., 2016).

PTSD prevalence rates also vary widely depending on age. Reports indicate that U.S. adolescents have a lifetime PTSD prevalence of 5% (8% in girls; Merikangas et al., 2010), which is a bit lower than the adult lifetime prevalence of 8.7% (American Psychiatric Association, 2013). Some studies conducted in the United States and United Kindom indicate lifetime rates of PTSD in children to be as low as 0.1% (Copeland et al., 2007; Ford, Goodman, & Meltzer, 2003). However, these rates most likely underestimate the occurrence of PTSD

and probably reflect difficulties in identifying PTSD in children. As we discuss below, developmentally sensitive criteria for identifying PTSD in children yield rates of PTSD more than three times higher than when the more traditional adult-based criteria for PTSD are used (Scheeringa, Myers, Putman, & Zeannah, 2012). Recent meta-analytic reviews suggest that 15.9% of youth develop PTSD following exposure to a PTE, with rates for girls (20.8%) nearly twice that of boys (11.1%; Alisic et al., 2014).

PTEs vary on several dimensions that affect the extent to which they are associated with PTSD in youth. First, traumatic events may be large scale (e.g., natural disasters, terrorism, war), or affect only a few individuals at a time (e.g., sexual maltreatment, medical trauma). Large-scale events, often referred to as disasters (e.g., Bonanno et al., 2010), affect entire communities and cause widespread distress, resulting in practical challenges for assessing and treating trauma-exposed youth. Second, PTEs may be an acute, single-occurrence event (e.g., a motor vehicle accident) or chronic (e.g., sexual abuse); in general, greater chronicity has been associated with more negative mental health outcomes (Danese & McEwen, 2012; Karam et al., 2014) and more complex forms of PTSD (Brewin et al., 2017). Third, PTEs that involve interpersonal violence have been associated with a higher risk for PTSD than nonviolent PTEs (Alisic et al., 2014). For example, the World Health Organization (WHO) Mental Health Surveys (Kessler et al., 2017) assessed over 68,000 adults from 24 countries and found the highest level of PTSD risk among those who experienced interpersonal violence (e.g., rape, other sexual assault). Among youth, child sexual abuse also has been associated with higher rates of PTSD compared to other PTEs (Deblinger, Mannarino, Cohen, Runyon, & Steer, 2011; McLean, Morris, Conklin, Jayawickreme, & Foa, 2014).

Diagnosis of PTSD in Youth

To date, most of the research on PTSD in youth is based on DSM-IV diagnostic criteria (American Psychiatric Association, 1994). However, present conceptualizations of PTSD are diverse and lack consensus, thus adding a layer of complexity to the assessment of PTSD in youth (La Greca & Danzi, 2019). Developmental issues surrounding the conceptualization of PTSD in youth further cloud the diagnostic picture (Danzi & La Greca, 2016, 2017; La Greca, Danzi, & Chan, 2017).

DSM-5

Briefly, DSM-5 (American Psychiatric Association, 2013) takes a broad approach to defining PTSD (Friedman, 2013) in order to capture the multiple clinical presentations observed with PTSD. DSM-5 uses a 20-symptom, four-factor model of PTSD, with symptoms clusters for reex-

periencing, avoidance, arousal, and cognitions/mood (newly added) (American Psychiatric Association, 2013; see Table 15.1); symptoms must last for a month or more and cause clinically significant distress or functional impairment.

This conceptualization of PTSD was based almost exclusively on research with adults, and its

TABLE 15.1. Key Symptoms and Clusters for the Diagnosis of PTSD Using DSM-5 and ICD-11

Clusters/symptoms	DSM-5 Adult criteria	DSM-5 Young child criteria	ICD-11 PTSD	ICD-11 Complex PTSD
Reexperiencing				
Intrusive memories	✓	✓	a	a
Nightmares	✓	✓	✓	✓
Flashbacks	✓	✓	✓	✓
Psychological distress	✓	✓		
Physiological reactions	✓	✓		
Avoidance				
Avoidance of internal cues (e.g., thoughts, memories)	✓		✓	✓
Avoidance of external cues	✓		✓	✓
Physical (e.g., activities, places)		✓		
Interpersonal (e.g., people, conversations)		✓		
Cognitions/mood				
Inability to recall trauma	✓			
Negative beliefs	✓			
Blame for event	✓			
Negative emotional state	✓	✓		
Anhedonia	✓	✓		
Detachment/estrangement	✓			
Inability to feel positive emotions	✓	✓		
Socially withdrawn play		✓		
Arousal				
Irritability/anger	✓	✓		
Reckless/self-destructive	✓			
Hypervigilance	✓	✓	✓	✓
Startle response	✓	✓	✓	✓
Concentration	✓	✓		
Insomnia	✓	✓		
Complex				
Affect dysregulation				✓
Beliefs about worthlessness/defeat				✓
Feelings of shame/guilt				✓
Difficulty sustaining relationships				✓
Difficulty feeling close to others				✓

Note. DSM-5 "Young Child" criteria are intended for *children 6 years and younger* but may be useful for older children as well.
aIntrusive memories must be vivid and accompanied by feelings of being immersed in the traumatic event in the present.

relevance to children has been questioned (e.g., Danzi & La Greca, 2016; La Greca et al., 2017). Most controversial are the symptoms that reflect negative alterations in cognitions and mood related to the trauma (Danzi & La Greca, 2016) such as extreme negative beliefs about oneself, others, or the world; distorted cognitions regarding blame for the traumatic event; persistent negative emotions; the inability to experience positive emotions; and feelings of detachment and estrangement from others. In addition, the symptom of "reckless or self-destructive behavior" was added to the arousal symptom cluster, although the relevance of this symptom for preadolescent youth is uncertain (La Greca et al., 2017). However, the DSM-5 conceptualization of PTSD does appear to perform well when used with adolescents (Hafstad, Dyb, Jensen, Steinberg, & Pynoos, 2014; Hafstad, Thoresen, Wentzel-Larson, Maercker, & Dyb, 2017).

For children age 6 years and younger, DSM-5 also provides "Young Child" criteria for diagnosing PTSD (American Psychiatric Association, 2013). These developmentally sensitive criteria require fewer symptoms for a diagnosis and deemphasize highly internalized or cognitively advanced symptoms that may be difficult for young children to report or for adults to observe (see La Greca & Danzi, 2019, for details). Although these criteria were developed in response to problems with DSM-IV and identify three to eight times more preschool youth as meeting criteria for PTSD than do adult-based criteria (Scheeringa, Weems, Cohen, Amaya-Jackson, & Guthrie, 2011; Scheering et al., 2012), the "fit" of the new DSM-5 "Young Child" criteria for preschool-age youth has yet to be fully evaluated.

Interestingly, DSM-5 "Young Child" criteria also may be useful for diagnosing or screening for PTSD in preadolescent youth ages 7–12 years. With preadolescents, rates of PTSD appear to double when using DSM-5 "Young Child" criteria compared to DSM-5 (adult-based) criteria recommended for this age group (Danzi & La Greca, 2017; Mikolajewski, Scheeringa, & Weems, 2017).

ICD-11

In contrast to DSM-5, ICD-11 takes a narrow approach to PTSD, designed to reduce the assessment burden and lessen overlap with other disorders (Friedman, 2013). ICD-11 focuses on three core PTSD clusters (reexperiencing the trauma in the present, avoidance of traumatic reminders, and a persistent sense of threat as manifested in arousal and hypervigilance) (Brewin et al., 2017),

and excludes symptoms shared with other psychological disorders (e.g., sleep difficulties, negative mood). Only three symptoms (one from each cluster) are needed for diagnosis; symptoms must be present for at least several weeks and cause functional impairment. See Table 15.1 for an overview of ICD-11 criteria for PTSD.

ICD-11 also includes criteria for complex PTSD (Brewin et al., 2017) to capture the posttraumatic reactions of individuals exposed to a chronic pattern of extreme traumatization (e.g., slavery, genocide, chronic physical or sexual abuse). In addition to all the criteria for PTSD, complex PTSD includes additional symptoms that reflect "disturbances in self-organization," such as severe problems with affect regulation, negative self-concept (e.g., feelings of shame, worthlessness, or failure), and pervasive difficulties in interpersonal relationships (Brewin et al., 2017; Karatzias et al., 2017; Sachser, Keller, & Goldbeck, 2017). These features of complex PTSD are thought to benefit from treatments that include emotion regulation strategies and efforts to improve interpersonal functioning (Cloitre et al., 2012). However, at present, there has been little study of complex PTSD in youth.

Research on ICD-11 continues to emerge since its release by the WHO in June 2018 (Buck, 2018). ICD-11 was adopted by the World Health Assembly in May 2019 and went into effect on January 1, 2020. The date for adoption by the United States will be sometime after January 2022.

Implications of PTSD Conceptualization for Assessment

The divergent conceptualizations of PTSD offered by DSM-5 and ICD-11 present a serious quandary for assessment. Which one(s) provide a valid assessment of PTSD? Which diagnostic model should be used with youth? At present, no single model emerges as the "best" for understanding (and therefore assessing) PTSD in youth.

Studies demonstrate that both DSM-5 and ICD-11 diagnostic models "fit" posttrauma responses in youth, but the overlap between the models is poor, and each model identifies youth who are "missed" by the other model (Danzi & La Greca, 2016; La Greca et al., 2017). For example, among children exposed to Hurricane Ike, only 45% of those meeting criteria for PTSD were identified by both DSM-5 and ICD-11 criteria (La Greca et al., 2017).

We expect that continued developments will emerge that bear on the developmental appropriateness of the various conceptualizations of PTSD in youth. For now, however, *we advocate the following diagnostic approach* to assessing PTSD in children and adolescents.

1. Use measures that assess the DSM-5 "Young Child" criteria with children age 6 years and younger.

2. Consider using measures that assess the DSM-5 "Young Child" criteria with preadolescent children (ages 7–12 years), particularly when screening youth for PTSD. The "Young Child" criteria identify substantially more preadolescents as having PTSD than do the adult-based criteria and are also likely to be inclusive of all the children who would have been identified by either DSM-5 adult criteria or ICD-11 (Danzi & La Greca, 2017). In other words, DSM-5 "Young Child" criteria are broader and more inclusive with this age group.

3. Otherwise, in general, it is advisable to use measures that assess both DSM-5 and ICD-11 criteria with preadolescents and adolescents (ages 7–18 years), at least until greater clarity is achieved on the "best" diagnostic model for PTSD for these age groups. Because some DSM-5-based measures contain symptoms consistent with both the DSM-5 and ICD-11 PTSD criteria, one measure might be used to obtain scores for both diagnostic models (although we recognize that this is not optimal). However, when time and resources are limited, the "shorter" ICD-11 criteria may be useful, as they still identify highly distressed children with central features of PTSD (Danzi & La Greca, 2016; La Greca et al., 2017).

4. For youth exposed to severe, chronic, or ongoing trauma, assessment measures that tap into aspects of complex PTSD would be advisable, as they become available.

Starter Kit of Assessment Measures for PTSD in Youth

Table 15.2 lists measures that might be included in a starter kit for PTSD assessment in youth. In general, the measures represent good examples of the rating scales and interviews used to evaluate youth for PTSD, and we discuss them in more detail in the sections that follow.

For school-age children and adolescents, the Child PTSD Symptom Scale for DSM-5 (CPSS-5) and the UCLA PTSD Reaction Index for DSM-5 (PTSD-RI-5) are the most widely used measures for assessing PTSD in youth. Both measures have been adapted recently for DSM-5, and either one

would be appropriate for a starter kit. The PTSD-RI-5 has multiple language versions and a caregiver report version, which could be especially useful, although caregiver report and multiple language versions of the CPSS-5 are likely to be developed (as was the case with the DSM-IV version of the CPSS). The child report measures take about 15 minutes to complete; the clinician interviews take about 30 minutes or more to administer.

For young children (ages 6 years and younger), caregiver reports typically have been used. The Young Child PTSD Checklist (YCPC) includes items that reflect DSM-5 criteria for young children, as well as items pertinent to ICD-11 criteria (see Table 15.1).

In addition to these measures, there have been efforts to develop a PTSD scale from the Child Behavior Checklist (CBCL; Ruggiero & McLeer, 2000), a well-validated, widely used, broad-based measure of childhood behavior problems (Achenbach & Rescorla, 2001). Much of the work on the validity of the CBCL PTSD scale has focused on sexually maltreated youth. At present, however, evidence for the validity of the CBCL PTSD scale for identifying trauma in youth exposed to sexual maltreatment is weak (Ruggiero & McLeer, 2000; Sim et al., 2005). There also have been mixed findings on the utility of the CBCL PTSD scale with preschool-age children (e.g., Dehon & Scheeringa, 2006; Loeb, Stettler, Gavila, Stein, & Chinitz, 2011). Nevertheless, some recent evidence suggests that the PTSD scale from the Youth Self-Report (YSR) may aid in the diagnosis of PTSD. Specifically, among 11- to 18-year-olds in a large outpatient sample, You, Youngstrom, Feeny, Youngstrom, and Findling (2017) compared the diagnostic accuracy of five PTSD measures to diagnoses obtained from structured interviews with the youth and caregiver. Youth YSR reports on the PTSD scale were more accurate than parent and teacher reports (on the parallel measure) in predicting a PTSD diagnoses; the youth trauma reports on the YSR also performed marginally better than their reports on the Child PTSD Symptom Scale in predicting PTSD. Thus, the YRS report of PTSD may be worth considering as an option for screening for PTSD among youth ages 11–18 years, especially if the YSR is already part of a clinic's standard assessment battery.

Finally, note that most measures in Table 15.2 reflect DSM-5 criteria for PTSD. The International Trauma Questionnaire (ITQ), based on ICD-11 criteria, has been developed and validated for use with adults (Cloitre et al., 2018; Karatzias et al.,

TABLE 15.2. Starter Kit of Measures for Screening and Assessing PTSD in Youth

Measure	Assesses	Versions	Ages	Comments/source
Child PTSD Symptom Scale for DSM-5 (CPSS-5)	• Trauma exposure (7 items) • PTSD symptoms (20 items) • Functioning (7 items) • Includes a screen for PTSD (6 items)	• Child self-report • Clinician interview • Caregiver report (in development) • English language • Multiple languages for DSM-IV version	8–18 years	Good correspondence between the versions; PTSD rates higher with child report Foa et al. (2018) *www.episcenter.psu.edu/sites/default/files/cpss-v%20 scoring%20%26%20psychometrics.pdf*
UCLA Child/Adolescent PTSD Reaction Index for DSM-5 (PTSD-RI-5)	• Trauma exposure (23 items) • PTSD symptoms (27 items) • Functioning (9 items) • Includes a dissociative subtype (4 items)	• Child self-report • Clinician interview • Caregiver report • English, Spanish, German, Arabic	7–18 years	Widely used measure of PTSD symptomatology; training video available at *www.nctsn.org/print/967* Elhai et al. (2013); Pynoos et al. (2015); Steinberg et al. (2013)
Young Child PTSD Checklist (YCPC)	• Trauma exposure (12 items) • PTSD symptoms (24 items) • Functioning (6 items)	• Caregiver report	1–6 years	*www.midss.org/content/young-child-ptsd-checklist* Scheering & Haslett (2010)
Child Behavior Checklist—Posttraumatic Stress Disorder Scale (CBCL-PTSD)	• PTSD symptoms (14-item version is recommended)	• Parent report • Youth report • (Teacher report not recommended)	11–18 years	Strongest support is for the Youth Self-Report version of this measure; mixed findings for this measure with preschool-age children Ruggiero & McLeer (2000); You et al. (2017)
International Trauma Questionnaire (ITQ)—Youth Version	• Adult-based ITQ has 12 items	• Youth report	11–18 years	Youth measure is currently under development; based on ICD-11 criteria for PTSD; adult-based ITQ is freely available Cloitre et al. (2018)

2017); initial studies of a youth version of the ITQ are currently ongoing. The adult-based ITQ is a 12-item, simply worded measure of the core features of PTSD. Until the ITQ has been validated for youth, clinicians and researchers might use the adult-based ITQ or relevant items from DSM-5 youth measures to approximate a score for PTSD using ICD-11 criteria (e.g., Danzi & La Greca, 2016, 2017). We note that this pragmatic approach is acceptable but not ideal, as the conceptualization of "intrusive memories" differs across DSM-5 and ICD-11 models.

Because measures of PTSD in youth based on the relatively new DSM-5 and ICD-11 diagnostic criteria are still evolving, we expect that further developments will emerge in the coming years. For this reason, in Table 15.3, we list several key resources for identifying trauma measures in youth. The websites listed will be useful to readers in identifying relevant measures for research and practice, and for keeping up with the psychometric support of various assessment instruments that are

currently being evaluated using recent DSM-5 and ICD-11 criteria.

Prediction: Initial Screening for Trauma Exposure and PTSD Using Rating Scales and Checklists

In general, our recommendations for assessing PTSD in youth are consistent with the "Practice Parameters for the Assessment and Treatment of Children and Adolescents with PTSD" developed by the American Academy of Child and Adolescent Psychiatry, as described by Cohen and the Workgroup on Quality Issues (2010). According to these practice parameters, in light of the high rates of children's trauma exposure, routine screening for PTSD is recommended during an initial mental health assessment. Specifically, clinicians should routinely ask children about their commonly experienced exposure to traumatic events (e.g., accidents, abuse, community violence) and

TABLE 15.3. Resources for Child and Adolescent Measures of PTSD and Trauma Exposure

Resource	Website	Type of information
National Center for PTSD	www.ptsd.va.gov/professional/assessment/child/index.asp	Includes information on a variety of measures assessing trauma and PTSD in youth. These measures are intended for use by qualified mental health professionals and researchers.
National Child Traumatic Stress Network	www.nctsn.org/treatments-and-practices/screening-and-assessments/measure-reviews	Measures database: Includes reviews of tools that measure children's experiences of trauma, their reactions to it, and other mental health and trauma-related issues.
International Society for Traumatic Stress Studies: Trauma Assessment Tools	www.istss.org/assessing-trauma.aspx	Trauma assessment tools: Includes test materials, treatment manuals, and other assessment resources, focused on PTSD assessment and treatment.
American Psychological Association	www.apa.org/ptsd-guideline/assessment/index.aspx	PTSD assessment instruments: Includes interview and self-report instruments used with adults. Includes DSM-5 versions of widely used measures.
National Center for Mental Health and Juvenile Justice	www.ncmhjj.com/resources/review-child-adolescent-trauma-screening-tools	Lists the profiles of 29 tools that screen youth for trauma, including the number of items, target age, accessibility, languages, and empirical support.
Evidence-Based Prevention and Support Center (PA Department of Human Services)	www.episcenter.psu.edu/newvpp/tfcbt/evaluation-tools#other%20clinical%20assessment%20tools	Lists a wide variety of clinical assessment tools relevant for evaluating trauma exposure and PTSD in youth and for monitoring comorbid symptomatology and risk factors for poor recovery.

screen for the presence of PTSD symptoms if trauma exposure is endorsed.

Children ages 7 years and older can provide their own report of trauma exposure and related symptoms; parent or caregiver report is the norm for youth ages 6 years and younger. When possible, both child and caregiver reports are preferred. The measures described below can be used for an initial evaluation of trauma exposure and PTSD symptoms in youth. If this initial evaluation reveals significant symptoms of PTSD, the clinician should conduct a formal evaluation (typically using a structured interview) to determine whether the youth meets criteria for PTSD; involving parents or other caregivers in the formal evaluation is desirable and customary (Cohen & the Workgroup on Quality Issues, 2010). (We focus in the next section on the use of structured interviews to determine a diagnosis of PTSD.)

Assessing Trauma Exposure

General Considerations

It is essential to know whether a youth has experienced a PTE before administering measures to assess symptoms of PTSD. Trauma exposure is necessary for the development of PTSD and is a primary component of both DSM and ICD models of PTSD. However, because there is variability in conceptualizations of what constitutes trauma exposure, we briefly elaborate on the conceptualization of trauma exposure here.

In DSM-IV, trauma was defined largely by the person's response to a traumatic event; the individual must respond with intense fear, helplessness, or horror (American Psychiatric Association, 1994). However, not all people who experience trauma and develop PTSD respond with fear, helplessness, or horror in the moment (Brewin, Lanius, Novac, Schnyder, & Galea, 2009). For example, survivors of sexual assault can present with a range of initial responses, such as numbness or flat affect (Chivers-Wilson, 2006). This may be especially true for children who experience sexual abuse, especially when the perpetrator is a parent or trusted adult, or if the abuse occurred when the child was very young and had a limited understanding of what was occurring (Adams, Mrug, & Knight, 2018; Cicchetti & Lynch, 1993). Thus, while it is useful to assess a person's response to potentially traumatic events, and questions about fear-inducing events provide a quick means of screening for

trauma exposure, the absence of an immediate or obvious fear response when confronted with a PTE does not rule out trauma exposure or PTSD.

Under DSM-5 guidelines, trauma involves exposure to actual or threatened death, injury, or sexual violence that is directly experienced or witnessed, or that happens to a close family member or friend (must be violent or accidental in cases of actual or threatened death of a family member or friend). DSM-5 clarifies that extreme exposure to traumatic events (e.g., as a first responder) counts as traumatic, whereas exposure through media does not (American Psychiatric Association, 2013). In contrast, ICD-11 leaves the construct of trauma largely to clinical judgment and only notes that the event must be extremely threatening or horrific (Brewin et al., 2017). These guidelines are helpful to keep in mind when assessing youth for trauma exposure.

Assessment Measures for Trauma Exposure

In routine clinical care, administering child- and parent-report measures assessing trauma exposure is a useful way of determining whether a youth has a trauma history. Some youth and parents find it easier to disclose trauma exposure by checking a box than by talking about the distressing event in detail.

As seen in Table 15.2, the most widely used PTSD ratings scales include items that assess trauma exposure. For example, the CPSS-5 contains items that ask about experiencing a severe natural disaster; being in a serious accident; having a frightening medical procedure; being the target of community or domestic violence; and so on. In most cases, it is desirable to obtain a broad, comprehensive assessment of trauma exposure, as a youth's trauma history may influence the chronicity of PTSD symptoms or the youth's response to treatment for a specific traumatic event (Self-Brown, Lai, Thompson, McGill, & Kelley, 2013). As such, the trauma screening items from the CPSS-5, the PTSD-RI-5, or the YCPC (for young children) can be very useful.

Rating Scales and Checklists for PTSD

After identifying the potentially traumatic event(s), the next step is to obtain the youth's reactions to the traumatic event(s). A youth might report stress-related reactions to a specific traumatic event (e.g., a hurricane that just occurred) or to the traumatic event that "bothers him or her the most now." Note that some measures (e.g., the PTSD-RI-5) ask youth to rate the event that bothers them the most, but others (e.g., the YCPC) ask the youth (or parent) to rate symptoms relevant for the totality of events they have experienced. Thus, in selecting an assessment measure, the clinician or researcher needs to determine which of the perspectives is desired.

The rating scales listed in Tables 15.2 and 15.4 represent the most widely used measures of PTSD symptomatology in youth, and all have psychometric support, at least based on DSM-IV criteria for PTSD (for details, see the systematic review by Eklund, Rossen, Koriakin, Chafouleas, & Resnick, 2018). We feature the CPSS-5 and the PTSD-RI-5 in Table 15.2 because the DSM-IV versions had strong psychometric support (including evidence of diagnostic classification accuracy; Eklund et al., 2018), and a DSM-5 version is available with strong initial empirical support. However, the other rating scales listed in Table 15.4 were widely used in earlier research and also may be useful to clinicians and researchers. Most scales have developed cutoff scores to identify youth with clinically significant levels of posttraumatic stress, and with a few exceptions, most are available for free. Note that an abbreviated, nine-item version of the PTSD-RI (based on DSM-IV) appears in the report on practice parameters (Cohen & the Workgroup on Quality Issues, 2010). Note also that some rating scales (e.g., the CPSS-5) have briefer "screening" versions that might precede use of the full rating scale if time is limited.

Because of diagnostic changes (DSM-5 and ICD-11) in definitions of PTSD, we expect that additional data will emerge regarding the various measures' diagnostic utility and predictive validity. We also expect the measures to be translated into diverse languages, as was the case with the DSM-IV-based measures of PTSD in youth, such as the PTSD-RI.

Ideally, clinicians would routinely obtain a child report (for school-age youth and adolescents) or parent report (for youth ages 6 and younger) of PTSD symptoms using one the measures listed in Tables 15.2 or 15.4. When possible, both child and parents reports are preferable. When youth (or parents) report elevated levels of posttraumatic stress, this initial assessment would be followed with a more detailed structured interview to determine whether the youth meets diagnostic criteria for PTSD (Cohen & the Workgroup on Quality Issues, 2010).

Informant Issues

Because it is difficult for young children (ages 6 years and younger) to report PTSD symptoms, parents or caregivers are typically the informants for young children. As seen in Tables 15.2 and 15.4, the measures that are developmentally appropriate for children 6 years of age and younger are exclusively parent/caregiver report measures. However, having parents or caregivers as the sole informants raises some concern about identifying PTSD in young children, as parents/caregivers have not been especially good reporters of PTSD symptoms in older youth.

For school-age youth (ages 7 years and older) or adolescents, the youth self-report is critical to evaluating PTSD symptoms. Parents seriously underestimate PTSD symptoms in their children, and this has been the case both for assessments conducted with PTSD rating scales and with diagnostic interviews. For example, among youth ages 11–18 years who had been hospitalized with injuries, Scheeringa, Wright, Hunt, and Zeanah (2006) found an almost ninefold increase in diagnostic rates of PTSD (37.5% rate) when using combined parent and child reports compared with only using parent reports (4.2% rate). Similar findings have been observed using PTSD ratings. For example, youth report many more PTSD symptoms than their parents (e.g., Korol, Green, & Gleser, 1999), and youth reports also outperform parent and teacher reports in identifying PTSD in youth ages 11–18 years (You et al., 2017). Essentially, children report more distress than parents, so it is critical to obtain the child's perspective.

In an ideal scenario, clinicians integrate information gathered from multiple informants, keeping in mind the previously described findings about parents potentially underreporting the youth's symptoms. If major discrepancies are observed between child and parent report, this is useful to know for treatment planning (e.g., clinicians may consider prioritizing parental psychoeducation or increasing communication in the family). Clinicians may also consider gathering information from other people in the child's life. This approach might be more helpful for some trauma types than for others, and it may be particularly fruitful if trauma reactions are occurring in settings outside the home. For example, observations of a child's functioning might be helpful to obtain from teachers for children exposed to a school shooting or from a medical treatment team

TABLE 15.4. Rating Scales and Checklist for Assessing PTSD in Children and Adolescents

Posttraumatic stress assessment measures	Informant	Trauma type	Cost/access	No. of items	Reference/source
Ages 7 years and above					
Child PTSD Symptom Scale for DSM-5 (CPSS-5-SR)	Child, parent/caregiver	Multiple types	Free	27	*www.nctsn.org/measures/child-ptsd-symptom-scale*
UCLA PTSD Reaction Index for Children/Adolescents for DSM-5 (PTSD-RI-5)	Child, parent/caregiver	Multiple types	Cost/contact authors	31	*www.ptsd.va.gov/professional/assessment/child/ucla_child_reaction_dsm-5.asp*
Child Trauma Screening Questionnaire (CTSQ)	Child	Mainly medical	Free	10	*www.nctsn.org/measures/child-trauma-screening-questionnaire* Kenardy, Spence, & Macleod (2006)
Children's Revised Impact of Events Scale (CRIES-8)	Child	War/disasters	Free	13	*www.childrenandwar.org/measures* Smith, Perrin, Dyregrov, & Yule (2002)
Trauma Symptoms Checklist for Children (TSCC)	Child	Multiple types	Cost/contact authors	54	*www.nctsn.org/measures/trauma-symptom-checklist-children* Briere (1996); Nilsson, Wadsby, & Svedin (2008)
Child's Reaction to Traumatic Events Scale—Revised	Child	Natural disasters; accident/fires	Free	23	*www.nctsn.org/measures/childs-reaction-traumatic-events-scale-revised* Based on the Horowitz Impact of Events Scale Jones, Fletcher, & Ribbe (2002); Napper et al. (2015)
Ages 6 years and younger					
Young Child PTSD Checklist (YCPC)[a]	Parent/caregiver	Multiple types	Free	42	*www.midss.org/content/young-child-ptsd-checklist*
Trauma Symptom Checklist for Young Children (TSCYC)	Parent/caregiver	Multiple types; grief/loss	Cost/contact author	90	*www.nctsn.org/measures/trauma-symptom-checklist-young-children* Briere (2005)

[a]Also a six-item screener version, as well as a version for older youth.

for medical trauma cases. As can be seen in Tables 15.2 and 15.4, measures designed for other informants are lacking, so clinicians could consider gathering impressions from other reporters informally. An integrated understanding of a child's perception of his or her symptoms, the parents' perspective, and (potentially) functioning across settings observed by other key adults would enrich case conceptualization and aid in treatment planning.

Assessing Comorbid Conditions

Although we discuss differential diagnosis in the section on clinical interviews, even early on in the assessment process it is important to be aware of several psychological conditions that frequently co-occur with PTSD. Most notably, these conditions include general anxiety, depression, and substance use (e.g., Bonanno et al., 2010; La Greca et al., 2013; Lai et al., 2013; Rowe, La Greca, & Alexandersson, 2010; also see La Greca & Danzi, 2019). Moreover, trauma exposure has been associated with symptoms of grief, depression, anxiety, stress-related health problems, and increases in substance use (Bonanno et al., 2010). For example, Kilpatrick and colleagues (2003) found that nearly 75% of the adolescents in a large national sample who met criteria for PTSD also met criteria for depression or substance use. Others find high comorbidity between PTSD and depression in youth who are affected by natural disasters, reside in refugee camps during war conflict, or survive physical abuse (e.g., Goenjian et al., 2005; Lai et al., 2013; Thabet, Abed, & Vostanis, 2004).

These comorbid conditions are important to assess because they contribute to the chronicity of youth PTSD (La Greca et al., 2013; Lai et al., 2013) and predict treatment resistance or poor treatment outcome (Jaycox et al., 2010). It is also possible that youth who are referred for an evaluation of depression, anxiety, or substance abuse have co-occurring symptoms of PTSD that have gone unrecognized. Thus, we recommend that readers review in this volume the chapters that cover the best measures for assessing conditions that frequently co-occur with PTSD in youth. Although the co-occurrence of behavior problems and PTSD has been less well studied, a comprehensive assessment should evaluate the presence of externalizing symptoms as well. For instance, PTSD symptoms of hyperarousal, such as trouble sleeping or concentrating, overlap with key symptoms of attention-deficit/hyperactivity disorder

(ADHD) (see Cohen & the Workgroup on Quality Issues, 2010).

Prescription: Using Interviews and Other Considerations to Guide Diagnosis and Treatment Planning

If initial screening of a youth reveals significant symptoms of PTSD, a formal assessment with a clinician-administered structured interview is indicated to confirm the presence of PTSD, and to evaluate the severity of the youth's PTSD symptoms and the extent to which functional impairment is evident (Cohen & the Workgroup on Quality Issues, 2010). Table 15.5, which lists a selection of key interviews that may be used for these purposes, is not intended to reflect a comprehensive list of all interviews that include an assessment of PTSD, but rather to provide a few of the most widely used and well-established diagnostic interviews that clinicians might consider using with youth. It is recommended that parents or other caregivers be involved in this process whenever possible (Cohen & the Workgroup on Quality Issues, 2010). Accordingly, many of the interviews in Table 15.5 include both child and parent/caregiver versions. Several of the interviews listed in Table 15.5 have been updated to reflect DSM-5 changes in diagnostic criteria for PTSD (e.g., Kiddie Schedule for Affective Disorders and Schizophrenia [K-SADS], PTSD-RI-5, Clinician-Administered PTSD Scale for DSM-5 [CAPS-CA-5]; psychometric evaluation of the DSM-5 versions are currently ongoing. All the interviews are intended for use by mental health professionals or trained research assistants, although they also can be administered by paraprofessionals with appropriate training. Below we discuss several important considerations in using clinical interviews for diagnostic purposes.

Assessing Trauma Exposure

General Considerations

Given that trauma exposure can be a sensitive or distressing topic for youth and parents, it is important to carefully consider how and when such questions should be asked. In most assessment situations, it is generally best to allow children and parents time to become comfortable with the assessment situation before broaching the topic of trauma. Importantly, clinicians also should keep in mind that the disclosure of some trauma types, such as child maltreat-

TABLE 15.5. Clinician-Administered Structured Interviews and Scales for Diagnosing PTSD in Children and Adolescents

Interviews	Informant	Ages	No. of Items	Reference/source/more details
Comprehensive diagnostic interviews with a PTSD module				
Schedule for Affective Disorders and Schizophrenia for School Age Children (K-SADS)	Child, parent/caregiver	6–18 years	18 PTSD items	See Weissman (2011) *https://en.wikipedia.org/wiki/kiddie_schedule_for_affective_disorders_and_schizophrenia*
Anxiety Disorders Interview Schedule, Child Version (ADIS-C)	Child, parent/caregiver	7–17 years	26 PTSD items	Silverman & Albano (1996)
Children's Interview for Psychiatric Symptoms (ChIPS)	Child, parent/caregiver	6–18 years	31 PTSD items	Weller et al. (1999); Young et al. (2016)
Diagnostic Infant and Preschool Assessment (DIPA)	Parent/caregiver	Age 6 and younger	46 PTSD items	Scheeringa (2004) *www.infantinstitute.com* *https://medicine.tulane.edu/node/18891*
Diagnostic interviews specific to PTSD				
UCLA PTSD Reaction Index for DSM-5 (PTSD-RI-5) (interview format)	Child, parent/caregiver	7–18 years	31	*www.ptsd.va.gov/professional/assessment/child/ucla_child_reaction_dsm-5.asp* The National Center for Child Traumatic Stress offers a training video administration and scoring of the PTSD Reaction Index for DSM-5, available at *www.nctsn.org/resources/administration-and-scoring-ucla-ptsd-reaction-index-dsm-5-video*
Children's PTSD Inventory (CPTSD-1)	Child	6–18 years	50	Saigh (2004) *www.nctsn.org/measures/childrens-ptsd-inventory*
Clinician-Administered PTSD Scale for DSM-5—Child/Adolescent Version (CAPS-CA-5)	Child	7–18 years	30	*www.ptsd.va.gov/professional/assessment/child/caps-ca.asp* Pynoos et al. (2015) Available from the National Center for PTSD at *www.ptsd.va.gov*

ment, require mandated reporting or have other legal or ethical obligations (e.g., Jackson, Kissoon, & Greene, 2015). As a routine procedure, families should be made aware of the limits of confidentiality at the start of the assessment process.

When asking youth and parents questions about trauma exposure and reactions, interviewers should be mindful of their own reactions to the content disclosed. Shock, outrage, pity, or distress are not appropriate responses to trauma disclosures. Instead, interviewers should remain calm, attentive, and supportive when discussing trauma exposure. Children should not be pressured to discuss their trauma exposure in great detail during the assessment process. With young children, interviewers may find it helpful to ask about trauma exposure while engaging the child in a distracting activity, such as playing a game or drawing.

Assessment When Trauma Exposure Is Known

In some cases, the clinician may have prior knowledge about the type(s) and extent of trauma exposure experienced by the youth (e.g., based on prior screening). Potential trauma exposure also may be obvious, for example, in the case of youth living in a community that just experienced a major disaster (e.g., fire, earthquake, flood) or youth admitted to a medical emergency care unit following a serious motor vehicle accident. In such cases, the trauma exposure portions of the clinical interview can be used both to obtain additional details about the index event and to evaluate whether the youth had additional exposure to PTEs that may be important to consider in treatment planning.

In situations in which the clinician is aware of trauma exposure (e.g., child referred for services due to a traumatic experience), clinical judgment should be used in determining how to involve the child in the assessment of trauma exposure. Specifically, when making this decision, clinicians might consider the developmental level of the child, the nature and severity of the traumatic experience, and the degree of avoidance/distress likely to be evoked by asking a child to discuss the experience during an initial evaluation. For a young child, the clinician might meet with the parent first to gain information about the traumatic experience, then later assess the child's reaction to it.

Assessment When Trauma Exposure Is Unknown

In many cases, youth may be referred for clinical services due to concerns other than trauma exposure. Thus, clinicians maybe unaware of whether a youth has been exposed to PTEs. Even if a rating scale or checklist was previously administered and no traumatic experiences were endorsed, it is recommended to briefly assess trauma exposure with the family during the clinical interview. In some instances, the youth may have been hesitant to disclose trauma exposure on a checklist or form, and may be more willing to disclose this type of information once rapport has been established with the clinician. In other instances, there may be reluctance to put particular labels on a traumatic experience—for example, it may be emotionally distressing for a teenager to classify a coercive sexual encounter as "rape" during an initial evaluation. Clinicians should be sensitive to these types of issues and briefly assess for trauma exposure during the clinical interview, even if trauma exposure was not endorsed on checklists or ratings forms.

For routine clinical care, when potential trauma exposure is not obvious, one might ask the youth (or parent) *whether they have experienced a frightening or stressful event.* Even when a child or parent does not report experiencing a frightening or stressful event, it is important to follow up with specific questions about exposure to different trauma types. Especially when the youth has chronic trauma exposure or when parents have their own trauma histories, the youth or parents may have difficulty identifying specific events as particularly frightening or traumatic. Furthermore, as noted earlier, parents have been shown to underestimate the impact of traumatic events on their children.

Thus, clinicians might provide examples of PTEs (e.g., serious motor vehicle accident, natural disaster, community violence, assault) and ask whether the youth has experienced any of these. Clinical interviews for assessing PTSD (see Table 15.5) typically include trauma exposure sections to aid the clinician in this process, with some interviews including more detailed items about trauma exposure than others. For clinicians interested in a thorough assessment of trauma exposure, the interview format of the PTSD-RI-5 includes 23 trauma types accompanied by questions a clinician might ask to assess for each trauma type, the youth's role in the traumatic experience (e.g., victim, witness), age(s) when the trauma was experienced, and details pertinent to each trauma type. Of the comprehensive diagnostic interviews listed in Table 15.5, the K-SADS provides the most extensive assessment of 13 different trauma types, each of which is accompanied by several recommended questions a clinician could ask to assess for each type of traumatic experience. The Anxiety Disorders Interview Schedule, Child Version (ADIS-C) offers a briefer assessment (nine items) of trauma exposure. Other interviews, such as the Children's Interview for Psychiatric Symptoms (ChIPS), only include general questions about trauma exposure and may be less useful for conducting a comprehensive assessment of trauma exposure across a variety of trauma types.

During the clinical interview, clinicians might consider using the trauma assessment sections from one of the previously mentioned clinical interviews to assess for trauma exposure as part of routine clinical practice (regardless of whether the child's initial presenting problem appears related to trauma). Clinicians can then decide whether to conduct a full clinical interview to assess for PTSD depending on whether trauma exposure was reported.

Clinical Interviews for Assessing PTSD

Clinical interviews are helpful to confirm a PTSD diagnosis and to obtain a precise and nuanced understanding of the youth's symptoms and functioning. Using a standardized interview, such as those listed in Table 15.5, ensures that the clinician asks a comprehensive set of questions and does not overlook a crucial aspect of the youth's psychological functioning. The reader is also referred to Leffler, Riebel, and Hughes (2015) for a review of general diagnostic interviews for youth.

Comprehensive Diagnostic Interviews with a PTSD Module

The selection of a clinical interview depends largely on the purpose of the assessment, the clinical context, and the time constraints involved. In most cases, a clinician might choose an interview that assesses a broad range of psychological disorders, including PTSD. This approach has the advantage of evaluating potential comorbid psychopathology, which in turn has implications for treatment planning. In addition, it may allow the clinician to rule out competing diagnoses (e.g., are the youth's symptoms more consistent with ADHD or PTSD?). Table 15.5 includes examples of comprehensive diagnostic interviews that include a PTSD module.

The K-SADS is a widely-used, semistructured interview for youth (ages 6–18 years) that includes a module for PTSD and also evaluates a wide variety of psychological concerns including mood disorders, anxiety disorders, disruptive behavior dis-

orders, psychotic disorders, eating disorders, and substance use (see Weissman, 2011). Clinicians could use the K-SADS by either administering the PTSD module or by assessing a full array of psychopathology. Similarly, the ADIS-C (Silverman & Albano, 1996) is another option that focuses on anxiety disorders, as well as a few of the most commonly co-occuring psychological disorders; it also includes a PTSD module. Other broad-based diagnostic interviews that have PTSD modules include the Diagnostic Interview for Children and Adolescents—Revised (Reich, 2000) and the Diagnostic Interview Schedule for Children–IV (Shaffer, Fisher, Lucas, Dulcan, & Schwab-Stone, 2000), although it is not clear whether DSM-5 versions of these structured interviews are currently available.

While it is ideal to understand co-occurring symptomatology when assessing for PTSD, this may not be feasible due to time and resource constraints. Clinicans interested in evaluating a wide range of psychopathology within in a limited time might consider using the ChIPS (Weller, Weller, & Rooney, 1999; Young, Bell, & Fristad, 2016), as this was designed as a brief but comprehensive diagnostic interview well suited to the time limitations of some clinical settings.

The aforementioned clinical interviews are designed for use with preadolescent children and adolescents. For younger children (i.e., ages 6 years and younger), clinicians might consider using the Diagnostic Infant and Preschool Assessment (DIPA; Scheeringa, 2004), which is a parent/caregiver report instrument that provides a developmentally sensitive assessment for an array of disorders most relevant for young children, including PTSD.

Diagnostic Interviews Specific to PTSD

Also available are clinical interviews developed specifically for use with trauma-exposed youth (see Table 15.5). For example, the CAPS-CA-5 is a 30-item clinical interview for youth ages 7 years and older (Pynoos et al., 2015); the items are designed to aid clinicians in determining whether youth meet DSM-5 diagnostic criteria for PTSD. Similarly, the Children's PTSD Inventory–1 (CPTSD-I; Saigh, 2004) assesses PTSD symptoms and functioning in youth ages 6–18 years.

Another clinician-administered interview that may be useful is the National Child Traumatic Stress Network (NCTSN) Child and Adolescent Needs and Strengths—Trauma Version (CANS–Trauma; Kisiel et al., 2011). This 110-item clinical interview for youth ages 0–18 years assesses trauma exposure and PTSD symptoms. However, in addition, this interview evaluates domains that are helpful for treatment planning, such as child strengths, life functioning, acculturation, risk, and caregiver needs and strengths.

Some of the rating scales mentioned in the previous section also have interview formats. For example, the PTSD-RI-5 can be administered as self-report and parent-report rating scales (see Tables 15.2 and 15.4), as well as through a structured interview format. The interview version has the advantage of allowing clinicians to use clinical judgment in determining whether endorsed PTSD symptoms are accompanied by clinically significant distress or functional impairment.

Overall, for a diagnosis of PTSD, youth must display significant PTSD symptoms, as well as functional impairment, and all the interviews in Table 15.5 can be used for this purpose. Even youth who do not meet threshold for a diagnosis of PTSD but display clinically elevated symptoms of PTSD may benefit from trauma-focused treatments (see La Greca & Danzi, 2019).

Considerations for Treatment Planning

For youth who meet diagnostic criteria for PTSD or have significant PTSS with functional impairment, treatment planning emerges as the next step in the assessment process. Assessing risk and protective factors and potential treatment moderators may facilitate treatment planning, as noted below. Table 15.6 summarizes these factors and some strategies for assessment; relevant measures also are listed on the website for the Evidence-Based Prevention and Support Center (see Table 15.3).

Risk and Resilience Factors and Treatment Moderators

Substantial research has documented risk and resilience factors associated with youth PTSD symptoms following trauma exposure (e.g., Bonanno et al., 2010; La Greca & Silverman, 2011). Assessing risk and protective factors identifies issues to consider in treatment because the issues are either important to address during intervention or they influence treatment outcome.

The risk and resilience factors associated with the development of PTSD can be conceptualized as falling within four categories: (1) preexisting youth characteristics, (2) trauma exposure, (3) characteristics of the posttrauma environment, and (4) the youth's psychological resources (La

Greca & Silverman, 2011). These risk and resilience factors can be evaluated as part of a comprehensive assessment of youth psychological functioning (see Table 15.6).

First, with respect to *preexisting characteristics*, youth age, gender, and ethnicity are associated with posttraumatic reactions, although these factors account for a small amount of variance in PTSS. Regarding age, children are more likely to exhibit psychological impairment than adults following traumatic events such as disasters, and younger children appear to be more vulnerable than older youth (Bonanno et al., 2010; Norris et al., 2002). Regarding gender, girls typically report more PTSD symptoms than boys (La Greca & Silverman, 2011). Moreover, minority ethnic/racial groups and youth of lower socioeconomic status (SES) often report higher levels of PTSD symptoms and are slower to recover over time than nonminority youth (Bonanno et al., 2010; La Greca & Silverman, 2011). Families from minority backgrounds might possess fewer financial or other resources to deal with trauma recovery, which could prolong the life disruption that ensues, especially after disasters (Bonanno et al., 2010). Youth from ethnic/racial minority groups may also experience additional stressors, including racial discrimination, that exacerbate PTSD symptoms (Chou, Asnaani, & Hofmann, 2012).

Overall, demographic factors do not appear to moderate treatment outcome for youth with PTSD, with one exception: Older youth may benefit more from cognitive-behavioral treatment (CBT) than younger youth (e.g., Morina, Koerssen, & Pollet, 2016). However, developmental issues in treatment delivery and effectiveness for youth with PTSD require further study.

Pretrauma psychosocial functioning in youth also predicts their stress reactions. For example, both pretrauma anxiety and depression are significant risk factors for PTSD symptoms (Bonanno et al., 2010). In fact, anxious children may be vulnerable to developing PTSD symptoms regardless of their levels of trauma exposure (e.g., La Greca, Silverman, & Wasserstein, 1998). Finally, *trauma history* may be a risk factor for the severity of posttraumatic reaction in youth. Trauma history also may moderate treatment outcome, as youth with more extensive trauma histories may be less responsive to treatment than youth with single-incident trauma exposure. (Note that we covered methods for assessing history of trauma exposure in youth in the descriptions of ratings scales, checklists, and interviews.)

TABLE 15.6. Risk and Resilience Factors and Potential Treatment Moderators for Youth with PTSD

Factor	Variable	Association with PTSD or treatment outcome	Assessment or treatment implications
Preexisting youth characteristics	Age	Younger more vulnerable than older youth	Demographic characteristics typically evaluated in routine clinical assessments.
	Gender	Girls report more PTSD symptoms than boys	Older youth may benefit more from cognitive-behavioral interventions than younger youth.
	Ethnicity	Minority youth report more PTSD than nonminority youth and may be slower to recover	
	Psychological functioning—anxiety and depression	Youth with preexisting anxiety and depression are related to greater PTSD after trauma exposure. Anxiety and depression commonly co-occur with PTSD (comorbidity) and could impede treatment outcome unless addressed.	Assess anxiety and depression as part of a comprehensive assessment either by use of checklist, rating scales, or comprehensive structured interviews (see Chapters 7 and 10, respectively, on depression and anxiety, this volume).
	Trauma history	Youth with prior trauma exposure may be more vulnerable to PTSD. Trauma history may influence treatment outcome.	See chapter sections on assessing trauma exposure by rating scales, checklists, or interviews. Also assess parental exposure to the same index traumatic event.
Trauma exposure	Life threat	Life threat may be critical to the emergence of PTSD. Greater life threat associated with PTSD severity in dose–response relationship.	These dimensions of trauma exposure are typically assessed by ratings scales and interviews for PTSD, as noted in this chapter.
	Loss/disruption	Loss and disruption are associated with youths' PTSD symptoms and interfere with recovery.	
Posttrauma environment	Social support	Important for mitigating the impact of trauma and reducing PTSD symptoms. Important moderator of treatment outcome.	Assess youths' social support from multiple sources using a validated checklist such as the Child and Adolescent Social Support Scale (Malecki & Demaray, 2002).

Parental distress and psychopathology	Parental functioning contributes to youth PTSD. When problematic, parental functioning could impede youth's treatment outcome (e.g., maternal depression associated with poorer treatment outcome for youth with PTSD; Dorsey et al., 2017).	Assess parental functioning as a routine part of a comprehensive assessment, especially if parent was exposed to the index trauma (e.g., shooting, terrorist attack, accident). The Patient Health Questionnaire–9 (PHQ-9; for parental depression), and the General Anxiety Disorder–7 (GAD-7; for parental anxiety) may be useful (see Kroenke et al., 2010).
Major life events	Youth who encounter major life stressors while recovering from a traumatic event have a slower recovery.	Assess and monitor major life events by asking child and parent about stressful events that have occurred recently, such as the death or illness of a family member, parental separation or divorce, etc. (see La Greca et al., 2010).
Youths' psychological resources	Coping strategies	Negative coping strategies, especially those reflecting poor emotion regulation, predict chronicity of PTSD symptoms. Positive coping could be promoted in treatment for PTSD.	Assess and monitor youths' coping strategies using developmentally appropriate measures such as the KidCope (Spirito et al., 1988).
Other potentially important treatment moderators	Comorbid elevations in anxiety, depression, or substance use	Common conditions comorbid with PTSD have implications for treatment planning. Current treatments for PTSD may have little impact on these co-occurring conditions.	Assess for comorbidity with PTSD by administering a comprehensive structured interview. Rating scales and checklists (as described in other chapters of this volume) also may be useful.
Conditions to rule out (differential diagnosis)	ADHD, specific phobia, bipolar disorder, physical disorders that mimic PTSD	N/A	Use of a comprehensive diagnostic interview should enable clinicians to rule in or rule out these diagnoses. Obtaining details about the onset and worsening of symptoms may help determine if symptoms are trauma-related.

Second, *aspects of traumatic exposure* also predict the emergence of PTSD symptoms in youth after trauma. In particular, the *presence or perception of life threat* may be critical. Youth who perceive that their lives (or the lives of loved ones) are threatened report greater PTSD symptoms (e.g., Bonanno et al., 2010; La Greca et al., 2010). Furthermore, the death (or threatened death) of a loved one, especially through a shooting or terrorist act, is strongly linked to development of PTSD symptoms in youth (e.g., Gurwitch, Sitterle, Young, & Pfefferbaum, 2002; Suomalainen, Haravuori, Berg, Kiviruusu, & Marttunen, 2011), as are natural disasters with substantial mass casualties (e.g., Furr et al., 2010). PTSD reactions arising from such events often are complicated by feelings of grief and guilt. For instance, youth who lose a loved one in a shooting or a terrorist attack must deal with bereavement and reconcile why they survived and the loved one did not; this could lead to impairing thoughts regarding whether they could have done more to prevent the death from occurring (La Greca & Silverman, 2011).

Trauma-related loss and life disruption is another key aspect of trauma exposure. After a disaster, for instance, youth and families often face a cascading series of life stressors that may last for months or years, such as the loss of one's home and/or possessions, a change of schools, shifts in parental employment and finances, friends moving away, altered leisure activities, and so on (La Greca & Silverman, 2011; La Greca, Silverman, Vernberg, & Prinstein, 1996; La Greca et al., 2010). Loss and disruption maintain PTSD symptoms and challenge youth adaptation and coping.

Pertinent to loss and disruption, clinicians should also consider aspects of the traumatic experience that might be ongoing (e.g., child abuse case in which custody issues are still being decided in court; medical trauma case in which treatments are ongoing or survival is uncertain). Traumatic experiences that are chronic or likely to re-occur present major impediments to recovery and should be handled carefully in treatment planning.

Importantly, trauma exposure can be influenced by the media, social media, or other forms of information technology. Studies repeatedly indicate that higher levels of media exposure to traumatic events (e.g., terrorist attack of 9/11, the Boston Marathon bombing; Comer et al., 2014; Holmes, Creswell, & O'Connor, 2007) are associated with greater PTSD symptoms, even for youth who live in areas remote from the event and did not lose a loved one.

Third, various *aspects of the posttrauma environment* (e.g., availability of social support, presence of parental psychopathology, occurrence of additional life stressors) can magnify or attenuate PTSD reactions in youth. (Table 15.6 notes measures that may be useful in this regard.) For example, *social support* from significant others mitigates the impact of natural disasters on youth PTSD symptoms (e.g., La Greca et al., 2010, 2013) and is an important moderator of postdisaster treatment outcome (e.g., Jaycox et al., 2010). Thus, assessing youth social support posttrauma is important, as are efforts to build social support during treatment.

In addition, *parents' psychological functioning* is important for youths' posttraumatic reactions and recovery (e.g., Gil-Rivas, Silver, Holman, McIntosh, & Poulin, 2007). In fact, in a meta-analysis of PTSD treatments for youth, Dorsey and colleagues (2017) found that greater maternal depressive symptoms were associated with poorer treatment outcomes for youth. Obtaining an evaluation of parental functioning is especially critical when youth and parents both are exposed to the same traumatic event (e.g., violent death of a loved one, natural disasters).

Finally, *major life events*, such as an illness or death in the family, or parental divorce or separation, occurring in the months following a traumatic event may significantly impede youths' recovery and predict greater persistence of PTSD symptoms over time (e.g., La Greca et al., 2010, 2013). Youth who experience major life events following a traumatic experience represent a high-risk group for chronic PTSD reactions (La Greca et al., 2013). As a result, ongoing monitoring of life events is useful when treating youth with PTSD.

Fourth and finally, youths' *psychological resources* also predict their reactions and recovery, and are important considerations for treatment. Specifically, youth who are found to have more negative *coping strategies* for dealing with stress, especially strategies that reflect poor emotion regulation (e.g., self-anger, blaming others), display higher levels of PTSD symptoms after natural disasters and evidence greater persistence of PTSD symptoms over time (La Greca et al., 1996, 2013). Thus, efforts to assess and promote adaptive coping may be useful for interventions with youth experiencing PTSD. (Note that trauma-focused treatments for youth with PTSD that have a strong evidence base typically address issues of child coping and emotion regulation; see de Arellano et al., 2014.)

Comorbidity and Implications for Treatment

As discussed earlier, several psychological conditions commonly co-occur with PTSD in youth, including anxiety, depression, and substance use, and should thus be evaluated in a comprehensive assessment of youth with PTSD. Because treatments for PTSD often have little impact on these comorbid symptoms (La Greca & Danzi, 2019), it is advisable to take comorbidity into account during treatment planning and consider using adjunct treatments that specifically target comorbid symptomatology in youth.

Conditions to Rule Out (Differential Diagnosis)

According to the "Practice Parameters for the Assessment and Treatment of PTSD" (Cohen & the Workgroup on Quality Issues, 2010), several psychological disorders have symptoms similar to those of PTSD; thus, is it important to differentiate these other disorders/symptoms from PTSD when conducting a comprehensive assessment. For example, the reexperiencing and avoidance symptoms of PTSD (e.g., restless, disorganized, or agitated activity or play) or arousal symptoms (e.g., difficulty sleeping or concentrating) are similar to symptoms of ADHD; here, a careful history of trauma exposure can help to evaluate whether a youth's symptoms are related to trauma onset or worsened with trauma exposure. Similarly, as discussed by Cohen and the Workgroup on Quality Issues (2010), clinicians should also rule out oppositional defiant disorder (which also features irritability and angry outbursts), specific phobia (which features avoidance of and hyperarousal to feared stimuli), and bipolar disorder (which features hypomania and hyperarousal symptoms, such as numbing and problems sleeping), among other possibilities. Some physical conditions, such as asthma, migraines, and seizure disorders, as well as prescription and nonprescription drug side effects (e.g., antipsychotics, antiasthmatics, antihistamines, diet pills, and cold medications), can produce symptoms similar to those of PTSD (Cohen & the Workgroup on Quality Issues, 2010). In all cases, taking a careful history that includes the onset and worsening of PTSD-like symptoms should help to differentiate these other conditions from PTSD.

Case Formulation and Treatment Planning

After completing a comprehensive assessment, determining that PTSD represents the primary diagnosis or key area of concern for a youth, and identifying any secondary conditions (or comorbid symptomatology) that may affect treatment, as well as risk and resilience factors that may influence recovery, the clinician may move on to case formulation and treatment planning. When PTSD or PTSS is conceptualized as the primary concern, treatment planning should begin with evidence-based treatment to reduce PTSD; adjunct treatments that address co-occurring symptomatology (e.g., anxiety, depression) or mitigate any areas of risk (e.g., lack of social support, poor coping) could be used to enhance the treatment for PTSD. These adjunct treatments might be incorporated into the PTSD treatment plan from the start or be activated later on if the initial PTSD treatment is not effective, or if the youth is slow to improve.

At present, CBT and trauma-focused CBT (TF-CBT) have the strongest evidence base for treating PTSD (or significant PTSS) in youth and are considered well established (de Arellano et al., 2014; Cohen & Mannarino, 2015; La Greca & Danzi, 2019). In fact, the practice parameters developed by the American Academy of Child and Adolescent Psychiatry (Cohen & the Workgroup on Quality Issues, 2010) recommend TF-CBT as the first line of treatment for children and adolescents with PTSD, as it is effective in treating a wide age range of youth (i.e., preschoolers through adolescents) with diverse types of trauma exposure. Some evidence also suggests that TF-CBT leads to reductions in co-occurring symptoms of depression (Lenz & Hollenbaugh, 2015) and other co-occuring problem areas (de Arellano et al., 2014). Moreover, TF-CBT has been adapted for multiple cultures and international populations (Cohen & Mannarino, 2015; Dorsey et al., 2017). Importantly, for youth who experience difficulty with the exposure-based elements of TF-CBT, CBT without a trauma focus also can be effective in reducing PTSS (La Greca & Danzi, 2019).

In terms of treatment delivery modalities, TF-CBT (and CBT) can be administered individually or in groups (for details on TF-CBT content and delivery, see Cohen & Mannarino, 2015; Cohen, Mannarino, & Deblinger, 2002, 2017). Individual TF-CBT typically is delivered to the parent and child. Group-based TF-CBT (especially in school settings) may be conducive to communitywide or large-scale traumatic events and may facilitate youths' access to and engagement in treatment relative to individual clinic-based treatment settings (e.g., Jaycox et al., 2010).

Other considerations for treatment planning include whether the youth displays comorbid conditions (especially anxiety, depression, ADHD, and substance use; Cohen & the Workgroup on Quality Issues, 2010), as such youth will likely need coordinated or adjunct treatment to address the co-occurring problem areas. Furthermore, because maternal depressive symptoms predict poorer child response to treatments for PTSD (Dorsey et al., 2017), treatment options for the youth's parent(s) may be an important consideration. Similarly, youth who have significant risk factors for poor recovery (e.g., lack of social support, stressful life events; see Table 15.6) will likely need an overall treatment plan that addresses these areas of risk.

The developmental stage of the youth is crucial to consider with treatment planning. The age of the child may influence the degree of parental involvement in treatment. Older adolescents (and especially those with trauma histories involving sexual assault) may prefer an increased sense of agency over their treatment and that the parent not be privy to sensitive details. For young children, parents should be highly involved in treatment; in fact, a major focus of treatment might be providing parent training around issues such as providing consistent positive attention, setting up a stable routine, modeling appropriate coping, and managing behavioral issues. In terms of developmental issues, some studies indicate that older youth age is related to better trauma treatment outcome (Lenz & Hollenbaugh, 2015; Morina et al., 2016), whereas others find that trauma treatment works better with younger youth (Goldbeck, Muche, Sachser, Tutus, & Rosner, 2016). As the PTSD treatment literature evolves, further attention to developmental issues, as well as key moderators of treatment outcome, will be critical.

Cultural issues and patient preferences need to be considered. For the most part, there has been little systematic study of cultural issues in the treatment of youth PTSD; however, TF-CBT, which has a strong evidence base, has been used with a wide range of trauma types and with youth from diverse cultures (see Cohen & Mannarino, 2015; Cohen et al., 2002, 2017). Clinicians should be sensitive to how different traumatic experiences may hold different meanings across diverse cultures. Clinicians should endeavor to educate themselves about culturally relevant factors when working with families of diverse backgrounds.

In terms of patient preferences, some literature suggests that youth or parents may have concerns about exposure-based therapies (e.g., Gola, Beidas, Antinoro-Burke, Kratz, & Fingerhut, 2015). They may express a desire to "move on" from the trauma and voice concerns that talking about it will make symptoms worse. This is an important issue to address when treatment planning. Many trauma-focused treatment manuals include components that provide psychoeducation for the family and a rationale for exposure work, along with recommendations for how the clinician might discuss these concerns with a family (see La Greca & Danzi, 2019). Some treatments, such as TF-CBT, start with strategies that are typically more acceptable to families (e.g., emotional awareness, relaxation techniques, coping skills) to allow family members time to become more comfortable with the treatment process and provide the child with skills to handle distressing content before beginning exposure work. Clinicians should work with their clients to address these concerns as they arise.

Finally, clinicians should remain vigilant about potential stressors or trauma reminders that may arise for the youth and incorporate these issues into treatment planning. For example, if a youth will be returning to school after a lengthy absence (e.g., due to a prolonged hospital stay after injury or school closure after a natural disaster), a clinician might prioritize coping skills to help the youth adjust to school or delay starting intense exposure work on the youth's first day back at school. During the intake and throughout treatment, the clinician should assess for upcoming life events and situations that could evoke trauma responses, in order to incorporate these into the treatment plan and support the family in preparing for them.

Progress, Process, and Outcome Measurement

Goal Measurement

Based on the foregoing discussion, clinicians may have multiple goals when treating youth with PTSD or significant PTSS. Treatment goals likely include (1) overall improvement in the youth's functioning; (2) reduction/improvement in PTSD symptoms, as reflected in a significant decline in PTSD symptom severity or loss of PTSD diagnosis; (3) reduction/improvement in any co-occurring area of concern (e.g., depression), as reflected in a significant decline in symptom severity or loss of comorbid diagnosis; and (4) improvements in areas of risk (e.g., low social support, poor coping, parental depression). In this chapter, we covered age-appropriate measures that assess PTSD symptoms and diagnosis, and also suggested some measures that may be useful for evaluating risk factors; other chapters in this volume cover the assessment of symptoms and diagnoses of potential comorbid psychological conditions. Assessing overall improvement in the youth's functioning is discussed below as an important strategy for monitoring treatment progress and outcome.

Monitoring Progress, Process, and Outcome

Monitoring Progress

It is critical to have a monitoring system in place during a youth's treatment for PTSD to guide the clinician in delivering effective treatment and to know when treatment termination is indicated. Treatment monitoring also is important because, in some cases, PTSD symptoms worsen before they improve. For example, parents might perceive that their child's symptoms have worsened if the child talks more about the traumatic event, even though the child is not avoiding traumatic reminders and this may be a sign of improvement (Salloum, Scheeringa, Cohen, & Storch, 2014). Thus, a monitoring system will be valuable to differentiate between minor worsening that reflects treatment effectiveness and significant worsening that could signal the need for a different or more intensive treatment.

To minimize assessment burden, brief rating measures such as the Clinical Global Impression—Improvement Scale (CGI-I; Busner & Targum, 2007; Guy, 1976) could be completed routinely (e.g., weekly) by the parent, clinician, and also the youth (if age 7 or older). Salloum and colleagues (2014) recommend a modified version of the CGI-I that has an 8-point scale of "improvement since the initial assessment" (1 = *free of symptoms*, 2 = *much improved*, 3 = *improved*, 4 = *minimally improved*, 5 = *no change*, 6 = *minimally worse*, 7 = *much worse*, 8 = *very much worse*). Ratings of 1–3 indicate a positive treatment response. Clinical worsening may be defined as three consecutive parent or clinician ratings of 6, or a single rating of 7 or 8 (Salloum et al., 2014); disagreements between parent, clinician, and youth ratings should be discussed and resolved. (Other chapters describe similar global rating scales, and the diagnostic interviews listed

in Table 15.5 also include ratings of improvement or overall symptom severity.)

If there is evidence of significant worsening, clinicians should consider implementing more intensive, alternative, or adjunct treatments. For example, youth who receive group-based TF-CBT and are worsening might need a more intensive individual treatment (Jaycox et al., 2010; Salloum et al., 2014). Moreover, to guide the clinician in selecting the best treatment options, it may be useful to readminister one of the recommended PTSD rating scales (see Table 15.2), as well as a rating scale that assesses any comorbid symptomatology (e.g., a depression rating scale if the youth is depressed). PTSD rating scales may help the clinician identify the types of symptoms that are most prominent, which could lead to an enhanced treatment strategy. For example, for youth with significant PTSD symptoms of reexperiencing or avoidance, trauma-focused exposure techniques might be most useful, whereas youth whose symptomatology is dominated by negative cognitions or alterations in mood might benefit from treatments that address depressive symptoms. Alternatively, youth with significant arousal symptoms might benefit most from relaxation and other mindfulness strategies (see La Greca & Danzi, 2019). Finally, for youth with significant comorbid symptomatology, adjunct treatments that address the co-occurring symptoms could be valuable.

Monitoring Process

In addition to a brief weekly evaluation of "treatment improvement," most evidence-based treatment manuals include measures that enable clinicians to evaluate treatment process (e.g., Cohen et al., 2017). In addition, brief versions of the PTSD symptom measures (e.g., those in Table 15.2) could be administered at the beginning of treatment sessions, to systematically track youths' improvement in relevant symptoms. Clinicians should be aware that symptom presentations may change over the course of treatment. For example, a child who is avoiding trauma reminders (e.g., refusing to attend school following a shooting) may report less distress in response to reminders during the intake but more distress once exposure activities start occurring during treatment. Readministering PTSD symptom scales (as described in Table 15.2) at different points throughout treatment allows the clinician to track these fluctuations over time and incorporate any new symptoms into the treatment plan.

Monitoring Treatment Outcome and Maintenance

Typical trauma-focused treatments for PTSD are 12–16 weeks in duration (Cohen & Mannarino, 2015), although some youth respond more rapidly to treatment than others (see de Arellano et al., 2014; La Greca & Danzi, 2019; Salloum et al., 2014, 2017). To determine whether a youth is an early treatment responder or whether the full treatment has been successful, it is useful to evaluate the youth's "responder status."

Multiple assessment methods can be used to evaluate responder status. First, global improvement on a measure such as the CGI-I can be useful to document overall improvement (as noted earlier). If the youth's overall functioning has improved for 2 consecutive weeks, as determined by both clinician and parent (and the child is age 7 or older), other measures can be administered to document a reduction in PTSD symptom severity and/or the loss of diagnosis. Specifically, rating scales discussed earlier in this chapter (see Tables 15.2 and 15.4) can be readministered to parents and youth at the end of treatment to evaluate reductions in PTSD symptom severity; here the goal would be scores below the clinical cutoffs for that measure, from both respondents. If significant symptom reduction is present, then "loss of diagnosis" can be confirmed by readministering the structured interview used to initially confirm the PTSD diagnosis (see Table 15.5) to the parent and youth. In cases where co-occurring symptomatology was present (e.g., anxiety, depression), the clinician also should assess for reductions in those symptoms (to below clinical cutoffs) on appropriate rating scale measures and/or for the loss of diagnosis on a structured interview, if the youth had previously achieved diagnostic levels. For example, in a stepped-care study of TF-CBT for preschool youth with PTSD, Salloum and colleagues (2014, 2017) defined "responder status" as children who had a score of 3 (improved), 2 (much improved), or 1 (free of symptoms) on the CGI-I for 2 consecutive weeks, and either a total score of 40 or less on the Trauma Symptom Checklist for Children or three or fewer PTSD symptoms on the Diagnostic Infant and Preschool Assessment, a semistructured interview administered to parents.

Clinicians should assess for "responder status" after treatment completion, although an earlier assessment of responder status might be indicated if the youth is rated as improved for 2 or more consecutive weeks of treatment. For example, in the studies by Salloum and colleagues (2014, 2017), youth were assessed for responder status at midtreatment, and those who were treatment responders were moved to the maintenance phase of treatment.

When youth do not meet responder status at the end of the specified treatment, the clinician must decide whether to continue treatment, initiate an alternative treatment, or to move to termination. A comprehensive reassessment of the youths's functioning that touches on all the specified treatment goals (e.g., improvement in functioning, reduction in PTSD symptoms, and symptoms of comorbid conditions) may assist the clinician in making a suitable determination.

In clinical practice, once treatment has been terminated, it is unusual to continue to monitor the youth's functioning. However, continued monitoring or a periodic reassessment may be useful in some situations (e.g., a youth who did not meet responder status at the time of treatment termination; a research protocol evaluating treatment maintenance). For example, in evaluating the impact of TF-CBT on sexually maltreated youths' symptoms of posttraumatic stress and co-occuring symptoms, Mannarino, Cohen, Deblinger, Runyon, and Steer (2012) conducted a comprehensive assessment (including rating scales and structured interview) at midtreatment, posttreatment, and at two subsequent follow-ups (6- and 12-months posttreatment).

Conclusions and Future Directions

Trauma assessment is extremely important, yet underutilized in most clinical settings. In this chapter, we have reviewed key measures of trauma exposure and posttraumatic stress for youth, as well as related assessment issues. This information should provide some guidance to clinicians and researchers interested in evaluating and understanding the impact of trauma on youth.

Before closing, we highlight several challenges in the area of trauma assessment. Perhaps foremost is the lack of consensus on what constitutes PTSD in youth (and adults) given the divergent orientations and diagnostic approaches of DSM-5 and ICD-11 (Danzi & La Greca, 2016; La Greca et al., 2017). Until greater consensus has been achieved across the classification systems, it may be advisable to assess youth PTSS in a manner that is congruent with both the narrow (e.g., ICD-11) and broad (e.g., DSM-5) approaches to conceptualizing PTSD. Moreover, regardless of the diagnostic approach, few measures that assess posttraumatic stress in youth have been updated to reflect these current conceptualizations of PTSD. Thus, the assessment of PTSD in youth should develop substantially over the next few years. (In this regard, resources provided in Table 15.3 may be useful.) Below we highlight several other critical areas for future research and practice.

Developmental Issues

Further study of developmental aspects of PTSD in youth is needed. Among young children (i.e., ages 6 years and younger), concern about the underrecognition of posttraumatic stress led to the emergence of developmentally sensitive diagnostic criteria that identify substantially more young children with PTSD than do adult-based criteria (Scheeringa et al., 2006). However, assessment measures based on these developmentally modified criteria are new and await further validation. Similarly, it has yet to be determined whether assessment measures being developed to assess ICD-11 criteria for PTSD in youth will also need modification for young children.

Among preadolescents (i.e., ages 7–12 years), a key issue for assessment research is whether youth in this age group should be evaluated using measures that reflect the "Young Child" criteria (noted earlier), or the more traditional adult-based criteria for PTSD. Current research indicates that the "Young Child" criteria identify about twice as many preadolescents with PTSD as adult-based PTSD criteria (Danzi & La Greca, 2017). Future studies may help to resolve this issue; meanwhile, it may be advisable to assess preadolescents using the "Young Child" criteria, especially for screening purposes, as these criteria are more inclusive.

Complex PTSD

At present, there has been little systematic research on complex PTSD in youth, and measures that assess complex PTSD (based on ICD-11 criteria) are under development. The features of complex PTSD that reflect disturbances in self-organization (e.g., problems with affect regulation and interpersonal relationships; negative self-concept) could have important implications for treatment planning, as they likely require treatments that address emotion regulation and interpersonal functioning (Cloitre et al., 2012). Until measures of complex PTSD are available, clinicians might rely on measures that tap emotion regulation and interpersonal functioning to supplement their assessment of PTSD when complex PTSD is suspected.

Cultural Issues

Cultural issues in the assessment of youth PTSD have received little systematic attention but are of high interest. Many of the measures listed in Table 15.2, for example, have been used internationally with youth from diverse cultures or with ethnically diverse youth within the United States. Yet culture shapes the subjective meaning of trauma and could influence symptom expression (Marsella & Christopher, 2004). Furthermore, among U.S. adults, there are ethnic differences in the kind and degree of PTSS reported by individuals of Hispanic backgrounds (compared to non-Hispanics; Marshall, Schell, & Miles, 2009). Thus, cultural diversity has the potential to impact the assessment of PTSS in youth and warrants systematic attention.

Assessment of Trauma Exposure and PTEs

In addition to refining measures of posttraumatic stress, further attention might be devoted to evaluating measures of trauma exposure in youth. Refining the assessment of trauma exposure is especially important for understanding differences in youth PTSD as a function of trauma type. Each of the measures listed in Tables 15.2, 15.4, and 15.5 has its own approach to categorizing and evaluating the types of trauma exposure; some are more comprehensive than others. Developing uniformity in the types of PTEs that are assessed would be useful. In this regard, the National Child Traumatic Stress Network's website (*www.nctsn.org/what-is-child-trauma/trauma-types*) may be instructive, as it defines multiple trauma types: bullying, community violence, complex trauma, disasters, domestic violence, early childhood trauma, medical trauma, physical abuse, refugee trauma, sexual abuse, terrorism and violence, and traumatic grief. Measures of trauma exposure might systematically include PTEs that reflect this comprehensive listing.

Furthermore, for some traumatic events (e.g., natural disasters, terrorist attacks), trauma exposure measures have been developed specifically for that type of event (e.g., Comer et al., 2014; La Greca et al., 2010). In other cases, such as medical trauma, clinical researchers have used different informal mixes of items to get at aspects of exposure (N. Kassam-Adams, personal communication, March 4, 2019). Ideally, all trauma exposure measures should assess perceived and actual life threat associated with the specific event. Having standard measures of trauma exposure designed for specific trauma types would facilitate a better understanding of the impact of certain traumatic events on youth.

In addition, most measures of trauma exposure predominantly focus on what happened during and after the event. Yet, at least with traumatic events that have some warning (e.g., hurricanes), emerging research suggests that perceptions of life threat and vulnerability during the buildup to the event can also contribute to youths' (and parents') posttraumatic stress (e.g., La Greca et al., 2019a, 2019b). Thus, further refinement in the standardization and scope of trauma-specific exposure measures may also be desirable.

Conclusions

As we noted at the beginning of this chapter, trauma exposure is a common experience among youth and leads to the development of PTSD or significant PTSS in a significant minority. Moreover, PTSD or PTSS often co-occur with other common psychological disorders, including anxiety, depression, and substance use (for older youth), yet evidence also indicates that PTSD is often underrecognized in youth. Consequently, it is important to assess for youths' trauma exposure and potential PTSS in routine clinical assessments, and certainly whenever youths' exposure to a potentially traumatic event is known. The measures surveyed in this chapter should help to guide the clinician and researcher through the trauma assessment process.

REFERENCES

Achenbach, T. M., & Rescorla, L. A. (2001). *Manual for the ASEBA school-age forms and profiles*. Burlington: Center for Children, Youth and Families, University of Vermont.

Adams, J., Mrug, S., & Knight, D. C. (2018). Characteristics of child physical and sexual abuse as predictors of psychopathology. *Child Abuse and Neglect, 86*, 167–177.

Alisic, E., Zalta, A. K., van Wesel, F., Larsen, S. E., Hafsted, G. S., Hassanpour, K., & Smid, G. E. (2014). Rates of post-traumatic stress disorder in trauma exposed children and adolescents: Meta-analysis. *British Journal of Psychiatry, 204*, 335–340.

American Psychiatric Association. (1994). *Diagnostic and statistical manual of mental disorders* (4th ed., text rev.). Washington, DC: Author.

American Psychiatric Association. (2013). *Diagnostic and statistical manual of mental disorders* (5th ed.). Arlington, VA: Author.

Bonanno, G. A., Brewin, C. R., Kaniasty, K., & La Greca, A. M. (2010). Weighing the costs of disaster: Consequences, risks, and resilience in individuals, families, and communities. *Psychological Science in the Public Interest, 11*(1), 1–49.

Brewin, C. R., Cloitre, M., Hyland, P., Shevlin, M., Maercker, A., Bryant, R. A., . . . Reed, G. M. (2017). A review of current evidence regarding the ICD-11 proposals for diagnosing PTSD and complex PTSD. *Clinical Psychology Review, 58*, 1–15.

Brewin, C. R., Lanius, R. A., Novac, A., Schnyder, U., & Galea, S. (2009). Reformulating PTSD for DSM-5: Life after Criterion A. *Journal of Traumatic Stress, 22*(5), 366–373.

Briere, J. (1996). *Trauma Symptom Checklist for Children (TSCC) professional manual*. Odessa, FL: Psychological Assessment Resources.

Briere, J. (2005). *Trauma Symptom Checklist for Young Children (TSCYC): Professional manual*. Odessa, FL: Psychological Assessment Resources.

Buck, C. (2018). ICD-11 codes released by WHO. Retrieved June 10, 2018, from *www.icd10monitor.com/news-alert-icd-11-codes-released-by-who*.

Busner, J., & Targum, S. D. (2007). The Clinical Global Impressions Scale: Applying a research tool in clinical practice. *Psychiatry (Edgmont), 4*(7), 28–37.

Centers for Disease Control and Prevention. (2008). CDC childhood injury report. Retrieved June 29, 2017, from *www.cdc.gov/safechild/child_injury_data.html*.

Chivers-Wilson, K. A. (2006). Sexual assault and posttraumatic stress disorder: A review of the biological, psychological, and sociological factors and treatments. *McGill Journal of Medicine, 9*, 111–118.

Chou, T., Asnaani, A., & Hofmann, S. G. (2012). Perception of racial discrimination and psychopathology across three U.S. ethnic minority groups. *Cultural Diversity and Ethnic Minority Psychology, 18*, 74–81.

Cicchetti, D., & Lynch, M. (1993). Toward an ecological/transactional model of community violence and child maltreatment: Consequences for children's development. *Psychiatry, 56*, 96–118.

Cloitre, M., Courtois, C. A., Ford, J. D., Green, B. L., Alexander, P., Briere, J., . . . van der Hart, O. (2012). The ISTSS Expert Consensus Treatment Guidelines for Complex PTSD in Adults. Retrieved December 1, 2018, from *www.istss.org/istss_main/media/documents/istss-expert-concesnsus-guidelines-for-complex-ptsd-updated-060315.pdf*.

Cloitre, M., Shevlin, M., Brewin, C. R., Bisson, J. I., Roberts, N. P., Maercker, A., . . . Hyland, P. (2018). The International Trauma Questionnaire: Development of a self-report measure of ICD-11 PTSD and complex PTSD. *Acta Psychiatrica Scandinavica, 138,* 536–546.

Cohen, J. A., & Mannarino, A. P. (2015). Trauma-focused cognitive behavior therapy for traumatized children and families. *Child and Adolescent Psychiatric Clinics of North America, 24*(3), 557–570.

Cohen, J. A., Mannarino, A. P., & Deblinger, E. (Eds.). (2002). *Trauma-focused CBT for children and adolescents: Treatment applications.* New York: Guilford Press.

Cohen, J. A., Mannarino, A. P., & Deblinger, E. (2017). *Treating trauma and traumatic grief in children and adolescents* (2nd ed.). New York: Guilford Press.

Cohen, J. A., & Workgroup on Quality Issues. (2010). Practice parameters for the assessment and treatment of children and adolescents with PTSD. *Journal of the American Academy of Child and Adolescent Psychiatry, 49,* 414–430.

Comer, J. S., Dantowitz, A., Chou, T., Edson, A. L., Elkins, R. M., Kerns, C., . . . Green, J. G. (2014). Adjustment among area youth after the Boston Marathon bombing and subsequent manhunt. *Pediatrics, 134,* 17–14.

Copeland, W. E., Keeler, G., Angold, A., & Costello, E. J. (2007). Traumatic events and posttraumatic stress in childhood. *Archives of General Psychiatry, 64,* 577–584.

Danese, A., & McEwen, B. S. (2012). Adverse childhood experiences, allostasis, allostatic load, and age-related disease. *Physiology and Behavior, 106,* 29–39.

Danzi, B. A., & La Greca, A. M. (2016). DSM-IV, DSM-5, and ICD-11: Identifying children with posttraumatic stress disorder after disasters. *Journal of Child Psychology and Psychiatry, 57,* 1444–1452.

Danzi, B. A., & La Greca, A. M. (2017). Optimizing clinical thresholds for PTSD: Extending the DSM-5 preschool criteria to school-aged children. *International Journal of Clinical and Health Psychology, 17,* 234–241.

de Arellano, M. A., Lyman, D. R., Jobe-Shields, L., George, P., Dougherty, R. H., Daniels, A. S., . . . Delphin-Rittmon, M. E. (2014). Trauma-focused cognitive-behavioral therapy for children and adolescents: Assessing the evidence. *Psychiatric Services (Washington, DC), 65*(5), 591–602.

Deblinger, E., Mannarino, A. P., Cohen, J. A., Runyon, M. K., & Steer, R. A. (2011). Trauma-focused cognitive behavioral therapy for children: Impact of the trauma narrative and treatment length. *Depression and Anxiety, 28,* 67–75.

Dehon, C., & Scheeringa, M. S. (2006). Screening for preschool posttraumatic stress disorder with the Child Behavior Checklist. *Journal of Pediatric Psychology, 31*(4), 431–435.

Dorsey, S., McLaughlin, K. A., Kerns, S. E. U., Harrison, J. P., Lambert, H. K., Briggs, E. C., . . . Amaya-Jackson, L. (2017). Evidence base update for psychosocial treatments for children and adolescents exposed to traumatic events. *Journal of Clinical Child and Adolescent Psychology, 46*(3), 303–330.

Eklund, K., Rossen, E., Koriakin, T., Chafouleas, S. M., & Resnick, C. (2018). Systematic review of trauma screening measures for children and adolescents. *School Psychology Quarterly, 33,* 30–43.

Elhai, J. D., Layne, C. M., Steinberg, A. S., Vrymer, M. J., Briggs, E. C., Ostrowski, S. A., & Pynoos, R. S. (2013). Psychometric properties of the UCLA PTSD Reaction Index: Part 2. Investigating factor structure findings in a national clinic-referred youth sample. *Journal of Traumatic Stress, 26,* 10–18.

Foa, E. B., Asnaani, A., Zang, Y., Capaldi, S., & Yeh, R. (2018.) Psychometrics of the Child PTSD Symptom Scale for DSM-5 for trauma-exposed children and adolescents. *Journal of Clinical Child and Adolescent Psychology, 47,* 38–46.

Ford, T., Goodman, R., & Meltzer, H. (2003). The British Child and Adolescent Mental Health Survey 1999: The prevalence of DSM-IV disorders. *Journal of the American Academy of Child and Adolescent Psychiatry, 42*(10), 1203–1211.

Friedman, M. J. (2013). Finalizing PTSD in DSM-5: Getting here from there and where to go next. *Journal of Traumatic Stress, 26*(5), 548–556.

Furr, J. M., Comer, J. S., Edmunds, J. M., & Kendall, P. C. (2010). Disasters and youth: A meta-analytic examination of posttraumatic stress. *Journal of Consulting and Clinical Psychology, 78*(6), 765–780.

Gil-Rivas, V., Silver, R. C., Holman, E. A., McIntosh, D. N., & Poulin, M. (2007). Parental response and adolescent adjustment to the September 11, 2001 terrorist attacks. *Journal of Traumatic Stress, 20*(6), 1063–1068.

Goenjian, A. K., Walling, D., Steinberg, A. M., Karayan, I., Najarian, L. M., & Pynoos, R. S. (2005). A prospective study of posttraumatic stress and depressive reactions among treated and untreated adolescents 5 years after a catastrophic disaster. *American Journal of Psychiatry, 162,* 2302–2308.

Gola, J. A., Beidas, R. S., Antinoro-Burke, D., Kratz, H. E., & Fingerhut, R. (2015). Ethical considerations in exposure therapy with children. *Cognitive and Behavioral Practice, 23*(2), 184–193.

Goldbeck, L., Muche, R., Sachser, C., Tutus, D., & Rosner, R. (2016). Effectiveness of trauma-focused cognitive behavioral therapy for children and adolescents: A randomized controlled trial in eight German mental health clinics. *Psychotherapy and Psychosomatics, 85*(3), 159–170.

Gurwitch, R. H., Sitterle, K. A., Young, B. H., & Pfefferbaum, B. (2002). The aftermath of terrorism. In A. M. La Greca, W. K. Silverman, E. M. Vernberg, & M. C. Roberts (Eds.), *Helping children cope with disasters and terrorism* (pp. 327–358). Washington, DC: American Psychological Association.

Guy, W. (1976). *ECDEU assessment manual for psy-*

chopharmacology. Washington, DC: Department of Health, Education, and Welfare.

Hafstad, G. S., Dyb, G., Jensen, T. K., Steinberg, A. M., & Pynoos, R. S. (2014). PTSD prevalence and symptom structure of DSM-5 criteria in adolescents and young adults surviving the 2011 shooting in Norway. *Journal of Affective Disorders, 169*, 40–46.

Hafstad, G. S., Thoresen, S., Wentzel-Larsen, T., Maercker, A., & Dyb, G. (2017). PTSD or not PTSD? Comparing the proposed ICD-11 and the DSM-5 PTSD criteria among young survivors of the 2011 Norway attacks and their parents. *Psychological Medicine, 47*, 1283–1291.

Holmes, E. A., Creswell, C., & O'Connor, T. G. (2007). Posttraumatic stress symptoms in London school children following September 11, 2001: An exploratory investigation of peri-traumatic reactions and intrusive imagery. *Journal of Behavior Therapy and Experimental Psychiatry, 38*, 474–490.

Jackson, A. M., Kissoon, N., & Greene, C. (2015). Aspects of abuse: Recognizing and responding to child maltreatment. *Current Problems in Pediatric and Adolescent Health Care, 45*, 58–70.

Jaycox, L. H., Cohen, J. A., Mannarino, A. P., Walker, D. W., Langley, A. K., Gegenheimer, K. L., . . . Schonlau, M. (2010). Children's mental health care following Hurricane Katrina: A field trial of trauma-focused psychotherapies. *Journal of Traumatic Stress, 23*(2), 223–231.

Jones, R. T., Fletcher, K., & Ribbe, D. R. (2002). *Child's Reaction to Traumatic Events Scale—Revised (CRTES-R): A self-report traumatic stress measure.* Blacksburg: Virginia Tech University.

Karam, E. G., Friedman, M. J., Hill, E. D., Kessler, R. C., McLaughlin, K. A., Petukhova, M., . . . Koenen, K. C. (2014). Cumulative traumas and risk thresholds: 12-month PTSD in the World Mental Health (WMH) surveys. *Depression and Anxiety, 31*, 130–142.

Karatzias, T., Cloitre, M., Maercker, A., Kazlauskas, E., Shevlin, M., Hyland, P., . . . Brewin, C. R. (2017). PTSD and Complex PTSD: ICD-11 updates on concept and measurement in the UK, USA, Germany and Lithuania. *European Journal of Psychotraumatology, 8*(Suppl. 7), 1418103.

Kenardy, J. A., Spence, S. H., & Macleod, A. C. (2006). Screening for posttraumatic stress disorder in children after accidental injury. *Pediatrics, 118*(3), 1002–1009.

Kessler, R. C., Aguilar-Gaxiola, S., Alonso, J., Benjet, C., Bromet, E. J., Cardoso, G., . . . Koenen, K. C. (2017). Trauma and PTSD in the WHO World Mental Health Surveys. *European Journal of Psychotraumatology, 8*(Suppl. 5), 1353383.

Kilpatrick, D. G., Ruggiero, K. J., Acierno, R., Saunders, B. E., Resnick, H. S., & Best, C. L. (2003). Violence and risk of PTSD, major depression, substance abuse/dependence, and comorbidity: Results from the Natural Survey of Adolescents. *Journal of Consulting and Clinical Psychology, 71*, 692–700.

Kisiel, C., Lyons, J. S., Blaustein, M., Fehrenbach, T., Griffin, G., Germain, J., . . . National Child Traumatic Stress Network. (2011). *Child and adolescent needs and strengths (CANS) manual: The NCTSN CANS Comprehensive—Trauma Version: A comprehensive information integration tool for children and adolescents exposed to traumatic events.* Chicago: Praed Foundation/Los Angeles, CA & Durham, NC: National Center for Child Traumatic Stress.

Korol, M., Green, B. L., & Gleser, G. C. (1999). Children's responses to a nuclear waste disaster: PTSD symptoms and outcome prediction. *Journal of the American Academy of Child and Adolescent Psychiatry, 38*, 368–375.

Kroenke, K., Spitzer, R. L., Williams, J. B. W., & Lowe, B. (2010). The Patient Health Questionnaire Somatic, Anxiety, and Depressive Symptom Scales: A systematic review. *General Hospital Psychiatry, 32*, 345–359.

La Greca, A. M., Brodar, K. E., Danzi, B. A., Tarlow, N., & Comer, J. S. (2019a, March). *Impact of disaster evacuation stressors on parents' mental health.* Presented at the 2019 International Convention of Psychological Science, Paris, France.

La Greca, A. M., Brodar, K. E., Danzi, B. A., Tarlow, N., Silva, K., & Comer, J. S. (2019b). Before the storm: Stressors associated with the Hurricane Irma evacuation process for families. *Disaster Medicine and Public Health Preparedness, 13*(1), 63–73.

La Greca, A. M., & Danzi, B. A. (2019). Posttraumatic stress disorder. In M. J. Prinstein, E. A. Youngstrom, E. J. Mash, & R. A. Barkley (Eds.), *Treatment of childhood disorders* (4th ed., pp. 495–538). New York: Guilford Press.

La Greca, A. M., Danzi, B. A., & Chan, S. F. (2017). DSM-5 and ICD-11 as competing models of PTSD in preadolescent children exposed to a natural disaster: Assessing validity and co-occurring symptomatology. *European Journal of Psychotraumatology, 8*, 1310591.

La Greca, A. M., Lai, B. S., Llabre, M. M., Silverman, W. K., Vernberg, E. M., & Prinstein, M. J. (2013). Children's postdisaster trajectories of PTS symptoms: Predicting chronic distress. *Child and Youth Care Forum, 42*(4), 351–369.

La Greca, A. M., & Silverman, W. S. (2011). Interventions for youth following disasters and acts of terrorism. In P. C. Kendall (Ed.), *Child and adolescent therapy: Cognitive-behavioral procedures* (4th ed., pp. 324–344). New York: Guilford Press

La Greca, A. M., Silverman, W., Lai, B., & Jaccard, J. (2010). Hurricane-related exposure experiences and stressors, other life events, and social support: Concurrent and prospective impact on children's persistent posttraumatic stress symptoms. *Journal of Consulting and Clinical Psychology, 78*, 794–805.

La Greca, A. M., Silverman, W. S., Vernberg, E. M., & Prinstein, M. J. (1996). Posttraumatic stress symptoms in children after Hurricane Andrew: A prospective study. *Journal of Consulting and Clinical Psychology, 64,* 712–723.

La Greca, A. M., Silverman, W. K., & Wasserstein, S. B. (1998). Children's predisaster functioning as a predictor of posttraumatic stress following Hurricane Andrew. *Journal of Consulting and Clinical Psychology, 66,* 883–892.

Lai, B. S., La Greca, A. M., Auslander, B. A., & Short, M. B. (2013). Children's symptoms of posttraumatic stress and depression after a natural disaster: Comorbidity and risk factors. *Journal of Affective Disorders, 146,* 71–78.

Leffler, J. M., Riebel, J., & Hughes, H. M. (2015). A review of child and adolescent diagnostic interviews for clinical practitioners. *Assessment, 22,* 690–703.

Lenz, S. A., & Hollenbaugh, K. M. (2015). Meta-analysis of trauma-focused cognitive behavioral therapy for treating PTSD and co-occurring depression among children and adolescents. *Counseling Outcome Research and Evaluation, 6*(1), 18–32.

Loeb, J., Stettler, E. M., Gavila, T., Stein, A., & Chinitz, S. (2011). The Child Behavior Checklist PTSD Scale: Screening for PTSD in young children with high exposure to trauma. *Journal of Traumatic Stress, 24,* 430–434.

Malecki, C. K., & Demaray, M. K. (2002). Measuring perceived social support: Development of the Child and Adolescent Social Support Scale. *Psychology in the Schools, 39,* 1–18.

Mannarino, A. P., Cohen, J. A., Deblinger, E., Runyon, M. K., & Steer, R. A. (2012). Trauma-focused cognitive-behavioral therapy for children: Sustained impact of treatment 6 and 12 months later. *Child Maltreatment, 17,* 231–241.

Marsella, A. J., & Christopher, M. A. (2004). Ethnocultural considerations in disasters: An overview of research, issues, and directions. *Psychiatric Clinics of North America, 27,* 521–539.

Marshall, G. N., Schell, T. L., & Miles, J. N. V. (2009). Ethnic differences in posttraumatic distress: Hispanics' symptoms differ in kind and degree. *Journal of Consulting and Clinical Psychology, 77,* 1169–1178.

McLaughlin, K. A., Koenen, K. C., Hill, E. D., Petukhova, M., Sampson, N. A., Zaslavsky, A. M., & Kessler, R. C. (2013). Trauma exposure and posttraumatic stress disorder in a national sample of adolescents. *Journal of the American Academy of Child and Adolescent Psychiatry, 52,* 815–830.

McLean, C. P., Morris, S. H., Conklin, P., Jayawickreme, N., & Foa, E. B. (2014). Trauma characteristics and posttraumatic stress disorder among adolescent survivors of childhood sexual abuse. *Journal of Family Violence, 29*(5), 559–566.

Merikangas, K. R., He, J. P., Burstein, M., Swanson, S. A., Avenevoli, S., Cui, L., . . . Swendsen, J. (2010). Lifetime prevalence of mental disorders in U.S. adolescents: Results from the National Comorbidity Survey Replication—Adolescent Supplement (NCS-A). *Journal of the American Academy of Child and Adolescent Psychiatry, 49*(10), 980–989.

Mikolajewski, A. J., Scheeringa, M. S., & Weems, C. F. (2017). Evaluating diagnostic and statistical manual of mental disorders, posttraumatic stress disorder diagnostic criteria in older children and adolescents. *Journal of Child and Adolescent Psychopharmacology, 27,* 374–382.

Morina, N., Koerssen, R., & Pollet, T. V. (2016). Interventions for children and adolescents with posttraumatic stress disorder: A meta-analysis of comparative outcome studies. *Clinical Psychology Review, 47,* 41–54.

Napper, L. E., Fisher, D. G., Jaffe, A., Jones, R. T., Lamphear, V. S., Joseph, L., & Grimaldi, E. M. (2015). Psychometric properties of the Child's Reaction to Traumatic Events Scale—Revised in English and Lugandan. *Journal of Child And Family Studies, 34*(5), 1285–1294.

Nilsson, D., Wadsby, M., & Svedin, C. G. (2008). The psychometric properties of the Trauma Symptom Checklist for Children (TSCC) in a sample of Swedish children. *Child Abuse and Neglect, 32,* 627–636.

Norris, F. H., Friedman, M. J., Watson, P. J., Byrne, C. M., Diaz, E., & Kaniasty, K. (2002). 60,000 disaster victims speak: Part I. An empirical review of empirical literature, 1981–2001. *Psychiatry: Interpersonal and Biological Processes, 65,* 207–239.

Price, J., Kassam-Adams, N., Alderfer, M. A., Christofferson, J., & Kazak, A. E. (2016). Systematic review: A reevaluation and update of the integrative (trajectory) model of pediatric medical traumatic stress. *Journal of Pediatric Psychology, 41*(1), 86–97.

Pynoos, R. S., Weathers, F. W., Steinberg, A. M., Marx, B. P., Layne, C. M., Kaloupek, D. G., . . . Kriegler, J. A. (2015). *Clinician-Administered PTSD Scale for DSM-5—Child/Adolescent Version.* Available from the National Center for PTSD at *www.ptsd.va.gov/professional/assessment/documents/caps-ca-5.pdf.*

Reich, W. (2000). Diagnostic Interview for Children and Adolescents (DICA). *Journal of the American Academy of Child and Adolescent Psychiatry, 39,* 59–66.

Rowe, C. L., La Greca, A. M., & Alexandersson, A. (2010). Family and individual factors associated with substance involvement and PTS symptoms among adolescents in greater New Orleans after Hurricane Katrina. *Journal of Consulting and Clinical Psychology, 78,* 806–817.

Ruggiero, K. J., & McLeer, S. V. (2000). PTSD scale of the Child Behavior Checklist: Concurrent and discriminant validity with non-clinic-referred sexually abused children. *Journal of Traumatic Stress, 13*(2), 287–299.

Sachser, C., Keller, F., & Goldbeck, L. (2017). Complex PTSD as proposed for ICD-11: Validation of a new disorder in children and adolescents and their response to trauma-focused cognitive behavioral therapy. *Journal of Child Psychology and Psychiatry,* 58(2), 160–168.

Saigh, P. A. (2004). *A structured interview for diagnosing posttraumatic stress disorder: Children's PTSD Inventory.* San Antonio, TX: PsychCorp.

Salloum, A., Scheeringa, M. S., Cohen, J. A., & Storch, E. A. (2014). Development of stepped care trauma-focused cognitive-behavioral therapy for young children. *Cognitive Behavioral Practice, 21,* 97–108.

Salloum, A., Small, B. J., Robst, J., Scheeringa, M. S., Cohen, J. A., & Storch, E. A. (2017). Stepped and standard care for childhood trauma: A pilot randomized clinical trial. *Research on Social Work Practice, 27,* 653–663.

Scheeringa, M. S. (2004). *Diagnostic Infant and Preschool Assessment (DIPA) (version 8/8/15).* Unpublished instrument. Retrieved February 26, 2019 from *https://medicine.tulane.edu/node/18891.*

Scheeringa, M. S., & Haslett, N. (2010). The reliability and criterion validity of the Diagnostic Infant and Preschool Assessment: A new diagnostic instrument for young children. *Child Psychiatry and Human Development, 41*(3), 299–312.

Scheeringa, M. S., Myers, L., Putnam, F. W., & Zeanah, C. H. (2012). Diagnosing PTSD in early childhood: An empirical assessment of four approaches. *Journal of Traumatic Stress, 25,* 359–367.

Scheeringa, M. S., Weems, C. F., Cohen, J. A., Amaya-Jackson, L., & Guthrie, D. (2011). Trauma-focused cognitive-behavioral therapy for posttraumatic stress disorder in three- through six-year-old children: A randomized clinical trial. *Journal of Child Psychology and Psychiatry, 52*(8), 853–860.

Scheeringa, M. S., Wright, M. J., Hunt, J. P., & Zeanah, C. H. (2006). Factors affecting the diagnosis and prediction of PTSD symptomatology in children and adolescents. *American Journal of Psychiatry, 163,* 644–651.

Self-Brown, S., Lai, B. S., Thompson, J. E., McGill, T., & Kelley, M. L. (2013). Posttraumatic stress disorder symptom trajectories in Hurricane Katrina affected youth. *Journal of Affective Disorders, 147,* 198–204.

Shaffer, D., Fisher, P., Lucas, C. P., Dulcan, M. K., & Schwab-Stone, M. E. (2000). NIMH Diagnostic Interview Schedule for Children Version IV (NIMH DISC-IV): Description, differences from previous versions, and reliability of some common diagnoses. *Journal of the American Academy of Child and Adolescent Psychiatry, 39*(1), 28–38.

Silverman, W. K., & Albano, A. M. (1996). *The Anxiety Disorders Interview Schedule for DSM–IV—Child and parent versions.* San Antonio, TX: Psychological Corporation.

Sim, L., Friedrich, W. N., Davies, W. H., Trentham, B., Lengua, L., & Pithers, W. (2005). The Child Behavior Checklist as an indicator of posttraumatic stress disorder and dissociation in normative, psychiatric, and sexually abused children. *Journal of Traumatic Stress, 18,* 697–705.

Smith, P., Perrin, S., Dyregrov, A., & Yule, W. (2002). Principal components analysis of the Impact of Event Scale with children in war. *Personality and Individual Differences, 34,* 315–322.

Spirito, A., Stark, L. J., & Williams, C. (1988). Development of a brief coping checklist for use with pediatric populations. *Journal of Pediatric Psychology, 13*(4), 555–574.

Steinberg, A. M., Brymer, M. J., Kim, S., Ghosh, C., Ostrowski, S. A., Gulley, K., . . . Pynoos, R. S. (2013). Psychometric properties of the UCLA PTSD Reaction Index: Part I. *Journal of Traumatic Stress, 26,* 1–9.

Suomalainen, L., Haravuori, H., Berg, N., Kiviruusu, O., & Marttunen, M. (2011). A controlled follow-up study of adolescents exposed to a school shooting: Psychological consequences after four months. *European Psychiatry, 26,* 490–497.

Thabet, A. A. M., Abed, Y., & Vostanis, P. (2004). Comorbidity of PTSD and depression among refugee children during war conflict. *Journal of Child Psychology and Psychiatry, 45,* 533–542.

Weissman, M. M. (2011). Standardized interviews for diagnostic assessments of children and adolescents in psychiatric research. *Journal of the American Academy of Child and Adolescent Psychiatry, 50,* 633–635.

Weller, E. B., Fristad, M. A., Weller, R. A., & Rooney, M. T. (1999). *Children's Interview for Psychiatric Syndromes: ChIPS.* Washington, DC: American Psychiatric Press.

You, D. S., Youngstrom, E. A., Feeny, N. C., Youngstrom, J. K., & Findling, R. L. (2017). Comparing the diagnostic accuracy of five instruments for detecting posttraumatic stress disorder in youth. *Journal of Clinical Child and Adolescent Psychology, 46*(4), 511–522.

Young, M. E., Bell, Z. E., & Fristad, M. A. (2016). Validation of a brief structured interview: The Children's Interview for Psychiatric Syndromes (ChIPS). *Journal of Clinical Psychology in Medical Settings, 23,* 327–340.

CHAPTER 16

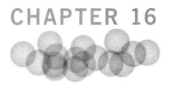

Life Events

Kathryn Grant, Jocelyn Smith Carter, Emma Adam, and Yo Jackson

Background and Overview

Stressful life experiences are the most well-established environmental predictor of mental health problems across the lifespan. Research focused on children and adolescents, in particular, has documented a powerful predictive relation between exposure to stressors and a range of psychological problems, including internalizing and externalizing disorders (Grant, Compas, Thurm, McMahon, & Gipson, 2004). Furthermore, there is evidence that stressors and mental health problems are reciprocally related and can lead to one another in ways that maintain and exacerbate psychopathology (Grant et al., 2004). For these reasons, assessment of stress exposure is crucial for understanding the manifestation and course of mental health problems and response to treatment (Epel et al., 2018).

State of the Field of Stress Measurement in Youth

Historically, stress measures have represented (1) stimulus (e.g., measures of events), (2) response (e.g., measures of distress in response to events), and (3) transactional perspectives (e.g., measures of events and responses combined) (Grant & McMahon, 2005; Schwarzer & Schulz, 2002). In recent years, leading developmental psychopathology researchers have recommended that stressful experiences be conceptualized and measured discretely, apart from the biological, cognitive, or emotional responses they elicit, to avoid confounding of stressors with response processes and to facilitate analysis of mediators and moderators across development (Grant et al., 2003; Herbert & Cohen, 1996; Monroe, 2008). This perspective is most consistent with a stimulus definition of stress (Cohen & Hamrick, 2003; Grant et al., 2003).

Given the historical association of the term *stress* with a wide array of psychological phenomena and definitions, we recommend use of the word *stressor* to refer to the environmental experiences that are the defining feature of stress research (Grant et al., 2003). The broader term *stress* is more useful as an inclusive term that refers not only to the environmental stressors themselves but also to the range of processes set in motion by exposure to environmental stressors. Thus, *stress research* refers to the body of literature that examines environmental stressors, as well as reciprocal and dynamic processes among stressors, mediators, moderators, and psychological symptoms.

Challenges across Methods

Beyond the various specific approaches to assessment, an overarching challenge applies across methods, and that is the lack of standardization of stressor measurement for children and adolescents. For example, a series of reviews of the stress literature conducted last decade (Grant et al., 2003, 2004, 2006; McMahon, Grant, Compas, Thurm, & Ey, 2003) revealed that few studies used comparable stressor measures. Approximately 60% used cumulative stressor checklists or interviews (as opposed to measures of specific stressors such as sexual abuse or exposure to a hurricane). Of these studies, fewer than 10% used a validated measure, and no single measure was used in more than 3% of studies (Grant et al., 2003). Forty-five percent of studies indicated that the authors developed their own measure of cumulative stressors. Psychometric data on most of these measures were not provided, and few of the authors who developed their own scales provided information about their method of measurement development or items included on their scales (Grant et al., 2004). In our current efforts to update these reviews, we continue to observe substantial variability in stress measurement.

This lack of standardization highlights a central difference between the state of the field of child and adolescent stressor measurement and the state of the field of child and adolescent psychopathology measurement. Specifically, taxonomies of child and adolescent psychopathology have been developed, but no such taxonomy exists for child and adolescent stressors. Several well-established taxonomies for child and adolescent psychopathology that have been developed include the DSM-5, the ICD-11, the Achenbach System of Empirically Based Assessment (ASEBA; Achenbach & Rescorla, 2001) and the Behavior Assessment System for Children (BASC, Reynolds & Kamphaus, 2004). Although DSM-5 and ICD-11 are generally regarded as the "gold standard" diagnostic systems in the United States and internationally (respectively), the ASEBA and the BASC have been used more frequently in stress research on children and adolescents. The development of these taxonomies represents an important achievement in the past half-century that has dramatically improved the ability of researchers and clinicians to communicate with one another about mental health problems affecting children and adolescents (Grant et al., 2004).

A standardized stressor measure would allow researchers across disciplines to compare results and replicate findings of environmental influences on developmental outcomes and to test theoretical models of the role of stressful life experiences in both normal and abnormal child development. A standardized measure would also allow researchers to determine whether (1) a certain magnitude of stress exposure is necessary for most children to learn to problem-solve and develop adaptive coping strategies and whether (2) a threshold exists above which exposure to stressful life experiences places most children at risk for negative learning and developmental outcomes.

A standardized measurement system would be equally beneficial to treatment. In clinical practice, stress measurement is further removed from empirical study, and assessment tools are even more variable and idiosyncratic. A standardized stressor measurement system would allow clinicians to better conceptualize and communicate environmental causes of disorder. Such information would also be useful to target coping and treatment efforts and could help clients understand and normalize their experiences. Such a system could also benefit prevention and education efforts. For example, a standardized stressor measurement system could be administered broadly (e.g., in schools, pediatricians' offices) to assist with the identification of children and adolescents at risk for negative developmental and learning outcomes, so that families are aware of risk and youth can receive prevention/intervention services.

In the sections below, we highlight progress toward the development of a stressor taxonomy and standardized stressor measurement system. We also review psychometrically sound stressor measures that are recommended until standardized measurement systems are developed.

Rating Scales, Checklists, Interviews, and Informants

Clinicians often inquire about current stressors as part of a social history, but clinicians do not routinely include formal stressor assessment (e.g., Sommers-Flanagan & Sommers-Flanagan, 2012). Although not yet part of a standardized stressor measurement system as described earlier, there are a number of validated stressor measures available to clinicians. We review those here.

General Stressors/Life Events Measures

Members of our research team published an exhaustive review of stress measures in 2004. At that time, advances had been made in the development and refinement of general stressor checklists for adolescents, but less progress had been made in the development of checklists for children. In particular, we identified 11 adolescent stressor measures as relatively well established (see Grant et al., 2004, for a review).

These general checklists are all similar in that they present respondents with a sample of negative and, in some cases, positive events that are representative of the types of events that researchers deem relevant. None of the inventories is designed to be exhaustive; rather, they are intended to offer a sufficiently broad sampling to be representative of stressful events and experiences in childhood and adolescence. We also found evidence of several well-established narrative stressor interviews with high interrater reliability (Adrian & Hammen, 1993; Garber, Robinson, & Valentiner, 1997; Rudolph & Hammen, 1999; Williamson et al., 2003). These interviews can be administered to adolescents and/or parents. In 2004, measures of cumulative life stressors had primarily been developed on European American middle-class samples (with some notable exceptions, e.g., Allison et al., 1999; Cheng, 1997; Gil, Vega, & Dimas, 1994; Nyborg & Curry, 2003; Richters & Martinez, 1993). These measures were criticized for lacking questions pertinent to youth of color (Miller, Webster, & MacIntosh, 2002).

Since our review, progress has been made in this area. For example, the measurement of acculturative stress has been refined to distinguish between acculturation stressors and discrimination, and the Hispanic Stress Inventory for Adolescents, a 91-item self-report measure with strong psychometric properties (Cervantes, Fisher, Córdova, Napper, & Napper, 2012; Cervantes, Goldbach, & Padilla, n.d.), has been developed. In addition, the construct of race-based traumatic stress injury provides a framework for organizing specific types of stressors related to racism, including racial discrimination, racial harassment, and discriminative harassment (Carter, 2007). To our knowledge, no measure has been developed to assess all three domains in youth, although measures of discrimination such as the Racism and Life Experiences Scale—Revised have been developed in adults and show adequate validity in adolescents (Flores et al., 2008; Smith-Bynum, Lambert, English, & Ialongo, 2014).

Additional advances in general stressor measurement since our 2004 review include work by George Slavich, PhD, to develop an online system for assessing life stressors that combines the depth of interview-based approaches with the efficiency of a self-report scale (Slavich & Sheilds, 2018). The Stress and Adversity Inventory (STRAIN) includes an extensive bank of stressor questions that cover both acute and chronic stressors, and which are administered using intelligent logic that prompts sets of follow-up questions when warranted. This allows the instrument to omit questions that would not apply to particular individuals (e.g., female reproductive questions for male) and to query identified stressors on various dimensions, including their chronicity and severity (similar to an interview format). The STRAIN has demonstrated excellent psychometric properties with adults (Slavich & Shields, 2018), and Slavich and his team are currently working to establish validity for an adolescent version that can be used with youth as young as 10 years old (G. Slavich, personal communication, August 24, 2018).

Our research team is working to validate a measure with analogous properties for young children. The Audio Computer-Assisted Self-Interview (ACASI) is administered on a laptop computer with audio support to parents (and can be administered to children as young as 8 years old). For example, in the Preschoolers' Adjustment and Intergenerational Risk project, a series of 47 serious life events (e.g., abuse, divorce, car accident, marital conflict) are administered visually on a computer screen while also being read aloud to support individuals with limited reading ability. The software uses skip logic to guide respondents through follow-up questions about each endorsed event to fully capture the range of important dimensions of stress exposure, including severity of the event, who was involved in the experience, and frequency of exposure.

Our team is also working to develop a series of taxonomically based stressor measures for adolescents that could serve as a basis for a standardized measurement system. Over the past 15 years, we have conducted six studies to lay the foundation for this system. The first of these was a longitudinal study of narrative stress interviews (Youth Life Stress Interview; Rudolph & Flynn, 2007) with a racially, ethnically, and socioeconomically diverse sample of adolescents that was designed to establish (1) a comprehensive list of objectively threatening major events (as well as the essential contextual descriptors associated with objective threat ratings) and (2) a taxonomic structure for organizing these events.

In this study, coders assessed the degree to which each stressor would pose threat or risk to an average adolescent (i.e., the "objective threat" rating). The chronicity, severity, and context of each stressful experience were used to make each determination of "objective threat." Once this quantitative analysis was complete, the coding team examined the stressors qualitatively (guided by the work of Strauss & Corbin, 1994), with the goal of condensing thousands of individual stressors and their relevant contextual descriptors to a list of (1) only stressors that are distinct from one another and (2) inclusive of relevant descriptors linked to objective threat ratings.

The next step was to place the distilled list of distinct, objectively threatening major events into a preliminary taxonomic structure using thematic analysis (Braun & Clarke, 2006). The goal of this analysis was to identify domains that cut across the various types of unique stressors. Theories guiding this analysis include those that designate stressors as interpersonal versus achievement events (Flynn & Rudolph, 2011; Lakey & Ross, 1994) and cumulative versus acute (Compas, 1987; Grant et al., 2004) emotion theory (Camras, 1992; Izard et al., 2011), Dohrenwend's (2000) six characteristics of events that contribute to impact (i.e., valence, source, unpredictability, centrality, magnitude, and potential to exhaust the individual physically), life-history theory dimensions of harsh versus unpredictable environmental risk (Brumbach, Figueredo, & Ellis, 2009; Ellis, Figueredo, Brumbach, & Schlomer, 2009), and Kendler, Hettema, Butera, Gardner, and Prescott's (2003) guidelines for contextual threat ratings of humiliation, entrapment, loss, and danger. The next step was to compare this list of stressors with those generated by a large, nationally representative sample of adolescents to ensure that it was not missing any important types of stressors affecting youth (Achenbach & Howell, 1995).

Results of these analyses are summarized in Appendix 16.1 (as cited in Grant et al., 2020). The essential contextual descriptors associated with objective threat ratings emerged as relatively similar across multiple major event categories and included (1) the degree of closeness with others involved in the event (as measured by centrality of relationship and time spent together), (2) the chronicity of the event or situation, (3) the predictability of the event or situation, (4) the amount of change in

daily living caused by the event or situation, and (5) (if an element of humiliation is involved) the extent to which the event, situation, or condition was public.

Next, we collected lists of systems and minor stressors from the narrative interviews conducted in the first study and compared them with one another, deleting redundancies, until a single list of unique stressors distinct from one another remained. Because youth generated relatively few systems level (e.g., racism, sexism) stressors, we then supplemented the systems level stressors (and essential contextual descriptors) with a review of the literature on theory and measures of systems level stressors (e.g., census and block data on exposure to violence, poverty, and segregation; observational measures of neighborhood decay; survey and observational measures and theory on exposure to racism, classism, sexism, and homophobia) to inform our list of stressors (Grant et al., 2020). Finally, we received feedback on this list from measurement- and/or systems-level stressor experts (Drs. Achenbach, Allison, Compas, Dohrenwend, Griffith, Hirsch, Kratochwill, Larson, Maton, Rudolph, Seidman, Tolan, Utsey, Watts).

To ensure stressors at the other end of the continuum were well represented, we examined daily diary data collected from three different samples of racially, ethnically, and socioeconomically diverse adolescents (ages 11–21) (Grant et al., 2020). Participants were instructed to identify events that were stressful throughout the day, and we condensed all of those generated to a list consisting only of minor stressors distinct from one another. Thematic analysis was again used to integrate systems and minor stressors and to identify essential contextual descriptors associated with those stressors identified as objectively threatening within the budding taxonomy.

Two essential contextual descriptors associated with objective threat ratings for systems level events emerged as relatively similar across systems level stressor domains: (1) pervasiveness of systems level event or situation across home, school, neighborhood, and nation; and (2) chronicity of event or situation (i.e., ongoing for longer than 6 months). In addition, four essential contextual descriptors associated with objective threat ratings for minor events emerged as relatively similar across minor stress domains: (1) the degree to which the events occur within the context of systemic conditions or major events associated with the domain, (2) the degree of closeness with others involved in the event (as measured by centrality of relationship and time spent together), (3) ongoing and frequent occurrence (i.e., weekly or daily), and (4) unpredictability (i.e., occurring without predictable pattern or timing). See Appendix 16.1.

Results of thematic analysis across major, systems, and minor events led to the selection of four primary taxonomic categories: (1) threat, (2) conflict, (3) loss (or lack), and (4) humiliation. These categories build on extant theory and research as outlined earlier (Brumbach et al., 2009; Camras, 1992; Compas, 1987; Dohrenwend, 2000; Ellis et al., 2009; Flynn & Rudolph, 2011; Grant et al., 2004; Izard et al., 2011; Kendler et al., 2003; Lakey & Ross, 1994) and are hypothesized to be specifically related to particular physiological, emotional, mental health, and learning outcomes (see Appendix 16.1). As part of this work, we also developed lab-based measures that are associated with these stressor domains including brief interviews that build upon Ewart and Kolodner's (1991) social competence interviews (see Appendix 16.2). We are currently working to establish psychometrics for interview, lab, and survey-based measures that build upon this taxonomic system.

The measures and measurement development work reviewed here has emanated from basic stress research. Despite great potential for clinical utility, these measures have yet to be applied to clinical settings to any great extent. Because the primary focus in clinical settings is on psychopathology, stressor measures used in these settings tend to focus on trauma as it relates to posttraumatic stress disorder (PTSD) symptoms. Below we provide the most up-to-date review of these measures.

Trauma Measures

Trauma treatment is not focused on changing the traumatic event but instead focuses on improving the child's and caretaker's adjustment following a traumatic event and/or assisting family members in managing the child's risk for exposure to any ongoing or future environmental challenges (e.g., Cohen, Mannarino, & Deblinger, 2017). Therefore, evidence-based assessment in the treatment of trauma exposure requires clinicians to attend to two goals: (1) measurement of the child and family members' trauma exposure history (i.e., the number and nature of events) and (2) measurement of the child and caretaker's reaction to trauma (e.g., psychological symptoms) both at the beginning and throughout the course of treatment. To

achieve these goals, there are several important issues that clinicians must consider.

First, trauma exposure may not be the original presenting problem for which children and families are referred for therapy. For example, Weinstein, Levine, Kogan, Harkavy-Friedman, and Miller (2000) provided evidence that trauma history, specifically child abuse, might not be disclosed until several months after therapy has begun. If trauma exposure is unknown to the clinician, it cannot be assessed or treated, nor can problems be conceptualized as possible trauma reactions. Additionally, even when therapists have knowledge of a child's traumatic experiences at the outset of therapy, the traumatic event(s) and concurrent symptoms may not always be the target of intervention (Shamseddeen et al., 2011). For example, most evidence-based treatment protocols for exposure to trauma suggest that intervention focus first on treating any concerns about disruptive or dangerous behavior (e.g., aggression, substance abuse, suicidal behavior) that may or may not be related to the child's trauma exposure (Child Sexual Abuse Task Force and Research & Practice Core, 2004). Furthermore, given that youth tend to experience multiple forms of trauma, what the parent (or child) may think is the most influential trauma may not actually be the most influential (Finkelhor, Turner, Shattuck, & Hamby, 2013).

Second, because there is no agreed-upon list of what constitutes a traumatic event, experiences considered traumatic for children can vary (Cohen, Mannarino, & Murray, 2011) and be intermittent. This means that practitioners must try to capture a moving target with commonly static (i.e., intake and posttreatment) assessment procedures.

Third, identification of the best informant of child traumatic event exposure is challenging for practitioners. For example, some clinicians may have concerns about a youth's ability to recall events accurately (Lieberman & Van Horn, 2004). Caretakers, however, may lack awareness of what the child has experienced or may wish to minimize the severity of events if their behavior partially contributed to the child's exposure (Cameron, Elkins, & Guterman, 2006). Additionally, there may be disagreement between the parent and the child when both are reporting on trauma exposure and symptomatology. For example, Stover, Hahn, Im, and Berkowitz (2010) found only moderate concordance (at most) between parent and child reports with regard to the type of trauma the child had experienced.

Fourth, psychopathology in trauma-exposed youth may not always be due to the initial trauma (Boney-McCoy & Finkelhor, 1996) but rather is related to other surrounding events such as what happened after the event (e.g., moving one's home after a natural disaster). This requires clinicians to parse out what aspects of youth's experiences are most distressing, often without the benefit of pre-trauma or baseline measurements of functioning.

Finally, if clinicians focus exclusively on treating behavioral or emotional problems and ignore the potential contribution exposure to trauma may have as the source of the maladjustment, the intervention may be less effective (Blizzard, 2006). Together, these issues highlight the challenge and the importance of assessing trauma exposure effectively in clinical settings.

Choosing Trauma Assessment Measures

Although it is important from a theoretical and empirical perspective to measure stressor exposure distinctly from emotional responses, from a practical perspective, it may be efficient for clinicians to measure the two together. For example, most measures of posttraumatic stress disorder (PTSD) combine measurement of stress exposure with responses to it.

The measures in Appendix 16.3 represent a collection of current tools across different methods, reporters, trauma types, and other psychological domains. A similar review was undertaken by Strand, Sarmiento, and Pasquale (2005) and Milne and Collin-Vézina (2015), and similar to the list provided by those researchers, the measures in Appendix 16.3 are divided into groups: (1) measures of events only, (2) measures of events and symptoms (nondiagnostic), (3) measures of symptoms of PTSD and related clinical disorders, and (4) those that capture multiple symptoms associated with trauma exposure (nondiagnostic).

The review provided here expands the list of tools in the previous reviews by including all tools published to date, now totaling over 65 measures on trauma exposure and related clinical outcomes for youth and families. Appendix 16.3 also provides, where available, the psychometric information for each tool. *Tool names in italics indicate a measure that has been documented in published research as useful for tracking change in symptoms or could be useful for ongoing assessment in treatment.* Appendix 16.3 is the most comprehensive list of measures for assessing trauma in youth to date.

Components of Trauma Measures

Method and Reporter

Most assessments of trauma exposure and reactions allow for school-age children or adolescents to self-report or have a caregiver report on a checklist or questionnaire (a few measures allow for day care provider or teacher report). Overall, there appear to be few measures designed for use with adolescents only and relatively few for preschool-age or younger youth, similar to the findings reported by Milne and Collin-Vézina (2015). Additionally, several semistructured interviews are available that can be used as tools for determining both the number and kinds of events, as well as associated diagnostic information for PTSD and other trauma-related disorders.

Trauma Type and Trauma Reactions

Although the majority of trauma assessment tools are broad and include a list of possible events one might experience, some assessment tools are designed for use with youth exposed to specific types of trauma (i.e., sexual abuse). Most tools query whether or not an incident has occurred but do not always query the frequency or severity of the experience. Therefore, event checklists can be beneficial for initial assessment of lifetime experiences but may require follow-up questions by clinicians for information about the chronicity and severity of the child's experiences.

Most tools targeting trauma reactions focus on identifying traumatic stress disorders in children and adolescents (e.g., reexperiencing, dissociation, avoidance, mood and anxiety symptoms) with the majority of tools designed to measure PTSD symptoms in youth. Because the items are often based on diagnostic criteria, the focus for assessment is often the child's reactions in general rather than the amount or level of trauma exposure.

Semistructured interviews, such as the Posttraumatic Stress Disorder Semi-Structured Interview and Observational Record (Scheeringa & Zeanah, 2005), combine questions about a child's exposure to traumatic events and the child's reactions to the event into one assessment. Such interviews allow clinicians to not only understand the type of trauma and the frequency of exposure, but also to connect specific events with specific reactions. It is important to remember that trauma symptomatology interviews tend to focus on internalizing symptoms, so additional interview questions may be necessary to rule out the presence of externalizing problems, social difficulties, or developmental delays related to trauma exposure.

Measures of Parent Stress

Although our focus in this chapter is assessment of life events affecting children and adolescents, we provide brief coverage of measures of parent stress here. Parenting stress can negatively impact treatment by making it difficult for parents to fully engage in therapy and provide support for their children (Friedberg & McClure, 2015; Murphy & Christner, 2012). For example, children with autism spectrum disorders who received cognitive-behavioral therapy for anxiety but did not respond to treatment had parents with higher levels of stress at baseline (Weiss, Viecili, & Bohr, 2015).

In some cases, parent stress is a recommended focus of treatment before beginning a manualized course of therapy as a method of increasing the efficacy of the treatment (Hastings & Beck, 2004). For example, a parent problem-solving module was designed for parents to complete before beginning evidence-based parent management training for children with aggression and conduct problems (Kazdin & Whitley, 2003). And, this parent problem-solving module is associated with more therapeutic change for both parents and children (Kazdin & Whitley, 2003).

The Parenting Stress Index (PSI) measures stress in the parenting role (Abidin, 2012) and is the most frequently used stress questionnaire in clinical practice (Barroso, Mendez, Graziano, & Bagner, 2018). The full parent-report measure includes 101 items, loading onto 12 subscales related to problems with the child and with parents. The PSI has several strengths: (1) strong internal and external validity (Haskett, Ahern, Ward, & Allaire, 2006); (2) a 36-item short form with strong psychometrics (Abidin, 1995); (3) validation in multiple populations, including parents of children with developmental disabilities and attention-deficit/hyperactivity disorder (Hutchinson, 2006); and (4) translations into multiple languages (Solis & Abidin, 1991; Tam, Chan, & Wong, 1994). The Stress Index for Parents of Adolescents (SIPA; Sheras, Abidin, & Konold, 1998) is the upward extension for adolescents and has similar psychometric properties. A recent meta-analysis revealed that parenting stress is highest in parents of children with autism spectrum disorder and developmental disabilities (Barroso et al., 2018).

Using Assessment to Guide Diagnosis, Case Formulation, and Treatment Planning

Engaging in evidence-based practice requires clinicians to also engage in evidence-based assessment by using empirically tested assessment tools, clinical expertise, and attention to client values to systematically determine both the mental health needs of clients and the outcomes of intervention (Hunsley & Mash, 2007; Roberts, Blossom, Evans, Amaro, & Kanine, 2017). In the case of life events assessment, stressors or traumas often represent an important cause of the onset or maintenance of symptoms and are therefore crucial to case conceptualization and treatment planning. Stressors can also serve as the primary target in treatment, as in the case of stress management therapies with youth (e.g., Cohen, Mannarino, Berliner, & Deblinger, 2000; Meichenbaum, 1985) and with families (e.g., Raviv & Wadsworth, 2010; Wadsworth et al., 2011). For these reasons, it is important to collect valid information about stressor exposure in children and families seeking mental health services. Given the challenges associated with assessing stressors and trauma described earlier, the following recommendations are provided to guide professionals in their efforts to conduct evidence-based assessment of life events as part of initial intakes and treatment planning.

Assessment of Stressor/Trauma History

First, clinicians should consider, no matter the referral issue, whether the youth's maladjustment is related to stressor/trauma exposure. Clinicians are encouraged to assess for stressors and traumas even when the presenting problem is not specific to an event in the youth's history given the impact that stressors and traumatic events can have as nonspecific risk factors for pathology and the evidence that untreated trauma can be teratogenic to positive treatment outcomes in youth (Pine & Cohen, 2002). Therefore, as a part of treatment conceptualization, we suggest that each case be reviewed for past and ongoing stress exposure and possible trauma history, and that the clinician include, as a part of the intake process, a measure that can provide information on these events.

Because we have yet to develop a definitive taxonomy of stressors and traumas, professionals should consider how the youth has adjusted to any significant experience in his or her history using the measures discussed earlier and in Appendices 16.1, 16.2, and 16.3 as a guide. For example, we recommend the Youth Life Stress Interview (Rudolph & Flynn, 2007) as an initial assessment tool, as this interview has demonstrated satisfactory psychometric properties, covers a wide range of episodic and chronic stressful life events, and can be administrated to parents and youth in approximately 30 minutes. We also recommend supplementing the existing domains in that measure with domains of Exposure to Racism/Discrimination, Acculturation Stressors, Exposure to Violence, and Sexuality/Body Image Stressors.

Recommended questionnaire options include the Juvenile Victimization Questionnaire (JVQ; Hamby, Finkelhor, Ormrod, & Turner, 2004) and the Childhood Trauma Questionnaire (CTQ; Bernstein et al., 1994). Both of these questionnaires assess for a diverse range of childhood traumas. The CTQ takes less time to complete, although it is limited primarily to adolescents. The JVQ can be administered to both school-age children and adolescents, but time to complete may be too long for clinicians with limited sessions.

Additionally, we recommend that clinicians make an effort to obtain a detailed history of the youth's exposure to stressors/traumatic experience from multiple informants (e.g., youth, parent, teacher), as the potential for bias or inaccuracy increases if just one informant reports on trauma exposure. For example, some youth may have been too young to know about certain forms of trauma exposure, such as neglect during infancy (Gilbert et al., 2009). Measures such as the Youth Life Stress Interview (Rudolph & Flynn, 2007) and Traumatic Events Screening Inventory (TESI; Edwards & Rogers, 1997; Ford et al., 2002; Ghosh-Ippen et al., 2002) provide options for administration to parents, as well as youth.

We also recommend that clinicians not solely rely on measures of PTSD symptoms to measure potential trauma exposure, as trauma exposure may be just as predictive of functioning as trauma symptoms. For example, Smith, Leve, and Chamberlain (2006) compared the predictive power between measures of PTSD symptoms and measures of trauma exposure in adolescents exposed to sexual abuse. They found that measurements of trauma exposure, as opposed to symptoms of PTSD, were better predictors of risky behavior.

We recommend that clinicians obtain information on not only the type of stressor/trauma exposure but also the severity and frequency of exposure, as these dimensions influence adjustment

and functioning (e.g., Jackson, Gabrielli, Fleming, Tunno, & Makanui, 2014; Manly, 2005). Therefore, information on these dimensions can help direct treatment development. Unfortunately, measures that capture all these dimensions have a long administration time (e.g., Jackson, Gabrielli, Tunno, & Hambrick, 2012). For this reason, clinicians with limited time may choose to begin with a brief survey measure and follow up with more extensive queries in an interview format.

Regardless of the manner in which stressors are assessed during the initial clinic visit, stressors are typically integrated into case conceptualizations that specify factors contributing to the problem presentation (Hoff et al., 2016). Beyond trauma-based disorders, stressors also impact broader internalizing and externalizing outcomes in evidence-based treatments for these disorders. In fact, the amount of stress a family reports can help identify the appropriate treatment modality, with high-adversity families benefiting more from individual than from group or family therapy (Lundahl, Risser, & Lovejoy, 2006).

Stressors predict treatment attendance and dropout, which in turn predict treatment outcome (e.g., Andra & Thomas, 1998; Kazdin & Wassell, 1998; Topham & Wampler, 2008). For these reasons, it is important to continue to assess for stress exposure throughout the course of treatment.

Process, Progress, and Outcome Measurement

As part of continued assessment or measurement-based care, clinicians must use their clinical judgment to balance assessment with time and financial constraints and not overburden the child or parent. For the ongoing measurement of children's trauma exposure and trauma-related symptoms, it is recommended that clinicians use measures that are short and have demonstrated adequate test–retest reliability. It is likely that a questionnaire format will work best to meet these demands, as interviews tend to take more time. For trauma-focused work, measures such as the Child PTSD Symptom Scale (Foa, Johnson, Feeny, & Treadwell, 2001) or the Child Stress Disorders Checklist (Saxe et al., 2003) may work well for clinicians, as both measures have shown satisfactory test–retest psychometrics and take less than 10 minutes to complete. More generally, brief stress interviews (see Appendix 16.2) can be readministered with an acknowledgment of past events using language such as "Last time I asked you these questions you told me. . . . Has anything else happened since then?"

Once ongoing assessment tools have been selected, clinicians are encouraged to systematize their assessment process. Assessment of stressors/traumas and their possible effects should occur at regular intervals during treatment. In this way, clinicians will have ongoing data to tailor the intervention to meet the mental health needs of their clients. Continuous assessment is also recommended because stressor/trauma exposure does not always have a specific stop and start, and youth may experience multiple stressful/traumatic events over the course of treatment. Fortunately, multiple studies have shown that repeatedly asking youth about their trauma history and trauma symptoms does not appear to impact youth negatively (e.g., Jackson et al., 2012).

Clinicians are also encouraged to track resilience, coping, and posttraumatic growth. Resilience can be tracked alongside symptomatology using comprehensive measures such as the ASEBA (Achenbach & Rescorla, 2001) and BASC systems (Reynolds & Kamphaus, 2004). Coping measures that are specific to particular stressors such as the Response to Stress Questionnaire (Connor-Smith, Compas, Wadsworth, Thomsen, & Saltzman, 2000) can be used to assess coping efficacy (i.e., appropriate matching of coping strategy with type of stressor). Posttraumatic growth can be measured using the Posttraumatic Growth Inventory for Children (Kilmer et al., 2009). Each of these measures has well-established psychometrics.

Regular systematic administration of empirically supported stress measures alongside symptom, resilience, coping, and growth measures provides the most comprehensive understanding of treatment progress. Such assessment also helps youth and parents see a "big picture" that goes far beyond diagnosis to include contextual circumstances that affect treatment and evidence of recovery and growth.

Summary and Conclusion

Stressful life experiences represent the most powerful environmental predictors of mental health problems in children and adolescents. Yet assessment and measurement of stressors have lagged far behind assessment and measurement of mental health problems. In this chapter, we have summarized the state of the field of stressor measurement for children and adolescents. In summary:

1. There has been growing agreement that stressors should be defined as environmentally based events or circumstances that are "objectively threatening" (i.e., independent raters agree they would pose threat to the average individual).
2. A number of well-validated stressor surveys and interviews have been developed for adolescents and a few have been developed for children.
3. Even the most well-validated measures have not been used consistently in stress research, and there is a lack of standardization of stressor measurement for children and adolescents.
4. In clinical practice, stressor measurement is further removed from empirical study, and assessment tools are even more variable and idiosyncratic.

We have summarized our efforts to develop an empirically based stressor taxonomy that could form the basis of a standardized stressor measurement system. See Appendix 16.1. We also have summarized existing stressor/trauma measures that have strong psychometrics and can be used in clinical practice until standardized measures are developed (see Appendix 16.3). In addition, we have provided recommendations for how the measures we have highlighted could be included in treatment planning and to what extent and how clinicians could/should monitor changes (e.g., new stressors) and processes and outcomes (e.g., coping, resilience, posttraumatic growth). In summary we recommend that

1. Clinicians measure a variety of stressors in both children and their parents/caregivers to guide case conceptualization and treatment recommendations.
2. Clinicians develop a systematic approach to integrating measures of stressors into ongoing treatment in ways that maximize contributions to therapy and minimize burden to clients.
3. Clinicians also include ongoing assessment of resilience, coping, and posttraumatic growth as a means of providing their clients with a "big picture" of treatment progress.

In conclusion, some form of stressor assessment is part of typical clinical practice, whether it be overt in the use of a specific tool or informal in the use of a clinical interview. For example, clinicians invariably collect histories that include an emphasis on stressor exposure as part of the intake process. It is also common for clinicians to collect information about barriers to treatment. Yet formal measurement of stressors has lagged behind the measurement of psychopathology, and the field does not yet have an empirically based stressor taxonomy with standardized measures to match. As a result, we do not yet have a common language for stressors the way we do for psychopathology. While researchers work to address this gap, we recommend that clinicians use those measures that have a strong empirical basis, so that they can effectively assess stressor exposure and response in service of treatment.

ACKNOWLEDGMENTS

This research was supported by grants from the Alfred P. Sloan Center on Parents, Children, and Work at the University of Chicago; DePaul University; the Institute for Policy Research at Northwestern University; the National Academy of Education; the National Alliance for Research on Schizophrenia and Depression; the National Institutes of Health (through OppNet and the National Institute on Alcohol Abuse and Alcoholism and the National Institute of Mental Health); the Social Sciences and Humanities Research Council of Canada; the Spencer Foundation; and the W. T. Grant Foundation.

REFERENCES

Abidin, R. R. (1995). *Parenting Stress Index, Third Edition*. Odessa, FL: Psychological Assessment Resources.

Abidin, R. R. (2012). *Parenting Stress Index, Fourth Edition*. Lutz, FL: Psychological Assessment Resources.

Achenbach, T. M., & Howell, C. T. (1995). Six-year predictors of problems in a national sample of children and youth: II. Signs of disturbance. *Journal of the American Academy of Child an Adolescent Psychiatry, 34*(4), 488–498.

Achenbach, T. M., & Rescorla, L. A. (2001). *Manual for the ASEBA School-Age Forms and Profiles*. Burlington: University of Vermont, Research Center for Children, Youth, and Families.

Adrian, C., & Hammen, C. (1993). Stress exposure and stress generation in children of depressed mothers. *Journal of Consulting and Clinical Psychology, 61*(2), 354–359.

Adverse childhood experiences (ACEs). (2015). Retrieved July 12, 2018, from *www.cdc.gov/violenceprevention/acestudy/index.html*.

Al-Yagon, M., & Mikulincer, M. (2004). Socioemotional and academic adjustment among children with learning disorders: The mediational role of attachment-based factors. *Journal of Special Education, 38*, 111–123.

Allison, K. W., Burton, L., Marshall, S., Perez-Febles, A., Yarrington, J., Kirsh, L. B., & Merriwether-DeVries, C. (1999). Life experiences among urban adolescents: Examining the role of context. *Child Development, 70*(4), 1017–1029.

Alloy, L. B., & Abramson, L. Y. (2004). *Life Events Interview manual*. Unpublished manuscript, Temple University, Philadelphia, PA.

Ammerman, R. T., Hersen, M., Van Hasselt, V. B., Lubetsky, M. J., & Sieck, W. R. (1994). Maltreatment in psychiatrically hospitalized children and adolescents with developmental disabilities: Prevalence and correlates, *Journal of the American Academy of Child and Adolescent Psychiatry, 33*(4), 567–576.

Andra, M. L., & Thomas, A. M. (1998). The influence of parenting stress and socioeconomic disadvantage on therapy attendance among parents and their behavior disordered preschool children. *Education and Treatment of Children, 21*, 195–208.

Athanasou, J. A. (2001). Young people in transition: Factors influencing the educational–vocational pathways of Australian school-leavers. *Education and Training, 43*(3), 132–138.

Barroso, N. E., Mendez, L., Graziano, P. A., & Bagner, D. M. (2018). Parenting stress through the lens of different clinical groups: A systematic review and meta-analysis. *Journal of Abnormal Child Psychology, 46*, 449–461.

Bernstein, D., & Fink, L. (1998). *Manual for the Childhood Trauma Questionnaire*. New York: The Psychological Corporation.

Bernstein, D. P., Fink, L., Handelsman, L., Foote, J., Lovejoy, M., Wenzel, K., . . . Ruggiero, J. (1995). Initial reliability and validity of a new retrospective measure of child abuse and neglect: Reply. *American Journal of Psychiatry, 152*(10), 1535–1537.

Bernstein, D. P., Fink, L., Handelsman, L., Foote, J., Lovejoy, M., Wenzel, K., . . . Ruggiero, J. (1994). Initial reliability and validity of a new retrospective measure of child abuse and neglect. *American Journal of Psychiatry, 151*, 1132–1136.

Birmaher, B., Khetarpal, S., Brent, D., Cully, M., Balach, L., Kaufman, J., & Neer, S. M. (1997). The screen for child anxiety related emotional disorders (SCARED): Scale construction and psychometric characteristics. *Journal of the American Academy of Child and Adolescent Psychiatry, 36*(4), 545–553.

Blake, D., Weathers, F., Nagy, L., Kaloupek, D., Klauminzer, G., Charney, D., & Keane, T. (1990). *Clinician-administered PTSD scale (CAPS)*. Boston: National Center for PTSD.

Blizzard, R. A. (2006). Prevention of intergenerational transmission of child abuse: A national priority. *Journal of Trauma and Disassociation, 7*, 1–6.

Boney-McCoy, S., & Finkelhor, D. (1996). Is youth victimization related to trauma symptoms and depression after controlling for prior symptoms and family relationships?: A longitudinal, prospective study. *Journal of Consulting and Clinical Psychology, 64,* 1406–1416.

Braun, V., & Clarke, V. (2006). Using thematic analysis in psychology. *Qualitative Research in Psychology, 3,* 77–101.

Briere, J. (1996). Psychometric review of Trauma Symptom Checklist 33 & 40. In B. H. Stamm (Ed.), *Measurement of stress, trauma, and adaptation* (pp. 381–383). Lutherville, MD: Sidran Press.

Briggs-Gowan, M., & Carter, A. S. (2008). Social-emotional screening status in early childhood predicts elementary school outcomes. *Pediatrics, 121*(5), 957–962.

Brumbach, B., Figueredo, A., & Ellis, B. (2009). Effects of harsh and unpredictable environments in adolescence on development of life history strategies. *Human Nature, 20*(1), 25–51.

Brymer, M. J., Steinberg, A. M., Watson, P. J., & Pynoos, R. S. (2012). Prevention and early intervention programs for children and adolescents. In J. G. Beck & D. M. Sloan (Eds.), *The Oxford handbook of traumatic stress disorders* (pp. 381–392). New York: Oxford University Press.

Cameron, M., Elkins, J., & Guterman, N. B. (2006). Assessment of trauma in children and youth. In N. B. Webb (Ed.), *Working with traumatized youth in child welfare* (pp. 53–66). New York: Guilford Press.

Carlson, E. (1997). *Trauma assessments: A clinician's guide.* New York: Guilford Press.

Carter, A. S., & Briggs-Gowan, M. J. (1998). *Child Life Events Screener.* New Haven, CT: Yale University.

Carter, R. T. (2007). Racism and psychological and emotional injury: Recognizing and assessing race-based traumatic stress. *The Counseling Psychologist, 35,* 13–105.

Cervantes, R. C., Fisher, D. G., Córdova, D., Napper, L. E., & Napper, L. (2012). The Hispanic Stress Inventory—Adolescent Version: A culturally informed psychosocial assessment. *Psychological Assessment, 24,* 187–196.

Cervantes, R. C., Goldbach, J. T., & Padilla, A. M. (2012). Using qualitative methods for revising items in the Hispanic Stress Inventory. *Hispanic Journal of Behavioral Sciences, 34,* 208–231.

Chaffin, M., & Shultz, S. K. (2001). Psychometric evaluation of the Children's Impact of Traumatic Events Scale—Revised. *Child Abuse and Neglect, 25,* 401–411.

Camras, L. A. (1992). Expressive development and basic emotions. *Cognition and Emotion, 6*(3–4), 269–283.

Chemtob, C. M., Nakashima, J., & Carlson, J. G. (2002). Brief treatment for elementary school children with disaster-related posttraumatic stress disorder: A field study. *Journal of Clinical Psychology, 58*(1), 99–112.

Cheng, C. (1997). Assessment of major life events for Hong Kong adolescents: The Chinese Adolescent Life Event Scale. *American Journal of Community Psychology, 25*(1), 17–33.

Child Sexual Abuse Task Force & Research & Practice Core, National Child Traumatic Stress Network. (2004). *How to implement trauma-focused cognitive behavioral therapy.* Durham, NC/Los Angeles, CA: National Center for Child Traumatic Stress.

Coddington, R. D. (1999). *Coddington Life Events Scales (CLES): Technical manual.* Toronto: Multi-Health Systems.

Cohen, J. A., & Mannarino, A. P. (1996). Factors that mediate treatment outcome of sexually abused preschool children. *Journal of American Academy of Child and Adolescent Psychiatry, 34,* 1402–1411.

Cohen, J. A., Mannarino, A. P., Berliner, L., & Deblinger, E. (2000). Trauma-focused cognitive behavioral therapy for children and adolescents: An empirical update. *Journal of Interpersonal Violence, 15*(11), 1202–1223.

Cohen, J. A., Mannarino, A. P., & Deblinger, E. (2017). *Treating trauma and traumatic grief in children and adolescents* (2nd ed.). New York: Guilford Press.

Cohen, J. A., Mannarino, A. P., & Murray, L. K. (2011). Trauma focused CBT for youth who experience ongoing traumas. *Child Abuse and Neglect, 35,* 637–646.

Cohen, S. (1988). Perceived stress in a probability sample of the United States. In S. Spacapan & S. Oskamp (Eds.), *The social psychology of health* (pp. 31–67). Thousand Oaks, CA: SAGE.

Cohen, S., & Hamrick, N. (2003). Stable individual differences in physiological response to stressors: Implications for stress-elicited changes in immune related health. *Brain, Behavior, and Immunity, 17,* 407–414.

Cohen, S., Kamarck, T., & Mermelstein, R. (1983). A global measure of perceived stress. *Journal of Health and Social Behavior, 24,* 385–396.

Compas, B. E. (1987). Coping with stress during childhood and adolescence. *Psychological Bulletin, 101*(3), 393–403.

Connor-Smith, J. K., Compas, B. E., Wadsworth, M. E., Thomsen, A. H., & Saltzman, H. (2000). Responses to stress in adolescence: Measurement of coping and involuntary stress responses. *Journal of Consulting and Clinical Psychology, 68,* 976–992.

Costello, E. J., Angold, A., March, J., & Fairbank, J. (1998). Life events and post-traumatic stress: The development of a new measure for children and adolescents. *Psychological Medicine, 28*(6), 1275–1288.

Dohrenwend, B. (2000). The role of adversity and stress in psychopathology: Some evidence and its implications for theory and research. *Journal of Health and Social Behavior, 41*(1), 1–19.

Edwards, J. H., & Rogers, K. C. (1997). The traumatic events screening inventory: Assessing trauma in children. In G. K. Kantor & J. L. Jasinski (Eds.), *Out of darkness: Contemporary perspectives on family violence* (pp. 113–118). Thousand Oaks, CA: SAGE.

Eisen, M. (1997). *The development and validation of a new measure of PTSD for young children.* Unpublished manuscript, Cal State Los Angeles, Los Angeles, CA.

Ellis, B., Figueredo, A., Brumbach, B., & Schlomer, G. (2009). Fundamental dimensions of environmental risk. *Human Nature, 20*(2), 204–268.

Epel, E. S., Crosswell, A. D., Mayer, S. E., Prather, A. A., Slavich, G. M., Puterman, E., & Mendes, W. B. (2018). More than a feeling: A unified view of stress measurement for population science. *Frontiers in Neuroendocrinology, 49*, 146–169.

Ewart, C. K., & Kolodner, K. B. (1991). Social competence interview for assessing physiological reactivity in adolescents. *Psychosomatic Medicine, 53*, 289–304.

Feindler, E., Rathus, J., & Silver, L. B. (2003). *Assessment of family violence: A handbook for researchers and practitioners.* Washington, DC: American Psychological Association.

Finkelhor, D., Ormrod, R. K., Turner, H. A., & Hamby, S. L. (2005). Measuring poly-victimization using the Juvenile Victimization Questionnaire. *Child Abuse and Neglect, 29*(11), 1297–1312.

Finkelhor, D., Turner, H. A., Shattuck, A., & Hamby, S. L. (2013). Violence, crime, and abuse exposure in a national sample of children and youth: An update. *JAMA Pediatrics, 167*, 614–621.

Finzi, R., Har-Even, D., Weizman, A., Tyano, S., & Shnit, D. (1996). The adaptation of the attachment style questionnaire for latency-aged children. *Psychologia: Israel Journal of Psychology, 5*, 167–177.

Fletcher, K. (1992). *When bad things happen.* Unpublished manuscript, Department of Psychiatry, University of Massachusetts Medical Center, Worcester, MA.

Fletcher, K. E. (1996a). Childhood posttraumatic stress disorder. In E. J. Mash & R. A. Barkley (Eds.), *Child psychopathology* (pp. 242–276). New York: Guilford Press.

Fletcher, K. E. (1996b). Psychometric review of the Parent Report of Child's Reaction to Stress. In B. H. Stamm (Ed.), *Measurement of stress, trauma, and adaptation* (pp. 225–227). Lutherville, MD: Sidran Press.

Flores, E., Tschann, J. M., Dimas, J. M., Bachen, E. A., Pasch, L. A., & de Groat, C. L. (2008). Perceived discrimination, perceived stress, and mental and physical health among Mexican-origin adults. *Hispanic Journal of Behavioral Sciences, 30*, 401–424.

Flynn, M., & Rudolph, K. D. (2011). Stress generation and adolescent depression: Contribution of interpersonal stress responses. *Journal of Abnormal Child Psychology, 39*(8), 1187–1198.

Foa, E., Johnson, K., Feeny, N., & Treadwell, K. R. (2001). The Child PTSD Symptom Scale: A preliminary examination of its psychometric properties. *Journal of Clinical Child Psychology, 30*, 376–384.

Ford, J. D., Racusin, R., Rogers, K., Ellis, C., Schiffman, J., Ribbe, D., . . . Edwards, J. (2002). *Traumatic Events Screening Inventory for Children (TESI-C) Version 8.4.* Dartmouth, VT: National Center for PTSD and Dartmouth Child Psychiatry Research Group.

Fox, N. A., & Leavitt, L. A. (1995). *The Violence Exposure Scale for Children—Revised (VEX-R).* College Park: Institute for Child Study, University of Maryland.

Foy, D. W., Wood, J. L., King, D. W., King, L. A., & Resnick, H. S. (1997). Los Angeles Symptom Checklist: Psychometric evidence with an adolescent sample. *Assessment, 4*, 377–384.

Friedberg, R. D., & McClure, J. M. (2015). *Clinical practice of cognitive therapy with children and adolescents: The nuts and bolts* (2nd ed.). New York: Guilford Press.

Friedrich, W. N., Grambsch, P., Damon, L., Hewitt, S., Koverola, C., Lang, R., . . . Broughton, D. (1992). Child Sexual Behavior Inventory: Normative and clinical comparisons. *Psychological Assessments, 4*, 303–311.

Friedrich, W. N., Lysne, M., Sim, L., & Shamos, S. (2004). Assessing sexual behavior in high-risk adolescents with the Adolescent Clinical Sexual Behavior Inventory (ACSBI). *Child Maltreatment, 9*, 239–250.

Garber, J., Robinson, N. S., & Valentiner, D. (1997). The relation between parenting and adolescent depression: Self-worth as a mediator. *Journal of Adolescent Research, 12*(1), 12–33.

Ghosh-Ippen, C., Ford, J., Racusin, R., Acker, M., Bosquet, K., Rogers, C., et al. (2002). *Traumatic Events Screening Inventory: Parent Report Revised.* San Francisco: Child Trauma Research Project of the Early Trauma Network and the National Center for PTSD Dartmouth Child Trauma Research Group

Gil, A. G., Vega, W. A., & Dimas, J. M. (1994). Acculturative stress and personal adjustment among Hispanic adolescent boys. *Journal of Community Psychology, 22*(1), 43–54.

Gilbert, R., Kemp, A., Thoburn, J., Sidebotham, P., Radford, L., Glaser, D., & MacMillan, H. L. (2009). Recognizing and responding to child maltreatment. *Lancet, 373*, 167–180.

Grant, K. E., Carter, J., Jackson, Y., Marshall, H., DeCator, D., Turek, C., . . . Achenbach, T. (2020). *A comprehensive, empirically-based stressor classification and measurement system for adolescents: Development and use to predict mental health outcomes.* Unpublished manuscript. DePaul University, Chicago, IL.

Grant, K. E., Compas, B. E., Stuhlmacher, A., Thurm, A. E., McMahon, S., & Halpert, J. (2003). Stressors and child and adolescent psychopathology: Moving from markers to mechanisms of risk. *Psychological Bulletin, 129*, 447–466.

Grant, K. E., Compas, B. E., Thurm, A. E., McMahon, S. D., & Gipson, P. (2004). Stressors and child and adolescent psychopathology: Measurement issues and prospective effects. *Journal of Clinical Child and Adolescent Psychology, 33*, 412–425.

Grant, K. E., Compas, B. E., Thurm, A. E., McMahon, S. Gipson, P. Campbell, A., . . . Westerholm, R. I.

(2006). Stressors and child and adolescent psychopathology: Evidence of moderating and mediating effects. *Clinical Psychology Review, 26,* 257–283.

Grant, K. E., & McMahon, S. (2005). Conceptualizing the role of stressors in the development of psychopathology. In B. L. Hankin & J. R. Z. Abela (Eds.), *Development of psychopathology: A vulnerability–stress perspective.* Thousand Oaks, CA: SAGE.

Gray, M. J., Litz, B. T., Hsu, J. L., & Lombardo, T. W. (2004). Psychometric properties of the life events checklist. *Assessment, 11*(4), 330–341.

Greenwald, R. (1999). *Lifetime Incidence of Traumatic Events–Parent Form (LITE-P).* Brookline, MA: Sidran Foundation.

Greenwald, R., & Rubin, A. (1999). Assessment of posttraumatic symptoms in children: Development and preliminary validation of parent and child scales. *Research on Social Work Practice, 9,* 61–75.

Gully, K. J. (2003). Expectations test: Trauma scales for sexual abuse, physical abuse, exposure to family violence, and posttraumatic stress. *Child Maltreatment, 8*(3), 218–229.

Hamada, R. S., Kameoka, V., Yanagida, E., & Chemtob, C. M. (2003). Assessment of elementary school children for disaster-related posttraumatic stress disorder symptoms: The Kauai recovery index. *Journal of Nervous and Mental Disease, 191*(4), 268–272.

Hamby, S. L., Finkelhor, D., Ormrod, R. K., & Turner, H. A. (2004). *The Juvenile Victimization Questionnaire (JVQ): Administration and scoring manual.* Durham, NH: Crimes Against Children Research Center.

Haskett, M. E., Ahern, L. S., Ward, C. S., & Allaire, J. C. (2006). Factor structure and validity of the Parenting Stress Index—Short Form. *Journal of Clinical Child and Adolescent Psychology, 35*(2), 302–312.

Hastings, R. P., & Beck, A. (2004). Practitioner review: Stress intervention for parents of children with intellectual disabilities. *Journal of Child Psychology and Psychiatry and Allied Disciplines, 45,* 1338–1349.

Herbert, T. B., & Cohen, S. (1996). Measurement issues in research on psychosocial stress. In H. B. Kaplan (Ed.), *Psychosocial Stress: Perspectives on structure, theory, life-course, and methods* (pp. 295–332). New York, NY: Academic Press.

Hoff, A. L., Swan, A. J., Mercado, R. J., Kagan, E. R., Crawford, E. A., & Kendall, P. C. (2016). Psychological therapy with children and adolescents: Theory and practice. In A. J. Consoli, L. E. Beutler, & B. Bongar (Eds.), *Comprehensive textbook of psychotherapy: Theory and practice* (2nd ed., pp. 267–283). Oxford, UK: Oxford University Press.

Horowitz, K., Weine, S., & Jekel, J. (1995). PTSD symptoms in urban adolescent girls: Compounded community trauma. *Journal of the American Academy of Child and Adolescent Psychiatry, 34,* 1353–1361.

Hunsley, J., & Mash, E. J. (2007). Evidence-based assessment. *Annual Review of Clinical Psychology, 3,* 29–51.

Hutchinson, M. E. (2006). *Does involvement in parent–child interaction therapy reduce parental stress?* Unpublished doctoral dissertation, California State University, Long Beach, CA.

Hyman, I. (1996). Psychometric reviews of My Worst Experience and My Worst School Experience Scale. In B. Stamm (Ed.), *Measurement of stress, trauma, and adaptation* (pp. 212–213). Lutherville, MD: Sidran Press.

Izard, C. E., Woodburn, E. M., Finlon, K. J., Krauthamer-Ewing, E. S., Grossman, S. R., & Seidenfeld, A. (2011). Emotion knowledge, emotion utilization, and emotion regulation. *Emotion Review, 3*(1), 44–52.

Jaberghaderi, N., Greenwald, R., Rubin, A., Zand, S. O., & Dolatabadi, S. (2004). A comparison of CBT and EMDR for sexually-abused Iranian girls. *Clinical Psychology and Psychotherapy, 11*(5), 358–368.

Jackson, Y., Gabrielli, J., Fleming, K., Tunno, A. M., & Makanui, P. K. (2014). Untangling the relative contribution of maltreatment severity and frequency to type of behavioral outcome in foster youth. *Child Abuse and Neglect, 38*(7), 1147–1159.

Jackson, Y., Gabrielli, J., Tunno, A. M., & Hambrick, E. P. (2012). Strategies for longitudinal research with youth in foster care: A demonstration of methods, barriers, and innovations. *Children and Youth Services Review, 34*(7), 1208–1213.

Jones, R. T. (1994). *Child's Reaction to Traumatic Events Scale (CRTES): A self-report traumatic stress measure.* Unpublished instrument, Department of Psychology, Virginia Polytechnic Institute and State University, Blacksburg, VA.

Jones, R. T. (1996). Psychometric review of Child's Reaction to Traumatic Events Scale (CRTES). In B. H. Stamm (Ed.), *Measurement of stress, trauma, and adaptation* (pp. 78–80). Lutherville, MD: Sidran Press.

Jones, R. T., Fletcher, K., & Ribbe, D. R. (2002). *Child's Reaction to Traumatic Events Scale—Revised (CRTES-R): A self-report traumatic stress measure.* Blacksburg, VA: Department of Psychology, Virginia Polytechnic Institute and State University, VA.

Kassam-Adams, N. (2006). The Acute Stress Checklist for Children (ASC-Kids): Development of a child self-report measure. *Journal of Traumatic Stress, 19,* 129–139.

Kaufman, J., Birmaher, B., Brent, D., Rao, U., Flynn, C., Moreci, P., . . . Ryan, N. (1997). Schedule for affective disorders and schizophrenia for school-age children-present and lifetime version (K-SADS-PL): Initial reliability and validity data. *Journal of the American Academy of Child and Adolescent Psychiatry, 36*(7), 980–988.

Kazdin, A. E., & Wassell, G. (1998). Treatment completion and therapeutic change among children referred for outpatient therapy. *Professional Psychology: Research and Practice, 29,* 332–340.

Kazdin, A. E., & Whitley, M. K. (2003). Treatment of parental stress to enhance therapeutic change among children referred for aggressive and antisocial behavior. *Journal of Consulting and Clinical Psychology, 71,* 504–515.

Keck Seeley, S. M., Perosa, S. L., & Perosa, L. M. (2004). A validation study of the Adolescent Dissociative Experiences Scale. *Child Abuse and Neglect, 28,* 755–769.

Kendler, K. S., Hettema, J. M., Butera, F., Gardner, C. O., & Prescott, C. A. (2003). Life event dimensions of loss, humiliation, entrapment, and danger in the prediction of onsets of major depression and generalized anxiety. *Archives of General Psychiatry, 60*(8), 789–796.

Kilmer, R. P., Gil-Rivas, V., Tedeschi, R. G., Cann, A., Calhoun, L. G., Buchanan, T., & Taku, K. (2009). Use of the revised Posttraumatic Growth Inventory for Children. *Journal of Traumatic Stress, 22,* 248–253.

King, L. A., King, D. W., Leskin, G., & Foy, D. W. (1995). The Los Angeles Symptom Checklist: A self-report measure of posttraumatic stress disorder. *Assessment, 2,* 1–17.

Lakey, B., & Ross, L. T. (1994). Dependency and self-criticism as moderators of interpersonal and achievement stress: The role of initial dysphoria. *Cognitive Therapy and Research, 18*(6), 581–599.

Lanktree, C. B., Gilbert, A. M., Briere, J., Taylor, N., Chen, K., Maida, C. A., & Saltzman, W. R. (2008). Multi-informant assessment of maltreated children: Convergent and discriminant validity of the TSCC and TSCYC. *Child Abuse and Neglect, 32*(6), 621–625.

Levendosky, A. A., Huth-Bocks, A., Semel, M. A., & Shapiro, D. L. (2002). Trauma symptoms in preschool-age children exposed to domestic violence. *Journal of Interpersonal Violence, 17,* 150–164.

Lieberman, A. F., & Van Horn, P. (2004). Assessment and treatment of young children exposed to traumatic events. In J. D. Osofsky (Ed.), *Young children and trauma: Intervention and treatment* (pp. 111–138). New York: Guilford Press.

Lundahl, B., Risser, H. J., & Lovejoy, M. C. (2006). A meta-analysis of parent training: Moderators and follow-up effects. *Clinical Psychology Review, 26,* 86–104.

Lyneham, H. J., Abbott, M. J., & Rapee, R. M. (2007). Interrater reliability of the Anxiety Disorders Interview Schedule for DSM-IV: Child and parent version. *Journal of the American Academy of Child and Adolescent Psychiatry, 46,* 731–736.

Manly, J. T. (2005). Advances in research definitions of child maltreatment. *Child Abuse and Neglect, 29*(5), 425–439.

McGee, R. A. (1990). *The Attribution for Maltreatment Interview.* Unpublished manuscript, University of Western Ontario.

McGee, R., Wolfe, D., & Olson, J. (2001). Multiple maltreatment, attribution of blame, and adjustment among adolescents. *Development and Psychopathology, 13,* 827–846.

McMahon, S. D., Grant, K. E., Compas, B. E., Thurm, A. E., & Ey, S. (2003). Stress and psychopathology in children and adolescents: Is there evidence of specificity? *Journal of Child Psychology and Psychiatry and Allied Disciplines: Annual Research Review, 44,* 107–133.

Meichenbaum, D. (1985). *Stress inoculation training.* Oxford, UK: Pergamon Press.

Miller, A., Enlow, M. B., Reiche, W., & Saxe, G. (2009). A diagnostic interview for acute stress disorder for children and adolescents. *Journal of Traumatic Stress, 22,* 549–556.

Miller, A. B., Saxe, G., Stoddard, F., Bartholomew, D., Hall, E., Lopez, C., . . . Reich, W. (2004). *Reliability and validity of the DICA-ASD.* Poster presented at the annual meeting of the International Society for Traumatic Stress Studies, New Orleans, LA.

Miller, D. B., Webster, S. E., & MacIntosh, R. (2002). What's there and what's not: Measuring daily hassles in urban African American adolescents. *Research on Social Work Practice, 12*(3), 375–388.

Milne, L., & Collin-Vézina, D. (2015). Assessment of children and youth in child protective services out-of-home care: An overview of trauma measures. *Psychology of Violence, 5*(2), 122–132.

Milner, J. S. (1986). The Child Abuse Potential Inventory: Manual, 2. Retrieved from *www.getcited.org/pub/102480769.*

Monroe, S. M. (2008). Modern approaches to conceptualizing and measuring human life stress. *Annual Review of Clinical Psychology, 4,* 33–52.

Muris, P., Meesters, C., van Melick, M., & Zwambag, L. (2001). Self-reported attachment style, attachment quality, and symptoms of anxiety and depression in young adolescents. *Personality and Individual Differences, 30,* 809–818.

Murphy, V. B., & Christner, R. W. (2012). A cognitive-behavioral case conceptualization for children and adolescents. In *Cognitive-behavioral interventions in educational settings: A handbook for practice* (2nd ed., pp. 81–114). Abingdon, UK: Routledge.

Nader, K. O. (1997). Assessing traumatic experiences in children. In J. P. Wilson & T. M. Keane (Eds.), *Assessing psychological trauma and PTSD* (pp. 291–348). New York: Guilford Press.

Nader, K. O., Newman, E., Weathers, F. W., Kaloupek, D. G., Kriegler, J. A., & Blake, D. D. (1998). *Clinician-Administered PTSD Scale for Children and Adolescents (CAPS-CA) interview booklet.* Los Angeles: Western Psychological Services.

Nyborg, V. M., & Curry, J. F. (2003). The impact of perceived racism: Psychological symptoms among African American boys. *Journal of Clinical Child and Adolescent Psychology, 32*(2), 258–266.

Overstreet, S., & Braun, S. (2000). Exposure to community violence and post-traumatic stress symptoms: Mediating factors. *American Journal of Orthopsychiatry, 70*(2), 263–271.

Pearlman, L. A. (2003). *Trauma and Attachment Belief Scale*. Los Angeles: Western Psychological Services.

Petty, J. (1990). *Checklist for Child Abuse Evaluations*. Odessa, FL: Psychological Assessment Resources.

Pine, D. S., & Cohen, J. A. (2002). Trauma in children and adolescents: Risk and treatment of psychiatric sequelae. *Biological Psychiatry, 51*, 519–531.

Putnam, F. W., & Peterson, G. (1994). Further validation of the Child Dissociative Checklist. *Dissociation, 7*, 204–211.

Raviv, T., & Wadsworth, M. E. (2010). The efficacy of a pilot prevention program for children and caregivers coping with economic strain. *Cognitive Therapy and Research, 34*(3), 216–228.

Reynolds, C. R., & Kamphaus, R. W. (2004). *BASC-2: Behavior Assessment System for Children, Second Edition Manual*. Circle Pines, MN: American Guidance Service.

Richters, J. E., & Martinez, P. (1993). The NIMH Community Violence Project: I. Children as victims of and witnesses to violence. *Psychiatry: Interpersonal and Biological Processes, 56*, 7–21.

Roberts, M. C., Blossom, J. B., Evans, S. C., Amaro, C. M., & Kanine, R. M. (2017). Advancing the scientific foundation for evidence-based practice in clinical child and adolescent psychology. *Journal of Clinical Child and Adolescent Psychology, 46*, 915–928.

Rodriguez, N., Steinberg, A. M., & Pynoos, R. S. (1999). *UCLA PTSD Index for DSM-IV*. Los Angeles: University of California at Los Angeles Trauma Psychiatry Service.

Rudolph, K. D., & Flynn, M. (2007). Childhood adversity and youth depression: Influence of gender and pubertal status. *Development and Psychopathology, 19*, 497–521.

Rudolph, K. D., & Hammen, C. (1999). Age and gender as determinants of stress exposure, generation, and reactions in youngsters: A transactional perspective. *Child Development, 70*(3), 660–677.

Saigh, P. A., Yasik, A. E., Oberfield, R. A., Green, B. L., Halamandaris, P. V., Rubenstein, H., . . . McHugh, M. (2000). The Children's PTSD Inventory: Development and reliability. *Journal of Traumatic Stress, 13*, 369–380.

Saxe, G., Chawla, N., Stoddard, F., Kassam-Adams, N., Courtney, D., Cunningham, K., . . . King, L. (2003). Child Stress Disorders Checklist: A measure of ASD and PTSD in children. *Journal of the American Academy of Child and Adolescent Psychiatry, 42*, 972–978.

Saylor, C. F., Swenson, C. C., Reynolds, S. S., & Taylor, M. (1999). The Pediatric Emotional Distress Scale: A brief screening measure for young children exposed to traumatic events. *Journal of Clinical Child Psychology, 28*, 70–81.

Scheeringa, M. S., & Zeanah, C. H. (2005). *PTSD semistructured interview and observational record for infants and young children*. New Orleans, LA: Department of Psychiatry and Neurology, Tulane University Health Sciences Center.

Scheeringa, M. S., Zeanah, C. H., Myers, L., & Putnam, F. W. (2003). New findings on alternative criteria for PTSD in preschool children. *Journal of the American Academy of Child and Adolescent Psychiatry, 42*, 561–570.

Schwarzer, R., & Schulz, U. (2003). The role of stressful life events. In A. M. Nezu, C. M. Nezu, & P. A. Geller (Eds.), *Comprehensive handbook of psychology: Vol. 9. Health psychology* (pp. 27–50). New York: Wiley.

Shaffer, D., Fisher, P., Lucas, C. P., Dulcan, M. K., & Schwab-Stone, M. E. (2000). NIMH Diagnostic Interview Schedule for Children Version IV (NIMH DISC-IV): Description, differences from previous versions, and reliability of some common diagnoses. *Journal of the American Academy of Child and Adolescent Psychiatry, 39*, 28–38.

Shahinfar, A., Fox, N. A., & Leavitt, L. A. (2000). Preschool children's exposure to violence: Relation of behavior problems to parent and child reports. *American Journal of Orthopsychiatry, 70*(1), 115–125.

Shamseddeen, W., Asarnow, J. R., Clarke, G., Vitiello, B., Wagner, K. D., Birmaher, B., . . . Brent, D. A. (2011). Impact of physical and sexual abuse on treatment response in the Treatment of Resistant Depression in Adolescent Study (TORDIA). *Journal of the American Academy of Child and Adolescent Psychiatry, 50*, 293–301.

Sheras, P. L., Abidin, R. R., & Konold, T. R. (1998). *Stress Index for Parents of Adolescents (SIPA)*. Odessa, FL: Psychological Assessment Resources.

Silverman, W. K., & Nelles, W. B. (1988). The Anxiety Disorders Interview Schedule for Children. *Journal of the American Academy of Child and Adolescent Psychiatry, 27*, 772–778.

Silverman, W. K., Saavedra, L. M., & Pina, A. A. (2001). Test–retest reliability of anxiety symptoms and diagnoses with the Anxiety Disorders Interview Schedule for DSM-IV: Child and Parent versions. *Journal of the American Academy of Child and Adolescent Psychiatry, 40*, 937–944.

Slavich, G. M., & Shields, G. S. (2018). Assessing lifetime stress exposure using the Stress and Adversity Inventory for Adults (Adult STRAIN): An overview and initial validation. *Psychosomatic Medicine, 80*, 17–27.

Smith, D. K., Leve, L. D., & Chamberlain, P. (2006). Adolescent girls' offending and health-risking sexual behavior: The predictive role of trauma. *Child Maltreatment, 11*, 346–353.

Smith-Bynum, M. A., Lambert, S. F., English, D., & Ialongo, N. S. (2014). Associations between trajectories of perceived racial discrimination and psychological symptoms among African American adolescents. *Development and Psychopathology, 26*, 1049–1065.

Solis, M. L., & Abidin, R. R. (1991). The Spanish Version Parenting Stress Index: A psychometric study. *Journal of Clinical Child Psychology, 20,* 372–378.

Sommers-Flanagan, J., & Sommers-Flanagan, R. (2012). *Clinical interviewing: 2012–2013 update.* New York: Wiley.

Spaccarelli, S. (1995). Measuring abuse stress and negative cognitive appraisals in child sexual abuse: Validity data on two new scales. *Journal of Abnormal Child Psychology, 23,* 703–727.

Spilsbury, J. C., Fletcher, K. E., Creeden, R., & Friedman, S. (2008). Psychometric properties of the Dimensions of Stressful Events Rating Scale. *Traumatology, 14,* 116–130.

Steinberg, A. M., Brymer, M. J., Decker, K. B., & Pynoos, R. S. (2004). The University of California at Los Angeles Post-Traumatic Stress Disorder Reaction Index. *Current Psychiatry Reports, 6*(2), 96–100.

Stover, C. S., & Berkowitz, S. (2005). Assessing violence exposure and trauma symptoms in young children: A critical review of measures. *Journal of Traumatic Stress, 18,* 707–717.

Stover, C. S., Hahn, H., Im, J. J., & Berkowitz, S. (2010). Agreement of parent and child reports of trauma exposure and symptoms in the early aftermath of a traumatic event. *Psychological Trauma: Theory, Research, Practice, and Policy, 2,* 159–168.

Strand, V. C., Sarmiento, T. L., & Pasquale, L. E. (2005). Assessment and screening tools for trauma in children and adolescents: A review. *Trauma, Violence, and Abuse, 6*(1), 55–78.

Strauss, A., & Corbin, J. (1994). *Grounded theory methodology: An overview.* Thousand Oaks, CA: SAGE.

Tam, K. K., Chan, Y. C., & Wong, C. K. M. (1994). Validation of the Parenting Stress Index among Chinese mothers in Hong Kong. *Journal of Community Psychology, 22,* 211–223.

Topham, G. L., & Wampler, K. S. (2008). Predicting dropout in a filial therapy program for parents and young children. *American Journal of Family Therapy, 36,* 60–78.

Wadsworth, M. E., Santiago, C. D., Einhorn, L., Etter, E. M., Rienks, S., & Markman, H. (2011). Preliminary efficacy of an intervention to reduce psychosocial stress and improve coping in low-income families. *American Journal of Community Psychology, 48,* 257–271.

Weinstein, B., Levine, M., Kogan, N., Harkavy-Friedman, J., & Miller, J. M. (2000). Mental health professionals' experiences reporting suspected child abuse and maltreatment. *Child Abuse and Neglect, 24,* 1317–1328.

Weiss, J. A., Viecili, M. A., & Bohr, Y. (2015). Parenting stress as a correlate of cognitive behavior therapy responsiveness in children with autism spectrum disorders and anxiety. *Focus on Autism and Other Developmental Disabilities, 30,* 154–164.

Williamson, D. E., Birmaher, B., Ryan, N. D., Shiffrin, T. P., Lusky, J. A., Protopapa, J., . . . Brent, D. A. (2003). The Stressful Life Events Schedule for Children and Adolescents: Development and validation. *Psychiatry Research, 119,* 225–241.

Wolfe, V., & Birt, J. (1993). *The Feelings and Emotions Experienced During Sexual Abuse Scale.* London, ON, Canada: London Health Sciences Center.

Wolfe, V. V., Gentile, C., Michienzi, T., Sas, L., & Wolfe, D. A. (1991). The Children's Impact of Traumatic Events Scale: A measure of post-sexual-abuse PTSD symptoms. *Behavioral Assessment, 13,* 359–383.

Wolfe, V. V., & Wolfe, D. A. (1986). *The Sexual Abuse Fear Evaluation (SAFE): A subscale for the Fear Survey Schedule for Children—Revised.* Unpublished questionnaire, Children's Hospital of Western Ontario, London, ON, Canada.

Yasik, A. E., Saigh, P. A., Oberfield, R. A., Green, B., Halamandaris, P., & McHugh, M. (2001). The validity of the Children's PTSD Inventory. *Journal of Traumatic Stress, 14*(1), 81–94.

APPENDIX 16.1. Empirically Based Stressor Taxonomy for Adolescents

TAXONOMIC DOMAIN 1: THREAT (of loss or humiliation; pressures and changes)

Stressor level	Contextual variables associated with objective threat	Interrater reliability
Systemic stressors		
Community violence; war; neighborhood tension resulting from income inequality and social diversity (these also constitute conflict events)	1. Pervasiveness of threat across home, school, neighborhood, and nation 2. Chronicity of threat (i.e., ongoing for longer than 1 month)	ICC range: .66–.85 ICC mean: .77
Major event stressors		
Threat of future loss or humiliation major events—see loss and humiliation major event lists; major changes (e.g., new parent, new sibling, new school, new language)	1. Experienced within the context of systemic events or conditions associated with this domain 2. Threat of high magnitude of negative change in usual activities (i.e., substantial change in daily activities) 3. Chronicity of threat (i.e., present for longer than 1 month—not applicable to changes) 4. Threat is unpredictable (i.e., event/s likely to occur without predictable pattern or timing) 5. Threat involves important attachment figures (e.g., parent, close friend) 6. For Threat of Humiliation Events: Event is likely to be highly visible (e.g., likely to occur in front of numerous peers)	ICC range: .65–.92 ICC mean: .75
Minor event stressors (lab protocol: threat of buzzer in timed achievement task)		
Threat of future loss or humiliation minor events—see loss and humiliation minor event lists (e.g., pop quizzes, public speaking requirements); minor changes (e.g., new teacher, new coach, new extracurricular activity)	1. Experienced within the context of systemic or major events associated with this domain 2. Ongoing and frequent occurrence of threat (i.e., weekly or daily) 3. Unpredictability (i.e., threats occur without predictable pattern or timing) 4. Involvement of important attachment figures in threat events (e.g., parent, close friend) 5. For Threat of Humiliation Events: Threats involve multiple witnesses (e.g., performance in front of numerous peers)	ICC range: .68–.73 ICC mean: .71

HYPOTHESIZED SPECIFICITY ASSOCIATIONS

Specific cognitive responses: hypervigilance, avoidance, or rumination

Specific emotional responses: anxiety or fear

Specific physiological responses: alert, geared up

Specific mental health or behavioral outcomes: anxiety symptoms and/or substance use symptoms (to blunt negative emotions)

Specific learning outcomes: when threat is related to learning foci, curvilinear relationship with anxiety; when threat is unrelated to learning foci, distracted, unfocused

Specific moderators: gender; interpersonal versus noninterpersonal (e.g., attachment vs. achievement); threat of loss versus threat of humiliation; personal versus impersonal (e.g., human violence vs. disaster)

Specific protective factors: worldview, philosophy or beliefs that provide meaning, acceptance, and/or hope in relation to the greatest possible threats

TAXONOMIC DOMAIN 2: LOSS (of achievement/status, attachment/relationship, autonomy/freedom) and **LACK** (of resources)

Stressor level	Contextual variables associated with objective threat	Interrater reliability
Systemic stressors		
Deprivation; low social capital; limited education, employment, health care, housing, public services, food, space, natural beauty; neglect	1. Pervasiveness of deprivation, neglect across home, school, neighborhood, and nation 2. Chronicity of deprivation, neglect (i.e., ongoing for longer than 1 month)	ICC range: .66–.85 ICC mean: .77
Major event stressors		
Death or separation involving central attachment figure(s); loss of means of living; loss of physical integrity; loss of primary status or identity; loss of central ideas or loss of trust in central attachment figure	1. Experienced within the context of systemic events or conditions associated with this domain 2. High magnitude of negative change in usual activities of the individual (i.e., substantial change in daily activities) 3. Chronicity of event or situation (i.e., ongoing for longer than 1 month) 4. Unpredictability (i.e., event/s occurred without predictable pattern or timing)	ICC range: .65–.92 ICC mean: .75

Minor event stressors (lab protocol: loss of money in rigged card game; additional options: cyberball (attachment), impossible "IQ" test (achievement), pretend punishment for rowdy behavior (autonomy))

Death or separation involving peripheral figure; minor separation involving major attachment figure; loss of material possession; minor reduction in status; loss of ideas that are not central to worldview or loss of trust in peripheral figure; hassles associated with deprivation (e.g., long wait for bus)	1. Experienced within the context of systemic and/or major events associated with this domain 2. Ongoing and frequent occurrence (i.e., weekly or daily) 3. Unpredictability (i.e., events occur without predictable pattern or timing)	ICC range: .68–.73 ICC mean: .71

HYPOTHESIZED SPECIFICITY ASSOCIATIONS

Specific cognitive responses: negative thoughts about the self, world, future; internal, stable, global attributions; hopelessness; helplessness; avoidant and/or ruminative coping

Specific emotional responses: sadness, sorrow, or despair

Specific physiological responses: slowed

Specific mental health or behavioral outcomes: depressive symptoms and/or substance use symptoms (to blunt negative emotions)

Specific learning outcomes: reduced engagement, reduced self-efficacy

Specific moderators: gender; interpersonal versus noninterpersonal; achievement versus attachment versus autonomy meaning domains; mental versus physical integrity; Kendler's external versus internal

Specific protective factors: physical and emotional comforting; positive events and relationships; exposure to growth mindsets that minimize attributions of fixed traits

TAXONOMIC DOMAIN 3: HUMILIATION

Stressor level	Contextual variables associated with objective threat	Interrater reliability
Systemic stressors		
Pervasive perfectionistic standards related to achievement or beauty; pervasive negative stereotypes (racism, classism, sexism, xenophobia, homophobia, ableism, and stereotypes about people who are fat)	1. For Standards and Stereotypes: Pervasiveness across home, school, neighborhood, and nation 2. For Standards and Stereotypes: Visibility (i.e., segregation, redlining, racial profiling, media representations) 3. For Standards and Stereotypes: Connection of stereotype to other stress domains (i.e., loss, conflict, change)	ICC range: .66–.85 ICC mean: .77
Major event stressors		
Physical debasement; sexual assault or abuse (these also constitute conflict and loss events); major failures and rejections (these also constitute loss events); major punishment (e.g., prison, expulsion; these also constitutes conflict and loss events)	1. Experienced within the context of systemic events or conditions associated with this domain 2. High magnitude of negative change in usual activities (i.e., substantial change in daily activities) 3. Chronicity of event or situation (i.e., ongoing for longer than 1 month) 4. Unpredictability (i.e., events occur without predictable pattern or timing) 5. Involvement of important attachment figures (e.g., parent, teacher, close friend, boyfriend, girlfriend) 6. Multiple witnesses (e.g., event or events occurred in front of numerous peers)	ICC range: .65–.92 ICC mean: .75
Minor event stressors (lab protocol: poorest performance in rigged oral reasoning task; additional option: TRIER public speaking task)		
Microaggressions related to stereotypes or standards listed earlier; verbal debasement (these also constitute conflict events); minor failures and rejections (these also constitute loss events); minor punishment (this also constitutes a conflict and loss event); falling short of social standards	1. Experienced within the context of systemic or major events associated with this domain 2. Ongoing and frequent occurrence (i.e., weekly or daily) 3. Unpredictability (i.e., events occur without predictable pattern or timing) 4. Involvement of important attachment figures (e.g., parent, teacher, close friend, boyfriend, girlfriend) 5. Multiple witnesses (e.g., event or events occur in front of numerous peers)	ICC range: .68–.73 ICC mean: .71

HYPOTHESIZED SPECIFICITY ASSOCIATIONS

Specific cognitive responses: negative thoughts about the self; internal, stable, global attributions; avoidant and/or ruminative coping

Specific emotional responses: shame

Specific physiological responses: slowed

Specific mental health or behavioral outcomes: depressive symptoms and/or substance use symptoms (to blunt negative emotions)

Specific moderators: loss of pride versus not measuring up; perfectionism regarding achievement versus appearance; stereotypes regarding racism versus classism versus sexism versus ableism versus homophobia versus xenophobia versus fat phobia

Specific learning outcomes: lowered expectations/aspirations for self in stereotyped areas; reduced engagement; reduced self-efficacy

Specific protective factors: exposure to positive beliefs about groups that are discriminated against and about diversity in general; exposure to growth mind-sets that minimize attributions of fixed traits

TAXONOMIC DOMAIN 4: CONFLICT/THWARTING OF GOALS/UNFAIR TREATMENT

Stressor level	Contextual variables associated with objective threat	Interrater reliability
Systemic stressors		
Dominance of one social group over another (e.g., segregation, oppression); pervasive community conflict; unjust laws and/or system of government	1. Pervasiveness of dominance, conflict, or unjust system(s) across home, school, neighborhood, and nation 2. Chronicity of dominance, conflict, or unjust system(s) (i.e., ongoing for longer than 1 month)	ICC range: .66–.85 ICC mean: .77
Major event stressors		
Major conflict; physical fight; other(s) thwart central goal(s); major unfair treatment of self or major attachment figure	1. Experienced within the context of systemic events or conditions associated with this domain 2. Centrality of relationship within which conflict occurs (e.g., parents) 3. High magnitude of negative change in usual activities related to the conflict (i.e., substantial change in daily activities) 4. Chronicity of event or situation (i.e., ongoing for longer than 1 month) 5. Unpredictability (i.e., conflict occurs without predictable pattern or timing)	ICC range: .65–.92 ICC mean: .75
Minor event stressors (lab protocol: confederates impede concentration through talking and cheat for reward for which participant strives)		
Minor conflict; other(s) thwart peripheral goals(s); minor unfair treatment of self or major attachment figure; major unfair treatment of peripheral figure; nonpersonal, temporary thwarting of goals (e.g., computer crashes, heavy traffic, bureaucracy)	1. Experienced within the context of systemic and/or major events associated with this domain 2. Centrality of relationship within which conflict occurs (e.g., parents) 3. Ongoing and frequent occurrence (i.e., weekly or daily) 4. Unpredictability (i.e., events occur without predictable pattern or timing)	ICC range: .68–.73 ICC mean: .71

HYPOTHESIZED SPECIFICITY ASSOCIATIONS

Specific cognitive responses: negative thoughts about others; hostile attribution bias; external, stable, global attributions

Specific emotional responses: annoyance, frustration, anger, or rage

Specific physiological responses: alert, geared up

Specific mental health or behavioral outcomes: oppositional defiant disorder or conduct disorder symptoms and/or substance use symptoms (to blunt negative emotions)

Specific learning outcomes: distracted, unfocused

Specific moderators: gender; personal versus impersonal thwarting of goals; conflict related to loss (or threat of loss) versus humiliation (or threat of humiliation); observed versus experienced

Specific protective factors: peaceful religiosity; gratitude; forgiveness; mindfulness; humility; organizing against injustice; exposure to growth mind-sets that minimize attributions of fixed traits

APPENDIX 16.2. Brief Stressor Interviews Modified from Ewart's Social Competence Interview (Ewart & Kolodner, 1991)

This tool can be used to collect information about stressor history and new events across the course of therapy, and also to monitor coping progress over time.

"I want to find out about stressful things that have happened to you. I will ask you about a type of stress and I want you to reexperience it, describing what happened just the way it did when it actually happened. If I start to ask about anything that you do not want to discuss, just let me know. If there is anything you wouldn't like to talk about, you don't have to.

"I may ask you questions as you talk, and it may sound like I am repeating a question or emphasizing a certain point. I won't be doing this to give you a hard time but to try to be sure that I understand what really happened to you.

"For the next 8 minutes, I want you to tell me about a specific type of stress. If you stop talking before the 8 minutes are up, I will prompt you to continue talking, and if you are still talking when 8 minutes are up, I will stop you.

"The type of stress we will be talking about is *threat*. I want you to describe an event in which you felt *threatened*. Threats can be against your body or your mind. For example, you might feel threatened for your safety because someone is following you home from school or telling you they are going to beat you up. You might also feel threatened by a friend who gets good grades because you don't want him or her to think that you are stupid or dumb. Think of an event in which you were threatened and tell me about it. What happened? Where did it happen? Who was involved?

"The type of stress we will be talking about is *loss*. I want you to describe a time in your life when you lost something. This could be a material thing like a cell phone or a person like your grandmother. Keep in mind that the person or thing does not have to be something that was lost forever. For example, you could have lost your father because he was sent to jail or lost your best friends because you moved to a different neighborhood. You might also think of things that you have lost that cannot be seen, like trust or a sense of safety. You may also choose to talk about something you are lacking because your family doesn't have enough money. I want you to tell me about a specific time when you lost something or were lacking something.

"The type of stress we will be talking about is *humiliation*. I want you to describe something that has happened in your life that was humiliating. You can think about the things that society or your family and friends think are important and a time when you have not met their standards or do not look or act the way others believe you should. Keep in mind that humiliation can be caused by something that you did or something that someone else did. If you cannot think of any specific thing that happened to you, you can talk about a specific time when a friend, family member, or other person you identify with experienced humiliation. But be sure it is someone with whom you deeply identify. Tell me what happened. Where did it happen? Who was involved?

"The type of stress we will be talking about is *conflict*. I want you to describe a time when you were treated unfairly, or someone or something stopped you from completing or doing something, or you had an argument with a family member, friend, or authority figure. You can think of one specific time or it could be something that continues to happen in your life that causes you to feel unfairly treated, blocked from doing or accomplishing something, or in a conflict. For example, your parent might not allow you to do something that is important to you or your coach might favor another player on the team over you, or your teacher might punish you when it was really someone else's fault. You could also think of arguments that you have had or seen between people who are important to you. I want you to focus on the conflict and what happened during this conflict. Now, tell me about a specific time when you experienced conflict whether it was resolved or is ongoing."

Cited in Grant et al. (2020).

APPENDIX 16.3. Comprehensive List of Trauma Measures for Children and Adolescents

Interviews

Measure	Content	Reporter	Administration time	Age range	Trauma type	Outcomes	Psychometrics/norms
Anxiety Disorders Interview Schedule for Children and Adolescents (PTSD section; Silverman & Nelles, 1988)	3 specific disorders or symptoms	Parent, child, adolescent	90 min (whole interview)	7–16	NA	PTSD, internalizing and externalizing disorders	Interrater reliability kappa = .43–.82 for the primary diagnosis, lower for the child interview than for the parent interview; Test–retest kappa = –.09–1.0. Lyneham, Abbott, & Rapee (2007); Silverman, Saavedra, & Pina (2001). No norm information published
Attributions for Maltreatment Interview (McGee, 1990)	4 multiple symptoms or reactions	Adolescent	NA	NA	Child maltreatment	Blame	Internal consistency range = .40–.84; test–retest reliability range = .68–.98. Feindler, Rathus, & Silver (2003); McGee, Wolfe, & Olson (2001). Clinical and nonclinical norms
Checklist for Child Abuse Evaluation (Petty, 1990)	2 events		NA	NA	Child maltreatment	NA	No information published
Child Abuse and Neglect Interview Schedule—Revised (Ammerman, Hersen, Van Hasselt, Lubetsky, & Sieck, 1994)	1 event and symptoms	Parent	45 min	NA	Family violence, child maltreatment	Parenting practices, child behavior, abuse, and violence exposure	High interrater reliability and low internal consistency[b]
Child and Adolescent Psychiatric Assessment (Costello, Angold, March, & Fairbank, 1998)	3 specific disorders or symptoms	Parent, child, adolescent	60 min	9–17	NA	PTSD	Kappa = .40–.79[b]. Clinical and nonclinical norms
Childhood PTSD Interview (Fletcher, 1996a)	4 multiple symptoms or reactions	Child, parent	30–40 min	7–18	NA	PTSD, internalizing and externalizing behaviors	High Kuder–Richardson–20 coefficients; high internal consistency; convergent validity with other measures developed by the author ranged from moderate to high; moderately correlated with the CBCL[b]. Carlson (1997). Clinical and nonclinical norms

Instrument	Reliability / norms	Scales / informant	Administration time	Age range	Trauma type	Construct(s) assessed
Children's Impact of Traumatic Events Scale—Revised (Wolfe, Gentile, Michienzi, Sas, & Wolfe, 1991)	Overall alpha = .69 (range = .56–79)[b] Chaffin & Shultz (2001) No norm information available	4 multiple symptoms or reactions Child, adolescent	10–40 min	8–16	Sexual abuse	PTSD, attributions, social reactions
Children's PTSD Inventory (Carter & Briggs-Gowan, 1988)	Test–retest = .86; internal consistency range = 53–89; interrater = .92 Saigh et al. (2000) Nonclinical norms	3 specific disorders or symptoms	20–45 min	7–18	NA	PTSD
Clinician-Administered PTSD Scale for Children and Adolescents (Nader, Newman, Weathers, Kaloupek, Kriegler, & Blake, 1998)	Internal consistency range = .64–.84; interrater range = .8–98 Saigh et al. (2000); Yasik et al. (2001) Clinical and nonclinical norms	3 Specific disorders or symptoms Child	30 min–2 hours	8–18	NA	Acute stress disorder, PTSD
Diagnostic Interview Schedule for Children (Shaffer, Fisher, Lucas, Dulcan, & Schwab-Stone, 2000)	Test–retest in clinical sample range = .42–96[b] No norm information	3 specific disorders or symptoms Child	70–120 min	6–17	NA	DSM-IV and ICD-10 disorders
Diagnostic Interview for Children and Adolescents Acute Stress Disorder Module (Miller, Enlow, Reiche, & Saxe, 2009)	Internal consistency = .85 (range = .76–93); interrater = 1.0 Miller et al. (2004) Clinical norms	3 specific disorders or symptoms Child	15 min	7–18	Medical, accidents, assault	Acute stress disorder, PTSD
Dimensions of Stressful Events (Spilsbury, Fletcher, Creeden, & Friedman, 2008)	Internal consistency = .62 Fletcher (1996a) No norm information	2 events	NA	2–28	Sexual abuse, community violence, disasters	Characteristics of the event(s), potential for PTSD
Expectations Test (Gully, 2003)	Test–retest = .68 (range = .38–98); internal consistency = .65 (range = .42–.82); interrater = .86 (range = .66–1)[b] Clinical and nonclinical norms	1 event and symptoms	15 min	7–14	Physical abuse, sexual abuse, domestic violence	Social expectations, trauma history
Kiddie Schedule for Affective Disorders and Schizophrenia for School-Age Children (Kaufman et al., 1997)	Inter-rater agreement range = .93–1.0; test-retest reliability kappa coefficients range = .63–1.0[b] Clinical and nonclinical norms	3 specific disorders or symptoms Parent, child, adolescent	35–75 min	6–18	NA	PTSD, internalizing and externalizing disorders
Life Events Interview (Alloy & Abramson, 2004)	No information available	2 events Child, adolescent, parent	NA	NA	Self-identified	NA

Measure name and anchor citation	Psychometric information available including norm information[a]	Type of information provided and reporter	Time to complete	Age	Type of trauma assessed	Clinical domains assessed
Los Angeles Symptom Checklist (King, King, Lesking, & Foy, 1995)	Reliability alpha = .95 total score, .94 PTSD symptoms; test–retest (2 weeks) = .90–.94[b] Foy, Wood, King, King, & Resnick (1997) Nonclinical norms	3 specific disorders or symptoms Adolescent	10–15 min	NA	NA	PTSD
Posttraumatic Symptom Inventory for Children (Eisen, 1997)	Construct validity: Trauma Symptom Checklist (r = .66), Child Dissociate Checklist and the Children's Perceptual Alteration Scale (r = .38)[b] Nonclinical norms	3 specific disorders or symptoms Child	30 min	4–8	NA	PTSD
Posttraumatic Stress Disorder Semi-Structured Interview and Observational Record (Scheeringa & Zeanah, 2005)	Interrater kappa = .29–1.0; kappa for the full diagnosis = .79 Scheeringa, Zeanah, Myers, & Putnam (2003) Clinical and nonclinical norms	3 specific disorders or symptoms Parent, caregiver	45 min	0–7	NA	PTSD
Stressful Life Events Schedule for Children and Adolescents (Williamson, Birmaher, Ryan, Shiffrin, Lusky, & Protopapa, 2003)	Interrater reliability kappa = .67–.84; test–retest reliability kappa = .68[b] Clinical and nonclinical norms	2 events Adolescent	NA	12–18	Changes, conflicts, loss	NA
Traumatic Events Screening Inventory (Edwards & Rogers, 1997)	Test–retest kappas = .50–.79 Stover & Berkowitz (2005)	2 events	20–30 min	6–18	Hospitalization, child maltreatment, domestic violence, community violence, disasters	NA
Violence Exposure Scale for Children—Revised (Fox & Leavitt, 1995)	Internal consistency range = 72–.86 Shahinfar, Fox, & Leavitt (2000) Nonclinical norms	2 events Child	20–25 min	4–10	Community and family violence	NA
Youth Life Stress Interview (Rudolph & Flynn, 2007)	High reliability was found for ratings of episodic stress impact (ICC = .95) and event content (Cohen's kappa = .92)[b] Nonclinical norms	2 events Child, parent	30 min	9–18	Family, academic, social	NA

Questionnaires

Measure	Psychometrics and norms	Format / Respondent	Administration time	Age range	Trauma type	Construct assessed
Abusive Sexual Exposure Scale (Spaccarelli, 1995)	No information available	2 events; Child, adolescent			Sexual abuse	NA
Acute Stress Checklist for Children (Kassam-Adams, 2006)	Internal consistency = .86; test-retest = .73	3 specific disorders or symptoms; Child	10 min	8–17	Injury/illness	Acute stress disorder
Adolescent Clinical Sexual Behavior Inventory (Friedrich, Lysne, Sim, & Shamos, 2004)	Self-report: internal consistency alpha = .68 (range = .45–.84); test–retest (1 week) r = .74; interrater r = .50; parent report: internal consistency = .68 (range = .39–.81); interrater = .50[b]; Clinical norms	4 multiple symptoms or reactions; Parent, adolescent	NA	12–18	Sexual abuse	Sexual behaviors
Adolescent Dissociative Experiences Scale–II (Keck Seeley, Perosa, & Perosa, 2004)	Cronbach's alpha = .93 (subscales = .72–.85); Keck Seeley et al. (2004); Strand, Sarmiento, & Pasquale (2006); Clinical and nonclinical norms	3 specific disorders or symptoms; Child, adolescent	NA	10–21	NA	Dissociative symptoms
Adolescent Self-Report Trauma Questionnaire (Horowitz, Weine, & Jekel, 1995)	Limited psychometrics; Nonclinical norms	1 event and symptoms; Child, adolescent	20 min	12–21	Community and domestic violence	PTSD
Attachment Questionnaire for Children (Muris, Meesters, Melick, & Zwambag, 2001)	Interrater reliability = .37; Muris, Meesters, van Melick, & Zwambag (2001); Nonclinical norms	4 multiple symptoms or reactions; Child, adolescent	5 min	9–18	NA	Attachment quality
Attachment Style Classification Questionnaire (Finzi, Har-Even, Weizman, Tyano, & Shnit, 1996)	Test–retest = .87–.95; internal consistency (alpha) = .69–.81[b]; Al-Yagon & Mikulincer (2004); Clinical and nonclinical norms	4 multiple symptoms or reactions; Child, adolescent	5 min	7–14	NA	Attachment quality
Child Abuse Potential Inventory (Milner, 1986)	Test–retest = .91; internal consistency = .97; Split-half reliability and internal consistency range = 92–96 (controls) and .95–.98 (abusers); Clinical and nonclinical norms	4 multiple symptoms or reactions; Parents	15 min	NA	Physical abuse, neglect, domestic violence	Parenting style, caregiver mood/anxiety symptoms, caregiver interaction style

Measure name and anchor citation	Psychometric information available including norm information[a]	Type of information provided and reporter	Time to complete	Age	Type of trauma assessed	Clinical domains assessed
Child Dissociative Checklist (Putnam & Peterson, 1994)	Moderate test–retest reliability; moderate to good internal reliability[b] Clinical and nonclinical norms	3 specific disorders or symptoms Parents	5 min	NA	NA	Dissociative symptoms
Child PTSD Symptom Scale (Foa, Johnson, Feeny, & Treadwell, 2001)	High internal consistency; moderate to good internal and test–retest reliability[b] Clinical and nonclinical norms	3 specific disorders or symptoms	15 min	8–18	NA	PTSD
Child Reaction to Traumatic Events Scale (Jones, 1994)	Acceptable Cronbach's alpha for total score; low alphas for intrusion and avoidance Jones (1996); Nader (1997) Clinical and nonclinical norms	3 specific disorders or symptoms Parents	10 min	NA	NA	PTSD
Child (Parent) Report of Post-Traumatic Symptoms (Greenwald & Rubin, 1999)	Excellent internal consistency; good concurrent validity between the both the CROPS and the PROPS and the Lifetime Incidence of Traumatic Events Scales[b] Jaberghaderi, Greenwald, Rubin, Zand, & Dolatabadi (2004) Clinical and nonclinical	3 specific disorders or symptoms Child, parent	5 min	6–18	NA	PTSD
Child Sexual Behavior Inventory (Friedrich et al., 1992)	Interrater reliability: between female primary caretaker and father ratings (r = .83), between mothers and psychiatric primary nurses (r = .43), and between mothers and teachers (r = .40); internal consistency alpha = .72 for the normative sample and .92 for the sexually abused sample; test–retest reliability = .91 (over 2 weeks) and = .85 (over 4 weeks) Clinical and nonclinical norms	4 multiple symptoms or reactions Parent, caregiver	NA	2–12	NA	Sexual behavior
Child Stress Disorders Checklist (Saxe et al., 2003)	Test–retest = .77; internal consistency = .84; interrater = .49 Clinical and nonclinical	1 event and symptoms Child, parent	5 min	2–18	Medical trauma, accidents, illness, assault	Acute stress disorder, PTSD, dissociation
Child's Reaction to Traumatic Events Scale—Revised (Jones, Fletcher, & Ribbe, 2002)	Internal consistency = .86 Clinical and nonclinical norms	3 specific disorders or symptoms Parents	3–10 min	6–18	NA	PTSD

Instrument	Psychometric properties / norms	Format	Time	Age	Content	Disorder
Childhood Trauma Questionnaire (Bernstein et al., 1994)	Cronbach's alpha = .95; Bernstein & Fink (1998); Bernstein et al. (1995); Clinical and nonclinical norms	2 events; Child, adolescent	5–10 min	12–18	Child maltreatment	NA
Children's Life Events Scale (Wolfe, Gentile, Michienzi, Sas, & Wolfe, 1991)	Test-retest kappa = .50–.78; interrater (mother–father) kappa = .40–.50; Briggs-Gowan & Carter (2008); Nonclinical norms	2 events; Child, adolescent, parent	NA	NA	Family, health, school, social	NA
Coddington's Life Events Scale for Adolescents (Coddington, 1999)	Test–retest = .69 (3 months); Athanasou (2001); Nonclinical norms	2 events; Child	15 min	13–19	Divorce, loss/death, moves, family changes	NA
(Screener for) Child Anxiety-Related Emotional Disorders (Birmaher et al., 1997)	Internal consistency alpha = .74–.93; test-retest reliability = .70–.90; discriminative validity (between anxiety and other disorders and within anxiety disorders); moderate parent–child agreement (r = .20–.47, $p < .001$, all correlations)[b]; Clinical norms	3 specific disorders or symptoms; Parent	10 min	NA	NA	Anxiety disorders
Feelings and Emotions Experienced during Sexual Abuse (Wolfe & Birt, 1993)	Internal consistency alpha range = .80–.95; predictive validity established by high trauma subscale scores and reports of dissociation; Feindler, Rathus, & Silver (2003); No norm information available	4 multiple symptoms or reactions; Child	NA	NA	Sexual abuse	Dissociation, feelings about abuse
History of Victimization Form (Feindler, Rathus, & Silver, 2003)	No information available	2 events; Child	NA	NA	Child maltreatment	NA
Juvenile Victimization Questionnaire (Hamby, Finkelhor, Ormrod, & Turner, 2004)	Test–retest = .59; internal consistency = .80; Finkelhor, Ormrod, Turner, & Hamby (2005); No norm information available	2 events; Child, adolescent	20 min	8–17	Child maltreatment, community violence, peer violence, assault	NA
Kauai Recovery Index (Hamada, Kameoka, Yanagida, & Chemtob, 2003)	Cronbach's alpha = .84; test-retest reliability = .50–.77 (over 28 days); Chemtob, Nakashima, & Carlson (2002); Nonclinical norms	3 specific disorders or symptoms; Child	15 min	6–15	Communitywide disasters (hurricanes)	PTSD

Measure name and anchor citation	Psychometric information available including norm information[a]	Type of information provided and reporter	Time to complete	Age	Type of trauma assessed	Clinical domains assessed
Life Events Checklist (Blake et al., 1990)	Test–retest (1 week) kappa range = .23–.84 Gray, Litz, Hsu, & Lombardo (2004) Nonclinical norms	2 events Child, adolescent	NA	8–18	Loss/death, family change	NA
Lifetime Incidence of Traumatic Events (Greenwald, 1999)	No information available	2 events Child, parent	NA	NA	Loss/death, accidents, maltreatment, disasters	NA
My Worst Experiences (Hyman, 1996)	Internal consistency: total score (.97) and subscales (.69–.94); test–retest reliability: total score (.88–.95) and subscales (median correlation = .77) Clinical and nonclinical norms	1 events and symptoms Child, adolescent	20–30 min	9–18	Disasters, maltreatment, loss, divorce, assault, school problems	PTSD, general maladjustment
Negative Appraisals of Sexual Abuse Scale (Spaccarelli, 1995)	Total scale internal consistency = .96 and subscales internal consistency = .78–.90; average intercorrelation between subscales = .53[b] Clinical norms	4 multiple symptoms Child	NA	11–18	Sexual abuse	Threat, harm, loss
Parent Emotional Reaction Questionnaire (Cohen & Mannarino, 1996)	Test–retest (.90); internal consistency (.87) Cohen & Mannarino (1996) Clinical and nonclinical norms	1 event and symptoms Parent	5–10 min	NA	Sexual abuse	Caregiver response/reaction to trauma
Parent Report of Children's Reaction to Stress (Fletcher, 1996b)	Internal consistency alphas = .89 (total), .81 (Criterion A), .86 (B), .70 (C), .81 (D); correlated (r = .93) with Childhood PTSD Interview—Parent Form; differentiated between traumatized and nontraumatized[b] Clinical and nonclinical norms	1 event and symptoms Parent	NA	NA	NA	PTSD

Measure	Reliability/norms	Format/Informant	Time	Age	Type	Outcome
Pediatric Emotional Distress Scale (Saylor, Swenson, Reynolds, & Taylor, 1999)	Test–retest (6–8 weeks) Pearson's range = .55–.61; internal consistency Cronbach's = .77 (range = .72–.85); interrater Pearson's = .59 (range = .47–.65). Clinical and nonclinical norms	4 multiple symptoms or reactions. Parent	10–15 min	2–10	NA	General maladjustment
Perceived Stress Scale (Cohen, Kamarck, & Mermelstein, 1983)	Internal reliability (4-item) r = .60, (10-item) r = .78. Cohen (1988). Nonclinical norms	4 multiple symptoms or reactions. Child, parent	5 min	NA	NA	General maladjustment
PTSD in Preschool Aged Children (Levendosky, Huth-Bocks, Semel, & Shapiro, 2002)	Limited psychometrics	3 specific disorders or symptoms. Parent, caregiver	10–15 min	2–5	NA	PTSD
Sexual Abuse Fear (Wolfe & Wolfe, 1986)	Internal reliability = .80. Feindler, Rathus, & Silver (2003). Clinical and nonclinical norms	4 multiple symptoms or reactions. Child	NA	11–19	Sexual abuse	Fear, discomfort
Stress Index for Parents of Adolescents (Sheras, Abidin, & Konold, 1998)	Internal consistency subscales > .80 and domains and Total Parenting Stress > .91. Clinical and nonclinical norms	1 event and symptoms. Parent, caregiver	20 min	11–19	Family stress, caregiver stress	General distress, parent–child relationship
Survey of Children's Exposure to Community Violence (Richters & Martinez, 1993)	Test–retest reliability = .81; internal consistency alpha = .83[b]. Overstreet & Braun (2000). Nonclinical norms	2 events. Parents	NA	6–10	Community violence	NA
Trauma and Attachment Belief Scale (Pearlman, 2003)	Internal consistency range = 67–96; test–retest reliability (1–2 weeks) range = .72–.75. Nonclinical norms	4 multiple symptoms or reactions. Adolescent	10–15 min	NA	NA	Cognitive distortions, interpersonal problems, self-efficacy, trauma-related attitudes

Measure name and anchor citation	Psychometric information available including norm information[a]	Type of information provided and reporter	Time to complete	Age	Type of trauma assessed	Clinical domains assessed
Trauma Symptom Checklist for Children (Briere, 1996)	Cronbach alpha range = .58–.89; coefficients for clinical scales range = .81–.86 (mean alpha = .84) Nonclinical norms	4 multiple symptoms or reactions	15–20 min	8–16	Child maltreatment, domestic violence, community violence, medical, assault	Anxiety, dissociation, PTSD, sexual concerns
Trauma Symptom Checklist for Young Children (Ford et al., 2002)	Internal consistency: total range = .73–.86, clinical scales range = .78–.93 Lanktree et al. (2008) Clinical and nonclinical norms	4 multiple symptoms or reactions Parent, caregiver	15–20 min	3–12	Child maltreatment, domestic violence, community violence, assault, war	PTSD, dissociation, mood/anxiety symptoms, sexual concerns
UCLA PTSD Index for DSM-IV (Rodriguez, Steinberg, & Pynoos, 1999)	Internal consistency Cronbach's alpha: Full Scale = .90; test–retest 6–28 days (Pearson's): Full Scale = .84 Brymer, Steinberg, Watson, & Pynoos (2012); Steinberg, Brymer, Decker, & Pynoos (2004)	1 event and symptoms Parent, child, adolescent	20–30 min	NA	Accident, maltreatment, disaster, medical	PTSD
Weekly Behavior Report (Cohen & Mannarino, 1996)	Test–retest (2 week) = .85 (range = .81–.88); internal consistency: sexually abused group (.80) and community comparison group (.76)[b] Clinical and nonclinical norms	3 specific disorders or symptoms Parent, caregiver	5–10 min	NA	Sexual abuse	PTSD
When Bad Things Happen (Fletcher, 1992a)	Internal consistency = .92 Fletcher (1996) Clinical and nonclinical norms	1 event and symptoms Child, adolescent	10–20 min	9–18	Family, academic, social	NA

Note. Published age ranges provided are for child or adolescent report versions of measures where applicable and available. Clinical domains are provided where applicable (i.e., not for event-only measures). 1, measures of events and symptoms (nondiagnostic); 2, measures of events only; 3, measures of symptoms of PTSD and related clinical disorders; and 4, measures of multiple symptoms associated with trauma exposure (nondiagnostic). Type of trauma assessed refers to either the kinds of samples on which the measure was created or has been used in published research. NA, no information available.

[a]Norm information is provided in example studies.
[b]Indicates anchor citation as the source of psychometric information.

CHAPTER 17

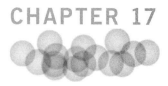

Assessing Bereavement and Grief Disorders

Christopher M. Layne and Julie B. Kaplow

There is clear evidence that close interpersonal relationships exert powerful beneficial effects on mental health, physical health, and longevity (Holt-Lunstad, Smith, & Layton, 2010), and are critically important in helping children and adolescents achieve normative developmental tasks (Steinberg, 2014). Conversely, as Umberson (2017) notes, social ties are a double-edged sword, as strained, conflicted, or lost social ties and damaged social networks can undermine health and well-being, increasing the risk for a variety of mental health difficulties (Layne et al., 2009). Indeed,

the frequency of bereavement-related experiences and their (until recently) lack of diagnostic and institutional recognition belies their seriousness as an underaddressed and underresourced social and public health issue (Mosher, 2018). For example, a survey of over 1,000 educators conducted by the American Federation of Teachers and New York Life Foundation (2012) found that although 70% had at least one student bereaved during the past year and 92% acknowledged childhood grief as a serious problem, only 1% had received bereavement training in university or graduate school. Furthermore, less than 3% reported that their school or district offered bereavement training, and 78% were unaware of any community bereavement supports.

Even more moderate distress reactions to bereavement can take a heavy toll on relationships, functioning, and health through a variety of pathways, including psychological, behavioral, social, and physiological processes (Umberson, 2017). Compared to nonbereaved youth, bereaved youth are at higher risk for a range of mental and behavioral health problems including depression, substance use, posttraumatic stress reactions, decreased academic performance, difficulties in relationships, suicide ideation, and early mortality (Brent, Melhem, Donohoe, & Walker, 2009;

Brent, Melhem, Masten, Porta, & Payne, 2012; Cerel, Fristad, Verducci, Weller, & Weller, 2006; Guldin et al., 2015; Hill et al., 2019; Kaplow, Saunders, Angold, & Costello, 2010; Keyes et al., 2014; Li et al., 2014; Oosterhoff, Kaplow, & Layne, 2018; Yu et al., 2017). In severe cases, untreated bereavement-related disorders can be chronic and debilitating conditions (e.g., Shear, 2015).

The risks that bereavement and ensuing grief reactions pose to health and mental well-being are increasingly attracting prominent public, medical, and political attention. Serendipitously, this chapter goes to press (April 2020) at the convergence of powerful developments that bring bereavement and grief into sharp relief as urgent global, psychiatric, legislative, and public health concerns. The first development, the rapidly escalating COVID-19 global epidemic—reminiscent of the 1918 Spanish flu epidemic—is currently wreaking havoc on the world's social institutions, economies, and social networks, with large cities and entire countries under lockdown and "social distancing" the new norm. The virus is so contagious and lethal (especially to high-risk groups), and hospital space so scarce in some regions, that loved ones of the seriously ill are not allowed to visit and care for them while they are dying and sometimes after they are dead. Given the extreme protocols enacted to protect medical workers, the seriously ill and dying are sequestered and largely isolated from human contact. Funerals and memorial services are being postponed and, in some cases, disbanded by police due to prohibitions against public gatherings. High mortality rates are resulting from such factors as inadequate precautions by government leaders; acute shortages of hospital beds, ventilators, healthcare workers, and medications; and reluctance by some members of the public to abide by public-health directives. Shortages of coffins and the continuing threat of contagion are leading to mass graves in some countries and large-scale cremations in others, even when the practice runs contrary to religious beliefs or cultural norms. As stated by adult grief researcher Katherine Shear, "Sadly, this pandemic is already associated with tremendous loss of lives worldwide. There are many aspects of COVID-19 that will increase the risk of grief derailers. Availability of effective grief therapy is more important than ever" (personal communication, March 23, 2020). We concur with this sobering admonition, but assert that it applies with equal force to making best-practice assessment tools and principles available in order to accurately, efficiently, and ef-

fectively identify and help those struggling in their grief—that is, *applying evidence-based assessment methods to provide bereavement-informed care* (see Youngstrom, Jenkins, Jensen-Doss, & Youngstrom, 2012).

The second development arises from the introduction of new bereavement-related disorders in diagnostic taxonomies, which are bringing renewed interest to the work of accurately identifying, efficiently assessing, and effectively treating bereaved youth. Recent advances include *persistent complex bereavement disorder,* a provisional diagnosis inserted in the appendix of DSM-5 (American Psychiatric Association, 2013) as an invitation for further study, and *prolonged grief disorder* in ICD-11 (scheduled for adoption by the World Health Organization in January 2022; Killikelly & Maercker, 2017). More recently, the APA has proposed *prolonged grief disorder* for inclusion in DSM-5-TR, expected for release by 2021. We discuss these three disorders here.

A third major development involves national attention by lawmakers to the persisting risks that bereavement imposes on siblings, spouses, and parents, thereby recognizing that all members of bereaved families are at risk and merit recognition and support. In a March 2020 letter to the U.S. House of Representatives, The Honorable Lloyd Doggett stated [citations added]:

> The lack of high-quality, consistent bereavement care following the death of a loved one is an urgent but invisible public health problem. Bereaved spouses [Christakis & Allison, 2006], parents [Li, Precht, Mortensen, & Olsen, 2003; Rostila, Saarela, & Kawachi, 2011], and siblings [Yu et al., 2017] are at risk of premature death as a result of their loss, and bereaved parents who lose a child *at any age* are more likely to suffer from cardiac problems [Li, Hansen, Mortensen, & Olsen, 2002], cancer [Li, Johansen, Hansen, & Olsen, 2002], psychiatric hospitalization [Li, Laursen, Precht, Olsen, & Mortensen, 2005], cognitive decline [Umberson, Donnelly, Xu, Farina, & Garcia, 2019], and other health complications [Umberson, Donnelly, & Farina, 2018]. These effects persist for an average of 18 years following the death [Rogers, Floyd, Seltzer, Greenberg, & Hong, 2008].

Other important developments conducive to bereavement work include growing public awareness of the damaging effects of childhood trauma and loss—including adverse childhood experiences (ACEs; Greeson et al., 2014), increasing regulatory requirements for systematic screening, increased availability of evidence-supported interventions (Chemtob et al., 2016), and efforts by many child service systems to adopt trauma-informed practices (Ko et al., 2008).

Bereavement: The "Exposure" Side of a Major and Often Silent Epidemic

Bereavement poses a double-barreled threat to young people, in that it is not only among the most common, but also the most distressing, form of trauma in both clinic-referred youth (Pynoos et al., 2014) and youth in the general population (Breslau et al., 1998; Kaplow, Saunders, Angold, & Costello, 2010). Tragically, the loss of a parent is a commonplace event in many childhoods: The United Nations Children's Fund (UNICEF; 2017) estimates that in 2015 nearly 140 million children worldwide had lost at least one parent, and 5.1 million had lost both parents. Using a hybrid of binomial probability and life table methods, the Childhood Bereavement Estimation Model (CBEM) estimates that 6.99% of children across the United States (approximately 1 in 14, or nearly 5.0 million) have or will have experienced the death of a parent or sibling by age 18. For youth up to age 25, these estimates more than double to almost 12.9 million (Burns, Griese, King, & Talmi, 2020). Self-report data from nationally representative studies of bereaved adolescents produce estimates ranging between 1.48 and 1.59% of adolescents reporting that their biological mother, and between 3.80 and 4.02% reporting that their biological father, is no longer living (Harris & Udry, 2008; Kessler, 2017). Regarding sibling bereavement, Hulsey, Hill, Layne, Gaffney, and Kaplow (2018) estimate that nearly 1% of U.S. youth experience the death of a sibling each year.

Even without factoring in grief reactions to the loss, bereavement per se as a stressful life event is cause for public health concern given its many associated risks (Feigelman, Rosen, Joiner, Silva, & Mueller, 2017). Compared to their nonbereaved peers, adolescents who have lost a parent are at heightened risk for an array of adjustment problems. These include lower self-esteem (Worden & Silverman, 1996); reduced resilience (Kennedy, Chen, Valdimarsdóttir, Montgomery, Fang, & Fall, 2018); lower grades and more school failures (Berg, Rostila, Saarela, & Hjern, 2014); and heightened risk for depression (Jacobs & Bovasso, 2009; Mack, 2001; Schoenfelder et al., 2011), suicide attempts (Jakobsen & Christiansen, 2011), suicide (Gulden et al., 2015), premature death due to any cause (Li

et al., 2014), drug abuse (von Sydow, Lieb, Pfister, Höfler, & Wittchen, 2002), violent crime involvement (Wilcox et al., 2010), youth delinquency (Draper & Hancock, 2011), and a greater number of, and more severe, psychiatric difficulties (Dowdney, 2000).

Recent reports from the Centers for Disease Control and Prevention (CDC) underscore that not only bereavement, but especially *bereavement under tragic and often traumatic circumstances*, is a major mental health concern and public health emergency. There were more than 2.8 million deaths in the United States in 2017—the most ever reported in a single year in over a century of government data collection. Although partly due to the growing sector of elderly adult Americans, these numbers especially reflect rising death rates among middle-aged and younger people. Too many American lives are being lost, too often and too early, to preventable causes, including drug overdose, suicide, motor vehicle accidents, and homicide (Redfield, 2018). For example, young people ages 16–24 made up 41% of all drivers involved in alcohol-related driving fatalities in 2016 (National Center for Statistics and Analysis, 2017). Furthermore, the suicide rate in 2017 was the highest in over 50 years, totaling more than 47,000 suicides nationwide—a 3.7% increase since 2016 (Hedegaard, Curtin, & Warner, 2018). Suicide has consistently ranked among the 10 leading causes of death over the past decade, having increased 35% between 1999 and 2018. The rate of increase has accelerated: The national suicide rate increased on average approximately 1% per year from 1999 to 2006, and by 2% per year from 2006 to 2018, with the 2018 suicide rate for males 3.7 times higher than for females (Hedegaard, Curtin, & Warner, 2020). The number of Americans aged 10 and older who took their lives in 2016 (nearly 45,000) was 30% higher than in 1999. Violent methods of suicide are also increasing: Gun-related deaths rose for a third consecutive year, totaling nearly 40,000 in 2017. About 60% of suicides in 2017 were by gun (Murphy, Xu, Kochanek, & Arias, 2018). Taken together, these statistics reflect a sobering global upward trend: Self-harm was the 14th leading cause of death worldwide in 2016 and is predicted to rise to the 11th leading cause of death by 2040 (Foreman et al., 2018). Drug overdose deaths are also rising, having increased over threefold during the past 18 years. Overdose fatalities hit a new high in 2017, reaching 70,237. Deaths from Fentanyl and its analogues have risen dramatically since 2013, with Americans of childbearing and childrearing age (25–54) being most likely to die from overdose (Hedegaard, Miniño, & Warner, 2018).

As a consequence of these converging threats, national life expectancy—a "thumb on the pulse" snapshot of overall U.S. population health that has climbed steadily for decades, typically rising a few months each year—dropped in 2015, leveled off in 2016, and dropped again in 2017 (Murphy et al., 2018). The last such protracted decline in national life expectancy occurred a full century ago, when World War I and the 1918 flu pandemic combined to kill over 500,000 Americans and over 50 million people worldwide (Arnold, 2018).

A grim reality of these sobering trends is that most child, adolescent, and family clinicians regularly encounter youth with significant loss histories. These histories may well include not only bereavement under normal circumstances (e.g., a grandparent dies of natural causes) but also multiple losses, often under tragic (e.g., a young parent dies of cancer or medical error), traumatic (auto accident), and potentially stigmatized circumstances (e.g., overdose, drunk driving, suicide, homicide, murder–suicide). For example, medical error was the third leading cause of death across the United States in 2013, accounting for some 251,000 deaths nationwide (Makary & Daniel, 2016). Many bereaved youth also have histories of other types of trauma, given that loss tends to co-occur in constellations of risk factors that accumulate and "travel" across development (Layne, Briggs-King, & Courtois, 2014; Pynoos et al., 2014), making the tasks of unpacking bereavement from trauma (as stressful life events), and grief from PTSD, depression, anxiety, and other distress reactions, much more challenging (Layne, Kaplow, Oosterhoff, Hill, & Pynoos, 2017). It thus behooves clinicians to equip themselves with the tools needed to accurately identify and effectively help bereaved and traumatically bereaved youth. These tools include guiding theory, developmentally and culturally appropriate assessment instruments, clinical knowledge and skills, and flexible interventions capable of addressing the varying effects of bereavement, traumatic bereavement, other co-occurring trauma, and their sequelae.

Accordingly, we begin our discussion with an overview of bereavement, including three bereavement-related disorders that reflect recent efforts by major health organizations to respond to growing public awareness and concern. We then provide a suggested "starter kit" for applying evidence-based assessment (EBA) methods and interweave our step-by-step application of a 12-step EBA method

with a case example (*Andre*) that illustrates many of the complexities inherent in assessing traumatically bereaved youth. We give special emphasis to traumatic bereavement in adolescence given growing evidence of the primacy of sudden loss as a potent causal risk factor for grief- and other stress-related disorders, as well as evidence that exposure to sudden loss is more likely to occur in adolescence than any other developmental period (Oosterhoff et al., 2018). In the second section of the chapter, *Prediction*, we work through the Andre case example by discussing rating scales, checklists, and the use of different informants to flesh out a broad ecological picture and guide clinical decision making. In the third section, *Prescription*, we demonstrate how assessment tools and decision-making heuristics can guide case formulation, diagnosis, and treatment planning. And in the fourth section, *Process*, we describe how developmentally sensitive grief theory and EBA principles can guide goal specification, tracking therapeutic process, monitoring therapeutic progress, and maintaining posttreatment gains.

The Nature, Developmental Timing, and Sequelae of Bereavement

Bereavement—especially sudden loss—and its sequelae have attracted considerable research attention in recent years as a major public health issue. These studies varyingly examine the nature of bereavement itself, including its circumstances, developmental timing and sequelae, risks for comorbidity, and its capacity to launch adverse developmental cascades.

Circumstances of the Death

Ways in which the specific circumstances of the death—especially tragic and traumatic deaths—can influence the clinical manifestations, course, and consequences of grief reactions are receiving increased clinical and research attention (Layne, Kaplow, Oosterhoff, et al., 2017). In their review of the literature on grief and bereavement after sudden and violent deaths, Kristensen, Weisæth, and Heir (2012) concluded that the sudden and violent loss of a loved one can adversely affect mental health and grief in a substantial proportion of bereaved individuals. Mental health disorders tended to be more elevated after sudden and violent losses than losses following natural deaths, and the trajectory of recovery more slow and protracted. The authors propose that a variety of circumstance-related risk factors (e.g., witnessing the death, finding the deceased, life threats, blaming others, being blamed for the death) are likely to influence the course of adjustment and to differentially relate to different outcomes, with some factors associating more strongly with PTSD and others with grief. The authors conclude that these differential relations highlight important distinctions between PTSD and grief, underscore the need to assess different outcomes (Van der Houwen et al., 2010), and call for individual treatment tailoring given that traumatic bereavement may require different intervention components than bereavement due to natural death (e.g., Saltzman et al., 2017). In a related study of children and caregivers bereaved by the loss of a parent/spouse under differing circumstances, Kaplow, Howell, and Layne (2014) found that children whose parent died due to prolonged illness reported higher levels of both maladaptive grief and posttraumatic stress symptoms than children who lost a caregiver to sudden natural death. The authors concluded that anticipated deaths may contain risk factors for both child PTSD and maladaptive grief.

Epidemiological studies of the correlates and consequences of traumatic bereavement underscore the importance of understanding the way in which a loved one died, developmental stages associated with highest risk for sudden loss, and developmental periods of maximum vulnerability to bereavement. Underscoring the "double-barreled" (highly prevalent, highly traumatogenic) nature of traumatic loss, Breslau and colleagues (1998) studied a representative sample of 2,181 Detroit citizens ages 18–45 years, of whom 60% reported the sudden unexpected death of a loved one. Although finding a low PTSD prevalence rate following exposure to any trauma (9.2%), among cases with PTSD, 31% reported a precipitating trauma of sudden unexpected death of a loved one. The authors concluded that although prior studies typically focused on combat, rape, and other assaultive violence as causes of PTSD, the sudden unexpected death of a loved one was a "far more important cause of PTSD in the community," accounting for nearly one-third of PTSD cases (p. 626).

Two studies used the Swedish National Patient Discharge Registry, including over 800,000 cases and over 30,000 bereaved children, to investigate correlates of parental loss. Berg, Rostila, and Hjern (2016) found that parental loss due to natural causes (i.e., diseases) during childhood is associated with a small increased risk of long-term con-

sequences for psychological health. In contrast, children bereaved by the death of a parent due to external causes (suicides, accidents, homicides) were at particular risk for hospitalizations due to depression, and preschool-age children who lost a parent regardless of cause were at risk for both hospitalization and outpatient care for depression. Furthermore, Rostila, Berg, Arat, Vinnerljung, and Hjern (2016) found that parental bereavement during childhood predicted self-inflicted injuries/poisoning in young adulthood by 30–40% for death from natural causes, and by a dramatic two- to threefold increase for parental deaths due to external causes or substance abuse. Risk of self-inflicting injuries was most prominent among both men and women who lost their father and among men who lost their mother during their preschool years. Compared to women, men were also more vulnerable to maternal loss due to natural causes during their preschool years.

Underscoring the importance of assessing both parental bereavement and the circumstances of the death, Guldin and colleagues (2015) followed a cohort of children who lost a parent before age 18 with a matched nonparentally bereaved cohort for up to 40 years. Using nationwide registers in three Scandinavian countries totaling over 7.3 million persons, the authors found that parental death in childhood, regardless of cause, doubled the risk of suicide; furthermore, having a parent die by suicide increased the risk of suicide nearly 3.5-fold. These risks persisted for at least 25 years. Suicide risk tended to be higher among children who lost a parent before age 6, and boys were at double the risk for suicide as girls.

Keyes and colleagues (2014) studied a large adult sample ($N = 27,534$) from the National Epidemiologic Survey on Alcohol and Related Conditions. The authors found that the unexpected death of a loved one (due to accident, murder, suicide, heart attack, terrorist attack) is the most *common* traumatic experience across the life course, endorsed by approximately half the sample, and that respondents were most likely to rate unexpected death as their *worst* lifetime experience. The age interval of 15–19 years carried the highest risk of exposure to first unexpected death. The authors found a dose–response relation between number of unexpected deaths and number of lifetime psychiatric disorders, observing an increased incidence after unexpected death at nearly every point across the life course for posttraumatic stress disorder, major depressive episode, and panic disorder. These findings add to earlier epidemiological evidence of heightened risk for conduct disorder, substance abuse, and impaired global functioning in bereaved youth (Kaplow, Saunders, Angold, & Costello, 2010).

Last, Oosterhoff, Kaplow, and Layne (2018) studied youth ($N = 10,148$) from the National Comorbidity Survey—Adolescent Supplement, a nationally representative adolescent survey. Sudden death (e.g., homicide, suicide, accident, overdose, stroke, infarction) was the most frequently reported traumatic event of all 18 traumatic events assessed, with a lifetime prevalence of 30%. Youth were most likely to have first experienced sudden death during middle adolescence (ages 15–16 years). After controlling for demographic variables and other trauma, sudden death was associated with five types of impaired academic functioning, including lower academic achievement, ability to concentrate and learn, enjoyment of school, perceived school belongingness, and belief that teachers treat youth fairly. The authors concluded that sudden death is common among adolescents and an important marker of risk for impaired school performance and that schools should routinely screen for bereavement and clinically assess bereaved youth to evaluate whether bereavement-informed mental health services are needed.

Cascading Developmental Consequences

A growing number of studies are tracking the longer-term consequences of bereavement and its aftermath by clarifying how the death of attachment figures can lead to distressing reminders, deprivations, secondary adversities (Layne et al., 2006), and lasting developmental impacts. Brent and colleagues (2012) found that parentally bereaved youth exhibited lower competence than nonbereaved controls in key developmental domains in later life, including success at work, career planning, peer attachment, and educational aspirations. The authors found no significant associations between youth age at time of death, gender of deceased parent, time elapsed since death, or cause of death and any developmental outcome. In contrast, youth functioning, family cohesion, and family adaptability mediated multiple paths linking parental death to impaired functioning in key developmental tasks.

Burrell, Mehlum, and Qin (2020) used data from over 370,000 Norwegians to study long-term developmental impacts of losing a parent. Compared to nonbereaved peers, parentally bereaved children were significantly *less* likely to complete

all educational levels—especially high school and university/college education—regardless of cause of death, gender of deceased, or age at bereavement. Premature school withdrawal and diminished interests in college attendance at Wave 1 predicted diminished academic accomplishments, persisting economic disadvantages, and, for females, a hesitancy to marry as they transitioned to adulthood. Other studies report such secondary adversities as financial insecurity, changing schools, and changing homes (Kaplow et al., 2010; Thompson, Kaslow, Price, Williams, & Kingree, 1998).

In a study of over 400,000 Swedish men who underwent military enlistment examinations in late adolescence, Kennedy and colleagues (2018) found that loss of a parent or sibling in childhood conferred a 49% increased risk of subsequent low stress resilience and an 8% increased risk of moderate stress resilience. These risks were highest in late adolescence and emerged regardless of cause of death or parent psychiatric hospitalization.

Comorbidity and Risky Behavior

Other studies underscore the risk for *comorbidity* (including posttraumatic stress disorder [PTSD]) after sudden loss. Atwoli and colleagues (2017) studied 19 World Mental Health surveys ($N = 78,023$) of both minors and adults, finding a PTSD prevalence rate after unexpected death (e.g., auto accident, murder, suicide, heart attack at young age) of 5.2%—a rate significantly higher than the 4% average found for 28 other lifetime traumatic events. Being female, believing one could have done something to prevent the death, prior history of trauma and of mental disorders, and relationship to the deceased were each significant predictors of PTSD. The final model demonstrated that PTSD can be accurately predicted using data collected in the immediate aftermath of trauma, including unexpected death. Underscoring the traumatogenic nature of sudden loss, 30.6% of all cases of unexpected death-related PTSD ranked in the top 5% of respondents with highest PTSD risk—a proportion six times greater than chance. The authors concluded that bereavement due to unexpected death is a major international public health issue given its high prevalence and high risk for PTSD.

Other nationally representative epidemiological studies have linked childhood bereavement to *risky behavior*, including suicide attempts in both adolescence (Thompson & Light, 2011) and later in life (e.g., Guldin et al., 2015) Layne,

Greeson, and colleagues (2014) examined relations between a history of up to 19 types of trauma and loss and adolescent risky behavior, finding a dose–response relation with nine types of high-risk adolescent behavior and functional impairment, including attachment difficulties, skipping school, running away from home, substance abuse, suicidality, criminality, self-injury, alcohol use, and sexual exploitation victimization. Hill and colleagues (2019) investigated hypothesized mediators of links between bereavement and suicide risk, including PCBD and two predictors of suicide ideation (*thwarted belongingness*—marked by a sense of loneliness, social isolation, low social connectedness, and poor social support) and *perceived burdensomeness to others*. The authors found a significant association between PCBD symptoms and thwarted belongingness—an important early marker of suicide risk.

Summary and Critique of Bereavement and Grief: The Missing Link

Considered as a whole, the extant literature links bereavement—especially tragic and traumatic death—to developmental disruption, functional impairment, risky behavior, early mortality, and increased risk for psychopathology across the life course. These studies shed light on ways in which prior losses can cascade forward into subsequent adversities, losses, compromised functioning, and risky behavior in ways that prolong distress, diminish achievement, and alter developmental trajectories (Layne, Greeson, et al., 2014; Layne & Hobfoll, 2020). These findings converge with those from the field of positive youth development that lack of childhood self-control (e.g., emotional dysregulation) is a potent predictor of adverse outcomes assessed decades later in young adulthood, including physical health, substance dependence, personal finances, criminal offending outcomes, and developmental derailment (school dropout, teenage pregnancy) (Moffitt et al., 2011). Taken together, these findings underscore the importance of risk screening for bereavement among children and adolescents, especially sudden loss in adolescence. More broadly, these findings also underscore the utility of integrating contextual variables into clinical assessment and case formulation. These include prior trauma history, current life stressors, comorbid conditions, caregiver health and functioning, and youth functioning in developmentally salient domains (McCormick, Kuo, & Masten, 2011), including school (Kaplow

et al., 2010; Oosterhoff et al., 2018), personal relationships, and future ambitions (Høeg et al., 2018, 2019).

Nevertheless, no study reviewed here—with the exception of Hill and colleagues (2019)—assessed grief reactions. This is a major design limitation, theory gap, and blind spot in the literature, given that attempting to study the nature and consequences of bereavement without grief reactions is analogous to studying the nature and consequences of trauma exposure without PTSD. Commendably, both the American Psychiatric Association (2013) with its fifth edition of the *Diagnostic and Statistical Manual of Mental Disorders* (DSM-5) and forthcoming DSM-5-TR, and the World Health Organization (2018) with its *International Classification of Disease, Eleventh Revision* (ICD-11), have taken major steps forward in recognizing the sizable proportion of bereaved individuals who exhibit serious adjustment problems and need mental health services. Both organizations are working to define and to find a place for bereavement-related disorders (including grief-related pathology) in their respective diagnostic taxonomies.

Preparation for Assessing Bereavement Consequences: Diagnoses, Prevalence, and a "Starter Kit"

A Tale of Three Disorders: Provisional, Pending, and Proposed Grief Diagnoses

This chapter goes to press at a momentous time, when three grief-related disorders are in play. Table 17.1 lists the three disorders to invite side-by-side comparisons. These disorders include (1) a nondiagnosable provisional disorder—*persistent complex bereavement disorder*, included in the appendix of DSM-5 (American Psychiatric Association, 2013) as an invitation for further research; (2) a proposed disorder—*prolonged grief disorder*, which is being put forth for public commentary as part of the American Psychiatric Association's procedures for adopting a new disorder in DSM-5-TR, expected to be released in 2021; and (3) a pending disorder—ICD-11 *prolonged grief disorder*, scheduled for official adoption by the World Health Organization in January 2022.

Persistent Complex Bereavement Disorder

DSM-5 (American Psychiatric Association, 2013) broke new ground by listing a provisional bereavement-related disorder—PCBD—in its appendix.

TABLE 17.1. Summary of diagnostic criteria for three grief-related diagnoses—provisional, proposed, and pending.

Provisional DSM-5 PCBD Criteria (2013)	Proposed DSM-5-TR PGD Criteria (2020)	Pending ICD-11 PGD Criteria (2022)*
A. Experienced the death of someone close	A. The death of a person close to the bereaved at least 12 months previously	A. Following the death of a partner, parent, child, or other person close to the bereaved
B. Since the death, experienced at least one of four B symptoms more days than not, to clinically significant degree, persisting at least 12 months after death in adults, 6 months in children:	B. Since the death, there has been a grief response characterized by intense yearning/longing for the deceased person or a preoccupation with thoughts or memories of the deceased person. This response has been present to a clinically significant degree nearly every day for at least the last month.	1. Persistent and pervasive longing for the deceased or 2. A persistent and pervasive preoccupation with the deceased
1. Persistent yearning/longing for deceased. (In young children, yearning may manifest in play and behavior, including behaviors that reflect being separated from, and also reuniting with, a caregiver or other attachment figure.) 2. Intense sorrow and emotional pain in response to death. 3. Preoccupation with deceased. 4. Preoccupation with circumstances of death. (In children, preoccupation with the death may be expressed through themes of play and behavior and may extend to preoccupation with possible death of close others.)		
C. Since the death, at least six symptoms are experienced on more days than not, to a clinically significant degree, have persisted for at least 12 months after the death in bereaved adults and 6 months for bereaved children:	C. As a result of the death, at least three of the following symptoms have been experienced to a clinically significant degree, nearly every day, for at least the last month: 1. Identity disruption (e.g., feeling as though part of oneself has died). 2. Marked sense of disbelief about the death. 3. Avoidance of reminders that the person is dead. 4. Intense emotional pain (e.g., anger, bitterness, sorrow) related to the death. 5. Difficulty moving on with life (e.g., problems engaging with friends, pursuing interests, planning for the future).	Accompanied by intense emotional pain (e.g., sadness, guilt, anger, denial, blame, difficulty accepting the death, feeling one has lost a part of oneself, inability to experience positive mood, emotional numbness, difficulty engaging with social or other activities).
Reactive distress to the death 1. Marked difficulty accepting the death. In children, this depends on child's capacity to comprehend the meaning and permanence of death. 2. Disbelief or emotional numbness over the loss. 3. Difficulty with positive reminiscing about the deceased. 4. Bitterness or anger related to loss. 5. Maladaptive appraisals about oneself in relation to the deceased or the death (e.g., self-blame).		

6. Excessive avoidance of reminders of the loss (e.g., avoidance of individuals, places, or situations associated with the deceased; in children, this may include avoidance of thoughts and feelings regarding the deceased).

Social/identity disruption
7. Desire to die to be with deceased.
8. Difficulty trusting others since death.
9. Feeling alone or detached from others since death.
10. Feeling life is meaningless or empty without deceased or belief that one cannot function without deceased.
11. Confusion about one's role in life or diminished sense of one's identity (e.g., feeling part of oneself died with deceased).
12. Difficulty or reluctance to pursue interests since the loss or to plan for the future (e.g., friendships, activities).

6. Emotional numbness.
7. Feeling that life is meaningless.
8. Intense loneliness (i.e., feeling alone or detached from others).

D. The disturbance causes clinically significant distress or impairment in social, occupational, or other important areas of functioning.

D. Disturbance causes clinically significant distress or impairment in social, occupational, or other important areas of functioning.

D. The disturbance causes significant impairment in personal, family, social, educational, occupational, or other important areas of functioning.

E. The bereavement reaction is out of proportion to or inconsistent with cultural, religious, or age-appropriate norms.

E. Duration of bereavement reaction clearly exceeds expected social, cultural, or religious norms for individual's culture and context.

E. Persisted for an abnormally long period of time (more than 6 months at a minimum): following the loss, clearly exceeding expected social, cultural, or religious norms for the individual's culture and context. Grief reactions that have persisted for longer periods that are within a normative period of grieving given the person's cultural and religious context are viewed as normal bereavement responses and are not assigned a diagnosis.

F. Symptoms not better explained by another mental disorder.

Specify if:
With traumatic bereavement: Bereavement due to homicide or suicide with persistent distressing preoccupations regarding the traumatic nature of the death (often in response to loss reminders), including the deceased's last moments, degree of suffering and mutilating injury, or malicious or intentional nature of the death.

Note. PCBD, persistent complex bereavement disorder; PGD, prolonged grief disorder; *Prolonged grief disorder (Killikelly & Maercker, 2017).

PCBD draws from evidence gathered by multiple teams of primarily adult bereavement researchers. These teams have utilized a variety of different theoretical viewpoints, assessment measures, and diagnostic criteria to identify a variety of types of maladaptive responses to bereavement, as reflected by such labels as *pathological, complicated, prolonged, traumatic, chronic,* and *morbid* grief (Wagner & Maercker, 2010). PCBD can be viewed as a complex amalgam of symptoms intended to integrate a variety of viewpoints regarding the essential nature and distinguishing features of maladaptive grief, and as an invitation for further study (Kaplow, Layne, & Pynoos, 2014). As discussed in an invited review (Kaplow, Layne, Pynoos, Cohen, & Lieberman, 2012) and a companion chapter focusing on treatment of PCBD (Kaplow, Layne, & Pynoos, 2019), PCBD Criterion A requires that the individual has experienced the death of a close person, and Criterion B includes one or more of four symptoms hypothesized to serve as gateways (early precursors through which the full disorder may eventually develop), including (1) persistent yearning/longing, (2) intense sorrow and emotional pain, (3) preoccupation with the deceased, and (4) preoccupation with the circumstances of the death. PCBD Criterion C symptoms are intended to flesh out the full disorder and are rationally partitioned into two clusters: *reactive distress to the death* and *social/identity disruption.* Criterion C requires that at least six of the 12 "C" symptoms be present for at least 12 months after the death for adults and 6 months for bereaved children. Unique to PCBD is a *with traumatic bereavement* specifier, restricted to cases of homicide or suicide linked to persisting distressing preoccupations with the traumatic nature of the death. To our knowledge, only one published study reports PCBD prevalence estimates in bereaved youth. Kaplow and colleagues (2018) found that 18% met provisional criteria for PCBD in a sample of referred youth.

Prolonged Grief Disorder in DSM-5-TR

As this chapter goes to press, the American Psychiatric Association is opening a window for public commentary on a new proposed diagnosis—*prolonged grief disorder*—for inclusion in DSM-5-TR, expected for release in 2021. Hereafter termed *PGD-5-TR,* this condition is simpler in composition and structure than its DSM-5 predecessor (PCBD). As shown in Table 17.1, Criterion A requires the death of a close person at least 12 months previously. Criterion B, a proposed gateway symptom, requires a grief response characterized by intense yearning/longing for the deceased person or a preoccupation with thoughts or memories of the deceased person, present to a clinically significant degree nearly every day for at least the last month. To meet Criterion C, three of eight grief symptoms must have been experienced to a clinically significant degree, nearly every day, for at least the last month. In contrast to PCBD in DSM-5, the Criterion C symptoms in PGD-5-TR are not partitioned into subtypes, nor is there a traumatic bereavement specifier. Although not included in these proposed PGD-5-TR criteria, a number of developmental modifications have been suggested (Layne, Oosterhoff, Pynoos, & Kaplow, 2020). These include a shortening of the Criterion A *time since death* requirement to 6 months to facilitate early risk detection and timely intervention, partitioning Criterion B into two symptoms to simplify assessment, and including preoccupation with the circumstances of the death as a Criterion B symptom. Any further modifications to PGD-5-TR will be made after the public commentary is reviewed, likely later in the year 2020.

Prolonged Grief Disorder in ICD-11

ICD-11, scheduled for official adoption in 2022, will also contain a prolonged grief disorder (hereafter PGD-ICD-11). As shown in Table 17.1, the symptom structure and method for endorsing symptoms of PGD-ICD-11 reflect the primary aim—*improving clinical utility*—that guided its development: to enhance communication, ease of use, and treatment planning (Killikelly & Maercker, 2017). PGD requires one of two "A" symptoms (persistent and pervasive longing for the deceased, or persistent and pervasive preoccupation with the deceased), and evidence of intense emotional pain ("B" symptoms; e.g., sadness, guilt, anger, denial, blame). The disorder must persist for an abnormally long period (minimum 6 months, depending on cultural factors); exceed social, cultural, or religious norms for the individual's culture and context; and cause significant impairment in important areas of functioning.

Barriers to Accurate Detection

Any effort to validly assess bereaved youth should begin with appreciating the social context and ramifications surrounding loss. If we do not ask, clients often do not tell (Mosher, 2018). Clients may remain silent due to traumatic avoidance, social stigma, cultural factors, shame, or guilt about the event or their response; lack of insight into how trauma and loss impair functioning at home, school, and with friends; fears of reprisal; desires to protect surviving caregivers from further distress; and perceiving the clinician as unready or reluctant to hear distressing material (Layne, Kaplow, Oosterhoff, et al., 2017). Youth and families may also be unaware that effective treatments exist. Furthermore, children rarely self-refer for treatment, but instead must rely on caregivers to be aware of their loss histories and consequent symptoms in order to receive appropriate mental health services. Clinicians may also feel discomfort with posing direct questions about a client's exposure histories, or may worry that obtaining detailed trauma histories will overly upset children and fragile caregivers. Training in structured or semistructured assessment tools also incurs significant time and training expense (Jensen-Doss, 2005).

Moreover, stress-related disorders such as PCBD, PGD, and PTSD pose a dual challenge beyond the complexities already inherent in child diagnostic assessment. This dual challenge centers on the need to accurately assess both sides of a cause–effect equation: *Exposure to stressful events* on the one hand, and *their causal consequences* on the other (Layne, Briggs-King, & Courtois, 2014) while recognizing that complex interplays and feedback loops between traumatic stress, grief reactions, and developmental disturbances can also arise (Layne, Kaplow, Oosterhoff, et al., 2017; Pynoos, Steinberg, & Wraith, 1995). A study exemplifies how assessment errors can arise on both sides of the equation, resulting in both underdetection of exposures and underdiagnosis of their effects. Chemtob and colleagues (2016) compared the accuracy of community clinicians (who used standard assessment practices) to trained study clinicians (who used structured assessment tools) in identifying trauma exposure and PTSD in 157 children. Four sobering findings emerged: (1) Clinic practitioners identified less than half (21.2%) of the youth identified by study clinicians as trauma-exposed (51.3%); (2) clinic practitioners identified only one-tenth of the cases of PTSD (1.9%) compared to those identified by study clinicians (19.1%); (3) although community clinicians had access to the structured assessment results located in each client's chart and made quarterly updates to their treatment plans, a 1-year follow-up chart review identified no changes in their clients' PTSD diagnosis; and finally (4) some

signs were apparent, as community clinicians and parents rated the underdiagnosed children as having emotional and behavioral problems and lower functioning. Given these findings, Chemtob and colleagues recommend the use of structured questions about specific life events and behavioral indicators rather than general inquiries, and that questions be asked at intake and throughout the course of treatment.

More generally, reliance on informal assessment tools (rather than checklist reminders and structured interviews) is linked to problems with both over- and underdiagnosis. Without structured instruments, clinicians tend to underestimate comorbidity and miss at least one diagnosis on average per client (Jensen-Doss, Youngstrom, Youngstrom, Feeny, & Findling, 2014). Similarly, children who receive a standard assessment in a community mental health clinic are more likely to receive both *a* diagnosis, and *only one* diagnosis, compared to children who complete a structured interview (Jensen & Weisz, 2002). Taken together, these findings raise several sobering questions as logical implications:

- Is there a deep disconnect between assessment and treatment in some practice settings?
- Namely, is there a tendency to adopt a "one and done" mentality, such that a search for diagnoses terminates once a first diagnosis is selected?
- Is there a tendency to "diagnose one, treat one" (mental disorder) when formulating a treatment plan, based on the assumption that any further assessment results are irrelevant once an initial diagnosis is logged in a client's chart?

EBA of Bereaved Youth

Despite its limitations, the extant bereavement literature provides useful guidance for EBA with bereaved youth that can address these sobering questions. In the remainder of this chapter we build on and extend beyond prior work (Kaplow et al., 2013, 2019; Layne, Kaplow, & Youngstrom, 2017) in adapting EBA methods for bereaved youth. In the next section, we suggest a list of assessment tools and invite the reader to accompany us in thinking through the complexities of risk screening, clinical assessment, case formulation, and treatment planning, using the case of a traumatically bereaved adolescent boy.

Conducting EBA with bereaved youth requires that clinicians not only be furnished with assessment tools that help them to accurately identify bereaved cases and generate useful initial diagnoses but be also trained and supported in their ongoing use throughout treatment. To date, solid advances have been made in creating developmentally appropriate assessment tools (Kaplow et al., 2018; 2019; Layne, Kaplow, & Youngstrom, 2017) and guidelines for child service systems (Ko et al., 2008) and evidence-based practice (DeRosa, Amaya-Jackson, & Layne, 2013). Nevertheless, two additional steps are sorely needed. First, EBA as a key tool for increasing the efficiency and effectiveness of evidence-based intervention (Hunsley & Mash, 2007). Second, clinicians must be furnished with critical reasoning tools, clinical training, and incentives needed to collect and use assessment data to guide *ongoing* diagnosis, case formulation, treatment planning, treatment delivery, and monitoring (Lambert, 2010). The following case example illustrates both sets of tools. It draws from such sources as EBA (Youngstrom et al., 2017); a bereavement training curriculum created by the authors; and the Core Curriculum on Childhood Trauma (Layne, Briggs-King, & Courtois, 2014)—a tool developed by the National Child Traumatic Stress Network to build foundational clinical knowledge and core skills in information gathering, critical reasoning, case conceptualization, and treatment planning.

EBA helps users to hit the assessment "sweet spot" (don't underassess or overassess; don't underdiagnose or overdiagnose) by offering a methodology to improve the chances that clinicians accurately identify and effectively help bereaved youth in need, while also improving their efficiency by matching the type and level of mental health resources to different types and levels of needs. EBA helps practitioners to work smarter with the assessment tools and clinical decision-making methods available to them (Youngstrom & Frazier, 2013). EBA does so by integrating psychology's traditional strengths of psychological assessment with evidence-based medicine's (EBM) rigorous focus on applying research and assessment findings to individual patients in a way that is both rapid and concretely linked to clinical decision making (Straus, Glasziou, Richardson, & Haynes, 2019). EBA works to sequence the evaluation process so that assessment tools are added only when they incrementally inform the diagnostic or treatment process (Youngstrom, 2013; Youngstrom & Frazier, 2013; Youngstrom et al., 2017). Indeed, too much testing, especially too early and when bereavement

rates are low, can produce high false-positive rates, poor treatment selection, and worse resource allocation (Kraemer, 1992; Straus et al., 2019). EBA's sequenced approach avoids redundancy in assessment batteries and prevents the selection of tests with low validity for the assessment question or hypothesis at hand.

What might an EBA framework look like as applied to the evaluation of bereavement or traumatic bereavement? Table 17.2 is a detailed adaptation of a 12-step model for applying EBA principles and practices developed by Youngstrom and colleagues (2017, Table 4) to community-based service settings that serve bereaved and traumatically bereaved youth, many of whom have other, co-occurring trauma. Our case example (Andre) unfolds in a school-based mental health clinic given that such a clinic serves as the primary point of access to mental health services for many youth living in underserved communities with high prevalence rates of violence and loss (Grassetti et

---

TABLE 17.2. EBA Implementation

Assessment phases
- Preparation phase
- Prediction phase
- Prescription phase
- Process phase

Steps 1 and 2: Preparation phase
- Step A: Plan for most common issues in clinic setting
- Step B: Benchmark base rates for issues

Steps 3–5: Prediction phase
- **Step C: Evaluate risk and protective factors and moderators**
- **Step D: Revise probabilities based on intake assessments**
- **Step E: Gather collateral, cross-informant perspectives**

Steps 6–9: Prescription phase
- Step F: Focused, incremental assessments
- Step G: Intensive methods to finalize diagnoses/case formulation
- Step H: Assess for treatment plan and goal setting
- Step I: Learn and use client preferences

Steps 10–12: Process/progress/outcome phase
- Step J: Goal setting: Milestones and outcomes
- Step K: Progress and process measures
- Step L: Wrapping up and maintaining gains

al., 2018). The 12-step process is organized around the Four P's of EBA across a broad arc of EBPs. These include *preparation* prior to seeing clients, *prediction* (e.g., diagnosis), *prescription* (e.g., case formulation, treatment planning), and *process* (e.g., monitoring treatment response, therapeutic alliance, posttreatment status). Steps in the process are lettered instead of numbered to emphasize their flexible nature and the key role of clinical judgment given that some clients may be served best by iterating (or resequencing) steps as needed. (Readers can access additional open-science/open-teaching resources by Googling "EBA Wikiversity.")

In the next section, we build on prior work (Layne, Kaplow, & Youngstrom, 2017) by applying the 12-step EBA process listed in Table 17.2 to a case example that interweaves two strands: the story of a traumatically bereaved adolescent, and an intern's efforts to adapt and implement EBA practices in a school-based mental health clinic setting. The case is divided into four sections corresponding with the four EBA phases (*preparation, prediction, prescription,* and *process*). Each section begins with an EBA commentary and overview, followed by their application.

Applying the EBA 12-Step Program to a Clinical Case Example (Andre)

Preparation: Organizing Assessment Materials to Address Common Issues

First Contact: Initial Referral

Bud Schindler is a clinical psychology intern working as a mental health counselor in a school-based mental health clinic located in a low-socio-economic-status (SES), high-risk suburban community outside a large southwestern city. Clinic staff members include a full-time psychologist, one school counselor, and two psychology interns. Bud receives a referral from an assistant principal for a student whom he had sent to detention for fighting. Andre is a 16-year-old African American sophomore with a "C" grade point average and no prior disciplinary problems. The assistant principal learned from Andre's teacher that his brother was killed in a gang-related shooting during the spring of last school year (6 months earlier) and that he has struggled in school since. Andre has parental permission on file to receive clinic services.

EBA Step A (Preparatory Work): Calculating "In-House" Prevalence Rates and Assembling a "Starter" Toolkit

Some preparatory work increases the chances of successfully adopting and applying EBA in a practice setting (Youngstrom et al., 2017). Although often time-consuming to set up, these steps can pay dividends many times over in saved time and improved results—as gauged by metrics such as increased rates of reliable improvers and reduced rates of premature dropouts, treatment nonresponders, and reliable deteriorators (Lambert, 2010). Thus, Step A in Table 17.2 involves identifying the most commonly observed referral questions and diagnostic issues in the practice setting. At its most informal, this could entail staff members jotting down lists from memory, then compiling them. Other alternatives include taking a census of files of cases seen within the past 6 months or reviewing the files of a random sample of cases seen during the past year and tallying the results. Electronic health records systems carry the added advantage of generating exact numbers, generating "snapshots" of specific time periods, and examining trends in presenting problems and diagnoses over time.

Step A Implementation

With his supervisor's support, Bud proposes a plan in a staff meeting to adopt EBA practices throughout the clinic, including administering trauma- and bereavement-informed measures such as the Persistent Complex Bereavement Disorder (PCBD) Checklist and the PTSD Reaction Index for DSM-5—Brief Form (RI-5-BF; Table 17.4 provides references). The plan is approved. Bud then conducts a chart review of clients seen during the past 6 months and tabulates prevalence rates of the most common (e.g., top 20%) disorders. He reports the following: (1) A chart review of clinical interviews revealed that around 46% of students reported at least one significant death; (2) of these bereaved students, 17% met full criteria for a (provisional) PCBD diagnosis; (3) clinicians were still using the PCBD Checklist to informally assess grief reactions in recently bereaved students from whom the 6-month postdeath minimum could not be met for Criteria B and C (of these, 36% met the remaining PCBD criteria); (4) 65% of students reported at least one potentially traumatic experience (which for some students consisted of the death of their loved one under traumatic circumstances), 19% of whom predicted positive for PTSD as measured by the RI-5-BF.

EBA Step B (Preparatory Work): Obtaining Useful Benchmarks—National, State, and County Prevalence Rates

Step B involves benchmarking the "in-house" prevalence rates gathered in Step A against those reported in similar settings (e.g., Merikangas, He, Brody, et al., 2010; Merikangas, He, Burstein, et al., 2010; Youngstrom, Choukas-Bradley, Calhoun, & Jensen-Doss, 2014). These external benchmarks enhance the accuracy of the "exposure side" challenge of assessing stress-related disorders described earlier by placing them within broader (national/ state/local) contexts. Their functions include (1) act as a self-evaluating validity check by comparing one's in-house rates to those reported in similar populations (How do our rates match up? Do they appear reasonable? Are these isolated cases or part of a larger trend?); (2) improve professional networking by connecting the clinic's work to other settings; (3) surveil public health trends and epidemics, and proactively prepare for emerging threats; and (4) supply staff with information to advocate for students' health needs.

Applying Step B involves comparing one's local clinic prevalence rates against external benchmarks as obtained from sources such as similar practice settings; published rates, including national epidemiological cohort and survey studies (e.g., Oosterhoff et al., 2018); and national, state, county, or city government epidemiological mortality and other relevant statistics (e.g., CDC databases such as the Web-Based Injury Statistics Query and Reporting System [WISQARS]). Different external benchmarks are useful for different purposes. For example, the NCTSN provides a useful benchmark for *similar practice settings*, in that it consists of a national clinic-referred dataset gathered from mental health clinics across the United States that provide trauma- and bereavement-focused services. Pynoos and colleagues (2014) reported that 78% of the over 14,000 youth seen in NCTSN-affiliated clinics reported at least one traumatic life event; approximately 31% reported at least one bereavement experience. Additional benchmarks that come from studies of youth receiving mental health services underscore the need to screen for bereavement and co-occurring trauma exposure. The rate of documented maltreatment in youth receiving care in community mental health clinics is approximately 46% (Lau & Weisz, 2003), whereas PTSD prevalence rates range from 13 to 28%, with substantial comorbidity in the form of comorbid diagnoses, risky behaviors, and impaired functioning in important life tasks (Mueser & Taub, 2008; Silva et al., 2000).

Other useful external benchmarks consist of *published rates from representative epidemiological studies*. A useful benchmark for gauging both the prevalence of sudden loss and its links to school performance comes from Oosterhoff and colleagues (2018). However, because the actual survey combined deaths involving human malice (e.g., murder) that pose special clinical risks and challenges (Layne, Kaplow, & Pynoos, 2017) with other deaths due to accidents and natural causes, the study carries limited utility as a benchmark for both the national prevalence and impact on functioning of cases that specifically involve homicide. Moreover, because Bud's school-based clinic is located in a low-SES, high-crime suburb of a large city, an additional (but little overlapping; Bud's school serves students ages 13–19) benchmark is the epidemiological work by Breslau and colleagues (1998) of over 2,000 Detroit citizens ages 18–45 years, which found that 60% of the sample reported the sudden unexpected death of a loved one. Further underscoring the clinical import of traumatic bereavement, a review of the literature on traumatic bereavement identified increased risks for multiple comorbid conditions including grief disorders, major depressive disorder, PTSD, alcohol and drug abuse/dependence, and suicidal ideation (Kristensen et al., 2012).

A third set of external benchmarks consist of *local, state, regional, or national epidemiological mortality statistics*. Hulsey and colleagues (2018) used the U.S. Bureau of the Census Current Population Survey (CPS) and the CDC WONDER database. The authors found that between 2012 and 2015, on average, 61,389 children per year were bereaved by the death of a sibling, producing a nationally representative prevalence estimate of .0832%. This suggests that almost 1% of youth across the United States are newly bereaved by the death of a sibling each year. The authors recommend the use of up-to-date CDC and other databases with narrow time windows to capture recent trends and emerging threats (e.g., recent surges in deaths due to synthetic opioids and suicide) (see Burns et al., 2020).

Step B Implementation

Bud first searches WISQARS for national prevalence rates and learns that unintentional injury, suicide, and homicide were the leading three causes of death (both nationally and across Texas) for 15- to 19-year-olds in 2016. Each cause can be further broken down into particular mechanism. For example, motor vehicle accidents, poisoning (including drug overdose), and drowning are the three leading causes of fatal unintentional injury. Searching WONDER, Bud learns that in Harris County, Texas, where the school is located, the prevalence rate (per 100,000) of all causes of death has increased from 50.5 in 2011 to 58.4 in 2017, making bereavement an increasingly prominent public health issue countywide. Bud signs up for e-mail updates to surveil national and regional trends, threats, and resources. (See Layne, Youngstrom, & Kaplow, Table 1 at Wikiversity for online resources offering automatic e-mail updates.)

Prediction: Routine Assessment—Developing a Core Risk Screening and Assessment Battery

EBA Step C: Initial Referral and Risk Screening for Primary Risk Factors and Associated Conditions

Step C focuses on ensuring that good assessment tools are available to cover the problems most likely to be seen in the practice setting. Gathering "in-house" prevalence rates in Step A, and external benchmarks in Step B, are valuable tools to guide risk screening for the most likely stressors (e.g., bereavement, traumatic bereavement, and other trauma exposures), co-occurring stressors (e.g., domestic violence, community violence), and primary conditions (e.g., PCBD, PTSD). These prevalence rates and benchmarks are also valuable in assisting with differential diagnosis, especially comorbid conditions (e.g., major depressive disorder, suicide ideation, panic disorder, alcohol and drug abuse, delinquent behavior) and functional impairment at school, home, and so forth (Kristensen et al., 2012; Muester & Taub, 2008).

Beyond reducing the underdetection problems described earlier, there are compelling advantages to using standardized assessment tools rather than clinician-generated diagnoses for stress-related disorders and to creating a clinic culture that views comprehensive and accurate diagnosis as an integral part of EBP (Norcross & Wampold, 2011). Timely risk assessment and diagnosis facilitates timely protective action (e.g., crisis intervention), and early intervention that carries greater opportunities to prevent serious functional impairment, risky behavior, and developmental disruption. Compared to open-ended questions, standardized tools exhibit higher interrater reliability, higher validity coefficients benchmarked against expert consensus, greater treatment engagement, greater reductions in internalizing symptoms (Jensen-Doss & Weisz, 2008), and more sensitive detection of trauma histories (Chemtob et al., 2016).

Given the widespread prevalence of bereavement, traumatic bereavement, and other trauma (as causal risk factors) and consequent distress reactions (e.g., grief, PTSD) documented in Steps A and B, a variety of search strategies can be used to identify useful trauma- and bereavement-focused measures. Options noted by Youngstrom and colleagues (2017) include special issues, edited handbooks on assessment, and professional practice parameters. More recent resources can be identified via focused electronic literature searches that pair the topic/disorder (e.g., bereavement or grief) AND the assessment function (e.g., risk screening or assessment). Because many journals publish papers online well before they are formally published, online engines such as Google Scholar can also be configured to send notifications when studies on a given topic (e.g., grief, bereavement) are newly posted. Another useful strategy is to review the *Measures Review Database* compiled by the NCTSN (*www.nctsn.org/resources/online-research/measures-review*). This no-cost service lists measures of potentially traumatic events, common distress reactions, and youth functioning. Descriptions of each measure also summarize details regarding test reliability, test validity, and how to obtain the measure.

The task of assembling a risk screening and clinical assessment battery for bereavement and trauma can be complex and multilayered. In contrast to disorders with a primarily endogenous or heavily biologically determined causal locus (e.g., schizophrenia, depression, mania), stress-related disorders such as bereavement and trauma are primarily exogenous in nature, in that they require evidence of exposure to an external stressor plus clinically significant distress and functional impairment. These cause–effect links can be conveyed through a broad range of intervening variables (mediating and moderating variables) located across different levels of the ecology. These intervening variables in turn can lead to highly variable response trajectories among individuals exposed to similar events, including *stress resistance, resilient recovery,* and *deterioration* (Layne et al., 2009; Layne & Hobfoll, 2020). Influential intervening variables may include child-intrinsic factors such as biological diatheses (genetic polymorphisms), temperament (emotional reactivity to negative stimuli), developmental level, prior history, and cognitive factors (degree of unexpectedness, finding meaning); and child-extrinsic factors such as the manner of death, the child's relationship to the deceased, culture, and socioenvironmental protective and vulnerability factors (institutional responses—was an arrest made?), the health of surviving caregivers, parenting practices, and social support (Kaplow & Layne, 2014; Layne, Kaplow, Oosterhoff, et al., 2017; Pynoos et al., 1995; Umberson, 2017). We thus recommend, as a general expectation, that practitioners who seek to assess stress-related disorders—especially in youth, for whom the health and functioning of adult caregiving systems is so vitally influential and important—should plan to at least double the number of ecological factors they typically assess for predominantly endogenous disorders. As we show later, sorting these factors into categories (*hypothesized causal risk factors, vulnerability factors,* and *protective factors*) across levels of the ecology systematizes and facilitates case formulation and treatment planning (Layne, Briggs-King, & Courtois, 2014).

Evidence that bereavement and trauma can be associated with a broad range of difficulties beyond PCBD/PGD, including PTSD, depression, somatic problems, and suicide ideation (Kristensen et al., 2012), also underscores the need for careful differential diagnosis. The importance of accurate differential diagnosis is underscored by evidence that grief reactions, depression, and posttraumatic stress reactions are related but empirically distinguishable diagnostic constructs in bereaved youth (Spuij et al., 2012). Furthermore, adolescence is a second critical period of heightened brain plasticity (i.e., capacity to be shaped by experience), second only to early childhood in its vulnerability to physical and psychological harms, including drugs, toxins, stress, trauma, and loss. Adolescence (which, from a neuroscience perspective, currently spans ages 10–25) is thus a developmental window of neural "rewiring" in which brain systems that manage rewards, relationships, self-regulation, and planning for the future each mature and are highly susceptible to disruptions (Steinberg, 2014), including developmental derailment following bereavement (Burrell et al., 2020). Prediction-phase

EBA with adolescents should thus focus on not only trauma and loss exposure and associated distress reactions but also signs of potential *functional impairment, risky behavior,* and *developmental disruption.* Indicators of developmental disruption can include decreased school performance, risky behavior and self-harm, pessimistic future outlook, negative alterations in self-concept, diminished sense of life purpose/meaning, disillusionment with the social contract, estrangements in close relationships, negative attitudes toward family life, and diminished or abandoned professional aspirations (see Module 4 Introduction in Saltzman et al., 2017). For example, parentally bereaved youth are at risk for low academic achievement and at higher risk for breakups in intimate relationships, especially when the parent died of suicide (Høeg et al., 2018, 2019). Accordingly, Table 17.3 lists 12 markers of risk for severe persisting distress, functional impairment, and developmental disruption (Layne, Pynoos, & Griffin, 2019; McCormick et al., 2011; Pynoos et al., 1995) to be used when assessing major stress-related disorders including PCBD and PTSD. These risk markers can be used as an unobtrusive mental or paper checklist (Gawande, 2009) to quickly gauge the overall clinical severity and complexity of the case, the breadth and pervasiveness of the stressors' impact, and the likelihood that specialized therapeutic services are needed. We divide the 12 P's into three periods (*Pre-exposure, Peri-exposure,* and *Post-exposure*) in relation to a focal stressor involving trauma, loss, or traumatic loss.

Risky Tetrads

Although many different types of trauma and loss can occur across development, it is especially important not to miss "double-barreled" life experiences that are both highly prevalent and highly impactful. Thus, instead of simply checking off risk markers like a summative checklist, be watchful for developmentally linked intersecting and compounding risks. A developmentally-informed EBA approach to risk assessment calls for special vigilance for *risky tetrads,* which are a synergistic convergence of risks formed by the intersection of four concepts. We define a risky tetrad as (1) *a developmental period with* (2) *increased risk for exposure to, and* (3) *increased vulnerability to the harmful effects of,* (4) *a specific stressor.*

For example, early adolescent girls (1: developmental period) are highly susceptible (3: increased vulnerability) to social aggression (4: a specific

TABLE 17.3. The 12 P's: 12 Markers of Risk for Impairment and Developmental Disruption

Risk for developmental disruption generally increases as a function of the following:

Preexposure factors

1. *Prenatal problems:* Intrauterine exposure to maternal psychological distress (e.g., PTSD) is linked to neuronal, immunological, and behavioral abnormalities in affected offspring (e.g., Breen et al., 2018).
2. *Prior history/polyvictimization:* Prior trauma history, especially repeated exposure to different trauma types, increases risk (e.g., Kerig, 2014).
3. *Parenting problems:* Youth whose caregivers have poor parenting skills (many of whom also have trauma histories) are at increased risk for major life adversities, harmful developmental cascades, and harmful intergenerational cascades (Bellis et al., 2013).
4. *Period:* The developmental *period* during which exposure occurs matters. Developmental *tasks* that are either currently under way (e.g., forming primary attachment relationships) or were recently acquired/consolidated, are at greater risk for disruption (e.g., regressive behavior) (McCormick et al., 2011). Development also applies to differing levels of *risk for exposure* (childhood carries greatest risk for maltreatment; adolescence, greater risk for motor accidents), and *vulnerability* to the effects of exposure if it occurs (young adolescent girls are highly susceptible to social aggression) (Teicher, Tomoda, & Andersen, 2006).

Periexposure factors

5. *Potency:* The greater the magnitude of the stressor (witnessing severe injury or death, life threat, weapon use, violation of bodily integrity, malicious threats), the greater the risk.
6. *Personal:* Interpersonal *trauma* that betrays core assumptions of care, protection, and safety— including malicious harm, abuse, or neglect (e.g., murder, parental suicide, sexual assault, physical abuse, exploitation)—increases risk (Kerig, 2014). Perpetration of harm toward others also increases risk (Kerig, Chaplo, Bennett, & Modrowski, 2015). Regarding *bereavement,* the more central, unique, emotionally intense, and indispensable one's relationship to the deceased was, the more devastating the loss (Smith et al., 2017).
7. *Peritraumatic distress:* Intense acute reactions, including catastrophic appraisals of threat, danger, harm, consequence (thinking life will never be the same), and intense physiological and emotional responses (dissociation, terror, horror, cold chills, heart bursting), increase risk.
8. *Persistence:* Stressors that extend or reoccur over a lengthy time (e.g., sexual abuse that

(continued)

extends for months or years), especially across sensitive developmental transitions and multiple developmental periods, increase risk.

Postexposure factors

9. *Pervasiveness:* The greater the number of developmental *domains* (family, friends, school, romantic relationships) and developmental *tasks* (ability to trust, self-concept, life aspirations, morality/conscience development) a stressor disrupts, the greater the risk.
10. *Protected place:* Safe places in a youth's ecology create opportunities for traumatized or bereaved youth to resiliently "bounce back" and recover, improve functioning, and make up for lost time by taking advantage of developmental opportunities (e.g., afterschool clubs, sports). In contrast, an absence of safe places after stress exposure increases risk.
11. *Impaired functioning:* Stressors that not only cause significant distress but also induce functional impairment in life domains where important developmental tasks are under way, increase risk. Marginally functioning youth ("C" or "D" grade students) are at greater risk for developmental underachievement (college rejection), disruption (held back a year), and derailment (school dropout) than high-functioning youth ("A" or "B" grade students).
12. *Perilous activities:* Risky or dangerous behavior (drug/alcohol use, fighting, promiscuity, reckless driving, criminal behavior), either before or after stress exposure, increases risk.

stressor) at an age when they have increased access to cell phones and computers, and create private lives away from adult supervision (2: increased risk for exposure) (Teicher, Tomoda, & Andersen, 2006). Another risky tetrad lies at the convergence of adolescence (1: developmental period) and traumatic bereavement (4: specific stressor) (Layne et al., 2017). This risky tetrad arises from a heightened risk of exposure to traumatic death via adolescents' large social networks; easy access to risky activities (e.g., cars, alcohol, drugs, weapons, gangs); high fatal accident, overdose, suicide, and homicide rates; increased autonomy from adult supervision (2: increased risk); and stress-sensitive developmental processes (3: increased vulnerability) (Steinberg, 2014).

Step C Implementation

Drawing on what he learned in Steps A and B, Bud assembles a list of measures to cover problems associated with bereavement and co-occurring trauma typically seen in school-based clinic settings, including comorbid conditions. During this process, Bud review the NCTSN Measures Review Database, looking for evidence of developmentally sensitive test construction and validation. Given his goal to accurately assess stress-related disorders following traumatic bereavement, he searches for both "exposure-side" and "consequences-side" measures. He thus searches for assessment tools that cover bereavement and other types of trauma exposure, likely diagnoses following traumatic bereavement (e.g., PCBD, PTSD), and signs of child behavior problems and functional impairment. Bud also conducts a literature review of candidate tools to assess PCBD. Table 17.4v (created for EBA Steps C and D in Table 17.2) matches common presenting problems with recommended assessment tools, including measures of maladaptive grief (PCBD), PTSD, depression, functional impairment at school and in relationships, suicidal ideation, and their intended use (*in italics*). (Measures are also briefly listed in Table 17.4.)

The list in Table 17.4 derives from multiple EBA considerations (Youngstrom et al., 2017), including intended population; reliability and validity evidence; developmental appropriateness; resources available (e.g., time, personnel, space, budget); and the degree to which the test facilitates continuity between assessment, case formulation, and treatment planning. For example, the PCBD Checklist can be scored to yield either a provisional PCBD diagnosis or subscale scores reflecting primary dimensions of multidimensional grief theory (described later) that facilitates bereavement-focused case formulation and treatment planning (Kaplow et al., 2013, 2019; Saltzman et al., 2017). Alternatives to measures listed in Table 17.4, some free of charge, may also be available depending on the intended uses and population (e.g., Beidas et al., 2015). Examples include the Adolescent Grief Inventory, which does not provide a PCBD or PGD diagnosis (Andriessen et al., 2018), and the Persistent Complex Bereavement Inventory (Lee, 2015), developed with college students and adults. Furthermore, although the Strengths and Difficulties Questionnaire (SDQ) has been used to support assessment-driven, modularized treatments (e.g., Chorpita et al., 2015, 2017; Herres et al., 2017),

TABLE 17.4. Matching Assessment Tools to Common Presenting Problems in the Clinic

Common presenting problem/condition	Assessment tool (intended application)
Bereavement and grief reactions (PBCD, etc.)	UCLA Persistent Complex Bereavement Disorder (PCBD) Checklist (Kaplow et al., 2018): risk screening and in-depth clinical assessment
Trauma exposure and PTSD symptoms • Witnessing murder • Direct life threat • Fear for other brother • Other trauma (accident)	UCLA PTSD Reaction Index for DSM-5 Brief Screening Form (RI-5-BF; Rolon-Arroyo et al., 2018): risk screening.
	UCLA PTSD Reaction Index for DSM-5 Self-Report Scale (RI-5; Kaplow et al., 2019; Pynoos & Steinberg, 2017): in-depth clinical assessment
	UCLA PTSD Reaction Index for DSM-5 Parent Report Scale (Pynoos & Steinberg, 2017b): collateral assessment
Depression symptoms	Short Mood and Feelings Questionnaire (SMFQ; Angold et al., 1995): risk screening
Level of functioning/disruptions in life domains	Strengths and Difficulties Questionnaire (SDQ) Self-Report Version (Goodman, Meltzer, & Bailey, 1998): in-depth assessment
	Brief Problem Checklist (BPC; Chorpita et al., 2010): in-depth assessment
	Top Problems (Weisz et al., 2011): in-depth assessment
	SDQ Parent/Teacher's Report Version (Goodman, 1997): collateral assessment
Suicide ideation/risky behavior (optional, as indicated)	Columbia–Suicide Severity Rating Scale (C-SSRS)—Adult Version (Posner et al., 2011): in-depth assessment, if indicated
Somatic symptoms (optional, as indicated)	Children's Somatization Inventory (CSI-24; Walker, Beck, Garber, & Lambert, 2008): optional risk screening, if indicated

more comprehensive broad-spectrum measures such as the Child Behavior Checklist (CBCL) and Youth Self-Report (YSR) may be preferable depending on time, personnel, and budget constraints. The CBCL and YSR also contain a Somatic Complaints subscale for assessing health-related complaints—a useful and more culturally sensitive tool for health clinic settings where referrals may come from students initially presenting with somatic complaints.

Second Contact: Risk Screening

After summoning Andre to the clinic, Bud first works on establishing rapport, then screens Andre for trauma exposure using the RI-5-BF (a trauma/PTSD screen) and assesses for bereavement and grief reactions using the PCBD Checklist. Andre's responses identify several "12 P" risk markers for severe persisting distress, functional impairment, and developmental disruption. These include a potent stressor (witnessing traumatic death) and functional impairment (school problems). Bud quickly rough-scores both instruments, noting that Andre scored in the moderate-to-high range on the RI-5-BF, the PCBD Checklist, and the Short Mood and Feelings Questionnaire (SMFQ). Providing feedback, Bud explains that Andre seems to be going through some difficulties with which Bud could help. He asks if they could schedule a follow-up visit to learn more about how. Andre assents, and they agree on a suitable time several days later. Noting that Andre's mother has already signed a consent form, Bud states that he could learn more about how to be helpful if he spoke with one of Andre's parents and a teacher who has known him longest. Andre assents, suggesting his mother and homeroom teacher as sources.

EBA Step D: Revising Probabilities Based on Intake Assessments

A Bayesian EBA framework adopts the best available prevalence estimates of impaired responses to bereavement as the *base rate* of bereavement-related disorders, which in turn serves as a starting point for client assessment. Given that his internal chart review in Step A produced a clinic bereavement-related prevalence rate of 46%, 17% of whom met full criteria for (provisional) PCBD, then 17% serves as the initial estimate of likelihood for PCBD for the next bereaved student seen at the beginning of the assessment process. Furthermore, because the chart review revealed that

65% of students reported at least one potentially traumatic experience, 19% of whom predicted positive for PTSD, 19% serves as the initial estimate of likelihood for PTSD for the next student who reports a traumatic experience (including traumatic bereavement).

Step D Implementation

Bud carefully scores and interprets the screening and assessment tools he administered to Andre. Andre scores well above the clinical cutoffs (score = 38) on the RI-5-BF (PTSD symptoms) and the PCBD Checklist (grief reactions), and just above the cutoff (i.e., 8; Angold et al., 1995) on the SMFQ (depression symptoms). Focusing first on the RI-5-BF (assessing PTSD as a concurrent diagnosis), Bud relies on a test validation study (Kaplow et al., 2019) to guide several clinical decisions. Using receiver operating characteristic (ROC) analyses (Youngstrom, 2014), the authors found that a cutoff score of 21 maximized sensitivity and specificity as benchmarked against a "gold standard" structured clinical interview. Because the base rate directly affects diagnostic accuracy, the study also employed two base rates to approximate *general outpatient* (15%) versus *specialty* clinic (32%) settings, respectively, when calculating posterior probabilities. The authors also computed multilevel diagnostic likelihood ratios (DLRs) to assess levels of PTSD risk based on RI-5 total scale scores (McGee, 2002; Straus et al., 2019). A DLR value for a given test score range is obtained by dividing the proportion of individuals with a diagnosis who score within that range by the proportion of cases without the diagnosis who score within the same range. DLRs < 1.0 lower the odds of a PTSD diagnosis; values near 1.0 indicate no change; values between 2 and 5 represent a moderate increase, those between 5 and 10 represent a large increase, and >10 are often clinically decisive odds changes (Straus et al., 2019). Referring to the general outpatient base rate of 15%, Bud notes that students with total scores between 36 and 44 (DLR = 14.94) carry the highest risk of PTSD (posterior probability = 73%). Andre's RI-5-BF score of 38 places him in the highest-risk category for PTSD.

Focusing on maladaptive grief reactions, Bud notes that a developmentally appropriate clinical assessment tool for assessing PCBD criteria has recently become available (Kaplow et al., 2018). He thus chooses to go with the provisional diagnosis furnished by the PCBD Checklist as his best available diagnostic prediction. Bud also retains the diagnostic estimate of the SMFQ screening tool. He makes a chart entry, stating that Andre screened positive for PTSD, provisional PCBD, and depression, and that an in-depth clinical assessment is scheduled.

Pragmatic Implementation

There are two ways of looking at lists: in a linear order, or as a set of things to accomplish in any order. Clinical reality is that the same dozen or so steps in doing good assessment will not always happen in the same order; nor do they need to. A recent study (Grassetti et al., 2018) informs decision making regarding risk screening, clinical assessment, and the decision whether and how to treat. Both an initial group-based risk screening and a subsequent individual clinical assessment proved useful for making different clinical decisions, including case identification, diagnosis, suitability for treatment, and attrition. To promote trauma- and bereavement-informed schools, the authors recommend that (1) school staff be trained to recognize both PTSD and maladaptive grief (PCBD or PGD) symptoms and refer as appropriate for trauma and bereavement-focused assessment; (2) use of universal screening and enhanced caregiver consent procedures can reduce false negatives; (3) for youth with histories of multiple exposures, use targeted treatment engagement, family engagement, and referrals for supplementary or alternative services; and (4) improve links between home and school contexts, especially for multiply traumatized, underserved youth with pressing mental health needs.

Table 17.5 presents an assessment planning guide (Layne, Briggs-King, & Courtois, 2014). The guide supports fact finding and hypothesis testing across a broad range of assessment activities, from risk screening to posttreatment follow-up. In contrast to the step-by-step EBA procedure described in Table 17.2, the method presented in Table 17.5 centers on *primary assessment questions and available information sources*. This method is designed to maximize both the rigor and informational yield of the assessment process, as well as the capacity of practitioners to adapt their work to the resource-poor, disrupted, unstable, uncoordinated, and often chaotic environments in which bereaved youth live. (Our caregiver participation rates have ranged from 100% in a randomized controlled trial to 0% in a juvenile justice setting.) The method orients the assessment process around a series of key questions or hypotheses (Column 1), and specific traits or constructs to assess (Column 2) in order to address those questions/hypotheses. The method aligns with assessment practices that value diversity in sources, methods, and the informative inferences that can be drawn from both converging and diverging reports between information sources (De Los Reyes, Thomas, Goodman, & Kundey, 2013). Given the barriers that practitioners frequently encounter throughout the assessment process (e.g., limited or irregular access to information sources), the method encourages practitioners to be highly opportunistic in seeking out the best available sources (Column 3; e.g., youth, parent, teacher), using diverse types of information (Column 4; e.g., self-report, observational report, structured interview, school archives), and utilizing multiple methods/procedures used to collect data (Column 5). Our case example presents an idealized scenario (in which Bud has access to four sources: a vice-principal, a student, his mother, and a teacher) to illustrate the incorporation of different perspectives and the value of both converging versus diverging reports across sources.

Application of EBA Steps E, F, and G (Collateral Sources)

Given Andre's assent, Bud calls his mother, Mrs. D., describes Andre's referral to the clinic and his professional role, and secures her consent to provide information. She also consents to Bud's collection of information from Andre's homeroom teacher and agrees to come to the clinic for an interview.

Third Contact: Andre's Teacher

Bud then calls Andre's homeroom teacher and asks her to serve as a source of information regarding Andre's school functioning before and after his brother's death. His teacher describes Andre as being a "funloving, easygoing kid" during most of his freshman year, but after his brother was killed in the spring, he missed some school and returned "looking very sad and withdrawn." Since then, "he doesn't joke around so much—he looks a lot more distracted and tuned out." His grades have suffered as well: "His other teachers tell me he often turns in assignments late and that his work quality has been pretty poor. They're worried he'll fail and have to repeat the year. His art class is an exception, in which he does well and seems to enjoy himself." She also completes the SDQ Parent/Teacher form. Applying SDQ scoring methods used in published studies (e.g., Chorpita et al., 2017), Bud notes concerns in multiple areas, including Emotional Symptoms (unhappy or downhearted; nervous/fearful), Conduct Problems (usually obedient, but got into a fight recently), Hyperactivity/Inattention (restless, fidgeting/squirming, distracted/wandering attention, leaves tasks unfinished), Peer Relationship Problems (more solitary, no good friends anymore, may be bullied), and low/average Prosocial Behavior (keeps to himself). His Total Difficulties score fell in the very high range. Andre's teacher observational report scores (on the Impact Supplement) reflect being upset or distressed, interference with peer relations, and interference with classroom learning.

Fourth Contact: In-Depth Clinical Assessment

Drawing on his knowledge of local prevalence rates and the increased posterior probabilities provided by the initial risk screening, Bud prepares a battery to assess for trauma and loss exposure, PTSD diagnostic status, and potential comorbidities, and to obtain baseline measures in case treatment is appropriate. During their second visit, Bud administers the RI-5 Self-Report (not the RI-5-BF he used for risk screening) to more thoroughly assess Andre's trauma history and PTSD diagnostic status, the SDQ (self-report), the Brief Problems Checklist (BPC; to assess which symptom clusters, internalizing or externalizing, are predominant), and the Columbia–Suicide Severity Rating Scale (C-SSRS; given possible suicide ideation). (He holds the Child Symptom Inventory [CSI-24; Walker, Beck, Garber, & Lambert, 2009] in reserve, should Andre report any somatic symptoms.) During the assessment, Bud notes that Andre has a history of traumatic bereavement (his brother's murder) and other trauma (being in a scary car accident, various types of community violence), is experiencing significant difficulties in school, and interpersonal difficulties (not getting along well with friends or at home). His BPC profile shows elevations in both internalizing and externalizing problems. Andre's suicide ideation scores are moderately elevated but below the cutoff. Bud decides that bereavement- and trauma-focused intervention is appropriate. He explained that the clinic offered services, including a group, for students who have been through difficult experiences like his. Using the RI-5 Trauma History Profile as a prompt, Bud gently reviews some of the events Andre has endorsed and invites him

to consider which experience is creating the most problems for him now so they can decide whether it would be helpful to work on (Layne, Pynoos, & Cardenas, 2001). Looking both apprehensive and relieved, Andre relates the following experience:

"My oldest brother, Marcus, got killed in front of me. It happened after he had just gotten out of jail. I think they [members of a rival gang] were looking for him. Me and my two brothers were walking to the cleaners at around 5 o'clock. Then a car drove up; they yelled 'Capone!' and shot three times. I was walking behind and threw myself down real quick. Marcus fell back against the fence. I saw blood on his chest and his eyes looked weird and his arms were shaking, like he was spastic. I thought, 'Oh, God, they killed him!' Then they jumped out of the car and started chasing us—my other brother and me. We scattered and ran home as fast as we could. I kept looking over my shoulder to make sure they weren't following me. When I didn't see them, I got scared that they were chasing my brother instead. My heart was beating so fast it felt like it was gonna explode. I finally reached home and my brother was already there calling 911. My mom was home, but at first we didn't want to tell her what happened, 'cause she'd been so happy to have Marcus back home. She started screaming and crying when she heard us talking to the 911 operator. She fell down and started screaming, 'Not my boy! My boy!' My brother called my dad at work and told him what happened. Then my brother and I went back to where Marcus got shot, but they had already come and took him away. There were still police there who had it taped off and they asked us questions. There was a chalk outline of his body and blood on the sidewalk. My brother and I went back home. My mom and dad were there and were calling all the hospitals—we didn't know where they took him and the cops didn't know either. My mom was crying so hard my dad had to do the talking. When they finally told us where he was, we went to the hospital, but they wouldn't tell us what happened. We just sat in the waiting room. Mom was crying and dad just sat there pounding his leg with his fist. I'd never seen him so angry. My cousin came, and the doctor told us my brother was dead. They let us go in the room where he was lying on a cart. It was weird seeing him lying there not moving. My mom was crying and talking to him like he was still alive. Then we went home and stayed up late. My cousin got drunk. Mom didn't stop cry-

TABLE 17.5. Planning for Assessment of Traumatic Bereavement: Focus on Bereavement, Trauma, and Developmental Impact

Question/hypothesis	Traits or constructs to assess	Sources of information	Types of information to gather	Methods (tools and procedures)	Assessment intervals (EBA phase)[a]
1. *Risk factor exposure:* Andre has been • Bereaved (by the death of his brother) • Traumatized (by witnessing his brother's murder) • Traumatized due to direct life threat (close physical proximity to the shooting) • Traumatized (fearing for his other brother's life as they fled)	• *Bereavement* (death of brother) • *Trauma exposure* (witnessed brother's violent death) • *Trauma exposure* (direct life threat during the shooting)	Collateral source: School clinic records and staff Collateral source: Andre's mother (if available) Andre (the client)	• Archival data (medical records) • Interview data (nurse) Informed consent Interview data (caregiver) Self-report screening test Self-report psychological test (If needed): Semi-structured clinical interview	• Review medical exam records • Interview school nurse Obtain caregiver informed consent Interview mother to verify Andre's bereavement, trauma exposure, other major life adversities Administer RI-5-BF trauma/loss exposure screen to verify bereavement (death of brother), trauma exposure (witnessing violent death, and via personal life threat due to close proximity to the shooting) Administer Reaction Index (RI-5) Trauma History Profile section to verify trauma, traumatic bereavement Administer CAPS-CA-5 Trauma History section to verify trauma exposure, traumatic bereavement	Preparation (Step A) Preparation (Step A) Baseline clinical assessment (Step E) Initial risk screening (Step C) Baseline clinical assessment (Step F) Baseline clinical assessment (Step G)

2. *Andre meets diagnostic criteria for*
• PCBD
• PTSD
• Differential/comorbid diagnosis—rule out:
• Depression
• High risk for suicide
• Normative cultural idioms of distress (e.g., somatic complaints, culturally specific mourning rituals)
	• PTSD
	• PCBD
	• Depression
	• Level of functioning/potential disruption in developmentally salient life domains
	  At school
	  With peers
	  With family
	• Risky behavior
	• Suicide risk
		Andre
		
		Andre
			Self-report screening test
			
			• Self-report psychological test battery assessing:
			  PCBD symptoms/ provisional diagnosis
			  PTSD symptoms/ diagnosis
			  Level of functioning
			  Suicide risk
			
			Clinical interview
				Administer:
				• RI-5-BF PTSD symptom screen
				• MFQ
				
				Administer:
				• RI-5 self-report full symptom scale
				• PCBD Checklist (full symptom scale)
				• SDQ (self-report of functioning)
				• C-SSRS (suicide risk)
				• (Optional) CSI-24 (somatic symptoms)
				• (Optional) BPC (evaluate whether internalizing vs. externalizing symptoms are predominant)
				
				• Conduct clinical/diagnostic interview to review completed battery and assess risky behavior
				• Top Problems (assess current functioning, individual treatment goals)
					Initial risk screening (Step C)
					
					Baseline clinical assessment /Dx (If appropriate for treatment, proceed to) pregroup clinical interview (Steps F, G, H)
					
					Baseline clinical assessment (Steps G, X)

492

Question	Informant	Test type	Administer / Assess	Assessment phase
	Mother	- Observational-report psychological test - Clinical interview	- (If needed) Administer CAPS-CA Symptom Section to verify symptoms, impairment, PTSD diagnosis Administer: - RI-5 (caregiver report) focusing on symptoms, functional impairment - SDQ (parent observational report focusing on distress, functional impairment) Assess concerns for her son, family functioning, need for referral to family services	Baseline clinical assessment (Step E)
	Teacher(s)	- (If needed) Observational-report psychological test - Interview	Administer SDQ (teacher observational report) Interview about Andre's current functioning (including before the event, if available)	Baseline clinical assessment (Step E)
3. *Is Andre responding favorably to trauma- and grief-focused treatment? Is he making sufficient progress and on track to reach therapeutic goals?*	Andre - PCBD - PTSD - Depression - Level of functioning - At school - With peers - With family	Self-report psychological test data	Administer: - RI-5-BF - PCBD Checklist - SDQ - Top Problems (idiographic) - Reliable change index for key measures Assess therapeutic progress as benchmarked against end-of-module "readiness to proceed" indicators	Midtreatment (Steps I, J)
4. *Has Andre made sufficient clinically significant improvement to warrant termination?*	Andre - PCBD - PTSD - Depression - Level of functioning - At school - With peers - With family - Risky behavior - Suicide risk	Self-report psychological test data	Administer: - RI-5 - PCBD Checklist - SDQ - Top Problems - C-SSRS	Posttreatment Follow-up (Steps J, K)
	Teacher	Observational-report psychological test	Administer SDQ (teacher observational report)	Posttreatment (Step J)

Note: BPC, Brief Problem Checklist; CAPS-CA-5, Clinician-Administered PTSD Scale for DSM-5—Child/Adolescent Version; C-SSRS= Columbia–Suicide Severity Rating Scale; CSI-24, Children's Somatization Inventory; Dx, clinical diagnosis; MFQ, Mood and Feelings Questionnaire; PCBD, persistent complex bereavement disorder; PTSD, posttraumatic stress disorder; RI-5, UCLA PTSD Reaction Index for DSM-5; RI-5-BF, UCLA PTSD Reaction Index for DSM-5—Brief Form; PCBD Checklist, Persistent Complex Bereavement Disorder Checklist; SDQ, Strengths and Difficulties Questionnaire.

aA detailed version of the 12-step evidence-based assessment procedure applied to bereaved children and adolescents can be found at Wikiversity.

ing that entire week, and dad almost didn't talk at all. He just sat staring. My older brother and I mostly just stayed in our rooms. Lots of people came to his funeral and cried a lot. I didn't. None of it felt real. It didn't even look like him in the casket.

"A few days later I went back to school. I just couldn't stand being home anymore. I was quiet and tried not to think about him. Mom cried whenever she talked about him for a few weeks after that. But then she and dad mostly stopped talking about him. About the only time they talk about Marcus now is when they're getting on our case, like 'don't make the same mistakes your brother did.' It makes me mad 'cause it's like he never did anything right, but he was a fun brother and he looked out for me. Now mom and dad don't get along. They either snap at each other or just barely talk and they're real moody. Mom lost her job last year, and I know they're worried about money. They try not to talk about it in front of us, but I hear them arguing in their bedroom. My brother and I don't hang around each other much anymore either. We don't hang much with our old friends anymore, 'cause they were Marcus's friends too and it's hard to be around them. People talk about us now, so we mostly keep to ourselves. Kids say stuff about Marcus at school and online, like 'He got what was coming to him for running with a gang.' It made me real mad, so I called one of them out [challenged him to fight]."

Listening attentively, Bud quietly identifies multiple "12 P" markers of risk for severe distress and disruption (from Table 17.3), suggesting a complex case presentation and need for intervention. When Andre finishes, Bud thanks him for sharing his story, saying he will review this information and get back to him soon. Bud then scores and interprets Andre's test protocols. Using the Kaplow and colleagues (2019) paper as a reference and its PTSD base rate of 15% (Bud's best guess is 19% in his clinic), Bud notes that Andre's RI-5 score of 40 places him above the diagnostic threshold of 35, with a DLR of 6.99 and posterior probability of 55%. Scoring Andre's Trauma History Profile reveals a childhood and adolescence free of significant trauma (creating a *protected place* for healthy development) until he was 14, when Andre and his family were involved in a serious car accident. Andre's SDQ self-report Total Difficulties score is in the moderate range (Emotional Symptoms, Conduct Problems, Hyperactivity/Inattention, and Peer Relationship Problems are elevated), suggest-

ing some functional impairment. Andre's C-SSRS score is slightly elevated but below the cutoff, suggesting mild suicide ideation. Bud reviews Andre's test results and local referral resources during his next supervision meeting.

Fifth Contact: Andre's Mother

In her visit to the clinic, Mrs. D. expresses concern for her son, noting that although she knew his midterm grades had dropped from last year, she was surprised and disappointed when Andre's teacher recently requested a meeting in which she expressed concern that Andre was showing little motivation, working below ability level, turning in some assignments late, and was often inattentive in class. Mrs. D was shocked when Andre was sent to detention recently for fighting. Bud invites her to complete several observational measures of Andre's adjustment, including the SDQ Parent/Teacher Report and the RI-5 Parent Report. A quick review of the measures reveals significant concerns about her son. Bud gently queries whether there might be a connection between how Andre is doing and the hard times their family has been going through. Nodding, Mrs. D. says, "I've been thinking that, too," and tearfully describes how happy their family was to have their eldest son back home after serving an 18-month prison sentence and their devastation over his murder. She explains that her husband grew up in a "very rough neighborhood" and had worked hard to raise their family in the suburbs where he believed they would be safer. She states that although "we're barely holding it together," she and her husband are committed to raising their two living sons as best they can. Both boys had looked up to their older brother, especially Andre, "who idolized him," and she and her husband are worried that they will be tempted to follow his example and "go down the same path." So although it pains them, they speak little of Marcus, and when they do, it is mostly to share updates of the police investigation (no arrest has been made) or warn their sons about making the same mistakes. She notes gratefully that they are close to extended family members "who help if things get rough."

Bud quickly reviews Mrs. D.'s completed protocols, noting significant elevations on both. Bud recognizes that parents' observational reports of their children's PTSD symptoms tend to correlate more strongly with the parent's self-reported PTSD symptoms than with their children's self-reported PTSD, especially when the parents carry a PTSD diagnosis themselves (e.g., Ghesquiere et al., 2008). Thus, Mrs. D.'s elevated scores on her observational report of her son's PTSD symptoms may be acting as a rough projective test of her own distress. Bud hypothesizes that Mrs. D. is also traumatically bereaved and at risk for serious health and mental health problems (e.g., Umberson, 2017). Respecting Andre's wish for some privacy, and adhering to confidentiality guidelines in their school clinic, Bud shares only general details of his interview with Andre and suggests that it will be helpful for Andre to join a school-based group that focuses on trauma and loss. Mrs. D. approves. After gently noting the difficulties her family is going through and her concerns about their children, Bud offers to refer the family to a local clinic that specializes in working with bereaved families. Mrs. D. accepts the referral.

Bud scores Mrs. D.'s two test forms, noting interreporter convergences with those of Andre's teacher in multiple domains, including SDQ Emotional Symptoms (unhappy or downhearted), Conduct Problems (fighting), and Hyperactivity/Inattention. Mrs. D. reported that Andre was solitary, had few friends (Peer Relationship Problems), and did some service work with his church youth group (Prosocial Behavior). Her Total Difficulties score falls in the high range, reflecting serious concerns. Her scores on the SDQ Impact Supplement show elevations in being upset/distressed and interference with home life, friendships, classroom learning, and leisure activities. Mrs. D.'s RI-5 observational report on PTSD symptoms has elevations in Intrusion (Criterion B: emotional distress/reactivity to reminders); Avoidance (Criterion C: avoidance of external reminders); Negative Alterations in Cognitions and Mood (Criterion D: negative affect; decreased interest in activities); and Alterations in Arousal and Reactivity (Criterion E: irritability and aggression; startle reaction) and meet minimum criteria for PTSD.

Prescription: Using Assessment to Guide Diagnosis, Case Formulation, and Treatment Planning

EBA Steps F, G, H, and I

Good clinical training covers mainstream advances in identifying factors that contribute to discrepancies between parents' observational reports and children's self-reports of children's behaviors and functioning and their meaning (e.g., De Los Reyes et al., 2013). Beyond this mainstream knowledge, however, *trauma-* and *bereavement-informed* clini-

cal training should cover how factors rooted in traumatic and loss-related life experiences can greatly compound the complexity and variability of family members' individual reactions to trauma and loss. Family members may perceive and react to the same stressful event in markedly different ways depending on such factors as differing levels and types of exposure (e.g., witnessing the event, life threat, physical injury, fear for others' safety), relationship to the deceased, psychological closeness to the deceased, developmental stage, prior history of trauma or loss, reactions to different sets of trauma and loss reminders, differences in coping strategies, cultural factors, differences in personality/temperament, and differing levels of access to mental health services and other resources (e.g., Kaplow et al., 2012; Kaplow & Layne, 2014; Layne et al., 2006; Pynoos et al., 1995). Family members' varying reactions and different adjustment trajectories (Layne & Hobfoll, 2020) can create powerful dissonances that disrupt family dynamics; create misunderstandings, estrangements, and losses of social support; and act as vulnerability factors that exacerbate and prolong distress (Layne et al., 2006; Saltzman, Pynoos, Lester, Beardslee, & Layne, 2013). Thus, assessment and therapeutic work with bereaved youth should take into account the functioning of child caregiving systems, including parent/caregiver health and well-being, parenting practices, parental facilitation of the child's grieving (Howell et al., 2016; Howell, Shapiro, Layne, & Kaplow, 2016; Kaplow, Layne, & Pynoos, 2014; Shapiro, Howell, & Kaplow, 2014; Wardecker, Kaplow, Layne, & Edelstein, 2017), and if relevant, the functioning of community leaders (e.g., administrators after a school shooting).

Considering Racial Disparities

On a societal level, studies have identified a range of racial disparities in risks that are relevant to EBA-based screening of minority youth and families (Umberson, 2017; Umberson et al., 2017, 2019). Black children and adolescents had the highest mortality rate in 2016, followed by Native Americans and non-Hispanic whites (Centers for Disease Control and Prevention, 2016). Umberson (2017) examined racial differences in lifetime exposure to the death of family members using nationally representative U.S. data sets. Compared to white youth, black youth were significantly more likely from childhood through midlife to be bereaved by the death of a mother, father, or sibling.

Bereaved adults are also at risk (Umberson et al., 2018): Compared to white adults, black adults are more likely to experience the death of a child and a spouse from young adulthood through later life. Black and Hispanic parents are also more likely to lose a child and to have lost multiple loved ones (Umberson et al., 2017). Regardless of race or sex, Umberson and her colleagues (2017, 2018) found that parents who lose a child before age 50 are at long-term risk for poor physical health, depression, disability, cardiovascular disease, dementia, and mortality, and that the health disparities gap between races nearly closes after differences in child loss are taken into account. The authors propose that racial disparities in bereavement—in which black individuals and families are exposed to earlier and more frequent deaths—contribute to cumulative disadvantage across the life course and to the intergenerational transmission of health disadvantage. Of relevance to school discipline problems, Black students are disproportionately more likely to be harassed, bullied, and disciplined by suspensions and expulsions than are other racial groups (U.S. Department of Education Office for Civil Rights, 2018).

Four Guiding Questions Instead of "Diagnose One, Treat One"

Taken together, the sheer number, potency, and complexity of factors to consider when working with traumatized and bereaved youth underscore the need for powerful fact-finding and hypothesis-generating heuristics that guide thoughtful, question-oriented assessment and case formulation (Hunsley & Mash, 2007). Clinical assessment, case formulation, and treatment planning for stress-related disorders such as PCBD/PGD and PTSD, especially in children and adolescents who are heavily dependent on caregiving systems, requires a high degree of ecological proficiency. We thus propose that instead of the simplistic "diagnose one, treat one" and "one and done" clinical decision-making heuristics suspected earlier, clients are better served by decision-making heuristics that prompt four pairs of probing questions. The first question focuses on negative outcomes: "What could it be? What else could it be?" is a maxim of evidence-based medicine (Groopman, 2007) that discourages premature closure in clinical decision making by encouraging a search for alternative explanations, diagnoses, and comorbid conditions. The second question focuses on factors hypothesized to lead to those diagnoses and

reflects the potent contributions of stressful life events and circumstances to many adjustment disorders and health conditions: "What could there be in this client's history that could help explain this? What else could there be in their history?" encourages a systematic search for a range of different impactful experiences across the client's developmental lifespan that either alone or in combination could explain the outcome of interest, including its course over time (Layne & Hobfoll, 2020). The third question, "When could it be in their history? When else could it be?" invites practitioners to consider the developmental periods during which stressful life events and circumstances took place, potential developmental tasks and transitions that could have been impacted, and potential developmental disruptions (McCormick et al., 2011; Pynoos et al., 2014). The fourth question, "Where could it be in their ecology? Where else could it be?" invites a search for different risk factors and beneficial resources (protective and promotive factors; see Layne, Steinberg, & Steinberg, 2014) across levels of the ecology. Used judiciously, these four pairs of questions can guide practitioners in assembling a working clinical theory out of interlocking conceptual pieces that span multiple developmental periods and multiple levels of the ecology, and integrate them into the case formulation and treatment plan.

Application of EBA Steps F, G, H, and I

Bud then integrates assessment data from his three sources and uses these to guide clinical diagnosis, case formulation, and treatment planning. He focuses specifically on six EBA tasks: (1) whether to add focused assessment tools; (2) identifying moderators (vulnerability and protective factors) that increase or decrease the likelihood of disorder, assist in building a working clinical theory, and may serve as sites for intervention; (3) finalize diagnosis, including differential diagnosis and comorbid conditions; (4) build a case formulation; (5) create a treatment plan including treatment goals; and (6) incorporate client preferences. To address steps (1) and (3), Bud considers the incremental utility of using a semistructured or structured diagnostic interview for PTSD (e.g., Pynoos et al., 2015). These methods have substantially higher reliability than unstructured interviews (Garb, 1998), increasing the accuracy of both diagnosis and ensuing treatment choices. Contrary to concerns that structured interviews damage therapeutic rapport, patients rate structured approaches favorably, reporting that they offer a more comprehensive understanding of patients and their situation (Bruchmüller, Margraf, Suppiger, & Schneider, 2011; Suppiger et al., 2009). Semistructured interviews allow clinicians added flexibility in considering developmental (e.g., Kaplow et al., 2012) and cultural factors that may change the clinical presentation or internal experience of distress reactions. Diagnostic interviews and self-report checklists can complement each other during in-depth clinical evaluation to inform both diagnosis and treatment goal setting (Layne Kaplow, Oosterhoff, et al., 2017).

Given multiple considerations, including (1) a confirmed history of traumatic bereavement, (2) Andre's history of other trauma exposures, (3) a >50% likelihood of a PTSD diagnosis, (4) clinically significant levels of depression, (5) Andre's willingness to participate in group-based treatment, and (6) evidence of positive treatment response and very few iatrogenic outcomes in a randomized controlled trial (Layne et al., 2008) of Trauma

and Grief Component Therapy for Adolescents (Saltzman et al., 2017), which addresses both trauma and bereavement, Bud decides that his primary treatment targets lie above the wait-test threshold and that he should actively intervene (Straus et al., 2019). He logs DSM-5 diagnoses of PTSD, adjustment disorder (provisional PCBD), and provisional major depressive disorder in Andre's school clinic chart.

To address EBA Task 2 (identifying moderators) listed earlier, Bud prepares for an upcoming supervision meeting by filling out the CHECKS Heuristic (for a case of a traumatized and bereaved adolescent girl, see Layne, Kaplow, & Youngstrom, 2017). Shown in Figure 17.1a, the CHECKS Heuristic is a path analytic model that comprises four elements: *causal risk factors* (hypothesized to exert direct causal effects on the outcome), two moderator variables—*vulnerability factors* (hypothesized to interact with the causal risk factor, intensifying, worsening, and/or prolonging its effects) and *protective factors* (hypothesized to interact with the

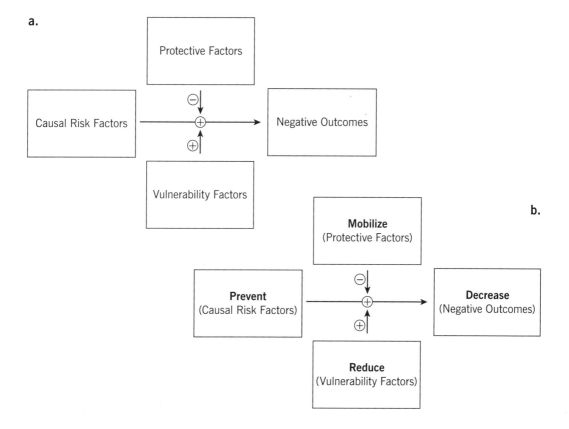

FIGURE 17.1. Using CHECKS (a) for case formulation and (b) for treatment planning.

risk factor, mitigating or buffering its effects)—and *negative outcomes* (hypothesized consequences of one or more causal risk factors) (Layne et al., 2009). CHECKS serves as both a case formulation tool by helping learners use causal reasoning skills to formulate a working clinical theory (Figure 17.1a), and as a treatment planning tool by leading learners to specify primary intervention objectives for each conceptual bin (Figure 17.1b; Layne, Steinberg, & Steinberg, 2014).

"CHECKS" is an acronym that prompts users to ask and answer six basic questions. The first four questions build case formulation skills: *What Caused the problem?* (identify causal risk factors); *What might Help the problem to get better?* (identify protective factors); *What might Exacerbate the problem?* (identify vulnerability factors); and *What is the most pressing Consequence?* (identify, prioritize negative outcomes). The last two questions build intervention planning skills: *What are the Key intervention objectives?* (specify treatment priorities); and *How do we know whether treatment is Successful?* (monitor treatment response).

CHECKS can be a useful therapeutic tool for case formulation, treatment planning, assessment planning, and engaging clients in making informed decisions about their care. It is highly adaptable, encouraging systematic simultaneous or sequential interventions according to which conceptual bins are therapeutically prioritized. For example, Bud may first emphasize *decreasing negative outcomes* and *mobilizing protective factors* by teaching emotional regulation skills to manage PTSD and PCBD symptoms, then focus on *preventing causal risk factors* by reducing risky behavior and *reducing vulnerability factors* by reducing social isolation. Users should recognize that different configurations of risk, protective, and vulnerability factors may be required to explain (and thus treat) different negative outcomes (e.g., PTSD, PCBD, depression). For example, being estranged from his brother and their friends (because they are trauma reminders) may act as potent causal risk factors for depression, but act as vulnerability factors for PTSD and PCBD/PGD. It may thus be necessary to reconfigure the model depending on which negative outcome (PTSD, PCBD/PGD, or depression) is prioritized for intervention. Bud lists four causal risk factors. He hypothesizes that the shooting contained at least three traumatic (PTSD Criterion A) events, including witnessing his brother's murder, direct life threat (being shot at and chased), and intense fear that his other brother would also be killed (threat to

a loved one). Bereavement (PCBD/PGD Criterion A) serves as a fourth causal risk factor. Bud also identifies multiple vulnerability factors and prioritizes/ranks them according to their hypothesized effectiveness in decreasing PTSD linked to his brother's death. Many vulnerability factors involve feelings of social isolation, interpersonal strains, and estrangements arising from the terrifying, horrific circumstances of the death and grief over the loss (Layne, Kaplow, Oosterhoff, et al., 2017).

Studying treatment models for traumatic bereavement, Bud learns that trauma-related intrusive, avoidance, and numbing symptoms can both exacerbate maladaptive grief reactions (e.g., feed desires for revenge) and encroach upon and interfere with adaptive grief reactions (e.g., stifle attempts to remember, reminisce, feel comforting connections to the deceased). Bud thus decides to focus on grief as a second therapeutic priority (after PTSD symptoms evoked by the traumatic death have receded). *Multidimensional grief theory* (Kaplow et al., 2013; Layne, Kaplow, Oosterhoff, et al., 2017; Saltzman et al., 2017) provides a useful framework for conceptualizing Andre's difficulties with grieving by proposing that individuals' grief reactions generally fall within three broad dimensions. These include *separation distress* (pining, yearning, and longing to be physically reunited with the deceased); *existential/identity distress* (feeling diminished, or losing a sense of purpose and meaning, due to the loss), and *circumstance-related distress* (thoughts, beliefs, assumptions, emotions, fantasies, and behavioral urges linked to the manner of death). Each dimension centers on a central coping challenge. For separation distress, it is to find ways to form healthy psychological and/or spiritual connections to the deceased. For existential/identity distress, it is to work through who I am as a person and the purpose of my existence and reasons for living. For circumstance-related distress, it is to come to terms with how the person died, including allowing distressing thoughts, assumptions, emotions, fantasies, and behavioral urges to recede over time; and to make one's life a positive response to how the loved one died. Each primary grief dimension spans a range of both adaptive/constructive and maladaptive/unhelpful responses to the death. The specific types of grief reactions that bereaved people manifest reflect how they are responding to and coping with the three domain-specific challenges. In turn, domain-specific grief reactions can be used to create an individualized grief profile and to individually tailor intervention, in that each grief dimension has its own therapeutic objectives and practice elements (Kaplow et al., 2019; Layne, Kaplow, Oosterhoff, et al., 2017).

Drawing on multidimensional grief theory and on his assessments with Andre and his mother, Bud hypothesizes that a lack of adult-facilitated opportunities to reminisce about his brother's positive influence in his life impedes Andre's desire to create a sense of psychological and spiritual connection with his brother, exacerbating his separation distress. This lack of attention to his brother's memory also frustrates Andre because he feels that the good parts of his brother's life and the positive legacy he left behind are ignored (exacerbating Andre's existential/identity distress, or ability to derive a sense of meaning and purpose from the loss). Andre's resentment may induce him to identify with his deceased brother more strongly by feeling obligated to champion and defend his brother's memory, perhaps heightening his parents' fears that he will "follow in the same path" and suffer a similar fate. Bud also hypothesizes that Andre's deceased brother's friends serve as *loss reminders*, evoking potent grief reactions by reminding him of his brother's continuing absence (Layne et al., 2006). Because interpersonal reminders can be especially potent cues in evoking PTSD and maladaptive grief reactions (Layne et al., 2010), Bud focuses especially on family factors he theorizes are contributing to Andre's difficulties. Bud hypothesizes that Andre and his brother serve as *trauma reminders* to one another, each serving as a cue to the other that evokes posttraumatic stress reactions (intrusive images, avoidance, etc.) to their respective terrifying experiences. Bud also hypothesizes that witnessing his parents' ongoing distress serves as an ongoing trauma reminder of witnessing their agony the day his brother was murdered. Andre appears to be highly reactive to both trauma and loss reminders and engages in avoidant coping—spending long hours alone in his room where he feels lonely, isolated, bored, depressed, and agitated. Although a common coping strategy, avoidance of trauma and loss reminders is generally maladaptive given its role in intensifying and prolonging distress (Howell et al., 2014).

Bud also hypothesizes that a confluence of conditions are contributing to Andre's deteriorating adjustment and problem behavior by undermining his ability and motivation to succeed in school, form healthy interpersonal relationships, and form positive future aspirations (Layne et al., 2001; Oosterhoff et al., 2018; Saltzman et al., 2017). Contributing symptom constellations include PTSD (hypervigilance; inability to sleep, concentrate, or relax; intense negative emotions; intrusive thoughts and mental images; pessimistic expectations that people can die easily anytime) and depressive reactions (e.g., feeling sad, lonely, isolated, agitated, and hopeless over his family's plight). Also prominent are Andre's grief reactions. These include separation distress (Andre misses his brother terribly and is frustrated at his lack of opportunities to remember, reminisce, and reconnect with his brother's memory) and existential/identity distress (e.g., feeling lost without his brother, life has lost its savor, blighted future outlook, diminished life ambitions). Circumstance-related distress is also prominent, in that the social stigma linked to his brother's death exacerbates Andre's distress (e.g., fear and rage that his brother's murderers are still at large, desires for revenge, feeling socially marginalized and estranged from others, resentment that his brother's memory is tainted by his stigmatized death), leaving him feeling defensive, angry, and alone. Bud hypothesizes that Andre is vigilant and reactive to cues of possible disrespect to his brother's memory, increasing his risk for getting into fights over perceived taunts at school and dismissive comments on social media.

Drawing on his working case formulation and knowledge of general treatment components utilized in bereavement-focused interventions (Kaplow, Layne, & Pynoos, 2019), Bud then reviews, as needed, NCTSN Intervention Fact Sheets (*www.nctsn.org/treatments-and-practices/trauma-treatments*) and other relevant evidence-based summaries (Straus et al., 2019), selects an evidence-based intervention, and creates a treatment plan. Given its modular focus on trauma/PTSD, bereavement/grief, adolescent risky behavior and developmental disruption, and flexibility in offering a group-based, individually based, or dual (individual + group) modality in school- or community-based settings, Bud selects *Trauma and Grief Component Therapy for Adolescents* (TGCTA; Saltzman et al., 2017). Table 17.6 lists the five CHECKS domains, the key therapeutic objectives of each domain, and the TGCTA modules and exercises therein that address them. Because Andre (and his fellow group members) are dealing with issues involving both trauma and bereavement, Bud chooses to implement a full course of TGCTA including Modules 1 (Skills Building), 2 (Trauma Processing), 3 (Loss Processing), and 4 (Promoting Adaptive Developmental Progression).

TABLE 17.6. Using the CHECKS Heuristic as a Planning Tool for Modularized Treatment

CHECKS domain	Key therapeutic objectives	TGCTA: module numbers and practice element(s) to emphasize
Causal risk factors	Prevent exposure to gang violence; promote safety	*Modules 1 and 4:* (a) Learn to discriminate between safe and unsafe places; (b) replace risky behavior with positive behaviors; (c) engage school resource officer in raising awareness regarding safety.
Protective factors	Mobilize protective factors	*Module 1:* (a) Teach adaptive coping skills, build group cohesion; (b) teach social support skills to recruit support from family, school, and community; (c) invite school resource officer to present at parent night about safety and resisting gang recruitment attempts.
Vulnerability factors	Reduce vulnerability factors	*Module 1:* (a) Reduce loneliness by strengthening group cohesion, teaching social support skills, positive activities scheduling; (b) reduce avoidance of reminders/bridge interpersonal estrangements; (c) refer family for trauma/grief-focused treatment; (d) advocate/present on bereavement at clinic/school staff meetings and parent night; offer to consult with staff on how to support traumatized and bereaved youth.
Negative outcomes	Decrease psychological distress, functional impairment, and risky behavior; correct and repair developmental disruption	*Module 2:* (a) Use trauma narrative construction to reduce PTSD symptoms linked to life threat, witnessing traumatic death, fear for other brother; (b) reduce PCBD symptoms (circumstance-related distress) by constructing a narrative of how his brother died, processing desires for revenge. *Module 3:* (c) Reduce PCBD symptoms including separation distress (facilitating positive connection to the deceased) and existential/identity distress (meaning building, legacy building). *Module 4:* (d) Promote positive life ambitions; (e) promote adaptive developmental progression; (f) strengthen commitment to the social contract through prosocial behavior (volunteering, acts of service).

Process: Using Assessment to Guide Process, Progress, and Outcome Measurement

Weaving Together EBA Steps I, J, and K

A variety of individual-level therapeutic tools have been used to facilitate treatment planning, monitoring treatment response (progress), and outcome assessment with TGCTA. Layne and colleagues (2008) used the Reliable Change Index (Tingey, Lambert, Burlingame, & Hansen, 1996) to assess pre- to posttreatment and pretreatment to follow-up outcomes in a randomized controlled trial comparing a full course (Modules 1–4) of TGCTA against a contrast group who received classroom-based skills and psychoeducation selected from Modules 1 and 4. The authors found good rates of reliable improvement in PTSD (58% at posttreatment, 81% at 4-month follow-up) and depression symptoms (23% at posttreatment, 61% at follow-up) in the treatment group, and higher odds of reliable improvement in PTSD at both posttreatment and 4-month follow-up. Few or no reliable deteriorators were found in either condition.

A school-based treatment outcome study of TGCTA (Herres et al., 2017) demonstrates the utility of integrating individualized (ideographic) ratings with standard nomothetic (general norm-based) measures to evaluate therapeutic progress, especially given evidence that clinicians strongly prefer ideographic (client-centered) measures over nomothetic measures (Jensen-Doss et al., 2018). Herres and colleagues (2017) used an ideographic Top Problems measure (Weisz et al., 2011) by inviting students to identify the top three problems for which help is currently needed, rated from 0 (*not at all a problem*) to 10 (*a huge problem*), at the start of each weekly group session. Student concerns included family health, distress symptoms (e.g., worry, difficulty concentrating), and school performance. Top Problem ratings decreased significantly across all three measured phases of treatment. The authors also found a treatment moderating effect, such that students with higher baseline *internalizing* symptoms showed less benefit in their Top Problems from Module 1 (psychoeducation/skills building components), and more benefit from Modules 2 and 3 (trauma- and loss-focused components), than students with higher baseline *externalizing* symptoms. The authors suggested that youth with predominantly externalizing problems may benefit more from abbreviated TGCTA (skills-building Modules 1 and 4); whereas youth with predominantly internalizing problems may benefit most from a full course of treatment including trauma (Module 2) and/or grief-processing work (Module 3).

Implementation of EBA Steps I, J, and K

Table 17.5 includes Bud's assessment plan for monitoring treatment response (via progress measures) during treatment, assessing posttreatment outcomes, and prescribed assessment intervals. Bud summons Andre to a pregroup individual interview (Saltzman et al., 2017) to invite him to the first group session, briefly review (and modify, as needed) his proposed treatment plan, including the traumatic event they plan to work on, and identify Andre's "top problems." Given Andre's history of multiple traumatic experiences and the underserved community in which he lives, Bud places extra emphasis on engagement. (If much time has elapsed since their in-depth assessment, it may be appropriate to re-administer key outcome measures (e.g., RI-5, PCBD Checklist, SMFQ, SDQ) to obtain a current baseline.

Along with standard monitoring tools (to track group cohesion, therapeutic alliance, and provide timely feedback; see Lambert, 2010), idiographic tools can also be built into flexibly delivered treatments to monitor client progress, assess the therapeutic process, surveil for new or recurring life stressors (a critically important therapeutic task when working with youth who live in dangerous communities), and tailor treatment accordingly. For example, TGCTA progress measures include a Personal Goals worksheet, in which youth specify their personal treatment goals early in Module 1, and a standard "Check-In" opening exercise for each session, in which clients report on whether they completed assigned practice exercises. Each of the four TGCTA modules contains an introduction and overview that specifies milestones

to evaluate therapeutic progress and gauge readiness to proceed (or to graduate after Module 4). For example, "readiness to proceed" benchmarks for Module 1 include the ability to identify at least one trauma or loss reminder and enact a coping plan when encountering it. Regarding therapeutic process, each session contains at least one therapeutic exercise that can be used to track client engagement (e.g., reporting on reminders encountered that week; a "check-out" exercise in which members describe what they found most valuable. Final sessions of Module 4 focus on relapse prevention and termination, including a "good good-bye" activity that helps members bereaved by sudden loss to discriminate between "good good-byes" and traumatic separations. Booster follow-up sessions (e.g., Fall of next school year) can also be scheduled to assess ongoing adjustment, surveil for new or recurring stressful life events, and catch up on one another's lives.

Conclusion

As death and taxes are the only two inevitables in life, it is peculiar that bereavement and grief are only now coming into their own as diagnostic, public health, and public policy concerns. Mental health training often overlooks bereavement, both in terms of detecting it and addressing its sequelae, including grief reactions, comorbid conditions, and its reverberating effects across the ecology and across development. We hope that our application of EBA will help to raise the standard of care for bereaved youth and their families. More broadly, we hope that this work will contribute to ongoing developments in public health, public policy, medicine, and mental health in recognizing bereavement as a major life stressor that is unique in its capacity to change the developmental trajectories of individuals, families, and societies.

ACKNOWLEDGMENTS

This work was supported in part by the New York Life Foundation (Julie B. Kaplow and Christopher M. Layne, Principal Investigators). We thank Eric Youngstrom for giving permission to adapt the 12-step evidence-based assessment process used in Table 17.2, Brooks Keeshin for his collegial review of a prior chapter draft, and Robert Pynoos and Alan Steinberg for enriching our discussion of developmental disruption.

AUTHOR DISCLOSURES

The authors are coauthors of *Trauma and Grief Component Therapy for Adolescents* (Saltzman, Layne, Pynoos, Olafson, Kaplow, & Boat, 2017) and the Persistent Complex Bereavement Disorder Checklist (Layne, Kaplow, & Pynoos, 2014).

REFERENCES

American Federation of Teachers and New York Life Foundation. (2012). Grief in the classroom: Nationwide survey among school teachers on childhood bereavement. Retrieved from *www.aft.org/sites/default/files/release_bereavement121012.pdf*.

American Psychiatric Association. (2013). *Diagnostic and statistical manual of mental disorders* (5th ed.). Arlington, VA: Author.

Andriessen, K., Hadzi-Pavlovic, D., Draper, B., Dudley, M., & Mitchell, P. B. (2018). The Adolescent Grief Inventory: Development of a novel grief measurement. *Journal of Affective Disorders, 240,* 203–211.

Angold, A., Costello, E. J., Messer, S. C., Pickles, A., Winder, F., & Silver, D. (1995). The development of a short questionnaire for use in epidemiological studies of depression in children and adolescents. *International Journal of Methods in Psychiatric Research, 5,* 237–249.

Arnold, C. (2018). *Pandemic 1918: Eyewitness accounts from the greatest medical holocaust in modern history.* New York: St. Martin's Press.

Atwoli, L., Stein, D. J., King, A., Petukhova, M., Aguilar-Gaxiola, S., Alonso, J., . . . Kessler, R. C. (2017). Posttraumatic stress disorder associated with unexpected death of a loved one: Cross-national findings from the world mental health surveys. *Depression and Anxiety, 34,* 315–326.

Beidas, R. S., Stewart, R. E., Walsh, L., Lucas, S., Downey, M. M., Jackson, K., . . . Mandell, D. S. (2015). Free, brief, and validated: Standardized instruments for low-resource mental health settings. *Cognitive and Behavioral Practice, 22,* 5–19.

Bellis, M. A., Lowey, H., Leckenby, N., Hughes, K., & Harrison, D. (2013). Adverse childhood experiences: Retrospective study to determine their impact on adult health behaviours and health outcomes in a UK population. *Journal of Public Health, 36,* 81–91.

Berg, L., Rostila, M., Saarela, J., & Hjern, A. (2014). Parental death and subsequent school performance. *Pediatrics, 133,* 682–689.

Breen, M. S., Wingo, A. P., Koen, N., Donald, K. A., Nicol, M., Zar, H. J., . . . Stein, D. J. (2018). Gene expression in cord blood links genetic risk for neurodevelopmental disorders with maternal psychological distress and adverse childhood outcomes. *Brain Behavior and Immunity, 73,* 320–330.

Brent, D., Melhem, N., Donohoe, M. B., & Walker, M. (2009). The incidence and course of depression in bereaved youth 21 months after the loss of a parent to suicide, accident, or sudden natural death. *American Journal of Psychiatry, 166,* 786–794.

Brent, D. A., Melhem, N. M., Masten, A. S., Porta, G., & Payne, M. W. (2012). Longitudinal effects of parental bereavement on adolescent developmental competence. *Journal of Clinical Child and Adolescent Psychology, 41,* 778–791.

Breslau, N., Kessler, R. C., Chilcoat, H. D., Schultz, L. R., Davis, G. C., & Andreski, P. (1998). Trauma and posttraumatic stress disorder in the community: The 1996 Detroit area survey of trauma. *Archives of General Psychiatry, 55,* 626–632.

Bruchmüller, K., Margraf, J., Suppiger, A., & Schneider, S. (2011). Popular or unpopular?: Therapists' use of structured interviews and their estimation of patient acceptance. *Behavior Therapy, 42,* 634–643.

Burns, M., Griese, B., King, S., & Talmi, A. (2020). Childhood bereavement: Understanding prevalence and related adversity in the United States. *American Journal of Orthopsychiatry.* [Epub ahead of print]

Burrell, L. V., Mehlum, L., & Qin, P. (2020). Educational attainment in offspring bereaved by sudden parental death from external causes: A national cohort study from birth and throughout adulthood. *Social Psychiatry and Psychiatric Epidemiology.* [Epub ahead of print]

Centers for Disease Control and Prevention, National Center for Health Statistics (2016). Naitonal Vital Statistics System. Retrieved from *www.cdc.gov/nchs/nvss/index.htm*.

Cerel, J., Fristad, M. A., Verducci, J., Weller, R. A., & Weller, E. B. (2006). Childhood bereavement: Psychopathology in the 2 years postparental death. *Journal of the American Academy of Child and Adolescent Psychiatry, 45,* 681–690.

Chemtob, C. M., Gudiño, O. G., Luthra, R., Yehuda, R., Schmeidler, J., Auslander, B., . . . Abramovitz, R. (2016). Child trauma exposure and posttraumatic stress disorder: Identification in community mental health clinics. *Evidence-Based Practice in Child and Adolescent Mental Health, 1,* 103–115.

Childhood Bereavement Estimation Model. (2018). Understanding childhood grief in the U.S. Retrieved January 31, 2019, from *www.judishouse.org/cbem*.

Chorpita, B. F., Daleiden, E. L., Park, A. L., Ward, A. M., Levy, M. C., Cromley, T., . . . Krull, J. L. (2017). Child STEPs in California: A cluster randomized effectiveness trial comparing modular treatment with community implemented treatment for youth with anxiety, depression, conduct problems, or traumatic stress. *Journal of Consulting and Clinical Psychology, 85,* 13–25.

Chorpita, B. F., Park, A., Tsai, K., Korathu-Larson, P., Higa-McMillan, C. K., & Nakamura, B. J. (2015). Balancing effectiveness with responsiveness: Therapist satisfaction across different treatment designs in the Child STEPs randomized effectiveness trial. *Journal of Consulting and Clinical Psychology, 83,* 709–718.

Christakis, N. A., & Allison, P. D. (2006). Mortality after the hospitalization of a spouse. *New England Journal of Medicine 354*(7), 719–730.

De Los Reyes, A., Thomas, S. A., Goodman, K. L., & Kundey, S. M. A. (2013). Principles underlying the use of multiple informants' reports. *Annual Review of Clinical Psychology, 9*, 123–149.

DeRosa, R. R., Amaya-Jackson, L., & Layne, C. M. (2013). From rifts to riffs: Evidence-based principles to guide critical thinking about next-generation child trauma treatments and training. *Training and Education in Professional Psychology, 7*, 195–204.

Dowdney, L. (2000). Annotation: Childhood bereavement following parental death. *Journal of Child Psychology and Psychiatry, 41*, 819–830.

Draper, A., & Hancock, M. (2011). Childhood parental bereavement: The risk of vulnerability to delinquency and factors that compromise resilience. *Mortality, 16*, 285–305.

Feigelman, W., Rosen, Z., Joiner, T., Silva, C., & Mueller, A. S. (2017). Examining longer-term effects of parental death in adolescents and young adults: Evidence from the National Longitudinal Survey of Adolescent to Adult Health. *Death Studies, 41*, 133–143.

Foreman, K. J., Marquez, M., Dolgert, A., Fukutaki, K., Fullman, N., McGaughey, M., . . . Murray, C. J. L. (2018). Forecasting life expectancy, years of life lost, and all-cause and cause-specific mortality for 250 causes of death: Reference and alternative scenarios for 2016–40 for 195 countries and territories. *Lancet, 392*, 2052–2090.

Garb, H. N. (1998). *Studying the clinician: Judgment research and psychological assessment.* Washington, DC: American Psychological Association.

Gawande, A. (2009). *The Checklist Manifesto: How to get things right.* New York: Holt.

Ghesquiere, A., Fan, M., Berliner, L., Rivara, F. P., Jurkovich, G. J., Russo, J., . . . Zatzick, D. F. (2008). Adolescents' and parents' agreement on posttraumatic stress disorder symptoms and functioning after adolescent injury. *Journal of Traumatic Stress, 21*, 487–491.

Goodman, R. (1997). The Strengths and Difficulties Questionnaire: A research note. *Journal of Child Psychology and Psychiatry, 38*, 581–586.

Goodman, R., Meltzer, H., & Bailey, V. (1998). The strengths and difficulties questionnaire: A pilot study on the validity of the self-report version. *European Child and Adolescent Psychiatry, 7*(3), 125–130.

Grassetti, S. N., Williamson, A. A., Herres, J., Kobak, R., Layne, C. M., Kaplow, J. B., . . . Pynoos, R. S. (2018). Evaluating referral, screening, and assessment procedures for middle school trauma/grief-focused treatment groups. *School Psychology Quarterly, 33*, 10–20.

Greeson, J., Briggs, E. C., Layne, C. M., Belcher, H. M. E., Ostrowski, S. A., Kim, S., . . . Fairbank, J. A. (2014). Traumatic childhood experiences in the 21st century: Broadening and building on the ACE Studies with data from the National Child Traumatic Stress Network. *Journal of Interpersonal Violence, 29*, 536–556.

Groopman, J. (2007). *How doctors think.* New York: Houghton Mifflin.

Guldin, M.-B., Li, J., Pedersen, H. S., Obel, C., Agerbo, E., Gissler, M., . . . Vestergaard, M. (2015). Incidence of suicide among persons who had a parent who died during their childhood: A population-based cohort study. *Journal of the American Medical Association Psychiatry, 72*, 1227–1234.

Harris, K. M., & Udry, J. R. (2008). *National Longitudinal Study of Adolescent to Adult Health (Add Health), 1994–2008.* Chapel Hill: Carolina Population Center, University of North Carolina/Ann Arbor, MI: Inter-university Consortium for Political and Social Research.

Hedegaard, H., Curtin, S. C., & Warner, M. (2018). *Suicide mortality in the United States, 1999–2017 (NCHS Data Brief No. 330).* Hyattsville, MD: National Center for Health Statistics.

Hedegaard, H., Curtin, S. C., & Warner, M. (2020). *Increase in suicide mortality in the United States, 1999–2018 (NCHS Data Brief No. 362).* Hyattsville, MD: National Center for Health Statistics.

Hedegaard, H., Miniño, A. M., & Warner, M. (2018). *Drug overdose deaths in the United States, 1999–2017 (NCHS Data Brief No. 329).* Hyattsville, MD: National Center for Health Statistics.

Herres, J., Williamson, A. A., Kobak, R., Layne, C. M., Kaplow, J. B., Saltzman, W. R., & Pynoos, R. S. (2017). Internalizing and externalizing symptoms moderate treatment response to school-based trauma and grief component therapy for adolescents. *School Mental Health, 9*, 184–193.

Hill, R., Oosterhoff, B., Layne, C. M., Rooney, E., Yudovich, S., Pynoos, R. S., & Kaplow, J. (2019). Multidimensional grief therapy: Pilot open trial of a novel intervention for bereaved children and adolescents. *Journal of Child and Family Studies, 28*, 3062–3074.

Høeg, B. L., Johansen, C., Christensen, J., Frederiksen, K., Dalton, S. O., Dyregrov, A., . . . Bidstrup, P. E. (2019). Early parental loss and intimate relationships in adulthood: A nationwide study. *Developmental Psychology, 54*(5), 963–974.

Høeg, B. L., Johansen, C., Christensen, J., Frederiksen, K., Dalton, S. O., Bøge, P., & Bidstrup, P. E. (2018). Does losing a parent early influence the education you obtain?: A nationwide cohort study in Denmark. *Journal of Public Health, 41*(2), 296–304.

Holt-Lunstad, J., Smith, T. B., & Layton, J. B. (2010). Social relationships and mortality risk: A meta-analytic review. *PLOS Medicine, 7*(7), e1000316.

Howell, K. H., Barrett-Becker, E. P., Burnside, A. N., Wamser-Nanney, R., Layne, C. M., & Kaplow, J. B. (2016). Children facing parental cancer versus parental death: The buffering effects of positive parenting and emotional expression. *Journal of Child and Family Studies, 25*(1), 152–164.

Howell, K. H., Kaplow, J. B., Layne, C. M., Benson, M. A., Compas, B. E., Katalinski, R., . . . Pynoos, R. (2014). Predicting adolescent posttraumatic stress in the aftermath of war: Differential effects of coping strategies across trauma reminder, loss reminder, and family conflict domains. *Anxiety, Stress, and Coping, 28,* 88–104.

Howell, K. H., Shapiro, D. N., Layne, C. M., & Kaplow, J. B. (2015). Individual and psychosocial mechanisms of adaptive functioning in parentally bereaved children. *Death Studies, 39,* 296–306.

Hulsey, E., Hill, R., Layne, C., Gaffney, D., & Kaplow, J. (2018). Calculating the incidence rate of sibling bereavement among children and adolescents across the United States: A proposed method. *Death Studies.* [Epub ahead of print]

Hunsley, J., & Mash, E. J. (2007). Evidence-based assessment. *Annual Review of Clinical Psychology, 3,* 29–51.

Jacobs, J., & Bovasso, G. (2009). Re-examining the long-term effects of experiencing parental death in childhood on adult psychopathology. *Journal of Nervous and Mental Disease, 197,* 24–27.

Jakobsen, I., & Christiansen, E. (2011). Young people's risk of suicide attempts in relation to parental death: A population-based register study. *Journal of Child Psychology and Psychiatry, 52,* 176–183.

Jensen, A. L., & Weisz, J. R. (2002). Assessing match and mismatch between practitioner-generated and standardized interviewer-generated diagnoses for clinic-referred children and adolescents. *Journal of Consulting and Clinical Psychology, 70,* 158–168.

Jensen-Doss, A. (2005). Evidence-based diagnosis: Incorporating diagnostic instruments into clinical practice. *Journal of the American Academy of Child and Adolescent Psychiatry, 44,* 947–952.

Jensen-Doss, A., Smith, A. M., Becker-Haimes, E. M., Ringle, V. M., Walsh, L. M., Nanda, M., . . . Lyon, A. R. (2018). Individualized progress measures are more acceptable to clinicians than standardized measures: Results of a national survey. *Administration and Policy in Mental Health and Mental Health Services Research, 45,* 392–403.

Jensen-Doss, A., & Weisz, J. R. (2008). Diagnostic agreement predicts treatment process and outcomes in youth mental health clinics. *Journal of Consulting and Clinical Psychology, 76,* 711–722.

Jensen-Doss, A., Youngstrom, E. A., Youngstrom, J. K., Feeny, N. C., & Findling, R. L. (2014). Predictors and moderators of agreement between clinical and research diagnoses for children and adolescents. *Journal of Consulting and Clinical Psychology, 82,* 1151–1162.

Kaplow, J. B., Howell, K. H., & Layne, C. M. (2014). Do circumstances of the death matter?: Identifying socioenvironmental risks for grief-related psychopathology in bereaved youth. *Journal of Traumatic Stress, 27,* 42–49.

Kaplow, J. B., & Layne, C. M. (2014). Sudden loss and psychiatric disorders across the life course: Toward a developmental lifespan theory of bereavement-related risk and resilience. *American Journal of Psychiatry, 171,* 807–810.

Kaplow, J. B., Layne, C. M., Oosterhoff, B., Goldenthal, H., Howell, K., Wamser-Nanney, R., . . . Pynoos, R. (2018). Validation of the Persistent Complex Bereavement Disorder (PCBD) Checklist: A developmentally informed assessment tool for bereaved youth. *Journal of Traumatic Stress, 31,* 244–254.

Kaplow, J. B., Layne, C. M., & Pynoos, R. S. (2014, January). Persistent complex bereavement disorder as a call to action: Using a proposed DSM-5 diagnosis to advance the field of childhood grief. ISTSS Trauma Blog.

Kaplow, J. B., Layne, C. M., & Pynoos, R. S. (2019). Diagnosis and treatment of persistent complex bereavement disorder in children and adolescents. In M. Prinstein, E. Youngstrom, E. J. Mash, & R. A. Barkley (Eds.), *Treatment of childhood disorders* (4th ed., pp. 560–590). New York: Guilford Press.

Kaplow, J. B., Layne, C. M., Pynoos, R. S., Cohen, J. A., & Lieberman, A. (2012). DSM-V diagnostic criteria for bereavement-related disorders in children and adolescents: Developmental considerations. *Psychiatry, 75,* 243–266.

Kaplow, J. B., Layne, C. M., Saltzman, W. R., Cozza, S. J., & Pynoos, R. S. (2013). Using multidimensional grief theory to explore effects of deployment, reintegration, and death on military youth and families. *Clinical Child and Family Psychology Review, 16,* 322–340.

Kaplow, J. B., Rolon-Arroyo, B., Layne, C. M., Rooney, E., Oosterhoff, B., Hill, R., . . . Pynoos, R. S. (2019). Validation of the UCLA PTSD Reaction Index for DSM-5 (RI-5): A developmentally-informed assessment tool for trauma-exposed youth. *Journal of the American Academy of Child and Adolescent Psychiatry.* [Epub ahead of print]

Kaplow, J. B., Saunders, J., Angold, A., & Costello, E. J. (2010). Psychiatric symptoms in bereaved versus nonbereaved youth and young adults: A longitudinal epidemiological study. *Journal of the American Academy of Child and Adolescent Psychiatry, 49,* 1145–1154.

Kennedy, B., Chen, R., Valdimarsdóttir, U., Montgomery, S., Fang, F., & Fall, K. (2018). Childhood bereavement and lower stress resilience in late adolescence. *Journal of Adolescent Health, 63,* 108–114.

Kerig, P. K. (2014). For better or worse: Intimate relationships as sources of risk or resilience for girls' delinquency. *Journal of Research on Adolescence, 24,* 1–11.

Kerig, P., Chaplo, S., Bennett, D., & Modrowski, C. (2016). "Harm as harm"—Gang membership, perpetration trauma, and posttraumatic stress symptoms among youth in the juvenile justice system. *Criminal Justice and Behavior, 43,* 635–652.

Kessler, R. C. (2017). *National Comorbidity Survey: Adolescent Supplement (NCS-A), 2001–2004.* Ann Arbor, MI: Inter-university Consortium for Political and Social Research.

Keyes, K. M., Pratt, C., Galea, S., McLaughlin, K. A.,

Koenen, K. C., & Shear, M. K. (2014). The burden of loss: Unexpected death of a loved one and psychiatric disorders across the life course in a national study. *American Journal of Psychiatry, 171*, 864–871.

Killikelly, C., & Maercker, A. (2017). Prolonged grief disorder for ICD-11: The primacy of clinical utility and international applicability. *European Journal of Psychotraumatology, 8*(Suppl. 6), 1476441.

Ko, S. J., Ford, J. D., Kassam-Adams, N., Berkowitz, S. J., Wilson, C., Wong, M., . . . Layne, C. M. (2008). Creating trauma-informed systems: Child welfare, education, first responders, health care, juvenile justice. *Professional Psychology: Research and Practice, 39*, 396–404.

Kraemer, H. C. (1992). *Evaluating medical tests: Objective and quantitative guidelines*. Newbury Park, CA: SAGE.

Kristensen, P., Weisæth, L., & Heir, T. (2012). Bereavement and mental health after sudden and violent losses: A review. *Psychiatry, 75*, 76–97.

Lambert, M. J. (2010). *Prevention of treatment failure: The use of measuring, monitoring, and feedback in clinical practice*. Washington, DC: American Psychological Association.

Layne, C. M., Briggs-King, E., & Courtois, C. (2014). Introduction to the Special Section: Unpacking risk factor caravans across development: Findings from the NCTSN Core Data Set. *Psychological Trauma: Theory, Research, Practice, and Policy, 6*(Suppl. 1), S1–S8.

Layne, C. M., Greeson, J. K. P., Kim, S., Ostrowski, S. A., Reading, S., Vivrette, R. L., . . . Pynoos, R. S. (2014). Links between trauma exposure and adolescent high-risk health behaviors: Findings from the NCTSN Core Data Set. *Psychological Trauma: Theory, Research, Practice, and Policy, 6*(Suppl. 1), S40–S49.

Layne, C. M., & Hobfoll, S. E. (2020). Understanding posttraumatic adjustment trajectories in school-age youth: Supporting stress resistance, resilient recovery, and growth. In E. Rossen (Ed.), *Supporting and educating traumatized students: A guide for school-based professionals* (2nd ed., pp. 75–97). New York: Oxford University Press.

Layne, C. M., Kaplow, J. B., Oosterhoff, B., & Hill, R. (2019, June). *Developmental perspectives on DSM-5-TR prolonged grief disorder criteria: Proposals for improvement*. Invited presentation at the Workshop on Developing Criteria for a Disorder of Pathological Grieving for DSM 5-TR, American Psychiatric Association, New York.

Layne, C. M., Kaplow, J. B., Oosterhoff, B., Hill, R., & Pynoos, R. S. (2017). The interplay between posttraumatic stress and grief reactions in traumatically bereaved adolescents: When trauma, bereavement, and adolescence converge. *Adolescent Psychiatry, 7*, 220–239.

Layne, C. M., Kaplow, J. B., & Pynoos, R. S. (2014). *Persistent Complex Bereavement Disorder (PCBD) Checklist—Youth Version 1.0: Test and administration manual*. Los Angeles: UCLA.

Layne, C. M., Kaplow, J. B., & Youngstrom, E. A. (2017). Applying evidence-based assessment to childhood trauma and bereavement: Concepts, principles, and practices. In M. A. Landholt, M. Cloitre, & U. Schnyder (Eds.), *Evidence based treatments for trauma-related disorders in children and adolescents* (pp. 67–96). Cham, Switzerland: Springer.

Layne, C. M., Olsen, J. A., Baker, A. Legerski, J. P., Isakson, B., Pašalić, A., . . ., & Pynoos, R. S. (2010). Unpacking trauma exposure risk factors and differential pathways of influence: Predicting post-war mental distress in Bosnian adolescents. *Child Development, 81*, 1053–1076.

Layne, C. M., Oosterhoff, B., Pynoos, R. S., & Kaplow, J. B. (2020, February). *Developmental Analysis of Draft DSM 5-TR criteria for prolonged grief disorder: Report from the Child and Adolescent Bereavement Subgroup*. Report submitted to the Panel on Developing Criteria for a Disorder of Pathological Grieving for DSM 5-TR, American Psychiatric Association.

Layne, C. M., Pynoos, R. S., & Cardenas, J. (2001). Wounded adolescence: School-based group psychotherapy for adolescents who sustained or witnessed violent interpersonal injury. In M. Shafii & S. Shafii (Eds.), *School violence: Contributing factors, management, and prevention* (pp. 163–186). Washington, DC: American Psychiatric Press.

Layne, C. M., Pynoos, R., & Griffin, D. (2019). *Trauma and development: Part 1. How to think development*. Los Angeles, CA, and Durham, NC: UCLA/Duke University National Center for Child Traumatic Stress. Retrieved from *https://learn.nctsn.org/course/view.php?id=94*.

Layne, C. M., Saltzman, W. R., Poppleton, L., Burlingame, G. M., Pašalić, A. Duraković-Belko, E., . . . Pynoos, R. S. (2008). Effectiveness of a school-based group psychotherapy program for war-exposed adolescents: A randomized controlled trial. *Journal of the American Academy of Child and Adolescent Psychiatry, 47*, 1048–1062.

Layne, C. M., Steinberg, J. R., & Steinberg, A. M. (2014). Causal reasoning skills training for mental health practitioners: Promoting sound clinical judgment in evidence-based practice. *Training and Education in Professional Psychology, 8*, 292–302.

Layne, C. M., Warren, J. S., Hilton, S., Lin, D., Pasalic, A., Fulton, J., . . . Pynoos, R. S. (2009). Measuring adolescent perceived support amidst war and disaster: The Multi-Sector Social Support Inventory. In B. K. Barber (Ed.), *Adolescents and war: How youth deal with political violence* (pp. 145–176). New York: Oxford University Press.

Layne, C. M., Warren, J. S., Saltzman, W. R., Fulton, J., Steinberg, A. M., & Pynoos, R. S. (2006). Contextual influences on post-traumatic adjustment: Retraumatization and the roles of distressing reminders, secondary adversities, and revictimization. In L. A. Schein, H. I. Spitz, G. M. Burlingame, & P. R. Muskin (Eds.), *Group approaches for the psychological effects of terrorist disasters* (pp. 235–286). New York: Haworth.

Lau, A. S., & Weisz, J. R. (2003). Reported maltreatment among clinic-referred children: Implications for presenting problems, treatment attrition, and long-term outcomes. *Journal of the American Academy of Child and Adolescent Psychiatry, 42,* 1327–1334.

Lee, S. A. (2015). The Persistent Complex Bereavement Inventory: A measure based on the DSM-5. *Death Studies, 39,* 399–410.

Li, J., Hansen, D., Mortensen, P. B., & Olsen, J. (2002). Myocardial infarction in parents who lost a child: A nationwide prospective cohort study in Denmark. *Circulation, 106*(13), 1634–1639.

Li, J., Johansen, C., Hansen, D., & Olsen, J. (2002). Cancer incidence in parents who lost a child. *Cancer, 95,* 2237–2242.

Li, J., Laursen, T. M., Precht, D. H., Olsen, J., & Mortensen, P. B. (2005). Hospitalization for mental illness among parents after the death of a child. *New England Journal of Medicine, 352*(12), 1190–1196.

Li, J., Precht, D. H., Mortensen, P. B., & Olsen, J. (2003). Mortality in parents after death of a child in Denmark: A nationwide follow-up study. *The Lancet, 361,* 363–367.

Li, J., Vestergaard, M., Cnattingius, S., Gissler, M., Bech, B. H., Obel, C., & Olsen, J. (2014). Mortality after parental death in childhood: A nationwide cohort study from three Nordic countries. *PlOS Medicine, 11*(7), e1001679.

Mack, K. Y. (2001). Childhood family disruptions and adult well-being: The differential effects of divorce and parental death. *Death Studies, 25,* 419–443.

Makary, M. A., & Daniel, M. (2016). Medical error—the third leading cause of death in the US. *British Medical Journal, 353,* i2139.

McCormick, C. M., Kuo, S. I-C., & Masten, A. S. (2011). Developmental tasks across the lifespan. In K. L. Fingerman, C. A. Berg, J. Smith, & T. C. Antonucci (Eds.), *Handbook of lifespan development* (pp. 117–140). New York: Springer.

McGee, S. (2002). Simplifying likelihood ratios. *Journal of General Internal Medicine, 17,* 646–649.

Merikangas, K. R., He, J. P., Brody, D., Fisher, P. W., Bourdon, K., & Koretz, D. S. (2010). Prevalence and treatment of mental disorders among US children in the 2001–2004 NHANES. *Pediatrics, 125,* 75–81.

Merikangas, K. R., He, J. P., Burstein, M., Swanson, S. A., Avenevoli, S., Cui, L., . . . Swendsen, J. (2010). Lifetime prevalence of mental disorders in U.S. adolescents: Results from the National Comorbidity Survey Replication—Adolescent Supplement (NCS-A). *Journal of the American Academy of Child and Adolescent Psychiatry, 49,* 980–989.

Moffitt, T. E., Arseneault, L., Belsky, D., Dickson, N., Hancox, R. J., Harrington, H., . . . Caspi, A. (2011). A gradient of childhood self-control predicts health, wealth, and public safety. *Proceedings of the National Academy of Sciences of the USA, 108,* 2693–2698.

Mosher, P. J. (2018). Everywhere and nowhere: Grief in child and adolescent psychiatry and pediatric clinical populations. *Child and Adolescent Psychiatric Clinics of North America, 27,* 109–124.

Mueser, K. T., & Taub, J. (2008). Trauma and PTSD among adolescents with severe emotional disorders involved in multiple service systems. *Psychiatric Services, 59,* 627–634.

Murphy, S. L., Xu, J. Q., Kochanek, K. D., & Arias, E. (2018). *Mortality in the United States, 2017* (NCHS Data Brief No. 328). Hyattsville, MD: National Center for Health Statistics.

National Center for Statistics and Analysis. (2017, October). *Alcohol impaired driving: 2016 data* (Traffic Safety Facts Report No. DOT HS 812 450). Washington, DC: National Highway Traffic Safety Administration.

Norcross, J. C., & Wampold, B. E. (2011). What works for whom: Tailoring psychotherapy to the person. *Journal of Clinical Psychology, 67,* 127–132.

Oosterhoff, B., Kaplow, J. B., & Layne, C. M. (2018). Links between bereavement due to sudden death and academic functioning: Results from a nationally representative sample of adolescents. *School Psychology Quarterly, 33,* 372–380.

Posner, K., Brown, G. K., Stanley, B., Brent, D. A., Yershova, K. V., Oquendo, M. A., . . . Mann, J. J. (2011). The Columbia-Suicide Severity Rating Scale: Initial validity and internal consistency findings from three multisite studies with adolescents and adults. *American Journal of Psychiatry, 168,* 1266–1277.

Pynoos, R., & Steinberg, A. M. (2017). *The UCLA PTSD Reaction Index for DSM-5.* Los Angeles: Department of Psychiatry and Biobehavioral Sciences, University of California, Los Angeles.

Pynoos, R., Steinberg, A. M., Layne, C. M., Liang, L.-J., Vivrette, R. L., Briggs, E. C., . . . Fairbank, J. (2014). Modeling constellations of trauma exposure in the National Child Traumatic Stress Network Core Data Set. *Psychological Trauma: Theory, Research, Practice, and Policy, 6,* S9–S17.

Pynoos, R., Steinberg, A., & Wraith, R. (1995). A developmental psychopathology model of childhood traumatic stress. In D. Cicchetti & D. J. Cohen (Eds.), *Manual of developmental psychopathology* (Vol. 2, pp. 72–95). New York: Wiley.

Pynoos, R., Weathers, S. W., Steinberg, A. M., Marx, B. P., Layne, C. M., Kaloupek, D. G., . . . Kriegler, J. A. (2015). *Clinician-Administered PTSD Scale for DSM-5 Child/Adolescent Version (CAPS-CA-5).* Washington, DC: National Center for PTSD.

Redfield, R. (2018, November 29). CDC Director's Media Statement on U.S. Life Expectancy. Retrieved from *www.cdc.gov/media/releases/2018/s1129-us-life-expectancy.html.*

Rogers, C. H., Floyd, F. J., Seltzer, M. M., Greenberg, J., & Hong, J. (2008). Long-term effects of the death of a child on parents' adjustment in midlife. *Journal of Family Psychology, 22*(2), 203–211.

Rolon-Arroyo, B., Arnold, D. H., Breaux, R. P., & Harvey, E. A. (2018). Reciprical relations between parenting behaviors and conduct disorder symptoms in preschool children. *Child Psychiatry and Human Development, 49,* 786–799.

Rostila, M., Berg, L., Arat, A., Vinnerljung, B., & Hjern, A. (2016). Parental death in childhood and self-inflicted injuries in young adults—a national cohort study from Sweden. *European Child and Adolescent Psychiatry, 25,* 1103–1111.

Rostila, M., Saarela, J., & Kawachi, I. (2011). Mortality in parents following the death of a child: A nationwide follow-up study from Sweden. *Journal of Epidemiology and Community Health, 66,* 927–933.

Saltzman, W. R., Layne, C. M., Pynoos, R. S., Olafson, E., Kaplow, J. B., & Boat, B. (2017). *Trauma and grief component therapy for adolescents: A modular approach to treating traumatized and bereaved youth.* Cambridge, UK: Cambridge University Press.

Saltzman, W. R., Pynoos, R. S., Lester, P., Beardslee, W. R., & Layne, C. M. (2013). Enhancing military family resilience through family narrative co-construction. *Clinical Child and Family Psychology Review, 16,* 294–310.

Schoenfelder, E., Sandler, I., Wolchik, S., & MacKinnon, D. (2011). Quality of social relationships and the development of depression in parentally-bereaved youth. *Journal of Youth and Adolescence, 40,* 85–96.

Shapiro, D. N., Howell, K. H., & Kaplow, J. B. (2014). Associations among mother–child communication quality, childhood maladaptive grief, and depressive symptoms. *Death Studies, 38,* 172–178.

Shear, M. K. (2015). Complicated grief. *New England Journal of Medicine, 372,* 153–160.

Silva, R. R., Alpert, M., Munoz, D. M., Singh, S., Matzner, F., & Dummit, S. (2000). Stress and vulnerability to posttraumatic stress disorder in children and adolescents. *American Journal of Psychiatry, 157,* 1229–1235.

Smith, A. J., Layne, C. M., Coyle, P., Kaplow, J., Brymer, M., Pynoos, R. S., & Jones, R. T. (2017). Predicting grief reactions one year following a mass university shooting: Evaluating dose–response and contextual predictors. *Violence and Victims, 32,* 1024–1043.

Spuij, M., Reitz, E., Prinzie, P., Stikkelbroek, Y., de Roos, C., & Boelen, P. A. (2012). Distinctiveness of symptoms of prolonged grief, depression, and posttraumatic stress in bereaved children and adolescents. *European Child and Adolescent Psychiatry, 21,* 673–679.

Steinberg, L. (2014). *The age of opportunity: Lessons from the new science of adolescence.* New York: Harcourt.

Straus, S. E., Glasziou, P., Richardson, W. S., & Haynes, R. B. (2019). *Evidence-based medicine: How to practice and teach EBM* (5th ed.). New York: Elsevier.

Suppiger, A., In-Albon, T., Hendriksen, S., Hermann, E., Margraf, J., & Schneider, S. (2009). Acceptance of structured diagnostic interviews for mental disorders in clinical practice and research settings. *Behavior Therapy, 40,* 272–279.

Teicher, M. H., Tomoda, A., & Andersen, S. L. (2006). Neurobiological consequences of early stress and childhood maltreatment: Are results from human and animal studies comparable? *Annals of the New York Academy of Sciences, 1071,* 313–323.

Thompson, M. P., Kaslow, N. J., Price, A. W., Williams, K., & Kingree, J. B. (1998). Role of secondary stressors in the parental death–child distress relation. *Journal of Abnormal Child Psychology, 26*(5), 357–366.

Thompson, M. P., & Light, L. S. (2011). Examining gender differences in risk factors for suicide attempts made 1 and 7 years later in a nationally representative sample. *Journal of Adolescent Health, 48*(4), 391–397.

Tingey, R., Lambert, M., Burlingame, G., & Hansen, N. (1996). Assessing clinical significance: Proposed extensions to method. *Psychotherapy Research, 6,* 109–123.

Umberson, D. (2017). Black deaths matter: Race, relationship loss, and effects on survivors. *Journal of Health and Social Behavior, 58,* 405–420.

Umberson, D., Donnelly, R. E., & Farina, M. (2018). Race, life course exposure to death of a family member, and health. *Innovation in Aging, 2*(Suppl. 1), 336.

Umberson, D., Donnelly, R., Xu, M., Farina, M., & Garcia, M. A. (2019). Death of a child prior to midlife, dementia risk, and racial disparities. *Journal of Gerontology: Social Sciences.* [Epub ahead of print]

Umberson, D., Olson, J. S., Crosnoe, R., Liu, H., Pudrovska, T., & Donnelly, R. (2017). Death of family members as an overlooked source of racial disadvantage in the United States. *Proceedings of the National Academy of Sciences of the USA, 114,* 915–920.

UNICEF (2017, June 16). Orphans [Press release]. Retrieved from *www.unicef.org/media/media_45279. html.*

U.S. Department of Education Office for Civil Rights. (2018). 2015–16 Civil Rights Data Collection, School Climate and Safety.

Van der Houwen, K., Stroebe, M., Stroebe, W., Schut, H., van den Bout, J., & Wijngaards-De Mej, L. (2010). Risk factors for bereavement outcome: A multivariate approach. *Death Studies, 34,* 195–220.

von Sydow, K., Lieb, R., Pfister, H., Höfler, M., & Wittchen, H. (2002). What predicts incident use of cannabis and progression to abuse and dependence?: A 4-year prospective examination of risk factors in a community sample of adolescents and young adults. *Drug and Alcohol Dependence, 68,* 49–64.

Wagner, B., & Maercker, A. (2010). The diagnosis of complicated grief as a mental disorder: A critical appraisal. *Psychologica Belgica, 50,* 27–48.

Walker, L. S., Beck, J. E., Garber, J., & Lambert, W. (2009). Children's Somatization Inventory: Psychometric properties of the Revised Form (CSI-24). *Journal of Pediatric Psychology, 34,* 430–440.

Wardecker, B. M., Kaplow, J. B., Layne, C. M., & Edelstein, R. S. (2017). Caregivers' positive emotional expression and children's psychological functioning after parental loss. *Journal of Child and Family Studies, 26,* 3490–3501.

Wardecker, B. M., Kaplow, J. B., Layne, C. M., & Edelstein, R. S. (2017). Caregivers' positive emotional expression and children's psychological functioning after parental loss. *Journal of Child and Family Studies, 26*, 3490–3501.

Weisz, J. R., Chorpita, B. F., Frye, A., Ng, M. Y., Lau, N., Bearman, S. K., . . . Hoagwood, K. E. (2011). Youth Top Problems: Using idiographic, consumer-guided assessment to identify treatment needs and to track change during psychotherapy. *Journal of Consulting and Clinical Psychology, 79*, 369–380.

Wilcox, H., Kuramoto, S., Lichtenstein, P., Långström, N., Brent, D., & Runeson, B. (2010). Psychiatric morbidity, violent crime, and suicide among children and adolescents exposed to parental death. *Journal of the American Academy of Child and Adolescent Psychiatry, 49*, 514–523.

Worden, W., & Silverman, P. (1996). Parental death and the adjustment of school aged children. *Omega, 33*, 91–102.

World Health Organziation. (2018). *International classification of diseases for mortality and morbidity statistics* (11th rev.). Geneva, Switzerland: Author.

Youngstrom, E. A. (2013). Future directions in psychological assessment: Combining evidence-based medicine innovations with psychology's historical strengths to enhance utility. *Journal of Clinical Child and Adolescent Psychology, 42*, 139–159.

Youngstrom, E. A. (2014). A primer on receiver operating characteristic analysis and diagnostic efficiency statistics for pediatric psychology: We are ready to ROC. *Journal of Pediatric Psychology, 39*, 204–221.

Youngstrom, E. A., Choukas-Bradley, S., Calhoun, C. D., & Jensen-Doss, A. (2014). Clinical guide to the evidence-based assessment approach to diagnosis and treatment. *Cognitive and Behavioral Practice, 22*, 20–35.

Youngstrom, E. A., & Frazier, T. W. (2013). Evidence-based strategies for the assessment of children and adolescents: Measuring prediction, prescription, and process. In D. J. Miklowitz, W. E. Craighead, & L. Craighead (Eds.), *Developmental psychopathology* (2nd ed., pp. 36–79). New York: Wiley.

Youngstrom, E. A., Jenkins, M. M., Jensen-Doss, A., & Youngstrom, J. K. (2012). Evidence-based assessment strategies for pediatric bipolar disorder. *Israel Journal of Psychiatry and Related Sciences, 49*, 15–27.

Youngstrom, E. A., Van Meter, A., Frazier, T. W., Hunsley, J., Prinstein, M. J., Ong, M.-L., & Youngstrom, J. K. (2017). Evidence-based assessment as an integrative model for applying psychological science to guide the voyage of treatment. *Clinical Psychology: Science and Practice, 24*, 331–363.

Yu, Y., Liew, Z., Cnattingius, S., Olsen, J., Vestergaard, M., Fu, B., . . . Li, J. (2017). Association of mortality with the death of a sibling in childhood. *Journal of the American Medical Association Pediatrics, 171*, 538–545.

CHAPTER 18

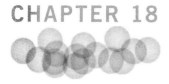

Child Maltreatment

Helen M. Milojevich and Vicky Veitch Wolfe

The study of child maltreatment, begun in earnest in the 1970s, is a relative latecomer in the field of childhood psychopathology. However, since that time, tremendous gains have been made in our understanding of this serious problem. The growing recognition of the extent of child maltreatment and concern about its lifelong effects have led to significant changes in law, social work, education, and mental health. Indeed, there is even evidence that our increased knowledge and efforts toward recognition, prevention, and intervention have led to overall reductions in the prevalence of several forms of maltreatment, including child sexual abuse and physical abuse (Finkelhor, 2008). The professions of psychology and the behavioral sciences have made enormous contributions toward understanding of the effects of child maltreatment and have led to great improvements in assessment, prevention, and treatment of maltreated children

and adolescents, and their families. These advancements have moved the field forward from the initial need to document and describe child maltreatment to advancements in understanding the specific ways that maltreatment affects children and results in psychological processes that often lead to lifelong adjustment difficulties.

We review in this chapter current issues related to child maltreatment, with the general assumption that from our core bases of knowledge, assessment methodology will grow. The chapter consists of four main parts: (1) an epidemiological overview of the problem of child maltreatment, including prevalence and incidence, characteristics of the abuse and perpetrators, child victims, their families, and communities, as well as a basic assessment kit to serve as a starting point for clinicians; (2) an in-depth review of assessment strategies and tools that have been developed especially for maltreatment victims and their families, and factors that attenuate and exacerbate the effects of maltreatment; (3) an overview of the impact of maltreatment on children and adolescents, and how the impact relates to assessment and treatment; and (4) an overview of how assessment informs diagnosis and treatment planning. Drawing from extant evidence-based methods, we make practical suggestions for clinical assessments. Of note, although we present assessments that cover a range of maltreatment subtypes, throughout the chapter, we emphasize child sexual abuse, as it is particularly difficult to assess clinically; therefore, clinicians may need extra scaffolding in the assessment of this form of maltreatment.

Background and "Starter Kit"

Definition of Child Maltreatment

In contrast to other chapters in this volume, this chapter focuses on a complex life experience—child maltreatment—and not on a diagnosis or disorder. *Child maltreatment* refers to all forms of abuse and neglect of a child under age 18 years by a parent, caregiver, or another person in a custodial role (Centers for Disease Control and Prevention, 2019). There are four primary subtypes of child maltreatment, including child sexual abuse (CSA), child physical abuse (CPA), neglect, and emotional abuse. Broadly speaking, CSA refers to sexual contact with a child that occurs under one of the following circumstances: "(1) when a large age or maturational difference exists between the partners; (2) when the partner is in a position of authority over or in a care-taking relationship with the child; (3) when the acts are carried out against the child by using violence or trickery" (Finkelhor, 1984, p. 101). A wide array of behaviors falls under the umbrella term *CSA*, including acts such as intercourse, oral–genital contact, fondling, exhibitionism or exposing children to adult sexual activity or pornography, and use of a child for prostitution or pornography.

Regarding the other subtypes of maltreatment, CPA refers to the intentional use of physical force against a child that results in, or has the potential to result in, physical injury (Leeb, Paulozzi, Melanson, Simon, & Arias, 2008). Examples include hitting, kicking, shaking, burning, or other shows of force against a child. Exposure to *neglect* is generally divided into two forms: failure to provide and failure to supervise. *Failure to provide* refers to failure by a caregiver to meet a child's basic physical, emotional, medical/dental, or educational needs—or combination thereof (Barnett, Manly, & Cicchetti, 1993). *Failure to supervise*, on the other hand, refers to failure by the caregiver to ensure a child's safety within and outside the home given the child's emotional and developmental needs. Finally, *emotional abuse*, also referred to as *psychological abuse*, is defined as "intentional caregiver behavior that conveys to a child that he/she is worthless, flawed, unloved, unwanted, endangered, or valued only in meeting another's needs"

(Leeb et al., 2008, p. 14). Emotional abuse includes behaviors such as blaming, belittling, intimidating, terrorizing, isolating, or otherwise behaving in ways that are harmful, potentially harmful, or insensitive to the child's developmental needs, or that can potentially damage the child psychologically or emotionally (Barnett, Manly, & Cicchetti, 1991).

Given the range of commission and omission acts that fall under the broad term of "child maltreatment," it is perhaps not surprising that maltreatment is associated with a host of outcomes, some specific to the abuse or neglect and others related more indirectly to the broader environmental context surrounding child maltreatment. Moreover, the specifics of the maltreatment exposure (e.g., type of maltreatment, age of the child, gender of the perpetrator, the number and frequency of the maltreatment experiences) all seem to exert some influence on these outcomes (Dunn, Nishimi, Powers, & Bradley, 2017; Lunkenheimer, Busuito, Brown, & Skowron, 2018; Manly, Kim, Rogosch, & Cicchetti, 2001; Putnam, 2003). As such, children exposed to maltreatment are an extremely heterogeneous group for whom few broad generalizations hold.

Prevalence

In 2017, approximately 3.5 million children were the subjects of at least one report to Child Protective Services (CPS) for suspected child maltreatment in the United States alone (U.S. Department of Health and Human Services [DHHS], 2019). Of those 3.5 million children, 17% were classified as victims with substantiated or indicated exposure to some form of abuse or neglect, while most of the remaining children received an alternative response. Nationally, in 2017, an estimated 674,000 victims of child maltreatment made the overall victim rate 9.1 victims per 1,000 children in the population. Broken down by maltreatment subtype, roughly 75% are neglected, 18% are physically abused, and 9% are sexually abused, with 7% having exposure to some other form of maltreatment. The same child can get counted in more than one category, and neglect plus physical abuse is the most common combination, affecting 5% of the cases. Demographically, children under age 1 year have the highest rate of victimization at 25.3 per 1,000 children of the same age in the national population. Other estimates indicate that approximately 13% of all U.S. children will experience a *confirmed* case of maltreatment by 18 years of age (Wildeman et al., 2014). Importantly, wide discrepancies exist in estimates of child maltreatment based on informant type, with official agency reports estimating far fewer victims than parent or self-reports (Gilbert et al., 2009). In fact, one study indicated that only 5% of children exposed to physical abuse and 8% of children who have been sexually abused come in contact with CPS (MacMillan, Jamieson, & Walsh, 2003).

For CSA, estimates range from 8 to 31% for girls and from 3 to 17% for boys worldwide (Barth, Bermetz, Heim, Trelle, & Tonia, 2013). Prevalence rates vary considerably depending on how sexual abuse is defined. For instance, studies that include noncontact forms of abuse and abuse by peers tend to yield high abuse estimates (Goldman & Padayachi, 2000). Due to the complicating factor of adolescent consensual sexual activity, definitions for adolescents tend to vary regarding the upper age limited considered as abuse, the age difference required between the victim and offender for non-coercive sexual contacts (typically increased to 10 years), and the ways that coercion and abuse of authority are defined. Survey questions about sexual abuse also vary across studies. Some studies include a general question about sexual abuse history as a gate to asking more detailed questions, sometimes using vague terms such as "unwanted sexual touching," whereas others ask about history of specific acts, without necessarily defining the acts as sexual abuse. The latter method tends to yield higher estimates of abuse because some respondents may not consider their experiences as abusive (e.g., young males abused by older females). Research suggests an advantage of more inclusive definitions when studying the impact of abuse because more victims who are affected by abuse are included (Long & Jackson, 1990).

Based on a review of 19 studies of adult retrospective reports of childhood experiences, Finkelhor (1994) concluded that approximately 20% of women and 5–10% of men had at least one episode of sexual abuse during their childhood. More recent studies yield similar estimates (Barth et al., 2013; Pereda, Guilera, Forns, & Gómez-Benito, 2009; Stoltenborgh, van IJzendoorn, Euser, & Bakermans-Kranenburg, 2011). A large-scale study of over 34,000 adults from a large, U.S., representative sample revealed a prevalence rate of child sexual abuse prior to age 18 of 10.14% (Pérez-Fuentes et al., 2013). Of that approximate 10%, 75.2% were women and 24.8% were men. In another large-scale, population-based study (N = 2,293), Finkelhor, Shattuck, Turner, and Hamby (2014)

found that, by age 17, the lifetime experience of sexual abuse was 26.6% for girls and 5.1% for boys. Of note, for girls, considerable risk for sexual abuse and assault was concentrated in late adolescence, as the rate rose from 16.8% for 15-year-old girls to 26.6% for 17-year-old girls. Although some have suggested that epidemiological studies overestimate prevalence, most studies indicate that even in anonymous studies, individuals tend to under-report CSA by at least 16–50% (Fergusson, Woodward, & Horwood, 2000; Goodman et al., 2003; Greenhoot, McCloskey, & Gisky, 2005; Widom & Morris, 1997; Williams, 1994). Overall, these statistics reveal that sexual victimization is higher among youth compared to adults. Indeed, Hashimi and Finkelhor (1999) reported that rates of abuse of adolescents ages 12–17 were 2.0–3.3 times higher than rates for young adults ages 18–24.

Incidence data reflect the number of cases made known to public agencies during a specified period of time. Incidence data grossly underestimate true rates of child maltreatment because most cases are never reported to official agencies. However, in addition to providing information about agency-reported maltreatment, incidence data may be used to detect epidemiological trends, including rates of disclosure to official agencies. Compared to prevalence studies, data on incidence rates of child maltreatment are relatively rare. Retrospective surveys estimate that between 5 and 12.0% of child maltreatment cases are reported to police or other authorities (MacMillan et al., 1997, 2003; Saunders, Villeponteaux, Lipovsky, Kilpatrick, & Veronen, 1992). However, Finkelhor (1994), combining prevalence and incidence estimates, calculated that approximately 30% of sexual abuse, for instance, is disclosed to official agencies during childhood. In some cases, abuse is disclosed to parents and peers but not to official agencies. Data from the National Survey of Adolescents, which included 1,958 girls ages 12–17 years, revealed that 48% of sexual abuse victims had disclosed their abuse to an adult, and an additional 25% had disclosed to a peer (Kogan, 2004). Hanson, Resnick, Saunders, Kilpatrick, and Best (1999), also reporting data from the National Survey of Adolescents, found that only half of those who disclosed their abuse to a relative, friend, or other confidant had also made a disclosure to an official agency. More recent data suggest that disclosure to authorities is relatively rare in cases of CSA. For example, in a sample of almost 2,000 Swedish adolescents who had experienced CSA, less than 7% had reported the abuse to official agencies (Priebe & Svedin,

2008). Moreover, upon reviewing the literature on disclosure, London, Bruck, Ceci, and Shuman (2013) concluded that only a small minority of CSA victims report their abuse to authorities during childhood.

Evidence based on both incidence and prevalence data suggests a decrease in most forms of child maltreatment during the past three decades. Findings from the Fourth National Incidence Study of Child Abuse and Neglect (NIS-4; Sedlak et al., 2010) indicated that the estimated number of sexually abused children decreased from 217,700 in 1993 to 135,300 in 2005–2006 (a 38% decrease in the number of sexually abused children and a 44% decrease in the rate of sexual abuse). Similarly, the rates of CPA and emotional abuse decreased 23 and 33%, respectively. Moreover, data from the National Child Abuse and Neglect Data System (NCANDS), which aggregates and publishes statistics from state child protection agencies, suggest that sexual abuse declined 6%, physical abuse declined 3%, and neglect declined 2% from 2007 to 2008 (Finkelhor, Jones, & Shattuck, 2010). Even more striking, reports of child maltreatment to official agencies decreased significantly from 1992 to 2008 (58% for CSA, 55% for CPA, and 10% for neglect). For CSA in particular, 1990 U.S. statistics indicated that sexual abuse cases comprised 17% of all confirmed or validated reports of maltreatment, whereas in 2004, CSA accounted for only 9.7% of reported maltreatment cases (DHHS, 2004; Sedlak & Broadhurst, 1996). Although there is some evidence that declines in incidence rates were in part due to changes in CPS procedures, verification, and recording methods, other evidence indicates that the trend appears to reflect actual declines in maltreatment. Positive effects of prevention programs, public awareness campaigns, and increased prosecution likely contribute to the decline (Finkelhor et al., 2010). Finkelhor and Jones (2004) argued that societal deterrents against sexual abuse have been particularly effective. Between 1986 and 1997, the number of persons incarcerated for sex crimes against children doubled (Finkelhor & Ormrod, 2001), and these data did not include the increased number of offenders who received nonincarceration penalties following sexual abuse charges (e.g., probation). Citing data collected in Illinois and Pennsylvania, Finkelhor and Jones highlighted significant declines in sexual abuse cases involving fathers. They argued that biological fathers, who may be the least compulsive of CSA offender types, may

be particularly deterred by the possibility of detection and prosecution.

Starter Kit

Numerous assessments of child maltreatment exist, including reports from caregivers and children, as well as information gleaned from official records. Although we describe many of these assessments in detail later in this chapter, here we highlight a potential "starter kit" of assessments as examples of commonly used, psychometrically sound rating scales and interviews that may be used to evaluate clients. We assume that your clinic is already using a broad assessment measure, such as the Achenbach System of Empirically Based Assessment (Achenbach & Rescorla, 2001), or the Behavior Assessment Scales for Children (Reynolds & Kamphaus, 2015). Surprisingly, most of these do not ask about traumatic events or abuse, focusing instead on behavior. Therefore, we recommend that a "starter kit" supplement them with an exposure measure and have a posttraumatic stress disorder (PTSD) measure available as well for follow-up (also see La Greca & Danzi, Chapter 15, this volume). Specifically, we recommend the brief version of the Traumatic Events Screening Inventory–Parent Report Revised (TESI-PRR; Ippen et al., 2002); the Childhood Trauma Questionnaire (CTQ; Bernstein et al., 1994), and the Trauma Symptoms Checklist for Young Children (TSCYC; Briere et al., 2001).

First, regarding exposure measures, the TESI-PRR is a 25-item instrument. The Parent Report version is designed to be completed by parents as a questionnaire or to be given as a semistructured interview to determine the exposure history of children to traumatic events (Ippen et al., 2002). Caregivers are presented with 24 potentially traumatic events and asked to respond (*yes, no, unsure*) to indicate whether the child has had exposure to these events. Events include sexual abuse, as well as physical abuse, domestic violence, community violence, accidents and injuries, and natural disasters. There is a structured interview version of the TESI for children ranging in age from 4 to 18 years. The TESI versions are free, and copies are available on Wikiversity.

Another well-designed option is the CTQ, a 70-item, Likert-like inventory that yields five subscales: Emotional Abuse, Physical Abuse, Emotional Neglect, Sexual Abuse, and Physical Neglect (Bernstein & Fink, 1998; Bernstein et al.,

1994). Although originally developed for adults, it has been used with youth as young as age 12 years and has demonstrated good sensitivity and specificity with known maltreatment information (Bernstein, Ahluvalia, Pogge, & Handelsman, 1997). Bernstein and colleagues (2003) have also created a shortened, 28-item version of the CTQ that demonstrates good convergent and discriminant validity. The CTQ is commercially distributed by Pearson.

The Stressful Life Events Screening Questionnaire—Revised (SLESQ-R), a free option that covers exposure (Goodman, Corcora, Turner, Yuan, & Green, 1998), has 13 items with multiple parts, including questions about sexual and physical abuse, as well as violence exposure and other potentially traumatic events. It is freely available, and also on Wikiversity.

To assess PTSD and other trauma-related symptoms in children, we recommend the TSCYC, which is a 90-item caregiver-report measure commercially distributed by Psychological Assessment Resources. As we discuss later in this chapter, CSA and other forms of child maltreatment place children at increased risk of a range of behavioral and mental health problems. Thus, when beginning to work with a client suspected of having experienced sexual abuse, it is crucial to assess not only his or her potential trauma exposure but also trauma-related symptoms that may need to be addressed during treatment. The TSCYC yields information about eight potential domains of symptoms: PTSD, anxiety, depression, anger, and abnormal sexual behavior. Of note, the TSCYC demonstrates psychometric strengths and has been studied extensively within a sexual abuse population (Pollio, Glover-Orr, & Wherry, 2008; Wherry, Corson, & Hunsaker, 2013; Wherry, Graves, & Rhodes King, 2008). A free, much shorter alternative is the Child PTSD Symptom Scale (CPSS-5; Foa, Asnaani, Zang, Capaldi, & Yeh, 2018), which focuses more specifically on symptoms of PSTD. This new version of the CPSS aligns with DSM-5 criteria. Also see La Greca and Danzi (Chapter 15, this volume) for more details about assessing acute stress reactions and PTSD.

Last, to assess general mental health functioning, for those not already using the Achenbach System of Empirically Based Assessment, we recommend the Child Behavior Checklist (CBCL), which is a widely used, 118-item caregiver-report measure. Respondents are asked to rate how likely various behaviors (e.g., crying or arguing) are reflective of their child. The CBCL is coded via standardized procedures that provide age- and gender-normed scores on the youth's adjustment. There are three primary scales: Internalizing, Externalizing, and Total Problems, as well as eight or nine statistically derived clinical syndrome scales (e.g., depressed, attention problems, aggressive behavior) and several DSM-oriented scales. The CBCL has excellent reliability and validity (Achenbach & Rescorla, 2001), and there are also teacher- and child-report versions for school-age children and adolescents. There are a variety of alternatives to the CBCL, but there also has been a lot of research looking to create new scales specifically to assess potential abuse or PTSD with the CBCL; thus, viewed from the lens of assessing for potential maltreatment, the CBCL has more research than most of its competitors.

In summary, these assessments provide a starting point to assess both maltreatment exposure and trauma-related problems in child clients. Of note, here we highlight measures that utilize different informants (i.e., caregiver, child, teacher). In clinical settings, it may not be possible at times to get information from a particular source. For example, when a child has been removed from the home, obtaining a parent report may not be feasible. Similarly, young children may not be able to report on their maltreatment history as accurately as older children (Ghetti, Goodman, Eisen, Qin, & Davis, 2002). Therefore, clinicians may have to rely more heavily on one or another of these assessments. As mentioned, however, these are only four of numerous assessment tools. Next, we describe the range of assessments in more detail.

Rating Scales, Checklists, and Different Informants

There are a variety of different referral questions that involve assessment of potential abuse and neglect. We concentrate on screening for abuse in a general clinical setting, and assessment for treatment planning when maltreatment is identified. Other referral questions, such as assessment of risk abuse, parental competence, or evaluating the perpetrator of abuse in a forensic context, involve additional legal and technical considerations (see Crooks & Wolfe, 2007, for an overview). Inherent in assessing a child who has been maltreated, particularly in cases of suspected sexual abuse, is obtaining accurate background information relevant not only to the maltreatment but also to other forms of trauma and adverse childhood events, along with other types of family-based adversities. Given that many youth experience multiple types of maltreatment and adversity, broad-based assessment of negative life events is important to gain an understanding of factors that might contribute to child adjustment problems and have a bearing on service delivery. Although there is growing awareness of the need to assess multiple forms of adversity (e.g., Sheridan & McLaughlin, 2014), less attention has been paid to the development of psychometrically sound assessment tools for these purposes, particularly tools that are appropriate and feasible for clinical settings (Hanson, Smith, Saunders, Swenson, & Conrad, 1995). Indeed, given the complexity of child maltreatment and the difficulty in obtaining such sensitive information on a large sample of children and youth, the task of developing these tools has been quite daunting, particularly because large sample sizes are required to address the many relevant issues adequately.

Due to unique risk factors and psychological outcomes, types of maltreatment need to be considered separately for both research and clinical purposes (Egeland & Sroufe, 1981; Higgins & McCabe, 2000). Many maltreated children experience multiple forms of abuse and adversity, and various combinations of different forms of abuse and adversity appear to have unique outcomes that are not accounted for by simply summing forms of maltreatment (Sheridan & McLaughlin, 2014). Thus, when assessing the effects of a specific form of maltreatment, it is necessary to assess and consider the impact other forms of maltreatment and adversity. As well, it is important to assess the specific aspects of that form of maltreatment, and to consider how that form of maltreatment interacts with other adversities to predict unique outcomes. Broad-based assessment strategies typically assess four types of maltreatment: sexual abuse, physical abuse, neglect, and emotional abuse (exposure to domestic violence is also sometimes categorized as child maltreatment). For each type of maltreatment, important details include the acts involved, the offender, the age when the events occurred and ended, the frequency and duration of the events, and whether there were any injuries and health, or developmental consequences directly linked with the maltreatment (Barnett et al., 1993; Hanson et al., 1995; Wolfe & Birt, 1997).

Developmental issues should also be considered, such as age of first maltreatment episode and con-tinuity of maltreatment across the preschool, elementary, and adolescent years. For sexual abuse, details about the disclosure process are important, including how the abuse was discovered, to whom the child disclosed (if at all), and whether any CPS, family, and/or criminal legal matters have occurred, are planned, or are in progress. To assess and control comprehensively for other forms of adversity, exposure to nonmaltreatment negative life events should be assessed, as well as family-based risk factors. Many maltreated children have complex and chaotic backgrounds that necessitate careful history taking; details about biological parents and stepparents, parental separations, past and current living arrangements, and school placements should all be assessed. Caregiver mental health, substance abuse problems, and history of criminal involvement have important implications for the adjustment of maltreatment victims and should also be assessed.

Whenever possible, it is wise to solicit historical data, and maltreatment and adversity information, from multiple sources. In many cases, maltreatment-related information reported by parents, medical personnel, CPS, and children themselves is consistent and reliable (Kaufman, Jones, Stielglitz, Vitulano, & Mannarino, 1994; McGee, Wolfe, Yuen, Wilson, & Carnochan, 1995). However, Kaufman and colleagues (1994) found that medical records and parent reports often yielded information about abuse severity and other forms of abuse that was not available in CPS files. For example, CPS files revealed that 77% of their sample of sexually abused children and adolescents had experienced emotional maltreatment; when medical, parent, and CPS records were all surveyed for each case, 98% of cases revealed evidence of emotional maltreatment. More recently, Everson and colleagues (2008) found that interviews with adolescents elicited prevalence rates of maltreatment four to six times higher than those found in CPS records. Moreover, 20 of 45 adolescents with CPS determinations of maltreatment failed to report maltreatment during the study interview. As such, it is important both to consider the source of maltreatment-related information and to attempt to obtain substantiation from multiple informants. Below we describe broad-based assessments that provide insight into sexual abuse exposure, as well as other forms of child maltreatment and trauma (Table 18.1). These assessments are gathered from three sources: caregivers, children, and official records.

TABLE 18.1. General Assessments of Child Maltreatment

Assessment	Cost	Informant	Ages	No. of items	Exposure subtypes	Additional information
Traumatic Events Screening Inventory—Revised—Brief Version (TESI-PRR)	Free	Caregiver	0–6	24	Types of traumas including CSA	Frequency, duration
Abuse Dimensions Inventory (ADI)	Request from author	Caregiver	7–12	54	CSA, CPA	Force/coercion, perpetrator, postdisclosure reaction
Child Abuse Potential Inventory (CAPI)	$ (Psychological Assessment Resources)	Caregiver	N/A[a]	160	CPA	Distress, rigidity, unhappiness, problems with child and self, problems with family, problems with others
Parent–Child Conflict Tactics Scale (CTSPC)	Free	Caregiver	0–18	35	Nonviolent discipline, psychological aggression, physical assault, weekly discipline, neglect, CSA	
Child Trauma Questionnaire (CTQ)	$ (Pearson)	Child	12–18	70	EM, CPA, EN, CSA, PN	
Juvenile Victimization Questionnaire (JVA)	Free	Child	8–18	37	Types of traumas, including forms of maltreatment (e.g., CSA)	
Traumatic Events Questionnaire—Adolescents (TEQ-A)	Request from author	Child	13–18	46	Types of traumas, including CSA	
Child and Adolescent Psychiatric Assessment (CAPA) Life Events Module	Free	Child	9–18	30	Types of life events, including CSA	Low- versus high-magnitude events
Violence Exposure Scale for Children (VEX-R)	Free	Child	4–10	25	Violence exposure in home, school, and neighborhood	Witness versus victim
Multidimensional Neglectful Behavior Scale—Child Report (MNBS-CR)	Free	Child	6–17	51	Neglect: emotional, cognitive, supervision, physical, abandonment, alcohol use, conflict exposure, general appraisal, depression	
Maltreatment Classification Scheme (MCS)[b]	Free	Official records	0–18	N/A	EM, PN, CPA, CSA	Six dimensions: (1) type, (2) severity, (3) frequency, (4) developmental period, (5) separation from caregivers, and (6) perpetrator
History of Victimization Form (HVF)	Request from author	Official records	0–18	N/A	CSA, CPA, neglect, EM, family violence	Severity, use of force, perpetrator, number of perpetrators

Note. EM, emotion maltreatment/abuse; PN, physical neglect; CPA, child physical abuse; CSA, child sexual abuse; EN, emotional neglect.
[a]The CAPI assesses parents' potential to physically abuse their children; therefore, the measure does not directly assess children.
[b]LONGSCAN's adapted version is referred to as the Modified Maltreatment Classification Scheme (MMCS).

Broad-Based Assessment of Child Maltreatment

Caregiver Reports

Most caregiver-report measures of child maltreatment are in fact broad-based questionnaires designed to assess a range of traumatic or abusive experiences of the child, with sexual abuse being one of the potential exposures. An example is the TESI-PRR, a 24-item, semistructured interview to determine the exposure history of children ages 6 years and younger to traumatic events (Ippen et al., 2002). As described previously, caregivers are asked to respond (*yes, no, unsure*) to indicate whether the child has been exposed to 24 potentially traumatic events, including sexual abuse, physical abuse, domestic violence, community violence, accidents and injuries, and natural disasters. Clinician and child-report versions of the TESI can be used for children ranging from ages 4 to 18 years.

Another semistructured caregiver interview, the Abuse Dimensions Inventory (ADI; Chaffin, Wherry, Newlin, Crutchfield, & Dykman, 1997), has subsequently been used to gather information from CPS workers (Silovsky & Niec, 2002). The ADI has six sections: physical abuse (12 items), sexual abuse (13 items), force or coercion used to gain submission to sexual abuse (nine items), force or coercion used to gain secrecy about either physical or sexual abuse (six items), role relationships between child and abuser (nine relationships identified), and postdisclosure reactions abusers might express regarding admission and blame (five items). Factor analyses of 136 ADIs yielded four factors: Sexual Abuse Severity and Coercion, Sexual Abuse Duration and Number of Events, Physical Abuse Severity and Coercion, and Physical Abuse Duration and Number of Events. Role relationship and abuser's reaction did not load heavily on any factor. In a subsequent study, ADI sexual abuse severity ratings correlated with child-reported PTSD symptoms (Chaffin & Shultz, 2001).

Additional caregiver-report measures to assess exposure to child maltreatment include the Child Abuse Potential Inventory (CAPI; Milner, 1986) and the Parent–Child Conflict Tactics Scale (CTSPC; Straus, Hamby, Finkelhor, Moore, & Runyan, 1998), although these measures primarily tap into exposure to physical abuse rather than sexual abuse. Specifically, the CAPI is a 160-item caregiver-report questionnaire designed to screen parents suspected of physically abusing their children. The CAPI assesses attitudes such as "Children should be seen but not heard" that do not directly ask about abusive behaviors but have been found in previous samples to be highly correlated with abusive behaviors (Milner, Charlesworth, Gold, Gold, & Friesen, 1988). Similarly, the CTSPC measures psychological and physical abuse and neglect of children by parents, in addition to nonviolent forms of discipline. The CTSPC also includes supplemental scales to assess neglect and sexual abuse (Straus et al., 1998).

Child and Adolescent Self-Reports

Large-scale epidemiological studies have necessitated the development of assessment tools for children and adolescents to determine prevalence of maltreatment, victimization, and adversity. As mentioned previously, perhaps the most commonly used self-report measure of childhood victimization is the CTQ, a 70-item, Likert-like inventory (Bernstein & Fink, 1998; Bernstein et al., 1994). The CTQ yields five subscales: Emotional Abuse, Physical Abuse, Emotional Neglect, Sexual Abuse, and Physical Neglect. Of note, the CTQ has been used with youth as young as age 12 years and has demonstrated good sensitivity and specificity with known maltreatment information (Bernstein et al., 1997). Bernstein and colleagues (2003) created a shortened, 28-item version of the CTQ that has demonstrated good convergent and discriminant validity.

The Juvenile Victimization Questionnaire (JVQ; Finkelhor, Ormrod, Turner, & Hamby, 2005; Hamby & Finkelhor, 2001, 2004) has been used as a self-report measure for children and youth ages 8 years and older. A caregiver version uses similar wording, so that it is directly comparable to the youth-report version and can be used for children under age 8. The JVQ assesses 34 offenses against youth in five areas: Conventional Crime (assaults, property crimes), Child Maltreatment (physical, sexual, and emotional abuse, neglect, family abduction/custodial interference), Peer and Sibling Victimization (assaults and property offenses), Sexual Assault (rape and sexual assaults attempted or completed, flashing, sexual harassment, and statutory sexual offenses), and Witnessing and Indirect Victimization (domestic violence, abuse of a sibling, community violence, civil disturbances and riots, and war-zone violence). The JVQ takes 20–30 minutes to complete, depending on the number of victimizations reported. Following screener questions, more in-depth information is obtained, including perpetrator characteristics, use of a weapon, injuries, and co-occurrence of the event with another reported event (in case one event falls into more than one category).

The Traumatic Events Questionnaire—Adolescents (TEQ-A; Lipschitz, Bernstein, Winegar, & Southwick, 1999), a 46-item self-report questionnaire, uses a multiple-choice format to elicit details about six forms of traumatic experiences: Witnessing Home Violence, Witnessing or Being the Victim of Community Violence, Accidental Physical Injuries, Physical Abuse, and Sexual Abuse. The TEQ-A defines "sexual abuse" as sexual contact between a minor and an adult 5 years older or a peer 2 years older. A two-level gating system is used, with two initial sexual abuse questions: "When you were growing up, did anyone try to have some kind of sexual contact with you in a way that made you feel uncomfortable?" and "If so, how old was the person who did this?" Details of each sexual incident are then obtained, including the age of onset, duration, identity of perpetrators, use of force, and exact nature of each traumatic experience. When adolescents' responses on the TEQ-A were compared to a best-estimate source (based on information from therapist interviews, chart reviews, and child welfare agencies), the agreement for sexual abuse was 88% (kappa = .75) and for physical abuse was 84% (kappa = .66). Comparisons between the TEQ-A and the CTQ revealed that although relatively comparable at more severe levels of sexual abuse, the CTQ is more sensitive than the TEQ-A in detecting sexual abuse of lesser severity.

Several available life events checklists include items reflecting childhood maltreatment, as well as other types of negative life events and adversities. The Child and Adolescent Psychiatric Assessment (CAPA) Life Events Module (Costello, Angold, March, & Fairbank, 1998) was developed for use with the Great Smoky Mountain Epidemiological Study. Both high- and low-magnitude negative life events are assessed, including physical and sexual abuse. Comparisons of parent and child completed versions yielded good intraclass correlations (.72 [child] and .83 [parent] for high-magnitude events, and .62 [child] and .58 [parent] for low-magnitude events). Other child-report measures of maltreatment, but not sexual abuse, include the Violence Exposure Scale for Children (VEX-R; Fox & Leavitt, 1995) and the Multidimensional Neglectful Behavior Scale—Child Report (MNBS-CR; Kantor et al., 2004).

Chart Reviews

In research settings, the most established maltreatment assessment tool for children is the Maltreatment Classification Scheme (MCS; Barnett et al., 1993), which has been adapted for use by Longitudinal Studies of Child Abuse and Neglect (LONGSCAN), a consortium of five longitudinal studies of child abuse and neglect conducted at several sites across the United States (Runyan et al., 1998). The MCS was originally developed to collect information from CPS records; LONGSCAN's adapted version is referred to as the Modified Maltreatment Classification Scheme (MMCS). The MCS assesses severity of incidents within each subtype of maltreatment, frequency and chronicity, length of CPS involvement, developmental period during which the events occurred, type and number of placements outside the home, and the perpetrators of the incident. Within the major forms of maltreatment, different subtypes are recorded. The MCS is available from Barnett and colleagues (1993), and the MMCS LONGSCAN version is available at *www.ndacan.cornell.edu*. Although, in a clinical setting, comprehensive coding of children's CPS records is not feasible, or perhaps even informative, a cursory review of a patient's chart or court records can provide valuable information about the maltreatment or trauma exposure of the child. For example, a review of a CPS chart can provide a clinician with information about past cases of alleged or substantiated maltreatment, including the type of maltreatment, age at exposure, and perpetrator. CPS files also often contain information about the child's family history, including parents' mental health and criminal records. As such, an initial chart review may highlight potential (or substantiated) trauma that needs further assessment or treatment.

Risk and Resiliency Factors

Considerable attention has been paid to understanding factors that place children at risk for maltreatment, as well as factors that protect children and promote resilience. For example, three child factors have repeatedly been linked to risk for child maltreatment: age, gender, and disabilities/intellectual ability (Brown, Cohen, Johnson, & Salzinger, 1998; Dubowitz et al., 2011; Hussey, Chang, & Kotch, 2006). Maltreatment rates are highest for infants and drop rapidly with age. The substantiated rates of maltreatment in the United States in 2017 were 15 per 1,000 children ages 0–3 years, 10 per 1,000 in 4- 7-year-olds, and 5 per 1,000 in 16- to 17- year-olds (DHHS, 2019). Neglect is more likely in single-parent families, families with financial strain, and when the caregiver is using alcohol or drugs.

The role of age in predicting risk of maltreatment seems somewhat dependent on the maltreatment subtype in question. For physical abuse, fatal cases of abuse are most common in children younger than age 2 years (Kirschner & Wilson, 2001; Kotch, Chalmers, Fanslow, Marshall, & Langley, 1993). In contrast, approximately 10% of sexually abused children are under age 6, with a slight increase in onset at ages 6–7 years, and a dramatic increase around age 10 (33%; Bagley & Mallick, 2000; Finkelhor, 1994; Vogeltanz et al., 1999). Indeed, data from the National Survey of Adolescents (Hanson et al., 2003) revealed that 60% of sexual abuse occurred between ages of 11 and 16. Because of the large age span considered under the umbrella of sexual abuse, the nature, impact, and etiology of sexual victimization vary at different developmental points (Black, Heyman, & Slep, 2001).

Similarly, gender differences are found for some, but not all, forms of maltreatment. Specifically, girls are at higher risk of sexual abuse, but differences in physical abuse and neglect generally are not reported (DHHS, 2019; Sedlak et al., 2010). In fact, girls are victims of CSA three to five times more often than boys (Boney-McCoy & Finkelhor, 1995; Fergusson, Lynskey, & Horwood, 1996; Sachs-Ericsson, Blazer, Plant, & Arnow, 2005; Sedlak & Broadhurst, 1996). Sexual abuse experiences differ for boys and girls (Gordon, 1990; Watkins & Bentovim, 1992), with girls generally describing their experiences more negatively (Fischer, 1991). This may be because girls tend to be younger at the onset of their abuse (Dong, Anda, Dube, Giles, & Felitti, 2003) and their perpetrators tend to be older (Romano & De Luca, 2001). Girls are abused by family members more often, and abuse perpetrated by family members tends to be more serious. Fergusson and colleagues (1996) reported that 61.3% of abuse perpetrated by family members included some form of intercourse, and that 71% of familial abuse involved more than one episode. Boys are more likely to be abused by adolescent males and by females (Dube et al., 2005; Finkelhor, Hotaling, Lewis, & Smith, 1990). They may perceive abuse by adolescent males as a form of sexual experimentation (Romano & De

Luca, 2001), and up to 20% of males describe sexual abuse by older females as either nonthreatening or pleasurable (Bagley & Thurston, 1996).

Children with developmental disabilities are at heightened risk for child maltreatment, with prevalence estimates two to three times greater than those of children without disabilities (Hershkowitz, Lamb, & Horowitz, 2007; Jones et al., 2012; Maclean et al., 2017; Sullivan & Knutson, 2000). Despite ample evidence that children with disabilities are more likely to be maltreated, less in known about the mechanisms underlying these associations. One potential mechanism that has received some attention is the additional emotional, physical, economic, and social demands placed on parents and caregivers (Hibbard, Desch, & Committee on Child Abuse and Neglect, 2007). These added demands place increased stress and strain on parents and caregivers, which may lead to increased use of corporal punishment as parents struggle to cope emotionally. Moreover, children with disabilities often experience greater physical and social isolation, increased dependence and lack of control over their lives and bodies (e.g., need for assistance when bathing, dressing, and toileting), and communication impairments that may increase risk of being selected by perpetrators, prevent reporting, and impede validation of abuse allegations (Westcott & Jones, 1999).

Numerous individual factors have also been investigated as potential sources of resilience in the face of maltreatment exposure. For example, longitudinal studies suggest that certain personality characteristics (e.g., ego resilience and ego overcontrol), self-esteem, temperament, and intellectual ability may serve to protect children from maltreatment sequelae and promote resilience (Afifi & MacMillan, 2011; Haskett, Nears, Ward, & McPherson, 2006). *Ego control* refers to the ability to master impulses, and "ego resilience" refers to the ability to modify ego control depending on context (Afifi & MacMillan, 2011). Both personality traits have been linked to greater resilience in children exposed to maltreatment (Flores, Cicchetti, & Rogosch, 2005). Evidence for the role of intellectual ability in resilient functioning, on the other hand, has been more mixed (Afifi & MacMillan, 2011; Jaffee, Caspi, Moffitt, Polo-Thomas, & Taylor, 2007).

Family Factors

Several interrelated family factors have been linked with risk of child maltreatment: maternal maltreatment history, unplanned pregnancy, low parental education, low family income, parental alcohol and drug abuse, parental mental illness, harsh discipline, parent–child relationship problems, maternal death, living with only one or with no natural parent, marital discord, separation, divorce, and maternal remarriage (Bagley & Mallick, 2000; Dong et al., 2003; Euser, van IJzendoorn, Prinzie, & Bakermans-Kranenburg, 2010; Gilbert et al., 2009; Hanson et al., 2006; Hussey et al., 2006; Turner, Finkelhor, & Ormrod, 2006; Sedlak et al., 2010; Walsh, MacMillan, & Jamieson, 2003; Zuravin & Fontanella, 1999). Simply put, increasing levels of family-related adversity correspond to increasing risk of child victimization (Gilbert et al., 2009; Hussey et al., 2006). Indeed, in a nationally representative sample of 4,053 children ages 2–17 and their caregivers, Turner and colleagues (2006) found, first, that exposure to multiple forms of maltreatment and victimization was common, with almost 66% of the sample reporting exposure to multiple forms of victimization (e.g., maltreatment, community violence, domestic violence). Second, greater child victimization was associated with higher levels of family-related adversity, such as low socioeconomic status and being in a single-parent household.

For CSA specifically, factors that negatively affect parental ability to monitor child safety appear to be particularly potent in predicting risk for abuse. Drawing from the National Survey of Adolescents, Hanson and colleagues (2006) found that not living with a biological parent increased the odds of sexual abuse by 1.8. As well, parental alcohol abuse, which affects parental availability and child monitoring, increased the odds of adolescent reports of extrafamilial sexual abuse by 1.7 and doubled the odds of multiple victimization (Hanson et al., 2006; Stevens, Ruggiero, Kilpatrick, Resnick, & Saunders, 2005). Finkelhor, Moore, Hamby, and Straus (1997) found that leaving a child at home alone without adequate supervision increased the odds of child sexual victimization by 3.4. Likewise, Fergusson and colleagues (1996) found that poor parental supervision, lack of knowledge about sexual abuse risk factors, and child exposure to risky social environments increased odds of sexual abuse.

Families can also serve as a source of protection and resilience in the aftermath of maltreatment exposure. The most commonly cited family-level protective factors include stable caregiving, parental support, and positive parent–child relationships (Afifi & MacMillan, 2011; Folger & Wright,

2013). For example, in a sample of 147 youth exposed to sexual abuse, satisfaction with caregiver support at the time of abuse disclosure was associated with less depression and better self-esteem in the youth 1 year later (Rosenthal, Feiring, & Taska, 2003). Similar findings have been reported regarding the presence of at least one stable caregiver (Herrenkohl, Herrenkohl, & Egolf, 1994) and less conflictual parent–child relationships (Daigneault, Hébert, & Tourigny, 2007).

Community and Social Factors

Studies that have examined race, culture, and ethnicity as risk factors for child maltreatment have been inconclusive (Kenny & McEachern, 2000). However, living in high-risk communities appears to increase maltreatment risk. Drake and Pandey (1996) found that communities with higher percentages of families in poverty (> 41%) had significantly higher rates of child sexual victimization compared to other communities. As well, Boney-McCoy and Finkelhor (1995) found that children from dangerous communities were at increased risk for child sexual victimization (odds ratio [OR] = 1.5) compared to children from other communities. Relatively little attention has been paid to potential community-level resilience factors, although some evidence has emerged for the role of socially cohesive neighborhoods (e.g., neighbors are trusting and helpful) and neighborhoods characterized by high levels of informal social control (e.g., adults monitor the behavior of neighborhood children; Jaffee et al., 2007). Next, we turn to the impact of maltreatment on children and adolescents, with an eye toward assessments that can be used to identify PTSD and mental health functioning in this population.

Impact of Maltreatment on Child Victims

Child maltreatment is not a disorder with a clearly delineated list of symptoms. Rather, abuse (or neglect) is best considered a negative life event that poses significant risk for the development of a broad spectrum of behavioral and emotional problems. Moreover, child sexual abuse, physical abuse, neglect, and domestic violence exposure are often experienced comorbidly and on frequent occasions (Berzenski & Yates, 2011; Cook et al., 2005; Dong et al., 2003; Finklehor, Turner, Ormrod, & Hamby, 2009). As a result, child maltreatment has the potential to affect numerous developmental processes negatively, setting the stage for a lifetime of sequelae. In some cases, the abuse or neglect was a defining event that led to maltreatment-related mental health concerns. However, many maltreatment victims had behavioral, emotional, and developmental problems before the maltreatment occurred, or lived within familial and/or community contexts that likely would have led to mental health problems even if the maltreatment had not occurred. Thus, evaluating the impact of child maltreatment per se can be quite complex, particularly given developmental issues that affect manifestation of symptoms for preschoolers, children, and adolescents. Below we outline maltreatment-related symptoms and provide brief descriptions of assessments that can be utilized to document such symptoms.

Attachment Issues

Attachment between a child and caregiver is a major influence on development. Warm, consistent parenting and secure dyadic attachment are protective or resilience factors, and insecure and particularly disorganized attachment styles are now established predictors of internalizing (Groh, Roisman, van IJzendoorn, Bakermans-Kranenburg, & Fearon, 2012; Madigan, Atkinson, Laurin, & Benoit, 2013) and externalizing problems (Fearon, Bakermans-Kranenburg, van IJzendoorn, Lapsley, & Roisman, 2010). Unfortunately, there is no easy-to-use, structured approach to evaluating attachment; most research is based on variations of the Strange Situation laboratory method. DSM-5 has two diagnoses that are relevant—reactive attachment disorder (RAD) and disinhibited social engagement disorder (DSED). These diagnoses focus on the child's behavior, not on the dyadic attachment per se. The Practice Parameter for the American Academy of Child and Adolescent Psychiatry notes that the prevalence of both of these conditions is low, with prevalence rate estimates of zero in pediatric clinics and very low in general practice settings (Zeanah, Cheshire, Boris, and the American Academy of Child & Adolescent Psychiatry Committee on Quality Issues, 2016). These conditions are most likely to be observed with children in institutionalized settings, or with a series of placements in foster care, and even then they do not affect the majority of youth in those settings. The clinical standard is not to assign these diagnoses in the absence of a clear history of severe trauma or deprivation, or institutional placement (Zeanah et al., 2016). When there is a history of significant deprivation, it makes sense to assess parenting, family interactions, and other risk and resilience factors before considering these diagnoses.

PTSD and Dissociation

The literature on PTSD provides an important clinical and research framework for conceptualizing maltreatment sequelae, particularly for victims of CSA. For example, the fifth edition of the *Diagnostic and Statistical Manual of Mental Disorders* (DSM-5; American Psychiatric Association, 2013) supports consideration of PTSD as a possible diagnosis for CSA victims; in fact, the definition of trauma includes developmentally inappropriate sexual experiences with or without threatened or actual violence or injury. A diagnosis of PTSD requires four conditions: (1) The person was exposed (either directly or indirectly) to death, threatened death, actual or threatened serious injury, or actual or threatened sexual violence; (2) the traumatic event is persistently reexperienced via memories, flashbacks, nightmares, emotional distress, or physical reactivity; (3) the person avoids trauma-related thoughts/feelings or external reminders; and (4) the presence of negative thoughts/feelings and arousal/reactivity that began or worsened after trauma. To be considered PTSD, these conditions need to last for more than 1 month, create distress or functional impairment, and not be due to medication, substance use, or other illness. La Greca and Danzi (Chapter 15, this volume) detail assessment methods when PTSD is a clinical concern.

Research consistently links exposure to CSA and other forms of abuse to the development of PTSD in children and adolescents (Bal, Van Oost, de Bourdeaudhuij, & Crombez, 2003; Boney-McCoy & Finkelhor, 1995, 1996; Cloitre et al., 2009; Cutajar et al., 2010; Danielson, de Arellano, Kilpatrick, Saunders, & Resnick, 2005; Hébert, Langevin, & Daigneault, 2016; Kilpatrick et al., 2003; Ullman, Najdowski, & Filipas, 2009). For example, in a prevalence study with a community sample of older adolescents, experiencing rape or CSA increased the odds of developing PTSD by 49% (Cuffe et al., 1998). Other studies of identified sexual abuse victims indicate that between 36 and 60% meet diagnostic criteria for PTSD (Alisic et al., 2014; Dubner & Motta, 1999; Kendall-Tackett, Williams, & Finkelhor, 1993; McLeer et al., 1998; V. Wolfe & Birt, 2005; D. Wolfe, Sas, & Wekerle, 1994). Compared with other negative life events in childhood and adolescence, such as serious accidents, natural and man-made disasters, and even physical abuse, sexual abuse is particularly potent in provoking PTSD symptomatology (Bal, Crombez, Van Oost, & Debourdeaudhuij, 2003; Bal, Van Oost, et al., 2003; Boney-McCoy & Finkelhor, 1996; Cuffe et al., 1998; Dubner & Motta, 1999). Despite relatively high rates of negative life events among clinic-referred children, PTSD is more prevalent among CSA victims than among other clinic-referred children and adolescents (McLeer et al., 1998; V. Wolfe & Birt, 2005) and as compared to those who experience other types of maltreatment (Runyon & Kenny, 2002). Even when prior mental health and quality of parent–child relationships were controlled, Boney-McCoy and Finkelhor (1996) found that sexually abused youth reported more PTSD symptoms than their nonabused peers, revealing a medium effect size.

Related to PTSD is the tendency for abuse victims to dissociate, which means that victims mentally disconnect from their thoughts, feelings, memories, or sense of identity (Bernstein & Putnam, 1986). Dissociation is an ephemeral phenomenon that has been difficult to study. In the face of trauma, dissociation can be considered a defensive process that enables a child to mentally avoid the ongoing trauma that he or she cannot avoid physically (Terr, 1991; van der Kolk, van der Hart, & Marmar, 1996). If traumatic events and dissociative reactions occur repeatedly or continuously, dissociation can become a habit-like, unconscious, and automatic response triggered by less severe day-to-day stressors, thereby affecting everyday information processing and functioning (Liotti, 1999; Post et al., 1998). Dissociation is thought to have its roots in early childhood trauma, particularly sexual abuse, physical abuse, and neglect (Briere & Runtz, 1989; Hagan, Hulette, & Lieberman, 2015; Hulette, Freyd, & Fisher, 2011; Ogawa, Sroufe, Weinfield, Carlson, & Egeland, 1997; Schimmenti & Caretti, 2016; Yeager & Lewis, 1996). In fact, one meta-analytic study demonstrated a strong association between sexual trauma and dissociative symptoms, with an effect size of 0.42 (van IJzendoorn & Schuengel, 1996).

Early childhood trauma may set the stage for dissociative disorders because of the extreme vulnerability of young children, who are more likely to experience extreme distress under frightening circumstances, or because young children appear to have innate dissociative abilities that dissipate as more effective coping strategies develop. The perpetuation and exacerbation of early dissociative processes disrupt normal processes that integrate different aspects of experience, resulting in the three main components of dissociation: memory disturbance, distortion of perceptions, and failure to develop a consistent and integrated sense of "self" and "identity" (Macfie, Cicchetti, & Toth, 2001; Perzow et al., 2013; Zayed, Wolfe, & Birt, 2006). Dissociation is generally considered to fall along a continuum from typical everyday occurrences (e.g., intense thought absorption, lapses in memory when driving) to the most extreme form of dissociation, dissociative identity disorder (Dorahy et al., 2014; Ross & Joshi, 1992).

General Functioning and Mental Health

Exposure to child maltreatment places children at increased risk for a range of negative behavioral and mental health outcomes (Brown, Cohen, Johnson, & Smailes, 1999; Cicchetti, 2016; Fergusson, Horwood, & Lynskey, 1996; Hillberg, Hamilton-Giachritsis, & Dixon, 2011; Jonson-Reid, Kohl, & Drake, 2012; Luster, Small, & Lower, 2002). In fact, as many as 80% of young adults exposed to maltreatment in childhood meet diagnostic criteria for at least one psychiatric disorder at age 21 (Silverman, Reinherz, & Giaconia, 1996). For example, numerous studies have indicated higher rates of depressive symptoms and mood disorders among maltreated youth compared to nonmaltreated community controls (Chen et al., 2010; Danielson et al., 2005; Dunn, McLaughlin, Slopen, Rosand, & Smoller, 2013; Howard & Wang, 2005; Kilpatrick et al., 2003; Kim & Cicchetti, 2010; Lindert et al., 2014; Luster et al., 2002; Maniglio, 2010; Naar-King, Silvern, Ryan, & Sebring, 2002; Romens & Pollak, 2012; Runyon, Faust, & Orvaschel, 2002). Even after controlling for prior adjustment and parent–child relationship, sexual abuse victims, for instance, show a fourfold increase in risk for depression subsequent to sexual abuse (Boney-McCoy & Finkelhor, 1996).

Numerous factors have been linked to increased risk of depression among maltreated youth. Unlike children, adolescents tend to have more depressive symptoms than PTSD symptoms (Feiring, Taska, & Lewis, 2002; Tebbutt, Swanston, Oates, & O'Toole, 1997). However, as in PTSD, girls show more symptoms of depression than do boys (Danielson et al., 2005; Feiring, Taska, & Lewis, 1999, 2002; Runyon et al., 2002). For CSA, a number of abuse-related factors have been linked to increased risk of depression, including abuse severity, physical coercion and assault during the sexual abuse, repeated episodes, and abuse by a family member

(Danielson et al., 2005; Feiring et al., 2002; Garnefski & Diekstra, 1997). Furthermore, continued contact with the offender, which is more common with intrafamilial cases, is associated with long-term problems with depression and self-esteem (Tebbutt et al., 1997).

Maltreatment also places individuals at elevated risks for suicidal ideation and gestures, as well as death by suicide (Cutajar et al., 2010; Dunn et al., 2013; Miller et al., 2017). In a review, Miller and colleagues (2013) concluded that findings by maltreatment subtype suggest that each form of maltreatment is independently associated with suicidal ideation and suicide attempts; however, CSA and emotional abuse may be more important in explaining suicidal behavior relative to physical abuse or neglect. Moreover, each maltreatment subtype seems to contribute unique variance in adolescent suicide attempts, suggesting an additive effect. Finally, the links between child maltreatment exposure and suicide tend to remain even after accounting for a range of covariates, such as child demographics, mental health, family functioning, and peer relations. Regarding CSA, sexually abused boys are twice as likely as sexually abused girls to report suicidal ideation (Garnefski & Diekstra, 1997). Risk factors for suicidal ideation and behaviors among sexual abuse victims include family dysfunction and socioeconomic adversity (Fergusson et al., 2000). Danielson and colleagues (2005) found that 70% of depressed youth with a history of both sexual and physical abuse experienced suicidal ideation.

Across childhood and adolescence, child maltreatment has also been linked with increased risk of externalizing behaviors and symptomatology, including anger, aggression, conduct problems, and substance use (Crea, Easton, Florio, & Barth, 2018; Jones et al., 2013; Keiley, Howe, Dodge, Bates, & Pettit, 2001; Kim & Cicchetti, 2010; Lewis, McElroy, Harlaar, & Runyan, 2016; Maikovich-Fong & Jaffee, 2010; Manly, Oshri, Lynch, Herzog, & Wortel, 2013; Milojevich, Russell, & Quas, 2018; Moylan et al., 2010; Oshri, Rogosch, Burnette, & Cicchetti, 2011; Simpson & Miller, 2002). For example, during the preschool and early primary school years, sexually abused children show increased anger and aggression, particularly among children who were very young when the abuse first occurred, and among those who experienced multiple types of maltreatment (English, Graham, Litrownik, Everson, & Bangdiwala, 2005; Lau et al., 2005). It is unclear, at times, whether these externalizing problems arise specifically from the maltreatment experiences or from the types of family stressors typical of children who show externalizing problems in general. In their nationally representative survey of children ages 2–17 years, Turner and colleagues (2006) documented relatively high rates of externalizing problems for sexual abuse victims. However, the increase in externalizing problems was accounted for by family dysfunction and other types of negative life events and adversities. Furthermore, in a longitudinal study examining the effects of physical abuse and domestic violence exposure in childhood on adolescent externalizing behaviors, although both physical abuse and domestic violence exposure were associated with externalizing outcomes at the bivariate level, only children with exposure to both forms of adversity were at elevated risk of externalizing behaviors after researchers controlled for additional stressors in the family and surrounding environment (Moylan et al., 2010).

Regarding CSA sequelae, both longitudinal and cross-sectional studies of sexual abuse victims indicate that sexual abuse prematurely sets in motion a series of sexual experiences that have serious lifelong consequences. Kendall-Tackett and colleagues (1993) estimated that approximately one-fourth of sexually abused children display sexual behavior problems, with the link between sexual behavior problems and CSA being strongest among preschool-age children (Johnson, 1988; see Friedrich, 1993, for a review). Overall, sexual abuse victims tend to be younger both when they begin consensual sexual activities and when they have their first consensual sexual intercourse experience (Fergusson, Horwood, & Lynskey, 1997; Lalor & McElvaney, 2010; Noll, Trickett, & Putnam, 2000), which places them at risk for early pregnancy (Noll, Shenk, & Putnam, 2008). Indeed, exposure to CSA significantly increases the odds of experiencing an adolescent pregnancy by 2.21-fold (Noll et al., 2008). Of note, early teenage pregnancy has important implications of intergenerational transmission of child maltreatment. Teenage mothers tend to leave school early, have fewer social and economic opportunities in life, suffer greater social disadvantage, be less competent and more punitive as parents, suffer more depression, and more often be the victims of spousal violence (Bardone, Moffitt, Caspi, & Dickson, 1996; Brooks-Gunn & Chase-Landsale, 1995; Woodward, Fergusson, & Horwood, 2001).

Adolescents who report a history of CSA and/or family violence are also more likely to engage in risky sexual behavior. For example, youth exposed to CSA are four times more likely than their peers to engage in sex without condoms, to have sex after drug use, and to have sex with multiple partners (Voisin, 2005). Furthermore, these risky behaviors are twice as prevalent among those who perceive that their peers engage in similar, risky sexual practices. Girls with a history of sexual abuse may find it particularly difficult to assert themselves in sexual situations, either to resist sexual advances or to ensure safe sexual practices (Brown, Kessel, Lourie, Ford, & Lipsitt, 1997; Johnsen & Harlow, 1996). Moreover, CSA victims are at high risk of revictimization, including sexual assaults during adolescence and adulthood (Barnes, Noll, Putnam, & Trickett, 2009; Classen, Palesh, & Aggarwal, 2005; Lalor & McElvaney, 2010; Scoglio, Kraus, Saczynski, Jooma, & Molnar, 2019). Considering this range of negative outcomes associated with maltreatment exposure, we provide examples of assessments to measure general functioning and mental health in maltreatment-exposed children and adolescents in Table 18.2.

Implications for Clinical Assessment

As is evident from this review, child maltreatment has numerous effects throughout the lifespan. Thus, the assessment of child maltreatment must be developmentally informed, multidimensional, and integrate historical and current contextual information with an array of emotional and behavioral symptoms and psychological processes. Child maltreatment sets in motion several negative mental health processes that have the capacity cumulatively to affect a broad range of adjustment concerns. Compared to other serious negative life events, abuse exposure is strongly linked to the development of depression and PTSD, and early childhood abuse appears to sow the seeds of dissociative processes and disorders. CSA, specifically, is linked with numerous sexuality problems, ranging from increased risk of sexual victimization to age-inappropriate interest in sexual activities. In the following section, we discuss ways to use assessment to guide diagnosis and treatment of children and adolescents exposed to maltreatment.

Using Assessment to Guide Diagnosis and Treatment

The World Health Organization (WHO; 2017) has released clinical guidelines for front-line workers

responding to children and adolescents who have been sexually abused. Within these guidelines are specific considerations for the assessment of maltreatment and other life traumas. We feel that these guidelines help set the stage for understanding the use of assessment to guide the diagnosis and treatment of children potentially exposed to maltreatment. The WHO (p. 3) states:

> In line with the principle of "do no harm," when the medical history is being obtained and, if needed, a forensic interview is being conducted, health-care providers should seek to minimize additional trauma and distress for children and adolescents who disclose sexual abuse. This includes: minimizing need to repeatedly tell their history; interviewing them on their own (i.e., separately from their caregivers), while offering to have another adult present as support; building trust and rapport by asking about neutral topics first; conducting a comprehensive assessment of their physical and emotional health, in order to facilitate appropriate decisions for conducting examinations and investigations, assessing injuries and providing treatment and/or referrals; asking clear, open-ended questions without repetitions; using language and terminology that is appropriate to age and non-stigmatizing; allowing the child or adolescent to respond in the manner of their choice, including, for example, by writing, drawing or illustrating with models.

Epidemiological findings also provide an important framework for conducting a comprehensive assessment of victims' physical and emotional health by identifying the types of background and contextual information relevant to clinical assessment. Most importantly, however, extant epidemiological data highlight the broad extent of child maltreatment and other life adversities, and relatively low rates of disclosures. For instance, although considerable attention has been given to false CSA reports, underreporting of CSA is more common (McElvaney, 2015), and its detection is essential for proper diagnosis and treatment. Thus, all clinicians working with children and youth, not just those who specialize in CSA and childhood trauma, should be mindful that many children who are identified for mental health service have undisclosed histories of CSA and other forms of maltreatment. Underreporting of CSA is most common among males, children with disabilities, and children who perceive either negative or ineffectual consequences to their disclosures (Alaggia, Collin-Vézina, & Lateef, 2019; Anderson, 2016). Adolescents tend to disclose to their peers rather than to adults (Priebe & Svedin, 2008). In many

TABLE 18.2. Assessments of General Functioning, Mental Health, and Trauma in Children and Adolescents

Assessment	Original author(s)	Informant	Description
Trauma Symptom Checklist for Young Children (TSCYC)	Briere et al. (2001)	Caregiver	90 items; assesses trauma-related symptoms in children; eight subscales: anxiety, depression, anger, and abnormal sexual behavior
Trauma Symptom Checklist for Young Children—Short Form (TSCYC-SF)	Wherry, Corson, & Hunsaker (2013)	Caregiver	32 items; assesses trauma-related symptoms in children
Achenbach System of Empirically Based Assessment (ASEBA)	Achenbach & Rescorla (2001)	Three informant versions: caregiver, teacher, or child; different versions for preschool and adult age groups	118 items; assesses behavioral and emotional problems in children but does not specifically ask about abuse or traumatic events
Diagnostic Interview Schedule for Children (DISC-IV)	Shaffer et al. (1996)	Clinician	Assesses 34 common psychiatric diagnoses of children and adolescents
Assessment Checklist for Children (ACC)	Tarren-Sweeney (2007)	Caregiver	120 items; assesses behaviors, emotional states, traits and relating to others, as manifested among children in care; 10 clinical scales and two self-esteem scales; free but restricted access; *www.childpsych.org.uk/obtainacc.html*
Brief Assessment Checklist for Children (BAC-C)	Tarren-Sweeney (2013b)	Caregiver	20 items; designed to screen/monitor emotional and behavioral difficulties experienced by children in out-of-home care; developed from 120-item Assessment Checklist; free; available at *www.childpsych.org.uk/bac-c_english(us).pdf*
Pediatric Emotional Distress Scale (PEDS)	Saylor, Swenson, Reynolds, & Taylor (1999)	Caregiver	21 items; assesses symptomatology in children following stressful and/or traumatic event
Trauma Play Scale (TPS)	Findling, Bratton, & Henson (2006)	Clinician	Observation-based measure of play behaviors in children exposed to trauma; five subscales: Intense Play, Repetitive Play, Play Disruption, Avoidant Play Behavior, and Expression of Negative Affect
Story Stem Assessment Profile (SSAP)	Hodges, Steele, Kaniuk, Hillman, & Asquith (2009)	Clinician	Assessment profile captures effects of abuse in young children; asked to continue a narrative; interview analyzed against specific themes
Dominic Interactive Assessment (DI)	Valla, Bergeron, & Smolla (2000)	Child	91 items; assesses psychiatric symptoms related to common mental health disorders based on seven DSM-III-R and DSM-IV diagnoses; uses a cartoon

			picture format to make it more engaging, with a version for ages 6–11 years and an age 12 and up version; also available as a Windows computer administered version, in English and French; $50 license and $6 per administration; *www.dominicinteractive.com*
Assessment Checklist for Adolescents (ACA)	Tarren-Sweeney (2013a)	Caregiver	120 items; assesses behaviors, emotional states, traits and manners of relating to others; includes 10 clinical scales and two self-esteem scales; for adolescents in out-of-home care (ages 12–17 years)
Brief Assessment Checklist for Adolescents (BAC-A)	Tarren-Sweeney (2013b)	Caregiver	20 items; brief screening tool for use by social or health professionals without child mental health qualification; for adolescents in out-of-home care (ages 12–17 years)
Solution-Focused Recovery Scale (SFRS)	Dolan (1991)	Child	36 items; Likert-style; positive coping skills specific to childhood sexual abuse
Child and Youth Resilience Measure–28 (CYRM-28)	Ungar & Liebenberg (2005)	Child	28 items; assesses resilience across cultural contexts; Likert scale
Child and Youth Resilience Measure–12 (CYRM-12)	Liebenberg, Ungar, & LeBlanc (2013)	Child	12 items; assesses resilience across cultural contexts
Minnesota Multiphasic Personality Inventory—Adolescent (MMPI-A)	Butcher et al. (1992)	Child	478 items; assesses psychopathology among youth; large range of clinical and supplementary scales included
Beck Self-Concept Inventory for Youth (BSCY-I)	Beck, Beck, Jolly, & Steer (2001)	Child	20 items; assesses competence and self-worth; Likert-style
Children's Global Assessment of Functioning Scale (CGAS)	Shaffer et al. (1983)	Clinician	Assesses global functioning among children and adolescents; comparable scoring to the Global Assessment of Functioning
Adolescent Clinical Sexual Behavior Inventory (ACSBI)	Friedrich, Lysne, Sim, & Shamos (2004)	Two versions: child and caregiver	45 items; assesses range of sexual behaviors among adolescents; scored on 3-point scale
Child Sexual Behavior Inventory (CSBI)	Friedrich (1998)	Caregiver	38 items; measure of the frequency of sexual behaviors in children ages 2–10 years

Note. Adapted from Denton, Frogley, Jackson, John, and Querstret (2017). DSM-IV, fourth edition of the *Diagnostic and Statistical Manual of Mental Disorders*; DSM-III-R, third revised edition of the *Diagnostic and Statistical Manual of Mental Disorders*.

cases, CSA is reported to caregivers, but caregivers do not inform official agencies. At the very least, it is important to screen for known histories of CSA, other forms of maltreatment, and other negative life events and adversities, through CPS records and/or caregiver reports. Consideration should also be given to routinely asking children about maltreatment experiences. Research demonstrates that most children do not disclose abuse unless prompted (London et al., 2013) and may have feelings of shame due to their abuse history (Deblinger & Runyon, 2005), so well planned, nonsuggestive interviews can provide a catalyst for disclosures that might not otherwise occur.

When screening for CSA specifically, clinicians need to discard some common myths. Although most consider sexual abuse to be perpetrated by adults, particularly parents and caregivers, abuse by siblings, older youth, and peers is quite common (Finkelhor et al., 2014; Krienert & Walsh, 2011). The way questions are asked about history of CSA is also important (Bottoms, Quas, & Davis, 2007; Lyon, Ahern, & Scurich, 2012; Stolzenberg & Lyon, 2014). Simply asking about CSA may not be sufficient because some children and parents may have a limited understanding of what CSA includes. Thus, more detailed questions without reference to "abuse" likely prompt more accurate information.

Epidemiological studies have also revealed the sad fact that for many maltreatment victims, *when it rains, it pours.* Child maltreatment often occurs in the midst of dysfunctional and inadequate caregiving that falls short in monitoring and protecting children, lacks the emotional sensitivity needed to detect child problems, and fails to nurture adequate communication needed to promote early disclosures (Elliott & Carnes, 2001; Finkelhor & Baron, 1986). Victims of CSA often experience other forms of childhood maltreatment, witness domestic violence, live in violent and impoverished communities, and experience other life adversities (Dong et al., 2003; Finkelhor et al., 2014; Pérez-Fuentes et al., 2013). They are also at increased risk of subsequent sexual victimization during their childhood, adolescence, and adult years (Barnes et al., 2009). Thus, in addition to documenting CSA and other adversities, it is important to obtain historical and current information about parenting, with the goal of identifying past and current risk factors. Given the high risk of revictimization, assessment strategies must identify current child, family, and community risks risk factors.

Disclosure of CSA and involvement in child welfare investigations expose children and youth to a host of family and system stressors. Family reactions to the disclosure are among the most potent predictors of child adjustment subsequent to CSA (Elliott & Carnes, 2001; Godbout, Briere, Sabourin, & Lussier, 2014). Caretakers' inability to provide protection from further maltreatment leads to children's placement outside of the home with relatives or in foster or group homes. Alternative care can be stressful for youth, who may perceive these protective actions as punishment for their disclosure (Greeson et al., 2011). Even when in alternative care, most youth continue to have contact with their families and in some cases have ongoing contact with the accused. Furthermore, most maltreated children in CPS care eventually return home (Albert, 2017). In many cases, child maltreatment, particularly CSA, leads to a number of criminal and child protection legal proceedings (Walsh, Jones, Cross, & Lippert, 2010). Although most children do not testify in criminal or child welfare proceedings, those who do often find the experience very stressful (Milojevich, Quas, & Yano, 2016; Quas & Goodman, 2012). Even when the child is not directly involved in the process, criminal and child protection legal proceedings create stress for those involved in the child's care, which is often communicated to the child. Thus, the assessment process should include an examination of how family, alternative care, and system stressors have affected the child, and how the family, child, and system adapt to these stressors. (See Figure 18.1 for a chart of the child welfare process.)

The Reason for Referral

The first consideration when assessing maltreatment victims is to determine the purpose of the assessment and the questions to be asked. In many cases, maltreatment victims are referred to identify how the abuse (or neglect) affected them and to provide direction for the types of interventions needed to help them recover. This typically occurs in the context of mental health services, but it can also occur in the context of legal proceedings, such as child welfare matters, custody and access disputes, civil litigation, and victim compensation applications. In most cases, adjustment problems have instigated the referral, but in some cases, caregivers and social workers want a "checkup" to determine the impact of the abuse and to explore ways to prevent future adjustment problems. In some cases, youth are referred for assessment be-

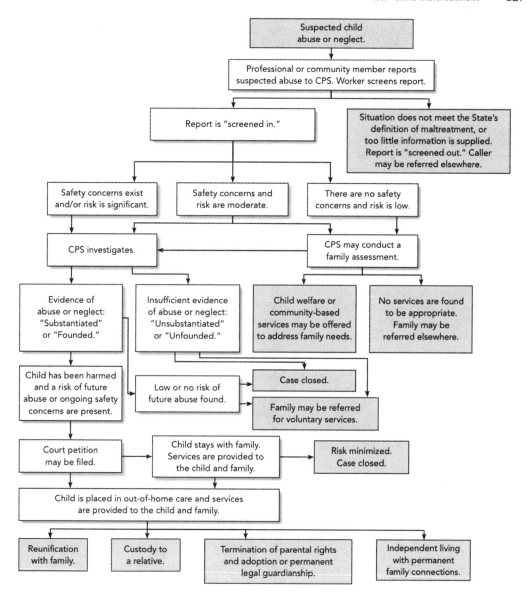

FIGURE 18.1. Flowchart of how the child welfare system works. From Child Welfare Information Gateway (2013).

cause of other problems, such as conduct problems or intentional self-harm. Because of the child's maltreatment history, questions arise as to whether the abuse contributed to the development or exacerbation of the problem. Thus, assessments for maltreatment may focus specifically on the effects of the abuse or be part of a broader assessment that addresses adjustment concerns.

Even if the original assessment was not intended for legal purposes, assessment reports are often requested or subpoenaed for criminal or civil proceedings. Prior to initiating an assessment, all parties should be informed of limits of confidentiality, particularly the possibility that the report might be subpoenaed by a judge. Other limits of confidentiality, including report of the abuse, should also be reviewed. Issues relevant to legal proceedings should be considered. For instance, if new details about maltreatment were reported by the youth during the course of the assessment, then care should be taken to document both the context of the disclosure and the youth's verbatim statements, and subsequent reports to CPS. This is important to avoid potential allegations that the disclosures were in some way "led" by assessment questions, misinterpreted by the assessor, or in some way mishandled in terms of child protection mandates. Care should also be taken to document all sources of information and to interpret assessment information in line with knowledge of maltreatment-related research.

Starting with Standard Good Assessment Strategies

Psychological assessment of children and youth require some basic components. As stated in the WHO (2017) guidelines, positive rapport is essential to all assessments, but it is particularly important for CSA victims and their families. Families who have undergone CPS and justice system investigations are often wary of mental health services (Davies, Seymour, & Read, 2000), and children may fear yet another interview about the abuse (Milojevich et al., 2016). Exploration of child and family concerns, and their goals at the outset of the assessment, may be helpful, and assessors should take time to explain the assessment process and how assessment information is used to assist with planning services. To understand the impact of maltreatment on children, it is best to assess the "whole child," not just the abuse, that is, taking time to learn about the children's interests, strengths, friends, and family. Although much of the focus of assessment is on mental health problems, the goals of mental health interventions include positive adjustment and personal growth. Knowing the child's strengths and interests identifies areas on which to build resilience and competence and helps the child and family members feel hopeful and balanced about mental health services. We have focused on maltreatment-specific types of information in this chapter. However, other basic information is required, including child developmental history, academic adjustment, and family and social relationships. Past efforts toward resolving problems should be explored, both within the family and through mental health services, including methods that have been successful and unsuccessful, and perceptions of the reasons behind these outcomes.

Building an Assessment Protocol

At the start of this chapter we recommended a starter kit for assessment; here, we provide additional considerations when building an assessment protocol. Individual assessors tend to establish preferred assessment methods and strategies. Our purpose in this chapter is to provide information about the assessment methods available for establishing an assessment protocol. Given the breadth and complexity of issues inherent in assessing maltreatment victims, an assessment approach is recommended that is multigating, multivariate, multi-informant, and multimethod. "Multigating" refers to using broad-band assessment tools to guide more specific areas of inquiry. Broad-band assessments include interviews, questionnaires, and personality measures that span multiple factors (see Table 18.2). For instance, the CBCL (Achenbach & Rescorla, 2001) provides an excellent overview of both child competencies and behavioral and emotional problems. Pairing the CBCL with a method that covers potential exposure, such as the SLESQ-R or TESI, ensures that the initial assessment covers the possibilities. As well, diagnostic interviews, such as the Diagnostic Interview for Children and Adolescents–IV (Reich, Welner, & Herjanic, 1997) and the Diagnostic Interview Schedule for Children (Shaffer, Fisher, Dulkan, & Davies, 1996), provide a thorough investigation of common mental health problems. Available computer-administered versions of these interviews for parent and adolescent completion enhance feasibility within clinical settings. Once specific mental health issues are identified from these broad-band assessments, more narrow-band evaluations can be conducted. That said, these broad-band assessment tools are often not sensitive to some of the specific effects of maltreatment. Thus, it is recommended that for identifying symptoms and for diagnostic purposes, broad-band assessment tools be supplemented with measures that independently assess PTSD and sexual problems (see Table 18.2; also see La Greca & Danzi, Chapter 15, this volume).

The multivariate aspects of assessment protocols refer to four domains: (1) background, (2) symptoms, (3) psychological processes, and (4) family and other social supports and stressors. By assessing these four domains, the child's problems may be conceptualized in terms of antecedents and consequences of the maltreatment and adversity and identified child and family factors may serve as objectives and goals for interventions. The multi-informant and multimethod aspects of an assessment protocol provide a layered strategy for ensuring a thorough evaluation and guard against biases stemming from different informants or methods. Assessment strategies should include the child and the child's primary caregivers, and when possible and relevant, information from social workers, therapists, and teachers. For background, it is often helpful to gather information from multiple sources (charts, CPS workers, parents, and sometimes the children themselves) because it is unlikely that any single source presents a full account of all relevant information. As well, inconsistencies from different sources are not uncommon and may call for clarification. Whenever CPS is involved in a case, it is often helpful to invite the primary worker to participate in the assessment process. CPS workers can clarify custodial status and provide supervisory orders and information about past and ongoing child welfare concerns, often with detail that is not readily available from CPS reports, which may not reflect the most recent events relevant to the case.

Although parents generally provide a good assessment of externalizing types of problems, parents with mental health problems sometimes overreport child problems and may underreport symptoms in other circumstances (e.g., during custody and access or child welfare proceedings (Friedrich, 2002; Sourander et al., 2006). Teacher reports can provide an unbiased alternative assessment of adjustment problems and additional information about the child's academic and social adjustment (Youngstrom, Loeber, & Stouthamer-Loeber, 2000). For sexual problems, parents are typically the best informants for sexualized behaviors of children (who may deny anything sexual; Larsson & Svedin, 2002), but adolescents are typically the better informants for themselves because parents are often unaware of their sexual activities, and adolescents are less hesitant than children to report sexual issues (Stanton et al., 2000). PTSD symptoms are best reported by the child or adolescent (Meiser-Stedman, Smith, Glucksman, Yule, & Dalgleish, 2007) because many symptoms are cognitive in nature. However, some youth may wish to avoid having their PTSD symptoms detected (as part of the avoidance aspect of PTSD); thus, caregiver reports provide an alternative source of information, particularly about the more observable aspects of PTSD. Likewise, youth tend to be the best informants of other internalizing symptoms (van der Ende, Verhulst, & Tiemeier, 2012), but some children may under- or overreport their symptoms (Friedrich, 2002). Varying assessment methods can help to ensure that information drawn from children is consistent and reliable. Whereas self-report measures are very helpful, supplementing the assessment protocol with pro-jective and observational tools may provide checks against method biases (Mihura, Meyer, Dumitrascu, & Bombel, 2013).

Assessment throughout the Intervention Process

Like the assessment process, interventions for maltreatment victims tend to be multidimensional to address multiple problems and often require long-term involvement (for an overview of interventions with CSA victims, see Wolfe, 2006). Assessment information is essential in developing an effective treatment and intervention plan and can help the clinician triage and prioritize treatment objectives. Because of the heterogeneous needs of maltreated children and their families, a "modular" treatment approach may be the most effective strategy for developing individualized treatment plans and for evaluating therapeutic effectiveness; that is, specific programs and techniques need to be developed and evaluated that address the particular abuse-specific sequelae exhibited by particular children. Clinicians can then prioritize treatment goals and systematically utilize proven interventions in a goal-oriented fashion. Particular abuse-specific goals should be established and monitored on a regular basis. Friedrich (1996) has described a goal attainment process that allows for continuous monitoring of therapeutic progress. Goals are individually established, with acceptable and desirable outcomes denoted.

More specifically, once a treatment plan is in place, it is important to monitor progress of specific objectives on an ongoing basis through tailored methods such as parent or child daily monitoring of symptoms and clinician sessional ratings of progress toward goals. Idiographic monitoring methods, such as the Top Problems approach (Weisz et al., 2011), are ways of tracking change (see Freeman & Young, Chapter 4, this volume, for more options). If the case formulation suggests that the internalizing or acting-out behaviors are sequelae to the maltreatment, then repeating symptom measures could provide midterm and outcome measures with normative benchmarks for clinically significant change (see Youngstrom & Prinstein, Chapter 1, this volume, and the Wikiversity pages for details). Once a specific set of goals is met, new goals and objectives may be set and monitored, with a continuation of the process until the child's mental health difficulties are addressed in full. For example, for a sexually abused child with sexual behavior problems, a treatment priority might be decreasing inappropriate sexual behaviors with other children. Multiple sessions are required to address those problems, and tailored monitoring strategies may be put in place until the sexualized problems are under control. At that point, other problems may be considered a second stage of intervention, such as addressing the child's PTSD symptoms, which also may be monitored until symptoms are resolved.

Summary and Conclusions

We have provided in this chapter an overview of issues related to maltreatment exposure, with special attention paid to CSA, including epidemiological findings, situational correlates of maltreatment, and the impact of maltreatment on victims. The findings reviewed provide a framework for assessing maltreated children for both clinical and research purposes. Child maltreatment is a serious negative life event that has great potential to set in motion a lifetime of adjustment problems. Numerous mental health problems are clearly linked with child maltreatment, including PTSD, dissociation, depression, sexuality problems, and risk for subsequent revictimization. Additional problems are likely not only influenced by the maltreatment experience but also linked with the emotional, familial, and social contexts associated with maltreatment. For example, behavioral and conduct problems have links with the sexual abuse, but the links are likely through depression and PTSD symptoms such as hyperarousal, as well as dysfunctional family and social contexts that often accompany sexual abuse.

There are clearly great individual differences in risk for developing mental problems subsequent to maltreatment exposure. Understanding the effects of child maltreatment requires consideration of many layers of contributing factors that are interrelated in complex ways. Child maltreatment itself constitutes a heterogeneous set of circumstances, including different acts, perpetrators, types of coercion, and frequencies and durations. Although these factors are related to maltreatment sequelae, research suggests that children's perceptions of maltreatment severity have much more to do with subsequent impact than specific maltreatment factors. Furthermore, children's perceptions of maltreatment severity do not necessarily correspond to the severity dimensions typically assessed by researchers (i.e., abusive acts, coercion, relationship to perpetrator). This suggests that either researchers have not yet found a way to define abuse se-

verity that reflects children's experiences, or that individual differences in the ways children experience negative life events such as sexual abuse have much to do with the child's resilience. It is possible that children's perceptions of their maltreatment are influenced by factors other than the abuse itself, such as postdisclosure stressors related to family reactions, involvement with CPS and the legal system, and the experience of other forms of adversity. It is also possible that children's ways of coping with maltreatment reflect premorbid coping tendencies; that is, well-adjusted children who have good coping skills and good family support may cope more effectively at the time of the maltreatment, perceive less threat and helplessness, act in effective ways to minimize the probability of further abuse or negative impact, and subsequently experience fewer negative mental health outcomes. But children with poor self-esteem, who rely on avoidant, internalizing, or externalizing forms of coping and have distant, nonsupportive familial relationships, may react at the time of the maltreatment with great horror and helplessness, may fail to disclose their abuse, and may therefore experience repeated episodes of abuse. Further longitudinal research is needed with large representative samples to investigate how premorbid adjustment and coping factors affect the impact of maltreatment. The good news on this front is the success of several large-scale research projects that have assessed both mental health and histories of negative life events, including sexual abuse, thus providing methodological templates for future prospective longitudinal studies. These findings have important implications for developing prevention programs that promote healthy coping when children face serious, negative life events, including but not limited to sexual abuse.

Over the past couple decades, the field has been enhanced by the development and refinement of tools to assess maltreatment victims. In particular, we now have a number of tools that assess PTSD, dissociation, and sexuality problems at different developmental points. As well, various tools that are now available assess both details about sexual abuse and details of other childhood maltreatment, adversities, and family-related problems. Our toolkit now also includes measures that assess children's perceptions and attributions about their maltreatment and their family situation. Clinically, these tools may be used as part of a more comprehensive assessment of victim adjustment that is multigating, multitrait, multimethod, multiinformant, ensuring that all appropriate symptoms are assessed, that results do not just reflect method variance, and that the perspectives of multiple people involved in a child's life are considered.

REFERENCES

Achenbach, T. M., & Rescorla, L. A. (2001). *Manual for the ASEBA School-Age Forms and Profiles*. Burlington: University of Vermont, Research Center for Children, Youth, and Families.

Afifi, T. O., & MacMillan, H. L. (2011). Resilience following child maltreatment: A review of protective factors. *Canadian Journal of Psychiatry, 56*, 266–272.

Alaggia, R., Collin-Vézina, D., & Lateef, R. (2019). Facilitators and barriers to child sexual abuse (CSA) disclosures: A research update (2000–2016). *Trauma, Violence, and Abuse, 20*, 260–283.

Albert, V. (2017). *From child abuse to permanency planning: Child welfare services pathways and placements.* New York: Routledge.

Alisic, E., Zalta, A. K., Van Wesel, F., Larsen, S. E., Hafstad, G. S., Hassanpour, K., & Smid, G. E. (2014). Rates of post-traumatic stress disorder in trauma-exposed children and adolescents: Meta-analysis. *British Journal of Psychiatry, 204*, 335–340.

American Psychiatric Association. (2013). *Diagnostic and statistical manual of mental disorders* (5th ed.). Arlington, VA: Author.

Anderson, G. D. (2016). The continuum of disclosure: Exploring factors predicting tentative disclosure of child sexual abuse allegations during forensic interviews and the implications for practice, policy, and future research. *Journal of Child Sexual Abuse, 25,* 382–402.

Bagley, C. C., & Mallick, K. (2000). Prediction of sexual, emotional, and physical maltreatment and mental health outcomes in a longitudinal cohort of 290 adolescent women. *Child Maltreatment, 5,* 218–226.

Bagley, C., & Thurston, W. E. (1996). *Understanding and preventing child sexual abuse: Vol. 2. Male victims, adolescents, adult outcomes and offender treatment.* Hampshire, UK: Ashgate.

Bal, S., Crombez, G., Van Oost, P., & Debourdeaudhuij, I. (2003). The role of social support in well-being and coping with self-reported stressful events in adolescents. *Child Abuse and Neglect, 27*, 1377–1395.

Bal, S., Van Oost, P., De Bourdeaudhuij, I., & Crombez, G. (2003). Avoidant coping as a mediator between self-reported sexual abuse and stress-related symptoms in adolescents. *Child Abuse and Neglect, 27,* 883–897.

Bardone, A. M., Moffitt, T., Caspi, A., & Dickson, N. (1996). Adult mental health and social outcomes of adolescent girls with depression and conduct disorder. *Development and Psychopathology, 8,* 811–829.

Barnes, J. E., Noll, J. G., Putnam, F. W., & Trickett, P. K. (2009). Sexual and physical revictimization among victims of severe childhood sexual abuse. *Child Abuse and Neglect, 33*(7), 412–420.

Barnett, D., Manly, J. T., & Cicchetti, D. (1991). Continuing toward an operational definition of psychological maltreatment. *Development and Psychopathology, 3,* 19–29.

Barnett, D., Manly, J. T., & Cicchetti, D. (1993). Defining child maltreatment: The interface between policy and research. In D. Cicchetti & S. Toth (Eds.), *Child abuse, child development, and social policy* (pp. 7–73). Norwood, NJ: Ablex.

Barth, J., Bermetz, L., Heim, E., Trelle, S., & Tonia, T. (2013). The current prevalence of child sexual abuse worldwide: A systematic review and meta-analysis. *International Journal of Public Health, 58*, 469–483.

Beck, J. S., Beck, A. T., Jolly, J., & Steer, R. A. (2001). *Manual for the Beck Youth Inventories of Emotional and Social Impairment* (2nd ed.). San Antonio, TX: Harcourt Assessment.

Bernstein, D. P., Ahluvalia, T., Pogge, D., & Handelsman, L. (1997). Validity of the Childhood Trauma Questionnaire in an adolescent psychiatric population. *Journal of the American Academy of Child and Adolescent Psychiatry, 36,* 340–348.

Bernstein, D. P., & Fink, L. (1998). *Childhood Trauma Questionnaire: A retrospective self-report.* San Antonio, TX: Psychological Corporation.

Bernstein, D. P., Fink, L., Handelsman, L., Foote, J., Lovejoy, M., Wenzel, K., . . . Ruggiero, J. (1994). Initial reliability and validity of a new retrospective measure of child abuse and neglect. *American Journal of Psychiatry, 15,* 1132–1136.

Bernstein, D. P., & Putnam, F. W. (1986). Development, reliability, and validity of a dissociation scale. *Journal of Nervous and Mental Disease, 174,* 727–735.

Bernstein, D. P., Stein, J. A., Newcomb, M. D., Walker, E., Pogge, D., Ahluvalia, T., . . . Zule, W. (2003). Development and validation of a brief screening version of the Childhood Trauma Questionnaire. *Child Abuse and Neglect, 27,* 169–190.

Berzenski, S. R., & Yates, T. M. (2011). Classes and consequences of multiple maltreatment: A person-centered analysis. *Child Maltreatment, 16,* 250–261.

Black, D. A., Heyman, R. E., & Slep, A. M. S. (2001). Risk factors for child sexual abuse. *Aggression and Violent Behavior, 6,* 203–229.

Boney-McCoy, S., & Finkelhor, D. (1995). Prior victimization: A risk factor for child sexual abuse and for PTSD-related symptomatology among sexually abused youth. *Child Abuse and Neglect, 19,* 1401–1421.

Boney-McCoy, S., & Finkelhor, D. (1996). Is youth victimization related to trauma symptoms and depression after controlling for prior symptoms and family relationships?: A longitudinal, prospective study. *Journal of Consulting and Clinical Psychology, 64,* 1406–1416.

Bottoms, B. L., Quas, J. A., & Davis, S. L. (2007). The influence of the interviewer-provided social support on children's suggestibility, memory, and disclosures.

In M.-E. Pipe, M. E. Lamb, Y. Orbach, & A.-C. Cederborg (Eds.), *Child sexual abuse: Disclosure, delay, and denial* (pp. 135–157). Mahwah, NJ: Erlbaum.

Briere, J., Johnson, K., Bissada, A., Damon, L., Crouch, J., Gil, E., . . . Ernst, V. (2001). The Trauma Symptom Checklist for Young Children (TSCYC): Reliability and association with abuse exposure in a multi-site study. *Child Abuse and Neglect, 25,* 1001–1014.

Briere, J., & Runtz, M. (1989). University males' sexual interest in children: Predicting potential indices of "pedophilia" in a nonforensic sample. *Child Abuse and Neglect, 13,* 65–75.

Brooks-Gunn, J., & Chase-Lansdale, P. L. (1995). Adolescent parenthood In M. H. Bornstein (Ed.), *Handbook of parenting: Vol. 3. Status and social conditions of parenting* (pp. 113–149). Hillsdale, NJ: Erlbaum.

Brown, J., Cohen, P., Johnson, J. G., & Salzinger, S. (1998). A longitudinal analysis of risk factors for child maltreatment: Findings of a 17-year prospective study of officially recorded and self-reported child abuse and neglect. *Child Abuse and Neglect, 22,* 1065–1078.

Brown, J., Cohen, P., Johnson, J. G., & Smailes, E. M. (1999). Childhood abuse and neglect: Specificity and effects on adolescent and young adult depression and suicidality. *Journal of the American Academy of Child and Adolescent Psychiatry, 38,* 1490–1496.

Brown, L. K., Kessel, S. M., Lourie, K. J., Ford, H., & Lipsitt, L. (1997). Influence of sexual abuse on HIV-related attitudes and behaviors in adolescent psychiatric inpatients. *Journal of the American Academy of Child and Adolescent Psychiatry, 36,* 316–322.

Butcher, J. N., Williams, C. L., Graham, J. R., Archer, R. P., Tellegen, A., Ben-Porath, Y. S., & Kaemmer, B. (1992). *The Minnesota Multiphasic Personality Inventory–Adolescent.* Oxford, UK: Pearson.

Centers for Disease Control and Prevention. (2019). Child abuse and neglect prevention. Retrieved from *www.cdc.gov/violenceprevention/childabuseandneglect/index.html.*

Chaffin, M., & Shultz, S. K. (2001). Psychometric evaluation of the Children's Impact of Traumatic Events Scale—Revised. *Child Abuse and Neglect, 25,* 401–411.

Chaffin, M., Wherry, J. N., Newlin, C., Crutchfield, A., & Dykman, R. (1997). The Abuse Dimensions Inventory: Initial data on a research measure of abuse severity. *Journal of Interpersonal Violence, 12,* 569–589.

Chen, L. P., Murad, M. H., Paras, M. L., Colbenson, K. M., Sattler, A. L., Goranson, E. N., . . . Zirakzadeh, A. (2010). Sexual abuse and lifetime diagnosis of psychiatric disorders: Systematic review and meta-analysis. *Mayo Clinic Proceedings, 85*(7), 618–629.

Cicchetti, D. (2016). Socioemotional, personality, and biological development: Illustrations from a multi-level developmental psychopathology perspective on child maltreatment. *Annual Review of Psychology, 67,* 187–211.

Classen, C. C., Palesh, O. G., & Aggarwal, R. (2005). Sexual victimization: A review of the empirical literature. *Trauma, Violence, and Abuse, 2,* 103–129.

Cloitre, M., Stolbach, B. C., Herman, J. L., Kolk, B. V. D., Pynoos, R., Wang, J., & Petkova, E. (2009). A developmental approach to complex PTSD: Childhood and adult cumulative trauma as predictors of symptom complexity. *Journal of Traumatic Stress, 22,* 399–408.

Cook, A., Spinazzola, J., Ford, J., Lanktree, C., Blaustein, M., Cloitre, M., . . . van der Kolk, B. (2005). Complex trauma in children and adolescents. *Psychiatric Annals, 35,* 390–398.

Costello, E. J., Angold, A., March, J., & Fairbank, J. (1998). Life events and post-traumatic stress: The development of a new measure for children and adolescents. *Psychological Medicine, 28,* 1275–1288.

Crea, T. M., Easton, S. D., Florio, J., & Barth, R. P. (2018). Externalizing behaviors among adopted children: A longitudinal comparison of preadoptive childhood sexual abuse and other forms of maltreatment. *Child Abuse and Neglect, 82,* 192–200.

Crooks, C. V., & Wolfe, D. A. (2007). Child abuse and neglect. In E. J. Mash & R. A. Barkley (Eds.), *Assessment of childhood disorders* (4th ed., pp. 639–684). New York: Guilford Press.

Cuffe, S. P., Addy, C. L., Garrison, C. Z., Waller, J. L., Jackson, K. L., McKeown, R. E., & Chilappagari, S. (1998). Prevalence of PTSD in a community sample of older adolescents. *Journal of the American Academy of Child and Adolescent Psychiatry, 37,* 147–154.

Cutajar, M. C., Mullen, P. E., Ogloff, J. R., Thomas, S. D., Wells, D. L., & Spataro, J. (2010). Psychopathology in a large cohort of sexually abused children followed up to 43 years. *Child Abuse and Neglect, 34,* 813–822.

Daigneault, I., Hébert, M., & Tourigny, M. (2007). Personal and interpersonal characteristics related to resilient developmental pathways of sexually abused adolescents. *Child and Adolescent Psychiatric Clinics of North America, 16,* 415–434.

Danielson, C. K., de Arellano, M. A., Kilpatrick, D. G., Saunders, B. E., & Resnick, H. S. (2005). Child maltreatment in depressed adolescents: Differences in symptomatology based on history of abuse. *Child Maltreatment, 10,* 37–48.

Davies, E., Seymour, F., & Read, J. (2000). Children's and primary caretakers' perceptions of the sexual abuse investigation process: A New Zealand example. *Journal of Child Sexual Abuse, 9,* 41–56.

Deblinger, E., & Runyon, M. K. (2005). Understanding and treating feelings of shame in children who have experienced maltreatment. *Child Maltreatment, 10,* 364–376.

Denton, R., Frogley, C., Jackson, S., John, M., & Querstret, D. (2017). The assessment of developmental trauma in children and adolescents: A systematic review. *Clinical Child Psychology and Psychiatry, 22,* 260–287.

Dolan, Y. M. (1991). *Resolving sexual abuse: Solution-focused therapy and Eriksonian hypnosis for adult survivors.* New York: Norton.

Dong, M., Anda, R. F., Dube, S. R., Giles, W. H., & Felitti, V. J. (2003). The relationship of exposure to childhood sexual abuse to other forms of abuse, neglect, and household dysfunction during childhood. *Child Abuse and Neglect, 27,* 625–639.

Dorahy, M. J., Brand, B. L., Şar, V., Krüger, C., Stavropoulos, P., Martínez-Taboas, A., . . . Middleton, W. (2014). Dissociative identity disorder: An empirical overview. *Australian and New Zealand Journal of Psychiatry, 48,* 402–417.

Drake, B., & Pandey, S. (1996). Understanding the relationship between neighborhood poverty and specific types of child maltreatment. *Child Abuse and Neglect, 20,* 1003–1018.

Dube, S. R., Anda, R. F., Whitfield, C. L., Brown, D. W., Felitti, V. J., Dong, M., & Giles, W. H. (2005). Long-term consequences of childhood sexual abuse by gender of victim. *American Journal of Preventive Medicine, 28,* 430–438.

Dubner, A. E., & Motta, R. W. (1999). Sexually and physically abused foster children and posttraumatic stress disorder. *Journal of Consulting and Clinical Psychology, 67,* 367–373.

Dubowitz, H., Kim, J., Black, M. M., Weisbart, C., Semiatin, J., & Magder, L. S. (2011). Identifying children at high risk for a child maltreatment report. *Child Abuse and Neglect, 35,* 96–104.

Dunn, E. C., McLaughlin, K. A., Slopen, N., Rosand, J., & Smoller, J. W. (2013). Developmental timing of child maltreatment and symptoms of depression and suicidal ideation in young adulthood: Results from the National Longitudinal Study of Adolescent Health. *Depression and Anxiety, 30,* 955–964.

Dunn, E. C., Nishimi, K., Powers, A., & Bradley, B. (2017). Is developmental timing of trauma exposure associated with depressive and post-traumatic stress disorder symptoms in adulthood? *Journal of Psychiatric Research, 84,* 119–127.

Egeland, B., & Sroufe, A. (1981). Attachment and early maltreatment. *Child Development, 52,* 44–52.

Elliott, A. N., & Carnes, C. N. (2001). Reactions of nonoffending parents to the sexual abuse of their child: A review of the literature. *Child Maltreatment, 6,* 314–331.

English, D. J., Graham, J. C., Litrownik, A. J., Everson, M., & Bangdiwala, S. I. (2005). Defining maltreatment chronicity: Are there differences in child outcomes? *Child Abuse and Neglect, 29,* 575–595.

Euser, E. M., van IJzendoorn, M. H., Prinzie, P., & Bakermans-Kranenburg, M. J. (2010). Prevalence of child maltreatment in the Netherlands. *Child Maltreatment, 15,* 5–17.

Everson, M. D., Smith, J. B., Hussey, J. M., English, D., Litrownik, A. J., Dubowitz, H., . . . Runyan, D. K. (2008). Concordance between adolescent reports of childhood abuse and child protective service determinations in an at-risk sample of young adolescents. *Child Maltreatment, 13,* 14–26.

Fearon, R. P., Bakermans-Kranenburg, M. J., van IJzendoorn, M. H., Lapsley, A. M., & Roisman, G. I. (2010). The significance of insecure attachment and disorganization in the development of children's externalizing behavior: A meta-analytic study. *Child Development, 81,* 435–456.

Feiring, C., Taska, L., & Lewis, M. (1999). Age and gender differences in children and adolescents adaptation to sexual abuse. *Child Abuse and Neglect, 23,* 115–128.

Feiring, C., Taska, L., & Lewis, M. (2002). Adjustment following sexual abuse discovery: The role of shame and attributional style. *Developmental Psychology, 38,* 79–92.

Fergusson, D. M., Horwood, J., & Lynskey, M. (1996). Childhood sexual abuse and psychiatric disorder in young adulthood: II. Psychiatric outcomes of childhood sexual abuse. *Journal of the American Academy of Child and Adolescent Psychiatry, 35,* 1365–1374.

Fergusson, D. M., Horwood, J., & Lynskey, M. (1997). Childhood sexual abuse, adolescent sexual behaviors and sexual revictimization. *Child Abuse and Neglect, 21,* 789–803.

Fergusson, D. M., Lynskey, M., & Horwood, J. (1996). Childhood sexual abuse and psychiatric disorder in young adulthood: I. Prevalence of sexual abuse and factors associated with sexual abuse. *Journal of the American Academy of Child and Adolescent Psychiatry, 34,* 1355–1364.

Fergusson, D. M., Woodward, L. J., & Horwood, L. J. (2000). Risk factors and life processes associated with the onset of suicidal behavior during adolescence and early adulthood. *Psychological Medicine, 30,* 23–39.

Findling, J. H., Bratton, S. C., & Henson, R. K. (2006). Development of the Trauma Play Scale: An observation-based assessment of the impact of trauma on play therapy behaviors of young children. *International Journal of Play Therapy, 15,* 7–36.

Finkelhor, D. (1984). *Child sexual abuse: New theory and research.* New York: Free Press.

Finkelhor, D. (1994). Current information on the scope and nature of child sexual abuse. *The Future of Children, 4,* 31–53.

Finkelhor, D. (2008). *Childhood victimization.* New York: Oxford University Press.

Finkelhor, D., & Baron, L. (1986). High risk children. In D. Finkelhor, S. Araji, L. Baron, A. Browne, S. Peters, & G. Wyatt (Eds.), *A sourcebook on child sexual abuse* (pp. 60–88). Beverly Hills, CA: SAGE.

Finkelhor, D., Hotaling, G., Lewis, I. A., & Smith, C. (1990). Sexual abuse in a national survey of adult men and women: Prevalence, characteristics, and risk factors. *Child Abuse and Neglect, 14,* 19–28.

Finkelhor, D., & Jones, L. M. (2004, January). Explanations for the decline in child sexual abuse cases. Retrieved April 26, 2006, from *www.ojp.usdoj.gov/ojjdp.*

Finkelhor, D., Jones, L. M., & Shattuck, A. (2010). *Up-*

dated trends in child maltreatment, 2008. Durham, NH: Crimes Against Children Research Center.

Finkelhor, D., Moore, D., Hamby, S. L., & Straus, M. A. (1997). Sexually abused children in a national survey of parents: Methodological issues. *Child Abuse and Neglect, 21,* 1–9.

Finkelhor, D., & Ormrod, R. K. (2001). *Offenders incarcerated for crimes against juveniles* (Bulletin). Washington, DC: U.S. Department of Justice, Office of Justice Programs, Office of Juvenile Justice and Delinquency Prevention.

Finkelhor, D., Ormrod, R. K., Turner, H. A., & Hamby, S. L. (2005). Measuring poly-victimization using the Juvenile Victimization Questionnaire. *Child Abuse and Neglect, 29,* 1297–1312.

Finkelhor, D., Shattuck, A., Turner, H. A., & Hamby, S. L. (2014). The lifetime prevalence of child sexual abuse and sexual assault assessed in late adolescence. *Journal of Adolescent Health, 55,* 329–333.

Finkelhor, D., Turner, H., Ormrod, R., & Hamby, S. L. (2009). Violence, abuse, and crime exposure in a national sample of children and youth. *Pediatrics, 124,* 1411–1423.

Fischer, G. J. (1991). Is lesser severity of child sexual abuse a reason more males report having liked it? *Annals of Sex Research, 4,* 131–139.

Flores, E., Cicchetti, D., & Rogosch, F. A. (2005). Predictors of resilience in maltreated and nonmaltreated Latino children. *Developmental Psychology, 41,* 338–351.

Foa, E. B., Asnaani, A., Zang, Y., Capaldi, S., & Yeh, R. (2018). Psychometrics of the Child PTSD Symptom Scale for DSM-5 for trauma-exposed children and adolescents. *Journal of Clinical Child and Adolescent Psychology, 47,* 38–46.

Folger, S. F., & Wright, M. O. D. (2013). Altering risk following child maltreatment: Family and friend support as protective factors. *Journal of Family Violence, 28,* 325–337.

Fox, N. A., & Leavitt, L. A. (1995). *The Violence Exposure Scale for Children—Revised (VEX-R).* College Park: University of Maryland.

Friedrich, W. N. (1993). Sexual victimization and sexual behavior in children: A review of recent literature. *Child Abuse and Neglect, 17,* 59–66.

Friedrich, W. N. (1996). Clinical considerations of empirical treatment studies of abused children. *Child Maltreatment, 1,* 343–347.

Friedrich, W. N. (1998). Behavioral manifestations of child sexual abuse. *Child Abuse and Neglect, 22,* 523–531.

Friedrich, W. N. (2002). *Psychological assessment of sexually abused children and their families.* Thousand Oaks, CA: SAGE.

Friedrich, W. N., Lysne, M., Sim, L., & Shamos, S. (2004). Assessing sexual behavior in high-risk adolescents with the Adolescent Clinical Sexual Behavior Inventory (ACSBI). *Child Maltreatment, 9,* 239–250.

Garnefski, N., & Diekstra, R. F. W. (1997). Child sexual abuse and emotional and behavioral problems in adolescence: Gender differences. *Journal of the American Academy of Child and Adolescent Psychiatry, 36,* 323–329.

Gateway. (2013). *How the child welfare system works.* Washington, DC: U.S. Department of Health and Human Services.

Ghetti, S., Goodman, G. S., Eisen, M. L., Qin, J., & Davis, S. L. (2002). Consistency in children's reports of sexual and physical abuse. *Child Abuse and Neglect, 26,* 977–995.

Gilbert, R., Widom, C. S., Browne, K., Fergusson, D., Webb, E., & Janson, S. (2009). Burden and consequences of child maltreatment in high-income countries. *Lancet, 373,* 68–81.

Godbout, N., Briere, J., Sabourin, S., & Lussier, Y. (2014). Child sexual abuse and subsequent relational and personal functioning: The role of parental support. *Child Abuse and Neglect, 38,* 317–325.

Goldman, J. D. G., & Padayachi, U. K. (2000). Some methodological problems in estimating incidence and prevalence in child sexual abuse research. *Journal of Sex Research, 37,* 305–314.

Goodman, G. S., Ghetti, S., Quas, J. A., Edelstein, R. S., Alexander, K. W., Redlich, A. D., . . . Jones, D. P. (2003). A prospective study of memory for child sexual abuse: New findings relevant to the repressed memory controversy. *Psychological Science, 14,* 113–118.

Goodman, L. A., Corcoran, C., Turner, K., Yuan, N., & Green, B. L. (1998). Assessing traumatic event exposure: General issues and preliminary findings for the Stressful Life Events Screening Questionnaire. *Journal of Traumatic Stress, 11,* 521–542.

Gordon, M. (1990). The family environment of sexual abuse: An examination of the gender effect. *Journal of Family Violence, 5,* 321–332.

Greenhoot, A. F., McCloskey, L. A., & Gisky, E. (2005). A longitudinal study of adolescents' recollections of family violence. *Applied Cognitive Psychology, 19,* 719–743.

Greeson, J. K., Briggs, E. C., Kisiel, C. L., Layne, C. M., Ake, G. S., Ko, S. J., & Fairbank, J. A. (2011). Complex trauma and mental health in children and adolescents placed in foster care: Findings from the National Child Traumatic Stress Network. *Child Welfare, 90,* 91–108.

Groh, A. M., Roisman, G. I., van IJzendoorn, M. H., Bakermans-Kranenburg, M. J., & Fearon, R. P. (2012). The significance of insecure and disorganized attachment for children's internalizing symptoms: A meta-analytic study. *Child Development, 83,* 591–610.

Hagan, M. J., Hulette, A. C., & Lieberman, A. F. (2015). Symptoms of dissociation in a high-risk sample of young children exposed to interpersonal trauma: Prevalence, correlates, and contributors. *Journal of Traumatic Stress, 28,* 258–261.

Hamby, S. L., & Finkelhor, D. (2001). *Choosing and*

using child victimization questionnaires (NCJ186027). Washington, DC: U.S. Department of Justice, Office of Juvenile Delinquency and Prevention.

Hamby, S. L., & Finkelhor, D. (2004). *The Comprehensive Juvenile Victimization Questionnaire*. Durham: University of New Hampshire.

Hanson, R. F., Kievit, L. W., Saunders, B. E., Smith, D. W., Kilpatrick, D. G., Resnick, H. S., & Ruggiero, K. J. (2003). Correlates of adolescent reports of sexual assault: Findings from the National Survey of Adolescents. *Child Maltreatment, 8*, 261–272.

Hanson, R. F., Resnick, H. S., Saunders, B. E., Kilpatrick, D. G., & Best, C. (1999). Factors related to the reporting of childhood rape. *Child Abuse and Neglect, 23*, 559–569.

Hanson, R. F., Seer-Brown, S., Fricker-Elhai, A. E., Kilpatrick, D. G., Saunders, B. E., & Resnick, H. S. (2006). The relations between family environment violence exposure among youth: Findings from the National Survey of Adolescents. *Child Maltreatment, 11*, 3–15.

Hanson, R., Smith, D., Saunders, B., Swenson, C., & Conrad, L. (1995). Measurement in child abuse research: A survey of researchers. *APSAC Advisor, 8*, 7–10.

Hashimi, P. Y., & Finkelhor, D. (1999). Violent victimization of youth versus adults in the National Crime Victimization Survey. *Journal of Interpersonal Violence, 14*, 799–820.

Haskett, M. E., Nears, K., Ward, C. S., & McPherson, A. V. (2006). Diversity in adjustment of maltreated children: Factors associated with resilient functioning. *Clinical Psychology Review, 26*, 796–812.

Hébert, M., Langevin, R., & Daigneault, I. (2016). The association between peer victimization, PTSD, and dissociation in child victims of sexual abuse. *Journal of Affective Disorders, 193*, 227–232.

Herrenkohl, E. C., Herrenkohl, R. C., & Egolf, B. (1994). Resilient early school-age children from maltreating homes: Outcomes in late adolescence. *American Journal of Orthopsychiatry, 64*, 301–309.

Hershkowitz, I., Lamb, M. E., & Horowitz, D. (2007). Victimization of children with disabilities. *American Journal of Orthopsychiatry, 77*, 629–635.

Hibbard, R. A., Desch, L. W., & Committee on Child Abuse and Neglect. (2007). Maltreatment of children with disabilities. *Pediatrics, 119*, 1018–1025.

Higgins, D. J., & McCabe, M. P. (2000). Relationships between different types of maltreatment during childhood and adjustment in adulthood. *Child Maltreatment, 5*, 261–272.

Hillberg, T., Hamilton-Giachritsis, C., & Dixon, L. (2011). Review of meta-analyses on the association between child sexual abuse and adult mental health difficulties: A systematic approach. *Trauma, Violence, and Abuse, 12*, 38–49.

Hodges, J., Steele, M., Kaniuk, J., Hillman, S., & Asquith, K. (2009). Narratives in assessment and research on the development of attachments in mal-

treated children. In N. Midgley, J. Anderson, E. Grainger, T. Nesic-Vuckovic, & C. Urwin (Eds.), *Child psychotherapy and research: New approaches, emerging findings* (pp. 200–213). New York: Routledge.

Howard, D. E., & Wang, M. Q. (2005). Psychosocial correlates of U.S. adolescents who report a history of forced sexual intercourse. *Journal of Adolescent Health, 36*, 372–379.

Hulette, A. C., Freyd, J. J., & Fisher, P. A. (2011). Dissociation in middle childhood among foster children with early maltreatment experiences. *Child Abuse and Neglect, 35*, 123–126.

Hussey, J. M., Chang, J. J., & Kotch, J. B. (2006). Child maltreatment in the United States: Prevalence, risk factors, and adolescent health consequences. *Pediatrics, 118*, 933–942.

Ippen, C. G., Ford, J., Racusin, R., Acker, M., Bosquet, M., Rogers, K., . . . Edwards, J. (2002). *Traumatic Events Screening Inventory—Parent Report Revised*. Hanover, NH: U.S. Department of Veterans Affairs, National Center for PTSD.

Jaffee, S. R., Caspi, A., Moffitt, T. E., Polo-Tomas, M., & Taylor, A. (2007). Individual, family, and neighborhood factors distinguish resilient from non-resilient maltreated children: A cumulative stressors model. *Child Abuse and Neglect, 31*, 231–253.

Johnsen, L. W., & Harlow, L. L. (1996). Childhood sexual abuse linked with adult substance use, victimization, and AIDS-risk. *AIDS Education and Prevention, 8*, 44–57.

Johnson, T. C. (1988). Child perpetrators—children who molest other children: Preliminary findings. *Child Abuse and Neglect, 13*, 571–585.

Jones, D. J., Lewis, T., Litrownik, A., Thompson, R., Proctor, L. J., Isbell, P., . . . Runyan, D. (2013). Linking childhood sexual abuse and early adolescent risk behavior: The intervening role of internalizing and externalizing problems. *Journal of Abnormal Child Psychology, 41*, 139–150.

Jones, L., Bellis, M. A., Wood, S., Hughes, K., McCoy, E., Eckley, L., . . . Officer, A. (2012). Prevalence and risk of violence against children with disabilities: A systematic review and meta-analysis of observational studies. *Lancet, 380*, 899–907.

Jonson-Reid, M., Kohl, P. L., & Drake, B. (2012). Child and adult outcomes of chronic child maltreatment. *Pediatrics, 129*, 839–845.

Kantor, G. K., Holt, M. K., Mebert, C. J., Straus, M. A., Drach, K. M., Ricci, L. R., . . . Brown, W. (2004). Development and preliminary psychometric properties of the Multidimensional Neglectful Behavior Scale—Child Report. *Child Maltreatment, 9*, 409–428.

Kaufman, J., Jones, B., Stieglitz, E., Vitulano, L., & Mannarino, A. P. (1994). The use of multiple informants to assess children's maltreatment experiences. *Journal of Family Violence, 9*, 227–248.

Keiley, M. K., Howe, T. R., Dodge, K. A., Bates, J. E., &

Pettit, G. S. (2001). The timing of child physical maltreatment: A cross-domain growth analysis of impact on adolescent externalizing and internalizing problems. *Development and Psychopathology, 13,* 891–912.

Kendall-Tackett, K. A., Williams, L. M., & Finkelhor, D. (1993). Impact of sexual abuse on children: A review and synthesis of recent empirical studies. *Psychological Bulletin, 113,* 164–180.

Kenny, M. C., & McEachern, A. G. (2000). Racial, ethnic, and cultural factors of childhood sexual abuse: A selected review of the literature. *Clinical Psychology Review, 20,* 905–922.

Kilpatrick, D. G., Ruggiero, K. J., Acierno, R., Saunders, D. E., Resnick, H. S., & Best, C. L. (2003). Violence and risk of PTSD, major depression, substance abuse/dependence, and comorbidity: Results from the National Survey of Adolescents. *Journal of Consulting and Clinical Psychology, 71,* 692–700.

Kim, J., & Cicchetti, D. (2010). Longitudinal pathways linking child maltreatment, emotion regulation, peer relations, and psychopathology. *Journal of Child Psychology and Psychiatry, 51,* 706–716.

Kirschner, R. H., & Wilson, H. (2001). Pathology of fatal child abuse. In R. M. Reece & S. Ludwig (Eds.), *Child abuse: Medical diagnosis and management* (2nd ed., pp. 467–516). Philadelphia: Lippincott, Williams & Wilkins.

Kogan, S. M. (2004). Disclosing unwanted sexual experiences: Results from a national sample of adolescent women. *Child Abuse and Neglect, 28,* 1–19.

Kotch, J. B., Chalmers, D. J., Fanslow, J. L., Marshall, S., & Langley, J. D. (1993). Morbidity and death due to child abuse in New Zealand. *Child Abuse and Neglect, 17,* 233–247.

Krienert, J. L., & Walsh, J. A. (2011). Sibling sexual abuse: An empirical analysis of offender, victim, and event characteristics in National Incident-Based Reporting System (NIBRS) Data, 2000–2007. *Journal of Child Sexual Abuse, 20,* 353–372.

Lalor, K., & McElvaney, R. (2010). Child sexual abuse, links to later sexual exploitation/high-risk sexual behavior, and prevention/treatment programs. *Trauma, Violence, and Abuse, 11,* 159–177.

Larsson, I., & Svedin, C. G. (2002). Teachers' and parents' reports on 3- to 6-year-old children's sexual behavior—a comparison. *Child Abuse and Neglect, 26,* 247–266.

Lau, A. S., Leeb, R. T., English, D., Graham, J. C., Briggs, E. C., Brody, K. E., & Marshall, J. M. (2005). What's in a name?: A comparison of methods for classifying predominant type of maltreatment. *Child Abuse and Neglect, 29,* 533–551.

Leeb, R. T., Paulozzi, L., Melanson, C., Simon, T., & Arias, I. (2008). *Child Maltreatment Surveillance: Uniform Definitions for Public Health and Recommended Data Elements, Version 1.0.* Atlanta, GA: Centers for Disease Control and Prevention, National Center for Injury Prevention and Control.

Lewis, T., McElroy, E., Harlaar, N., & Runyan, D. (2016). Does the impact of child sexual abuse differ from maltreated but non-sexually abused children?: A prospective examination of the impact of child sexual abuse on internalizing and externalizing behavior problems. *Child Abuse and Neglect, 51,* 31–40.

Liebenberg, L., Ungar, M., & LeBlanc, J. C. (2013). The CYRM-12: A brief measure of resilience. *Canadian Journal of Public Health, 104,* 131–135.

Lindert, J., von Ehrenstein, O. S., Grashow, R., Gal, G., Braehler, E., & Weisskopf, M. G. (2014). Sexual and physical abuse in childhood is associated with depression and anxiety over the life course: Systematic review and meta-analysis. *International Journal of Public Health, 59,* 359–372.

Liotti, G. (1999). Disorganization of attachment as a model for understanding dissociative psychopathology. In J. Solomon & C. George (Eds.), *Attachment disorganization* (pp. 291–317). New York: Guilford Press.

Lipschitz, D. S., Bernstein, D. P., Winegar, R. K., & Southwick, S. M. (1999). Hospitalized adolescents' reports of sexual and physical abuse: A comparison of two self-report measures. *Journal of Traumatic Stress, 12,* 641–654.

London, K., Bruck, M., Ceci, S. J., & Shuman, D. W. (2013). Disclosure of child sexual abuse: A review of the contemporary empirical literature. In M.-E. Pipe, Lamb, M. E., Orbach, Y., & Cederborg, A. C. (Eds.), *Child sexual abuse: Disclosure, delay, and denial* (pp. 11–40). New York: Psychology Press.

Long, P. J., & Jackson, J. L. (1990, November). *Defining childhood sexual abuse.* Poster presented at the annual meeting of the Association for Advancement of Behavior Therapy, San Francisco.

Lunkenheimer, E., Busuito, A., Brown, K. M., & Skowron, E. A. (2018). Mother–child coregulation of parasympathetic processes differs by child maltreatment severity and subtype. *Child Maltreatment, 23,* 211–220.

Luster, T., Small, S. A., & Lower, R. (2002). The correlates of abuse and witnessing abuse among adolescents. *Journal of Interpersonal Violence, 17,* 1323–1340.

Lyon, T. D., Ahern, E. C., & Scurich, N. (2012). Interviewing children versus tossing coins: Accurately assessing the diagnosticity of children's disclosures of abuse. *Journal of Child Sexual Abuse, 21,* 19–44.

Macfie, J., Cicchetti, D., & Toth, S. L. (2001). The development of dissociation in maltreated preschool-age children. *Development and Psychopathology, 13,* 233–254.

Maclean, M. J., Sims, S., Bower, C., Leonard, H., Stanley, F. J., & O'Donnell, M. (2017). Maltreatment risk among children with disabilities. *Pediatrics, 139,* e20161817.

MacMillan, H. L., Fleming, J. E., Trocmé, N., Boyle, M. H., Wong, M., Racine, Y. A., . . . Offord, D. R. (1997). Prevalence of child physical and sexual abuse in the community: Results from the Ontario Health Supplement. *Journal of the American Medical Association, 278,* 131–135.

MacMillan, H. L., Jamieson, E., & Walsh, C. A. (2003). Reported contact with child protection services among those reporting child physical and sexual abuse: Results from a community survey. *Child Abuse and Neglect, 27,* 1397–1408.

Madigan, S., Atkinson, L., Laurin, K., & Benoit, D. (2013). Attachment and internalizing behavior in early childhood: A meta-analysis. *Developmental Psychology, 49,* 672–689.

Maikovich-Fong, A. K., & Jaffee, S. R. (2010). Sex differences in childhood sexual abuse characteristics and victims' emotional and behavioral problems: Findings from a national sample of youth. *Child Abuse and Neglect, 34,* 429–437.

Maniglio, R. (2010). Child sexual abuse in the etiology of depression: A systematic review of reviews. *Depression and Anxiety, 27,* 631–642.

Manly, J. T., Kim, J. E., Rogosch, F. A., & Cicchetti, D. (2001). Dimensions of child maltreatment and children's adjustment: Contributions of developmental timing and subtype. *Development and Psychopathology, 13,* 759–782.

Manly, J. T., Oshri, A., Lynch, M., Herzog, M., & Wortel, S. (2013). Child neglect and the development of externalizing behavior problems: Associations with maternal drug dependence and neighborhood crime. *Child Maltreatment, 18,* 17–29.

McElvaney, R. (2015). Disclosure of child sexual abuse: Delays, non-disclosure and partial disclosure: What the research tells us and implications for practice. *Child Abuse Review, 24,* 159–169.

McGee, R. A., Wolfe, D. A., Yuen, S. A., Wilson, S. K., & Carnochan, J. (1995). The measurement of maltreatment: A comparison of approaches. *Child Abuse and Neglect, 19,* 233–249.

McLeer, S., Dixon, J. F., Henry, D., Ruggiero, K., Escovitz, K., Niedda, T., & Scholle, R. (1998). Psychopathology in non-clinically referred sexually abused children. *Journal of the American Academy of Child and Adolescent Psychiatry, 37,* 1326–1333.

Meiser-Stedman, R., Smith, P., Glucksman, E., Yule, W., & Dalgleish, T. (2007). Parent and child agreement for acute stress disorder, post-traumatic stress disorder and other psychopathology in a prospective study of children and adolescents exposed to single-event trauma. *Journal of Abnormal Child Psychology, 35,* 191–201.

Mihura, J. L., Meyer, G. J., Dumitrascu, N., & Bombel, G. (2013). The validity of individual Rorschach variables: Systematic reviews and meta-analyses of the comprehensive system. *Psychological Bulletin, 139,* 548–605.

Miller, A. B., Eisenlohr-Moul, T., Giletta, M., Hastings, P. D., Rudolph, K. D., Nock, M. K., & Prinstein, M. J. (2017). A within-person approach to risk for suicidal ideation and suicidal behavior: Examining the roles of depression, stress, and abuse exposure. *Journal of Consulting and Clinical Psychology, 85,* 712–722.

Miller, A. B., Esposito-Smythers, C., Weismoore, J. T., & Renshaw, K. D. (2013). The relation between child maltreatment and adolescent suicidal behavior: A systematic review and critical examination of the literature. *Clinical Child and Family Psychology Review, 16,* 146–172.

Milner, J. S. (1986). *The Child Abuse Potential Inventory: Manual* (2nd ed.). DeKalb, IL: Psytec.

Milner, J. S., Charlesworth, J. R., Gold, R. G., Gold, S. R., & Friesen, M. R. (1988). Convergent validity of the Child Abuse Potential Inventory. *Journal of Clinical Psychology, 44,* 281–285.

Milojevich, H. M., Quas, J. A., & Yano, J. Z. (2016). Children's participation in legal proceedings: Immediate and long-term consequences. In M. K. Miller & B. H. Bornstein (Eds.), *Advances in psychology and law* (Vol. 1, pp. 185–216). New York: Springer.

Milojevich, H. M., Russell, M. A., & Quas, J. A. (2018). Unpacking the associations among maltreatment, disengagement coping, and behavioral functioning in high-risk youth. *Child Maltreatment, 23,* 355–364.

Moylan, C. A., Herrenkohl, T. I., Sousa, C., Tajima, E. A., Herrenkohl, R. C., & Russo, M. J. (2010). The effects of child abuse and exposure to domestic violence on adolescent internalizing and externalizing behavior problems. *Journal of Family Violence, 25,* 53–63.

Naar-King, S., Silvern, L., Ryan, V., & Sebring, D. (2002). Type and severity of abuse as predictors of psychiatric symptoms in adolescence. *Journal of Family Violence, 17,* 133–149.

Noll, J. G., Shenk, C. E., & Putnam, K. T. (2008). Childhood sexual abuse and adolescent pregnancy: A meta-analytic update. *Journal of Pediatric Psychology, 34,* 366–378.

Noll, J. G., Trickett, P. K., & Putnam, F. W. (2000). Social network constellation and sexuality of sexually abused and comparison girls in childhood and adolescence. *Child Maltreatment, 5,* 323–337.

Ogawa, J. R., Sroufe, L. A., Weinfield, N. S., Carlson, E. A., & Egeland, B. (1997). Development and the fragmented self: Longitudinal study of dissociative symptomatology in a nonclinical sample. *Development and Psychopathology, 9,* 855–879.

Oshri, A., Rogosch, F. A., Burnette, M. L., & Cicchetti, D. (2011). Developmental pathways to adolescent cannabis abuse and dependence: Child maltreatment, emerging personality, and internalizing versus externalizing psychopathology. *Psychology of Addictive Behaviors, 25,* 634–644.

Pereda, N., Guilera, G., Forns, M., & Gómez-Benito, J. (2009). The prevalence of child sexual abuse in community and student samples: A meta-analysis. *Clinical Psychology Review, 29,* 328–338.

Pérez-Fuentes, G., Olfson, M., Villegas, L., Morcillo, C.,

Wang, S., & Blanco, C. (2013). Prevalence and correlates of child sexual abuse: A national study. *Comprehensive Psychiatry, 54,* 16–27.

Perrin, S., Meiser-Stedman, R., & Smith, P. (2005) The Children's Revised Impact of Event Scale (CRIES): Validity as a screening instrument for PTSD. *Behavioural and Cognitive Psychotherapy, 33,* 487–498.

Perzow, S. E., Petrenko, C. L., Garrido, E. F., Combs, M. D., Culhane, S. E., & Taussig, H. N. (2013). Dissociative symptoms and academic functioning in maltreated children: A preliminary study. *Journal of Trauma and Dissociation, 14,* 302–311.

Pollio, E. S., Glover-Orr, L. E., & Wherry, J. N. (2008). Assessing posttraumatic stress disorder using the trauma symptom checklist for young children. *Journal of Child Sexual Abuse, 17,* 89–100.

Post, R. M., Weiss, S. R. B., Li, H., Smith, M. A., Zhang, E. X., Xing, G., . . . McCann, U. D. (1998). Neural plasticity and emotional memory. *Development and Psychopathology, 10,* 829–856.

Priebe, G., & Svedin, C. G. (2008). Child sexual abuse is largely hidden from the adult society: An epidemiological study of adolescents' disclosures. *Child Abuse and Neglect, 32,* 1095–1108.

Putnam, F. W. (2003). Ten-year research update review: Child sexual abuse. *Journal of the American Academy of Child and Adolescent Psychiatry, 42,* 269–278.

Quas, J. A., & Goodman, G. S. (2012). Consequences of criminal court involvement for child victims. *Psychology, Public Policy, and Law, 18,* 392–414.

Reich, W., Welner, Z., & Herjanic, B. (1997). *Diagnostic Interview for Children–IV (DICA-IV).* Toronto: Multi-Health Systems.

Reynolds, C. R., & Kamphaus, R. (2015). *Behavior Assessment System for Children (BASC)* (3rd ed.). Bloomington, MN: Pearson.

Romano, E., & De Luca, R. V. (2001). Male sexual abuse: A review of effects, abuse characteristics, and links with latter psychological functioning. *Aggression and Violent Behavior, 6,* 55–78.

Romens, S. E., & Pollak, S. D. (2012). Emotion regulation predicts attention bias in maltreated children at-risk for depression. *Journal of Child Psychology and Psychiatry, 53,* 120–127.

Rosenthal, S., Feiring, C., & Taska, L. (2003). Emotional support and adjustment over a year's time following sexual abuse discovery. *Child Abuse and Neglect, 27,* 641–661.

Ross, C., & Joshi, S. (1992). Schneiderian symptoms and childhood trauma in the general population. *Comprehensive Psychiatry, 33,* 269–273.

Runyan, D. K., Curtis, P., Hunter, W., Black, M., Kotch, J., Bangdiwala, K., . . . Landsverk, J. (1998). LONGSCAN: A consortium for longitudinal studies of maltreatment and the life course of children. *Aggression and Violent Behavior, 3,* 275–285.

Runyon, M. K., Faust, J., & Orvaschel, H. (2002). Differential symptom patterns of post-traumatic stress disorder (PTSD) in maltreated children with and without concurrent depression. *Child Abuse and Neglect, 26,* 39–53.

Runyon, M. K., & Kenny, M. C. (2002). Relationship of attributional style, depression, and posttraumatic distress among children who suffered physical or sexual abuse. *Child Maltreatment, 7,* 254–264.

Sachs-Ericsson, N., Blazer, D., Plant, E. A., & Arnow, B. (2005). Childhood sexual and physical abuse and the 1-year prevalence of medical problems in the National Comorbidity Survey. *Health Psychology, 24,* 32–40.

Saunders, B., Villeponteaux, L., Lipovsky, J., Kilpatrick, D., & Veronen, L. (1992). Child sexual abuse as a risk factor for mental disorders among women: A community survey. *Journal of Interpersonal Violence, 7,* 189–204.

Saylor, C. F., Swenson, C. C., Reynolds, S. S., & Taylor, M. (1999). The Pediatric Emotional Distress Scale: A brief screening measure for young children exposed to traumatic events. *Journal of Clinical Child Psychology, 28,* 70–81.

Schimmenti, A., & Caretti, V. (2016). Linking the overwhelming with the unbearable: Developmental trauma, dissociation, and the disconnected self. *Psychoanalytic Psychology, 33,* 106–128.

Scoglio, A. A., Kraus, S. W., Saczynski, J., Jooma, S., & Molnar, B. E. (2019). Systematic review of risk and protective factors for revictimization after child sexual abuse. *Trauma, Violence, and Abuse.* [Epub ahead of print]

Sedlak, A. J., & Broadhurst, D. D. (1996). *The Third National Incidence Survey of Child Abuse and Neglect.* Washington, DC: U.S. Department of Health and Human Services.

Sedlak, A. J., Mettenburg, J., Basena, M., Peta, I., McPherson, K., & Greene, A. (2010). *Fourth National Incidence Study of Child Abuse and Neglect (NIS-4).* Washington, DC: U.S. Department of Health and Human Services.

Shafer, D., Gould, M. S., Brasic, J., Ambrosini, P., Fisher, P., Bird, H., & Aluwahlia, S. (1983). A children's global assessment scale (CGAS). *Archives of General Psychiatry, 40,* 1228–1231.

Shaffer, D., Fisher, P., Dulkan, M. K., & Davies, M. (1996). The NIMH Diagnostic Interview Schedule for Children: Description, acceptability, prevalence rates and performance in the MECA study. *Journal of the American Academy of Child and Adolescent Psychiatry, 35,* 865–877.

Sheridan, M. A., & McLaughlin, K. A. (2014). Dimensions of early experience and neural development: Deprivation and threat. *Trends in Cognitive Sciences, 18,* 580–585.

Silovsky, J. F., & Niec, L. (2002). Characteristics of young children with sexual behavior problems: A pilot study. *Child Maltreatment, 7,* 187–197.

Silverman, A. B., Reinherz, H. Z., & Giaconia, R. M. (1996). The long-term sequelae of child and adolescent abuse: A longitudinal community study. *Child Abuse and Neglect, 20,* 709–723.

Simpson, T. L., & Miller, W. R. (2002). Concomitance between childhood sexual and physical abuse and substance use problems: A review. *Clinical Psychology Review, 22,* 27–77.

Sourander, A., Pihlakoshi, L., Aromaa, M., Rautara, P., Helenius, H., & Sillanpää, M. (2006). Early predictors of parent- and self-reported global psychological difficulties among adolescents: A prospective cohort study from age 3 to age 15. *Social Psychiatry and Psychiatric Epidemiology, 41,* 173–182.

Stanton, B. F., Li, X., Galbraith, J., Cornick, G., Feigelman, S., Kaljee, L., & Zhou, Y. (2000). Parental underestimates of adolescent risk behavior: A randomized, controlled trial of a parental monitoring intervention. *Journal of Adolescent Health, 26,* 18–26.

Stevens, T. N., Ruggiero, K. J., Kilpatrick, D. G., Resnick, H. S., & Saunders, B. E. (2005). Variables differentiating singly and multiply victimized youth: Results from the National Survey of Adolescents and implications for secondary prevention. *Child Maltreatment, 10,* 211–223.

Stoltenborgh, M., van IJzendoorn, M. H., Euser, E. M., & Bakermans-Kranenburg, M. J. (2011). A global perspective on child sexual abuse: Meta-analysis of prevalence around the world. *Child Maltreatment, 16,* 79–101.

Stolzenberg, S. N., & Lyon, T. D. (2014). How attorneys question children about the dynamics of sexual abuse and disclosure in criminal trials. *Psychology, Public Policy, and Law, 20,* 19–30.

Straus, M. A., Hamby, S. L., Finkelhor, D., Moore, D. W., & Runyan, D. (1998). Identification of child maltreatment with the Parent–Child Conflict Tactics Scales: Development and psychometric data for a national sample of American parents. *Child Abuse and Neglect, 22,* 249–270.

Sullivan, P. M., & Knutson, J. F. (2000). Maltreatment and disabilities: A population-based epidemiological study. *Child Abuse and Neglect, 24,* 1257–1273.

Tarren-Sweeney, M. (2007). The Assessment Checklist for Children—ACC: A behavioral rating scale for children in foster, kinship and residential care. *Children and Youth Services Review, 29,* 672–691.

Tarren-Sweeney, M. (2013a). The Assessment Checklist for Adolescents—ACA: A scale for measuring the mental health of young people in foster, kinship, residential and adoptive care. *Children and Youth Services Review, 35,* 384–393.

Tarren-Sweeney, M. (2013b). The Brief Assessment Checklists (BAC-C, BAC-A): Mental health screening measures for school-aged children and adolescents in foster, kinship, residential and adoptive care. *Children and Youth Services Review, 35,* 771–779.

Tebbutt, J., Swanston, H., Oates, R. K., & O'Toole, B. I. (1997). Five years after child sexual abuse: Persisting dysfunction and problems of prediction. *Journal of the American Academy of Child and Adolescent Psychiatry, 35,* 330–339.

Terr, L. C. (1991). Childhood traumas: An outline and overview. *American Journal of Psychiatry, 148,* 10–20.

Turner, H. A., Finkelhor, D., & Ormrod, R. (2006). The effect of lifetime victimization on the mental health of children and adolescents. *Social Sciences and Medicine, 62,* 13–27.

Ullman, S. E., Najdowski, C. J., & Filipas, H. H. (2009). Child sexual abuse, post-traumatic stress disorder, and substance use: Predictors of revictimization in adult sexual assault survivors. *Journal of Child Sexual Abuse, 18,* 367–385.

Ungar, M., & Liebenberg, L. (2005). The International Resilience Project: A mixed methods approach to the study of resilience across cultures. In M. Ungar (Ed.), *Handbook for working with children and youth: Pathways to resilience across cultures and contexts* (pp. 211–226). Thousand Oaks, CA: SAGE.

U.S. Department of Health and Human Services. (2004). *Child Maltreatment 2002: Reports from the States to the National Child Abuse and Neglect Data Systems—National Statistics on Child Abuse and Neglect.* Washington, DC: Author.

U.S. Department of Health and Human Services, Administration for Children and Families, Administration on Children, Youth and Families, Children's Bureau. (2019). *Child Maltreatment 2017.* Available from *www.acf.hhs.gov/cb/research-data-technology/statistics-research/child-maltreatment.*

Valla, J. P., Bergeron, L., & Smolla, N. (2000). The Dominic-R: A pictorial interview for 6- to 11-year-old children. *Journal of the American Academy of Child and Adolescent Psychiatry, 39,* 85–93.

van der Ende, J., Verhulst, F. C., & Tiemeier, H. (2012). Agreement of informants on emotional and behavioral problems from childhood to adulthood. *Psychological Assessment, 24,* 293–300.

van der Kolk, B. A., van der Hart, O. V., & Marmar, C. R. (1996). Dissociation and information processing in posttraumatic stress disorder. In B. A. van der Kolk, A. C. McFarlane, & L. Weisaeth (Eds.), *Traumatic stress: The effects of overwhelming experience on mind, body, and society* (pp. 303–327). New York: Guilford Press.

van IJzendoorn, M. H., & Schuengel, C. (1996). The measurement of dissociation in normal and clinical populations: Meta-analytic validation of the Dissociative Experiences Scale (DES). *Clinical Psychology Review, 16,* 365–382.

Vogeltanz, N. D., Wilsnack, S. C., Harris, T. R., Wilsnack, R. W., Wonderlich, S. A., & Kristjanson, A. F. (1999). Prevalence and risk factors for childhood sexual abuse in women: National survey findings. *Child Abuse and Neglect, 23,* 579–592.

Voisin, D. R. (2005). The relationship between violence exposure and HIV sexual risk behavior: Does gender matter? *American Journal of Orthopsychiatry, 75,* 497–506.

Walsh, C., MacMillan, H. L., & Jamieson, E. (2003).

The relationship between parental substance abuse and child maltreatment: Findings from the Ontario Health Supplement. *Child Abuse and Neglect, 27,* 1409–1425.

Walsh, W. A., Jones, L. M., Cross, T. P., & Lippert, T. (2010). Prosecuting child sexual abuse: The importance of evidence type. *Crime and Delinquency, 56,* 436–454.

Watkins, B., & Bentovim, A. (1992). The sexual abuse of male children and adolescents: A review of current research. *Journal of the American Academy of Child and Adolescent Psychiatry, 33,* 197–248.

Weisz, J. R., Chorpita, B. F., Frye, A., Ng, M. Y., Lau, N., Bearman, S. K., . . . Hoagwood, K. E. (2011). Youth Top Problems: Using idiographic, consumer-guided assessment to identify treatment needs and to track change during psychotherapy. *Journal of Consulting and Clinical Psychology, 79,* 369–380.

Westcott, H. L., & Jones, D. P. H. (1999). Annotation: The abuse of disabled children. *Journal of Child Psychology and Psychiatry, 40,* 497–506.

Wherry, J. N., Corson, K., & Hunsaker, S. (2013). A short form of the Trauma Symptom Checklist for Young Children. *Journal of Child Sexual Abuse, 22,* 796–821.

Wherry, J. N., Graves, L. E., & Rhodes King, H. M. (2008). The convergent validity of the Trauma Symptom Checklist for Young Children for a sample of sexually abused outpatients. *Journal of Child Sexual Abuse, 17,* 38–50.

Widom, C. S., & Morris, S. (1997). Accuracy of adult recollections of childhood victimization: Part 2. Childhood sexual abuse. *Psychological Assessment, 9,* 34–46.

Wildeman, C., Emanuel, N., Leventhal, J. M., Putnam-Hornstein, E., Waldfogel, J., & Lee, H. (2014). The prevalence of confirmed maltreatment among US children, 2004 to 2011. *JAMA Pediatrics, 168,* 706–713.

Williams, L. M. (1994). Recall of childhood trauma: A prospective study of women's memories of child sexual abuse. *Journal of Consulting and Clinical Psychology, 62,* 1167–1176.

Wolfe, D. A., Sas, L., & Wekerle, C. (1994). Factors associated with the development of post-traumatic stress disorder among child victims of sexual abuse. *Child Abuse and Neglect, 18,* 37–50.

Wolfe, V. V. (2006). Child sexual abuse. In E. J. Mash &

R. A. Barkley (Eds.), *Treatment of childhood disorders* (3rd ed., pp. 569–623). New York: Guilford Press.

Wolfe, V. V., & Birt, J. (1997). Child sexual abuse. In E. J. Mash & L. Terdal (Eds.), *Assessment of childhood disorders* (3rd ed., pp. 569–623). New York: Guilford Press.

Wolfe, V. V., & Birt, J. H. (2005). *The Children's Impact of Traumatic Events Scale—Revised (CITES-R): Scale structure, internal consistency, discriminant validity, and PTSD diagnostic patterns.* Unpublished manuscript. (Available from V. V. Wolfe, London Health Sciences Centre, 346 South St., London ON N6A 4G5 or *vicky.wolfe@lhsc.on.ca*.)

Woodward, L., Fergusson, D. M., & Horwood, L. J. (2001). Risk factors and life processes associated with teen pregnancy: Results of a prospective study from birth to 20 years. *Journal of Marriage and the Family, 63,* 1170–1184.

World Health Organization. (2017). *Responding to children and adolescents who have been sexually abused: WHO clinical guidelines.* Geneva, Switzerland: Author.

Yeager, C. A., & Lewis, D. O. (1996). The intergenerational transmission of violence and dissociation. *Child and Adolescent Psychiatric Clinics of North America, 5,* 393–430.

Youngstrom, E., Loeber, R., & Stouthamer-Loeber, M. (2000). Patterns and correlates of agreement between parent, teacher, and male adolescent ratings of externalizing and internalizing problems. *Journal of Consulting and Clinical Psychology, 68,* 1038–1050.

Zayed, R., Wolfe, V. V., & Birt, J. (2006). *Child Dissociation Checklist: Psychometric properties of parent- and child-report versions.* Unpublished manuscript. (Available from V. V. Wolfe, PhD, London Health Sciences Centre, 346 South Street, London, ON, N6A 2L2 Canada.

Zeanah, C. H., Chesher, T., Boris, N. W., & American Academy of Child and Adolescent Psychiatry Committee on Quality. (2016). Practice parameter for the assessment and treatment of children and adolescents with reactive attachment disorder and disinhibited social engagement disorder. *Journal of the American Academy of Child and Adolescent Psychiatry, 55,* 990–1003.

Zuravin, S. J., & Fontanella, C. (1999). Parenting behaviors and perceived parenting competence of child sexual abuse survivors. *Child Abuse and Neglect, 23,* 623–632.

PART VII

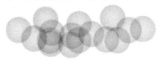

Problems of Adolescence and Emerging Adulthood

CHAPTER 19

Substance Use Problems

Tammy A. Chung and Frances L. Wang

Experimentation with substance use typically begins in adolescence, with a subset of youth transitioning to regular use, of whom a small proportion become addicted (Fergusson, Boden, & Horwood, 2008). Developmental changes that occur during adolescence, a period that spans roughly ages 10–19 (World Health Organization [WHO], 2014), contribute to increased risk for onset and escalation of substance use. Specifically, rapid physical maturation, ongoing brain development, and a normative increase in sensation seeking and risk taking during adolescence contribute to risk for substance use (Jordan & Andersen, 2017). Greater reliance on peers, relative to family, as sources of information and influence, and increasing independence (e.g., obtaining a driver's license), also set the stage for adolescent substance use (Brown et al., 2008; Hall et al., 2016). Heavy substance use during adolescence is cause for concern due to its impact on neuropsychological functioning (Lisdahl, Shollenbarger, Sagar, & Gruber, 2018; Spear, 2018) and increased risk for progression to substance use disorder (SUD; Hingson, Heeren, & Winter, 2006; Jordan & Andersen, 2017).

Given significant harm associated with adolescent substance use, evidence-based assessment (EBA) provides a framework for selecting and sequencing measures to guide treatment and monitor its progress (Youngstrom et al., 2017). This chapter follows the steps outlined in an EBA framework, and its emphasis on developing rapport and a collaborative relationship to actively engage the adolescent as a partner in the assessment process. Developing rapport is especially critical when discussing stigmatizing and sensitive topics such as substance use, and when working with substance-using youth, who may have histories of trauma. A full understanding of adolescent substance use requires a "whole-person" approach to assessment, which covers multiple domains (e.g., mental and physical health, family, school), including personal strengths, as well as the adolescent's recovery environment (e.g., system of supports in the community) (National Institute on Drug Abuse [NIDA], 2014). The assessment also needs to be tailored to ensure sensitivity to gender, race/ethnicity, and culture (Council of National Psychological Associations for the Advancement of Ethnic Minority Interests, 2016). Reliable and valid assessment of psychiatric diagnoses provides the foundation for determining estimates of treatment need, understanding etiology, and monitoring clinical course (Robins & Guze, 1970).

We begin by reviewing definitions of SUD in the *Diagnostic and Statistical Manual of Mental Disorders* (DSM; American Psychiatric Association, 2000, 2013) and *International Classification of Diseases* (ICD; WHO, 2018). Next, the prevalence of SUD is reviewed to provide benchmarks for conditions that are most likely to be seen in a given setting, and that warrant consideration during comprehensive assessment. To prepare for the assessment process, we outline a substance use assessment "starter kit" (Table 19.1), which covers recommended measures for screening, time-limited intensive assessment, and comprehensive assessment. We then review the prediction phase of EBA, which involves the use of screening tools, collateral informants, and assessment of risk and protective factors to aid case identification. Following screening, an important clinical decision point often involves determining appropriate level of care, based on more in-depth assessment (see Table 19.1: "initial" [time-limited] or "comprehensive" assessment). Comprehensive assessment corresponds to the prescription phase of EBA, which we discuss next, and which covers selected measures that can be used to determine SUD diagnosis and severity, identify the adolescent's strengths and service needs, and develop the treatment plan. A brief description of methods to monitor treatment progress and outcomes follows. Finally, future directions for EBA of adolescent substance use and SUD are discussed.

Preparation: Organizing the Assessment Materials to Address Common Issues

Diagnosis of SUD

The fourth (DSM-IV; American Psychiatric Association, 2000) and fifth (DSM-5, American Psychiatric Association, 2013) editions of the DSM both define SUD as recurrent use of a substance that causes significant impairment in functioning or subjective distress. DSM-IV included the diagnostic categories of substance abuse and dependence (Table 19.2). DSM-IV substance abuse required that individuals meet one of four criteria representing repeated substance-related interpersonal problems (e.g., physical fights, relationships ended due to substance use); impairment in major role obligations at school, home, or work (e.g., school grades dropped or missed school due to substance use); legal problems (e.g., charged for substance-related disorderly conduct or assault); or hazardous use (e.g., driving while intoxicated). For a DSM-IV substance dependence diagnosis, three of seven criteria representing the broad domains of physiological dependence (i.e., tolerance, withdrawal), impaired control over substance use (e.g., difficulty limiting, cutting down, or stopping substance use), and high priority of substance use in the person's life (e.g., much time spent using the drug, use despite psychological problems caused by use) were required.

In contrast to DSM-IV's two SUD diagnoses and separate criterion sets, DSM-5 uses a single set of 11 criteria (Table 19.2) to determine a diagnosis of SUD, based on extensive literature reviews and empirical data (Hasin et al., 2013). DSM-5 also excludes legal problems as a criterion and has added craving and marijuana withdrawal as SUD criteria (Hasin et al., 2013). Similar to DSM-IV, however, DSM-5 SUD criteria represent the broad domains of physiological dependence (tolerance, withdrawal), impaired control over substance use, high priority of substance use in the individual's life, hazardous use, and certain substance-related negative consequences (e.g., substance-related interpersonal problems). Individuals who endorse two or more of the criteria within a 12-month period meet the threshold for a DSM-5 SUD diagnosis. DSM-5 SUD diagnoses are scaled on a continuum of severity as *mild* (2–3 criteria met), *moderate* (4–5 criteria met), or *severe* (6 or more criteria met), reflecting an important departure from the categorical approach to SUD diagnosis in DSM-IV. Overall, despite differences between DSM-IV and DSM-5 SUD criteria sets, the two classification systems generally show good agreement in identifying the same cases as meeting criteria for a diagnosis, with some differences (Bartoli, Carra, Crocamo, & Clerici, 2015; Chung, Cornelius, Clark, & Martin, 2017).

The 11th edition of the ICD (ICD-11; WHO, 2018) recognizes two main SUD diagnoses: substance dependence and harmful use. ICD-11 diagnoses of substance dependence and harmful use are organized hierarchically and are mutually exclusive, with dependence representing the more severe disorder. ICD-11 substance dependence represents a disorder in self-regulation of substance use, with a strong internal drive to engage in sub-

TABLE 19.1. Assessment Starter Kit

	Substance use	Mental health	Time (min)	Format	Cost
Brief screen (5–10 min)					
S2BI	X		5	Questionnaire	Free
BSTAD	X		5	Questionnaire	Free
CRAFFT	X		5	Questionnaire	Free
GAIN Short Screen	X	X	5	Questionnaire	$100 to use GAIN paper measures for 5 years
Initial asssessment (20–45 min)					
Teen-ASI	X	X	20–45	Semistructured interview	Free
GAIN Quick	X	X	20–30	Structured interview	See GAIN above
Comprehensive diagnostic assessment (1–2 hr)					
DISC	X	X	60–120	Structured interview	Paper: copy/mailing fee
GAIN Initial	X	X	90–120	Semistructured interview	See GAIN above
K-SADS	X	X	90–120	Semistructured interview	Free for certain uses
Teen-ASI	X	X	20–45	Structured interview	Free
Lifetime Drug Use History	X		10	Interview	Paper: copy/mailing fee
Timeline Followback (TLFB)	X		10–15	Interview	Free
Rutgers Alcohol/Marijuana Adolescent Problems Index (RAPI/MAPI)	X		10	Questionnaires	Free
Motives for Alcohol and Drug Use	X		10	Questionnaires	Free
Readiness Ruler, Contemplation Ladder	X		1	Questionnaire	Free
Urine/saliva drug screen	X		10	Biological	Lab testing fee
Outcome evaluation (45–90 min)					
CASI	X	X	45–90	Semistructured interview	Free paper version

Note: Brief screen: Identify individuals who may benefit from further assessment; *Initial assessment:* Determine need for brief advice, brief intervention or referral for comprehensive assessment or treatment; *Comprehensive assessment:* Identify problem areas and strengths across multiple domains of functioning for treatment planning; *Outcome evaluation:* Assess substance use and mental health to evaluate response to treatment.

TABLE 19.2. SUD symptoms for DSM-IV, DSM-5, and ICD-11

	DSM-IV	DSM-5	ICD-11
A1. Role impairment	Abuse	SUD	(Dependence[a])
A2. Hazardous use	Abuse	SUD	—
A3. Legal problems	Abuse	—	—
A4. Interpersonal problems	Abuse	SUD	(Dependence[a])
D1. Tolerance	Dependence	SUD	Dependence
D2. Withdrawal	Dependence	SUD	Dependence
D3. Use more or longer than intended (larger/longer)	Dependence	SUD	Dependence
D4. Repeated attempts or strong desire to reduce or stop use (quit/cut down)	Dependence	SUD	Dependence
D5. Much time spent using	Dependence	SUD	Dependence
D6. Reduce activities in order to use	Dependence	SUD	Dependence
D7. Psychological or physical problems due to use	Dependence	SUD	Harmful use
Craving	—	SUD	Dependence

Note: DSM, *Diagnostic and Statistical Manual of Mental Disorders*; ICD, *International Classification of Diseases*; A1–A4 refer to the four DSM-IV substance abuse criteria (one of four needed for diagnosis of DSM-IV substance abuse); D1–D7 refer to the seven DSM-IV substance dependence criteria (three or more of seven needed for diagnosis of DSM-IV substance dependence). DSM-5 SUD symptoms are A1, A2, A4, D1–D7 and craving; two symptoms or fewer = no DSM-IV SUD; two to three symptoms = mild disorder; four to five symptoms = moderate disorder; six or more symptoms = severe disorder. [a]The impairment or substance-related problem needs to be due to a pattern of compulsive substance use for the criterion to be met.

stance use as a core feature. Similar to DSM-IV substance dependence in the domains covered, ICD-11 is notable for its particular emphasis on impaired control over substance use as a defining feature of dependence. ICD-11 (WHO, 2018) does not specify a minimum number of dependence criteria needed for a diagnosis, but it does state that features are typically present for at least 12 months, or at least 1 month in the context of heavy (e.g., daily) use. The second ICD-11 SUD diagnosis, harmful pattern of substance use, refers to substance use that causes recurrent damage to physical (e.g., alcohol-related injury) or mental (e.g., depressive disorder due to drug use) health, or that has resulted in behavior leading to harm to the health of others (e.g., substance-related interpersonal violence). Preliminary results suggest that ICD-11 SUD criteria, compared to DSM-5 criteria, identify more youth as having an alcohol or marijuana use disorder (Chung, Cornelius, et al., 2017). ICD-11 and DSM-5 also differ in the specific cases that are identified as meeting SUD criteria (Lago, Bruno, & Degenhardt, 2016). Cross-system differences in case identification highlight the evolving status of SUD definitions and the importance of careful assessment of diagnostic criteria, particularly among adolescents, who may misinterpret diagnostic symptom queries (Chung & Martin, 2005).

Prevalence of Substance Use and SUD in Adolescents

Alcohol is the substance consumed most often by adolescents, followed by marijuana and nicotine (Johnston et al., 2018). The prevalence of substance use increases with age during adolescence, according to the Monitoring the Future (MTF) national school-based survey of 8th, 10th, and 12th graders. For example, among 8th, 10th, and 12th graders in the MTF (past 30 days), there were increases across these grades in alcohol use (8.0, 19.7, 33.2%, respectively), marijuana use (5.5, 15.7, 22.9%, respectively), and any cigarette use (1.9, 5.0, 9.7%, respectively) (Johnston et al., 2018). Regarding higher levels of substance use consumption in MTF, the prevalence of heavy or "binge" alcohol use (i.e., consuming five or more drinks in a row in the past 2 weeks) increased from 13.3% in 8th grade to 31.5% in 12th grade, and daily marijuana use increased from 0.8% in 8th grade to 5.9% in 12th grade (Johnston et al., 2018). Emerging drug trends among adolescents in MTF involving prescription drug misuse and vaping (including e-cigarettes, Juul) also warrant attention, with 4.9% of high school seniors reporting any prescription drug misuse in the past 30 days and 11.0% reporting vaping nicotine in the past month (Johnston et al., 2018).

According to the 2016 National Survey on Drug Use and Health (NSDUH), 4.3% of 12- to 17-year-olds met criteria for a DSM-IV SUD in the past year; specifically, 2.0% met criteria for alcohol use disorder, and 3.2% for an illicit drug use disorder, most often due to cannabis (2.3%; Center for Behavioral Health Statistics and Quality [CBHSQ], 2017). SUD prevalence peaks in young adulthood at ages 18–25 (CBHSQ, 2017), emphasizing the importance of halting the progression of substance-related problems in adolescence in order to reduce rates of SUD in young adulthood. Among adolescents with SUD, most (up to 90%) meet criteria for one or more co-occurring psychiatric conditions, such as conduct disorder, depression, or attention-deficit/hyperactivity disorder (ADHD) (Chan, Dennis, & Funk, 2008), signaling the importance of comprehensive assessment. With regard to gender differences in SUD prevalence, females have higher rates of SUD than males in early adolescence; however, by late adolescence and early adulthood, males have higher rates of SUD (CBHSQ, 2017). Sexual-minority youth, relative to their heterosexual counterparts, are at greater risk for substance use, possibly due to discrimination and minority stress (Kidd, Jackman, Wolff, & Veldhuis, 2018).

SUD prevalence differs across settings (e.g., primary care, mental health, or school-based clinic). Understanding the base rate of SUD in a specific setting provides a benchmark for determining the likelihood that an individual will meet criteria for a SUD, which can help to minimize errors in diagnostic assessment (e.g., by prompting further probing). For example, a relatively large study showed varying rates of DSM-IV SUD among adolescents receiving services in the following public sectors of care: alcohol and drug treatment (82.6%), juvenile justice (62.1%), mental health setting (40.8%), public school-based services for youth with serious emotional disturbance (23.6%), and child welfare (19.2%) (Aarons, Brown, Hough, Garland, & Wood, 2001). Homeless youth, in particular, show high rates of SUD, ranging from 44 to 86.1% (Ginzler, Garrett, Baer, & Peterson, 2007; Medlow, Klineberg, & Steinbeck, 2014; Slesnick & Prestopnik, 2005). In contrast, in a primary care sample of youth screened for past-year DSM-5 alcohol or marijuana use disorder, 3.6% had an alcohol use disorder and 13.6% had a cannabis use disorder (D'Amico et al., 2016). Differences in SUD prevalence across settings reflect local demographics and referral patterns and highlight the importance of preparing an assessment battery that will efficiently cover the most common conditions at a given setting as a starting point.

Substance Use Assessment Starter Kit

Assessment typically progresses according to a sequence that begins first with screening to identify youth who might benefit from more intensive evaluation, then employs more comprehensive forms of assessment to determine appropriate level of care, treatment needs, and treatment plans. Table 19.1 outlines recommended measures that can serve as a starting point for assessment. The measures, outlined briefly below and reviewed in later sections, cover substance use screening (5–10 minutes), initial assessment (20–45 minutes), and more comprehensive substance use assessment (1–2 hours).

Two brief substance use screens (<2 minutes), Screening to Brief Intervention (S2BI; Levy et al., 2014) and Brief Screener for Tobacco, Alcohol, and Other Drugs (BSTAD; Kelly et al., 2014), are recommended for use with adolescents ages 12–17. If further assessment is indicated, and time is limited (20–45 minutes), the Teen Addiction Severity Index (T-ASI; Kaminer, Bukstein, & Tarter, 1991) efficiently covers multiple areas of functioning that may be affected by substance use (e.g., school, family). The T-ASI can be used to support decisions regarding treatment referral and planning.

Comprehensive assessment involves in-depth evaluation of substance use, SUD, and co-occurring psychopathology, typically for treatment planning or research. For comprehensive assessment of mental health conditions, structured interview options include the Diagnostic Interview Schedule for Children (DISC; Shaffer, Fisher, Lucas, Dulcan, & Schwab-Stone, 2000) updated for DSM-5 or Global Appraisal of Individual Needs—Initial (GAIN-I; Dennis, White, Titus, & Unsicker, 2008). A semistructured interview option is the Kiddie Schedule for Affective Disorders and Schizophrenia (K-SADS; Kaufman, Birmaher, et al., 2016). Details on recent frequency and quantity of substance use can be obtained by completing a calendar-based Timeline Followback (TLFB; Lewis-Esquerre et al., 2005), which can be used to initiate a discussion of typical contexts of use (e.g., with friends or alone, usual places where use occurs) to inform treatment planning. Questionnaire measures, such as the Rutgers Alcohol Problems Index and Marijuana Adolescent Problem Inventory (RAPI/MAPI; Knapp et al., 2018; White & Labouvie, 1989) can be used to evaluate severity of alcohol- and marijuana-related problems (e.g., alcohol-related blackouts) that are not captured well by diagnostic criteria. Other measures that can inform treatment planning include readiness to change (Moyers, Martin, Houck, Christopher, & Tonigan, 2009), and reasons for substance use (Kuntsche & Kuntsche, 2009; Simons, Correia, Carey, & Borsari, 1998). The breadth and depth of measures included in a comprehensive assessment battery depend on the purpose of the assessment, as well as available time and resources.

Validity of Youth Self-Report of Substance Use

Validity of self-reported sensitive information such as substance use, substance-related negative consequences, and illegal activity is increased when adolescents understand the assessment process (e.g., the purpose of the assessment, what will be asked, how long it will take), how the information will be used, and who will have access to the information provided (Boruch, Dennis, & Cecil, 1996; Del Boca & Darkes, 2003). Youth self-reports of substance use have shown validity when obtained in certain contexts, for example, when there is assurance of confidentiality and minimal risk of consequences associated with disclosure (e.g., research setting) (Winters, Stinchfield, Henly, & Schwartz, 1990). In a clinic, treatment, or juvenile justice setting, youth may minimize disclosure of substance use for fear of associated consequences (e.g., penalties, impending legal action, referral to unwanted services) (Buchan, Dennis, Tims, & Diamond, 2002). Methods to increase the validity of self-report include developing rapport with the adolescent, for example, by using motivational interviewing techniques (see below) (O'Leary Tevyaw, Spirito, Colby, & Monti, 2018), conducting the assessment in a private space, and discussing the limits of confidentiality (Del Boca, Darkes, & McRee, 2016; Winters et al., 1990). Research generally demonstrates the validity of self-report of substance use against biological measures of substance use (e.g., urine drug screen, saliva test) when collected in specific circumstances, such as assurance of confidentiality (Dillon, Turner, Robbins, & Szapocznik, 2005; Winters et al., 1990).

Biological measures of substance use and collateral informants (e.g., caretakers) can be used as external checks on the validity of self-reported information, but they have limitations of their own (see relevant sections below). Other sources of information, obtained with appropriate consent (e.g., medical, school, treatment, and legal records) can fill in gaps regarding an adolescent's history. The use of multimodal assessment and integration of findings across sources constitutes a "best estimate" diagnostic process.

Motivational Interviewing Techniques

Motivational interviewing (MI; Miller & Rollnick, 2012) is an empathic, nonjudgmental, therapeutic style that has shown some efficacy in reducing substance use with youth (Tanner-Smith & Lipsey, 2015). An MI approach, which uses a nonconfrontational and concerned stance (O'Leary Tevyaw et al., 2018), may help increase validity of self-report of sensitive information, for example, by enhancing rapport. The main MI techniques include expressing empathy, developing discrepancy, avoiding argumentation, rolling with resistance, and supporting self-efficacy (Miller & Rollnick, 2012). Empathy can be expressed, for example, through reflective listening and being attentive to the adolescent's needs (e.g., taking short breaks). Discrepancy can be developed by asking about personal goals, and how substance use plays a role in achieving those goals. The MI techniques of avoiding arguments and rolling with resistance can be used to minimize defensiveness and maintain the adolescent's active engagement in the interview. Self-efficacy can be supported by reflecting back to the adolescent past successes in attaining goals. Skillful use of MI techniques can facilitate a collaborative relationship in which adolescent and interviewer work together as partners during the assessment. Importantly, empathic, nonjudgmental assessment conducted in a MI style, provided with constructive feedback, can constitute an intervention in itself (O'Leary Tevyaw et al., 2018).

Prediction: Screening, Risk Assessment, and Protective Factors

In the prediction phase of EBA, two brief substance use screens, S2BI and BSTAD, are recommended for initial identification of youth who might benefit from further evaluation. In general, substance use risk ranges on a continuum from *low risk* (experimental or nonproblematic use) to *moderate risk* (more regular use, some associated problems) to *high risk* (more frequent or heavy use and associated problems) (Levy et al., 2014). Notably, most youth prefer computerized screening over interview format, even when they know that the computerized results will be given to a health care provider (Kelly et al., 2014). Screening results are typically reviewed with the adolescent in the context of a brief motivational enhancement discussion (O'Leary Tevyaw et al., 2018), focusing on reinforcing current healthy behaviors and reducing substance-related harms. Web versions of the S2BI and BSTAD screening tools include recommended action steps based on screening results (e.g., further assessment and referral, brief intervention) to guide clinical practice. To minimize substance-related harm, indicated prevention may be useful when risk factors for substance use (e.g., friends who drink), reviewed below, are found to be present prior to the onset of substance use (National Research Council & Institute of Medicine, 2009).

Brief Screens: S2BI, BSTAD, CRAFFT, GAIN-SS

The S2BI screen is based on a single question that asks about past-year frequency of use separately for eight substances (e.g., alcohol, marijuana, tobacco, prescription drugs, cocaine), with six fixed response options that range from *never* to *daily*. In a pediatric sample (ages 12–17), the S2BI had good sensitivity and specificity in discriminating between youth who reported no past year substance use (excluding tobacco) versus any use (sensitivity: 100%, specificity: 84%), and detecting any past-year DSM-5 SUD (sensitivity: 90%, specificity: 94%) (Levy et al., 2014). S2BI had higher sensitivity and specificity for identifying DSM-5 severe SUD (100 and 94%, respectively) (Levy et al., 2014). S2BI's single frequency item had high sensitivity and specificity in discriminating between the four categories of *no past-year use, use with no SUD, mild/moderate SUD*, and *severe SUD* for each of the eight substances examined (Levy et al., 2014).

The BSTAD uses questions on friends' substance use and frequency of substance use to identify youth with past-year DSM-5 SUD. For 12- to 14-year-olds, screening starts by asking about friends' substance use (which youth may be more comfortable discussing than their own use), followed by questions on personal frequency of substance use (e.g., "In the past year, on how many days did you use [substance]?"). For 15- to 17-year-olds, and 14-year-olds in high school, the question order is reversed. Using only the frequency of use item to screen for past-year DSM-5 SUD, the BSTAD had high sensitivity and specificity for alcohol use disorder (sensitivity = 0.96; specificity = 0.85), marijuana use disorder (sensitivity = 0.80; specificity = 0.93), and tobacco use disorder (sensitivity = 0.95; specificity = 0.97) in a large pediatric sample (92.8% African American) (Kelly et al., 2014). Although the screening performance of the peer substance use item was not evaluated, personal frequency of substance use, especially when assessed by computer, provides an efficient empirically based brief substance use screen.

CRAFFT, a six-item substance use screening tool, is available in an online interactive format that can identify youth ages 12–18 at high risk for SUDs who could benefit from further evaluation (Knight, Sherritt, Shrier, Harris, & Chang, 2002; Mitchell et al., 2014). Each letter of CRAFFT cues a screening item. Screening starts with three items that query frequency of alcohol, marijuana, and other drug use in the past year (i.e., "During the past year, on how many days did you use [substance]?"). If no substance use was reported, only the first screening question ("Car") is asked: "Have you ever ridden in a Car driven by someone (including yourself) who was "high" or had been using alcohol or drugs?" The other screening items are: Do you ever use alcohol or drugs to Relax, feel better about yourself, or fit in? Do you ever use alcohol or drugs while you are by yourself, Alone? Do you ever Forget things you did while using alcohol or drugs? Do your Family or friends ever tell you that you should cut down on your drinking or drug use? Have you ever gotten into Trouble while you were using alcohol or drugs? A positive response to two or more items indicates increased risk for SUD and that further assessment is warranted. CRAFFT had high sensitivity (0.91) and specificity (0.93) in identifying DSM-5 mild SUD among 12- to 17-year-olds (92.0% African American) in primary care (Mitchell et al., 2014).

The Global Assessment of Individual Needs—Short Screener (GAIN-SS; Dennis, Feeney, Stevens, & Bedoya, 2006) was developed to identify behavioral health problems that warrant further evaluation or referral to treatment among youth ages 10 and older. The GAIN-SS, available in paper and computer-administration formats, includes 20 items that comprise four five-item subscales: Internalizing Disorders (depression, anxiety), Externalizing Disorders (conduct problems, ADHD), Substance Use Disorders, and Crime/Violence. The "minimal" version of the GAIN-SS uses a past-year time frame (Dennis et al., 2008) with subscales summed to compute a total score, or each subscale can be used as a separate five-item screen (Sacks et al., 2007). The Substance Use Disorders subscale includes five questions that cover frequency of substance use (one item: last used alcohol or drugs weekly), increasing priority of substance use in the adolescent's life (two items), and substance-related problems (two items). The GAIN-SS has high internal consistency (alpha = .96), and its subscales are highly correlated with their respective main scales on the full GAIN interview (r = .84–.94) (Dennis, Chan, & Funk, 2006). GAIN-SS total score and subscores have high sensitivity (>90%) and specificity (>92%) for identifying the presence of a behavioral disorder (Dennis, Chan, & Funk, 2006). The GAIN-SS covers both mental health and substance use problems in a developmentally appropriate tool for use in schools and clinics (Substance Abuse and Mental Health Services Administration [SAMHSA], 2011).

Cross-Informant Assessment: Youth and Caregiver Reports

To supplement adolescent self-report, collateral informants (e.g., parents, peers, and teachers) may be contacted for information (with appropriate consent) about the youth's substance use and behavior. Parents often have limited knowledge regarding details (e.g., frequency and quantity) of their child's substance use (Burleson & Kaminer, 2006; Fisher Sherri et al., 2006), and generally underreport substance use relative to the adolescent's self-report (Winters, Anderson, Bengston, Stinchfield, & Latimer, 2000). Parents, however, can provide important information on their relationship with the adolescent and may be able to report more observable behavior (e.g., changes in mood, sleep) (Wish, Hoffman, & Nemes, 1997). Research indicates that youth in treatment, compared to collateral informants, reported more days of any substance use in the past 3 months, but slightly fewer days of alcohol use (on average, roughly 7 vs. 8 days) (Dennis et al., 2008). In addition, although youth and collateral informants reported a similar number of substance-related symptoms in the past year (an average of four to five symptoms), collateral informants reported different symptoms compared to youth (Dennis et al., 2008). Although collateral informants may be likely to underreport some types of substance use relative to the adolescent, the inclusion of collat-

eral informants as part of the assessment process can increase the validity of adolescent self-report (i.e., as an external "check" for self-report), provide a more complete clinical picture of changes in the adolescent's daily functioning, and engage supportive caregivers early in the treatment process.

Psychosocial Risk and Protective Factors

Identifying an adolescent's personal risk factors for substance use is critical to understanding how substance use began and how it can be reduced, whereas assessment of protective factors (e.g., an adolescent's coping skills, parental warmth) identifies strengths that can be emphasized and leveraged in treatment. Risk and protective factors associated with substance use include individual factors (e.g., genetic risk, co-occurring psychopathology, history of trauma), interpersonal factors (e.g., family and peer relations), and environmental factors (e.g., availability and access to substances, neighborhood conditions) (Hawkins, Catalano, & Miller, 1992; Stone, Becker, Huber, & Catalano, 2012). According to a bioecological model of youth development (Bronfenbrenner & Morris, 2006), there is a nested structure of risk and protection, such that individuals are nested within families, which in turn reside in neighborhoods, which are nested within communities. These nested social systems interact to amplify or reduce risk as youth mature (Bronfenbrenner & Morris, 2006). Each level, from the individual to community, has a unique profile of risk and protection associated with propensity for substance use (Bronfenbrenner & Morris, 2006). Risk factors can cluster within an individual (e.g., conduct problems, poor academic performance, affiliation with deviant peers) in a "problem behavior syndrome" (Donovan & Jessor, 1985). A greater number of risk factors, rather than any single type of risk factor, contributes to risk for youth substance use (Hawkins et al., 1992). The effect of risk and protective factors on adolescent substance use also may be modified by factors such as age, gender, and race/ethnicity (Stone et al., 2012).

At the individual level, assessment of personality traits and co-occurring psychopathology can identify youth who may benefit from specialized or more intensive intervention. In particular, the personality traits of impulsivity and sensation seeking are robustly associated with adolescent substance use (Conrod, 2016; Fergusson et al., 2008). The Substance Use Risk Profile Scale (SURPS; Woicik, Stewart, Pihl, & Conrod, 2009) covers four major personality-based risk factors for youth substance use: anxiety sensitivity, hopelessness, impulsivity, and sensation seeking, which can be linked to intervention content (Conrod, 2016).

In addition to personality-based risk factors, two broad types of psychopathology have been found to precede and predict substance use in adolescence: internalizing (e.g., depression, anxiety, trauma-related) and externalizing (e.g., conduct problems, inattention, hyperactivity) disorders (Carliner, Gary, McLaughlin, & Keyes, 2017; Fergusson et al., 2008; Hussong, Ennett, Cox, & Haroon, 2017). Internalizing and externalizing behaviors can be assessed by questionnaire, such as the Youth Self-Report (Achenbach, 2009), or by interview (see structured and semistructured interviews, below). Experiences of abuse (physical, sexual, emotional) and neglect (Felitti et al., 1998; Finkelhor, Shattuck, Turner, & Hamby, 2013), and other types of stressful life events (e.g., homelessness, bullying), also increase risk for adolescent substance use (Carliner et al., 2016), possibly through the use of substances to cope with negative affect (Conrod, Stewart, Comeau, & Maclean, 2006). In this regard, the Difficulties in Emotion Regulation Scale (DERS; Gratz & Roemer, 2004) score has shown positive correlations with substance use in youth (Weinberg & Klonsky, 2009), and a DERS short form (18 items) shows preliminary evidence of concurrent validity (Kaufman, Xia, et al., 2016). Internalizing and externalizing disorders also may share, to some extent, an underlying deficit in emotion regulation (Neumann, van Lier, Gratz, & Koot, 2010), suggesting the potential of emotion regulation as a treatment target for certain youth.

A family history of addiction can confer genetic risk (Hines, Morley, Mackie, & Lynskey, 2015). The family environment, however, can powerfully shape an individual's beliefs and attitudes toward substance use. For example, as early as 3 years of age, some children appear to be able to identify alcoholic beverages based on responses to the Appropriate Beverage Task (Jones & Gordon, 2017; Zucker, Kincaid, Fitzgerald, & Bingham, 1995), suggesting their early exposure to and knowledge of alcohol in their immediate environment. Parents and siblings could serve as models for the use of substances and provide access (possibly inadvertently) to substances in the home (e.g., beer in the refrigerator). Conflict within the family (Fergusson, Horwood, & Lynskey, 1994), and poor parent–child relationship quality (Cablova, Pazderkova, & Miovsky, 2014) also increase risk for youth substance use. Parenting behaviors associated with increased risk for youth substance use include parenting styles such as harsh or inconsistent discipline (Brown et al., 2008; Windle et al., 2008) and low monitoring of youth behavior (Lac & Crano, 2009). In contrast, strong positive bonds in the family, clear rules against substance use, and authoritative parenting style (i.e., a balance of warmth with fair, consistent discipline) reduce risk for substance use (Brown et al., 2008).

Affiliation with substance-using or delinquent (e.g., gang membership) peers is one of the most robust risk factors for adolescent substance use (Fergusson et al., 2008; Stone et al., 2012). In recent years, the roles of both in-person and online peers and social media in risk for substance use have become increasingly important (Huang et al., 2014). In-person peers can provide actual access to substances, whereas online peers increase an adolescent's network of contacts and can influence behaviors, for example, by providing information or advice, or through social norms encouraging substance use (Hoorn, Crone Eveline, & Leijenhorst, 2016). Importantly, a higher proportion of substance users in an adolescent's social network (in-person) is associated with increased risk for substance use (Chung et al., 2015). Both in-person and online peers can influence an adolescent's attitudes toward substance use and contribute to perceived norms about the prevalence of substance use among one's peers (Huang et al., 2014). A meta-analysis of 19 studies indicated that greater alcohol-related social media engagement (e.g., posting, liking, commenting, viewing of alcohol-related social media content) is correlated (moderate effect sizes) with both greater self-reported drinking and alcohol-related problems among young adults (Curtis, Lookatch, McKay, Feinn, & Kranzler, 2018). Furthermore, exposure to social media posts that depict drinking behavior increased risk for alcohol use 1-year later among high school students (Nesi, Rothenberg, Hussong, & Jackson, 2017). Assessment of an adolescent's peer relations, both in-person and online, can help to identify not only risky peers but also potential supportive peers to facilitate recovery and maintain recovery.

Environmental factors such as availability and access to substances (Collins, Johnson, & Becker, 2007; Jessor, Costa, Krueger, & Turbin, 2006; Martins et al., 2016), neighborhood conditions (Fagan, Wright, & Pinchevsky, 2015), and social norms that are tolerant of use (Jackson et al., 2014; Reed, Lange, Ketchie, & Clapp, 2007) have been associated with adolescent substance use (Brown et al., 2008; Fergusson et al., 2008). Adolescents at risk for substance use also show low commitment or bonding to the school (e.g., poor relations with teachers and students, little feeling of belonging, not feeling safe at school) (Fletcher, Bonell, & Hargreaves, 2008). Assessment of environmental factors can be used in treatment planning to identify recovery supports and strengths in the youth's environment on which to build.

Prescription: Using Assessment to Guide Diagnosis, Case Formulation, and Treatment Planning

After identifying youth with suspected or known substance use through screening, the prescription phase of EBA uses structured or semistructured interviews as the primary tools to finalize diagnoses and evaluate SUD severity. The decision to use a structured or semistructured interview depends on factors such as resources for interviewer training and maximizing the reliability and validity of assessment. Structured interviews, which can be administered by trained lay interviewers, require minimal interviewer training because questions are read verbatim and answers are recorded as stated. Although reliability may be high for structured interviews, validity may be compromised because interviewers cannot explain or elaborate on the meaning of questions. In contrast, semistructured interviews require greater interviewer training and understanding of diagnostic concepts because interviewers have some flexibility in probing symptoms and clarifying what is being asked to accommodate a respondent's level of understanding (Dennis et al., 2008). There is a trade-off between reliability and validity, however, such that attempts to increase validity in a semistructured interview (e.g., by probing more) could reduce reliability (i.e., lower agreement in ratings) due to differences in how symptoms are queried. A semistructured interview typically requires ongoing supervision to minimize drift in ratings and could incur greater cost than a structured interview. More generally, when selecting a specific type of interview, one needs to consider the appropriateness of the measure for a specific setting, associated costs, diagnostic coverage, and administration time.

The aim of more intensive assessment following screening is to cover the full scope of problems experienced by the adolescent in order to determine placement in the appropriate level of care, identify specific service needs, and guide treatment planning. To support decisions regarding placement in level of care, the American Society of Addiction Medicine (ASAM) recommends assessment of six domains (Table 19.3), based on a "whole-person" approach to treatment. The six ASAM domains include Addiction Severity, Mental Health (e.g., co-occurring psychopathology) and Competencies/Skills (e.g., cooking, computing, music, dance, sports, hobbies, recreational activities), Medical Conditions (e.g., sexually transmitted infection [STI]/HIV, pain), Readiness to Change (Prochaska & DiClemente, 1983), Risk for Relapse, and Recovery Environment (e.g., parent's involvement in the youth's treatment).

Assessment of problem severity and level of functioning across the six ASAM (2013) domains guides decisions regarding placement in one of five levels of care (Table 19.3): brief intervention (usually one session delivered in a medical setting) (O'Leary Tevyaw et al., 2018), outpatient treatment (most common level of care for adolescents), intensive outpatient treatment and partial hospitalization, residential or inpatient treatment, and medically managed intensive inpatient treatment (e.g., medical management of acute withdrawal syndrome). Recommendation of placement in a specific level of care takes into consideration prior treatment history and response to treatment; current severity of SUD; mental and physical health conditions; and placement in the least restrictive level of care that will best serve the adolescent's needs (ASAM, 2013). Certain circumstances, however, such as single-episode use of a substance such as heroin or crystal meth, and very early use (e.g., early childhood or early adolescence) represent significant risk that warrants intervention (Winters, Latimer, & Stinchfield, 2002). Matching youth to services based on specific needs tends to result in better outcomes than providing generic "one size fits all" programming (Taxman & Caudy, 2015).

We describe in the sections below two types of in-depth assessment, a briefer "initial assessment" (20–45 minutes), and a longer "comprehensive" diagnostic assessment (1–2 hours), which can be used after screening or to evaluate an adolescent with suspected or known substance use. Recommended "initial" and "comprehensive" diagnostic interviews are reviewed below. Comprehensive reviews of substance use and psychiatric diagnostic interview measures can be found elsewhere (Leffler, Riebel, & Hughes, 2015; Vincent, 2011; Winters, Botzet, & Lee, 2018; Wright, 2018). Online

TABLE 19.3. ASAM Assessment Domains and Levels of Care

Six ASAM assessment domains
used to determine appropriate level of care

1. Severity of substance use, acute intoxication, and withdrawal potential (current and past)

2. Current and lifetime medical conditions (e.g., STI, HIV)

3. Mental health conditions (e.g., depression, conduct problems, trauma history, suicidality)

4. Readiness to change: precontemplation (not yet thinking about reducing substance use); contemplation; taking action; maintaining reductions in substance use or abstinence

5. Risk for relapse and potential for continuing substance use (e.g., craving, compulsion to use)

6. Environment for recovery (e.g., family and living situation, school and community resources)

Five levels of care

Assessment of the six ASAM domains informs recommendation for a specific level of care. Ongoing assessment supports recommendations regarding change in level of care.

1. *Brief intervention.* Brief intervention is typically for adolescents with lower levels of substance use severity (e.g., no SUD). Brief intervention can provide psychoeducation regarding the health risks of substance use and motivational enhancement to reduce substance use.

2. *Outpatient treatment.* Outpatient treatment is the most common level of care for adolescents.

3. *Intensive outpatient treatment (IOP) and partial (day) hospitalization.* IOP involves treatment up to 20 hours per week (e.g., three 3-hour sessions per week) with average duration of 6–8 weeks. Partial hospitalization involves 4–6 hours of treatment per day for 5 days per week, usually after inpatient or residential treatment, as part of continuing care.

4. *Residential or inpatient treatment.* Youth with severe SUD, who typically have needs in multiple areas (e.g., mental health, family, medical), may benefit from intensive treatment in a residential setting to stabilize acute mental and physical health conditions before transitioning to a less intensive level of care.

5. *Medically managed intensive inpatient treatment.* This setting provides 24-hour medical care, for example, to manage acute alcohol withdrawal syndrome.

Note. From American Society of Addiction Medicine (2013).

resources that include other relevant measures include PhenX (*phenxtoolkit.org*), NIH Toolkit (*nihtoolbox.org*), and Patient-Reported Outcomes Measurement Information Systems (PROMIS) health measures (*www.healthmeasures.net/explore-measurement-systems/promis*).

Initial Assessment

The relatively brief "initial assessment" (20–45 minutes) is suited for settings where time is limited, and brief intervention and referrals to behavioral health treatment are the main services provided. Two "initial assessment" measures—the T-ASI (Kaminer et al., 1991) and Global Appraisal of Individual Needs—Quick (GAIN Quick; Titus et al., 2013) —are reviewed.

The T-ASI (Kaminer et al., 1991) is a semistructured interview that covers seven domains of functioning: substance use, school performance (e.g., suspension), employment, family relations, legal status (e.g., juvenile detention, probation, drug court), peer and interpersonal relationships, and psychiatric status (e.g., medication, treatment utilization). In addition to obtaining patient perceptions of impairment in each domain rated on a 5-point scale (*not at all* to *always*), each domain is rated by the clinician in terms of treatment need on a 5-point scale (*no problem, treatment not indicated* to *extreme problem, treatment absolutely necessary*; interrater reliability $r = .78$) (Kaminer, Wagner, Plummer, & Seifer, 1993).

The GAIN Quick (Titus et al., 2013) is recommended for use in targeted or at-risk populations (e.g., student assistance programs, correctional settings) to provide an initial, efficient overview of the adolescent's functioning across multiple domains. The GAIN Quick consists of nine separate screeners, each 4–10 items long (210 items total), which cover substance use, mental health (Internalizing and Externalizing Disorder subscales), school problems, work problems, physical health, sources of stress, risk behaviors for infectious diseases (e.g., STI, HIV), and crime and violence. GAIN Quick screens had good internal consistency and reliability in a clinical sample of adolescents: SUD screen alpha = .76 and total disorder screener alpha = .90 (Titus et al., 2013). The GAIN Quick substance use screen (five items) had high sensitivity (0.88) and specificity (1.00) in identifying SUD in a clinical sample of adolescents; the total problem score also had high sensitivity (0.98) and specificity (0.87) in detecting a behavioral disorder (Titus et al., 2013).

Comprehensive Diagnostic Assessment

Comprehensive assessment obtains detailed diagnostic and life-history information across the six ASAM domains for the purposes of determining appropriate level of care, case formulation, and treatment planning. Ideally, multiple sources of information are integrated, including adolescent self-report, collateral informant (e.g., caretaker) reports, biological testing (e.g., urine drug testing), and external records (e.g., school, medical, court, prior treatment) in order to identify the adolescent and family's strengths and needs, determine and prioritize treatment goals, and select intervention components. We end this section with a brief example of how the measures described below might be used in a comprehensive assessment session.

Assessing Substance Use and SUD: General Considerations

Substance use assessment often covers lifetime history and recent pattern of use, typically using different measures. Although different measures are used, due to the different timescales involved (e.g., years vs. days), the discussion that occurs during assessment of both lifetime and recent patterns of substance use can be integrated, in some cases, as part of treatment in a seamless process. Notably, actively engaging the adolescent in a nonjudgmental discussion of pattern of substance use can sometimes help him or her gain insight into the perceived benefits and costs of substance use, as well as identify contexts and reasons for use that can determine skills to develop and strengths to leverage (O'Leary Tevyaw et al., 2018).

A lifetime history of substance use records the age of onset of each type of substance, onset of regular use of the substance (e.g., age at which the substance was used at least once per month for at least 6 months), frequency and quantity of use, mode of use (if applicable, e.g., injection of heroin, bong for cannabis, vape nicotine or cannabis), and primary substance used (Skinner, 1984; Skinner & Sheu, 1982). Ten commonly assessed classes of substances include alcohol (e.g., usual quantity consumed per occasion, frequency of heavy drinking episodes: consumption of >4/5 drinks per occasion by females/males), cannabis, nicotine (e.g., cigarettes, e-cigs, Juul), hallucinogens, inhalants, opioids (e.g., misuse of prescription opiates), sedatives and anxiolytics, stimulants (e.g., misuse of prescription medication), caffeine, and "other" substances (e.g., bath salts, synthetic cannabis, caffeinated alcoholic beverages). An important goal is to determine when changes in pattern of substance use occurred (i.e., increases, decreases, extended periods of abstinence), and what explained the changes in use (e.g., met a drug-using friend; stopped use while in treatment), to the extent that an adolescent has insight into factors associated with changes in substance use (Skinner, 1984). An understanding of what drives the changes in an adolescent's substance use helps identify substance-specific coping skills and vulnerabilities (e.g., triggers for substance use), and characteristics of the adolescent's recovery environment (e.g., substance use in the household) that can guide the selection of treatment components.

Most often, recent substance use (e.g., the past month) is of greatest interest, and can be assessed using a calendar-based method such as the TLFB (Sobell & Sobell, 1995). An initial step in completing the TLFB involves identifying personally relevant "anchor" dates (e.g., holidays, birthdays, significant events such as vacations) during the time frame of interest (e.g., past month) that can cue the recall of drinking and substance use episodes on specific days. Information on overall frequency of use (e.g., weekly vs. daily) for each type of drug used is sought, followed by more detailed information on whether use tended to occur on weekdays or weekends (if use was not daily). Usual quantity consumed per day, and whether a greater quantity was consumed on certain days (e.g., weekday vs. weekend, or on certain occasions, such as holidays) is assessed. Note that for alcohol, quantity is typically assessed as a "standard drink," which represents one 12-ounce regular beer (5% alcohol), one 5-ounce glass of wine (12% alcohol), or one 1.5-ounce shot of liquor (40% alcohol) (National Institute on Alcohol Abuse and Alcoholism [NIAAA], 2016). Cannabis quantity is typically reported as joints, blunts, hits, or grams; however, no standard cannabis quantity unit exists. Discussion of recent pattern of use can lead to exploration of specific topics, based on what is reported. For example, a relatively long stretch of abstinence might reveal a recent successful attempt to limit use, perceived benefits of abstinence, and strategies used to limit substance use. The TLFB has shown validity among adolescents for reports of alcohol, cannabis (frequency of use), and cigarettes (Dennis, Funk, Godley, Godley, & Waldron, 2004; Lewis-Esquerre et al., 2005).

When determining the presence of DSM and ICD SUD diagnoses in adolescents, assessment needs to take into account that development of SUD criteria was based on clinical experience with adults. Compared to their adult counterparts, adolescent substance users typically have shorter histories of substance use and tend to show a pattern of less frequent consumption, but consumption of a higher quantity per occasion, on average, especially for alcohol (i.e., binge drinking) (Chung, Creswell, Bachrach, Clark, & Martin, 2018). Adolescents, compared to adults, are more likely to have milder SUD, differ in the type of negative consequences reported (e.g., more likely to report alcohol poisoning or drug overdose due to inexperience), and are less likely to report withdrawal as a result of heavy substance use (Deas, Riggs, Langenbucher, Goldman, & Brown, 2000). Adolescents are also more likely than adults to be polysubstance users (e.g., report alcohol, marijuana, nicotine use) (Deas et al., 2000).

In the context of these developmental differences, assessment of SUD criteria, particularly those representing impaired control over use, need to be probed carefully to ensure that difficulties in controlling substance use among adolescents reflect a compulsion to engage in use rather than, for example, impulsivity or peer influences to engage in use (Chung & Martin, 2005). Furthermore, adolescent substance use can have effects on physical health that include, for example, substance-related injury, STI, HIV, pregnancy, poor nutrition, and disrupted sleep. Other substance-related consequences that warrant assessment and therapeutic intervention include trauma (e.g., physical, sexual, emotional) (Fergusson, McLeod, & Horwood, 2013; Tonmyr & Shields, 2017). The adolescent's legal status (e.g., court-mandated treatment, probation) needs to be assessed, and appropriate referrals and services addressed, even though substance-related legal problems are no longer a DSM-5 SUD criterion. In addition, because co-occurring psychopathology may predate, be exacerbated by, or develop as a result of substance use, assessment needs to determine the temporal ordering of co-occurring conditions to understand the adolescent's level of functioning prior to substance use onset. Information regarding the adolescent's level of functioning prior to the onset of substance use provides a context for setting reasonable treatment goals and expectations regarding short- and long-term treatment outcomes.

Other general considerations include sensitivity during the assessment to gender differences and sexual orientation in mental health symptom profiles, and cultural factors that influence how symptoms are reported. Specifically, adolescent females in substance use treatment, compared to males, are more likely to report mental health symptoms (both internalizing and externalizing disorders) and prior mental health treatment, but less illegal activity (Dennis, White, & Ives, 2009). Gender differences in mental health symptom profiles and legal involvement underscore the importance of assessing experiences of victimization (e.g., bullying) and abuse, homelessness, and exposure to violence (e.g., witness a shooting, a fight), as well as involvement in illegal activity, which may be associated with substance use. Although little is known regarding mental health profiles of sexual-minority youth in substance use treatment, high rates of stressful life events, and experiences of discrimination and trauma in this at-risk group, urge coverage of these topics to guide treatment planning (Mereish, Gamarel, & Operario, 2018). Assessment also needs to be tailored to accommodate cultural factors that, for example, affect how symptoms are reported or experienced (e.g., reporting depression as physical complaints) (Council of National Psychological Associations for the Advancement of Ethnic Minority Interests, 2016).

To summarize this section, comprehensive assessment needs to be tailored to accommodate personal factors such as age, gender, sexual orientation, and race/ethnicity that can affect the type of symptoms experienced, how symptoms are reported, and how questions are interpreted. Three comprehensive diagnostic assessment instruments are reviewed below: the DISC, a structured interview, and two semistructured interviews, the GAIN-I and the K-SADS.

Diagnostic Interviews

The Diagnostic Interview Schedule for Children (DISC; Fisher et al., 1993; Shaffer et al., 2000), a structured interview, available in computer format, covers 36 DSM-IV and ICD-10 psychiatric diagnoses for lifetime, past year, and past month time frames. Recent work updated the DISC to assess DSM-5 SUD by including a craving item and revising the scoring algorithm (Spirito et al., 2016). Youth-report (ages 9–17) and parent-report (of youth ages 6–17) versions of the DISC are available. The DISC assesses psychiatric conditions in modules, providing flexibility in which conditions are covered. Most questions are answered "yes" or "no" to simplify responding and minimize coding errors. Skip outs are used to minimize administration time. The DISC has high sensitivity for psychiatric disorders, including SUD (0.73–1.0) (Fisher et al., 1993). Test–retest reliability of youth report was generally fair to excellent for disruptive behavior disorders and SUD (kappa = .46–.80), with the exception of alcohol abuse (kappa = .32), likely due to needing to meet only one criterion for this DSM-IV diagnosis) (Shaffer, Fisher, & Lucas, 2004).

The GAIN—Initial (GAIN-I; Dennis, White, Titus, & Unsicker, 2008), a semistructured interview, can be used to assess diagnoses of SUD, aid the determination of level-of-care placement based on the ASAM's Patient Placement Criteria (Mee-Lee, Shulman, Fishman, Gastfriend, & Miller, 2013), and support individualized treatment planning. The GAIN-I includes and expands on the same nine subscales included in the GAIN-SS (described earlier), as well as additional modules that assess victimization and traumatic stress, illegal activities, social support, recovery environment risk (e.g., household members using drugs, social supports available to help manage stress), treatment motivation and self-efficacy, and cognitive impairment. Among adolescents in substance use treatment, the GAIN's General Individual Severity Scale (the measure's total composite score) and the four subscales that comprise the composite severity score (i.e., the 16-item Substance Problem Scale, 43-item Internal Mental Distress Scale [e.g., depression, anxiety, suicidal ideation], 33-item Behavior Complexity Scale [e.g., inattention, hyperactivity, conduct problems], and 31-item Crime/Violence Scale) had internal consistency reliabilities >.90 (Dennis et al., 2008). A test–retest study of lifetime SUD diagnosis resulted in fair agreement (kappa = .55; 40 vs. 44% for lifetime dependence diagnosis) (Dennis et al., 2002). GAIN self-reports of substance use were consistent with parent reports and urine tests for tetrahydrocannabinol (THC; kappa = .7–.9) among youth in an outpatient treatment setting (Dennis et al., 2002), and showed fair agreement with collateral report and urine testing for THC (kappa = .53–.69) among youth entering residential treatment (Godley, Godley, Dennis, Funk, & Passetti, 2002). Overall, GAIN-I demonstrates sound psychometric characteristics across a range of clinical settings with substance-using youth.

The Kiddie Schedule for Affective Disorders and Schizophrenia for School-Age Children (K-SADS; Kaufman, Birmaher, et al., 2016), a semistructured interview, is used with youth and their parents that covers most major present (past year) and lifetime DSM-5 diagnoses. Disorders are covered in modules, which begin with screening questions that determine skip outs if a minimum threshold of problem severity is not met, in order to shorten administration time (Leffler et al., 2015). Symptoms and diagnoses are rated on a 4-point scale (0 = no information, 1 = not present, 2 = subthreshold, 3 = meets threshold). The modular format allows for flexible selection of specific disorders to be assessed. The original version of the K-SADS showed high interrater agreement for symptom and diagnostic ratings (kappa: .93–1.00) (Kaufman et al., 1997). Although the K-SADS assesses DSM-5 SUD, details regarding recent pattern of substance use could be collected using a calendar-based measure such as the TLFB, as needed, to complement diagnostic assessment.

Alcohol- and Marijuana-Related Problems

To supplement assessment of SUD criteria by structured or semistructured diagnostic interview, questionnaires provide another method of querying substance-related problems. Questionnaire or computer-administered items, relative to interview, may result in greater disclosure of sensitive information. Alternatively, however, questionnaires could result in careless or inconsistent responses, especially if the measure does not include an internal validity check (e.g., a subscale to check consistency of responses). The Rutgers Alcohol Problems Index (RAPI; White & Labouvie, 1989) is a widely used, 18-item (originally 23-item) scale, with some items that overlap with DSM and ICD criteria (e.g., went to school drunk, neglected responsibilities), and others that are distinct (e.g., passed out, black out). RAPI items are rated on a 5-point Likert scale (0 = never to 4 = more than 10 times in the past year). The 18-item measure shows unidimensional structure, and multiple studies in adolescent samples have shown concurrent and predictive validity of RAPI scores (Neal, Corbin, & Fromme, 2006). A score >8 on the 18-item version suggests greater need for treatment (Neal et al., 2006).

The Marijuana Adolescent Problem Inventory (MAPI; Knapp et al., 2018), which is based on the RAPI, includes 23 similar items, also rated on a 5-point Likert scale. MAPI items were found to represent a single factor, with high internal consistency reliability (alpha = .89) among adolescent cannabis users in outpatient treatment (Knapp et al., 2018). MAPI scores demonstrated concurrent validity through significant associations with cannabis diagnoses and frequency of cannabis use in an adolescent treatment sample (Knapp et al., 2018).

Reasons for Substance Use

Individuals generally use substances for rewarding effects (positive reinforcement) or to relieve distress (negative reinforcement) (Cox & Klinger, 1988). Understanding an individual's reasons for substance use can reveal triggers and cues for substance use that can inform the development of a relapse prevention plan to strengthen substance-specific coping skills. The Drinking Motives Questionnaire (DMQ), a widely used measure of reasons for alcohol use, assesses four drinking motives: social reasons for drinking, drinking to enhance positive mood, drinking to cope, and drinking to conform with peers (Cooper et al., 2008; Kuntsche & Kuntsche, 2009). Among the DMQ's four factors, drinking to cope had the strongest associations with alcohol-related problems in adolescents (Cooper et al., 2008). The Marijuana Motives Questionnaire (MMQ; Simons et al., 1998), a 25-item measure based on the DMQ, assesses five motives for marijuana use: Enhancement of Positive Mood, Coping, Social, Conformity, and Expansion (i.e., increasing experiential awareness) (Simons et al., 1998). Among the marijuana motives, coping and enhancement reasons for use have been associated with more frequent use and marijuana-related problems (Simons et al., 1998). An alternative measure, the Comprehensive Marijuana Motives Questionnaire (CMMQ; Blevins, Banes, Stephens, Walker, & Roffman, 2016; Lee, Neighbors, Hendershot, & Grossbard, 2009) consists of 12 factors that assess the following reasons for use: Enjoyment, Conformity, Coping, Experimentation, Boredom, Alcohol, Celebration, Altered Perception, Social Anxiety, Relative Low Risk, Sleep/Rest, and Availability. Boredom and Sleep/Rest, two scales not included in the MMQ, were associated with greater frequency of marijuana use (Lee et al., 2009), and may be especially useful when assessing youth who often report difficulties with boredom and sleep.

Readiness to Change Substance Use

Youth referred for substance use evaluation or treatment typically express ambivalence regarding readiness to change substance use behavior (Den-

nis et al., 2002; Jensen et al., 2011). Assessment of how motivated an adolescent is to change can help determine, for example, whether a motivational enhancement intervention may be useful (Jensen et al., 2011), or whether the adolescent would benefit from strengthening relapse prevention and coping skills to maintain reductions in use that have already been initiated (Slavet et al., 2006). Motivation for treatment has been associated with treatment attendance and positive therapeutic working alliance (Joe, Knight, Becan, & Flynn, 2014), which in turn predicted positive outcome at 1-year follow-up. Two single item measures, the Contemplation Ladder (Biener & Abrams, 1991; Slavet et al., 2006) and Readiness Ruler (Moyers et al., 2009), have been used to assess readiness to change with adolescent substance users.

The Contemplation Ladder (Biener & Abrams, 1991) consists of 11 rungs (0–11) that are associated with statements such as no desire to change ("No thought about quitting"), ambivalence ("I often think about changing the way that I use drugs, but I have not planned to change it yet"), and taking action ("I have changed my drug use") that cover the continuum of change. Among incarcerated adolescents, ladder score shortly after incarceration was positively associated with treatment engagement and predicted marijuana use 3 months after incarceration (Slavet et al., 2006). As an alternative measure, the Readiness Ruler (Moyers et al., 2009), is a visual analog scale ranging from 1–10 (1 = *not ready to change*; 5 = *unsure*; 10 = *taking action*), on which adolescents indicate readiness to quit or cut down on specific substances. The Readiness Ruler for alcohol and marijuana, which is brief and easy to administer, showed good concurrent and predictive validity in a sample of treated adolescents based on hypothesized associations with substance use severity (Maisto et al., 2011a, 2011b).

Executive Cognitive Functioning

Risk for substance use has been associated with poor academic performance (Townsend, Flisher, & King, 2007), and lower executive functioning, which includes cognitive abilities such as response inhibition and working memory (Gustavson et al., 2017). Furthermore, heavy substance use appears to impact executive functioning in adolescents (Lisdahl et al., 2018). Assessment of executive functioning could provide general information to aid the selection and tailoring of treatment components to accommodate an adolescent's ability to absorb, retain, and implement intervention materials. The Behavior Rating Inventory of Executive Function (BRIEF; Gioia, Isquith, Guy, & Kenworthy, 2000; Roth, Erdodi, McCulloch, & Isquith, 2015), an 80-item questionnaire with youth- and parent-report forms, assesses the adolescent's executive cognitive functioning in daily activities. The BRIEF's eight scales, which can be combined to create a global composite score, assess Emotion Regulation, Impulse Control, Flexibility, Planning, Organization, Working Memory, Task Completion, and Self-Monitoring (Gioia et al., 2000). In cross-sectional analyses, the BRIEF global executive dysfunction score was correlated with SUD risk factors, such as externalizing behaviors, and substance use in adolescents (Clark et al., 2017). Youth with a suspected or known learning disability, or other type of cognitive impairment, would benefit from evaluation by a specialist (Wright, 2018).

Biological Testing

Biological testing can be used as an objective measure to detect recent drug use, typically to supplement self-report of substance use. Informing the adolescent at the beginning of the assessment that a biological assay will be administered can increase the validity of self-report, based on the adolescent's understanding that self-report will be checked against an objective standard (Winters, Stinchfield, Henly, & Schwartz, 1990). Urine drug screen and breathalyzer are commonly used biological assays at the initial substance use evaluation and for ongoing monitoring during treatment (American Society of Addiction Medicine, 2013; Hadland & Levy, 2016). Urine drug screens can typically detect drug use within hours to days (up to 3 days of last use) depending on the type of substance, and the intensity and duration of use (American Society of Addiction Medicine, 2013). Breathalyzers can detect alcohol for several hours after consumption, depending on factors such as the quantity consumed. Other types of biological assays test bodily fluids such as saliva and blood, or tissue such as hair and fingernail clippings (Hadland & Levy, 2016). Limitations of biological assays, such as the time window for detection of substance use, whether qualitative (positive vs. negative test result) or quantitative test results are generated, and the accuracy of the specific test need to be considered (American Society of Ad-

diction Medicine, 2013; Hadland & Levy, 2016). Other considerations include cost (e.g., for test kits, lab processing), invasiveness of testing (e.g., obtaining a blood or hair sample), and vulnerability of the sample to tampering (Winters, Fahnhorst, & Botzet, 2007). Wearable sensors, such as SCRAM ankle monitor and WrisTAS wristband, both of which are used to monitor alcohol use, have mostly been used for forensic (SCRAM) or research purposes (WrisTAS, SCRAM) (Greenfield, Bond, & Kerr, 2014).

Comprehensive Assessment Example

The session begins with an explanation of the purpose of the assessment (e.g., to determine level of care), estimated time to complete the assessment, and limits of confidentiality. The adolescent is informed that a biological test of recent substance use is to be obtained, the purpose of the test, the type of test used (e.g., urine drug screen, saliva drug screen, breathalyzer), what substances the test would cover, when test results would be returned, and who would be notified of the biological test results. Biological testing can be done at any time after the explanation of the test procedure and obtaining consent. Comprehensive assessment includes assessment of lifetime and recent history of substance use with measures such as the Lifetime History of Drug Use and the TLFB. Coverage of the six ASAM domains could be completed with the GAIN-I or the DISC and K-SADS in combination with the T-ASI and measures of readiness to change. Other measures, for example, family functioning (e.g., Family Environment Scale; Moos & Moos, 1986) are used as needed to assess specific treatment needs. Information from collateral informants and other sources (e.g., prior treatment, medical and court records) can be integrated to develop a coherent history of the adolescent's functioning to determine level-of-care recommendation, guide treatment planning, and prioritize treatment goals. A recommendation regarding placement into level of care takes into consideration factors such as severity of substance-related problems, concurrent psychiatric and medical conditions, coping skills, family environment, and response to prior treatment (American Society of Addiction Medicine, 2013). Treatment goals are ideally set, with input from the adolescent and others (e.g., family, court), and negotiated in an ongoing, collaborative manner through clinician-facilitated discussions to actively engage the adolescent as an active partner in therapy (Douaihy, Kelly, & Gold, 2014).

Process, Progress, and Outcome Measurement

For youth admitted to publicly funded substance use treatment, problems related to marijuana and alcohol use together accounted for 87% of admissions (SAMHSA, 2017). The court/criminal justice system is the largest source of youth referrals to publicly funded substance use treatment, followed by family/self-referral (20%), school referrals (13%), and other community-based referral sources (24%) (SAMHSA, 2017). Since many youth are referred to treatment by external sources (e.g., juvenile justice), motivational enhancement approaches can help increase readiness to change substance use (Jensen et al., 2011; O'Leary Tevyaw et al., 2018). During treatment, the adolescent's personal profile of risk and protective factors is continually updated to reflect new information (initial disclosure of past abuse) and changes in the adolescent's behavior and social environment. Persistent difficulty in maintaining agreed-upon treatment goals (e.g., goal to reduce or stop use of a specific substance) can result in a recommended adjustment of the treatment plan to a higher level of care (American Society of Addiction Medicine, 2013).

Measuring Treatment Progress and Outcomes

During treatment, assessment plays a key role in monitoring treatment response. Measures need to be brief due to repeated administration (e.g., across multiple treatment sessions), demonstrate reliability and validity, and be sensitive to change (Youngstrom et al., 2017). The most commonly used measures to monitor substance use during treatment include urine drug screens and self-report measures such as the calendar-based TLFB. Importantly, urine drug screens need to be administered by personnel trained in the interpretation of the test results given the possibility of false-positive and false-negative results, varying time windows to detect substance use, and varying sensitivities of the assays used (Jarvis et al., 2017). Training in the TLFB is available online (e.g., YouTube: CTN Webinar Timeline Followback). TLFB forms can be found at *www.nova.edu/gsc/forms/timeline-followback-forms.html*.

Response to motivational enhancement intervention, in terms of "readiness to change," which can fluctuate during treatment, can be tracked with brief measures such as the Readiness Ruler and the Contemplation Ladder (Maisto et al., 2011a; Slavet et al., 2006). In addition to the Ruler and Ladder, other brief measures have been used in naturalistic treatment outcome research to monitor change in motivation to abstain from substance use across treatment sessions in adolescents. For example, single-item measures of motivation and confidence to abstain ask "How motivated are you to abstain from marijuana?" and "How confident are you that you can abstain from marijuana?", with each rated on a 10-point scale (1 = *not motivated/confident* to 10 = *very motivated/confident*) (Chung & Maisto, 2016; see Appendix 19.1). Results from adolescents who completed these items after their intensive outpatient sessions indicated that confidence and motivation to abstain from marijuana generally increased during treatment (Chung & Maisto, 2016). Single-item measures of motivation and confidence to abstain are sensitive to change at the session level (e.g., week to week) and at longer intervals (e.g., monthly) (Chung & Maisto, 2016), and have shown good concurrent and predictive validity (Amodei & Lamb, 2004; King, Chung, & Maisto, 2009), suggesting their potential utility in monitoring progress, although data are currently limited regarding their use as a therapeutic tool in working with patients.

Following treatment, abstinence can be challenging to maintain, with rates of return to substance use reaching 60% or more in the first year after treatment (Buckheit, Moskal, Spinola, & Maisto, 2018; Chung & Maisto, 2006). The Relapse Review (RR; Brown, Myers, Mott, & Vik, 1994), a structured interview, typically used for research purposes, aims to characterize the context and cues associated with an adolescent's return to substance use. Importantly, the RR can be used as part of treatment to provide structured discussion of relapse precipitants and the context of substance use to strengthen coping and prevention strategies. The RR first asks the adolescent to provide a detailed description of the relapse episode, defined as the first use of any amount of alcohol or drugs following treatment. The adolescent is then asked a series of structured questions about thoughts, feelings, and behaviors before, during, and after the relapse episode. Relapse triggers are coded according to Marlatt's taxonomy (Marlatt, 1996) and include categories such as Negative Emotion (e.g., frustration, anger, sadness), Other Emotion (e.g., positive feeling, craving), and Negative Interpersonal Situation (e.g., argument). Treated youth reported two broad classes of reasons for relapse, "positive feelings and social reasons for use" and "negative interpersonal situation and being offered the drug," with roughly half of youth reporting a different reason for their next relapse, suggesting the need for a varied repertoire of substance-specific coping skills to maintain abstinence over time (Ramo, Prince, Roesch, & Brown, 2012).

In addition to substance use, evaluation of treatment outcome needs to consider an adolescent's functioning across the six ASAM domains that are used to determine a recommendation for level of care. In this regard, dimensional measures of change (e.g., symptom counts, rating scales) and cutoff points facilitate clinical decision making and can be aligned to placement criteria, which in turn can be linked to evidence-based practice (American Society of Addiction Medicine, 2013). The GAIN measures (described earlier) and Comprehensive Adolescent Severity Inventory (Meyers, McLellan, Jaeger, & Pettinati, 1995) are two instruments that are recommended for evaluation of adolescent treatment outcome.

The Comprehensive Adolescent Severity Inventory (CASI; Meyers et al., 1995) is a 45- to 90-minute semistructured interview (training required for administration) used to inform treatment planning and evaluate treatment outcome. Development of the CASI's 10 modules was based on theory and clinical experience in treating adolescent substance use, and cover Alcohol and Drug Use, Stressful Life Events, Mental Health, Family Relations, Peer Relations, Legal Involvement, Education, Physical Health, Use of Free Time, and Sexual Behavior. To track changes over time, questions ask about the onset of specific behaviors, and occurrence of behaviors within specific time frames (e.g., the past month, the other 11 months of the past year). In a sample of adolescent substance users in treatment, CASI subscales were represented by four higher-order dimensions: Chemical Dependency, Psychosocial Functioning, Delinquency, and Risk Behavior, each of which had high internal consistency (alpha = .78–.96) and test–retest reliability (intraclass correlation coefficients: .88–.96) (Meyers et al., 2006). CASI dimensions showed concurrent validity based on substantial associations with relevant scores on the Brief Symptom Inventory (Meyers et al., 2006). In support of predictive validity, CASI dimensions assessed in treatment predicted posttreatment functioning among adolescent substance users (Meyers et al., 2006).

Future Directions

As a transdiagnostic framework that can be used in parallel with DSM and ICD, Research Domain Criteria (RDoC) provide a complementary, dimensionally based conceptualization of psychopathology (Cuthbert & Insel, 2013). RDoC covers five major domains of functioning, which include negative valence systems (e.g., stress response), positive valence systems (e.g., sensitivity to reward), cognitive systems (e.g., executive functioning), social processes, and arousal systems (e.g., sleep). Each RDoC domain of functioning reflects a continuum of severity, similar to DSM-5 SUD. An important RDoC goal is to characterize each domain at levels of analysis that range from genes and brain circuits through behavior. The three RDoC domains that are most relevant for addictive behaviors include positive valence (reward sensitivity), negative valence (negative emotionality and stress response), and cognitive systems (executive functioning) (Kwako, Momenan, Litten, Koob, & Goldman, 2016; Litten et al., 2015). These RDoC domains play important roles in an influential neurobiological model of addiction in which high reward sensitivity increases risk for early initiation and escalation of substance use, and cognitive (e.g., executive functioning) and negative valence systems (e.g., stress, withdrawal syndrome) contribute to heavy substance use and relapse risk (Koob & Volkow, 2016). RDoC and DSM-5 signal a shift toward more dimensional conceptualizations of psychopathology.

The Addictions Neuroclinical Assessment (ANA) has been proposed to assess the three RDoC domains most relevant to addiction (Kwako et al., 2016). Using a personalized medicine approach to assessment, the ANA includes self-report, computerized tasks, and neuroimaging measures to determine an individual's unique profile of strengths and needs for the purpose of tailoring treatment. Much work remains to be done to refine the ANA battery, but the potential for using assessment to select neurocognitive and other interventions to address specific impairments is high (Diamond, 2012; Riggs, 2015).

A rapidly developing area, digital health, involves the use of mobile phones, apps, and wearable devices to collect data in real time to monitor changes in mood, cognition, behavior, and substance use (Carreiro et al., 2018; Mohr, Zhang, & Schueller, 2017). Some research demonstrates the feasibility of using smartphones to provide recovery support among adolescents, with one study finding that youth who accessed (vs. those who did not) mobile intervention components reported lower rates of substance use in the following week (32 vs. 43%) (Dennis, Scott, Funk, & Nicholson, 2015). Another study, which tested a text message smoking cessation intervention found that readiness to stop smoking mediated the intervention's effects on reducing cigarette use, but only among adolescents who had fewer smoking friends (Mason, Mennis, Way, & Campbell, 2015). However, the feasibility of using mobile phones with youth in substance use treatment remains an issue (e.g., some youth have limited access to phones when in treatment, phones may not be in service). These initial studies suggest the transformative potential of mobile phones for real-time assessment of substance use and substance use intervention among adolescents, with some caveats.

Conclusion

Reliable and valid assessment is essential for case identification, and understanding etiology, course, and treatment response. The EBA strengths-based approach to screening and comprehensive assessment covers multiple areas of functioning (e.g., six ASAM domains) in order to understand the "whole person" in the context of the broader recovery environment (e.g., family, peer, and community support systems). Due to the possible sanctions and stigma associated with reporting substance use, methods to enhance the validity of self-report, such as developing rapport through the use of an MI style and clear discussion of the limits of confidentiality are recommended. More generally, measures that are tailored to age, gender, race/ethnicity, and culture can help adolescents feel that their experiences are acknowledged and increase engagement during the assessment. Decisions regarding the specific measure to use for a given purpose (e.g., screening, referral differential diagnosis, treatment planning) depend on factors such as required training, administration time, and psychometrics. Assessment is an ongoing process that integrates information across multiple informants and sources of information to refine case formulation and update treatment priorities in line with evolving strengths and needs. The collaborative dialogue that develops during assessment can be an intervention in itself, and in some cases, woven into treatment.

Emerging results regarding the effects of heavy alcohol and marijuana use on adolescent brain structure and functioning (Lisdahl et al., 2018), newer modes of substance use (e.g., vaping, e-cigs), and recent trends in substance use (e.g., decline in cigarette use, and increase in vaping) highlight the importance of keeping substance use measures up to date. High rates of co-occurring psychopathology, which often predate substance use onset and can complicate its treatment, compel comprehensive assessment to identify the full range of treatment needs. Importantly, diagnostic assessment is at an important crossroad. Traditional systems, such as DSM-5 and ICD-11, are now being used in parallel with alternative, more dimensional systems, such as RDoC and the proposed multimodal ANA (Kwako et al., 2016), which is under development. In addition, computerized assessment tools, smartphone and social media data collection, wearable and other biosensors, combined with advanced analytic methods (e.g., adaptive testing, big data analysis methods) promise to provide personalized "just in time" intervention when and where support is needed (Carreiro et al., 2018; Mohr et al., 2017). However, issues of privacy, confidentiality, and the psychometrics of these new measures, as well as the acceptability and feasibility of these novel tools across age ranges and different settings remain to be addressed. Regardless of the specific tools, the central goal of assessment is to connect with the strengths of the adolescent and family in collaborating on a treatment plan that meets the adolescent's identified needs.

REFERENCES

Aarons, G. A., Brown, S. A., Hough, R. L., Garland, A. F., & Wood, P. A. (2001). Prevalence of adolescent substance use disorders across five sectors of care. *Journal of the American Academy of Child and Adolescent Psychiatry, 40,* 419–426.

Achenbach, T. M. (2009). *The Achenbach System of Empirically Based Assessemnt (ASEBA): Development, findings, theory, and applications.* Burlington: University of Vermont Research Center for Children, Youth, and Families.

American Psychiatric Association. (2000). *Diagnostic and statistical manual of mental disorders* (4th ed., text rev.). Washington, DC: Author.

American Psychiatric Association. (2013). *Diagnostic and statistical manual of mental disorders* (5th ed.). Arlington, VA: Author.

American Society of Addiction Medicine. (2013). The ASAM criteria: Treatment criteria for addictive, substance-related, and co-occurring conditions. Retrieved from *www.asam.org/publications/the-asam-criteria.*

Amodei, N., & Lamb, R. J. (2004). Convergent and concurrent validity of the Contemplation Ladder and URICA scales. *Drug and Alcohol Dependence, 73*, 301–306.

Bartoli, F., Carra, G., Crocamo, C., & Clerici, M. (2015). From DSM-IV to DSM-5 alcohol use disorder: An overview of epidemiological data. *Addictive Behaviors, 41*, 46–50.

Biener, L., & Abrams, D. B. (1991). The Contemplation Ladder: Validation of a measure of readiness to consider smoking cessation. *Health Psychology, 10*, 360–365.

Blevins, C. E., Banes, K. E., Stephens, R. S., Walker, D. D., & Roffman, R. A. (2016). Motives for marijuana use among heavy-using high school students: An analysis of structure and utility of the Comprehensive Marijuana Motives Questionnaire. *Addictive Behaviors, 57*, 42–47.

Boruch, R., Dennis, M. L., & Cecil, J. (1996). Fifty years of empirical research on privacy and confidentiality in research settings. In G. Stanley, J. Sieber, & G. Melton (Eds.), *Research ethics* (pp. 129–173). Lincoln: University of Nebraska Press.

Bronfenbrenner, U., & Morris, P. A. (2006). The bioecological model of human development. In W. Damon & R. M. Lerner (Eds.), *Handbook of child psychology: Vol. 1. Theoretical models of human development* (6th ed., pp. 793–828). New York: Wiley.

Brown, S. A., McGue, M., Maggs, J., Schulenberg, J., Hingson, R., Swartzwelder, S., . . . Murphy, S. (2008). A developmental perspective on alcohol and youths 16 to 20 years of age. *Pediatrics, 121*(Suppl. 4), S290–S310.

Brown, S. A., Myers, M. G., Mott, M. A., & Vik, P. W. (1994). Correlates of success following treatment for adolescent substance abuse. *Applied and Preventive Psychology, 3*, 61–73.

Buchan, B. J., Dennis, M., Tims, F. M., & Diamond, G. S. (2002). Cannabis use: Consistency and validity of self-report, on-site urine testing and laboratory testing. *Addiction, 97*, 98–108.

Buckheit, K. A., Moskal, D., Spinola, S., & Maisto, S. A. (2018). Clinical course and relapse among adolescents presenting for treatment of substance use disorders: Recent findings. *Current Addiction Reports, 5*, 174–191.

Burleson, J. A., & Kaminer, Y. (2006). Adolescent alcohol and marijuana use: Concordance among objective, self, and collateral reports. *Journal of Child and Adolescent Substance Abuse, 16*, 53–68.

Cablova, L., Pazderkova, K., & Miovsky, M. (2014). Parenting styles and alcohol use among children and adolescents: A systematic review. *Drugs: Education, Prevention, and Policy, 21*, 1–13.

Carliner, H., Gary, D., McLaughlin, K. A., & Keyes, K. M. (2017). Trauma exposure and externalizing disorders in adolescents: Results from the National Comorbidity Survey Adolescent Supplement. *Journal of the American Academy of Child and Adolescent Psychiatry, 56*, 755–764.

Carliner, H., Keyes, K. M., McLaughlin, K. A., Meyers, J. L., Dunn, E. C., & Martins, S. S. (2016). Childhood trauma and illicit drug use in adolescence: A population-based National Comorbidity Survey Replication–Adolescent Supplement Study. *Journal of the American Academy of Child and Adolescent Psychiatry, 55*, 701–708.

Carreiro, S., Chai, P. R., Carey, J., Lai, J., Smelson, D., & Boyer, E. W. (2018). mHealth for the detection and intervention in adolescent and young adult substance use disorder. *Current Addiction Reports, 5*(2), 110–119.

Center for Behavioral Health Statistics and Quality, Substance Abuse and Mental Health Services Administration. (2017). *2016 National Survey on Drug Use and Health: Detailed tables.* Rockville, MD: Author.

Chan, Y. F., Dennis, M. L., & Funk, R. R. (2008). Prevalence and comorbidity of major internalizing and externalizing problems among adolescents and adults presenting to substance abuse treatment. *Journal of Substance Abuse Treatment, 34*, 14–24.

Chung, T., Cornelius, J., Clark, D., & Martin, C. (2017). Greater prevalence of proposed ICD-11 alcohol and cannabis dependence compared to ICD-10, DSM-IV, and DSM-5 in treated adolescents. *Alcoholism: Clinical and Experimental Research, 41*, 1584–1592.

Chung, T., Creswell, K. G., Bachrach, R., Clark, D. B., & Martin, C. S. (2018). Adolescent binge drinking: Developmental context and opportunities for prevention. *Alcohol Research: Current Reviews, 39*, 5–15.

Chung, T., & Maisto, S. A. (2006). Relapse to alcohol and other drug use in treated adolescents: Review and reconsideration of relapse as a change point in clinical course. *Clinical Psychology Review, 26*, 149–161.

Chung, T., & Maisto, S. A. (2016). Time-varying associations between confidence and motivation to abstain from marijuana during treatment among adolescents. *Addictive Behaviors, 57*, 62–68.

Chung, T., & Martin, C. S. (2005). What were they thinking?: Adolescents' interpretations of DSM-IV alcohol dependence symptom queries and implications for diagnostic validity. *Drug and Alcohol Dependence, 80*, 191–200.

Chung, T., Sealy, L., Abraham, M., Ruglovsky, C., Schall, J., & Maisto, S. A. (2015). Personal network characteristics of youth in substance use treatment: Motivation for and perceived difficulty of positive network change. *Substance Abuse, 36*, 380–388.

Clark, D. B., Chung, T., Martin, C. S., Hasler, B. P., Fitzgerald, D. H., Luna, B., . . . Nagel, B. J. (2017). Adolescent executive dysfunction in daily life: Relationships to risks, brain structure and substance use. *Frontiers in Behavioral Neuroscience, 11*, 223.

Collins, D., Johnson, K., & Becker, B. J. (2007). A meta-analysis of direct and mediating effects of community coalitions that implemented science-based substance abuse prevention interventions. *Substance Use and Misuse, 42,* 985–1007.

Conrod, P. J. (2016). Personality-targeted Interventions for substance use and misuse. *Current Addiction Reports, 3,* 426–436.

Conrod, P. J., Stewart, S. H., Comeau, N., & Maclean, A. M. (2006). Efficacy of cognitive-behavioral interventions targeting personality risk factors for youth alcohol misuse. *Journal of Clinical Child and Adolescent Psychology, 35,* 550–563.

Cooper, M. L., Krull, J. L., Agocha, V. B., Flanagan, M. E., Orcutt, H. K., Grabe, S., . . . Jackson, M. (2008). Motivational pathways to alcohol use and abuse among Black and White adolescents. *Journal of Abnormal Psychology, 117,* 485–501.

Council of National Psychological Associations for the Advancement of Ethnic Minority Interests. (2016). *Testing and assessment with persons and communities of color.* Washington, DC: American Psychological Association.

Cox, W. M., & Klinger, E. (1988). A motivational model of alcohol use. *Journal of Abnormal Psychology, 97,* 168–180.

Curtis, B. L., Lookatch, S. D. R., McKay, J., Feinn, R., & Kranzler, H. (2018). Meta-analysis of the association of alcohol-related social media use with alcohol consumption and alcohol-related problems in adolescents and young adults. *Alcoholism: Clinical and Experimental Research, 42,* 978–986.

Cuthbert, B. N., & Insel, T. R. (2013). Toward the future of psychiatric diagnosis: The seven pillars of RDoC. *BMC Medicine, 11,* 126.

D'Amico, E. J., Parast, L., Meredith, L. S., Ewing, B. A., Shadel, W. G., & Stein, B. D. (2016). Screening in primary care: What is the best way to identify at-risk youth for substance use? *Pediatrics, 138*(6), e20161717.

Deas, D., Riggs, P., Langenbucher, J., Goldman, M., & Brown, S. (2000). Adolescents are not adults: Developmental considerations in alcohol users. *Alcoholism: Clinical and Experimental Research, 24,* 232–237.

Del Boca, F. K., & Darkes, J. (2003). The validity of self-reports of alcohol consumption: State of the science and challenges for research. *Addiction, 98*(Suppl. 2), 1–12.

Del Boca, F. K., Darkes, J., & McRee, B. (2016). Self-report assessments of psychoactive substance use and dependence. In K. Sher (Ed.), *Oxford handbook of substance use disorders* (pp. 430–465). New York: Oxford University Press.

Dennis, M. L., Chan, Y. F., & Funk, R. R. (2006). Development and validation of the GAIN Short Screener (GAIN-SS) for psychopathology and crime/violence among adolescents and adults. *American Journal on Addictions, 15,* 80–91.

Dennis, M. L., Feeney, T., Stevens, L. H., & Bedoya, L. (2006). *Global Appraisal of Individual Needs—Short Screener (GAIN-SS): Administration and Scoring Manual, Version 2.0.1.* Bloomington, IL: Chestnut Health Systems.

Dennis, M. L., Funk, R., Godley, S. H., Godley, M. D., & Waldron, H. (2004). Cross-validation of the alcohol and cannabis use measures in the Global Appraisal of Individual Needs (GAIN) and Timeline Followback (TLFB; Form 90) among adolescents in substance abuse treatment. *Addiction, 99*(Suppl. 2), 120–128.

Dennis, M. L., Scott, C. K., Funk, R. R., & Nicholson, L. (2015). A pilot study to examine the feasibility and potential effectiveness of using smartphones to provide recovery support for adolescents. *Substance Abuse, 36,* 486–492.

Dennis, M., Titus, J. C., Diamond, G., Donaldson, J., Godley, S. H., Tims, F. M., . . . Scott, C. K. (2002). The Cannabis Youth Treatment (CYT) experiment: Rationale, study design and analysis plans. *Addiction, 97*(Suppl. 1), 16–34.

Dennis, M. L., White, M. K., & Ives, M. L. (2009). Individual characteristics and needs associated with substance misuse of adolescents and young adults in addiction treatment. In C. Leukefeld, T. Gullotta, & M. Stanton Tindall (Eds.), *Handbook on adolescent substance abuse prevention and treatment: Evidence-based practice* (pp. 45–72). New London, CT: Child and Family Agency Press.

Dennis, M. L., White, M., Titus, J. C., & Unsicker, J. (2008). *Global Appraisal of Individual Needs: Administration guide for the GAIN and related measures.* Normal, IL: Chestnut Health Systems.

Diamond, A. (2012). Activities and programs that improve children's executive functions. *Current Directions in Psychological Science, 21,* 335–341.

Dillon, F. R., Turner, C. W., Robbins, M. S., & Szapocznik, J. (2005). Concordance among biological, interview, and self-report measures of drug use among African American and Hispanic adolescents referred for drug abuse treatment. *Psychology of Addictive Behaviors, 19,* 404–413.

Donovan, J. E., & Jessor, R. (1985). Structure of problem behavior in adolescence and young adulthood. *Journal of Consulting and Clinical Psychology, 53,* 890–904.

Douaihy, A., Kelly, T. M., & Gold, M. A. (2014). *Motivational Interviewing: A guide for medical trainees.* New York: Oxford University Press.

Fagan, A. A., Wright, E. M., & Pinchevsky, G. M. (2015). Exposure to violence, substance use, and neighborhood context. *Social Science Research, 49,* 314–326.

Felitti, V. J., Anda, R. F., Nordenberg, D., Williamson, D. F., Spitz, A. M., Edwards, V., . . . Marks, J. S. (1998). Relationship of childhood abuse and household dysfunction to many of the leading causes of death in adults: The Adverse Childhood Experiences (ACE) Study. *American Journal of Preventive Medicine, 14,* 245–258.

Fergusson, D. M., Boden, J. M., & Horwood, L. J. (2008). The developmental antecedents of illicit drug use: Evidence from a 25-year longitudinal study. *Drug and Alcohol Dependence, 96*, 165–177.

Fergusson, D. M., Horwood, L. J., & Lynskey, M. T. (1994). Parental separation, adolescent psychopathology, and problem behaviors. *Journal of the American Academy of Child and Adolescent Psychiatry, 33*, 1122–1131; discussion 1131–1133.

Fergusson, D. M., McLeod, G. F., & Horwood, L. J. (2013). Childhood sexual abuse and adult developmental outcomes: Findings from a 30-year longitudinal study in New Zealand. *Child Abuse and Neglect, 37*, 664–674.

Finkelhor, D., Shattuck, A., Turner, H., & Hamby, S. (2013). Improving the adverse childhood experiences study scale. *JAMA Pediatrics, 167*, 70–75.

Fisher, P. W., Shaffer, D., Piacentini, J. C., Lapkin, J., Kafantaris, V., Leonard, H., & Herzog, D. B. (1993). Sensitivity of the Diagnostic Interview Schedule for Children, 2nd edition (DISC-2.1) for specific diagnoses of children and adolescents. *Journal of the American Academy of Child and Adolescent Psychiatry, 32*, 666–673.

Fisher, S. L., Bucholz, K. K., Reich, W., Fox, L., Kuperman, S., Kramer, J., . . . Bierut, L. J. (2006). Teenagers are right—parents do not know much: An analysis of adolescent–parent agreement on reports of adolescent substance use, abuse, and dependence. *Alcoholism: Clinical and Experimental Research, 30*, 1699–1710.

Fletcher, A., Bonell, C., & Hargreaves, J. (2008). School effects on young people's drug use: A systematic review of intervention and observational studies. *Journal of Adolescent Health, 42*, 209–220.

Ginzler, J. A., Garrett, S. B., Baer, J. S., & Peterson, P. L. (2007). Measurement of negative consequences of substance use in street youth: An expanded use of the Rutgers Alcohol Problem Index. *Addictive Behaviors, 32*, 1519–1525.

Gioia, G. A., Isquith, P. K., Guy, S., & Kenworthy, L. (2000). *BRIEF: Behavior Rating Inventory of Executive Function*. Odessa, FL: Psychological Assessment Resources.

Godley, M. D., Godley, S. H., Dennis, M. L., Funk, R., & Passetti, L. L. (2002). Preliminary outcomes from the assertive continuing care experiment for adolescents discharged from residential treatment. *Journal of Substance Abuse Treatment, 23*, 21–32.

Gratz, K. L., & Roemer, L. (2004). Multidimensional assessment of emotion regulation and dysregulation: Development, factor structure, and initial validation of the Difficulties in Emotion Regulation Scale. *Journal of Psychopathology and Behavioral Assessment, 36*, 41–54.

Greenfield, T. K., Bond, J., & Kerr, W. C. (2014). Biomonitoring for improving alcohol consumption surveys: The new gold standard? *Alcohol Research: Current Reviews, 36*, 39–45.

Gustavson, D. E., Stallings, M. C., Corley, R. P., Miyake, A., Hewitt, J. K., & Friedman, N. P. (2017). Executive functions and substance use: Relations in late adolescence and early adulthood. *Journal of Abnormal Psychology, 126*, 257–270.

Hadland, S. E., & Levy, S. (2016). Objective testing: Urine and other drug tests. *Child and Adolescent Psychiatric Clinics of North America, 25*, 549–565.

Hall, W. D., Patton, G., Stockings, E., Weier, M., Lynskey, M., Morley, K. I., & Degenhardt, L. (2016). Why young people's substance use matters for global health. *Lancet Psychiatry, 3*, 265–279.

Hasin, D. S., O'Brien, C. P., Auriacombe, M., Borges, G., Bucholz, K., Budney, A., . . . Grant, B. F. (2013). DSM-5 criteria for substance use disorders: Recommendations and rationale. *American Journal of Psychiatry, 170*, 834–851.

Hawkins, J. D., Catalano, R. F., & Miller, J. Y. (1992). Risk and protective factors for alcohol and other drug problems in adolescence and early adulthood: Implications for substance abuse prevention. *Psychological Bulletin, 112*, 64–105.

Hines, L. A., Morley, K. I., Mackie, C., & Lynskey, M. (2015). Genetic and environmental interplay in adolescent substance use disorders. *Current Addiction Reports, 2*, 122–129.

Hingson, R. W., Heeren, T., & Winter, M. R. (2006). Age at drinking onset and alcohol dependence: Age at onset, duration, and severity. *Archives of Pediatric and Adolescent Medicine, 160*, 739–746.

Hoorn, J., Crone Eveline, A., & Leijenhorst, L. (2016). Hanging out with the right crowd: Peer influence on risk-taking behavior in adolescence. *Journal of Research on Adolescence, 27*, 189–200.

Huang, G. C., Unger, J. B., Soto, D., Fujimoto, K., Pentz, M. A., Jordan-Marsh, M., & Valente, T. W. (2014). Peer influences: The impact of online and offline friendship networks on adolescent smoking and alcohol use. *Journal of Adolescent Health, 54*, 508–514.

Hussong, A. M., Ennett, S. T., Cox, M. J., & Haroon, M. (2017). A systematic review of the unique prospective association of negative affect symptoms and adolescent substance use controlling for externalizing symptoms. *Psychology of Addictive Behaviors, 31*, 137–147.

Jackson, K. M., Roberts, M. E., Colby, S. M., Barnett, N. P., Abar, C. C., & Merrill, J. E. (2014). Willingness to drink as a function of peer offers and peer norms in early adolescence. *Journal of Studies on Alcohol and Drugs, 75*, 404–414.

Jarvis, M., Williams, J., Hurford, M., Lindsay, D., Lincoln, P., Giles, L., . . . Safarian, T. (2017). Appropriate use of drug testing in clinical addiction medicine. *Journal of Addiction Medicine, 11*, 163–173.

Jensen, C. D., Cushing, C. C., Aylward, B. S., Craig, J. T., Sorell, D. M., & Steele, R. G. (2011). Effectiveness of motivational interviewing interventions for adolescent substance use behavior change: A meta-analytic review. *Journal of Consulting and Clinical Psychology, 79,* 433–440.

Jessor, R., Costa, F. M., Krueger, P. M., & Turbin, M. S. (2006). A developmental study of heavy episodic drinking among college students: The role of psychosocial and behavioral protective and risk factors. *Journal of Studies on Alcohol, 67,* 86–94.

Joe, G. W., Knight, D. K., Becan, J. E., & Flynn, P. M. (2014). Recovery among adolescents: Models for post-treatment gains in drug abuse treatments. *Journal of Substance Abuse Treatment, 46,* 362–373.

Johnston, L. D., Miech, R. A., O'Malley, P. M., Bachman, J. G., Schulenberg, J. E., & Patrick, M. E. (2018). *Monitoring the Future national survey results on drug use: 1975–2017: Overview, key findings on adolescent drug use.* Ann Arbor: Institute for Social Research, University of Michigan.

Jones, S. C., & Gordon, C. S. (2017). A systematic review of children's alcohol-related knowledge, attitudes and expectancies. *Preventive Medicine, 105,* 19–31.

Jordan, C. J., & Andersen, S. L. (2017). Sensitive periods of substance abuse: Early risk for the transition to dependence. *Developmental Cognitive Neuroscience, 25,* 29–44.

Kaminer, Y., Bukstein, O., & Tarter, R. E. (1991). The Teen Addiction Severity Index: Rationale and reliability. *International Journal on Addictions, 26,* 219–226.

Kaminer, Y., Wagner, E., Plummer, B., & Seifer, R. (1993). Validation of the Teen Addiction Severity Index (T-ASI): Preliminary findings. *American Journal on Addiction, 2,* 221–224.

Kaufman, E. A., Xia, M., Fosco, G., Yaptangco, M., Skidmore, C. R., & Crowell, S. E. (2016). The Difficulties in Emotion Regulation Scale Short Form (DERS-SF): Validation and Replication in Adolescent and Adult Samples. *Journal of Psychopathology and Behavioral Assessment, 38,* 443–445.

Kaufman, J., Birmaher, B., Axelson, D., Perepletchikova, F., Brent, D., & Ryan, N. (2016). *K-SADS-PL DSM-5.* Pittsburgh, PA: Authors.

Kaufman, J., Birmaher, B., Brent, D., Rao, U. M. A., Flynn, C., Moreci, P., . . . Ryan, N. (1997). Schedule for Affective Disorders and Schizophrenia for School-Age Children—Present and Lifetime Version (K-SADS-PL): Initial reliability and validity data. *Journal of the American Academy of Child and Adolescent Psychiatry, 36,* 980–988.

Kelly, S. M., Gryczynski, J., Mitchell, S. G., Kirk, A., O'Grady, K. E., & Schwartz, R. P. (2014). Validity of brief screening instrument for adolescent tobacco, alcohol, and drug use. *Pediatrics, 133,* 819–826.

Kidd, J., Jackman, K. B., Wolff, M., Veldhuis, C. H., & Hughes, T. L. (2018). Risk and protective factors for substance use among sexual and gender minority youth: A scoping review. *Current Addiction Reports, 5,* 158–173.

King, K. M., Chung, T., & Maisto, S. A. (2009). Adolescents' thoughts about abstinence curb the return of

marijuana use during and after treatment. *Journal of Consulting and Clinical Psychology, 77,* 554–565.

Knapp, A. A., Babbin, S. F., Budney, A. J., Walker, D. D., Stephens, R. S., Scherer, E. A., & Stanger, C. (2018). Psychometric assessment of the marijuana adolescent problem inventory. *Addictive Behaviors, 79,* 113–119.

Knight, J. R., Sherritt, L., Shrier, L. A., Harris, S. K., & Chang, G. (2002). Validity of the CRAFFT substance abuse screening test among adolescent clinic patients. *Archives of Pediatric and Adolescent Medicine, 156,* 607–614.

Koob, G. F., & Volkow, N. D. (2016). Neurobiology of addiction: A neurocircuitry analysis. *Lancet Psychiatry, 3,* 760–773.

Kuntsche, E., & Kuntsche, S. (2009). Development and validation of the Drinking Motive Questionnaire Revised Short Form (DMQ–R SF). *Journal of Clinical Child and Adolescent Psychology, 38,* 899–908.

Kwako, L. E., Momenan, R., Litten, R. Z., Koob, G. F., & Goldman, D. (2016). Addictions neuroclinical assessment: A neuroscience-based framework for addictive disorders. *Biological Psychiatry, 80,* 179–189.

Lac, A., & Crano, W. D. (2009). Monitoring matters: Meta-analytic review reveals the reliable linkage of parental monitoring with adolescent marijuana use. *Perspectives in Psychological Science, 4,* 578–586.

Lago, L., Bruno, R., & Degenhardt, L. (2016). Concordance of ICD-11 and DSM-5 definitions of alcohol and cannabis use disorders: A population survey. *Lancet Psychiatry, 3,* 673–684.

Lee, C. M., Neighbors, C., Hendershot, C. S., & Grossbard, J. R. (2009). Development and preliminary validation of a comprehensive marijuana motives questionnaire. *Journal of Studies on Alcohol and Drugs, 70,* 279–287.

Leffler, J. M., Riebel, J., & Hughes, H. M. (2015). A review of child and adolescent diagnostic interviews for clinical practitioners. *Assessment, 22,* 690–703.

Levy, S., Weiss, R., Sherritt, L., Ziemnik, R., Spalding, A., Van Hook, S., & Shrier, L. A. (2014). An electronic screen for triaging adolescent substance use by risk levels. *JAMA Pediatrics, 168,* 822–828.

Lewis-Esquerre, J. M., Colby, S. M., Tevyaw, T. O., Eaton, C. A., Kahler, C. W., & Monti, P. M. (2005). Validation of the timeline follow-back in the assessment of adolescent smoking. *Drug and Alcohol Dependence, 79,* 33–43.

Lisdahl, K. M., Shollenbarger, S., Sagar, K. A., & Gruber, S. A. (2018). The neurocognitive impact of alcohol and marijuana use on the developing adolescent and young adult brain. In P. M. Monti, S. M. Colby, & T. O'Leary Tevyaw (Eds.), *Brief interventions for adolescent alcohol and substance abuse* (pp. 50–82). New York: Guilford Press.

Litten, R. Z., Ryan, M. L., Falk, D. E., Reilly, M., Fertig, J. B., & Koob, G. F. (2015). Heterogeneity of alcohol use disorder: Understanding mechanisms to advance personalized treatment. *Alcoholism: Clinical and Experimental Research, 39,* 579–584.

Maisto, S. A., Krenek, M., Chung, T., Martin, C. S., Clark, D., & Cornelius, J. (2011a). A comparison of the concurrent and predictive validity of three measures of readiness to change alcohol use in a clinical sample of adolescents. *Psychological Assessment, 23,* 983–994.

Maisto, S. A., Krenek, M., Chung, T., Martin, C. S., Clark, D., & Cornelius, J. (2011b). Comparison of the concurrent and predictive validity of three measures of readiness to change marijuana use in a clinical sample of adolescents. *Journal of Studies on Alcohol and Drugs, 72,* 592–601.

Marlatt, G. A. (1996). Taxonomy of high-risk situations for alcohol relapse: Evolution and development of a cognitive-behavioral model. *Addiction, 91,* S37–S49.

Martins, S. S., Mauro, C. M., Santaella-Tenorio, J., Kim, J. H., Cerda, M., Keyes, K. M., . . . Wall, M. (2016). State-level medical marijuana laws, marijuana use and perceived availability of marijuana among the general U.S. population. *Drug and Alcohol Dependence, 169,* 26–32.

Mason, M., Mennis, J., Way, T., & Campbell, L. F. (2015). Real-time readiness to quit and peer smoking within a text message intervention for adolescent smokers: Modeling mechanisms of change. *Journal of Substance Abuse Treatment, 59,* 67–73.

Medlow, S., Klineberg, E., & Steinbeck, K. (2014). The health diagnoses of homeless adolescents: A systematic review of the literature. *Journal of Adolescence, 37,* 531–542.

Mee-Lee, D., Shulman, G. D., Fishman, M. J., Gastfriend, D., & Miller, M. M. (Eds.). (2013). *The ASAM Criteria: Treatment criteria for addictive, substance-related, and co-occurring conditions* (3rd ed.). Carson City, NV: Change Companies.

Mereish, E. H., Gamarel, K. E., & Operario, D. (2018). Understanding and addressing alcohol and substance use in sexual and gender minority youth. In P. M. Monti, S. M. Colby, & T. O'Leary Tevyaw (Eds.), *Brief interventions for adolescent alcohol and substance abuse* (pp. 305–327). New York: Guilford Press.

Meyers, K., Hagan, T. A., McDermott, P., Webb, A., Randall, M., & Frantz, J. (2006). Factor structure of the Comprehensive Adolescent Severity Inventory (CASI): Results of reliability, validity, and generalizability analyses. *American Journal of Drug and Alcohol Abuse, 32,* 287–310.

Meyers, K., McLellan, A. T., Jaeger, J. L., & Pettinati, H. M. (1995). The development of the Comprehensive Addiction Severity Index for Adolescents (CASI-A): An interview for assessing multiple problems of adolescents. *Journal of Substance Abuse Treatment, 12,* 181–193.

Miller, W. R., & Rollnick, S. (2012). *Motivational interviewing: Preparing people for change* (3rd ed.). New York: Guilford Press.

Mitchell, S. G., Kelly, S. M., Gryczynski, J., Myers, C. P., O'Grady, K. E., Kirk, A. S., & Schwartz, R. P. (2014). The CRAFFT cut-points and DSM-5 criteria for alcohol and other drugs: A reevaluation and reexamination. *Substance Abuse, 35,* 376–380.

Mohr, D. C., Zhang, M., & Schueller, S. M. (2017). Personal sensing: Understanding mental health using ubiquitous sensors and machine learning. *Annual Review of Clinical Psychology, 13,* 23–47.

Moos, R. H., & Moos, B. S. (1986). *Family Environment Scale manual* (2nd ed.). Palo Alto, CA: Consulting Psychologists Press.

Moyers, T. B., Martin, J. K., Houck, J. M., Christopher, P. J., & Tonigan, J. S. (2009). From in-session behaviors to drinking outcomes: A causal chain for motivational interviewing. *Journal of Consulting and Clinical Psychology, 77,* 1113–1124.

National Institute on Alcohol Abuse and Alcoholism. (2016). *Rethinking drinking* (NIH Publication No. 15-3770). Rockville, MD: Author.

National Institute on Drug Abuse. (2014). *Principles of Adolescent substance use disorder treatment: A research-based guide* (NIH Publication No. 14-7953). Bethesda, MD: Author.

National Research Council & Institute of Medicine. (2009). *Preventing mental, emotional, and behavioral disorders among young people: Progress and possibilities.* Washington, DC: National Academies Press.

Neal, D. J., Corbin, W. R., & Fromme, K. (2006). Measurement of alcohol-related consequences among high school and college students: Application of item response models to the Rutgers Alcohol Problem Index. *Psychological Assessment, 18,* 402–414.

Nesi, J., Rothenberg, W. A., Hussong, A. M., & Jackson, K. M. (2017). Friends' alcohol-related social networking site activity predicts escalations in adolescent drinking: Mediation by peer norms. *Journal of Adolescent Health, 60,* 641–647.

Neumann, A., van Lier, P. A., Gratz, K. L., & Koot, H. M. (2010). Multidimensional assessment of emotion regulation difficulties in adolescents using the Difficulties in Emotion Regulation Scale. *Assessment, 17,* 138–149.

O'Leary Tevyaw, T., Spirito, A., Colby, S. M., & Monti, P. M. (2018). Motivational enhancement in medical settings for adolescent substance use. In P. M. Monti, S. M. Colby, & T. O'Leary Tevyaw (Eds.), *Brief interventions for adolescent alcohol and substance abuse* (pp. 153–187). New York: Guilford Press.

Prochaska, J. O., & DiClemente, C. C. (1983). Stages and processes of self-change of smoking: Toward an integrative model of change. *Journal of Consulting and Clinical Psychology, 51,* 390–395.

Ramo, D. E., Prince, M. A., Roesch, S. C., & Brown, S. A. (2012). Variation in substance use relapse episodes among adolescents: A longitudinal investigation. *Journal of Substance Abuse Treatment, 43,* 44–52.

Reed, M., Lange, J., Ketchie, J., & Clapp, J. (2007). The relationship between social identity, normative information, and college student drinking. *Social Influence, 2,* 269–294.

Riggs, N. R. (2015). Translating developmental neuroscience to substance use prevention. *Current Addiction Reports, 2,* 114–121.

Robins, E., & Guze, S. B. (1970). Establishment of diagnostic validity in psychiatric illness: Its application to schizophrenia. *American Journal of Psychiatry, 126,* 983–986.

Roth, R. M., Erdodi, L. A., McCulloch, L. J., & Isquith, P. K. (2015). Much ado about norming: The Behavior Rating Inventory of Executive Function. *Child Neuropsychology, 21,* 225–233.

Sacks, S., Melnick, G., Cohen, C., Banks, S., Friedmann, P. D., Grella, C., . . . Zlotnick, C. (2007). CJDATS Co-Occurring Disorders Screening Instrument (CODSI) for Mental Disorders (MD): A validation study. *Criminal Justice and Behavior, 34,* 1198–1215.

Shaffer, D., Fisher, P., & Lucas, C. P. (2004). Diagnostic Interview Schedule for Children (DISC). In M. J. Hilsenroth & D. L. Segal (Eds.), *Comprehensive handbook of psychological assessment: Vol. 2. Personality assessment* (pp. 256–270). Hoboken, NJ: Wiley.

Shaffer, D., Fisher, P., Lucas, C. P., Dulcan, M. K., & Schwab-Stone, M. E. (2000). NIMH Diagnostic Interview Schedule for Children Version IV (NIMH DISC-IV): Description, differences from previous versions, and reliability of some common diagnoses. *Journal of the American Academy of Child and Adolescent Psychiatry, 39,* 28–38.

Simons, J., Correia, C. J., Carey, K. B., & Borsari, B. E. (1998). Validating a five-factor marijuana motives measure: Relations with use, problems, and alcohol motives. *Journal of Counseling Psychology, 45,* 265–273.

Skinner, H. A. (1984). Instruments for assessing alcohol and drug problems. *Bulletin of the Society of Psychologist in Addictive Behaviors, 3,* 21–33.

Skinner, H. A., & Sheu, W.-J. (1982). Reliability of alcohol use indices: The Lifetime Drinking History and the MAST. *Journal of Studies on Alcohol and Drugs, 43,* 1157–1170.

Slavet, J. D., Stein, L. A. R., Colby, S. M., Barnett, N. P., Monti, P. M., Golembeske, C., Jr., & Lebeau-Craven, R. (2006). The Marijuana Ladder: Measuring motivation to change marijuana use in incarcerated adolescents. *Drug and Alcohol Dependence, 83,* 42–48.

Slesnick, N., & Prestopnik, J. (2005). Dual and multiple diagnosis among substance using runaway youth. *American Journal of Drug and Alcohol Abuse, 31,* 179–201.

Sobell, L. C., & Sobell, M. B. (1995). *Alcohol Timeline Followback users' manual.* Toronto: Addiction Research Foundation.

Spear, L. P. (2018). Effects of adolescent alcohol consumption on the brain and behaviour. *Nature Reviews Neuroscience, 19,* 197–214.

Spirito, A., Bromberg, J. R., Casper, T. C., Chun, T. H., Mello, M. J., Dean, J. M., & Linakis, J. G. (2016). Reliability and validity of a two-question alcohol screen in the pediatric emergency department. *Pediatrics, 138,* e20160691.

Stone, A. L., Becker, L. G., Huber, A. M., & Catalano,

R. F. (2012). Review of risk and protective factors of substance use and problem use in emerging adulthood. *Addictive behaviors, 37,* 747–775.

Substance Abuse and Mental Health Services Administration. (2011). *Identifying mental health and substance use problems of children and adolescents: A guide for child-serving organizations* (HHS Publication No. SMA 12-4670). Rockville, MD: Author.

Substance Abuse and Mental Health Services Administration. (2017). *Treatment Episode Data Set (TEDS): 2005–2015: National Admissions to Substance Abuse Treatment Services* (BHSIS Series S-91, HHS Publication No. SMA 17-5037). Rockville, MD: Author.

Tanner-Smith, E. E., & Lipsey, M. W. (2015). Brief alcohol interventions for adolescents and young adults: A systematic review and meta-analysis. *Journal of Substance Abuse Treatment, 51,* 1–18.

Taxman, F. S., & Caudy, M. S. (2015). Risk tells us who, but not what or how. *Criminology and Public Policy, 14,* 71–103.

Titus, J. C., Feeney, T., Smith, D. C., Rivers, T. L., Kelly, L. L., & Dennis, M. L. (2013). *GAIN-Q3 3.2: Administration, clinical interpretation, and brief intervention.* Normal, IL: Chestnut Health Systems, Retrieved from *http://gaincc.org/GAINQ3.*

Tonmyr, L., & Shields, M. (2017). Childhood sexual abuse and substance abuse: A gender paradox? *Child Abuse and Neglect, 63,* 284–294.

Townsend, L., Flisher, A. J., & King, G. (2007). A systematic review of the relationship between high school dropout and substance use. *Clinical Child and Family Psychology Review, 10,* 295–317.

Vincent, G. M. (2011). *Screening and assessment in juvenile justice systems: Identifying mental health needs and risk of reoffending.* Washington, DC: Technical Assistance Partnership for Child and Family Mental Health.

Weinberg, A., & Klonsky, E. D. (2009). Measurement of emotion dysregulation in adolescents. *Psychological Assessment, 21,* 616–621.

White, H. R., & Labouvie, E. W. (1989). Towards the assessment of adolescent problem drinking. *Journal of Studies on Alcohol, 50,* 30–37.

Windle, M., Spear, L. P., Fuligni, A. J., Angold, A., Brown, J. D., Pine, D., . . . Dahl, R. E. (2008). Transitions into underage and problem drinking: Developmental processes and mechanisms between 10 and 15 years of age. *Pediatrics, 121*(Suppl. 4), S273–S289.

Winters, K. C., Anderson, N., Bengston, P., Stinchfield, R. D., & Latimer, W. W. (2000). Development of a parent questionnaire for use in assessing adolescent drug abuse. *Journal of Psychoactive Drugs, 32,* 3–13.

Winters, K. C., Botzet, A., & Lee, S. (2018). Assessing adolescent substance use problems and other areas of functioning: State of the art. In P. M. Monti, S. M. Colby, & T. O'Leary Tevyaw (Eds.), *Brief interventions for adolescent alcohol and substance abuse* (pp. 83–107). New York: Guilford Press.

Winters, K. C., Fahnhorst, T., & Botzet, A. (2007).

Adolescent substance use and abuse. In E. J. Mash & R. A. Barkley (Eds.), *Assessment of childhood disorders* (4th ed., pp. 184–209). New York: Guilford Press.

Winters, K. C., Latimer, W. W., & Stinchfield, R. (2002). Clinical issues in the assessment of adolescent alcohol and other drug use. *Behavior Research and Therapy, 40,* 1443–1456.

Winters, K. C., Stinchfield, R. D., Henly, G. A., & Schwartz, R. H. (1990). Validity of adolescent self-report of alcohol and other drug involvement. *International Journal of the Addictions, 25,* 1379–1395.

Wish, E. D., Hoffman, J. A., & Nemes, S. (1997). The validity of self-reports of drug use at treatment admission and at followup: Comparisons with urinalysis and hair assays. *NIDA Research Monograph, 167,* 200–226.

Woicik, P. A., Stewart, S. H., Pihl, R. O., & Conrod, P. J. (2009). The Substance Use Risk Profile Scale: A scale measuring traits linked to reinforcement-specific substance use profiles. *Addictive Behaviors, 34,* 1042–1055.

World Health Organization. (2014). *Health for the world's adolescents: A second chance in the second decade.* Geneva, Switzerland: Author.

World Health Organization. (2018). *International classification of diseases* (11th ed.). Geneva, Switzerland: Author.

Wright, A. J. (2018). Comprehensive assessment of substance abuse and addiction risk in adolescence. In T. MacMillan & A. Sisselman-Borgia (Eds.), *New directions in treatment, education, and outreach for mental health and addiction* (pp. 25–55). Cham, Switzerland: Springer International.

Youngstrom, E. A., Van Meter, A., Frazier, T. W., Hunsley, J., Prinstein, M. J., Ong, M. L., & Youngstrom, J. K. (2017). Evidence-based assessment as an integrative model for applying psychological science to guide the voyage of treatment. *Clinical Psychology: Science and Practice, 24,* 331–363.

Zucker, R. A., Kincaid, S. B., Fitzgerald, H. E., & Bingham, C. R. (1995). Alcohol schema acquisition in preschoolers: Differences between children of alcoholics and children of nonalcoholics. *Alcoholism: Clinical and Experimental Research, 19,* 1011–1017.

APPENDIX 19.1. Motivation and Confidence to Stop Using Drugs

A. How <u>MOTIVATED</u> are you to <u>ABSTAIN</u> (*not use at all*) from . . .

	Not at all				Somewhat			Very motivated		
Alcohol	1	2	3	4	5	6	7	8	9	10
Marijuana	1	2	3	4	5	6	7	8	9	10
Tobacco	1	2	3	4	5	6	7	8	9	10
Other drug (specify):	1	2	3	4	5	6	7	8	9	10

B. How <u>CONFIDENT</u> are you that you will be able to <u>ABSTAIN</u> (*not use at all*) from . . .

	Not at all				Somewhat			Very confident		
Alcohol	1	2	3	4	5	6	7	8	9	10
Marijuana	1	2	3	4	5	6	7	8	9	10
Tobacco	1	2	3	4	5	6	7	8	9	10
Other drug (specify):	1	2	3	4	5	6	7	8	9	10

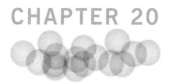

CHAPTER 20

Early-Onset Schizophrenia

Aditi Sharma and Jon M. McClellan

Schizophrenia is a complex neurodevelopmental disorder characterized by disruptions in cognition, perception, affect, and sociality. The illness typically presents in late adolescence and early adulthood and affects approximately 21 million people worldwide (Charlson et al., 2018). Affected individuals often suffer substantial long-term morbidity and mortality, with an increased risk of suicide, substance abuse, and other health problems. The global burden of disease is substantial (Gore et al., 2011).

We review in this chapter the clinical presentation and assessment of early-onset schizophrenia, which is defined as schizophrenia with onset prior to 18 years of age. Childhood-onset schizophrenia is defined by onset prior to age 13 and is rare. Schizophrenia in children and adolescents is diagnosed using the same DSM-5 (American Psychiatric Association, 2013) or ICD-11 (World Health Organization [WHO], 2018) criteria used to diagnose the illness in adults.

Epidemiology, Diagnostic Criteria, and Phenomenology

Epidemiology

Schizophrenia generally first presents during middle to late adolescence, with the age of onset peaking between 15 and 30 years of age. Onset prior to age 13 years is rare and often difficult to diagnose. The diagnostic validity of schizophrenia in very young children has not been established (McClellan, Stock, & American Academy of Child and Adolescent Psychiatry Committee on Quality Issues, 2013).

A recent meta-analysis of 129 global datasets estimated the worldwide age-adjusted point prevalence of schizophrenia to be 0.28%. The prevalence estimates did not vary widely across countries or regions. Although, historically, the illness was thought to be slightly more common in males, this analysis did not find any overall significant gender differences (Charlson et al., 2018).

Diagnostic Criteria

Early-onset schizophrenia and childhood-onset schizophrenia are diagnosed using the same criteria as for adult-onset. The diagnosis of schizophrenia per DSM-5 criteria requires at least two of five core symptoms: delusions, hallucinations, disorganized speech, grossly disorganized or catatonic behavior, and negative symptoms (American Psychiatric Association, 2013). At least one of the two symptoms must include delusions, hallucinations, or disorganized speech. Active positive symptoms (delusions, hallucinations and/or thought disorganization) must persist for at least 1 month unless successfully treated. Evidence of the illness must be present for at least 6 months, with an associated decrease in level of functioning, as compared with functioning prior to onset of illness.

ICD-11 criteria are similar to DSM-5 criteria, with at least two of the following symptoms required to make the diagnosis: disruptions in thinking, perceptions (e.g., hallucinations), self-experience (e.g., the belief that one's feelings thoughts or behaviors are under the control of someone else), cognition, volition, affect, and behavior. At least one core symptom must be present, defined as persistent delusions, persistent hallucinations, thought disorder, and/or experiences of influence, passivity, or control. In contrast to DSM-5, ICD-11 only requires 1 month of persistent symptoms to make the diagnosis (WHO, 2018).

Screening during the Interview

Screening for potential psychotic symptoms is part of standard psychiatric assessment, including inquiry about possible hallucinations and thought problems, as well as changes in behavior. When evaluating a child or adolescent's report of psychotic-like symptoms, it is important to assess for objective findings on mental status examination, such as disorganized speech, evidence of internal preoccupation, and odd beliefs and behaviors. The diagnosis of psychosis is made based on clinical evidence of psychotic thinking, not just on the report of psychotic-like symptoms on a symptom checklist.

Diagnostic Issues and Differential Diagnostic Considerations

Once it is clear to the evaluator that the patient is experiencing a psychotic illness, the next step is to identify the underlying cause. Psychotic symptoms are the key features of schizophrenia spectrum disorders, but they also occur with mood disorders and other medical conditions (e.g., intoxication, autoimmune conditions, delirium, genetic disor-

ders, neoplasms, medication effects [corticosteroids, stimulants, sedatives], and neurodegenerative disorders; McClellan, 2018; Staal, Panis, & Schieveld, 2019). Differentiating the cause for psychosis is critical, as treatments vary depending on the underlying condition.

The first step in any assessment of psychotic-like symptoms is to establish the validity of symptoms, that is, to determine whether they represent true psychosis as part of an overall psychotic illness. A substantial portion of children and adolescents (17 and 8%, respectively) report psychotic-like symptoms (Kelleher, Connor, et al., 2012). These typically involve reports suggestive of hallucinations or odd beliefs. The majority of children and adolescents reporting such experiences do not have a psychotic disorder, although many have other mental health conditions (Jeppesen et al., 2015; Kirli et al., 2019).

Clinical Presentation

Symptoms of schizophrenia are often characterized by three broad domains: positive symptoms, negative symptoms, and disorganization (McClellan et al., 2013).

Hallucinations and delusions are referred to as the positive symptoms of schizophrenia. These are often most apparent in the acute phases of illness. Hallucinations are sensory experiences that are generated by a person's mind rather than something in the environment. Common examples include hearing voices or seeing things. A delusion is a fixed, false belief that may be irrational or bizarre and is not part of a shared cultural or religious understanding.

Deficits in thinking and function, such as social withdrawal, flattened affect, and apathy, are referred to as negative symptoms. Compared with positive symptoms, negative symptoms are often chronic rather than episodic and typically do not respond as well to antipsychotic medication therapy (Leucht et al., 2017). Distinguishing negative symptoms from depression can be difficult given overlapping symptoms of apathy and social withdrawal.

Individuals with schizophrenia also present with disorganized speech, bizarre and unpredictable behaviors, and cognitive deficits, all of which have a significant impact on functioning.

Some affected persons develop catatonia, which is characterized by a general lack of response to one's environment (stupor, mutism, negativism), odd mannerisms, stereotypic movements, agitation, and echolalia (i.e., repeating words or sounds without regard for their meaning) or echopraxia (i.e., involuntarily repeating or mimicking movements of others) (American Psychiatric Association, 2013). Catatonia by itself is not diagnostic of schizophrenia and may represent a variety of psychiatric, neurological, and medical conditions (Sorg, Chaney-Catchpole, & Hazen, 2018).

Course of Illness

The course of illness in schizophrenia generally consists of four phases: prodromal phase, acute phase, recuperative phase, and residual phase (McClellan et al., 2013). Depending on when the patient is evaluated during the course of illness, the presentation may be quite varied.

During the prodromal phase, a person experiences functional deterioration, with the beginning signs of evolving psychosis. Prodromal symptoms can be difficult to distinguish from other disorders, such as depression, given several overlapping problems, including social withdrawal, isolation, and decreased functioning. Changes in functioning may be subtle and may involve the development of odd beliefs and behaviors. A decrease in self-care, including declining hygiene, can occur. The prodrome may be obscured by preexisting (or baseline) symptoms of social and cognitive difficulties. The duration of the prodrome is variable, from days to weeks, to a more gradual insidious onset.

During the acute phase of illness, positive symptoms are most apparent. It is during this phase that patients present with overt hallucinations, delusions, and bizarre behaviors. Because of the more overtly observable quality of these symptoms, it is often during the acute phase that the disorder is identified. The preponderance of positive symptoms can also lead to challenges with diagnosis given the overlap with other disorders that present similarly.

Following the resolution of the acute phase, the patient enters the recuperative or recovery phase. Negative symptoms are often more apparent during this period. Depression may also occur following resolution of the acute phase of illness. Improvement in functioning has a variable time course, with some patients responding to treatment better than others. Whereas some patients may recover from their episodes completely, others suffer chronic long-term impairment.

Affected individuals can have extended periods (several months or more) during which they do not experience significant positive symptoms.

During these residual phases, many patients continue to have some difficulties with negative symptoms. Unfortunately, not all patients improve to the point that positive psychotic symptoms resolve. Some remain chronically symptomatic despite treatment.

Assessments for Initial Evaluation and Diagnosis
Starter Kit of Assessments

As with any standard psychiatric evaluation, it is important to take a thorough history and to assess a broad range of potential symptoms and differential diagnosis. General screens for childhood psychopathology can be useful, such as the Strengths and Difficulties Questionnaire (*www.sdqinfo.com*) (Goodman, Ford, Simmons, Gatward, & Meltzer, 2000). The Achenbach System of Empirically Based Assessment (Achenbach & Rescorla, 2003) includes a Thought Problems scale that assesses hallucinations and strange ideas and behaviors but is not diagnostically specific (Salcedo et al., 2018). Similarly, the Child and Adolescent Symptom Inventory includes a set of questions based on DSM criteria for psychosis. In general, these questionnaires capture reports of unusual experiences and perceptions but need to be considered in the context of other clinical findings, since most such reports are false positives (Rizvi et al., 2019). These checklists may be completed ahead of the first interview, online or in the waiting room, then reviewed with the family during the interview.

The Brief Psychiatric Rating Scale for Children (BPRS-C) is a clinician-driven rating scale that can be used clinically to measure a number of different aspects of psychopathology, including psychotic symptoms. It is useful for evaluating and monitoring symptoms of psychosis, as well as symptoms associated with behavioral, mood, and anxiety disorders. It goes into more depth than most of the broad checklists and incorporates clinical judgment into the assessment.

There are more specific tools available to screen for patients at risk for psychosis. Kelleher, Harley, Murtagh, and Cannon (2011) found the Adolescent Psychotic Symptom Screener (APSS; a seven-item screening tool) to have good sensitivity and specificity for identifying psychotic-like symptoms. However, it is important to note that in this small study, none of the subjects had a psychotic illness based on diagnosis following a structured interview. This highlights the limitations of reliance on screening tools for diagnosis. The diagnosis of psychosis requires more than endorsement of symptoms on a checklist and ultimately is based on reported symptoms plus changes in mental status, behavior and function.

Based on the initial screen, if a psychotic illness is suspected, there are measures specifically designed to assess the presence and severity of psychotic symptoms, and structured diagnostic interviews, as described in the following section.

Psychotic Symptom Rating Scales

When psychotic symptoms are present, standardized rating scales are useful for assessing the severity of key symptoms. Commonly used scales include the Positive and Negative Syndrome Scale (PANSS), and the Scales for the Assessment of Positive and Negative Symptoms (SAPS and SANS).

The PANSS, is a 33-item, clinician-administered measure. Each item is scored on an 8-point scale. In addition to measuring positive and negative symptoms, it also provides a measure of general psychopathology (Kay, Fiszbein, & Opler, 1987).

The SAPS and the SANS are clinician-administered scales. The SAPS consists of 34 items, rated on a 6-point scale of 0–5 (Andreason, 1984). The SANS is 25 items, also rated on a 6-point scale (Andreasen, 1983).

Different Informants and Collateral Information

Evidence of a psychotic disorder is often observable to others. This may include changes in behavior, odd preoccupations, and unusual thinking. Observations should be sought from multiple informants. Given that schizophrenia often includes paranoia, the person with the illness may deny all symptoms. Conversely, youth who are anxious, somatic, overly imaginative, and/or engaging in negative attention-seeking behaviors may overreport symptoms. In general, since children typically have no natural understanding of psychosis, they may misunderstand or misinterpret the question and respond about experiences that are more developmentally appropriate (e.g., imaginary friends, make-believe).

Information from parents and other caretakers is important to document changes in the youth's thinking and behavior. A youth suffering from psychosis often does not share internal experiences, so the diagnostician must rely on family members and others to provide information regarding symptoms, including observations of responding to internal stimuli, odd or unusual beliefs, social withdrawal, and bizarre or unpredictable behaviors. Direct observations of overt changes in thinking and behavior are better predictors of diagnosis than the report of symptoms suggestive of psychosis in the absence of other mental status or behavioral changes.

Collateral information also should be sought from schools regarding both overall functioning and any potential observable features of psychosis. Screening questionnaires, such as the SDQ, are helpful for assessing broad domains of psychopathology. To assess more specific reports of possible psychosis, it is often helpful for the evaluator to speak with the informant directly.

Finally, given that psychotic symptoms often include bizarre and unpredictable behaviors, other sources of information may be available, such as medical records from other providers, emergency room evaluations, and interactions with law enforcement. Any credible observation of unexpected, bizarre changes in behavior and mental status requires a thorough evaluation, even if the person is no longer experiencing such symptoms (or denies that such symptoms ever occurred.)

Risk and Protective Factors

A number of different environmental exposures have been identified as potential risk factors for schizophrenia, including early neurodevelopmental insults, obstetrical complications, viral infections, nutritional deficits, cannabis use, social defeat and childhood trauma (Davis et al., 2016). These exposures confer risk for many different developmental, medical, and psychiatric problems, and definitive mechanisms specifically linking these factors to schizophrenia have yet to be established. Causal pathways are likely complex and interactive and depend on the cumulative impact of genetic and environmental insults at key points in brain development.

The early accurate identification of individuals at risk to develop psychotic illnesses remains an important public health need. As it stands, there is often a significant lag between the first onset of symptoms, and proper diagnosis and treatment. A longer duration of untreated psychosis is associated with worse symptomatic outcomes, greater positive and negative symptom severity, lower likelihood of remission, and poorer social functioning and global outcomes (Penttila, Jaaskelainen, Hirvonen, Isohanni, & Miettunen, 2014).

Criteria for identifying individuals at high clinical risk for developing schizophrenia generally involve attenuated (e.g., subthreshold) psychotic symptoms, psychotic symptoms that are brief and self-limiting, and/or a significant decline in functioning associated with strong familial risk. In research studies, these criteria are generally predictive of the eventual development of schizophrenia (Fusar-Poli et al., 2013). However, most adolescent youth classified as being at clinically high risk for psychosis do not develop a psychotic illness over 2-year follow-up (Addington et al., 2019). In studies of adolescents in the general population who are either admitted to psychiatric hospitals or seeking psychiatric services, high-risk status is not a strong predictor for eventual conversion to psychosis (the rates of which are low in this age group) (Lindgren et al., 2014; Therman et al., 2014).

Since duration of untreated psychosis is a potentially targetable risk factor, community-based programs have been developed to provide early identification and intervention services. By design, early intervention services provide targeted psychosocial and psychopharmacological treatments using a multidisciplinary integrated team approach. In a meta-analytic review, Correll and colleagues (2018) found that patients enrolled in early intervention programs had greater improvements in positive and negative symptoms, fewer hospitalizations, and better overall functioning, as compared to those receiving treatment as usual, over follow-up periods up to 2 years.

Once the diagnosis of early-onset schizophrenia is established, predictors of poor outcome include poorer premorbid functioning, greater severity of negative symptoms, and lower IQ (McClellan et al., 2013). Other clinical features that worsen the prognosis include comorbid substance abuse and poor compliance with treatment. Factors that potentially improve outcomes include family and community support, and access to intensive effective academic, occupational, and psychosocial services and programming. These factors are the basis for the design of treatment protocols in early intervention programs.

Diagnostic Process

A comprehensive evaluation, sometimes requiring multiple assessments, is needed in order to accurately make the diagnosis of schizophrenia or other psychotic illnesses. The differential diagnosis is complicated, and the clinical presentation can shift over time (Bromet et al., 2011; Castro-Fornieles et al., 2011). Misdiagnosis of early-onset schizophrenia is common (McClellan et al., 2013).

Endorsement of hallucinations alone is not sufficient to diagnose psychosis. Subjectively reported symptoms need to be considered in the context of objective signs and data (Ulloa et al., 2000).

Prescription: Using Assessment to Guide Diagnosis, Case Formulation, and Treatment Planning

Assessing for early-onset schizophrenia should consist of an interview, developmental history, mental status examination, and clinically relevant medical workup.

Interview

The diagnostic interview generally includes time with the caregivers and child together and with each separately. In addition to the standard elements of a psychiatric assessment, the evaluation focuses specifically on the nature, timing, and functional impact of suspected psychotic symptoms. Psychotic illnesses have characteristic patterns of symptom presentation and course of illness. For example, historically, schizophrenia is characterized by premorbid and prodromal symptoms, which evolve into periods of acute psychosis. The illness is associated with a significant decline in function and often has a waxing and waning course. In contrast, psychotic mood disorders, particularly bipolar disorder, are more often characterized by cyclical episodes of disturbances in mood, energy, thinking, and sleep. Although presentations vary, and symptoms between different psychotic conditions overlap, the skilled diagnostician looks for and recognizes unique patterns of illness across the lifespan, not simply a cross-sectional view of the patient's functioning and symptom reports at the time of referral.

Similarly, psychotic symptoms have characteristic qualitative features. Changes in thinking and behavior are generally observable to family members, friends, teachers, and other members of the community. True psychotic symptoms typically are not situational, that is, only reported in the context of behavioral outbursts or emotional dysregulation, or only at specific times of day (e.g., bedtime) (Hlastala & McClellan, 2005). Psychosis is generally associated with confusion, disorganized thinking and behaviors, and disruptions in social functioning and personal health care. The more detailed, elaborate, and situationally specific the reports of psychotic-like symptoms, and/or the more such reports occur in the absence of other, associated psychotic phenomena, the less likely such reports represent true psychosis.

Thus, the mental status exam is a key part of the assessment. Understanding the child or adolescent's cognitive functioning, as well as speech and language skills, is critical in interpreting symptom reports that are suggestive of psychosis. For example, a 15-year-old child with a developmental delay may express fantastical ideas, but these may not necessarily be related to psychosis. Similarly, a youth with impaired language skills may appear to exhibit features of paucity of thought, or thought blocking, when in fact the deficit is in expressive language.

Careful examination of premorbid functioning and developmental history is also an important element of the assessment. There are patterns of premorbid functioning that are suggestive of schizophrenia (e.g., social awkwardness and isolation, learning difficulties), although these historical features by themselves do not confirm the diagnosis. Premorbid functioning also helps predict future functioning and identifies issues important to address in treatment planning (e.g., histories of aggression, substance abuse). The developmental history may indicate other diagnoses that are either comorbid or mimic the symptoms of schizophrenia (e.g., autism or genetic disorders with associated developmental delays). Ultimately, historical information must be integrated with the current history and observations from the mental status exam to make an accurate diagnostic formulation.

Structured and Semistructured Interviews

Semistructured or structured interviews can be useful in assessing youth with symptoms suggestive of a psychotic disorder. Research studies addressing early-onset schizophrenia in children and adolescents generally use one of the following:

• The *Kiddie Schedule for Affective Disorders and Schizophrenia* (K-SADS; Kaufman et al., 1997, 2016), based on the adult Schedule for Affective Disorders and Schizophrenia (SADS), is a widely used semistructured interview conducted with parent and child separately. It has several sections for different diagnoses that can be administered depending on the patient's responses in the general interview. There are a variety of different versions that vary somewhat in terms of range of anchors and specific symptoms covered (see Galanter,

Hundt, Goyal, Le, & Fisher, 2012, for review and discussion). The new DSM-5 version also has a computer-assisted administration format available. Because of the flexibility in asking questions and probing responses, the K-SADS is best suited for interviewers with some clinical experience.

• The *Structured Clinical Interview for DSM-IV Childhood Disorder* (Kid-SCID; Matzner, Silva, Silvan, Chowdhury, & Nastasi, 1997) is based on the widely used Structured Clinical Interview for DSM-IV, a structured interview developed for use in adults. With the publication of DSM-5, a new version of the SCID is now in use, the SCID-5. A revised version of the Kid-SCID for DSM-5 has not yet been published.

• The *Mini-International Neuropsychiatric Interview for Children and Adolescents* (MINI-KID), adapted from the Mini-International Neuropsychiatric Interview (MINI) for use in children, is a structured diagnostic interview that is shorter than the K-SADS and has been found to be similarly reliable (Sheehan et al., 2010). The increased structure makes it easier for less clinically experienced interviewers to use. A DSM-5 version is now available.

• For evaluating an individual who is suspected of being in a prodromal state, the Structured Interview for Prodromal Symptoms (SIPS) can be used (Kelleher, Murtagh, et al., 2012).

In general, these diagnostic tools inquire about a broad array of potential symptoms, with positive responses triggering a more focused interview addressing specific diagnostic entities. Patient and family reports provided during diagnostic interviews are generally combined with information from other sources (e.g., medical records) and integrated into a consensus diagnosis. This approach models good diagnostic practices to follow in routine care and highlights the importance of supplementing clinical judgment with standardized measures when making a diagnosis.

Differential Diagnosis

Bipolar disorder with psychosis, schizoaffective disorder, autism spectrum disorder, posttraumatic stress disorder (PTSD), emerging personality disorders, substance use disorders, and medical conditions may all present with symptoms similar to schizophrenia. A careful evaluation, with longitudinal reassessment, is often necessary to clarify the diagnosis.

Mood Disorders

Mood disorders can present with psychosis. If psychotic symptoms are present only during a depressive, manic, or mixed episode, then the diagnosis is most consistent with the respective mood disorder with psychotic features. If the person has persistent psychosis, meeting the core symptom criteria for schizophrenia, while also suffering from intermittent major mood episodes that overall are present for the majority of the duration of the illness, then the best-fitting diagnosis is schizoaffective disorder (American Psychiatric Association, 2013). Differentiating between psychotic mood disorders and schizophrenia can be a challenge, especially during the early course of the illness. Long-term follow-up is often needed to clarify the diagnosis (Bromet et al., 2011).

Medical Conditions

Underlying medical conditions are important and potentially reversible causes of psychotic symptoms and need to be ruled out in any case of new-onset psychosis. Clinical indicators, such as physical exam findings, severity, and time course of functional decline, can guide the extensiveness of the workup. Medical conditions that potentially cause psychosis include delirium, central nervous system infections, toxic exposures, endocrine disturbances, autoimmune disorders, genetic syndromes, and neoplasms. Prescription drugs can cause psychosis, with an increased risk of doing so when used in excess. Prescription medications with known associations with psychosis include psychostimulants, steroids, dextromethorphan, antihistamines, anticholinergics, and barbiturates ("Drugs that may cause psychiatric symptoms," 2008).

In general, other than substance-induced psychosis, most medical illnesses associated with psychosis are rare. Potential warning signs that psychotic symptoms might be due to a physical ailment include fluctuations in mental status exam, fever, neurological problems, and exposures to known toxins/substances of abuse. Youth being evaluated for psychosis should also be referred for basic pediatric care, with more extensive evaluations as indicated, based on the presenting symptoms and history.

Substances of Abuse

A number of different substances of abuse can cause psychosis (e.g., cocaine, cannabis, amphetamines, inhalants, hallucinogens, and synthetic recreational drugs; Wilson, Szigeti, Kearney, & Clarke, 2018). The increased availability of high-potency cannabis is a public health concern given that its daily use is associated with higher rates of first-episode psychosis (Di Forti et al., 2019). Because substance abuse is a common comorbidity in youth (and adults) with psychotic disorders and psychotic-like symptoms, it can be difficult to determine whether substances are the causative or contributing agents, especially if there is not a sustained period of sobriety (Stentebjerg-Olesen, Pagsberg, Fink-Jensen, Correll, & Jeppesen, 2016). The risk of developing a primary psychotic disorder secondary to substance abuse is presumed to be heightened in some individuals who harbor genetic or other risk factors (Khokhar, Dwiel, Henricks, Doucette, & Green, 2018).

Trauma

Children and adolescents with a history of maltreatment report hallucinations and other psychotic-like symptoms at a higher rate than those without a trauma history (Kelleher et al., 2013). A systematic review of 35 studies (28 independent samples) of children with broadly defined psychotic symptoms, including affective psychoses and unspecified psychotic disorders, found a 34% rate of comorbidity of PTSD (Stentebjerg-Olesen et al., 2016). Although the association between childhood trauma and development of psychotic symptoms is well established, these studies generally focus on psychotic symptoms broadly rather than on the narrower diagnostic criteria required for schizophrenia. Histories of child abuse and neglect are common in youth reporting atypical psychotic symptoms in the absence of more overt signs of thought disorder or bizarre behaviors (McClellan, 2018). Of course, the presence of trauma does not preclude a diagnosis of schizophrenia. Many individuals with serious mental health disorders have histories of significant trauma. The important issue to clarify is whether the symptoms represent psychosis or posttraumatic experiences.

Developmental Disorders and Autism

The similarities between core features of autism spectrum disorders and diagnostic criteria of schizophrenia create challenges when assessing symptoms suggestive of psychosis in this population. Lack of social and emotional reciprocity, restricted, fixated interests, and perseverative idiosyncratic beliefs—all common features of autism—mirror symptoms of the social withdrawal and disordered thinking in schizophrenia. Children with autism spectrum disorders sometimes communicate utilizing complex scripts that can resemble descriptions of psychotic symptoms. Examples include parroting movies, other learned phrases, or fascination with video games or other fictional media figures—all of which need to be distinguished from delusional beliefs. Considering the patient's developmental age can help distinguish reports of psychotic-like symptoms from true psychotic symptoms. What may sound like a delusion in an adolescent with a developmental delay could be a description of an imaginary experience, similar to what might be seen in a younger, typically developing child. This highlights the importance of taking a developmental perspective when assessing potential psychotic-like symptoms in children and adolescents.

Deterioration from baseline is a key component of psychotic illness. Core features of autism represent long-standing baseline patterns of language, interests, and behavior, whereas the onset of schizophrenia represents a marked deviation from the person's baseline level of functioning. Distinguishing these patterns can be a challenge, however, in persons with baseline developmental problems that worsen during adolescence. Children with diagnoses of autism spectrum disorder are at higher risk for developing psychotic symptoms (Sullivan, Rai, Golding, Zammit, & Steer, 2013). Both conditions stem from early disruptions in neurodevelopment, and some genetic errors are associated with both illnesses (McClellan & King, 2010). To make the diagnosis of schizophrenia in a person with autism, prominent hallucinations or delusions must be present (American Psychiatric Association, 2013).

Aspects to Consider in Case Formulation and Treatment Planning

Once the diagnosis is made, the goal is to educate the patient and family about treatment options, both psychopharmacological and psychosocial interventions. Incorporating patient and family preferences in treatment planning builds the alliance and helps improve outcomes by improving adherence (McClellan et al., 2013).

Comorbidity

Individuals with schizophrenia have a high rate of comorbid substance use disorders, medical conditions, and psychosocial difficulties. Identifying these related problems is important for the provision of effective treatment.

Comorbid learning disorders and behavioral problems are common, and often predate the onset of schizophrenia. It is not clear whether such premorbid difficulties are early manifestations of the underlying neurodevelopmental insult that ultimately evolves into schizophrenia (Rapoport, Giedd, & Gogtay, 2012). In some cases, patients with schizophrenia have a known underlying genetic syndrome that is associated with both the illness and other medical complications. For example, velocardiofacial syndrome, which is caused by a microdeletion on chromosome 22q11.2 and is the greatest known genetic risk factor for schizophrenia, is associated with cardiac defects, cleft palate, immune problems, growth and feeding issues, and delayed development (Van, Boot, & Bassett, 2017).

Substance use is common in individuals with schizophrenia, with approximately one-half of affected individuals experiencing some type of substance abuse or dependence during their lifetime (Khokhar et al., 2018). The substances most often abused include alcohol, cannabis, and nicotine. Comorbid substance abuse has been associated with a number of different problems in this population, including treatment noncompliance, greater symptom severity, higher rates of hospitalization, impaired functioning, and suicide. Thus, addressing substance abuse is an important part of treatment planning.

Several population cohort studies have found elevated rates of premorbid cannabis use in patients who later develop schizophrenia, or more broadly in persons who report psychotic-like symptoms. The relationship between substance use and the development of psychosis appears to be bidirectional, since the report of psychotic-like symptoms also predicts the later use of substances (Degenhardt et al., 2018). Genetic factors may increase the risk for both substance abuse and schizophrenia, with the concurrence of both disorders potentially representing shared vulnerability (Khokhar et al., 2018). Further research is needed to define genetic and neurobiological factors that mediate the risk between the two conditions.

Long term, schizophrenia is associated with significant medical morbidity and a substantially shortened lifespan (Laursen, Nordentoft, & Mortensen, 2014). Compared to the general population, individuals with schizophrenia are more likely to have cardiovascular and metabolic illnesses, including hypertension, diabetes, and coronary artery disease. There are a number of different potential contributing risk factors. The risk of antipsychotic medications, particularly second-generation agents, for metabolic side effects is well established (Hirsch et al., 2017). In addition, persons with schizophrenia often do not receive adequate health care. Many do not follow healthy lifestyle habits, such as proper diet, exercise, and the avoidance of substances (including tobacco) (Laursen et al., 2014). Finally, it may be that some genetic and neurobiological factors underlying schizophrenia also contribute to cardiovascular and metabolic problems.

In addition, persons with schizophrenia have a much higher rate of suicide as compared to the general population (Hettige, Bani-Fatemi, Sakinofsky, & De Luca, 2018). Several risk factors have been implicated, including higher rates of stressful events, the potential impact of psychotic symptoms on suicidal behaviors, and the overall impact of the illness on functioning and quality of life. Ongoing, systematic monitoring for suicidality in affected persons is a necessary part of treatment.

Diagnostic Shifts

For psychotic illnesses, the diagnosis needs to be reassessed over time. Multiple community studies have shown that diagnostic presentations can change over time in young patients with early psychotic symptoms. Diagnostic stability appears to improve as time elapses from initial diagnosis (Bromet et al., 2011). A small study of 24 patients with first-episode, early-onset psychosis showed a significant improvement in agreement between diagnosis at between 1- and 2-year follow-up compared with diagnosis at onset and 1-year follow-up (Fraguas et al., 2008). Over long-term follow-up, some youth originally diagnosed as having schizophrenia turn out to have other psychotic conditions (e.g., bipolar disorder), whereas others have issues related to posttraumatic phenomena and personality disorders (McClellan et al., 2013).

Assessment for Services

Determining the services needed to support an individual with early-onset schizophrenia is an important part of the diagnostic assessment. Outcomes rely on more than the treatment of psychotic symptoms. For example, the recognition of cognitive deficits and learning disorders can guide appropriate school accommodations and help

with qualification for state services. Similarly, the identification of comorbid conditions such as substance abuse, helps define intervention needs and decreases the risk of noncompliance and treatment failures.

Prognostic Indicators

For youth with early-onset schizophrenia, modifiable prognostic indicators include lack of access to services and duration of untreated psychosis. Early identification community-based programs that provide a comprehensive array of evidence-based pharmacological and psychosocial serves are designed to address these factors. Unfortunately, some risk factors, such as lower baseline intellectual functioning, higher rates of premorbid problems, earlier onset, and greater negative symptoms are difficult to modify. However, youth with these concerns can be targeted for more intensive services.

Cultural Considerations and Patient Preferences

Psychiatric symptoms must be assessed within the context of the culture of the patient and family. Beliefs and behaviors that may seem unusual to the evaluator may be a normal part of the patient's culture and thus not reflect true psychosis. For this reason, it is important to ask about the background of apparently unusual beliefs. For example, a youth who believes God has a special plan for him or her may be experiencing religious delusions or may be describing something he or she learned in Sunday school. Other examples included shared family or group beliefs in paranormal activities, such as ghosts or extraterrestrial beings. Such beliefs are common in the general population, and care is needed to avoid misdiagnosing such beliefs as psychosis (Pechey & Halligan, 2011).

Conversely, in some cultures, psychiatric illnesses are conceptualized as demonic possession, for example, the belief that someone's mental illness is caused by witchcraft (Campbell et al., 2017). In this example, while the belief in bewitchment is cultural, the person may still have a mental illness and require treatment.

Other cultural considerations include choice of treatment. Cultural factors impact a patient's and family's decision making about whether to take antipsychotic medication, their willingness to accept risks of adverse effects, and their engagement with psychosocial services. The clinician should explore the patient's cultural background and preferences when developing a treatment plan. In a study of adult patients (N = 100) with recently diagnosed schizophrenia, a survey of patient preferences found two groups: one that prioritized functional outcomes, and another that prioritized clinical outcomes (Bridges et al., 2018). Understanding these preferences improves patient rapport and potentially enhances treatment compliance and outcomes.

Appropriate access to services also often has cultural implications. For example, in a multisite study of community-based care for first-episode psychosis, African American participants in the treatment-as-usual arm had higher ratings of psychotic symptoms and were less likely to receive key services. In the intensive community-based treatment arm, there were no racial differences in symptom ratings (Oluwoye et al., 2018). Thus, differences in illness severity and treatment response, at least in this study, were due not to racial or ethnic differences but to whether the participants had access to more effective treatment and support services.

Process, Progress, and Outcome Measurement

Individuals with schizophrenia often experience chronic impairment and morbidity, and as a result, require long-term monitoring and care. Even if patients recover completely, some periodic monitoring is warranted given the risk for recurrent episodes of psychosis. In the short term, once treatment goals have been established with the patient and family, and the patient is receiving treatment, it is useful to monitor for symptom recurrence, improvement in functioning, and medication adherence.

Outcome Measurement

Symptoms can be measured over time by using standardized rating scales. The same measures that are used to assess symptom severity and frequency at baseline (SAPS, SANS, PANSS, and/or BPRS-C) may also be used to measure symptom severity over time. Each of these tools has been used in clinical trials assessing the efficacy of antipsychotic mediations, with the PANSS probably the most widely used.

Monitoring of Overall Functioning

Systematic treatment should address functional outcomes in addition to the core symptoms of schizophrenia. In youth with early-onset schizophrenia, it is important to assess functional measures such as school attendance, participation in school, recreational and leisure activities, and basic self-care. Some individuals with early-onset schizophrenia need additional support, such as special education programs, occupational training, and assisted transition into adult services (e.g., independent living skills support).

Medication Adherence

Poor medication adherence is a major problem in the treatment of schizophrenia. In the Clinical Antipsychotic Trials of Intervention Effectiveness (CATIE) study, 74% of the 1,432 adult patients who received antipsychotic medications discontinued the medication before 18 months of treatment (Lieberman et al., 2005). Younger age was associated with earlier discontinuation of medications.

In the Treatment of Early-Onset Schizophrenia Study (TEOSS), only 12% of children and adolescents with schizophrenia spectrum disorders remained on the original randomized antipsychotic medication through the first 12 months of treatment (Findling et al., 2010). Reasons for stopping the medication included lack of efficacy, side effects, and noncompliance.

Education for Relapse Prevention

Tracking medication adherence and providing information regarding relapse prevention are important components of effective treatment. Early identification of relapse symptoms can also lead to earlier intervention in such situations and potentially reduce the severity of relapse.

Clinical Case Examples

Zoe

Presentation

Zoe is a 12-year-old girl referred to an early psychosis clinic for an evaluation. She and her family recently moved across the country. Since that time, Zoe has been complaining of headaches and stomachaches and has missed several days of school due to not feeling well. She saw her pediatrician and, after a medical workup that was largely negative, was referred to a mental health clinic. Prior to this, Zoe had never been in mental health treatment.

She has a normal IQ and no learning problems. Her academic and social functioning are normal.

At intake, she and her parents completed several rating scales, including the Child Behavior Checklist (CBCL) and Youth Self-Report (YSR). On the YSR, Zoe endorsed many features of anxiety, sleep problems, and hearing voices. On the CBCL, her mother also reported concerns about anxiety and sleep problems. However, in reviewing the findings, her parents were alarmed to learn that Zoe endorsed hearing voices and expressed the fear that she might have schizophrenia.

At the initial interview with the mental health evaluator, Zoe reports that she sees two figures who speak to her. Their names are "Kyle" and "Janie." She describes them vividly and feels their presence more strongly when she feels anxious and when she goes to school.

A diagnostic feedback session was scheduled 3 weeks after the initial appointment. At the return visit, her parents report that Zoe has been talking more about the voices. She told her parents that "Janie tells me to do things" and "Kyle is mean to me" and that the voices are much more bothersome when she is at school. Given her concerns, her parents have kept Zoe home from school. Her parents are extremely distressed and are inquiring about an antipsychotic medication that they have read about online.

On interview, Zoe is well groomed and well spoken. She does not appear internally preoccupied. Her speech and thoughts are organized. Zoe is able to tell the examiner her birthday, the current date, and her new address. She has a euthymic affect when describing her hallucinations. She reports missing her old school and friends and is quite anxious about attending the new school and meeting new people. When the clinician suggests that she cannot miss more school, Zoe starts crying.

Analysis

In this case, although the patient endorses hallucinations on a questionnaire, the following clinical interview and historical features are not consistent with a primary psychotic disorder:

- Age (onset of true psychosis below age 13 years is rare)
- High premorbid and current functioning (no learning disorders, no social problems)
- Organized thinking on the mental status exam
- Articulate and organized speech and behaviors
- Intact self-care (good grooming and hygiene)

- Highly organized description of the hallucinations
- Report of hallucinations that are situationally specific (e.g., being worse with anxiety and when she goes to school)

The more likely explanation is that Zoe is experiencing a difficult adjustment after the move and has significant anxiety (commonly manifesting with physical symptoms in children and young adolescents). Her experience of hallucinations is not in dispute, as only she can know what her own sensory experiences are. However, it is fair to tell the parents that the hallucinations are unlikely to be related to a disorder such as schizophrenia and that they may be explained as part of an active imagination or overvalued thought. A hallmark of anxiety disorders is the experience of distressing thoughts, and these may be described as visual/auditory hallucinations by children (especially if such reports are reinforced by adults). There appears to be a behavioral function to Zoe's report of hallucinations: Her parents allow her to stay home from school when she reports that the voices are bothering her, so she does not have to face the main trigger to her anxiety (her new school).

Treatment Course

Zoe enrolls in cognitive-behavioral therapy (CBT) for anxiety, and her therapist implements a graded return-to-school plan. She also sees a psychiatrist who prescribes a selective serotonin reuptake inhibitor (SSRI) to treat her anxiety. Zoe is not prescribed an antipsychotic. Her parents are coached to interpret reports of hearing voices as a sign of distress, and to encourage Zoe to use her coping skills rather than focusing on the content of the perceptual experiences. After 6 weeks, Zoe reports some improvement in school attendance and decreased awareness of the voices. After 12 weeks, she has completed her CBT and is back in school full time.

Dan

Presentation

Dan, a 17-year-old young man with a history of attention-deficit/hyperactivity disorder (ADHD) is brought to the pediatrician by his mother because he has become more withdrawn and isolated over the past 6 months. He rarely engages with friends and seems to go days without speaking to his parents. Dan's grades have deteriorated, and he is no longer completing homework assignments. His grandmother, visiting from out of state, has noticed that his hair seems greasy and wonders if he has been changing his clothes. Dan seems to be awake late at night and spends a lot of time playing video games on his computer and reading message boards online.

On initial interview, Dan speaks quietly and makes little eye contact. He is disheveled and wearing clothes that are quite wrinkled. He answers questions briefly using one- to two-word answers and endorses feeling depressed, with decreased interest in previously enjoyed activities and low energy.

Dan's pediatrician diagnoses him with depression and prescribes fluoxetine, an antidepressant medication. The pediatrician asks him to follow up in 6 weeks. At the follow-up visit, Dan appears more disheveled and is slightly malodorous. He makes little eye contact and seems distracted. He takes a long time to answer questions. Some of the conversation is hard to follow because Dan's sentences do not always make sense. He does not always seem to register what others say to him. His affect is flat. Dan's weight is down 4 pounds since the initial visit. His mother shares that at the parent–teacher conference, his teacher commented that when he comes into the classroom, he seems confused and often takes a while to find his seat. Dan has been observed talking and laughing to himself at home and in school. His mother asks if his antidepressant needs to be increased or changed.

Analysis

On initial presentation, it makes sense that Dan's pediatrician is concerned about depression. He is more withdrawn, endorses anhedonia and sadness, and appears to have decreased motivation based on declining grades. However, there are features of the mental status exam at the initial assessment that suggest evolving psychosis. A marked deterioration in functioning, social relatedness, and self-care are all hallmark prodromal symptoms of psychosis. On the mental status exam, Dan's paucity of speech and lack of engagement is a sign of developing thought disorder, and also might represent some degree of paranoia.

At the follow-up visit, both history and exam provide a clearer picture of psychosis. Disorganized thought is demonstrated by Dan's difficulty finding his seat in class and on exam by his speech pat-

tern. Delayed responses to questions may reflect thought blocking. More overt signs include others seeing Dan talking to himself, weight loss, and further decline in self-care.

Treatment Course

Dan's pediatrician refers him to the emergency room, where he becomes agitated. He is admitted to a psychiatric unit. At intake, the treatment team completes a PANSS, and Dan's initial score is 95, with positive responses for several domains of psychosis, including hallucinations, persecutory beliefs, conceptual disorganization, social withdrawal, blunted affect, lack of spontaneity, and stereotyped thinking. He is prescribed risperidone, an atypical antipsychotic medication. Over the next 2 weeks, Dan slowly starts to exhibit improvements in thinking and self-care. He continues to be quiet and isolative. He is eventually discharged home and follows up with an early-onset psychosis program.

Conclusion

The diagnosis of early-onset schizophrenia is based on a comprehensive assessment, using screening tools and standardized ratings scales as adjuncts to clinical judgment based on interview, examination, and collateral information. Use of structured interview tools can improve diagnostic accuracy in assessing this commonly misdiagnosed condition. Systematic monitoring over time using standardized measures may improve diagnostic accuracy and treatment outcomes. Accurate, early diagnosis is important to ensure proper treatment and monitoring, which in turn may lead to improved outcomes for patients.

REFERENCES

Achenbach, T. M., & Rescorla, L. A. (2003). Manual for the ASEBA Adult Forms and Profiles. Burlington: University of Vermont.

Addington, J., Stowkowy, J., Liu, L., Cadenhead, K. S., Cannon, T. D., Cornblatt, B. A., . . . Woods, S. W. (2019). Clinical and functional characteristics of youth at clinical high-risk for psychosis who do not transition to psychosis. Psychological Medicine, 49(10), 1670–1677.

American Psychiatric Association. (2013). Diagnostic and statistical manual of mental disorders (5th ed.). Arlington, VA: Author.

Andreasen, N. C. (1983). *The Scale for the Assessment of Negative Symptoms (SANS)*. Iowa City: University of Iowa.

Andreasen, N. C. (1984). *The Scale for the Assessment of Positive Symptoms (SAPS)*. Iowa City: University of Iowa.

Bridges, J. F., Beusterien, K., Heres, S., Such, P., Sanchez-Covisa, J., Nylander, A. G., . . . de Jong-Laird, A. (2018). Quantifying the treatment goals of people recently diagnosed with schizophrenia using best–worst scaling. *Patient Preference and Adherence, 12,* 63–70.

Bromet, E. J., Kotov, R., Fochtmann, L. J., Carlson, G. A., Tanenberg-Karant, M., Ruggero, C., & Chang, S. W. (2011). Diagnostic shifts during the decade following first admission for psychosis. *American Journal of Psychiatry, 168,* 1186–1194.

Campbell, M. M., Sibeko, G., Mall, S., Baldinger, A., Nagdee, M., Susser, E., & Stein, D. J. (2017). The content of delusions in a sample of South African Xhosa people with schizophrenia. *BMC Psychiatry, 17,* 41.

Castro-Fornieles, J., Baeza, I., de la Serna, E., Gonzalez-Pinto, A., Parellada, M., Graell, M., . . . Arango, C. (2011). Two-year diagnostic stability in early-onset first-episode psychosis. *Journal of Child Psychology and Psychiatry, 52,* 1089–1098.

Charlson, F. J., Ferrari, A. J., Santomauro, D. F., Diminic, S., Stockings, E., Scott, J. G., . . . Whiteford, H. A. (2018). Global epidemiology and burden of schizophrenia: Findings From the Global Burden of Disease Study 2016. *Schizophrenia Bulletin, 44*(6), 1195–1203.

Correll, C. U., Galling, B., Pawar, A., Krivko, A., Bonetto, C., Ruggeri, M., . . . Kane, J. M. (2018). Comparison of early intervention services vs treatment as usual for early-phase psychosis: A systematic review, meta-analysis, and meta-regression. *JAMA Psychiatry, 75,* 555–565.

Davis, J., Eyre, H., Jacka, F. N., Dodd, S., Dean, O., McEwen, S., . . . Berk, M. (2016). A review of vulnerability and risks for schizophrenia: Beyond the two hit hypothesis. *Neuroscience and Biobehavioral Reviews, 65,* 185–194.

Degenhardt, L., Saha, S., Lim, C. C. W., Aguilar-Gaxiola, S., Al-Hamzawi, A., Alonso, J., . . . WHO World Mental Health Survey Collaborators. (2018). The associations between psychotic experiences and substance use and substance use disorders: Findings from the World Health Organization World Mental Health surveys. *Addiction, 113,* 924–934.

Di Forti, M., Quattrone, D., Freeman, T. P., Tripoli, G., Gayer-Anderson, C., Quigley, H., . . . Group, E.-G. W. (2019). The contribution of cannabis use to variation in the incidence of psychotic disorder across Europe (EU-GEI): A multicentre case–control study. *Lancet Psychiatry, 6*(5), 427–436.

Drugs that may cause psychiatric symptoms. (2008). *Medical Letter on Drugs and Therapeutics, 50*(1301), 100–103.

Findling, R. L., Johnson, J. L., McClellan, J., Frazier, J. A., Vitiello, B., Hamer, R. M., . . . Sikich, L. (2010). Double-blind maintenance safety and effectiveness findings from the Treatment of Early-Onset Schizophrenia Spectrum (TEOSS) study. *Journal of the American Academy of Child and Adolescent Psychiatry, 49,* 583–594; quiz 632.

Fraguas, D., de Castro, M. J., Medina, O., Parellada, M., Moreno, D., Graell, M., . . . Arango, C. (2008). Does diagnostic classification of early-onset psychosis change over follow-up? *Child Psychiatry and Human Development, 39,* 137–145.

Fusar-Poli, P., Borgwardt, S., Bechdolf, A., Addington, J., Riecher-Rossler, A., Schultze-Lutter, F., . . . Yung, A. (2013). The psychosis high-risk state: A comprehensive state-of-the-art review. *JAMA Psychiatry, 70,* 107–120.

Galanter, C. A., Hundt, S. R., Goyal, P., Le, J., & Fisher, P. W. (2012). Variability among research diagnostic interview instruments in the application of DSM-IV-TR criteria for pediatric bipolar disorder. *Journal of the American Academy of Child and Adolescent Psychiatry, 51,* 605–621.

Goodman, R., Ford, T., Simmons, H., Gatward, R., & Meltzer, H. (2000). Using the Strengths and Difficulties Questionnaire (SDQ) to screen for child psychiatric disorders in a community sample. *British Journal of Psychiatry, 177,* 534–539.

Gore, F. M., Bloem, P. J., Patton, G. C., Ferguson, J., Joseph, V., Coffey, C., . . . Mathers, C. D. (2011). Global burden of disease in young people aged 10–24 years: A systematic analysis. *Lancet, 377,* 2093–2102.

Hettige, N. C., Bani-Fatemi, A., Sakinofsky, I., & De Luca, V. (2018). A biopsychosocial evaluation of the risk for suicide in schizophrenia. *CNS Spectrums, 23,* 253–263.

Hirsch, L., Yang, J., Bresee, L., Jette, N., Patten, S., & Pringsheim, T. (2017). Second-generation antipsychotics and metabolic side effects: A systematic review of population-based studies. *Drug Safety, 40,* 771–781.

Hlastala, S. A., & McClellan, J. (2005). Phenomenology and diagnostic stability of youths with atypical psychotic symptoms. *Journal of Child and Adolescent Psychopharmacology, 15,* 497–509.

Jeppesen, P., Clemmensen, L., Munkholm, A., Rimvall, M. K., Rask, C. U., Jorgensen, T., . . . Skovgaard, A. M. (2015). Psychotic experiences co-occur with sleep problems, negative affect and mental disorders in preadolescence. *Journal of Child Psychology and Psychiatry, 56,* 558–565.

Kaufman, J., Birmaher, B., Axelson, D., Perepletchikova, F., Brent, D., & Ryan, N. (2016). Schedule for Affective Disorders and Schizophrenia for School-Age Children—Present and Lifetime DSM-5. Retrieved April 25, 2019, from *www.kennedykrieger.org/sites/default/files/community_files/ksads-dsm-5-screener.pdf.*

Kaufman, J., Birmaher, B., Brent, D., Rao, U., Flynn, C., Moreci, P., . . . Ryan, N. (1997). Schedule for Affective Disorders and Schizophrenia for School-Age Children—Present and Lifetime Version (K-SADS-PL): Initial reliability and validity data. *Journal of the American Academy of Child and Adolescent Psychiatry, 36,* 980–988.

Kay, S. R., Fiszbein, A., & Opler, L. A. (1987). The Positive and Negative Syndrome Scale (PANSS) for schizophrenia. *Schizophrenia Bulletin, 13,* 261–276.

Kelleher, I., Connor, D., Clarke, M. C., Devlin, N., Harley, M., & Cannon, M. (2012). Prevalence of psychotic symptoms in childhood and adolescence: A systematic review and meta-analysis of population-based studies. *Psychological Medicine, 42,* 1857–1863.

Kelleher, I., Harley, M., Murtagh, A., & Cannon, M. (2011). Are screening instruments valid for psychotic-like experiences?: A validation study of screening questions for psychotic-like experiences using in-depth clinical interview. *Schizophrenia Bulletin, 37,* 362–369.

Kelleher, I., Keeley, H., Corcoran, P., Ramsay, H., Wasserman, C., Carli, V., . . . Cannon, M. (2013). Childhood trauma and psychosis in a prospective cohort study: Cause, effect, and directionality. *American Journal of Psychiatry, 170,* 734–741.

Kelleher, I., Murtagh, A., Molloy, C., Roddy, S., Clarke, M. C., Harley, M., & Cannon, M. (2012). Identification and characterization of prodromal risk syndromes in young adolescents in the community: A population-based clinical interview study. *Schizophrenia Bulletin, 38,* 239–246.

Khokhar, J. Y., Dwiel, L. L., Henricks, A. M., Doucette, W. T., & Green, A. I. (2018). The link between schizophrenia and substance use disorder: A unifying hypothesis. *Schizophrenia Research, 194,* 78–85.

Kirli, U., Binbay, T., Drukker, M., Elbi, H., Kayahan, B., Keskin Gokcelli, D., . . . van Os, J. (2019). DSM outcomes of psychotic experiences and associated risk factors: 6-year follow-up study in a community-based sample. *Psychological Medicine, 49*(8), 1346–1356.

Laursen, T. M., Nordentoft, M., & Mortensen, P. B. (2014). Excess early mortality in schizophrenia. *Annual Review of Clinical Psychology, 10,* 425–448.

Leucht, S., Leucht, C., Huhn, M., Chaimani, A., Mavridis, D., Helfer, B., . . . Davis, J. M. (2017). Sixty years of placebo-controlled antipsychotic drug trials in acute schizophrenia: Systematic review, Bayesian meta-analysis, and meta-regression of efficacy predictors. *American Journal of Psychiatry, 174,* 927–942.

Lieberman, J. A., Stroup, T. S., McEvoy, J. P., Swartz, M. S., Rosenheck, R. A., Perkins, D. O., . . . Clinical Antipsychotic Trials of Intervention Effectiveness. (2005). Effectiveness of antipsychotic drugs in patients with chronic schizophrenia. *New England Journal of Medicine, 353,* 1209–1223.

Lindgren, M., Manninen, M., Kalska, H., Mustonen, U., Laajasalo, T., Moilanen, K., . . . Therman, S. (2014). Predicting psychosis in a general adolescent psychiatric sample. *Schizophrenia Research, 158,* 1–6.

Matzner, F., Silva, R., Silvan, M., Chowdhury, M., &

Nastasi, L. (1997). *Preliminary test–retest reliability of the KID-SCID.* Paper presented at the annual meeting of the American Psychiatric Association.

McClellan, J. (2018). Psychosis in children and adolescents. *Journal of the American Academy of Child and Adolescent Psychiatry, 57,* 308–312.

McClellan, J., & King, M. C. (2010). Genomic analysis of mental illness: A changing landscape. *Journal of the American Medical Association, 303,* 2523–2524.

McClellan, J., Stock, S., & American Academy of Child and Adolescent Psychiatry Committee on Quality Issues. (2013). Practice parameter for the assessment and treatment of children and adolescents with schizophrenia. *Journal of the American Academy of Child and Adolescent Psychiatry, 52,* 976–990.

Oluwoye, O., Stiles, B., Monroe-DeVita, M., Chwastiak, L., McClellan, J. M., Dyck, D., . . . McDonell, M. G. (2018). Racial–ethnic disparities in first-episode psychosis treatment outcomes from the RAISE-ETP study. *Psychiatric Services, 69*(11), 1138–1145.

Pechey, R., & Halligan, P. (2011). The prevalence of delusion-like beliefs relative to sociocultural beliefs in the general population. *Psychopathology, 44,* 106–115.

Penttila, M., Jaaskelainen, E., Hirvonen, N., Isohanni, M., & Miettunen, J. (2014). Duration of untreated psychosis as predictor of long-term outcome in schizophrenia: Systematic review and meta-analysis. *British Journal of Psychiatry, 205,* 88–94.

Rapoport, J. L., Giedd, J. N., & Gogtay, N. (2012). Neurodevelopmental model of schizophrenia: Update 2012. *Molecular Psychiatry, 17,* 1228–1238.

Rizvi, S. H., Salcedo, S., Youngstrom, E. A., Freeman, L. K., Gadow, K. D., Fristad, M. A., . . . Findling, R. L. (2019). Diagnostic accuracy of the CASI-4R Psychosis subscale for children evaluated in pediatric outpatient clinics. *Journal of Clinical Child and Adolescent Psychology, 48*(4), 610–621.

Salcedo, S., Rizvi, S., Freeman, L. K., Youngstrom, J. K., Findling, R. L., & Youngstrom, E. A. (2018). Diagnostic efficiency of the CBCL thought problems and DSM-oriented psychotic symptoms scales for pediatric psychotic symptoms. *European Child and Adolescent Psychiatry, 27,* 1491–1498.

Sheehan, D. V., Sheehan, K. H., Shytle, R. D., Janavs, J., Bannon, Y., Rogers, J. E., . . . Wilkinson, B. (2010). Reliability and validity of the Mini International Neuropsychiatric Interview for Children and Adolescents (MINI-KID). *Journal of Clinical Psychiatry, 71,* 313–326.

Sorg, E. M., Chaney-Catchpole, M., & Hazen, E. P. (2018). Pediatric catatonia: A case series-based review of presentation, evaluation, and management. *Psychosomatics, 59*(6), 531–538.

Staal, M., Panis, B., & Schieveld, J. N. M. (2019). Early warning signs in misrecognized secondary pediatric psychotic disorders: A systematic review. *European Child and Adolescent Psychiatry, 28*(9), 1159–1167.

Stentebjerg-Olesen, M., Pagsberg, A. K., Fink-Jensen,

A., Correll, C. U., & Jeppesen, P. (2016). Clinical characteristics and predictors of outcome of schizophrenia-spectrum psychosis in children and adolescents: A systematic review. *Journal of Child and Adolescent Psychopharmacology, 26,* 410–427.

Sullivan, S., Rai, D., Golding, J., Zammit, S., & Steer, C. (2013). The association between autism spectrum disorder and psychotic experiences in the Avon Longitudinal Study of Parents and Children (ALSPAC) birth cohort. *Journal of the American Academy of Child and Adolescent Psychiatry, 52,* 806–814.

Therman, S., Lindgren, M., Manninen, M., Loewy, R. L., Huttunen, M. O., Cannon, T. D., & Suvisaari, J. (2014). Predicting psychosis and psychiatric hospital care among adolescent psychiatric patients with the Prodromal Questionnaire. *Schizophrenia Research, 158,* 7–10.

Ulloa, R. E., Birmaher, B., Axelson, D., Williamson, D.

E., Brent, D. A., Ryan, N. D., . . . Baugher, M. (2000). Psychosis in a pediatric mood and anxiety disorders clinic: Phenomenology and correlates. *Journal of the American Academy of Child and Adolescent Psychiatry, 39,* 337–345.

Van, L., Boot, E., & Bassett, A. S. (2017). Update on the 22q11.2 deletion syndrome and its relevance to schizophrenia. *Current Opinion in Psychiatry, 30,* 191–196.

Wilson, L., Szigeti, A., Kearney, A., & Clarke, M. (2018). Clinical characteristics of primary psychotic disorders with concurrent substance abuse and substance-induced psychotic disorders: A systematic review. *Schizophrenia Research, 197,* 78–86.

World Health Organization. (2018). *The ICD-11 classification of mental and behavioural disorders: Clinical descriptions and diagnostic guidelines.* Geneva, Switzerland: Author.

CHAPTER 21

Eating and Feeding Disorders

Anna M. Bardone-Cone and Kristin M. von Ranson

Eating and feeding disorders capture a diverse array of psychological disorders that require diverse assessment tools and approaches to best capture the physical, behavioral, and cognitive aspects of these disorders. Although the fifth edition of the *Diagnostic and Statistical Manual of Mental Disorders* (DSM-5; American Psychiatric Association, 2013a) calls this category "Feeding and Eating Disorders," our focus is largely on eating disorders. In this chapter, we first provide background information on the different disorders, including descriptions of key symptoms (e.g., binge eating) and diagnoses, as well as prevalence data. We next follow the prediction, prescription, and process approach to assessment by focusing on screening tools and diagnostic aids (prediction), followed by interview assessments to finalize diagnoses (prescription), then measures for assessing progress and process (process). We include information related to cross-informant assessment, risk and pro-

tective factors, treatment moderators, goal setting and measurement, and additional considerations in case conceptualization and treatment planning.

Preparation

Eating and Feeding Disorder Diagnoses

Eating disorders involve persistent, abnormal eating-related behaviors that are typically accompanied by prominent body weight and shape concerns, and significantly diminish one's health or functioning. By contrast, *feeding disorders* include recurrent, abnormal eating behaviors not accompanied by body weight and shape concerns and encompass behaviors such as extremely picky eating or repeatedly eating nonfood substances (World Health Organization, 2018). Feeding disorders are diagnosed only when symptoms are not developmentally appropriate, do not reflect a culturally normative practice, and are not fully explained by another health condition. Until recently, most people seeking treatment for an eating disorder—and therefore experiencing significant, troubling symptoms—did not meet the narrow diagnostic criteria for anorexia nervosa (AN) and bulimia nervosa (BN) (Uher & Rutter, 2012), which helped spur the recent jump in number of specific feeding and eating disorders from two to six. Another reason for the increased number of eating disorders is that, contrary to assumptions, research has shown that eating disorder symptom patterns deemed "subthreshold" are actually more common and have more adverse effects than initially believed (e.g., Thomas, Vartanian, & Brownell, 2009).

Although feeding disorders were always thought to first occur exclusively in infancy and childhood, it is now recognized that these problems can begin in adulthood as well. Eating disorders and feeding disorders have been merged into a single diagnostic category in both major psychiatric diagnostic systems, DSM-5 (American Psychiatric Association, 2013a) and the *International Classification of Diseases* (ICD-11; Watson, Ellickson-Larew, Stanton, & Levin-Aspenson, 2016). In DSM-5, the category of feeding and eating disorders includes AN, BN, binge-eating disorder (BED), avoidant/restrictive food intake disorder (ARFID), pica, and rumination disorder, as well as other specified feeding or eating disorder (OSFED) and unspecified feeding or eating disorder (UFED). The latter two are residual categories for feeding and eating disorder-like symptom presentations involving clinically significant distress or impaired functioning in which symptoms do not fit the criteria for another specific diagnosis. We describe each disorder below, as well as key symptoms. Note that these DSM-5 diagnoses are largely consistent with those appearing in ICD-11.

Feeding Disorders and Symptoms

Pica is the frequent, developmentally inappropriate eating of non-nutritive, nonfood substances (e.g., soil, clay, chalk, paper, hair, ice, plastic, or metal) for at least 1 month in individuals at least 2 years old (American Psychiatric Association, 2013a). The behavior must not be socially or culturally normative. Pica often occurs in individuals with developmental disabilities or autism, and also may occur in individuals with schizophrenia or pregnant women. Pica onsets most often during childhood, but it may also occur in adulthood, particularly in individuals with an intellectual disability.

Rumination disorder ("rumination–regurgitation disorder" in ICD-11) involves the repeated regurgitation of food over a 1-month period (American Psychiatric Association, 2013a) among individuals of any age, including infancy. The regurgitated food may be chewed or swallowed again or spit out. The behavior must not occur exclusively during the course of AN, BN, BED, or ARFID. Rumination may be experienced as enjoyable or

soothing (Nicholls & Bryant-Waugh, 2009), or as a form of self-stimulation among individuals with neurodevelopmental disorders, particularly those with intellectual disability (American Psychiatric Association, 2013a).

Pica and rumination differ from AN and BN in that they do not stem from body image disturbance or a desire to lose, or avoid gaining, weight. To date, little systematic research exists on pica and rumination disorder (but see Wade, 2017). In the remainder of this chapter, we focus on AN, BN, BED, and ARFID, as defined in DSM-5.

Eating Disorder Symptoms

Three symptoms commonly found in various eating disorders are binge eating, compensatory behaviors, and overvaluation of weight and shape.

Binge Eating

Binge eating is a commonly reported eating disorder symptom that is characteristic of BN and BED, and also may occur in AN and OSFED. It is defined identically regardless of which eating disorder is being considered. Binge eating involves two elements: (1) eating an unusually large amount of food in a limited period of time (i.e., within 2 hours) and (2) experiencing a sense of loss of control over eating (i.e., over what or how much food is eaten, or perceiving oneself as unable to stop eating) (American Psychiatric Association, 2013a). To determine whether an amount of food eaten is unusually large requires one to consider the context (i.e., eating a "definitely" greater amount of food than most people would eat in a similar time period and under similar circumstances). For instance, because overeating at a holiday meal is a common experience, it would likely not meet the "unusually large amount" criterion for a binge-eating episode. Note that it is impossible to remove all subjectivity when determining whether a given eating episode is definitely large. No minimum calorie requirement has been specified for binge-eating episodes.

Because sometimes individuals feel a loss of control over eating even when they have not consumed an objectively large amount of food, a useful distinction can be made between objective and subjective binge episodes. For instance, one might feel a loss of control while eating a small amount of food—although it may be more than one would normally eat—or while eating the size of a normal meal. Accordingly, an "objective binge episode" is defined as a binge-eating episode that involves an objectively large amount of food, and a "subjective binge episode" is defined as an eating episode that involves a subjective loss of control but consumption of less than an objectively large amount of food (Fairburn, 2008).

Among children, perceived loss of control over eating may be more important than the actual amount of food eaten (American Psychiatric Association, 2013b; Tanofsky-Kraff, Goossens, et al., 2007), as children and adolescents tend to have less control over their access to food than adults do (Hoste, Labuschagne, & Le Grange, 2012). Research criteria for loss-of-control eating in children specify that episodes must include a sense of lack of control over eating, as well as food seeking in the absence of hunger or after satiation (Tanofsky-Kraff, Marcus, Yanovski, & Yanovski, 2008). According to these research criteria for loss-of-control eating, episode frequency must average at least twice a month for 3 months, and episodes must involve three or more of the following characteristics: eating in response to negative affect; secrecy regarding the episode; feelings of numbness or lack of awareness while eating; the perception of eating more than others; and/or negative affect following eating.

Compensatory Behaviors

Compensatory behaviors are motivated by a desire to avoid weight gain related to binge-eating episodes. Note that compensatory behaviors span purging behaviors, such as self-induced vomiting and laxative misuse, as well as nonpurging behaviors, such as fasting (e.g., not eating for > 24 hours) and excessive exercise with associated functional impairment, such as exercising despite illness, injury, or its interference with important activities (American Psychiatric Association, 2013a). The most frequently reported compensatory behavior in BN is self-induced vomiting (Mitchell, Hatsukami, Eckert, & Pyle, 1985).

Overvaluation of Weight and Shape

The core psychopathology of AN and BN includes the overvaluation of weight and shape, or judging oneself or one's worth largely or entirely based on one's body shape and weight rather than the full range of domains valued by those without eating disorders (e.g., relationships, school, or work) (Fairburn & Harrison, 2003). It is believed that overvaluation of weight and shape drives eating-disordered behaviors, as well as the frequent diagnostic crossover that occurs among eating disorders over time, particularly from restrictive eating to binge eating (Eddy et al., 2008).

Definitions of Eating Disorders

Avoidant/Restrictive Food Intake Disorder

Before 2013, problems similar to ARFID were described by a diagnosis of "feeding disorder of infancy or early childhood," in which infants and children were not growing as expected (American Psychiatric Association, 1994). However, this diagnosis was rarely used, and very little research was available on it. Consultations with experts who treated feeding problems in children and teenagers led to the current conceptualization of ARFID (Walsh, Attia, & Sysko, 2016).

As defined in DSM-5, ARFID involves avoidance or restriction of food intake that results in an individual's failure to meet nutritional or energy needs through eating (American Psychiatric Association, 2013a). This problem is demonstrated by at least one of the following features: clinically significant weight loss or, in children, faltering growth in height or weight; nutritional deficiency; reliance on feeding through a means other than food (i.e., enteral [tube] feedings or meal-replacement drinks); or psychosocial impairment. In contrast to AN, individuals with ARFID do not experience disturbance in their body image. In ARFID, the eating disturbance is not better explained by inadequate access to food, a culturally sanctioned practice (i.e., religious fasting or dieting), or developmentally normal behaviors (i.e., picky eating in children that is not severe and impairing), and significant eating problems persist beyond the food neophobia often seen between ages 2 and 6 (Norris, Spettigue, & Katzman, 2016).

Three causes of an individual's restricted diet in ARFID proposed in DSM-5 are sensory sensitivity, lack of interest in food or eating, and fear of aversive consequences of eating. Sensitivity to the color, appearance, smell, texture, temperature, or taste of foods may be described, as well as refusal to eat new foods or to tolerate the smell of food others are eating. Sometimes an individual develops ARFID after having had an aversive experience related to eating, such as choking or recurrent vomiting, which he or she wishes to avoid.

ARFID occurs similarly often in male and female infants and young children, but when comorbid with autism, those with ARFID are predominantly male (American Psychiatric Association, 2013a). ARFID may cause delays in both the growth and the cognitive development of younger children, whereas social functioning is more often affected among older children, adolescents, and adults with ARFID.

Anorexia Nervosa

AN has been described fairly consistently since the 19th century (Gull, 1874; Lasègue, 1873). In DSM-5, AN includes three required symptoms: restricted energy intake resulting in significantly low body weight; fear of gaining weight or becoming fat, or ongoing behavior interfering with weight gain; and body image disturbance, overreliance on weight or shape in one's self-evaluation, or lack of recognition of the gravity of one's current low weight (American Psychiatric Association, 2013a).

DSM-5 criteria for AN are broader and more inclusive than those in previous DSM editions. Although DSM-IV criteria for AN included the requirement that an individual's body weight fall below 85% of expected weight, and that, in women, amenorrhea be present (American Psychiatric Association, 2013b), ultimately research evidence did not support the validity of these criteria (Thomas et al., 2009). The presence of amenorrhea in AN is a clinical indicator of severely poor nutritional status, but research has not supported its usefulness in the AN diagnosis (Attia & Roberto, 2009). The hallmark symptom of "significantly low weight" is interpreted in the context of age, sex, developmental trajectory, and physical health, and is defined as less than is minimally normal or (in children and adolescents) expected. A specific body weight cutoff was purposely excluded from DSM-5 criteria for AN because it is acknowledged to be arbitrary; instead, a contextual approach is recommended in determining whether an individual has "significantly low weight."

AN has two subtypes: restricting type and binge-eating/purging type. In the restricting type, weight loss occurs through food restriction (i.e., dieting or fasting). Weight loss may also involve excessive exercise. In contrast, the binge-eating/purging type is characterized by recurrent episodes of binge eating, purging, or both, in addition to food restriction. Purging involves self-induced vomiting or misuse of laxatives, diuretics, enemas, or other substances; these behaviors are undertaken with the goal of compensating for food eaten, whether or not this belief is accurate (it often is not). Less common, and potentially dangerous,

purging methods involve the misuse of thyroid hormone or, among those with type 1 diabetes, reducing or omitting insulin doses to inhibit the metabolism of foods eaten during a binge-eating episode. Some individuals engage in a pattern of purging after eating small amounts of food. AN subtypes often change over time, typically from restricting type to binge-eating/purging type, or to BN (Eddy et al., 2008).

Bulimia Nervosa

BN involves three key features: recurrent binge eating, recurrent inappropriate compensatory behaviors, and overvaluation of body weight and shape (American Psychiatric Association, 2013a). For a DSM-5 diagnosis of BN, binge eating and compensatory behaviors must occur, on average, at least once weekly for 3 months. This frequency was reduced from twice weekly in DSM-IV on the basis of evidence that those who engaged in bulimic symptoms once weekly did not differ in eating pathology or general psychopathology from those who engaged in bulimic symptoms more often (Thomas et al., 2009). DSM-5 specifies no subtypes of BN.

Binge-Eating Disorder

BED involves binge eating at least once weekly over 3 months, on average, without regular compensatory behaviors (American Psychiatric Association, 2013a). Marked distress regarding binge eating must also be endorsed, as well as three of the following five binge-eating episode features: eating much more rapidly than normal; eating until uncomfortably full; eating when not physically hungry; eating alone because of embarrassment over how much one is eating; and feeling disgusted with oneself, depressed, or very guilty after binge eating.

Other Specified Feeding or Eating Disorder

This diagnostic category partially replaced DSM-IV's "not otherwise specified" category. It encompasses symptoms that do not meet full criteria for any of the preceding feeding or eating disorders and are clinically significant due to impairment or distress. It includes the word "specified," as one is to specify the precise type of symptoms following "OSFED" (e.g., "other specified feeding or eating disorder, atypical anorexia nervosa"). The following examples are provided in DSM-5, and include variants of AN, BN, and BED, as well as other, previously characterized eating-related syndromes.

1. *Atypical AN:* All AN criteria are met except that despite significant weight loss, one's weight is within or above the normal range.
2. *BN (of low frequency and/or limited duration):* All BN symptoms are met, except binge eating and compensatory behaviors occur < once a week or for < 3 months, on average.
3. *BED (of low frequency and/or limited duration):* All BED symptoms are met, except binge eating occurs < once a week or for < 3 months, on average.
4. *Purging disorder:* Recurrent purging behavior in the absence of objective binge-eating episodes.
5. *Night eating syndrome:* Recurrent nighttime eating, such as eating after awakening or excessive eating after the evening meal, that causes significant distress or impaired functioning and is not attributable to external influences, social norms, another mental or medical disorder, or medication.

Unspecified Feeding or Eating Disorder

UFED partially replaced DSM-IV's "not otherwise specified" category. Like OSFED, UFED represents symptoms that do not meet full criteria for any of the preceding feeding or eating disorders and are clinically significant due to impairment or distress. It differs from OSFED in that the clinician chooses not to specify why criteria are not met for a specific feeding or eating disorder, or when there is insufficient information to make a specific diagnosis, such as in a hospital emergency department.

Epidemiology of Eating Disorders

Prevalence

Population-based prevalence studies of childhood and adolescent eating disorders have provided variable estimates of AN, BN, and BED. In a U.S. representative sample of 9- and 10-year-old children, the prevalence of DSM-5 eating disorders was 1.4% overall, with prevalence of specific eating disorders as follows: OSFED 0.7%, AN 0.1%, BN 0%, and BED 0.6% (Rozzell, Moon, Klimek, Brown, & Blashill, 2019). They observed no gender differences. When studies are considered together, the prevalence of clinically significant eating disorders is estimated as approximately

6–13% in community-dwelling adolescents under 19 years, with lifetime prevalence of AN 0.8–1.7%, BN 0.8–2.6%, BED 2.3–3.0%, and subthreshold or atypical eating disorders in the rest (Mairs & Nicholls, 2016; Stice, Marti, & Rohde, 2013; Swanson, Crow, Le Grange, Swendsen, & Merikangas, 2011). According to epidemiological research, AN incidence is greatest among girls between ages 15 and 19 years, and BN incidence is greatest among women between ages 20 and 24 years (Jaite, Hoffmann, Glaeske, & Bachmann, 2013).

Lifetime prevalence estimates (DSM-IV) based on a nationally representative sample of 10,123 U.S. adolescents ages 13–18 years from the National Comorbidity Survey were as follows: AN 0.3%, BN 0.9%, subthreshold AN 0.8%, BED 1.6%, and subthreshold BED 2.5%, for an overall prevalence of 5.2% (Swanson et al., 2011). Girls reported higher rates of BN, BED, and subthreshold AN than did boys, but rates across genders of AN and subthreshold BED were similar. Compared to these population estimates, and using DSM-5 criteria, substantially higher rates of eating disorders were reported in a community sample of 496 high school girls who were interviewed prospectively eight times over 7 years (Stice et al., 2013). By age 20, lifetime prevalence for any feeding or eating disorder was 13.1%, with the following prevalence rates for specific disorders: AN 0.8%, BN 2.6%, BED 3.0%, atypical AN 2.8%, subthreshold BN 4.4%, subthreshold BED 3.6%, purging disorder 3.4%, and other feeding and eating disorders 11.5%. These latter findings suggest that many teenage girls may experience eating disorders not fitting DSM-5 categories.

Emerging prevalence estimates of ARFID, which vary according to the sample and measurement context, suggest that ARFID may be roughly as common as AN and BN. In a sample of 1,444 Swiss 8- to 13-year-old schoolchildren, 3.2% screened positive for current ARFID via self-report questionnaire (Kurz, van Dyck, Dremmel, Munsch, & Hilbert, 2015). An Australian, population-based survey of individuals ages 16 and older reported a 3-month prevalence of 0.3% for ARFID, using the question, "Are you currently avoiding or restricting eating any foods to the degree that you have lost a lot of weight and/or become lacking in nutrition (e.g., have low iron) and/or had problems with family, friends or at work?" (Hay et al., 2017, p. 21). Participant responses indicated ARFID only if they were not attributable to weight or shape concerns, cultural reasons, or another medical condition. North American reports indicate that a significant minority of those seeking outpatient treatment for an eating disorder (5–12%) and day treatment for younger adolescents with eating disorders (~23%) have ARFID (Brigham, Manzo, Eddy, & Thomas, 2018).

Age at Onset

Among teenage National Comorbidity Survey participants, the median age at onset of AN, BN, BED, and subthreshold BED ranged from 12.2 to 12.6 years (Swanson et al., 2011). However, for adult participants ages 18 and older in the same study, who were interviewed later in their lives about their lifetime eating disorder history, the median age at eating disorder onset ranged from 18 to 21 years (Hudson, Hiripi, Pope, & Kessler, 2007). Memory biases might partially account for these different findings. AN was found to onset only between ages 10 and 20 years, whereas a later (age 15 years) and much wider span of age at onset was reported for disorders involving binge eating (e.g., BN, BED, and subthreshold BED; Hudson et al., 2007). In the study of 496 teenage girls (mentioned earlier), the peak age of onset for binge eating was 16 years and that for purging, 18 years (Stice, Killen, Hayward, & Taylor, 1998). Overall, clinical studies in pediatrics, adolescent medicine, and eating disorder treatment settings suggest that, relative to patients with AN and BN, patients with ARFID tend to be younger, are more often male and have a co-occurring medical condition, and present for treatment later in their illness (Brigham et al., 2018; Eddy et al., 2015; Fisher et al., 2014; Norris et al., 2016).

Benchmarks in Clinical Settings

Two studies have examined the prevalence of eating disorders in mental health settings, both in inpatient settings. In an interview study, Feenstra, Busschbach, Verhuel, and Hutsebaut (2011), using DSM-IV criteria, reported that 12.5% of 257 teenagers referred to an inpatient program for complex personality psychopathology refractory to outpatient treatment had an eating disorder. This total prevalence figure included 4.3% with AN, 1.6% with BN, and 6.6% with eating disorder not otherwise specified. Another study found that 3.8% of 208 consecutively admitted adolescent inpatients had a self-reported eating disorder, and 22.1% had clinically significant shape/weight concerns (Dyl, Kittler, Phillips, & Hunt, 2006). In an emergency department setting, 16% of 942

patients ages 14–20 years, more than one-fourth (26.6%) of whom were male, screened positive for an eating disorder (Dooley-Hash, Banker, Walton, Ginsburg, & Cunningham, 2012).

Rates of eating disorders tend to be elevated in certain groups. For instance, youth with difficulties related to eating, feeding, and growth are often referred to gastroenterologists and other physicians. The base rate of ARFID among 8- to 18-year-olds in a chart review study of 2,231 consecutive referrals to 19 pediatric gastroenterology practices in an American city was 1.5%; two-thirds (67%) of these youth were male (Eddy et al., 2015). Another 2.4% of youth in this sample met at least one ARFID criterion, indicating that only a small minority had an eating disorder. Another at-risk group is athletes, especially in sports that emphasize leanness. Among adolescent and adult athletes, a review indicated that 6–45% of females and 0–45% of males had disordered eating or an eating disorder (Bratland-Sanda & Sundgot-Borgen, 2013). A third at-risk group is youth with type 1 diabetes, who may skip or reduce the amount of insulin taken to control their weight (Neumark-Sztainer et al., 2002). A 7-year prospective study of 71 girls with type 1 diabetes, starting at approximately age 11 years, 10 months, indicated that by age 23.7 years, 32.4% met the criteria for a current eating disorder and another 8.5% met criteria for a subthreshold eating disorder (Colton et al., 2015).

Starter Kit

In this chapter, we include recommended measures in the text and tables, but for an assessment battery that would serve especially well as a "starter kit," see Table 21.1. In selecting these core measures, we generally prioritized measures with good psychometric properties and accessibility (i.e., free) and sought to recommend a combination of measures that would provide broad coverage of the diversity of eating disorder pathology. For the prediction phase of assessment, we recommend the self-report measures of the Eating Disorder Examination Questionnaire (EDE-Q; Fairburn & Beglin, 2008) for adolescents and the Children's Eating Attitudes Test (ChEAT; Maloney, McGuire, & Daniels, 1988) for children when screening for anorexic and bulimic pathology, and the parental report measure of the Behavioral Pediatrics Feeding Assessment Scale (BPFAS; Crist & Napier-Phillips, 2001) when screening for feeding concerns from infancy through early childhood. For the prescription phase, where diagnoses are solidified, the De-

TABLE 21.1. Eating and Feeding Disorders Assessment Starter Kit

Prediction	Prescription	Process
For broad anorexic, bulimic, and binge-eating disorder pathology: Eating Disorder Examination Questionnaire (EDE-Q)—for adolescents Children's Eating Attitudes Test (ChEAT) — for children *For feeding concerns for infants/young children (parental report):* Behavioral Pediatrics Feeding Assessment Scale (BPFAS)	*For eating disorders:* Development and Well-Being Assessment (DAWBA) *For feeding disorders:* Pica, ARFID, and Rumination Disorder Interview (PARDI)	Clinical Impairment Assessment (CIA) Motivational Stages of Change for Adolescents Recovering from an Eating Disorder (MSCARED)

Note: Copyright © 2019 Bardone-Cone and Ransom; CC-BY 4.0.

velopment and Well-Being Assessment (DAWBA; Goodman, Ford, Richards, Gatward, & Meltzer, 2000) is recommended for confirmation of cases of AN, BN, and BED. For establishing feeding disorder diagnoses (e.g., ARFID), the Pica, ARFID, and Rumination Disorder Interview (PARDI; Bryant-Waugh et al., 2019) is recommended. To assess progress and process, we recommend the Clinical Impairment Assessment (CIA; Bohn & Fairburn, 2008) and the Motivational Stages of Change for Adolescents Recovering from an Eating Disorder (MSCARED; Gusella, Butler, Nichols, & Bird, 2003).

Prediction

Screening Tools and Diagnostic Aids

Given that eating disorders reflect a wide array of behaviors and cognitions, there is much to cover in screening tools and diagnostic aids. Some measures aim to provide this broad coverage, and others are more focused. Clinicians might consider use of both a broad measure and a selection of tailored measures for the behaviors/cognitions that seem most likely based on base rates and initial information gathered. It is important to remember that the role of screening measures is to identify those whose level of symptoms suggest the need for additional assessment; they are not intended to arrive at a diagnosis.

In the eating disorder field, when measures developed in child/adolescent samples are not available, it is common for measures originally developed for use in adults to be used with older adolescents and sometimes children, either as is or

with modifications. We include some unmodified measures developed in adults in this review, but only if they have psychometric support in youth (defined as below age 18). Especially when unmodified measures are used, assessors must pay attention to the complexity and comprehensibility of assessment item language when administering tests to children. Note that some eating disorder criteria are not simple for children of all ages to comprehend.

Overview of Screening Measures

Table 21.2 provides an overview of measures commonly used to screen for eating disorder pathology among children and adolescents. Table 21.3 lists key psychometric properties as reported in samples of children and adolescents (and parents of children/adolescents) for these measures (e.g., reliability, test–retest reliability, construct validity). We additionally summarize the limited data from receiver operating characteristics (ROC) analyses; there are scant findings from this approach among eating disorder measures for children and adolescents.

Screening measures providing broad coverage of anorexic and bulimic eating pathology include the 26-item ChEAT (Maloney et al., 1988), the EDE-Q (Fairburn & Beglin, 2008), the Minnesota Eating Behaviors Survey (MEBS; von Ranson, Klump, Iacono, & McGue, 2005), the Eating Disorder Inventory–3 (EDI-3; Garner, 2004), the SCOFF questionnaire (Morgan, Reid, & Lacey, 1999), the 26-item Eating Attitudes Test (EAT-26; Garner, Olmsted, Bohr, & Garfinkel, 1982), and the Eating Disorder Diagnostic Scale (EDDS;

Stice, Telch, & Rizvi, 2000)—which, despite its name, should be considered a screener not a diagnostic tool.

Measures that have a more focused rather than broad approach include measures that capture ARFID symptomatology and feeding concerns. For infants through very young children, these are often parental reports, including the Children's Eating Behaviour Questionnaire (CEBQ; Wardle, Guthrie, Sanderson, & Rapoport, 2001), the BPFAS (Crist & Napier-Phillips, 2001), and the Montreal Children's Hospital Feeding Scale (MCHFS; Ramsay, Martel, Porporino, & Zygmuntowicz, 2011). Additionally, the Eating Disturbances in Youth—Questionnaire (EDY-Q; Kurz et al., 2015) assesses ARFID symptoms by self-report among 8- to 13-year-olds. The Questionnaire of Eating and Weight Patterns—Adolescent form (QEWP-A; Johnson, Grieve, Adams, & Sandy, 1999) focuses on BED, as well as identifying binge eating, overeating, and loss-of-control eating in youth, while the Eating in the Absence of Hunger Questionnaire for Children and Adolescents (EAH-C; Tanofsky-Kraff, Ranzenhofer, et al., 2008) and the Emotional Eating Scale Adapted for Children and Adolescents (EES-C; Tanofsky-Kraff, Theim, et al., 2007) ask about conditions under which one eats, with a focus on eating in the absence of hunger (or in the presence of satiety) or in response to negative affect experiences. Examples of measures that uniquely assess aspects of body image include the Children's Body Image Scale (CBIS; Truby & Paxton, 2002), developed for young children, and the Drive for Muscularity Scale (DMS; McCreary & Sasse, 2000), developed in adolescent male samples. More related to process (discussed later), we also include the CIA (Bohn & Fairburn, 2008), which highlights when eating disorder symptoms are impairing, and the Anorexia Nervosa Stages of Change Questionnaire (ANSOCQ; Rieger et al., 2000) and the MSCARED (Gusella et al., 2003), both of which set eating disorders in the context of stage of readiness for change.

Almost all the measures listed in Table 21.2 are free; this was intentional, in that we wanted to identify measures to which most people would have access. One exception is the EDI-3 (Garner, 2004), which we retained because of the widespread use of it and its precursors (EDI-2 and EDI—with the latter's items published in Garner, Olmsted, & Polivy, 1983), and its inclusion of both eating pathology subscales (Drive for Thinness, Bulimia, Body Dissatisfaction) and related factors (e.g., Perfectionism, Ineffectiveness). There is also a cost for the MEBS (von Ranson et al., 2005), but it has good psychometrics across a broad age range; it contains items from the EDI and other existing measures but is significantly shorter than the EDI-3.

We note that some measures focus on very young children (e.g., toddlers), with these being parental reports. The majority, however, have been used and have psychometric data across childhood (e.g., ages 7–12), adolescence (e.g., ages 13–18), or both. In some cases, a measure has been widely used in adolescents, although it was developed in adult samples and has much more established psychometric properties in adult samples than in adolescent samples (e.g., EDE-Q, EAT-26). Although variations of the EDE-Q have been proposed for children and adolescents, in practice, the version used for adults is used for adolescents, and psychometric data support this as appropriate use.

Measures also differ in item length. Some of the very short measures (e.g., SCOFF) are especially appropriate for primary care settings, while longer measures may sometimes be considered an intermediate step between a short screener such as the SCOFF and a confirmatory structured or semistructured interview.

In addition to the traditional psychometric properties listed in Table 21.3, a handful of measures have some reports of ROC analyses in youth samples. More such studies have been done with adult samples; these are not reviewed here. As an example of measures with these ROC findings in child/adolescent samples, for the ChEAT, using a large sample of 10- to 15-year-olds, Chiba and colleagues (2016) reported the area under the ROC curve (AUC) as .83; with a cutoff score of 18, sensitivity was 69%, and specificity was 93%. However, Colton, Olmsted, and Rodin (2007) cautioned against the use of a cutoff based on their sample of 9- to 13-year-olds. They could not identify a cutoff score on the ChEAT that demonstrated adequate sensitivity and specificity; for example, a cutoff of 20 (typically used for adults to indicate a probable eating disorder) yielded 20% sensitivity and 98% specificity. Furthermore, the AUC was .75, which would be fairly good in a clinically realistic comparison but underwhelming in a sample with a lot of healthy controls. More consistency has been found for the SCOFF, in which a cutoff score of 2 is recommended (e.g., Lichtenstein, Hemmingsen, & Stoving, 2017; sensitivity of 77% and specificity of 72%).

TABLE 21.2. Questionnaires: Descriptive Information of Selected Youth Eating and Feeding Disorder Measures

Measure	No. of items	Description	Age	Reporter	Cost	Where to obtain
Anorexia Nervosa Stages of Change Questionnaire (ANSOCQ)	20	Respondents rate items representing specific anorexic symptoms, selecting which of five statements (representing precontemplation, contemplation, preparation, action, maintenance) best reflects their current attitudes regarding changing the symptoms.	14–19 years	Adolescent	None	Rieger et al. (2002); items in Appendix *cedd.org.au/wordpress/wp-content/uploads/2014/09/Anorexia-Nervosa-Stages-of-Change-Questionnaire-ANSOCQ.pdf*
Behavioral Pediatrics Feeding Assessment Scale (BPFAS)	35	Respondents report on the frequency of their child's eating behaviors (25 items) on a 5-point scale from *never* to *always*, as well as ways they respond to the behavior (feelings, strategies) (10 items) using the same 5-point scale. Additionally, parents provide a yes–no response for each item, indicating whether or not it is a problem for them. Typically reported as four scores: child behavior frequency, child behavior problems, parent feelings/strategies frequency, parent feelings/strategies problems.	9 mo.–7 years	Parent	None	*www.childrenshospitalvanderbilt.org/files/sites/default/files/drupalfiles/2018-08/behavioral-pediatrics-feeding-assessment-scale.pdf*
Children's Body Image Scale (CBIS)	2	The CBIS, a pictorial scale that can be used to measure body perception and satisfaction in children, comprises separate scales for males and females.	7–12 years	Child	None, if used for research	*www.monash.edu/medicine/base/research/clinical-research/childrens-body-image-scale* Contact the author, *helen.truby@monash.edu*
Children's Eating Attitudes Test (ChEAT)	26	Respondents rate items reflecting attitudes and behaviors related to AN and BN on a 6-point scale (*never* to *always*). The ChEAT was developed from the 26-item Eating Attitudes Test (EAT; Garner, Olmsted, Bohr, & Garfinkel, 1982) using simpler synonyms. No single agreed-upon factor structure has been identified, and the total score is most often used.	8–13 years	Child	None	*www.1000livesplus.wales.nhs.uk/sitesplus/documents/1011/cheat.pdf*
Children's Eating Behaviour Questionnaire (CEBQ)	35	Respondents rate the frequency of a child's eating behaviors/style on a 5-point scale from *never* to *always*. Eight subscales are generated via averaging subscale items: Food Responsiveness, Enjoyment of Food, Emotional Overeating, Desire to Drink, Satiety Responsiveness, Slowness in Eating, Emotional Undereating, and Fussiness.	3–9 years	Parent	None	*www.midss.org/content/child-eating-behaviour-questionnaire-cebq* Wardle, Guthrie, Sanderson, & Rapoport (2001); items in Table 2
Clinical Impairment Assessment (CIA)	16	This measure assesses the severity of psychosocial impairment due to eating disorder features. Respondents use a 4-point scale (*not at all*, *a lot*) to rate the extent to which their eating	15+ years	Adolescent	None	*www.credo-oxford.com/pdfs/Clinical_Impairment_Questionnaire_CIA_3.0.pdf*

habits, exercising, or feelings about shape, weight, or eating have impacted their lives in the past 28 days (e.g., interfered with relationships with others).

Measure	Items	Description	Age	Developmental stage	Bias	Source
Drive for Muscularity Scale (DMS)	15	Respondent rates items about attitudes and behaviors related to preoccupation with increasing muscularity using a 6-point response scale (*Always* to *Never*)	13+ years	Adolescent	None	McCreary & Sasse (2000); items in Table 1, with attention to rewording per table note
Eating in the Absence of Hunger Questionnaire for Children and Adolescents (EAH-C)	14	Respondents report on how often they eat past satiation or absent hunger in response to seven cues reflecting emotion and external cues. Ratings are on a 5-point scale (*never* to *always*). The EAH-C generates three subscales (External Eating, Negative Affect, and Fatigue/Boredom), as well as a total score.	6–19 years	Child/adolescent	None	Contact the author, *marian.tanofsky-kraff@usuhs.edu*
Eating Attitudes Test-26 (EAT-26)	26	This measure was originally developed to identify those with anorexic symptoms, but it can also be considered a measure of broad eating pathology (attitudes and behaviors). Items address body image, weight concerns, dieting, purging, and preoccupation with food, with a 6-point response scale (*never* to *always*). A clinical cutoff has generally been proposed as 20 for adults, but it is not clear whether this is appropriate for youth.	11+ years	Adolescent	None	*https://psychology-tools.com/test/eat-26* Online at *www.eat-26.com*
Eating Disorder Diagnostic Scale (EDDS)	22	The EDDS assesses symptoms related to AN, BN, and BED as defined in DSM-IV. Respondents are asked about body image, eating behaviors, and compensatory behaviors over the past 3–6 months and they respond using a variety of formats (7-point scale, yes–no, frequency reports). Note that a DSM-5 version of the EDDS has been developed (and is available at no cost at the same website as the EDDS), but as of this writing it has not yet been validated.	13+ years	Adolescent	None	*www.ori.org/sticemeasures*
Eating Disorder Examination Questionnaire (EDE-Q 6.0)	28	The EDE-Q is based on the Eating Disorders Interview, and items assess disordered eating thoughts and behaviors over the past 4 weeks (28 days). Yields a total score and four theorized subscales (dietary restraint eating concern, weight concern, and shape concern, with the latter two often combined), but there is inconsistent empirical support for the subscales in adolescent samples. Responses are either frequencies or on a 7-point scale. Scores (subscales or global) ≥ 4 are considered clinically significant. Earlier versions of the EDE-Q 6.0 (e.g., EDE-Q 4.0) may be used, since changes did not substantially affect the items included in computing total and subscale scores.	11–18+ years	Adolescent	None	*https://www.credo-oxford.com/pdfs/EDE-Q_6.0.pdf*

(continued)

TABLE 21.2. *(continued)*

Measure	No. of items	Description	Age	Reporter	Cost	Where to obtain
Eating Disorder Inventory–3 (EDI-3)	91	Assesses symptoms associated with eating disorders, with 12 primary scales: Drive for Thinness, Bulimia, Body Dissatisfaction, Low Self-Esteem, Personal Alienation, Interpersonal Insecurity, Interpersonal Alienation, Interoceptive Deficits, Emotional Dysregulation, Perfectionism, Asceticism, and Maturity Fears. The first three capture eating disorder pathology, and the others reflect psychological traits related to eating disorders. Respondents select one of six response options for each item.	13+ years	Adolescent	Yes	Pearson Assessment Resources *www.parinc.com/products/pkey/103*
Eating Disturbances in Youth—Questionnaire (EDY-Q)	14	Screen for ARFID, including its three variants: food avoidance emotional disorder, selective eating, and functional dysphagia. Other items inquire about pica and rumination disorder. There are also exclusion criteria for ARFID as part of this measure, namely, requiring scores < 3 on items reflecting distorted cognitions about weight or shape. Each item is rated on a 7-point scale (*Never true, Always true*).	8–13 years	Child	None	*http://nbn-resolving.de/ urn:nbn:de:bsz:15-qucosa-197246*
Emotional Eating Scale Adapted for Children and Adolescents (EES-C)	25	This measure assesses a child's urge to deal with (primarily) negative affect by eating. Respondents review a list of emotions and indicate the strength of their desire to eat in response using a 5-point scale (from *no desire to eat* to *very strong desire to eat*). Adapted from the EES developed for adults, with modifications including simpler instructions, a sample question and response, and simpler synonyms. (The EES-C also contains the emotion "happy," but this was not included in factor-analytic work or in the measure's subscales.) The measure generates three subscales: (1) Depression, (2) Anger, Anxiety, and Frustration, and (3) Feeling Unsettled, as well as a total summed score. The EES-C also added a column to report on the average number of days per week the child eats due to feeling this way.	8–17 years	Child/ adolescent	None	Tanofsky-Kraff, Theim, et al. (2007); items in Appendix
Minnesota Eating Behavior Survey (MEBS)	30	Respondents rate disordered eating attitudes and behaviors. There are two response formats: True–False for younger children (<13 years) and Definitely True/Probably True/Probably False/	10+ years	Child/ adolescent	Yes	Items available in von Ranson, Klump, Iacono, & McGue (2005)

Measure	#	Description	Age	Respondent	Norms	Source
		Definitely False for individuals 13 years+, which can be simplified to T–F. Yields a total score and four subscale scores (Body Dissatisfaction, Weight Preoccupation, Binge Eating, Compensatory Behaviors).				*But permission is needed from Pearson Assessment Resources*
Montreal Children's Hospital Feeding Scale (MCHFS)	14	The respondent (ideally the primary feeder of the child) rates each item on the frequency or difficulty level of the indicated behavior or the level of parental concern, using a 7-point scale, yielding a total summed score. Areas covered include oral motor, oral sensory, appetite, parental concerns about feeding, mealtime behaviors, parental strategies, and family reactions to the child's feeding. Scoring sheet provides translation to T-scores and categories of mild, moderate, and severe difficulties.	6 mo.–6 years	Parent	None	Ramsay, Martel, Porporino, & Zygmuntowicz (2011); items in Appendix
Motivational Stages of Change for Adolescents Recovering from an Eating Disorder (MSCARED)	9	This readiness to change measure was developed for adolescents and refers to eating disorders broadly. It uses the transtheoretical model of change with stages of precontemplation, contemplation, preparation, action, maintenance, and recovery. Although initially developed to focus on motivation to change in a global manner, authors of the MSCARED modified it to apply the same stage model to discrete behaviors (e.g., motivation to give up dieting, to give up binge eating). This measure also asks about what proportion of the day revolves around eating disorder issues as well as for whom adolescents are making steps to change (e.g., themselves, others). Note that this was designed as a brief interview but has also been used in a self-administered format.	12+ years	Adolescent	None	Contact the author, *joanne.gusella@gmail.ca*
Questionnaire on Eating and Weight Patterns—Adolescent form (QEWP-A)	12	Respondents rate items capturing BED symptomatology, yielding categories of BED, nonclinical binge eating (NCB), and no diagnosis (ND). Criteria for categories are reported in Johnson et al. (1999). Can also be used to categorize those endorsing binge eating (BE), overeating (OE), or no episodes of disordered eating (NE), as well as loss-of-control eating. Items come from the adult-developed QEWP but with simpler synonyms and two items combined into a two-part question.	10–18 years	Child/adolescent	None	Johnson, Grieve, Adams, & Sandy (1999); items in Appendix
SCOFF	5	This brief, simple screen involves five "yes" or "no" questions. Scoring ≥ 2 positive responses indicates risk for an eating disorder (AN, BN, BED).	10+ years	Child/adolescent	None	*www.bmj.com/content/319/7223/1467*

TABLE 21.3. Psychometric Properties of Youth Eating and Feeding Disorder Measures Based on Samples of Children and/or Adolescents

Measure	Citation(s)	Internal consistency (alpha)	Test–retest reliability (r)	Construct validity (e.g., r)
Anorexia Nervosa Stages of Change Questionnaire (ANSOCQ)	Pauli et al. (2017) Rieger et al. (2000) Rieger et al. (2002) Serrano et al. (2004)	.76–.94	.89–.90 across 1 week	.72 with drive for thinness; .85 with self-efficacy; .31 with active coping style; higher scores on attitudes/feelings scores protective against dropping out of treatment and predictive of weight gain.
Behavioral Pediatrics Feeding Assessment Scale (BPFAS)	Crist et al. (1994) Crist & Napier-Phillips (2001)	.74–.84	.82–.85 across 2 years	–.40 to –.54 with caloric intake; clinical sample from a feeding and nutrition clinic had significantly higher scores than a normative sample.
Children's Body Image Scale (CBIS)	Truby & Paxton (2002, 2008)	n/a	.67–.87 across 3 weeks	48% of girls wanted a thinner body, and 10% wanted a larger body, while 36% of boys wanted a thinner body and 20% wanted a larger body; correlations between perceived ideal discrepancy from the CBIS were –.27 to –.37 for body esteem and .22–.23 for dieting
Children's Eating Attitudes Test (ChEAT)	Lommi et al. (2019) Maloney et al. (1988, 1989) Smolak & Levine (1994)	.76–.87	.77 across 4–6 weeks	.36 with weight management behaviors; .39 with body dissatisfaction; higher scores for those with disordered eating per the SCOFF compared to those without disordered eating.
Children's Eating Behaviour Questionnaire (CEBQ)	Carnell & Wardle (2007) Wardle et al. (2001)	.72–.91	.52–.87 across 2 weeks	Betas for average total energy intake across 4–5 days were .42 for satiety responsiveness, .28 for food responsiveness, and .40 for enjoyment of food
Clinical Impairment Assessment (CIA)	Becker et al. (2010) Bohn & Fairburn (2008)	.93	n/a	.46 with EDE-Q global score; .32 with depressive symptoms
Drive for Muscularity Scale (DMS)	Brunet et al. (2010) McCreary & Sasse (2000) Yamamiya et al. (2019)	.84–.86	n/a	.24 with frequency of weight training; .61 with muscular/athletic internalization; boys scored higher than girls
Eating in the Absence of Hunger Questionnaire for Children and Adolescents (EAH-C)	Madowitz et al. (2014) Tanofsky-Kraff, Ranzenhofer, et al. (2008)	.80–.89	.65–.70 across a mean interval of 150 days (range = 5–565 days)	.23–.34 with depression; .25–.37 with anxiety; higher scores for patients with loss-of-control eating per interview compared to those without loss-of-control eating.

Measure	Citations	Internal consistency	Test–retest	Validity/Notes
Eating Attitudes Test (EAT-26)	Fortes et al. (2014), Garner et al. (1982), Kang et al. (2017), Pinus et al. (2017)	.82–.92	.82	EAT-26 scores predicted remission at follow-up in a female adolescent inpatient sample; correlations with EDI total scores ranged from .45 to .74 across eating disorder diagnostic groups.
Eating Disorder Diagnostic Scale (EDDS)	Lee et al. (2007), Stice et al. (2000, 2004)	.90	.87 across 1 week	Kappas for agreement between eating disorder groupings from the EDDS and diagnoses from the SCID: .93 for AN, .81 for BN, .74 for BED; correlations with global EDE-Q scores were .67–.75.
Eating Disorder Examination Questionnaire (EDE-Q 6.0)	Jennings & Phillips (2017), Machado et al. (2014), Penelo et al. (2013)	.72–.96	.87–.90 across 2 weeks	.70 with drive for thinness; .50 with body dissatisfaction; .38 with bulimic symptoms; .64 with SCOFF.
Eating Disorder Inventory–3 (EDI-3)	Cumella (2006), Fan et al. (2010), Garner (2004), Lichtenstein et al. (2017)	.73–.81	n/a	Scores on the eating disorder subscales (Drive For Thinness, Bulimia, Body Dissatisfaction) in the expected directions compared to healthy controls; review of manual (Cumella, 2006) reports good convergent validity with six established measures of eating disorder behaviors/issues.
Eating Disturbances in Youth—Questionnaire (EDY-Q)	Kurz et al. (2015, 2016), Murray et al. (2018)	Overall score: .62; subscales: .42–.52	n/a	EDY-Q diagnostic items for ARFID were not correlated; EDY-Q mean scores were weakly correlated (.21–.23) with items on dietary restraint, fear of weight gain, and dissatisfaction with weight; underweight children scored higher on the EDY-Q ARFID diagnostic items than normal- and overweight children.
Emotional Eating Scale Adapted for Children and Adolescents (EES-C)	Tanofsky-Kraff, Theim, et al. (2007), Vannucci et al. (2012)	.83–.95	.59–.74 across a mean interval of 3.35 months (range = .39–11.6 months)	Higher scores for participants with loss-of-control eating than for those not reporting loss-of-control eating; higher premeal state negative affect associated with more total energy intake at subsequent meals.
Minnesota Eating Behavior Survey (MEBS)	von Ranson et al. (2005)	.86–.89	.59–.61 across 3 years	.78–.83 with the EDE-Q global score

(continued)

TABLE 21.3. *(continued)*

Measure	Citation(s)	Internal consistency (alpha)	Test–retest reliability (*r*)	Construct validity (e.g., *r*)
Montreal Children's Hospital Feeding Scale (MCHFS)	Ramsay et al. (2011) Rogers et al. (2018)	.90	.85–.92 across 7–10 days	–.65 with enjoyment of food (CEBQ); .56 with fussiness (CEBQ); higher scores for clinical samples than normative sample.
Motivational Stages of Change for Adolescents Recovering from an Eating Disorder (MSCARED)	Bustin et al. (2013) Gusella et al. (2003)	n/a	.92 across 1 week	.64 with mother's rating of child's stage of change; .79 with interviewer's rating of stage of change; those in the action stage of change had less body dissatisfaction and less drive for thinness than those in earlier motivational stages; from start to end of treatment, girls moved up one motivational stage; initial stage of change associated with outcomes of better body image, more hopefulness, and more motivation (*r* = .54–.69); correlation of –.56 for change in stage of change scores and change in ChEAT scores; stage of change scores significantly higher at discharge.
Questionnaire on Eating and Weight Patterns—Adolescent form (QEWP-A)	Johnson et al. (1999, 2001)	n/a	Phi –.42 across 3 weeks (based on nonclinical binge eating and no diagnosis groups due to small numbers in BED group)	Participants categorized with BED had significantly higher depression and ChEAT-26 scores than those with nonclinical binge eating or with no diagnosis.
SCOFF	Estecha Querol et al. (2016) Lichtenstein et al. (2017) Rueda Jaimes et al. (2005)	.44–.64	n/a	.57–.71 with EDI eating pathology subscales (Drive for Thinness, Bulimia, Body Dissatisfaction); high-scoring girls had significantly lower daily energy intake than low scorers; kappa = .55 for clinical interview findings.

Cross-Informant Assessment

Although cross-informant assessment is considered a *sine qua non* of the assessment of children and adolescents, it takes on additional importance in the context of eating disorders due to the denial or misunderstanding of the seriousness of symptoms and minimization that is common in children and adolescents with AN (Couturier & Lock, 2006). Thus, obtaining parental reports of youths' behaviors are important to shore up potential unreliability of youth report due to minimization, denial, or lack of insight (Lock & La Via, 2015). That said, there are also circumstances in which a parent may not have the information to provide accurate reports, such as information on bulimic behaviors that tend to be secretive. Using birth cohort data (thus not selected for eating disorder symptoms), Swanson and colleagues (2014) found the greatest discrepancy between presence of vomiting: 4.9% according to adolescents versus 0.3% according to parents. Interestingly, there was a greater discrepancy in reports of presence of fasting for older adolescents (age 16; 13.2% by adolescent report vs. 1.6% by parent report) than for 14-year-olds (6.7% by adolescent report vs. 4.7% by parent report), which may be due to the greater autonomy that is typical of older adolescents, including their presence at fewer family meals. Parents were more likely than adolescents to assess them as thin (Swanson et al., 2014), which may reflect different perspectives or highlight potential denial by youth.

Collection of parental report can take several forms, although it should be noted that, in practice, there are few parental reporting measures for eating disorders. In some cases, there are parent versions of child/adolescent measures (e.g., Eating in the Absence of Hunger Questionnaire for Children/Adolescents—Parent Report [EAH-P; Madowitz et al., 2014]; QEWP-P [Johnson et al., 1999]) that were modified from child versions. In other cases, parent forms were created from the outset, and this is particularly true for assessing ARFID and feeding behaviors of very young children (e.g., BPFAS [Crist & Napier-Phillips, 2001]; CEBQ [Wardle et al., 2001]; MCHFS [Ramsay et al., 2011]). In cases in which a parent version of a child self-report measure is administered, findings are mixed in terms of psychometric properties. For example, the EAH-P had demonstrated good internal consistency (.88 for the total score), but parent–child agreement has been relatively low (r = .34 for the total score) (Madowitz et al., 2014).

However, given that this measure refers to identifying when children eat absent hunger or when sated, it makes sense that parents may not be as aware of their children's internal states. The level of agreement is also on par with parent–youth agreement about how the youth is doing in general (see Youngstrom & Prinstein, Chapter 1, this volume). That said, parents of children who engaged in loss-of-control eating endorsed significantly greater tendencies for eating motivated by negative affect or fatigue/boredom than did parents of youth without disordered eating (Shomaker et al., 2010). For the QEWP-P, Steinberg and colleagues (2004) report a kappa for parent–child agreement of only .19. There was agreement of 81.6% for no diagnosis, 15.5% for nonclinical binge eating, and 25.0% for BED, yielding 20% sensitivity and 80% specificity. For this measure, the difficulty may be that binge-eating behavior is often concealed out of shame and guilt; parents may not be able to identify binge-eating behavior easily because it is hidden.

Although parents are the most typical collateral informant, coaches are another potential informant for youth involved in sports. Coaches may notice whether an athlete is looking "too thin," may be concerned about weight loss after observing a trend of poorer performance (e.g., less stamina in long-distance running), and may have the opportunity to observe eating patterns during team meals. Some researchers have capitalized on the unique positions of coaches by providing training in detecting eating disorder symptoms (Whisenhunt, Williamson, Drab-Hudson, & Walden, 2008). Although the work by Whisenhunt and colleagues was to make coaches agents of change by fostering changes in the sports climate (e.g., reducing pressure related to weight) and coaching behaviors, we note that trained coaches could be well positioned to provide accurate assessments of youth on their teams. However, we did not identify any collateral measures of eating pathology geared toward coaches.

How is information from multiple informants used? Swanson and colleagues (2014) proposed four analytic approaches: (1) Use data from just one informant, regardless of whether there were multiple informants (in this case, a decision would need to be made as to which informant's data to use); (2) use data from both informants but as separate findings for consideration; (3) for cases of presence–absence of a symptom, create a single report using the "or" rule, so that a symptom is recorded as present if either the adolescent or the parent endorsed it for the adolescent; and (4) jointly model the responses of the multiple informants (see Fitzmaurice, Laird, Zahner, & Daskalakis, 1995; Horton & Fitzmaurice, 2004). The latter is ideal, since it makes efficient use of multiple informants' data but would require tailored algorithms for practical use.

Risk and Protective Factors

Our focus on risk and protective factors is on factors relevant to eating disorders given the minimal research on these factors for feeding disorders. Eating disorders are arguably best understood in a biopsychosocial model, and from these different domains (biology, psychological, social context) come potential risk and protective factors. Of note, most research on risk and protective factors, and eating disorders in general, has focused on white girls, so much less is known about boys and youth of color.

There is support for heritability of eating disorders, with evidence for genetics conferring risk via both twin studies (e.g., Kortegaard, Hoerder, Joergensen, Gillberg, & Kyvik, 2001) and adoption studies (e.g., Klump, Suisman, Burt, McGue, & Iacono, 2009). Klump and colleagues (2009) note that environmental factors (shared and nonshared) may play a role in their interaction with genetic factors. Furthermore, the balance of the impact of genetic and environmental factors on disordered eating may vary across development, with some research showing that shared environment is critical during younger developmental stages (e.g., prior to puberty; Klump, Perkins, Burt, McGue, & Iacono, 2007).

Using a prospective high-risk design, Stice, Gau, Rohde, and Shaw (2017) identified risk factors predicting onset of DSM-5 eating disorders in adolescent girls and young women. Notably, impaired psychosocial functioning and negative affect predicted onset of AN, BN, BED, and purging disorder, thus emerging as transdiagnostic risk factors. Additionally, low body mass index (BMI) predicted onset of AN. Thin ideal internalization, thinness expectancies, and dieting predicted BN, BED, and purging disorder (Stice et al., 2017), and longitudinal work with community samples of adolescent girls highlighted extreme dieting via fasting as a risk factor for bulimic pathology (Stice, Davis, Miller, & Marti, 2008). Other longitudinal work has identified the following predictors of disordered eating for girls: negative affect and depressive symptoms (Ferreiro, Seoane, & Senra, 2012;

Leon, Fulkerson, Perry, Keel, & Klump, 1999), body dissatisfaction, and perfectionism (Ferreiro et al., 2012). Low social support predicted disordered eating for boys, and high BMI predicted disordered eating for both girls and boy (Ferreiro, Seoane, & Senra, 2012). In a meta-analysis that included both adolescent and adult mostly female samples, perfectionism was found to predict increases in bulimic symptoms (Kehayes, Smith, Sherry, Vidovic, & Saklofske, 2019). In terms of social context, there is some evidence that participation in "leanness" sports (e.g., gymnastics, swimming, track, wrestling) may be prospectively associated with elevated disordered eating compared to participation in nonleanness sports (e.g., basketball, soccer) (Tamminen, Holt, & Crocker, 2012), often motivated by the belief that being leaner will improve sports performance.

Less work has been done on factors that may reduce risk for developing an eating disorder in youth. In their review, Littleton and Ollendick (2003) highlight positive family relationships as the protective factor with the most empirical support in guarding against eating disorder pathology. Furthermore, in their review on family meals, Skeer and Ballard (2013) found a consistent relationship between the frequency of family members' meals together and reduced disordered eating risk for adolescents; this relationship appeared to be most relevant to girls. In terms of individual factors, longitudinal work in adolescence supports self-esteem as a protective factor against body dissatisfaction (Beato-Fernández, Rodríguez-Cano, Belmonte-Llario, & Martínez-Delgado, 2004). Last, self-compassion has been found to be a robust protective factor against eating pathology and negative body image (Braun, Park, & Gorin, 2016). Although this has not been examined specifically in children or adolescents, self-compassion warrants additional research as a protective factor to assess and amplify.

Treatment Moderators

Little published work exists on moderators of treatment outcome (Murray, Loeb, & Le Grange, 2015), with most of what there is focused on family-based treatment. Some moderators reflect individual factors, namely, psychopathology severity. Ciao, Accurso, Fitzsimmons-Craft, and Le Grange (2015) found that younger adolescents and those with more severe levels of purging at baseline fared better with family-based treatment than with supportive psychotherapy. Le Grange and colleagues

(2012) found that both eating-related obsessionality and severity of eating disorder pathology acted as moderators at end of treatment for family-based treatment for AN, but not at follow-up, and Lock, Couturier, Bryson, and Agras (2006) identified comorbid psychiatric disorders as predictive of lower likelihood of remission for adolescents with AN in family-based treatment (FBT). Treatment outcome was better when a longer course of FBT for AN was applied in cases of elevated eating-related obsessionality in adolescents and single-parent homes (Lock, Agras, Bryson, & Kraemer, 2005). Thus, consideration should be given to assessing obsessionality related to eating disorders, for example, with the Yale–Brown–Cornell Eating Disorders Scale Self-Report Questionnaire (YBC-EDS-SRQ; Bellace et al., 2012) which assesses eating-disorder-related preoccupations and rituals, and comorbidity with a diagnostic interview such as the Schedule for Affective Disorders and Schizophrenia for School-Age Children (K-SADS; Kaufman et al., 1997).

Other moderators with support reflect family factors. Problematic family functioning predicted poorer outcome for adolescents with AN in FBT (Lock et al., 2006), and parental warmth was associated with good outcomes (Le Grange, Hoste, Lock, & Bryson, 2011). Findings are mixed regarding parental criticism as a moderator related to treatment dropout and poor outcomes. Interestingly, FBT with the youth and parents seen separately appears to be more effective than conjoint FBT in the context of high parental criticism toward the patient (Eisler et al., 2000).

In work on BN and BED, lower levels of overvaluation of weight/shape at baseline and shorter duration of the eating disorder predicted better outcomes across both enhanced cognitive-behavioral therapy (CBT-E) and interpersonal psychotherapy (IPT) in a female sample that included older adolescents/young adults (Cooper et al., 2016). Similarly, lower levels of overvaluation of weight/shape at baseline predicted remission at end of treatment in adolescents with BN (Le Grange, Crosby, & Lock, 2008).

A fairly reliable moderator of treatment outcome for both AN and BN is rapid response to treatment. For example, early weight gain (by the fifth session) predicted remission at end of treatment in FBT of adolescents with AN (Hughes, Sawyer, Accurso, Singh, & Le Grange, 2019). Doyle, Le Grange, Loeb, Doyle, and Crosby (2010) applied ROC analyses to find that a 2.88% weight gain or greater early on (by the fourth session)

best predicted end-of-treatment remission (AUC = .67, p = .02) for adolescents with AN in FBT. In the context of BN, "rapid response" refers to reductions in bulimic behaviors early in treatment. Based on ROC curves, rapid response defined as 65–70% reduction in binge eating by the fourth treatment session was associated with remission (Grilo, White, Wilson, Gueorguieva, & Masheb, 2012), and other work has specified that a 50–70% reduction in purging at around the fourth-week mark is most strongly related to remission from BN at end of treatment (Thompson-Brenner, Shingleton, Sauer-Zavala, Richards, & Pratt, 2015). In a sample of adolescents with BN, Le Grange, Doyle, Crosby, and Chen (2008) found that an 85% reduction of binge–purge symptoms by the sixth session most strongly predicted remission at end of treatment (AUC = .81, sensitivity = .78, specificity = .77) regardless of treatment (FBT or individual). In a review of aspects of therapeutic process in the treatment of eating disorders, Brauhardt, de Zwaan, and Hilbert (2014) concluded that rapid response is associated with better outcomes among adolescents, highlighting the need both to assess symptom change early in treatment and identify factors that predict early response.

Prescription

Semistructured and Structured Interviews

We recommend the use of a semistructured or structured interview to determine diagnoses suggested from the use of screeners or diagnostic aids. Table 21.4 lists diagnostic interviews frequently used in assessing eating and feeding disorders in children and adolescents.

The Eating Disorder Examination (EDE; Fairburn & Cooper, 1993) and the Children's Eating Disorder Examination (ChEDE; Bryant-Waugh, Cooper, Taylor, & Lask, 1996) yield both a global score and scores on four subscales: Restraint, Eating Concern, Weight Concern, and Shape Concern. These are the same scores reported on the EDE-Q, which was derived from the EDE. Additionally, and critical to the prescription phase, the EDE and ChEDE include diagnostic items that permit the diagnoses of eating disorders (AN, BN, BED).

The EDE is frequently used with adolescents, even though data about psychometrics for the EDE in this age group are limited. In order to adapt the EDE to make it suitable for younger individuals, two main modifications were made (Bryant-Waugh

TABLE 21.4. Structured and Semistructured Interviews for Diagnosing Eating and Feeding Disorders in Youth

Diagnostic interview	Citation(s)	Age	Version(s)	Structured or semistructured	Time to complete	Reliability of diagnoses	Where to obtain	Cost
Children's Eating Disorder Examination—Child (ChEDE)	Bryant-Waugh et al. (1996) Hilbert et al. (2013) Wade et al. (2008) Watkins et al. (2005)	8–16 years	Child	Semistructured	Mean of 1 hour (45–75 min)	Interrater reliability: .91–1.00. Children not receiving an AN diagnosis per the EDE had subscale scores similar to EDE norms for normative adult groups	www.phenxtoolkit.org/protocols/view/230101; Contact the author, r.bryant-waugh@ucl.ac.uk	No
Development & Well-Being Assessment (DAWBA)	Goodman et al. (2000) House et al. (2008)	11–18 years	Child/adolescent; parent	Structured (intended as an online assessment)	10–20 min for the eating disorder module	kappa = .59 with clinical diagnoses from a multidisciplinary team	www.DAWBA.info	No
Eating Disorder Examination (EDE)	Fairburn & Cooper (1993) House et al. (2008) Loeb et al. (2011)	16+ years (although in practice has been used through early adolescence (i.e., 12 years)	Adolescent	Semistructured	45–75 min	kappa = .10 with clinical diagnoses from a multidisciplinary team. Adolescents with AN are less likely to attain diagnostic thresholds for psychological aspects of AN compared to adults	www.credo-oxford.com/pdfs/EDE_17.0Dpdf	No
Pica, ARFID, and Rumination Disorder Interview (PARDI)	Bryant-Waugh et al. (2019) Bryant-Waugh & Cooke (2017)	2–22 years	Multi-informant: different versions depending on age of client, with parallel parent versions	Semistructured	Mean of 39 min	kappa = 0.75 for interrater reliability for ARFID diagnosis. Diagnoses from PARDI concurred with clinical judgment across age groups	Contact the author, r.bryant-waugh@ucl.ac.uk	No

et al., 1996). First, in order to assess overvaluation of weight/shape, instead of asking this question, children are directed to make a list of things that are important to how they see/think about themselves. These different domains are written on separate pieces of paper that the child then organizes in order of importance; this sort task is then interpreted in relation to overvaluation of weight/shape. The other modification involves rewording to focus on intent rather than actual behavior; this was developmentally appropriate since, for example, it is often difficult for children to go 8 or more hours without eating (an EDE item) without a parent intervening, even though they may want to and would if they could. For both the EDE and the ChEDE, some questions refer to the past 28 days and others refer to the past 3 months; thus, writing down a timetable of events to help orient to the time period is important. Even with this aid, children may have difficulties with chronology and reliable reporting over these time periods, and parental assistance may be requested in establishing a timetable prior to the assessment. For both the EDE and ChEDE, authors indicate that training is needed; furthermore, a detailed guide is provided (*www.credo-oxford.com/pdfs/ede_17.0d.pdf*).

The DAWBA (Goodman et al., 2000) was developed as a comprehensive assessment of a variety of psychiatric diagnoses, including the eating disorders AN, BN, and BED (under the module "dieting, weight and body shape"). Online administration of the DAWBA is recommended to ensure that screener/skip rules are applied correctly; provisional diagnoses are made by computer algorithm that are then reviewed and confirmed or modified by the clinician (e.g., based on additional informants). Youth ages 11–17 provide self-report, and there is also an interview for parents of youth ages 5–17 years. A clinician rater's manual is provided on the DAWBA website.

Compared to the EDE and ChEDE, the DAWBA is briefer and requires less administrator training. Additionally, data indicate that the DAWBA identifies a higher percentage of eating disorder cases than does the EDE (House, Eisler, Simic, & Micali, 2008), perhaps due to the online version providing a sense of anonymity and freeing up youth to be more open about symptoms. Since this module is embedded in a more comprehensive assessment (including anxiety disorders, mood disorders, and externalizing disorders), for those interested in also assessing comorbidity (recommended), the full DAWBA may be a useful tool. For these reasons, when interested in diagnosing AN, BN, or BED, the DAWBA is recommended.

For children who may have ARFID or a feeding disorder, the PARDI (Bryant-Waugh et al., 2019) is recommended. Although only preliminary data are available for the PARDI, its strengths are its currency and comprehensiveness in permitting the diagnosis of DSM-5-defined ARFID, pica, and rumination disorder for children and adolescents (ages 2–22 years), as well as its development by a well-established team of researchers and clinicians focused on feeding disorders. The PARDI assesses presence and severity of common features of ARFID and groups them into profiles of sensory sensitivity, lack of interest in eating, and fear of aversive consequences, in addition to applying an algorithm that allows for the diagnosis of ARFID, pica, and rumination disorder. For younger children, there is a version of the PARDI administered to parents; for ages 8 and older, there are also self-report versions for youth.

Additional Considerations in Case Formulation and Treatment Planning

An accurate diagnosis is a key aspect of case conceptualization that then informs treatment planning, but it is not the only factor. Given the complexity and multifaceted nature of eating disorders, working within a model that provides guidance on collecting additional data and how to organize it is useful. One broad model that takes a holistic, atheoretical approach to understanding the cognitions, affect, and behaviors of a psychological disorder is the temporal/contextual model (Zubernis, Snyder, & Neale-McFall, 2017), which is informed by the ecological systems work of Bronfenbrenner (1981) and includes an inner circle of personality, self-concept, biology, symptoms, life roles, readiness for change, and strengths, as well as an outer circle of environmental influences, such as culture, relationships, and societal influences, with interrelationships between these constructs and reciprocal influences posited. The temporal/contextual model is displayed as a diagram that may be useful to both assessor and client, and includes a timeline that can highlight how past experiences may have contributed to the development of symptoms, how present conditions may maintain symptoms, and what the client hopes the future will look like. Although this model was not developed for youth, we believe its core components are relevant to a rich assessment of eating disorders among children and adolescents and that gathering information across these various domains will be useful to multidisciplinary teams often involved in the treatment of eating disorders.

Three core areas included in this model that are especially relevant to eating disorders and/or youth are biology, relationships, and societal influences.

Physical Assessment

To address biological aspects relevant to eating disorders, a physical assessment is imperative, as is being connected to a physician for medical assessment and monitoring. The two main eating-disorder-related aspects to assess are height/weight/BMI (relevant to AN) and electrolyte imbalance (relevant to any purging behaviors), as these factors are important considerations in determining level of care. Additionally, concerns about bone density and body composition can be evaluated with dual-energy X-ray absorptiometry (DEXA), potential cardiac irregularities can be examined with electrocardiograms, and pubertal status can be determined via a physical exam to examine testicular volume (boys) and breast development (girls) (Tanner, 1981). Alternatively, there are self- and parent-report questionnaires for pubertal stage that are reasonably accurate and easier to use in outpatient mental health (Petersen, Crockett, Richards, & Boxer, 1988).

BMI on its own is not considered appropriate for children (Cole, Flegal, Nicholls, & Jackson, 2007). Instead, BMI percentiles are viewed as developmentally good alternatives, with a BMI lower than the 10th percentile mapping onto the level of malnutrition of AN (Lock & La Via, 2015). Another option involves examining deviations from prior growth trajectories, which places weight changes in the context of the individual's developmental history and can be more powerful for the youth and parents than comparison to a clinical cutoff point (Zucker, Merwin, Elliott, Lacy, & Eichen, 2009). By plotting a youth's height and weight history against Centers for Disease Control and Prevention (CDC) growth charts (www.cdc.gov/growthcharts/clinical_charts.htm), both intraindividual and interindividual contrasts emerge.

Additionally, a complete physical assessment is needed for differential diagnosis purposes. For example, significant weight loss could be due to the development of type 1 diabetes, thyroid disease, or celiac disease (Lock & La Via, 2015; Zucker et al., 2009). Last, related to the biological domain, a nutritional assessment may be warranted to understand energy intake. A dietary intake assessment can be done with dietary food records (which can be tailored for younger children with the use of images, or which parents of young children can help document) or via interviewer-assisted dietary recalls. For the latter, the interviewer can probe for more details and use models of food types and amounts as a way to obtain an accurate recounting.

Family Relationships

Family factors such as parental warmth and family functioning can act as moderators of treatment outcome and are therefore helpful to assess as part of treatment planning. Being able to bolster familial support and improve family functioning should be an asset to the recovery process. Furthermore, given that recommended treatment for youth with AN is FBT, assessing family functioning is important. This assessment can help identify familial difficulties that may need to be addressed in the context of FBT or to determine whether functioning concerns are so severe that another modality of treatment should be considered. The Family Assessment Device (FAD) is recommended for measuring family functioning. This 60-item measure contains seven subscales: Problem Solving, Communication, Responsiveness, Affective Involvement, Roles, Behavioral Control, and General Functioning (Epstein, Baldwin, & Bishop, 1983). The FAD can be completed by the youth and parents and has cutoff points that differentiate between healthy and pathological family functioning (Miller, Epstein, Bishop, & Keitner, 1985). In addition to assessing family functioning, a review of parental psychiatric history and attitudes/behaviors toward their bodies and eating provides important context for the youth's eating disorder.

It is generally understood that poor family functioning is more a result of a family member having an eating disorder than a cause of the eating disorder (Ciao, Accurso, Fitzsimmons-Craft, Lock, & Le Grange, 2015). It is extremely taxing to parent a child with an eating disorder, with particular strain when the eating disorder is AN due to the heightened morbidity and the role parents play in FBT for AN. Thus, another family-related factor to consider in treatment planning is caregiver strain. The Caregiver Strain Questionnaire—Short Form 7 (CGSQ-SF7; Brannan, Athay, & Vides de Andrade, 2012) was developed for families of youth with emotional/behavioral disorders, so it is not eating-disorder-specific. It assesses both objective strain (e.g., missed work/duties) and subjective internalized strain (e.g., worried about the child's future) to capture "the demands, responsibilities, and negative psychic consequences" of caring for children/adolescents with mental, emotional, and behavioral problems (Brannan, Heflinger, & Bickman, 1997). Although we could not find studies of eating disorders that used this measure, it would be worth consideration as part of an initial assessment of family factors and via repeated administration as a way of monitoring caregiver strain, especially prior to embarking on FBT.

Societal Context

Last, societal influences may be especially relevant for adolescents, and a thorough inquiry into friends, peers, school, extracurricular activities (e.g., sports), and social media use is recommended, as well assessment of socially related cognitions/behaviors, such as social comparison and the pressure to be thin. The sociodevelopmental aspect of eating disorder behaviors is displayed in data demonstrating that from early to middle adolescence (middle school to high school; puberty occurs for most girls during this transition), extreme weight control strategies jump from being endorsed by 9% to endorsement by 18%, and from middle to late adolescence (high school to post-high school) from 15 to 24% (Neumark-Sztainer, Wall, Eisenberg, Story, & Hannan, 2006). Thus, key transition periods marked by biological and/or social changes are associated with eating disorder pathology and should be assessed for a sense of context.

We additionally highlight three concepts included in the temporal/contextual model that may not be automatically considered in the assessment of eating disorders but would aid in case conceptualization and treatment planning. Immediately below we discuss culture and strengths, and in the section on process, we review the construct of and assessments for readiness to change.

Race/Ethnicity

Race and ethnicity are core aspects of culture that are relevant to eating disorders. Research among females finds that rates of eating disorders do not differ significantly across race/ethnicity when African Americans, Latino/as, Asian Americans, and non-Latino/a European Americans were examined (Bardone-Cone, Higgins Neyland, & Lin, 2017; Marques et al., 2011). In an adolescent sample, rates of fasting and diet pill use were similar across Latino/as, non-Hispanic African Americans, and non-Hispanic European Americans, but Latino/as reported more purging via vomiting or laxative use (Hazzard, Hahn, & Sonneville, 2017). In general, rates of eating disorders and eating disorder symptoms are similar across race/ethnicity, yet racial/ethnic minorities with eating disorder symptoms are routinely underdiagnosed. For example, in a vignette study, clinicians were more likely to identify disordered eating when the client was Latina or non–Latina European American (40–44%) than when the client was African American (17%) (Gordon, Brattole, Wingate, & Joiner, 2006). Furthermore, ethnic minority undergraduates appear to be less likely to be assessed for eating disorders or referred for further evaluation when disordered eating concerns are expressed than are European American college students (Becker, Franko, Speck, & Herzog, 2003; Franko, 2007). Thus, evidence for a racial/ethnic disparity in evaluation and referral appears to exist, and assessors must guard against this bias. The consequence of this disparity in assessment conclusions is not inconsequential; racial/ethnic minorities are often diagnosed only after symptoms have become more severe and, thus, more difficult to treat (Gordon, Perez, & Joiner, 2002). Using rating scales and semistructured interviews helps guard against bias.

Strengths

Eating disorder behaviors are generally conceptualized as coping strategies for dealing with negative affect and distress (e.g., binge eating to escape overwhelming negative emotions) or a sense of loss of control (e.g., dietary restriction to enhance a sense of control). In the context of this conceptualization, identifying strengths is especially important: What internal strengths or external supports are available to the client that can cultivate alternative responses to negative affect and feeling out of control in aspects of life? Assessment of factors such as coping skills, positive and uplifting peer relationships, and past examples of resilience is recommended as part of providing a holistic picture that is not solely pathology-focused and guiding intervention in terms of aspects to be bolstered. Both the youth and parents/family can contribute examples of the client's strengths. Explicitly referring to strengths as part of assessment can also counter the hopelessness and fear that often accompany an eating disorder.

Establishing Goals and Integrating Client Preferences

As with any psychological intervention, goals should be operationalized, so that they are measurable and may be assessed multiple times to evaluate progress. In general, goals should be established collaboratively with the youth and, as applicable, the parents. Eating disorders are unique, however, in that there is a place for goal setting that may be done without much consultation with the youth and family—this is in regard to weight in cases of AN. Due to the high lethality of AN related to low weight, goals related to weight gain are usually best established by physicians and nutritionists on a multidisciplinary team, but their rationale should be communicated to the youth and family.

Other goals include reduction of eating disorder behaviors and cognitions. The administration of a measure of readiness to change that taps into different disordered eating components may shed light on a temporal ordering of goals based on readiness. For example, Geller and colleagues (2008) found that their adolescent sample had highest action scores (i.e., taking action to change the behavior) for binge eating and highest precontemplation scores (i.e., not ready to change the behavior) for restriction and compensatory behaviors. This information from an individual client could be discussed to get a better sense of the "why" for the different stages of change, to establish buy-in for goals of reducing binge frequency, to help establish a hierarchy related to the client's preferences, and to open up a conversation on how restriction can serve to maintain binge eating, which may help increase motivation for reducing restriction. Furthermore, a readiness to change assessment may serve as a springboard to discuss what it would take to advance forward a stage (Gusella et al., 2003).

Goals involving reduction of disordered eating behavior may be operationalized in different ways. Obtaining a baseline frequency of typical rates of binge eating and vomiting, for example, can lead to an initial goal of *any* amount of decrease to provide a boost of self-efficacy, followed by more tailored behavioral goals, such as starting to disentangle linked behaviors by increasing the number of times a binge is *not* followed by compensatory behavior. Given evidence that significant reduction in bulimic behaviors early in treatment is predictive of good outcome (e.g., Le Grange, Doyle, et al., 2008), developing a treatment plan and strategies to greatly decrease these behaviors is impor-

tant. In conjunction with these goals of behavior reduction should be goal setting that is related to more adaptive behaviors the client will turn to for coping, for example, having a goal to go for a leisurely walk, turn to a favorite hobby (e.g., drawing, watching an engrossing program), or call a trusted friend when experiencing a strong urge to binge or restrict. Or the goal might be to practice mindfulness and distress tolerance in the face of negative affect instead of responding with an eating disorder behavior. The key is to have the goals be clear and measurable (e.g., a decrease in binge eating; engagement in a mindfulness activity).

Goals involving reduction of disordered eating cognitions may be operationalized using the EDE-Q, which assesses a dietary restraint mind-set, as well as concerns related to eating, weight, and shape, traditionally by inquiring about the past 28 days. For more frequent assessments, the time frame could be adjusted to the previous 14 days to get a sense of change; indeed, this has been done before in adolescent samples (e.g., Carter, Stewart, & Fairburn, 2001). Goals related to cognitions might include scores on the EDE-Q subscales or global scale moving to within 1 SD of age-matched community norms. This presents a goal that is reasonable (i.e., the goal is not for zero disordered eating thoughts) and meaningful (i.e., cognitions in a normative range). The consideration of the reliable change index and clinically significant change would also be appropriate in setting goals related to eating disorder cognitions as captured in the EDE-Q.

As part of goal setting, clinicians should consider a functional assessment of the eating disorder behaviors. Binge eating may temporarily provide an escape from negative affect and aversive self-awareness (Heatherton & Baumeister, 1991), and extreme dietary restriction may provide a sense of control (Serpell, Treasure, Teasdale, & Sullivan, 1999). Children and adolescents may not have the insight needed to connect their disordered eating behaviors to situational events, in which case collateral reports from parents and observations may be needed. A common assessment approach to facilitate functional analysis is self-monitoring, recording the occurrence of clearly defined target behaviors, along with their antecedents (e.g., affect, cognitions) and consequences. Use of technology (e.g., smartphones) makes this assessment approach easier, and the data collected can be reviewed in a therapy session to help the youth identify patterns that may be maintaining their disordered eating behaviors and develop goals.

Process

Goal and Progress Measurement

We focus here on goals that are closely tied to eating disorder pathology but note that the treatment provider should consider related goals as well in a full case conceptualization (e.g., mood, social support). Goals related to eating disorders may be grouped in terms of physical, behavioral, and cognitive goals. Physical goals in terms of rate of weight gain and absolute weight should be developed in tandem with physicians and nutritionists. Gregertsen, Mandy, Kanakam, Armstrong, and Serpell (2019) suggest that in the context of a treatment team, the therapist focus on psychotherapy aims, with another team member monitoring weight. This "division of labor" is congruent with a therapeutic objective of developing a sense of self distinct from one's weight by avoiding having the therapist play a dual role. Other perspectives, however, argue for regular weighing by the therapist. For example, in FBT, weekly weighing with only the youth and therapist present gets communicated to the parents, with the opportunity for the family to process any misinterpretations about weight fluctuations (Zucker et al., 2009). Whether a clinician directly assesses weight or receives reports from a physician or treatment team, a goal of early weight gain is recommended given that such weight gain by the fourth or fifth session predicts remission at end of treatment among youth with AN (Doyle et al., 2010; Hughes et al., 2019).

Target behaviors for goals to consider include loss-of-control eating, objective binge eating, dietary restriction, fasting, excessive exercise, and purging behaviors (e.g., vomiting and laxative use). Self-monitoring is a good way to track progress related to behavioral change. For example, youth may fill out daily records of behaviors they are working on, in addition to the context of the behavior (time, location), any environmental triggers, and the emotional, cognitive, and physiological precedents (e.g., sadness, self-doubt, hunger). Of note, optimal use of daily records requires clear definitions of the behaviors to be monitored (e.g., what constitutes a binge) and, for young children, simple language or visuals should be considered. Not only does self-monitoring help identify patterns and progress but it also permits the development of hypotheses that can be discussed and tested. For example, if the daily monitoring assessment shows that binge eating occurs primarily on weekends and after feeling lonely, therapist and

client can tailor a plan to address these high-risk scenarios.

As with early weight gain in AN, early reduction in binge-eating and purging behaviors (fourth to sixth sessions) in the context of BN predicts end-of-treatment remission in youth and thus should be a goal, with benchmarks available regarding what constitutes rapid response in bulimic behaviors (Grilo, Pagano, et al., 2012; Le Grange, Crosby, et al., 2008; Thompson-Brenner et al., 2015). Although a clear goal is the early and substantial decrease in eating disorder behaviors, it is important to set realistic expectations, so that clients do not expect to go from regular bulimic behaviors to none. Also, since "slips" are common (e.g., after a couple of weeks without binges, the occurrence of a binge), it is imperative that clients be prepared for such an eventuality and know that a lapse does not need to spiral down into a full-fledged return of eating pathology. Among eating disorder behaviors, excessive exercise is conceptually different in terms of reduction goals; although its driven quality is a focus of change, reduction of exercise itself to zero is generally not the goal.

In terms of goals related to eating disorder cognitions, repeated administration of the EDE-Q can provide data on progress toward decreasing disordered eating thinking. Although these questionnaires are set up for reporting on the past 28 days, the time period can be truncated to focus on shorter time periods if intended to be used frequently (e.g., biweekly) or it can be used for reporting on the past 28 days at the start of treatment, a halfway point, and end of treatment. One straightforward benchmark for progress may be moving into within 1 standard deviation of age-matched community norms on the EDE-Q/ChEDE-Q subscales. Progress can also be measured via examination of clinically significant change on the EDE-Q; Ekeroth and Birgegård (2014) recommend combining clinically significant (CS) change and the reliable change index (RCI), so that individuals passing the clinically significant cutoff and indexing positive reliable change can be considered remitted. They found a combined CS/RCI preferable to diagnostic change in a sample of adolescents with eating disorder; for example, the "remission" and "improved" categories based on diagnostic change were larger than the remission, improved, and probably improved CS/RCI categories, and of patients who improved diagnostically, 54% were categorized as "no change" on the CS/RCI. This research supports the application of CS/RCI to

EDE-Q scores to avoid false-positive outcomes from treatment when only diagnostic change is considered (Ekeroth & Birgegård, 2014). Given that physical and behavioral features of eating disorders improve earlier than cognitive/psychological ones (Clausen, 2004), long-term assessment of progress requires a focus on the measure of cognitive symptoms.

Another perspective regarding goals for eating disorder cognitions has to do with not only decreasing maladaptive thoughts but also increasing adaptive ones. To this end, the use of the Body Appreciation Scale–2 (BAS-2; Tylka & Wood-Barcalow, 2015) and the Intuitive Eating Scale–2 (IES-2; Tylka & Kroon Van Diest, 2013) may be appropriate for adolescents. These measures assess the degree to which one accepts and feels positively toward one's body and uses physiological cues more than emotional cues to drive eating, respectively. The goal of increases in these positive constructs related to body image and eating is an option worth considering in conjunction with decreases in maladaptive behaviors and cognitions; it could also provide a sense of hopefulness.

For a more visual assessment of cognitive change that may be especially appropriate for children, a pie chart approach can be used with the youth, indicating by size of the sectors of the circle what is most important to them from a list including body appearance (weight/shape), school, friends, and so forth. This assessment taps into overvaluation of weight/shape, a core eating disorder construct. With repeated pie charts across treatment, therapist and youth get a visual representation of the shrinking of the piece of the pie focused on weight/shape and can observe which domains grow or develop to take its place.

Related to but distinct from physical, behavioral, and cognitive symptoms of eating disorders is psychosocial impairment due to eating disorders. As progress is met in physical, behavioral, and cognitive goals, reduced impairment can also be expected. The CIA (Bohn & Fairburn, 2008) is a 16-item measure examining impairment in personal (mood, self-perception), social (interpersonal functioning, work performance), and cognitive domains affected by eating disorders and yields an overall score based on the past 28 days. Importantly, it is appropriate for repeated administration to gauge progress. Although developed in adult samples, it has been used in adolescents and has psychometric support among youth as well as older adolescents (e.g., college-age; Reas, Ro, Kapstad, & Lask, 2010). When modifications have been made for younger samples, they have included things such as replacing references to "work" with "school/schoolwork." The authors note that the CIA does not assess physical impairment secondary to eating disorders and recommend that a physician track physical progress while a psychologist/therapist tracks psychological and psychosocial progress.

Process Measurement

In a review of aspects of therapeutic process in the treatment of eating disorders, Brauhardt and colleagues (2014) found that both higher motivation and better therapeutic alliance were associated with better outcomes in adolescent samples. Given these findings, they suggest that patient motivation and therapeutic alliance be assessed, so that clinicians may intervene to bolster these important process variables if need be.

Readiness to Change

Before launching into treatment, it is valuable to know how ready the client feels to make changes and move toward recovery. This is perhaps especially important in the context of AN, which can be understood as ego-syntonic (Vitousek, Watson, & Wilson, 1998) given that the attainment of thinness and perceived control over eating via food restriction often aligns with youths' values about thinness and control. Indeed, the disorder often becomes part of their identity, of who they "are," and youth may be, at best, ambivalent about change, making it more challenging to give up the eating disorder for recovery and possibly contributing to treatment dropout. Of note, the readiness to change construct is part of the earlier temporal/contextual model related to case conceptualization (Zubernis et al., 2017).

In a youth sample, Bustin, Lane-Loney, Hollenbeak, and Ornstein (2013) found that stage of change advanced across treatment and was correlated with end-of-treatment eating disorder symptoms. Importantly, initial stage of change was not associated with outcome scores but change in motivation was. In samples of adolescents with eating disorders, motivational stage of change predicted short-term outcome, with those with higher motivation needing shorter residential treatment stays to reach an adequate discharge weight (McHugh, 2007). Additionally, motivational stage has been used to identify when youth are ready for stepped-down care (Touyz, Thornton, Rieger, George, & Beumont, 2003).

The Readiness and Motivation Interview (RMI; Geller, Cockell, & Drab, 2001), a semistructured interview developed in an adult sample, yields three motivational stage scores (precontemplation, contemplation, and action) for four symptom domains (restriction, binge eating, compensatory behaviors, and cognitions), in addition to a global motivation stage score and an internality score (i.e., making changes for themselves vs. others). The RMI has partial psychometric support for its use in adolescents; assessment of precontemplation and action stages appear reliable and valid, but in its current state, the contemplation and internality assessments should not be used in adolescents (Geller et al., 2008).

As shorter alternatives, the MSCARED (Gusella et al., 2003) and the ANSOCQ (Rieger et al., 2000) are brief, self-report questionnaires assessing stages of change in relation to eating disorder recovery: precontemplation, contemplation, preparation, action, maintenance, and recovery. The ANSOCQ was designed for individuals with AN and is therefore most appropriate for those individuals; however, discreet items may be broadly applicable to other eating disorders (e.g., motivation related to changing standards used to evaluate shape/weight). The MSCARED was developed for adolescents and provides both a global picture and how stage of change may vary depending on the specific eating disorder behavior (e.g., dieting, binge eating, purging).

For measuring progress, the brief measures may be most appropriate. Both the ANSOCQ and the MSCARED can be administered at multiple points along the course of treatment to assess movement in stage of change overall and for specific target behaviors (Gusella et al., 2003). Both can also open up a dialogue related to goal selection. We recommend the MSCARED for its ability to address motivation related to a broader array of eating disorder symptoms, but when working with a client with AN, the ANSOCQ would also be appropriate.

Therapeutic Alliance

"Therapeutic alliance" refers to the collaborative relationship between therapist and client, generally including emotional connection/bond, agreement on goals, and cooperation on tasks to achieve the goals (Zaitsoff, Pullmer, Cyr, & Aime, 2015). In their review of therapeutic alliance for adolescents with eating disorders, Zaitsoff and colleagues (2015) found that parent and adolescent reports are linked to different aspects of treatment; parent-rated alliance predicted dropout from FBT and adolescent-rated alliance predicted remission. Interestingly, in the literature on adult samples, only about half of alliance studies link higher therapeutic alliance to better outcomes; however, therapeutic alliance in the context of FBT consistently predicts better outcome for adolescents and their parents (Brauhardt et al., 2014). Therapeutic alliance has been posited as a mediator of early change and treatment outcome, the idea being that early successes (e.g., reduction in binge eating) may strengthen the therapeutic alliance at the start of therapy, which facilitates further progress (McFarlane, MacDonald, Royal, & Olmsted, 2013; Raykos, Watson, Fursland, Byrne, & Nathan, 2013; Turner, Bryant-Waugh, & Marshall, 2015).

Posttreatment Monitoring of Maintenance and Relapse Prevention

More research is needed on factors predicting relapse given few consistent findings and minimal research on youth. In a 6-year prospective study of women (including older adolescents/young adults) who had remitted from BN or eating disorder not otherwise specified (EDNOS), Grilo, Pagano, and colleagues (2012) found that higher stress predicted relapse. In particular, both work stress (for youth, this could be school stress) and social stress (e.g., a serious fight with a friend) acted as triggers. To the degree that similar stressors may increase risk for relapse in youth, relapse prevention plans that focus on coping skills for responding to stressful life events are warranted.

It is critical that therapist and youth and, as appropriate, parents develop short-term and long-term maintenance plans that are mindful of problem areas and early warning signs of a lapse. Short-term plans may lay out strategies for what to do and not do in relation to challenges—for example, regarding dietary restriction, youth can be reminded to eat regularly (recommended every 4 hours) and to not practice food avoidance. The short-term plan can be considered a succinct reminder of goals and strategies. The long-term plan may focus on minimizing situations of increased risk for disordered eating and identifying warning signs of lapses (e.g., restarting/increasing body comparison, urges to binge or vomit) and strategies for responding. In both cases, maintenance plans should be tailored to the youth's experiences and minor lapses should be expected, with the focus being on problem-solving what happened and getting back on track. For examples of short-term and long-term maintenance plans developed by Fairburn and colleagues, visit *www.credo-oxford.com/ pdfs/t12.1_short-term_maintenance_plan.pdf* and *www.credo-oxford.com/pdfs/t12.2_long-term_maintenance_plan.pdf*.

Conclusion

Applying a prediction/prescription/process framework to the assessment of eating and feeding disorders yields an efficient approach to assessment. Prediction tools help identify who seems most likely to meet criteria for an eating or feeding disorder. Clinicians may want to start with one of the screeners that provide broad coverage of eating pathology and follow up from there, as needed, with a more targeted screener or directly, with the prescription tool of a structured or semistructured interview to arrive at a diagnosis. While prediction and prescription measures reflect the start of assessment and intervention, assessment should continue throughout an intervention—and beyond, to track outcome. Process measures include those that monitor progress across treatment, with the focus of psychologists being behavioral and cognitive changes and related (lessening) impairment/interference. Progress monitoring should be framed with realistic expectations of possible behavioral slips (e.g., a period without binge eating interrupted by a binge) and ideally include the assessment of longer-term outcomes to better understand recovery as an outcome and as a dynamic experience. Process measures may also include aspects that can facilitate progress, including readiness to change and therapeutic alliance. The measures included in this chapter cut across these assessment steps, provide both broad and more tailored coverage of a variety of eating and feeding disorders and symptoms, include a range of item lengths so that clinicians can consider brevity of assessment, have psychometric support in child and/or adolescent samples (although how much psychometric examination varies), and are, for the most part, available at no cost.

Based on this review, it is clear to us that the eating disorder field would benefit from more research to validate youth measures of eating and feeding disorders. This would include making sure that measures developed in adults that are being used with children/adolescents (with or without modifications) have robust psychometric support.

One particular gap in the eating and feeding disorder assessment literature is the very limited body of work applying ROC statistics to data from youth samples. More work is needed to statistically generate meaningful cutoff points that will optimize sensitivity and specificity. As that body of research increases, an important next step would be meta-analytic work to see what can be concluded with most confidence regarding assessment tools.

Another observation from this review is a critique that is applied to research in the eating disorder field in general: a lack of diversity of study participants. This is definitely a limitation in terms of race/ethnicity given that extant eating disorder and feeding assessments have been validated in primarily white samples. For measures geared toward adolescents, there is also the bias of psychometric studies focusing on females. Fortunately, there are measures that attend to concerns that may be especially relevant to male youths, including the DMS. Any new development of assessments of eating and feeding disorders should take into consideration aspects of diversity such as race, ethnicity, and gender identity, and existing ones warrant additional psychometric examination in diverse samples.

Last, there are some relatively recent developed measures that we believe are promising but did not include in the tables, since we were unable to find psychometric support for them in child or adolescent samples. The Eating Pathology Symptoms Inventory (EPSI; Forbush et al., 2013), a 45-item questionnaire, generates eight subscales: Body Dissatisfaction, Binge Eating, Cognitive Restraint, Purging, Restricting, Excessive Exercise, Negative Attitudes toward Obesity, and Muscle Building. The EPSI is commendable for its breadth of coverage and its inclusion of eating-disorder-related aspects not regularly included in broad assessments, such as weight-related stigma and muscularity focus. It has impressive psychometrics in adult samples (including college-age samples) (Forbush, Wildes, & Hunt, 2014; Forbush et al., 2013) but awaits psychometric investigation in adolescents.

The Stanford–Washington University Eating Disorders Screen (SWED; Graham et al., 2019) also deserves mention. The SWED is a brief assessment tool that is deliverable online through the National Eating Disorders Awareness (NEDA) website (*www.nationaleatingdisorders.org/screening-tool*). The use of technology to provide more equitable access to this screener, the clear algorithms applied to determine risk categories (possible AN, possible clinical or subclinical eating disorder other than AN, high risk for an eating disorder, low risk for an eating disorder), and the recommendation/referral follow-up information based on risk categories are all important directions for eating disorder assessment. The SWED was developed in college samples and has good psychometrics in those samples (e.g., Fitzsimmons-Craft et al., 2019; Graham et al., 2019). Although the NEDA screener indicates that it is appropriate for youth ages 13 and older, we were unable to find psychometric reports outside of college-age samples.

Last, the Eating Disorder Assessment for DSM-5 (EDA-5; Sysko et al., 2015) shows promise as a possible prescriptive tool. The EDA-5 was developed in adults and designed so that limited training is needed for administration and it can be administered electronically, reducing administration time (Sysko et al., 2015). As a diagnostic tool, it focuses on more recent information regarding frequencies of behavior—for example, asking about binge eating frequencies in the prior week, then asking if this was consistent across the past 3 months and, if not, how the frequency differed. This is different from the timeline followback used in the EDE and the ChEDE. The EDA-5 provides broad diagnostic coverage of the eating and feeding disorders, allowing for the diagnosis of AN, BN, BED, ARFID, pica, rumination disorder, OSFED, and USFED. A youth version of the EDA-5 is listed on the website for the assessment (*eda5.org*), but we were only able to find published psychometrics of the EDA-5 in adult samples.

In summary, the field of eating and feeding disorders has an array of assessments that fit well into the prediction/prescription/process model and include screeners for both broad pathology and more focused symptoms. More psychometric work in youth samples is needed for measures developed in adults that are applied to youth, including more sophisticated analyses, such as ROC analyses that could generate meaningful cutoff points. Additionally, more assessment research is needed for ARFID and feeding disorders, diagnoses that are new to DSM-5, and for promising measures developed in young adults that need psychometric examination in children and adolescents.

REFERENCES

American Psychiatric Association. (1994). *Diagnostic and statistical manual of mental disorders* (4th ed.). Washington, DC: Author.

American Psychiatric Association. (2013a). *Diagnostic and statistical manual of mental disorders* (5th ed.). Arlington, VA: Author.

American Psychiatric Association. (2013b). Feeding and eating disorders. Retrieved from *www.dsm5.org/documents/eating%20disorders%20fact%20sheet.pdf*.

Attia, E., & Roberto, C. A. (2009). Should amenorrhea be a diagnostic criterion for anorexia nervosa? *International Journal of Eating Disorders, 42,* 581–589.

Bardone-Cone, A. M., Higgins Neyland, M. K., & Lin, S. L. (2017). Eating disorders in racial/ethnic minorities. In J. Fries & V. Sullivan (Eds.), *Eating disorders in special populations: Medical, nutritional, and psychological treatments.* London: Taylor & Francis Group.

Beato-Fernández, L., Rodríguez-Cano, T., Belmonte-Llario, A., & Martínez-Delgado, C. (2004). Risk factors for eating disorders in adolescents: A Spanish community-based longitudinal study. *European Child and Adolescent Psychiatry, 13*(5), 287–294.

Becker, A. E., Franko, D. L., Speck, A., & Herzog, D. B. (2003). Ethnicity and differential access to care for eating disorder symptoms. *International Journal of Eating Disorders, 33*(2), 205–212.

Becker, A. E., Thomas, J. J., Bainivualiku, A., Richards, L., Navara, K., Roberts, A. L., . . . Striegel-Moore, R. H. (2010). Adaptation and evaluation of the Clinical Impairment Assessment to assess disordered eating related distress in an adolescent female ethnic Fijian population. *International Journal of Eating Disorders, 43,* 179–186.

Bellace, D. L., Tesser, R., Berthod, S., Wisotzke, K., Crosby, R. D., Crow, S. J., . . . Halmi, K. A. (2012). The Yale–Brown–Cornell Eating Disorders Scale Self-Report Questionnaire: A new, efficient tool for clinicians and researchers. *International Journal of Eating Disorders, 45,* 856–860.

Bohn, K., & Fairburn, C. G. (2008). The Clinical Impairment Assessment Questionnaire (CIA 3.0) [Appendix]. In C. G. Fairburn (Ed.), *Cognitive behavior therapy and eating disorders* (pp. 315–318). New York: Guilford Press.

Brannan, A. M., Athay, M. M., & Vides de Andrade, A. R. (2012). Measurement quality of the Caregiver Strain Questionnaire-Short Form 7 (CGSQ-SF7). *Administration and Policy in Mental Health and Mental Health Services Research, 39*(1–2), 51–59.

Brannan, A. M., Heflinger, C. A., & Bickman, L. (1997). The Caregiver Strain Questionnaire: Measuring the impact on the family of living with a child with serious emotional disturbance. *Journal of Emotional and Behavioral Disorders, 5*(4), 212–222.

Bratland-Sanda, S., & Sundgot-Borgen, J. (2013). Eating disorders in athletes: Overview of prevalence, risk factors and recommendations for prevention and treatment. *European Journal of Sport Science, 13,* 499–508.

Brauhardt, A., de Zwaan, M., & Hilbert, A. (2014). The therapeutic process in psychological treatments for eating disorders: A systematic review. *International Journal of Eating Disorders, 47*(6), 565–584.

Braun, T. D., Park, C. L., & Gorin, A. (2016). Self-compassion, body image, and disordered eating: A review of the literature. *Body Image, 17,* 117–131.

Brigham, K. S., Manzo, L. D., Eddy, K. T., & Thomas, J. J. (2018). Evaluation and treatment of avoidant/restrictive food intake disorder (ARFID) in adolescents. *Current Pediatrics Reports, 6*(2), 107–113.

Bronfenbrenner, U. (1981). *The ecology of human development: Experiments by nature and design.* Cambridge, MA: Harvard University Press.

Brunet, J., Sabiston, C. M., Dorsch, K. D., & McCreary, D. R. (2010). Exploring a model linking social physique anxiety, drive for muscularity, drive for thinness and self-esteem among adolescent boys and girls. *Body Image, 7*(2), 137–142.

Bryant-Waugh, R., & Cooke, L. (2017). Development of the PARDI (Pica, ARFID, Rumination Disorder Interview): A structured assessment measure and diagnostic tool for feeding disorders. *Archives of Disease in Childhood, 102*(3), A29.

Bryant-Waugh, R. J., Cooper, P. J., Taylor, C. L., & Lask, B. D. (1996). The use of the Eating Disorder Examination with children: A pilot study. *International Journal of Eating Disorders, 19,* 391–397.

Bryant-Waugh, R., Micali, N., Cooke, L., Lawson, E. A., Eddy, K. T., & Thomas, J. J. (2019). Development of the Pica, ARFID, and Rumination Disorder Interview, a multi-informant, semi-structured interview of feeding disorders across the lifespan: A pilot study for ages 10–22. *International Journal of Eating Disorders, 52,* 378–387.

Bustin, L. A., Lane-Loney, S. E., Hollenbeak, C. S., & Ornstein, R. M. (2013). Motivational stage of change in young patients undergoing day treatment for eating disorders. *International Journal of Adolescent Medicine and Health, 25*(2), 151–156.

Carnell, S., & Wardle, J. (2007). Measuring behavioural susceptibility to obesity: Validation of the Child Eating Behaviour Questionnaire. *Appetite, 48*(1), 104–113.

Carter, J. C., Stewart, D. A., & Fairburn, C. G. (2001). Eating Disorder Examination Questionnaire: Norms for young adolescent girls. *Behaviour Research and Therapy, 39,* 625–632.

Chiba, H., Nagamitsu, S., Sakurai, R., Mukai, T., Shintou, H., Koyanagi, K., . . . Matsuishi, T. (2016). Children's Eating Attitudes Test: Reliability and validation in Japanese adolescents. *Eating Behaviors, 23,* 120–125.

Ciao, A. C., Accurso, E. C., Fitzsimmons-Craft, E. E., & Le Grange, D. (2015). Predictors and moderators of psychological changes during the treatment of adolescent bulimia nervosa. *Behaviour Research and Therapy, 69,* 48–53.

Ciao, A. C., Accurso, E. C., Fitzsimmons-Craft, E. E., Lock, J., & Le Grange, D. (2015). Family functioning in two treatments for adolescent anorexia nervosa. *International Journal of Eating Disorders, 48*(1), 81–90.

Clausen, L. (2004). Time course of symptom remission in eating disorders. *International Journal of Eating Disorders, 36*(3), 296–306.

Cole, T. J., Flegal, K. M., Nicholls, D., & Jackson, A. A. (2007). Body mass index cut offs to define thinness in children and adolescents: International survey. *British Medical Journal, 335*(7612), 194.

Colton, P. A., Olmsted, M. P., Daneman, D., Farquhar, J. C., Wong, H., Muskat, S., & Rodin, G. M. (2015). Eating disorders in girls and women with type 1 diabetes: A longitudinal study of prevalence, onset, remission, and recurrence. *Diabetes Care, 38*(7), 1212–1217.

Colton, P. A., Olmsted, M. P., & Rodin, G. M. (2007). Eating disturbances in a school population of preteen girls: Assessment and screening. *International Journal of Eating Disorders, 40,* 435–440.

Cooper, Z., Allen, E., Bailey-Straebler, S., Basden, S., Murphy, R., O'Connor, M. E., & Fairburn, C. G. (2016). Predictors and moderators of response to enhanced cognitive behaviour therapy and interpersonal psychotherapy for the treatment of eating disorders. *Behaviour Research and Therapy, 84,* 9–13.

Couturier, J. L., & Lock, J. (2006). Denial and minimization in adolescents with anorexia nervosa. *International Journal of Eating Disorders, 39*(3), 212–216.

Crist, W., McDonnell, P., Beck, M., Gillespie, C. T., Barrett, P., & Mathews, J. (1994). Behavior at mealtimes and the young child with cystic fibrosis. *Developmental and Behavioral Pediatrics, 15,* 157–161.

Crist, W., & Napier-Phillips, A. (2001). Mealtime behaviors of young children: A comparison of normative and clinical data. *Journal of Developmental and Behavioral Pediatrics, 22*(5), 279–286.

Cumella, E. J. (2006). Review of the Eating Disorder Inventory–3. *Journal of Personality Assessment, 87*(1), 116–117.

Dooley-Hash, S., Banker, J. D., Walton, M. A., Ginsburg, Y., & Cunningham, R. M. (2012). The prevalence and correlates of eating disorders among emergency department patients aged 14–20 years. *International Journal of Eating Disorders, 45*(7), 883–890.

Doyle, P. M., Le Grange, D., Loeb, K., Doyle, A. C., & Crosby, R. D. (2010). Early response to family-based treatment for adolescent anorexia nervosa. *International Journal of Eating Disorders, 43*(7), 659–662.

Dyl, J., Kittler, J., Phillips, K. A., & Hunt, J. I. (2006). Body dysmorphic disorder and other clinically significant body image concerns in adolescent psychiatric inpatients: Prevalence and clinical characteristics. *Child Psychiatry and Human Development, 36*(4), 369–382.

Eddy, K. T., Dorer, D. J., Franko, D. L., Tahilani, K., Thompson-Brenner, H., & Herzog, D. B. (2008). Diagnostic crossover in anorexia nervosa and bulimia nervosa: Implications for DSM-V. *American Journal of Psychiatry, 165,* 245–250.

Eddy, K. T., Thomas, J. J., Hastings, E., Edkins, K., Lamont, E., Nevins, C. M., . . . Becker, A. E. (2015). Prevalence of DSM-5 avoidant/restrictive food intake disorder in a pediatric gastroenterology healthcare network. *International Journal of Eating Disorders, 48*, 464–470.

Eisler, I., Dare, C., Hodes, M., Russell, G., Dodge, E., & Le Grange, D. (2000). Family therapy for adolescent anorexia nervosa: The results of a controlled comparison of two family interventions. *Journal of Child Psychology and Psychiatry and Allied Disciplines, 41*(6), 727–736.

Ekeroth, K., & Birgegård, A. (2014). Evaluating reliable and clinically significant change in eating disorders: Comparisons to changes in DSM-IV diagnoses. *Psychiatry Research, 216*(2), 248–254.

Epstein, N. B., Baldwin, L. M., & Bishop, D. S. (1983). The McMaster Family Assessment Device. *Journal of Marital and Family Therapy, 9*(2), 171–180.

Estecha Querol, S., Fernandez Alvira, J. M., Mesana Graffe, M. I., Nova Rebato, E., Marcos Sanchez, A., & Moreno Aznar, L. A. (2016). Nutrient intake in Spanish adolescents SCOFF high-scorers: The AVENA study. *Eating and Weight Disorders, 21*, 589–596.

Fairburn, C. G. (2008). Eating Disorder Examination (16.0D). In C. G. Fairburn (Ed.), *Cognitive behavior therapy and eating disorders* (pp. 265–308). New York: Guilford Press.

Fairburn, C. G., & Beglin, S. J. (2008). Eating Disorder Examination Questionnaire (6.0) [Appendix]. In C. G. Fairburn (Ed.), *Cognitive behavior therapy and eating disorders* (pp. 309–314). New York: Guilford Press.

Fairburn, C. G., & Cooper, Z. (1993). The eating disorder examination. In C. G. Fairburn & G. T. Wilson (Eds.), *Binge eating: Nature, assessment, and treatment* (12th ed., pp. 317–360). New York: Guilford Press.

Fairburn, C. G., & Harrison, P. J. (2003). Eating disorders. *Lancet, 361*, 407–416.

Fan, Y., Li, Y., Liu, A., Hu, X., Ma, G., & Xu, G. (2010). Associations between body mass index, weight control concerns and behaviors, and eating disorder symptoms among non-clinical Chinese adolescents. *BMC Public Health, 10*, 314.

Feenstra, D. J., Busschbach, J. J., Verheul, R., & Hutsebaut, J. (2011). Prevalence and comorbidity of Axis I and Axis II disorders among treatment refractory adolescents admitted for specialized psychotherapy. *Journal of Personality Disorders, 25*(6), 842–850.

Ferreiro, F., Seoane, G., & Senra, C. (2012). Gender-related risk and protective factors for depressive symptoms and disordered eating in adolescence: A 4-year longitudinal study. *Journal of Youth and Adolescence, 41*(5), 607–622.

Fisher, M. M., Rosen, D. S., Ornstein, R. M., Mammel, K. A., Katzman, D. K., Rome, E. S., . . . Walsh, B. T. (2014). Characteristics of avoidant/restrictive food intake disorder in children and adolescents: A "new disorder" in DSM-5. *Journal of Adolescent Health, 55*(1), 49–52.

Fitzmaurice, G. M., Laird, N. M., Zahner, G. E., & Daskalakis, C. (1995). Bivariate logistic regression analysis of childhood psychopathology ratings using multiple informants. *American Journal of Epidemiology, 142*, 1194–1203.

Fitzsimmons-Craft, E. E., Balantekin, K. N., Eichen, D. M., Graham, A. K., Monterubio, G. E., Sadeh-Sharvit, S., . . . Wilfley, D. E. (2019). Screening and offering online programs for eating disorders: Reach, pathology, and differences across eating disorder status groups at 28 U.S. universities. *International Journal of Eating Disorders, 52*(10), 1125–1136.

Forbush, K. T., Wildes, J. E., & Hunt, T. K. (2014). Gender norms, psychometric properties, and validity for the Eating Pathology Symptoms Inventory. *International Journal of Eating Disorders, 47*(1), 85–91.

Forbush, K. T., Wildes, J. E., Pollack, L. O., Dunbar, D., Luo, J., Patterson, K., . . . Bright, A. (2013). Development and validation of the Eating Pathology Symptoms Inventory (EPSI). *Psychological Assessment, 25*(3), 859–878.

Fortes, L., Kakeshita, I. S., Almeida, S. S., Gomes, A. R., & Ferreira, M. E. C. (2014). Eating behaviours in youths: A comparison between female and male athletes and non-athletes. *Scandinavian Journal of Medicine and Science in Sports, 24*, e62–e68.

Franko, D. L. (2007). Race, ethnicity, and eating disorders: Considerations for DSM-V. *International Journal of Eating Disorders, 40*(Suppl.), S31–S34.

Garner, D. M. (2004). *Eating Disorder Inventory–3: Professional manual*. Lutz, FL: Psychological Assessment Resources.

Garner, D. M., Olmsted, M. P., Bohr, Y., & Garfinkel, P. (1982). The Eating Attitudes Test: Psychometric features and clinical correlates. *Psychological Medicine, 12*, 871–878.

Garner, D. M., Olmsted, M. P., & Polivy, J. (1983). Development and validation of a multidimensional eating disorder inventory for anorexia nervosa and bulimia. *International Journal of Eating Disorders, 2*, 15–34.

Geller, J., Brown, K. E., Zaitsoff, S. L., Menna, R., Bates, M. E., & Dunn, E. C. (2008). Assessing readiness for change in adolescents with eating disorders. *Psychological Assessment, 20*, 63–69.

Geller, J., Cockell, S. J., & Drab, D. L. (2001). Assessing readiness for change in the eating disorders: The psychometric properties of the Readiness and Motivation Interview. *Psychological Assessment, 13*(2), 189–198.

Goodman, R., Ford, T., Richards, H., Gatward, R., & Meltzer, H. (2000). The development and well-being assessment: Description and initial validation of an integrated assessment of child and adolescent psychopathology. *Journal of Child Psychology and Psychiatry, 41*(5), 645–655.

Gordon, K. H., Brattole, M. M., Wingate, L. R., & Joiner, T. E., Jr. (2006). The impact of client race on clinician detection of eating disorders. *Behavior Therapy, 37*(4), 319–325.

Gordon, K. H., Perez, M., & Joiner, T. E., Jr. (2002).

The impact of racial stereotypes on eating disorder recognition. *International Journal of Eating Disorders, 32*(2), 219–224.

Graham, A. K., Trockel, M., Weisman, H., Fitzsimmons-Craft, E. E., Balantekin, K. N., Wilfley, D. E., & Taylor, C. B. (2019). A screening tool for detecting eating disorder risk and diagnostic symptoms among college-age women. *Journal of American College Health, 67,* 357–366.

Gregertsen, E. C., Mandy, W., Kanakam, N., Armstrong, S., & Serpell, L. (2019). Pre-treatment patient characteristics as predictors of drop-out and treatment outcome in individual and family therapy for adolescents and adults with anorexia nervosa: A systematic review and meta-analysis. *Psychiatry Research, 271,* 484–501.

Grilo, C. M., Pagano, M. E., Stout, R. L., Markowitz, J. C., Ansell, E. B., Pinto, A., . . . Skodol, A. E. (2012). Stressful life events predict eating disorder relapse following remission: Six-year prospective outcomes. *International Journal of Eating Disorders, 45*(2), 185–192.

Grilo, C. M., White, M. A., Wilson, G. T., Gueorguieva, R., & Masheb, R. M. (2012). Rapid response predicts 12-month post-treatment outcomes in binge-eating disorder: Theoretical and clinical implications. *Psychological Medicine, 42*(4), 807–817.

Gull, W. W. (1874). Anorexia nervosa. *Transactions of the Clinical Society of London, 7,* 22–28.

Gusella, J., Butler, G., Nichols, L., & Bird, D. (2003). A brief questionnaire to assess readiness to change in adolescents with eating disorders: Its applications to group therapy. *European Eating Disorders Review, 11,* 58–71.

Hay, P., Mitchison, D., Collado, A. E. L., Gonzalez-Chica, D. A., Stocks, N., & Touyz, S. (2017). Burden and health-related quality of life of eating disorders, including Avoidant/Restrictive Food Intake Disorder (ARFID), in the Australian population. *Journal of Eating Disorders, 5,* 21.

Hazzard, V. M., Hahn, S. L., & Sonneville, K. R. (2017). Weight misperception and disordered weight control behaviors among US high school students with overweight and obesity: Associations and trends, 1999–2013. *Eating Behaviors, 26,* 189–195.

Heatherton, T. F., & Baumeister, R. F. (1991). Binge eating as escape from self-awareness. *Psychological Bulletin, 110*(1), 86–108.

Hilbert, A., Buerger, A., Hartmann, A. S., Spenner, K., Czaja, J., & Warschburger, P. (2013). Psychometric evaluation of the Eating Disorder Examination adapted for children. *European Eating Disorders Review, 21,* 330–339.

Horton, N. J., & Fitzmaurice, G. M. (2004). Regression analysis of multiple source and multiple informant data from complex survey samples. *Statistics in Medicine, 23,* 2911–2933.

Hoste, R. R., Labuschagne, Z., & Le Grange, D. (2012).

Adolescent bulimia nervosa. *Current Psychiatry Reports, 14,* 391–397.

House, J., Eisler, I., Simic, M., & Micali, N. (2008). Diagnosing eating disorders in adolescents: A comparison of the Eating Disorder Examination and the Development and Well-Being Assessment. *International Journal of Eating Disorders, 41*(6), 535–541.

Hudson, J. I., Hiripi, E., Pope, H. G., Jr., & Kessler, R. C. (2007). The prevalence and correlates of eating disorders in the National Comorbidity Survey Replication. *Biological Psychiatry, 61*(3), 348–358.

Hughes, E. K., Sawyer, S. M., Accurso, E. C., Singh, S., & Le Grange, D. (2019). Predictors of early response in conjoint and separated models of family-based treatment for adolescent anorexia nervosa. *European Eating Disorders Review, 27*(3), 283–294.

Jaite, C., Hoffmann, F., Glaeske, G., & Bachmann, C. J. (2013). Prevalence, comorbidities and outpatient treatment of anorexia and bulimia nervosa in German children and adolescents. *Eating and Weight Disorders, 18*(2), 157–165.

Jennings, K. M., & Phillips, K. E. (2017). Eating Disorder Examination–Questionnaire (EDE–Q): Norms for clinical sample of female adolescents with anorexia nervosa. *Archives of Psychiatric Nursing, 31*(6), 578–581.

Johnson, W. G., Grieve, F. G., Adams, C. D., & Sandy, J. (1999). Measuring binge eating in adolescents: Adolescent and parent versions of the Questionnaire of Eating and Weight Patterns. *International Journal of Eating Disorders, 26*(3), 301–314.

Johnson, W. G., Kirk, A. A., & Reed, A. E. (2001). Adolescent version of the Questionnaire of Eating and Weight Patterns: Reliability and gender differences. *International Journal of Eating Disorders, 29*(1), 94–96.

Kang, Q., Chan, R. C. K., Li, X., Arcelus, J., Yue, L., Huang, J., . . . Chen, J. (2017). Psychometric properties of the Chinese version of the Eating Attitudes Test in young female patients with eating disorders in mainland China. *European Eating Disorders Review, 25,* 613–617.

Kaufman, J., Birmaher, B., Brent, D., Rao, U. M. A., Flynn, C., Moreci, P., . . . Ryan, N. (1997). Schedule for Affective Disorders and Schizophrenia for School-Age Children—Present and Lifetime version (K-SADS-PL): Initial reliability and validity data. *Journal of the American Academy of Child and Adolescent Psychiatry, 36,* 980–988.

Kehayes, I.-L. L., Smith, M. M., Sherry, S. B., Vidovic, V., & Saklofske, D. H. (2019). Are perfectionism dimensions risk factors for bulimic symptoms?: A meta-analysis of longitudinal studies. *Personality and Individual Differences, 138,* 117–125.

Klump, K. L., Perkins, P. S., Burt, S. A., McGue, M., & Iacono, W. G. (2007). Puberty moderate genetic influences on disordered eating. *Psychological Medicine, 37,* 627–634.

Klump, K. L., Suisman, J. L., Burt, S. A., McGue, M., & Iacono, W. G. (2009). Genetic and environmental influences on disordered eating: An adoption study. *Journal of Abnormal Psychology, 118,* 797–805.

Kortegaard, L. S., Hoerder, K., Joergensen, J. G., Gillberg, C., & Kyvik, K. O. (2001). A preliminary population-based twin study of self-reported eating disorder. *Psychological Medicine, 31,* 361–365.

Kurz, S., van Dyck, Z., Dremmel, D., Munsch, S., & Hilbert, A. (2015). Early-onset restrictive eating disturbances in primary school boys and girls. *European Child and Adolescent Psychiatry, 24*(7), 779–785.

Kurz, S., van Dyck, Z., Dremmel, D., Munsch, S., & Hilbert, A. (2016). Variants of early-onset restrictive eating disturbances in middle childhood. *International Journal of Eating Disorders, 49,* 102–106.

Lasègue, E. C. (1873). De l'anorexie hystérique. *Archives Generales de Médicine, 21,* 385–403.

Le Grange, D., Crosby, R. D., & Lock, J. (2008). Predictors and moderators of outcome in family-based treatment for adolescent bulimia nervosa. *Journal of the American Academy of Child and Adolescent Psychiatry, 47*(4), 464–470.

Le Grange, D., Doyle, P., Crosby, R. D., & Chen, E. (2008). Early response to treatment in adolescent bulimia nervosa. *International Journal of Eating Disorders, 41*(8), 755–757.

Le Grange, D., Hoste, R. R., Lock, J., & Bryson, S. W. (2011). Parental expressed emotion of adolescents with anorexia nervosa: Outcome in family-based treatment. *International Journal of Eating Disorders, 44,* 731–734.

Le Grange, D., Lock, J., Agras, W. S., Moye, A., Bryson, S. W., Jo, B., & Kraemer, H. C. (2012). Moderators and mediators of remission in family-based treatment and adolescent focused therapy for anorexia nervosa. *Behaviour Research and Therapy, 50*(2), 85–92.

Lee, S. W., Stewart, S. M., Striegel-Moore, R. H., Lee, S., Ho, S., Lee, P. W. H., . . . Lam, T. (2007). Validation of the Eating Disorder Diagnostic Scale for use with Hong Kong adolescents. *International Journal of Eating Disorders, 40,* 569–574.

Leon, G. R., Fulkerson, J. A., Perry, C. L., Keel, P. K., & Klump, K. L. (1999). Three to four year prospective evaluation of personality and behavioral risk factors for later disordered eating in adolescent girls and boys. *Journal of Youth and Adolescence, 28*(2), 181–196.

Lichtenstein, M. B., Hemmingsen, S. D., & Støving, R. K. (2017). Identification of eating disorder symptoms in Danish adolescents with the SCOFF Questionnaire. *Nordic Journal of Psychiatry, 71*(5), 340–347.

Littleton, H. L., & Ollendick, T. (2003). Negative body image and disordered eating behavior in children and adolescents: What places youth at risk and how can these problems be prevented? *Clinical Child and Family Psychology Review, 6*(1), 51–66.

Lock, J., Agras, W. S., Bryson, S., & Kraemer, H. C. (2005). A comparison of short- and long-term family therapy for adolescent anorexia nervosa. *Journal of the American Academy of Child and Adolescent Psychiatry, 44*(7), 632–639.

Lock, J., Couturier, J., Bryson, S., & Agras, S. (2006). Predictors of dropout and remission in family therapy for adolescent anorexia nervosa in a randomized control trial. *International Journal of Eating Disorders, 39,* 639–647.

Lock, J., & La Via, M. C. (2015). Practice parameter for the assessment and treatment of children and adolescents with eating disorders. *Journal of the American Academy of Child and Adolescent Psychiatry, 54*(5), 412–425.

Loeb, K. L., Jones, J., Roberto, C. A., Gugga, S. S., Marcus, S. M., Attia, E., & Walsh, B. T. (2011). Adolescent–adult discrepancies on the Eating Disorder Examination: A function of developmental stage or severity of illness? *International Journal of Eating Disorders, 44,* 567–572.

Lommi, S., Viljakainen, H. T., Weiderpass, E., & de Oliveira Figueiredo, R. A. (2019). Children's Eating Attitudes Test (ChEAT): A validation study in Finnish children. *Eating and Weight Disorders.* [Epub ahead of print]

Machado, P. P. P., Martins, C., Vaz, A. R., Conceição, E., Bastos, A. P., & Gonçalves, S. (2014). Eating Disorder Examination Questionnaire: Psychometric properties and norms for the Portuguese population. *European Eating Disorders Review, 22*(6), 448–453.

Madowitz, J., Liang, J., Peterson, C. B., Rydell, S., Zucker, N. L., Tanofsky-Kraff, M., . . . Boutelle, K. N. (2014). Concurrent and convergent validity of the eating in the absence of hunger questionnaire and behavioral paradigm in overweight children. *International Journal of Eating Disorders, 47*(3), 287–295.

Mairs, R., & Nicholls, D. (2016). Assessment and treatment of eating disorders in children and adolescents. *Archives of Disease in Childhood, 101*(12), 1168–1175.

Maloney, M. J., McGuire, J. B., & Daniels, S. R. (1988). Reliability testing of a children's version of the Eating Attitude Test. *Journal of the American Academy of Child and Adolescent Psychiatry, 27,* 541–543.

Maloney, M. J., McGuire, J., Daniels, S., & Specker, B. (1989). Dieting behavior and eating attitudes in children. *Pediatrics, 84,* 482–489.

Marques, L., Alegria, M., Becker, A. E., Chen, C. N., Fang, A., Chosak, A., & Diniz, J. B. (2011). Comparative prevalence, correlates of impairment, and service utilization for eating disorders across US ethnic groups: Implications for reducing ethnic disparities in health care access for eating disorders. *International Journal of Eating Disorders, 44,* 412–420.

McCreary, D. R., & Sasse, D. K. (2000). An exploration of the drive for muscularity in adolescent boys and girls. *Journal of American College Health, 48*(6), 297–304.

McFarlane, T. L., MacDonald, D. E., Royal, S., & Olmsted, M. P. (2013). Rapid and slow responders to eating disorder treatment: A comparison on clinically relevant variables. *International Journal of Eating Disorders, 46*(6), 563–566.

McHugh, M. D. (2007). Readiness for change and short-term outcomes of female adolescents in residential treatment for anorexia nervosa. *International Journal of Eating Disorders, 40,* 602–612.

Miller, I. W., Epstein, N. B., Bishop, D. S., & Keitner, G. I. (1985). The McMaster Family Assessment Device: Reliability and validity. *Journal of Marital and Family Therapy, 11,* 345–356.

Mitchell, J. E., Hatsukami, D., Eckert, E. D., & Pyle, R. L. (1985). Characteristics of 275 patients with bulimia. *American Journal of Psychiatry, 142,* 482–485.

Morgan, J. F., Reid, F., & Lacey, J. H. (1999). The SCOFF questionnaire: Assessment of a new screening tool for eating disorders. *British Medical Journal, 319*(7223), 1467–1468.

Murray, H. B., Thomas, J. J., Hinz, A., Munsch, S., & Hilbert, A. (2018). Prevalence in primary school youth of pica and rumination behavior: The understudied feeding disorders. *International Journal of Eating Disorders, 51,* 994–998.

Murray, S. B., Loeb, K. L., & Le Grange, D. (2015). Moderators and mediators of treatments for youth with eating disorders. In M. Maric, P. J. M. Prins, & T. H. Ollendick (Eds.), *Moderators and mediators of youth treatment outcomes* (pp. 210–229). New York: Oxford University Press.

Neumark-Sztainer, D., Patterson, J., Mellin, A., Ackard, D. M., Utter, J., Story, M., & Sockalosky, J. (2002). Weight control practices and disordered eating behaviors among adolescent females and males with type 1 diabetes: Associations with sociodemographics, weight concerns, familial factors, and metabolic outcomes. *Diabetes Care, 25*(8), 1289–1296.

Neumark-Sztainer, D., Wall, M., Eisenberg, M. E., Story, M., & Hannan, P. J. (2006). Overweight status and weight control behaviors in adolescents: Longitudinal and secular trends from 1999 to 2004. *Preventive Medicine, 43*(1), 52–59.

Nicholls, D., & Bryant-Waugh, R. (2009). Eating disorders of infancy and childhood: Definition, symptomatology, epidemiology, and comorbidity. *Child and Adolescent Psychiatric Clinics of North America, 18,* 17–30.

Norris, M. L., Spettigue, W. J., & Katzman, D. K. (2016). Update on eating disorders: Current perspectives on avoidant/restrictive food intake disorder in children and youth. *Neuropsychiatric Disease and Treatment, 12,* 213–218.

Pauli, D., Aebi, M., Metzke, C. W., & Steinhausen, H.-C. (2017). Motivation to change, coping, and self-esteem in adolescent anorexia nervosa: A validation study of the Anorexia Nervosa Stages of Change Questionnaire (ANSOCQ). *Journal of Eating Disorders, 5,* 11.

Penelo, E., Negrete, A., Portell, M., & Raich, R. M. (2013). Psychometric properties of the Eating Disorder Examination Questionnaire (EDE-Q) and norms for rural and urban adolescent males and females in Mexico. *PLOS ONE, 8*(12), e83245.

Petersen, A. C., Crockett, L., Richards, M., & Boxer, A. (1988). A self-report measure of pubertal status: Reliability, validity, and initial norms. *Journal of Youth and Adolescence, 17,* 117–133.

Pinus, U., Canetti, L., Bonne, O., & Bachar, E. (2019). Selflessness as a predictor of remission from an eating disorder: 1–4 year outcomes from an adolescent day-care unit. *Eating and Weight Disorders, 24*(4), 777–786.

Ramsay, M., Martel, C., Porporino, M., & Zygmuntowicz, C. (2011). The Montreal Children's Hospital Feeding Scale: A brief bilingual screening tool for identifying feeding problems. *Paediatrics and Child Health, 16*(3), 147–151, e16–e17.

Raykos, B. C., Watson, H. J., Fursland, A., Byrne, S. M., & Nathan, P. (2013). Prognostic value of rapid response to enhanced cognitive behavioral therapy in a routine clinic sample of eating disorder outpatients. *International Journal of Eating Disorders, 46*(8), 764–770.

Reas, D. L., Ro, O., Kapstad, H., & Lask, B. (2010). Psychometric properties of the Clinical Impairment Assessment: Norms for young adult women. *International Journal of Eating Disorders, 43,* 72–76.

Rieger, E., Touyz, S. W., & Beumont, P. J. V. (2002). The Anorexia Stages of Change Questionnaire (ANSOCQ): Information regarding its psychometric properties. *International Journal of Eating Disorders, 32,* 24–38.

Rieger, E., Touyz, S., Schotte, D., Beumont, P., Russell, J., Clarke, S., . . . Griffiths, R. (2000). Development of an instrument to assess readiness to recover in anorexia nervosa. *International Journal of Eating Disorders, 28*(4), 387–396.

Rogers, S., Ramsay, M., & Blissett, J. (2018). The Montreal Children's Hospital Feeding Scale: Relationships with parental report of child eating behaviours and observed feeding interactions. *Appetite, 125,* 201–209.

Rozzell, K., Moon, D. Y., Klimek, P., Brown, T., & Blashill, A. J. (2019). Prevalence of eating disorders among us children aged 9 to 10 years: Data from the Adolescent Brain Cognitive Development (ABCD) study. *JAMA Pediatrics, 173*(1), 100–101.

Rueda Jaimes, G., Martínez, L. D., Barajas, D. O., Plata, C. P., Martínez, J. R., & Afanador, L. C. (2005). Validación del cuestionario SCOFF para el cribado dè los trastornos del comportamiento alimentario en adolescentes escolarizadas [Validation of the SCOFF questionnaire for screening the eating behaviour disorders of adolescents in school]. *Atención Primaria, 35*(2), 89–94.

Serpell, L., Treasure, J., Teasdale, J., & Sullivan, V. (1999). Anorexia nervosa: Friend or foe? *International Journal of Eating Disorders, 25*(2), 177–186.

Serrano, E., Castro, J., Ametller, L., Martinez, E., & Toro, J. (2004). Validity of a measure of readiness to recover in Spanish adolescent patients with anorexia nervosa. *Psychology and Psychotherapy: Theory, Research, and Practice, 77,* 91–99.

Shomaker, L. B., Tanofsky-Kraff, M., Elliott, C., Wolkoff, L. E., Columbo, K. M., Ranzenhofer, L. M., . . . Yanovski, J. A. (2010). Salience of loss of control for pediatric binge episodes: Does size really matter? *International Journal of Eating Disorders, 43*(8), 707–716.

Skeer, M. R., & Ballard, E. L. (2013). Are family meals as good for youth as we think they are?: A review of the literature on family meals as they pertain to adolescent risk prevention. *Journal of Youth and Adolescence, 42*(7), 943–963.

Smolak, L., & Levine, M. P. (1994). Psychometric properties of the Children's Eating Attitudes Test. *International Journal of Eating Disorders, 16,* 275–282.

Steinberg, E., Tanofsky-Kraff, M., Cohen, M. L., Elberg, J., Freedman, R. J., Semega-Janneh, M., . . . Yanovski, J. A. (2004). Comparison of the child and parent forms of the Questionnaire on Eating and Weight Patterns in the assessment of children's eating-disordered behaviors. *International Journal of Eating Disorders, 36*(2), 183–194.

Stice, E., Davis, K., Miller, N. P., & Marti, C. (2008). Fasting increases risk for onset of binge eating and bulimic pathology: A 5-year prospective study. *Journal of Abnormal Psychology, 117,* 941–946.

Stice, E., Fisher, M., & Martinez, E. (2004). Eating Disorder Diagnostic Scale: Additional evidence of reliability and validity. *Psychological Assessment, 16*(1), 60–71.

Stice, E., Gau, J. M., Rohde, P., & Shaw, H. (2017). Risk factors that predict future onset of each DSM-5 eating disorder: Predictive specificity in high-risk adolescent females. *Journal of Abnormal Psychology, 126,* 38–51.

Stice, E., Killen, J. D., Hayward, C., & Taylor, C. B. (1998). Age of onset for binge eating and purging during late adolescence: A 4-year survival analysis. *Journal of Abnormal Psychology, 107,* 671–675.

Stice, E., Marti, C. N., & Rohde, P. (2013). Prevalence, incidence, impairment, and course of the proposed DSM-5 eating disorder diagnoses in an 8-year prospective community study of young women. *Journal of Abnormal Psychology, 122,* 445–457.

Stice, E., Telch, C. F., & Rizvi, S. L. (2000). Development and validation of the Eating Disorder Diagnostic Scale: A brief self-report measure of anorexia, bulimia, and binge-eating disorder. *Psychological Assessment, 12,* 123–131.

Swanson, S. A., Aloisio, K. M., Horton, N. J., Sonneville, K. R., Crosby, R. D., Eddy, K. T., . . . Micali, N. (2014). Assessing eating disorder symptoms in adolescence: Is there a role for multiple informants? *International Journal of Eating Disorders, 47*(5), 475–482.

Swanson, S. A., Crow, S. J., Le Grange, D., Swendsen, J., & Merikangas, K. R. (2011). Prevalence and corre-lates of eating disorders in adolescents: Results from the National Comorbidity Survey Replication Adolescent Supplement. *Archives of General Psychiatry, 68,* 714–723.

Sysko, R., Glasofer, D. R., Hildebrandt, T., Klimek, P., Mitchell, J. E., Berg, K. C., . . . Walsh, B. T. (2015). The Eating Disorder Assessment for DSM-5 (EDA-5): Development and validation of a structured interview for feeding and eating disorders. *International Journal of Eating Disorders, 48*(5), 452–463.

Tamminen, K. A., Holt, N. L., & Crocker, P. R. E. (2012). Adolescent athletes: Psychosocial challenges and clinical concerns. *Current Opinion in Psychiatry, 25*(4), 293–300.

Tanner, J. M. (1981). Growth and maturation during adolescence. *Nutrition Reviews, 39*(2), 43–55.

Tanofsky-Kraff, M., Goossens, L., Eddy, K. T., Ringham, R., Goldschmidt, A., Yanovski, S. Z., . . . Yanovski, J. A. (2007). A multisite investigation of binge eating behaviors in children and adolescents. *Journal of Consulting and Clinical Psychology, 75,* 901–913.

Tanofsky-Kraff, M., Marcus, M. D., Yanovski, S. Z., & Yanovski, J. A. (2008). Loss of control eating disorder in children age 12 years and younger: Proposed research criteria. *Eating Behaviors, 9,* 360–365.

Tanofsky-Kraff, M., Ranzenhofer, L. M., Yanovski, S. Z., Schvey, N. A., Faith, M., Gustafson, J., & Yanovski, J. A. (2008). Psychometric properties of a new questionnaire to assess eating in the absence of hunger in children and adolescents. *Appetite, 51*(1), 148–155.

Tanofsky-Kraff, M., Theim, K. R., Yanovski, S. Z., Bassett, A. M., Burns, N. P., Ranzenhofer, L. M., . . . Yanovski, J. A. (2007). Validation of the Emotional Eating Scale adapted for use in children and adolescents (EES-C). *International Journal of Eating Disorders, 40*(3), 232–240.

Thomas, J. J., Vartanian, L. R., & Brownell, K. D. (2009). The relationship between eating disorder not otherwise specified (EDNOS) and officially recognized eating disorders: Meta-analysis and implications for DSM. *Psychological Bulletin, 135,* 407–433.

Thompson-Brenner, H., Shingleton, R. M., Sauer-Zavala, S., Richards, L. K., & Pratt, E. M. (2015). Multiple measures of rapid response as predictors of remission in cognitive behavior therapy for bulimia nervosa. *Behaviour Research and Therapy, 64,* 9–14.

Touyz, S., Thornton, C., Rieger, E., George, L., & Beumont, P. (2003). The incorporation of the stage of change model in the day hospital treatment of patients with anorexia nervosa. *European Child and Adolescent Psychiatry, 12*(Suppl. 1), i65–i71.

Truby, H., & Paxton, S. J. (2002). Development of the Children's Body Image Scale. *British Journal of Clinical Psychology, 41*(2), 185–203.

Truby, H., & Paxton, S. J. (2008). The Children's Body Image Scale: Reliability and use with international standards for body mass index. *British Journal of Clinical Psychology, 47,* 119–124.

Turner, H., Bryant-Waugh, R., & Marshall, E. (2015).

The impact of early symptom change and therapeutic alliance on treatment outcome in cognitive-behavioural therapy for eating disorders. *Behaviour Research and Therapy, 73,* 165–169.

Tylka, T. L., & Kroon Van Diest, A. M. (2013). The Intuitive Eating Scale–2: Item refinement and psychometric evaluation with college women and men. *Journal of Counseling, 60,* 137–153.

Tylka, T. L., & Wood-Barcalow, N. (2015). The Body Appreciation Scale–2: Item refinement and psychometric evaluation. *Body Image, 12,* 53–67.

Uher, R., & Rutter, M. (2012). Classification of feeding and eating disorders: Review of evidence and proposals for ICD-11. *World Psychiatry, 11*(2), 80–92.

Vannucci, A., Tanofsky-Kraff, M., Shomaker, L. B., Ranzenhofer, L. M., Matheson, B. E., Cassidy, O. L., . . . Yanovski, J. A. (2012). Construct validity of the emotional eating scale adapted for children and adolescents. *International Journal of Obesity, 36*(7), 938–943.

Vitousek, K., Watson, S., & Wilson, G. T. (1998). Enhancing motivation for change in treatment-resistant eating disorders. *Clinical Psychology Review, 18*(4), 391–420.

von Ranson, K. M., Klump, K. L., Iacono, W. G., & McGue, M. (2005). The Minnesota Eating Behavior Survey: A brief measure of disordered eating attitudes and behaviors. *Eating Behaviors, 6*(4), 373–392.

Wade, T. (2017). *Encyclopedia of feeding and eating disorders.* Singapore: Springer.

Wade, T. D., Byrne, S., & Bryant-Waugh, R. (2008). The Eating Disorder Examination: Norms and construct validity with young and middle adolescent girls. *International Journal of Eating Disorders, 41,* 551–558.

Walsh, B. T., Attia, E., & Sysko, R. (2016). Classification of eating disorders. In B. T. Walsh, R. Sysko, & D. R. Glasofer (Eds.), *Handbook of assessment and treatment of eating disorders* (pp. 3–20). Arlington, VA: American Psychiatric Publishing.

Wardle, J., Guthrie C. A., Sanderson, S., & Rapoport, L. (2001). Development of the Children's Eating Behaviour Questionnaire. *Journal of Child Psychology and Psychiatry, 42,* 963–970.

Watkins, B., Frampton, I., Lask, B., & Bryant-Waugh, R. (2005). Reliability and validity of the child version of the Eating Disorder Examination: A preliminary investigation. *International Journal of Eating Disorders, 38,* 183–187.

Watson, D., Ellickson-Larew, S., Stanton, K., & Levin-Aspenson, H. (2016). Personality provides a general structural framework for psychopathology: Commentary on "Translational applications of personality science for the conceptualization and treatment of psychopathology." *Clinical Psychology: Science and Practice, 23,* 309–313.

Whisenhunt, B. L., Williamson, D. A., Drab-Hudson, D. L., & Walden, H. (2008). Intervening with coaches to promote awareness and prevention of weight pressures in cheerleaders. *Eating and Weight Disorders, 13*(2), 102–110.

World Health Organization. (2018). Feeding and eating disorders, ICD-11 for mortality and morbidity statistics. Retrieved from *https://icd.who.int/browse11/l-m/en#/http%3a%2f%2fid.who.int%2ficd%2fentity%2f1412387537.*

Yamamiya, Y., Shroff, H., Schaefer, L. M., Thompson, J. K., Shimai, S., & Ordaz, D. L. (2019). An exploration of the psychometric properties of the SATAQ-4 among adolescent boys in Japan. *Eating Behaviors, 32,* 31–36.

Zaitsoff, S., Pullmer, R., Cyr, M., & Aime, H. (2015). The role of the therapeutic alliance in eating disorder treatment outcomes: A systematic review. *Eating Disorders, 23*(2), 99–114.

Zubernis, L., Snyder, M., & Neale-McFall, C. (2017). Case conceptualization: Improving understanding and the treatment with the temporal/contextual model. *Journal of Mental Health Counseling, 39,* 181–194.

Zucker, N., Merwin, R., Elliott, C., Lacy, J., & Eichen, D. (2009). Assessment of eating disorder symptoms in children and adolescents. In J. L. Matson, F. Andrasik, & M. L. Matson (Eds.), *Assessing childhood psychopathology and developmental disabilities* (pp. 401–443). New York: Springer Science + Business Media.

CHAPTER 22

Adolescent Body Dysmorphic Disorder

Berta J. Summers, Ilana E. Ladis, Hilary Weingarden,
and Sabine Wilhelm

Background and Example "Starter Kit"

Description and Diagnostic Classification

Body dysmorphic disorder (BDD) is a distressing and debilitating psychiatric condition characterized by an excessive preoccupation with an imagined or slight flaw in one's physical appearance (most commonly skin, hair, and/or facial features; American Psychiatric Association, 2013). Specific appearance concerns in BDD are often heterogeneous and may shift over time. Individuals with BDD also engage in time-consuming, repetitive, appearance-focused rituals in response to their concerns, such as compulsive mirror checking, camouflaging appearance (e.g., with makeup, clothing, or careful body positioning), excessive grooming or skin picking, reassurance seeking, and behavioral avoidance. These rituals and avoidance behaviors may offer short-term relief of appearance-related anxiety, but they are thought to maintain pathology in the long term by reinforcing concerns and preventing opportunities to challenge and disconfirm one's maladaptive beliefs about appearance (e.g., Summers & Cougle, 2018; Veale et al., 1996; Wilhelm, Phillips, & Steketee, 2013).

The diagnostic classification of BDD has changed substantially since its first introduction in the third edition of the *Diagnostic and Statistical Manual of Mental Disorders* (DSM-III; American Psychiatric Association, 1980), where it was referred to as "dysmorphohobia." BDD was classified as a somatoform disorder in the DSM-III-R through DSM-IV-TR (American Psychiatric Association, 1987). Most recently in DSM-5, BDD was reclassified as an obsessive–Compulsive and related disorder, due to its phenomenological similarities to obsessive–compulsive disorder (OCD). Consistent with DSM-IV, DSM-5 diagnostic criteria specify that an individual present with preoccupations with his or her physical appearance (i.e., spending an hour or more each day thinking about perceived flaws in appearance) and clinically significant functional impairment or distress. DSM-5 criteria additionally specify the presence of repetitive behaviors (e.g., excessive mirror checking, grooming) for a BDD diagnosis. To this end, both BDD and OCD are defined by the presence of distressing intrusive thoughts and performance of related rituals or compulsions. However, BDD is distinct from OCD in that obsessions and rituals focus more narrowly on appearance, whereas in OCD symptoms focus on wide-ranging content (e.g., contamination, harm, symmetry, scrupulosity).

Epidemiology

BDD typically develops in adolescence, with a mean age at onset of just under 17 years, and follows a chronic course when untreated (Bjornsson et al., 2013). BDD affects males and females at roughly equal rates (Phillips & Diaz, 1997; Schneider, Turner, Mond, & Hudson, 2017) and is relatively common, with point prevalence rates in adolescent samples ranging from 1 to 2% (Mayville, Katz, Gipson, & Cabral, 1999; Rief, Buhlmann, Wilhelm, Borkenhagen, & Brahler, 2006; Schneider et al., 2017). One study found higher rates of BDD among older, compared to younger, adolescents (Schneider et al., 2017). Prevalence rates are also higher in studies examining only college student samples (ranging from 2 to 13%; Biby, 1998; Bohne et al., 2002; Cansever, Uzun, Donmez, & Ozsahin, 2003) or adolescent psychiatric inpatient samples (ranging from 6 to 14%; Dyl, Kittler, Phillips, & Hunt, 2006; Grant, Kim, & Crow, 2001). Adolescent-onset BDD is associated with greater symptom severity and greater likelihood of suicide attempts, compared to adult-onset BDD (Bjornsson et al., 2013). Adolescent-onset BDD may also disrupt normative developmental processes (Phillips, Didie, et al., 2006). For example, it may contribute to school avoidance or early dropout (see the next section of this chapter; Albertini & Phillips, 1999), as well as avoidance of social activities (e.g., extracurricular participation, dating). At its most severe, individuals with BDD can become housebound due to their symptoms. The disorder's early onset, severity, and chronic course underscore the importance of assessing BDD among adolescents.

Associated Clinical Features

When establishing a BDD diagnosis, clinicians should also consider whether the individual's presentation warrants the assignment of a diagnostic specifier to better characterize symptoms, as subgroups can have implications for prognosis and treatment considerations (i.e., level of insight; muscle dysmorphia). Classification to BDD subgroups can be determined during initial assessment, utilizing measures referenced later in this chapter.

Insight

Many individuals with BDD lack insight and fixedly believe that their appearance concerns are true (Eisen, Phillips, Coles, & Rasmussen, 2004). DSM-5 categorizes insight into three subgroups: (1) "With good or fair insight"; (2) "With poor insight"; and (3) "With absent insight/delusional beliefs," which refers to individuals who are completely convinced of their erroneous beliefs about their appearance (American Psychiatric Association, 2013). In one adolescent BDD sample ($N = 33$), 59% had current delusional symptoms and 83% had lifetime delusional BDD symptoms (Phillips, Didie, et al., 2006). Moreover, 42% of adolescents with BDD reported delusions/ideas of reference (i.e., beliefs that others were paying special attention to their appearance concern and subsequently mocking, judging, or rejecting them because of how they look). Rates of delusionality were higher in adolescents compared to adults with BDD in this study (Phillips, Menard, Pagano, Fay, & Stout, 2006). Delusionality is important to assess, as it has been linked with more severe BDD symptoms, higher likelihood of drug abuse and suicide attempts, and more severe social impairment (Phillips, Menard, et al., 2006). See the next section of this chapter for details on the Brown Assessment of Beliefs Scale (Eisen et al., 1998) which is the "gold standard" semistructured clinical interview used to evaluate degree of insight in patients with BDD.

Muscle Dysmorphia

Muscle dysmorphia (MD) is another subtype of BDD. Individuals with MD are primarily concerned with their body muscle composition or muscle mass (Pope, Gruber, Choi, Olivardia, & Phillips, 1997), generally worrying that they are too small or lack sufficient muscularity. In fact, individuals with MD are frequently above average in terms of strength and muscularity (Pope, Katz, & Hudson, 1993). In addition to traditional BDD symptoms such as mirror checking, MD is associated with excessive exercise (Leone, Sedory, & Gray, 2005), steroid abuse (Mosley, 2009), and dieting (Leone et al., 2005) to influence body composition. Like delusionality, presence of MD has been associated with more severe outcomes, including higher rates of substance use and suicidality (Pope et al., 2005).

Challenges in Detection and Assessment

One challenge associated with assessment of BDD is that patients are often secretive about their concerns and reluctant to report their symptoms to clinicians or other health care providers unless directly asked (Buhlmann, 2011; Grant et al., 2001; Marques, Weingarden, LeBlanc, & Wilhelm, 2011). This reluctance may stem from feelings of shame or from concerns about seeming superficial and vain. As a result, patients may be in treatment for depression, while their undiagnosed BDD is creating the most distress and impairment. Thus, it is imperative that clinicians directly ask about appearance concerns when working with adolescent patients.

Another challenge is that individuals with BDD typically do not recognize their appearance concerns as artifacts of a psychological illness; thus, they often seek out nonpsychiatric solutions for their appearance concerns, such as plastic surgery or other cosmetic procedures (Ribeiro, 2017). In a recent meta-analysis of 33 studies, Ribeiro found that 15% of adult plastic surgery patients (ranging from 2 to 57%), and 13% of dermatology patients (ranging from 5 to 35%) had BDD. Seeking nonpsychiatric medical treatments is not unique to adults with BDD. In a sample of 39 children and adolescents with BDD (Phillips, Grant, Siniscalchi, & Albertini, 2001), 41% had sought nonpsychiatric treatments for BDD (e.g., cosmetic surgeries, dentistry, dermatological treatments). The high prevalence of plastic surgery and cosmetic treatments in BDD is particularly concerning given that dissatisfaction after surgery, as well as the desire to seek additional surgery, are both common outcomes. This is because the root of the illness is not the individual's actual physical appearance but his or her distorted perception of his or her appearance (Veale, De Haro, & Lambrou, 2003). Poor success rates for plastic surgery are complicated by the fact that many plastic surgeons are unfamiliar with BDD and are therefore less likely to identify BDD in cosmetic surgery candidates or offer appropriate referrals for psychiatric intervention (Joseph et al., 2017).

Another challenge in BDD assessment is determining the potential validity of the patient's appearance concern(s). To obtain a diagnosis of BDD, an individual's body part(s) of concern must be objectively within the range of normal appearance (i.e., not a result of a birth defect, medical condition, or injury/accident). In fact, many individuals with BDD are objectively good-looking. It is also important to differentiate between normative appearance concerns and pathological appearance concerns, as most adolescents and adults can identify aspects of their appearance with which they are dissatisfied. Specifically, clinicians must determine the extent to which appearance concerns cause distress (e.g., self-dislike, suicidality) and/or functional impairment (e.g., make it difficult for the adolescent to engage socially, go to school, or participate in family events). Often, parents have trouble recognizing the severity of their adolescent's body image disturbance and only initiate treatment for their adolescent once he or she refuses to go to school or verbalizes suicidal thoughts anchored to dislike of their appearance.

Furthermore, appearance preoccupation should not be better accounted for by the presence of another disorder, such as concern about being too fat in the context of an eating disorder (e.g., anorexia nervosa, although eating disorders and BDD may co-occur). In a similar vein, symptoms of BDD can be mistaken for other psychiatric conditions if differential diagnoses are not carefully considered. See the third section of this chapter for detailed information on differential diagnosis for this condition. Finally, clinicians should consider certain risk factors that are known to complicate the presentation and course of BDD, including substance use and suicidality. These topics are discussed in greater depth below.

Starter Kit of Assessment Measures

There are many useful measures and rating scales to detect the presence and clinical features of BDD. As most measures have not been developed or validated specifically for children or adolescents, tools may need to be adapted for use in young patients. See Table 22.1 for a list of recommended assessment tools to use when evaluating BDD as a potential diagnosis. BDD-specific measures are described in greater detail below.

Screening Tools, Different Informants, and Assessment of Risk

We cover in this section the measures used to screen for BDD in adolescents. We also describe the context in which cross-informants may be useful in aiding diagnosis and assessment of ado-

TABLE 22.1. Recommended Tools for Assessing BDD

Assessment tool	Administration	Described further
Screening measures		
Body Dysmorphic Disorder Questionnaire—Adolescent Version (BDDQ-A; Phillips, 1996)	Self-report	Pages 622–623
Body Image Questionnaire—Child and Adolescent Version (BIQ-C; Veale, 2009)	Self-report	Page 623
Dysmorphic Concerns Questionnaire (DCQ; Mancuso, Knoesen, & Castle, 2010)	Self-report	Page 623
Diagnostic measures		
BDD module of the Structured Clinical Interview for DSM-5 (SCID-5; First, Williams, Karg, & Spitzer, 2015)	Clinician-rated semistructured interview	Page 625
Body Dysmorphic Disorder Examination (BDDE; Rosen & Reiter, 1996)	Clinician-rated semistructured interview	Page 626
Differential diagnoses		
Schedule for Affective Disorders and Schizophrenia for School-Age Children—Present and Lifetime Version (K-SADS-PL; Kaufman et al., 1997)	Clinician-rated semistructured interview	Pages 627–629
Mini-International Neuropsychiatric Interview for Children and Adolescents (MINI-KID; Sheehan et al., 2010)	Clinician-rated structured interview	Pages 627–629
BDD severity, symptoms, and insight		
BDD-Yale–Brown Obsessive Compulsive Scale—Adolescent Version (BDD-YBOCS-A; Phillips et al., 1997)	Clinician-rated semistructured interview	Pages 626–627
BDD Symptom Scale (BDD-SS; Wilhelm, Greenberg, Rosenfield, Kasarskis, & Blashill, 2016)	Self-report	Page 626
Brown Assessment of Beliefs Scale—Adolescent Version (BABS; Eisen et al., 1998)	Clinician-rated semistructured interview	Page 627

lescent BDD. Furthermore, we discuss risk factors specific to adolescent BDD that require careful attention by an assessor.

Screening Tools and Diagnostic Aids

Clinicians who wish to screen for the possibility that an adolescent has BDD in advance of conducting a diagnostic assessment can select from among several screening tools: the Body Dysmorphic Disorder Questionnaire—Adolescent Version (BDDQ-A; Phillips, 1996), the Body Image Questionnaire—Child and Adolescent Version (BIQ-C; Veale, 2009), and the Dysmorphic Concerns Questionnaire (DCQ; Mancuso, Knoesen,

& Castle, 2010; Oosthuizen, Lambert, & Castle, 1998).

Body Dysmorphic Disorder Questionnaire— Adolescent Version

The BDDQ-A is a brief, dichotomous self-report screening measure for BDD based on DSM-IV diagnostic criteria. It consists of four "yes" or "no," multiple-choice, and free-response items aimed at capturing the presence and description of one's appearance preoccupation(s) and the effect of the preoccupation in terms of distress, interference, and time. For example, the BDDQ-A asks, "Are you very worried about how you look?" This is followed by "If yes, do you think about your appearance problems a lot and wish you could think about them less?" The BDDQ-A also aims to screen out individuals whose appearance concerns may be better accounted for by an eating disorder (i.e., primary preoccupations surround being too fat). The BDDQ (original adult version) has high sensitivity (100%) and specificity (89–93%) for detecting BDD in adult psychiatric samples (Phillips, Atala, & Pope, 1995). The BDDQ-A has been used successfully in adolescent samples (e.g., Schneider et al., 2017), but no sensitivity or specificity data have been established, nor has further validation been carried out within adolescent samples specifically.

Body Image Questionnaire—Child and Adolescent Version

The BIQ-C (Veale, 2009) is a screening, severity, and outcome measure for BDD symptoms in children and adolescents. The BIQ-C is a slight adaptation from the original adult BIQ (Veale, 2009). The first item serves as an initial screener that assesses for the presence of appearance concerns. If an individual selects "yes" for this item, he or she completes all subsequent questions. The BIQ-C includes 12 Likert items ranging from 0 to 8 that capture severity of common symptoms and features of BDD (e.g., mirror checking, preoccupations with appearance, social interference due to appearance concern). For example, the measure evaluates the extent to which the adolescent believes his or her physical feature is ugly by asking, "How much do you feel your feature(s) is ugly, unattractive, or 'not right'?" A response of 0 corresponds to *Extremely ugly or "not right"* and 8 corresponds to *Not at all unattractive*. A total score can be generated by summing Likert items (with some reverse-scored items). Total scores range from 0 to 96, with higher scores indicating greater likelihood of a BDD diagnosis and more severe symptoms. Among adults, a BIQ score of 59 indicates probable BDD. However, the BIQ-C has not yet been validated in a youth sample. Thus, no BIQ-C clinical cutoff scores have been empirically determined for children or adolescents.

Dysmorphic Concerns Questionnaire

The DCQ (Oosthuizen et al., 1998) is a seven-item screening tool for BDD that also captures severity of BDD symptoms (Mancuso et al., 2010). The measure asks respondents to rate their degree of concerns about physical appearance compared to others (e.g., "Have you ever been very concerned about some aspect of your appearance?"; "Have you ever spent a lot of time covering up defects in your appearance/bodily functioning?"), with responses ranging from 0 (*not at all*) to 3 (*much more than most people*). The total score, which comprises summing all items, ranges from 0 to 21. The DCQ has strong internal consistency across a range of adult and adolescent clinical and nonclinical samples (Enander et al., 2018). A cutoff score of 9 on the DCQ has been shown to accurately categorize 96% of individuals with BDD in a combined adult BDD and nonclinical college sample in which 21% of the total sample met criteria for BDD, balancing strong sensitivity (96%) and specificity (91%) (Mancuso et al., 2010). Of note, sensitivity and specificity may be somewhat lower in a more complex, "real-world" sample not comprised of either treatment-seeking adults with BDD or nonclinical college students. A slightly modified version of the DCQ was further validated in three Swedish population-based adolescent and adult twin samples, in which 1–3% of each sample met criteria for a likely diagnosis of BDD (Enander et al., 2018). Using a more stringent cutoff score of ≥17, the DCQ accurately categorized 96% of individuals with BDD, with moderate sensitivity (56%) and strong specificity (99%).

Cross-Informant Assessment

Adolescents with BDD may be reluctant to disclose body image concerns to clinicians, due to embarrassment or shame (Weingarden & Renshaw, 2015). Therefore, it may be helpful for clinicians to obtain information from additional informants about patients' BDD symptoms. Specifically, parents may provide useful supplemental information about how much time their child may be spending engaged in BDD rituals (e.g., trying to "fix" appearance concerns, excessive mirror checking, camouflaging appearance concerns with clothing or makeup), or the extent of their child's avoidance of school or social activities due to appearance concerns. Parents may also shed light on family members' accommodation of the adolescent's BDD symptoms (e.g., spending excessive money on makeup or clothing for the adolescent, allowing the adolescent to skip activities due to distress, providing excessive reassurance to the adolescent that his or her appearance looks OK). Accommodation by parents is usually well intentioned, with the aim of lowering the adolescent's immediate distress. In the long run, however, parent accommodation maintains the adolescent's

BDD symptoms and should gradually be incorporated into treatment as a target to reduce.

Guidance counselors may also provide helpful additional information about an adolescent's BDD symptoms. Given the degree of shame associated with BDD, it may make sense to only seek input from counselors if the adolescent is comfortable with this. Counselors may specifically be able to speak to the extent to which the child appears distracted during school, is leaving to use the bathroom (potentially to engage in excessive mirror checking or other rituals throughout the day), or is disengaged socially, each of which may indicate interference due to BDD.

Risk Factors

Risk Factors for BDD Development

Relatively little research has examined potential risk factors in the development of BDD. Most existing research on the etiology of BDD has involved comparing rates of retrospectively recalled childhood events among adult BDD, control, or psychiatric comparison samples. These studies consistently point to childhood teasing and bullying as a potential risk factor for BDD development, particularly when teasing was focused on one's appearance (Buhlmann, Cook, Fama, & Wilhelm, 2007; Osman, Cooper, Hackmann, & Veale, 2004; Veale et al., 2015). It is important to note that due to reliance on retrospective recall, these studies cannot disentangle whether individuals with BDD truly experienced higher rates of teasing and bullying during childhood compared to control samples, or whether individuals with BDD recall these events more readily due to their heightened interpersonal sensitivity compared to control samples.

Studies also point to higher rates of retrospectively reported childhood abuse in adult BDD versus comparison samples (Buhlmann, Marques, & Wilhelm, 2012; Veale et al., 2015). While childhood abuse may heighten one's risk for developing BDD, abuse events should not be considered specific risk factors for BDD, as elevated rates of childhood abuse are documented across a wide range of psychiatric illnesses (Silverman, Reinherz, & Giaconia, 1996). Finally, some conceptual and empirical work on the etiology of BDD suggests that cultural and media-driven messages about the importance of beauty, in addition to family values that emphasize the importance of beauty, may contribute to development of BDD (Cororve

& Gleaves, 2001; Weingarden, Curley, Renshaw, & Wilhelm, 2017; Wilhelm, 2006).

Taken together, when clinicians are working with adolescent patients with BDD, it is beneficial to screen for bullying and abuse experiences, and to discuss with patients how they perceive and interpret family, cultural, and media values surrounding physical appearance. Moreover, it may be beneficial in treatment to identify whether the patient has developed unhelpful or distorted beliefs about him- or herself as a result of experiences such as bullying or abuse, and to teach patients (via cognitive skills) to objectively evaluate and challenge those distorted beliefs.

High-Risk Outcomes Associated with BDD

Research on the phenomenology and clinical correlates of BDD in adolescents is scarce and consists largely of case reports and case series. However, existing data suggest that several high-risk outcomes are common among adolescents with BDD and should be carefully assessed. See Hankin and Cohen (Chapter 7), Millner and Nock (Chapter 9), and Chung and Wang (Chapter 19) in this volume for approaches to assessing depression, suicide risk, and substance use, respectively, in adolescent patients.

Suicide

Risk for suicide is markedly high in adolescents with BDD and must be carefully and frequently assessed. It is also important to convey information about suicide risk to parents of adolescents with BDD. In a sample of 33 children and adolescents with BDD, lifetime suicide attempts were reported by 21% of participants (Albertini & Phillips, 1999). In a second study of 36 adolescents with BDD, 81% reported lifetime suicidal ideation, and 44% reported a lifetime suicide attempt (Phillips et al., 2006). This suicide attempt rate was significantly higher than that of an adult BDD sample (Phillips & Menard, 2006). Suicide risk in adolescent BDD is also substantially elevated compared to rates documented in related disorders, such as adolescent OCD (Storch et al., 2015).

Academic and Social Impairment

Adolescents with BDD are at very high risk of falling behind academically or socially as a result of avoidance and impairment due to BDD. In 36 adolescents with BDD, 100% reported academic and social interference resulting from BDD (Phillips, Didie, et al., 2006). Early dropout from school is documented in 18–22% of adolescents with BDD (Albertini & Phillips, 1999; Phillips et al., 2006), and 14% of adolescents in one sample reported becoming housebound for at least one week due to BDD (Phillips, Didie, et al., 2006).

Comorbid Depression, Anxiety, and Substance Use Disorders

Rates of comorbid psychiatric illnesses are also very high in BDD. See the third section of this chapter for more detailed information on diagnostic assessment of BDD and its differential diagnosis. In one adolescent sample, 84% had a comorbid mood disorder (73% major depression), 70% had a comorbid anxiety disorder, and 44% had a comorbid substance use disorder (31% alcohol use disorder, 39% other substance use disorder; Phillips, Didie, et al., 2006). Rates of substance use disorders were higher among adolescents than among adults with BDD in this study (Phillips, Didie, et al., 2006). A second study of substance use disorders in adolescents and adults with BDD documented lifetime substance use disorders in 49% and current substance use disorders in 17% of subjects (Grant, Menard, Pagano, Fay, & Phillips, 2005). Most common substances of abuse or dependence include alcohol (lifetime rates of 43%) and cannabis (lifetime rates of 30%). Participants who presented with comorbid substance use disorders were at significantly higher risk for suicide attempts, psychiatric hospitalization due to BDD, and social and occupational dysfunction due to BDD (Grant et al., 2005). Taken together, clinicians treating adolescents with BDD must regularly assess for changes in depression, anxiety, and substance use, and incorporate reduction of risk for these outcomes into treatment as appropriate.

Using Assessment to Guide Diagnosis, Case Formulation, and Treatment Planning

This section covers measures and diagnostic considerations for thorough assessment and treatment planning for patients with BDD. The two most commonly used clinician-rated interviews to establish a BDD diagnosis are the BDD module of the Structured Clinical Interview for DSM-5 (SCID-5; First, Williams, Karg, & Spitzer, 2015) and the Body Dysmorphic Disorder Examination (BDDE; Rosen & Reiter, 1996), though these measures have predominantly been used in adult populations. Once diagnosis has been established, BDD-specific symptoms, severity, and insight can be better characterized via the following measures, respectively: the BDD-Symptom Scale (BDD-SS; Wilhelm et al., 2016), the Yale–Brown Obsessive Compulsive Scale Modified for BDD—Adolescent Version (BDD-YBOCS-A; Phillips et al., 1997), and the Brown Assessment of Beliefs Scale—Adolescent Version (BABS; Eisen et al., 1998). This section also provides information about differential diagnostic considerations, which is particularly important when evaluating symptoms of BDD that overlap with other, more widely known psychiatric conditions. Finally, this section offers insight into treatment planning, establishing goals, and integrating patients' preferences into treatment.

Diagnostic Interviews

BDD Module of the Structured Clinical Interview for DSM-5

The SCID-5 (First et al., 2015) is a semistructured clinical interview designed to assess DSM-5 diagnostic criteria for a range of psychiatric disorders, including BDD. The SCID-5 can also be employed to evaluate comorbid and differential conditions. It is recommended that the SCID-5 be completed by an assessor who has clinical training and thorough understanding of DSM-5 diagnostic criteria. Previous versions of the SCID (those prior to SCID-5) are not recommended for determining BDD diagnosis, as the SCID-5 includes important features of the condition that map onto its current conceptualization as an obsessive–compulsive and related disorder (i.e., presence of appearance-related rituals). Questions assess duration and content of appearance concerns, corresponding compulsive rituals, and distress and functional impairment associated with symptoms. The BDD module also contains a question to ascertain whether appearance concerns are better accounted for by eating disorder-related concerns (i.e., concerns limited to weight and shape, and fears of being fat) along with scoring for specifiers (MD, degree of insight into symptoms). The BDD module of the SCID-5 can be completed in less than 10 minutes and has demonstrated excellent interrater (kappa = .95) and test–retest reliability (kappa = 1.00; Tolin et al., 2018). It is important to note that currently the SCID-5 is only validated for use in adults and thus must be adapted for use in adolescent populations.

Body Dysmorphic Disorder Examination

The BDDE (Rosen & Reiter, 1996) is a 34-item, semistructured clinical interview that was developed to measure severe body image disturbance and associated symptoms. Items evaluate the individual's preoccupation with physical appearance, self-consciousness, importance assigned to appearance, avoidance behaviors, and appearance-related compulsive symptoms, such as body checking/inspection and camouflaging the disliked body area(s). Six items are included solely for the purpose of providing more information to the interviewer and are not included in the total score. The remaining 28 items assess thoughts and behaviors anchored to the patient's most prominent appearance concern over the past 4 weeks. These items are rated from 0 to 6; a score of 0 indicates that the feature in question has not been present in the past month, while scores of 1–6 reflect the frequency and intensity of each symptom within this time period (with higher scores indicating more severe pathology).

Criteria for probable BDD include scores ≥4 (indicating that the feature was present on at least half of the days or was at least "moderate" in severity) on items measuring preoccupation with appearance (Q9), self-consciousness or embarrassment (Q10, Q11), overvaluation of the importance of appearance (Q18); negative self-evaluation due to appearance (Q19), and any item assessing distress/impairment/avoidance associated with appearance concern (Q13, Q23, Q24, Q25, or Q26). Of note, interviewers should also consider compulsive and repetitive behaviors anchored to patients' appearance concerns, as this diagnostic criterion was newly introduced in DSM-5, and the BDDE development was based on DSM-IV criteria. Total scores on the BDDE range from 0 to 168. The authors do not identify a clinical cutoff for the full score, as individuals may score high on the measure without meeting all DSM criteria. The BDDE has been shown to distinguish between clinical and nonclinical patients (Rosen & Reiter, 1996). In adult samples, this measure has also demonstrated adequate internal consistency (alphas from .81 to .93 for different populations), test–retest (r = .94), and interrater reliability (nonclinical intraclass coefficient [ICC] = .99, clinical ICC = .86), and has been adapted for use in several languages (Jorge et al., 2008). The BDDE has also been modified for self-report with strong internal consistency (alpha = .94; Boroughs, Krawczyk, & Thompson, 2010). Full psychometric data are not

yet available for the use of the BDDE in adolescent samples.

Assessment of Symptoms, Severity, and Insight

BDD Symptom Scale

The BDD-SS (Wilhelm, Greenberg, Rosenfield, Kasarkis, & Blashill, 2016) is a self-report measure that comprises 54 common BDD symptoms grouped into seven separate symptom clusters representing (1) checking rituals, (2) grooming rituals, (3) shape/weight rituals, (4) hair-pulling/skin-picking rituals, (5) behavioral avoidance, (6) surgery/dermatology seeking, and (7) BDD-related maladaptive cognitions. Patients are first asked to endorse (yes–no) the individual symptoms they experienced during the past week, after which they rate the overall/combined severity of their symptoms within each cluster from 0 (*no problem*) to 10 (*very severe*). The BDD-SS thus yields two total scores reflecting symptom count (ranging from 0 to 54) and severity (ranging from 0 to 70). The BDD-SS can be used to describe the nature and severity of the patient's symptoms at the initial assessment and to track progress across treatment. Additionally, the BDD-SS can serve as a useful treatment guide. For example, the measure can be used to highlight a patient's most prominent cognitions, avoidance behaviors, and rituals, which can then be explicitly targeted with treatment strategies such as cognitive restructuring or exposure with ritual prevention. The BDD-SS has been used in adolescent treatment studies (Greenberg, Mothi, & Wilhelm, 2016) and has demonstrated good convergent and discriminant validity, as well as adequate internal consistency for both symptom (internal consistency [KR-20] = .81) and severity scores (alpha = .75; Wilhelm et al., 2016) in adult populations.

Yale–Brown Obsessive Compulsive Scale Modified for BDD—Adolescent Version

The BDD-YBOCS-A (Phillips et al., 1997), a 12-item, semistructured measure of BDD severity over the past week, was adapted from the adult BDD-YBOCS (Phillips et al., 1997) and the child version of the Yale–Brown Obsessive Compulsive Scale (Scahill et al., 1997). Items examine obsessional preoccupations with the perceived appearance flaw (items 1–5), BDD-related repetitive/compulsive behaviors (6–10), insight into appearance beliefs (11), and behavioral avoidance due to cognitions or behaviors (12). Items are rated on a 5-point Likert scale from 0 (*no symptomatology*) to 4 (*extreme symptomatology*); scores on this measure range from 0 to 48, with higher scores indicative of more severe BDD symptoms. Though the BDD-YBOCS is not recommended as a stand-alone diagnostic tool, a total score of ≥20 is suggestive of probable BDD (e.g., Phillips, 2006). The BDD-YBOCS has demonstrated excellent interrater reliability (ICC = .97), test–retest reliability (*r* = .93), internal consistency (alpha =.92), sensitivity (90%), and specificity (86%; Phillips, Hart, & Menard, 2014). Using these metrics along with the standard deviation of the full sample (*SD* = 10.15; Phillips et al., 2014), the reliable change index (RCI-Diff; 90% confidence interval) is ±6.66 points (Jacobson & Truax, 1991). In addition to using this measure to evaluate severity of BDD presentation at an initial assessment, it also is commonly used to evaluate symptom change over the course of treatment (Phillips et al., 2014).

Brown Assessment of Beliefs Scale

The BABS (Eisen et al., 1998) is a seven-item, semistructured measure that clinicians may use to assesses a patient's current level of insight and delusionality related to BDD beliefs. This measure has been tailored for use in adolescents (Phillips, 2017) from the adult BABS (Eisen et al., 1998). During the interview, patients are asked to describe in their own words how they feel about their appearance to establish an overarching, global appearance-related belief (e.g., "I am ugly") that is referenced in each item. The first six items assess individuals' degree of conviction in this belief, their perception of others' view of this belief, their explanation of any discrepancy between their view and others' views, fixity of the belief, attempts to disprove the belief, and attributions about the cause of this belief (e.g., psychiatric/psychological vs. a reflection of true appearance concerns). These items are scored from 0 to 4 and summed to create a total score (0 to 24), with higher scores reflecting poorer insight/greater delusionality. Total scores can be used to categorize individuals as having *excellent* (0–3), *good* (4–7), *fair* (8–12), *poor* (13–17), or *absent* (≥18) insight. The seventh item, which is not included in the total score, assesses ideas/delusions of reference (i.e., the degree to which the individual believes that others are taking special notice because of his or her belief). In adult populations, the BABS has demonstrated high interrater reliability (ICC = .96), test–retest

reliability (range for individual items = .79–.98, median = .95), and internal consistency (alpha = .87) in patients with BDD, and also excellent sensitivity (100%) and good specificity (86%) for categorizing level of insight (i.e., *excellent, good, fair, poor, absent*) and can be used as a measure of progress over the course of treatment (Phillips, Hart, Menard, & Eisen, 2013). Though this measure has been used with adolescents (Greenberg et al., 2016), full psychometric data are not yet available for the use of the BABS in adolescent populations.

Differential Diagnosis

Careful differential diagnostic assessment is imperative for this population, as certain features of BDD (e.g., compulsive behaviors, social avoidance, body-focused repetitive behaviors, body image concerns, feelings of hopelessness, delusional beliefs) could lead clinicians to misdiagnose patients with BDD with a more widely recognized disorder. BDD is also highly comorbid with other psychiatric conditions (as discussed previously), though the majority of the comorbidity literature is based on research with adult populations. The SCID-5 (First et al., 2015) is commonly used to evaluate differential diagnoses in adults, though it has not yet been validated for use in adolescents and is currently being adapted for this purpose. The SCID-5 contains modules assessing each of the following key differential disorders that share overlapping features with BDD: OCD, excoriation/skin picking disorder, trichotillomania, social anxiety disorder (SAD), eating disorders (EDs), depression, and psychotic disorders.

Given that the SCID-5 has yet to be formally validated for use in adolescent populations, the Schedule for Affective Disorders and Schizophrenia for School-Age Children—Present and Lifetime Version (K-SADS-PL; Kaufman et al., 1997) or the Mini-International Neuropsychiatric Interview for Children and Adolescents (MINI-KID; Sheehan et al., 2010) would be more appropriate for assessing many of the previously listed diagnoses, though it is important to note that these interviews do not include modules for BDD, excoriation disorder, or trichotillomania. The K-SADS-PL is a semistructured, 82-item screening interview for parents and children/adolescents (ages 6–17) assessing current and past psychopathology (Kaufman et al., 1997). The MINI-KID (Sheehan et al., 2010) is a more structured diagnostic interview, also designed to assess psychiatric disorders in individuals ages 6–17. The MINI-KID can be administered with or without parents present; a separate version just for parents is also available. Below are comorbidity and differential diagnostic considerations that are important when evaluating a patient with possible BDD. See other chapters of this volume for more detailed descriptions of clinician-administered diagnostic assessments for adolescents, as well the first section of this chapter for further information about challenges in detection and assessment of BDD.

BDD and OCD

BDD and OCD share core symptoms, including repetitive intrusive thoughts and compulsions performed in order to ameliorate distressing thoughts or beliefs. Recurrent thoughts and compulsions in BDD are anchored to concerns about, and desire to fix or hide, a perceived defect in a patient's physical appearance (e.g., skin, hair, facial features). Target concerns in OCD can span a wider array of content (e.g., excessive doubt, contamination fear, fear of bringing harm to oneself or others, need for order or exactness, concern about immoral behavior). Therefore, it is critical when differentiating between diagnoses of BDD and OCD to clearly evaluate the focus and content of the patient's obsessions. Another clinical feature that can be used to differentiate BDD from OCD is level of insight. Individuals with OCD are often better able to recognize that their thoughts and behaviors are excessive and/or illogical, whereas individuals with BDD may exhibit lower insight into their condition and believe their concerns are valid (Phillips et al., 2012). Of note, however, children with OCD may not be insightful about the excessive nature of symptoms. The MINI-KID and K-SADS-PL can be used to diagnose OCD in adolescents.

BDD and Body-Focused Repetitive Behaviors

Excoriation (skin picking) disorder is characterized by compulsive picking of one's skin that results in tissue damage; similarly, trichotillomania is characterized by compulsive hair pulling that results in visible hair loss in the affected area. Both skin picking and hair pulling can be symptoms of BDD, but these conditions can also represent separate diagnoses. Indeed, skin-picking disorder and trichotillomania were recently added to the DSM-5, under the obsessive–compulsive and related disorders diagnostic category. When conducting a differential diagnostic assessment, it is important to determine the function or purpose of the compulsive behaviors in patients exhibiting these symptoms. Individuals with BDD may pick their skin or pull out hairs; however, the intention is often to change or "fix" their appearance concern (i.e., smooth the texture of their skin in the context of skin concerns, remove stray facial hairs or make their hairline more symmetrical in the context of hair concerns; Phillips & Taub, 1995). In excoriation disorder or trichotillomania, the function of the behavior is not solely to change/improve one's appearance; it may also serve a wide range of other functions (e.g., to regulate emotions, to serve an activating role when understimulated, to generate positive physical sensations; Woods & Houghton, 2014). Hair pulling and skin picking in the context of trichotillomania and excoriation disorder are also often performed outside of a patient's conscious awareness (e.g., while "zoning out"; Woods & Houghton, 2014), in contrast to the highly focused nature of picking or pulling in BDD to "fix" a flaw. The SCID-5 modules corresponding to these diagnoses can be used to assess for these conditions, although they should be tailored for younger populations, as the SCID-5 has not yet been validated for use in adolescents.

BDD and SAD

SAD is characterized by excessive fear of being embarrassed, judged, rejected, or otherwise negatively evaluated by others in social situations. SAD and BDD are often comorbid and share similar clinical features. In particular, SAD and BDD both involve fear of negative evaluation, as well as avoidance of feared situations (Fang & Hofmann, 2010). In determining whether a primary diagnosis of SAD or BDD may be more appropriate, it is necessary to understand the nature of the fears driving avoidance behaviors. Feared situations in SAD frequently involve a performance aspect such as public speaking or meeting new people, with concerns of being judged as stupid or incompetent (American Psychiatric Association, 2013). For children to obtain a diagnosis of SAD, anxiety surrounding social situations must include peer interactions (as opposed to just interactions with adults; American Psychiatric Association, 2013). In BDD, on the other hand, fears surrounding social interactions are primarily driven by concerns about being judged critically or rejected due to the way one looks (American Psychiatric Association, 2013). The MINI-KID or the K-SADS-PL can be utilized to assess adolescents for a diagnosis of SAD.

BDD and ED

Both BDD and EDs—particularly anorexia nervosa—are characterized by body image distortions (Dingemans,Van Rood, De Groot, & Van Furth, 2012; Grant, Kim, & Eckert, 2002; Jolanta & Tomasz, 2000). Body image concerns in EDs primarily focus on body weight and shape, whereas they tend to focus on specific features in BDD (e.g., skin, hair, facial features, breasts, genitals; American Psychiatric Association, 2013). Furthermore, shape and weight concerns experienced in the context of an ED (but not necessarily BDD) are accompanied by additional ED symptoms, such as disordered eating behavior (e.g., calorie restriction, bingeing or purging behaviors), low weight, and excessive exercise. It is important to note that MD is a subtype of BDD that shares clinical features of EDs (e.g., unusual eating, excessive exercise), as it is characterized by fears that the individual is too small and not muscular enough. BDD occurs in men and women at roughly equal rates, although the MD subtype, specifically, is most commonly displayed in men. On the other hand, the majority of individuals with EDs are female. Differentiating between these body image disorders can be quite complicated, and these illnesses can be comorbid. The MINI-KID or K-SADS-PL can be utilized to assess EDs in adolescents.

BDD and Major Depressive Disorder

Symptoms of major depressive disorder (MDD) and BDD have some notable overlap, as both conditions can be characterized by low mood, poor self-esteem, sensitivity to rejection, guilt, and feelings of unworthiness and defectiveness. Self-dislike in MDD may include dislike of one's appearance; however, this is typically in the context of more global feelings of defectiveness. Individuals with BDD, on the other hand, present with more prominent and specific appearance concerns that lead them to feel defective. Though MDD and BDD may not necessarily be mistaken for one another in a diagnostic interview, there is a risk of a clinician diagnosing MDD and overlooking a comorbid diagnosis of BDD due to not asking about significant appearance concerns at the interview, or due to dismissing a patient's admission of appearance concerns as normative. To this end, when evaluating an adolescent presenting with depression, it is important to inquire about the presence of appearance concerns and the effect of these concerns on a patient's functioning and distress. Patients with BDD often report that their comorbid depressive symptoms are exacerbated by their appearance concerns and associated symptoms; thus, the patient's perception of factors contributing to his or her depressive symptoms should be considered. Furthermore, assessing MDD in adolescents with BDD is crucial given the high risk for suicidal ideation and attempts in this population (Phillips & Menard, 2006). The MINI-KID and K-SADS-PL can be utilized to assess for the presence of MDD in adolescents.

BDD and Psychotic Disorders

Patients with BDD who have poor insight or delusional beliefs may be mistaken for patients having a psychotic disorder (Toh et al., 2017). In contrast to psychotic disorders, delusional symptoms in BDD focus specifically and solely on beliefs about one's physical appearance (e.g., "I look deformed," "I look monstrous"). Additionally, individuals with BDD may present with ideas or delusions of reference. As with other delusional beliefs in BDD, ideas of reference specifically focus on appearance (e.g., "The store clerk is taking special notice of me because of how deformed my nose looks"). Patients with BDD in the absence of a psychotic disorder do *not* present with other psychotic symptoms, such as hallucinations. On the other hand, in the context of schizophrenia or schizoaffective disorder, psychotic symptoms will be more wide ranging, potentially spanning additional types of delusions, hallucinations, bizarre behavior, and/or negative symptoms (American Psychiatric Association, 2013; Fang & Wilhelm, 2015). The MINI-KID and K-SADS-PL can be utilized to assess for the presence of psychotic disorders in adolescents.

Case Formulation and Planning

Establishing Goals for Treatment

Currently, cognitive-behavioral therapy (CBT) is regarded as the most efficacious psychotherapeutic treatment for BDD in adolescents (e.g., Greenberg et al., 2016; Mataix-Cols et al., 2015) and adults (e.g., Wilhelm et al., 2014). CBT for BDD involves psychoeducation in the form of an individualized case conceptualization, cognitive restructuring, exposure and response prevention, mindfulness exercises and perceptual retraining, core belief work, and relapse prevention (see detailed description below). Typical goals for adolescent BDD treatment include reducing suicide risk and targeting safety concerns, resuming school attendance in cases of school refusal, BDD symptom reduction, comorbid depressive symptom reduction (if applicable), improved insight, changes in beliefs about the importance of appearance, and improvements in the patient's general quality of life and global functioning. Decreasing functional impairment and avoidance anchored to symptoms in this population is critical, as adolescents with BDD may isolate themselves from their peers and have difficulty attending school, focusing in school, or doing their homework, or have problems at home due to their appearance concerns. Thus, it is imperative that the clinician spend time identifying and understanding the specific ways in which BDD symptoms are impacting the adolescent's social, school, and home life, in order to develop concrete goals to work toward across these contexts. Safety and risk concerns should also be thoroughly assessed, as adolescents with BDD often experience suicidal ideation. When safety is a concern, treatment should initially focus on safety planning and stabilization. It is important to consult with parents at the stage of goal establishment, particularly when the patient's insight into the illness and associated impairment is low. The younger the patient is, the more important it is to involve the parents in assessment and treatment, particularly as parents can provide encouragement and structure at home as the adolescent completes homework and fades out maladaptive behaviors. Another common treatment goal is to reduce the patient's reliance on rituals and safety behaviors (e.g., mirror checking, compulsive grooming, skin picking, comparing self to others, camouflaging perceived flaws, reassurance seeking, surgery seeking, parental accommodation, substance use), as these behaviors may offer short-term relief from appearance-related distress but function to maintain the illness in the long term. Thus, the clinician should work with the patient to identify key behaviors and rituals that are likely serving to reinforce maladaptive cognitions and behaviors and develop a plan for fading out these behaviors over the course of treatment. The BDD-SS (Wilhelm et al., 2016), described earlier in this section, can be a useful self-report instrument for gathering a comprehensive picture of a patient's symptoms—cognitions, avoidance behaviors, and rituals—to be targeted as goals in treatment.

Learning and Integrating Client Preferences

CBT treatment typically begins with psychoeducation about body image disturbance and factors that may lend themselves to the development of BDD (childhood events, social/societal expectations, genetic/biological disposition). During this introduction, the clinician also discusses the cognitive-behavioral model (Veale et al., 1996; Wilhelm et al., 2013), of BDD with the patient to better understand the idiosyncratic factors that maintain the patient's individual presentation (e.g., bullying experiences, familial expectations, social media, cognitive errors about the importance and consequence of appearance, negative interpretive biases, compulsive beauty rituals, avoidance behaviors). Given the heterogeneous nature of the disorder, development of the patient's personal model of BDD is key, as it integrates the patient's perception of his or her condition and offers a shared framework to understand patient-specific maintenance factors and treatment targets.

It is helpful to begin with some motivational interviewing (MI) techniques at the outset of treatment, as patients are typically eager to seek cosmetic interventions and thus are often skeptical and have reservations about a psychologically oriented program of treatment. MI allows the patient to identify his or her own reasons for engaging in treatment (e.g., values) and changing certain thoughts and behaviors that maintain body image concerns. Early in treatment, the clinician introduces the concept of "automatic thoughts" or "cognitive errors" (e.g., all-or-nothing thinking, mind reading, catastrophizing, emotional reasoning), and the role of these distortions in the disorder (i.e., fueling avoidance, strengthening beliefs about the importance and consequence of appearance). Once the patient is able to identify these problematic cognitions, he or she is taught ways of challenging and remediating them by evaluating evidence, conducting behavioral experiments to test the accuracy of the thoughts, and generating alternative, more helpful ways of thinking. Later treatment sessions (i.e., after behavioral work and perceptual retraining have been introduced and practiced) might also involve more advanced cognitive strategies. Specifically, the clinician might work with the adolescent to identify and challenge more deeply held core beliefs that maintain body image disturbance and negative affect (e.g., "I am defective," "I am unlovable," "I am worthless").

Once the patient has an initial foundation of cognitive restructuring techniques, treatment begins to incorporate exposure and response prevention. In these sessions, it is necessary to integrate patients' preferences for how to approach behavioral experiments and exposure exercises, as these components of treatment can be quite challenging and aversive. Thus, it is important to develop an exposure hierarchy (i.e., rank-ordered list of challenging situations) collaboratively with the patient and work through these goals in a systematic, graded fashion to facilitate the patient's ability and willingness to face fears associated with his or her appearance concerns (more on this topic below). Similarly, hierarchies can be developed to structure plans of fading-out rituals and safety behaviors that are time consuming and serve to maintain the patient's appearance concerns. As exposure and ritual prevention can be highly challenging and patients' insight may be poor, it is often beneficial for clinicians to incorporate motivation enhancement strategies or rewards throughout treatment, and particularly as exposure and ritual prevention are incorporated into treatment.

Perceptual retraining is also an important component of treatment in which patients are taught to have a healthier, more functional relationship with mirrors (i.e., not avoiding or getting "stuck" in the mirror for extended periods of time scrutinizing features). Patients with BDD tend to selectively attend to areas of their appearance they perceive to be defective, and this reinforces their distorted self-image. Perceptual retraining involves teaching patients to mindfully describe their physical features in the mirror in an objective, nonjudgmental manner, and view their appearance as a whole rather than hyperfocusing on perceived flaws. Perceptual retraining is often a challenging treatment component for patients with BDD. Therefore, the clinician may need to tailor the exercise to be less challenging at first, so that the patient will be willing to try it. For example, the patient could initially stand far away from the mirror and gradually move closer (i.e., to an arms-length distance away) with subsequent practice.

Treatment components (MI, cognitive restructuring, exposure and response prevention, and perceptual retraining) should be developmentally tailored and differentially emphasized, depending on the patient's needs and preferences. For example, younger adolescents might prefer more parental involvement, external rewards for their participation (e.g., a gift card or a toy) and behavioral interventions. Alternatively, older adolescents whose cognitive skills are more developed, might prefer less parental involvement, more cognitive interventions, and other types of rewards (e.g., privileges to use the car). Treatment may also include optional modules depending on the adolescent's presentation, such as sessions focusing on compulsive skin picking or weight, shape, and muscularity concerns.

Progress, Process, and Outcome Measurement

Goal Measurement: Defining Milestones and Outcomes

As briefly reviewed in the section on case formulation and treatment planning, common goals for treatment progress in this population include BDD symptom/severity reduction, improved insight, reduction in comorbid depressive symptoms, improved quality of life, and improved global functioning (i.e., social, school, and home life). We offer in this section suggestions for how to track and evaluate progress over the course of treatment using established self-report and clinician-rated measures (see "Progress Measures"). We also discuss process measures to consider when working with patients with BDD, such as patients' expectancies for treatment, homework compliance, in- and out-of-session exposure efforts (i.e., progress made on exposure hierarchy), and "subjective units of distress" ratings during exposure exercises (see "Process Measures"). Finally, we review tips for relapse prevention and retention of treatment gains posttreatment.

Progress Measures

BDD Symptoms, Severity, and Beliefs

Progress in BDD symptoms and severity can be monitored over the course of treatment via the BDD-SS and the BDD-YBOCS-A (psychometric properties were described earlier). The BDD-SS (Wilhelm et al., 2016) assesses number and severity of individual BDD symptoms and serves as a descriptive measure of disorder presentation. Broadly, any symptom group with a severity level of at least 5 (moderate) warrants clinical attention, whereas items with a severity level of 0 do not need to be addressed in treatment (Wilhelm et al., 2013).

Thus, the BDD-SS can be used to identify patient-specific treatment targets (maladaptive cognitions, rituals, avoidance behaviors) and track the nature and specificity of symptom improvement over the course of sessions. The BDD-YBOCS-A (Phillips et al., 1997) is regarded as the "gold standard" measure of past-week BDD symptom severity in both clinical and research contexts. Items map onto the diagnostic criteria (preoccupation, compulsive behaviors, associated distress and impairment), and the measure shows sensitivity to change over time. Patients are considered "treatment responders" once they experience at least a 30% reduction in BDD-YBOCS scores from baseline; this corresponds to clinician ratings of *much improved* on the Clinical Global Impressions (CGI) scale (Phillips et al., 2014; Wilhelm et al., 2014). Using this cut-off score, the BDD-YBOCS has demonstrated 90% sensitivity (i.e., 10% of patients rated as *much improved* on the CGI were not classified as responders on the BDD-YBOCS; Phillips et al., 2014). Clinicians might wish to administer these measures periodically (e.g., every 4–6 weeks) to evaluate symptom improvement. It is also recommended that the clinician monitor changes in insight/delusionality and beliefs about the importance of appearance. Insight can be evaluated using the BABS (psychometric properties reviewed earlier; Eisen et al., 1998).

Comorbid Depressive Symptoms

Depressive symptoms reflect an important facet of a patient's clinical presentation, as symptoms commonly co-occur with—and can be exacerbated by—BDD symptoms. Severity of depressive symptoms also may have implications for self-harm and suicide risk in this population. It is thus recommended that depressive symptoms, including suicide risk, be monitored closely over the course of treatment alongside BDD symptoms. One measure that may be useful for evaluating change in depressive symptoms is the Beck Depression Inventory for Youth (BDI-Y; Beck, Beck, & Jolly, 2001), which is a 20-item self-report assessment of the presence and severity of individual depressive symptoms. Clinicians could also use the Patient Health Questionnaire (PHQ-9; Kroenke & Spitzer, 2002), which is a nine-item self-report tool used to monitor the severity of depressive symptoms in response to treatment. See Hankin and Cohen (Chapter 7, this volume) for a detailed description of the assessment of depression and suicide risk among adolescents.

Quality of Life and Functional Disability

The clinician should assess the extent to which the patient's symptoms inhibit his or her ability to participate in and enjoy different aspects of life. One questionnaire that can be used to evaluate quality of life associated with body image concerns is the 19-item Body Image Quality of Life Inventory (BIQLI; Cash & Fleming, 2002), which quantifies the way in which body image influences the following domains of the individual's life: sense of self, social functioning, emotional well-being, eating, exercise, and grooming. Scores on the BIQLI range from −3 to +3, with score valence interpreted as body image having a positive, neutral (score of 0), or negative impact on the individual's quality of life. The BIQLI has demonstrated strong internal consistency (alpha = .93–95), test–retest reliability (.79; Cash & Fleming, 2002; Cash, Jakatdar, & Williams, 2004), and predictive validity across social, affective, and behavioral correlates in an ecological momentary assessment study with adult populations (Heron, Mason, Sutton, & Myers, 2015). However, this measure has not yet been validated in younger samples.

Adolescents with BDD may experience notable difficulty with relationships (e.g., difficulty engaging with peers, tension within the family) and school (e.g., inability to focus in class or on homework, an urge to avoid school) due to appearance concerns. A common measure used to evaluate functional disability anchored to specific psychiatric symptoms is the Sheehan Disability Scale (SDS; Sheehan, Harnett-Sheehan, & Raj, 1996), which assesses impairment across social, school, and family/home settings. Patients rate the extent to which their BDD symptoms have interfered in each of the three domains on a 10-point Likert scale, with higher scores reflecting greater functional impairment due to symptoms. Generally, a score of 5 (*moderate interference*) or higher on any specific domain warrants clinical attention (Sheehan et al., 1996).

Process Measures

One potential predictor of treatment outcome that should be considered is the patient's expectancies at the outset of therapy. After orienting a patient to treatment components and rationale, the patient can complete the four-item self-report Credibility/Expectancy Questionnaire (Borkovec & Nau, 1972) to gauge his or her impression of the credibility, expectancy of change, and treatment acceptability. This measure has demonstrated good reliability (alpha = .81–.86) and ability to differentiate between differing treatment rationales (Devilly & Borkovec, 2000).

Exposure hierarchies can be used to define—and outline a plan for achieving—meaningful treatment milestones in this population. Specifically, the patient and clinician can jointly generate a list of situations the patient avoids due to appearance concerns (e.g., social activities that require face-to-face interactions, being seen without makeup). These situations are organized in a hierarchical fashion by having patients assign a subjective units of distress (SUDs) rating from 0 to 100, according to how anxiety provoking each situation is. The hierarchy can serve as a road map for graded exposure exercises completed both in and out of session, over the course of treatment. Percentage of feared situations/stimuli faced, as well as reductions in SUDs ratings over repeated exposure trials can be valuable measures of progress. Patients should also be completing homework between each session to maximize treatment gains (e.g., cognitive-restructuring worksheets, out-of-session exposure exercises). Patients' homework compliance should be monitored, as it can reflect their level of investment and buy-in. When homework compliance is low, it is important to collaboratively consider and troubleshoot barriers with the patient (e.g., situational factors, low motivation, problems with the pacing of exposures) and for the clinician to incorporate motivation enhancement strategies.

Posttreatment Monitoring for Maintenance and Relapse Prevention

It is recommended that adolescent patients, and their parents, continue to monitor symptoms once treatment is terminated. Disorder sequelae tend to be aggravated during times of transition and stress (e.g., moving, attending a new school); thus, it may be particularly important to monitor symptoms during these periods. For example, it can be useful to teach patients how to monitor and document time and distress associated with preoccupations and rituals, as well as any increases in avoidance behaviors, parental accommodations, or other risky behaviors (e.g., substance use) weekly. Self-report measures can also be used to track more formally the presence and severity of individual symptoms (e.g., BDD-SS). Patients and their parents can examine trends over time to detect any significant upticks in symptoms. Depressive symp-

toms and suicidal ideation should also be monitored after termination of treatment.

The concept of monitoring can be practiced throughout sessions and further emphasized in late stages of treatment, when session frequency is being tapered, such that the patient monitors his or her own symptom changes on off-weeks and brings this information back to the next therapy session to review. Symptom monitoring for relapse prevention can be facilitated with a basic worksheet that also asks the patient to set a new CBT goal for the upcoming week and to report on how completion of the prior week's goal went. Goals can include practice of any relevant CBT skills, such as cognitive restructuring, exposure, and ritual prevention. Parents can be included in the relapse prevention plan and may be helpful for facilitating problem solving when a patient faces challenges.

Conclusion

BDD is a common yet underrecognized psychiatric illness that frequently onsets in adolescence. BDD is a debilitating disorder that is associated with elevated rates of depression, suicide risk, school and peer interference, and housebound avoidance. Therefore, it is critical for clinicians to effectively assess for BDD among adolescent patients.

At an initial clinical encounter with a new adolescent patient, clinicians may choose to incorporate a brief self-report screening tool into their introductory assessment battery. Screening tools such as the BDDQ-A and DCQ can detect possible signs of BDD, clueing the clinician in to the need for further, more detailed assessment. Following a positive screen, the clinician should further evaluate whether a patient meets diagnostic criteria for BDD using the SCID-5 BDD module. The clinician should conduct a careful differential assessment of conditions with overlapping features, including OCD, excoriation disorder, trichotillomania, SAD, ED, depression, and psychosis, using SCID-5 modules adapted for use in adolescents, the K-SADS-PL, or the MINI-KID.

Once a diagnosis of BDD has been established, it is useful to gauge the patient's current baseline symptom severity (BDD-YBOCS-A), degree of insight and possible delusionality of appearance concerns (BABS), and general constellation of BDD symptoms (BDD-SS). These baseline measures are also useful in subsequent goal setting and treatment planning. At the initial evaluation stage, it may also be useful to consider incorporating secondary informants, such as an adolescent's parent(s) or guidance counselor. These secondary sources may offer supplemental information about the patient's degree of functional interference due to BDD at home and at school, as well as information about the degree to which others' (family, school environment) are accommodating the patient's BDD symptoms. As accommodation maintains BDD symptoms in the long run, this information is also useful for informing treatment targets to incorporate gradually into the patient's exposure hierarchy. Finally, in the initial evaluation, it is critical to assess common risk factors associated with adolescent BDD, including comorbid diagnoses, levels of depression (BDI-Y), suicide risk, and substance use behaviors (K-SAD-PL, MINI-KID).

At the conclusion of this initial evaluation, the clinician will be ready to provide the patient and his or her parents with information about the BDD diagnosis and treatment, and to propose a general treatment plan. Across treatment, changes in BDD symptoms (BDD-YBOCS-A), insight (BABS), comorbid depression (BDI-Y), suicide risk, and reliance on safety behaviors, parental accommodation, or illicit substances should be monitored regularly and targeted in treatment as needed. Toward the end of treatment, the clinician should instruct the patient about how to monitor for changes in his or her own symptoms as part of a comprehensive relapse prevention plan, supported by the patient's parent(s).

REFERENCES

Albertini, R., & Phillips, K. (1999). Thirty-three cases of body dysmorphic disorder in children and adolescents. *Journal of the American Academy of Child and Adolescent Psychiatry, 38,* 453–459.

American Psychiatric Association. (1980). *Diagnostic and statistical manual of mental disorders* (3rd ed.). Washington, DC: Author.

American Psychiatric Association. (1987). *Diagnostic and statistical manual of mental disorders* (3rd ed., rev.). Washington, DC: Author.

American Psychiatric Association. (2013). *Diagnostic and statistical manual of mental disorders* (5th ed.). Arlington, VA: Author.

Beck, J. S., Beck, A. T., & Jolly, J. B. (2001). *Beck Youth Inventories of Emotional and Social Impairment: Depression Inventory for Youth, Anxiety Inventory for Youth, Anger Inventory for Youth, Disruptive Behavior Inventory for Youth, Self-Concept Inventory for Youth: Manual.* San Antonio, TX: Psychological Corporation.

Biby, E. L. (1998). The relationship between body dysmorphic disorder and depression, self-esteem, somatization, and obsessive–compulsive disorder. *Journal of Clinical Psychology, 54,* 489–499.

Bjornsson, A. S., Didie, E. R., Grant, J. E., Menard, W., Stalker, E., & Phillips, K. A. (2013). Age at onset and clinical correlates in body dysmorphic disorder. *Comprehensive Psychiatry, 54,* 893–903.

Bohne, A., Wilhelm, S., Keuthen, N. J., Florin, I., Baer, L., & Jenike, M. A. (2002). Prevalence of body dysmorphic disorder in a German college student sample. *Psychiatry Research, 109,* 101–104.

Borkovec, T. D., & Nau, S. D. (1972). Credibility of analogue therapy rationales. *Journal of Behavior Therapy and Experimental Psychiatry, 3,* 257–260.

Boroughs, M. S., Krawczyk, R., & Thompson, J. (2010). Body dysmorphic disorder among diverse racial/ethnic and sexual orientation groups: Prevalence estimates and associated factors. *Sex Roles, 63,* 725–737.

Buhlmann, U. (2011). Treatment barriers for individuals with body dysmorphic disorder: An internet survey. *Journal of Nervous and Mental Disease, 199,* 268–271.

Buhlmann, U., Cook, L. M., Fama, J. M., & Wilhelm, S. (2007). Perceived teasing experiences in body dysmorphic disorder. *Body Image, 4,* 381–385.

Buhlmann, U., Marques, M. L., & Wilhelm, M. S. (2012). Traumatic experiences in individuals with body dysmorphic disorder. *Journal of Nervous and Mental Disease, 200,* 95–98.

Cansever, A., Uzun, O., Donmez, E., & Ozsahin, A. (2003). The prevalence and clinical features of body dysmorphic disorder in college students: A study in a Turkish sample. *Comprehensive Psychiatry, 44,* 60–64.

Cash, T. F., & Fleming, E. C. (2002). The impact of body image experiences: Development of the Body Image Quality of Life Inventory. *International Journal of Eating Disorders, 31,* 455–460.

Cash, T. F., Jakatdar, T. A., & Williams, E. F. (2004). The Body Image Quality of Life Inventory: Further validation with college men and women. *Body Image, 1,* 279–287.

Cororve, M. B., & Gleaves, D. H. (2001). Body dysmorphic disorder: A review of conceptualizations, assessment, and treatment strategies. *Clinical Psychology Review, 21,* 949–970.

Devilly, G. J., & Borkovec, T. D. (2000). Psychometric properties of the credibility/expectancy questionnaire. *Journal of Behavior Therapy and Experimental Psychiatry, 31,* 73–86.

Dingemans, A. E., Van Rood, Y. R., De Groot, I., & Van Furth, E. F. (2012). Body dysmorphic disorder in patients with an eating disorder: Prevalence and characteristics. *International Journal of Eating Disorders, 45,* 562–569.

Dyl, J., Kittler, J., Phillips, K. A., & Hunt, J. I. (2006). Body dysmorphic disorder and other clinically significant body image doncerns in adolescent psychiatric inpatients: Prevalence and clinical characteristics. *Child Psychiatry and Human Development, 36,* 369–382.

Eisen, J. L., Phillips, K. A., Baer, L., Beer, D. A., Atala, K. D., & Rasmussen, S. A. (1998). The Brown Assessment of Beliefs Scale: Reliability and validity. *American Journal of Psychiatry, 155,* 102–108.

Eisen, J. L., Phillips, K. A., Coles, M. E., & Rasmussen, S. A. (2004). Insight in obsessive compulsive disorder and body dysmorphic disorder. *Comprehensive Psychiatry, 45,* 10–15.

Enander, J., Ivanov, V. Z., Mataix-Cols, D., Kuja-Halkola, R., Ljótsson, B., Lundström, S., . . . Rück, C. (2018). Prevalence and heritability of body dysmorphic symptoms in adolescents and young adults: A population-based nationwide twin study. *Psychological Medicine, 48,* 2740–2747.

Fang, A., & Hofmann, S. G. (2010). Relationship between social anxiety disorder and body dysmorphic disorder. *Clinical Psychology Review, 30,* 1040–1048.

Fang, A., & Wilhelm, S. (2015). Clinical Features, cognitive biases, and treatment of body dysmorphic disorder. *Annual Review of Clinical Psychology, 11,* 187–212.

First, M. B., Williams, J., Karg, R. S., & Spitzer, R. L. (2015). *User's guide for the Structured Clinical Interview for DSM-5 Disorders, Clinician Version (SCID-5-CV):* Arlington, VA: American Psychiatric Publishing.

Grant, J. E., Kim, S. W., & Crow, S. J. (2001). Prevalence and clinical features of body dysmorphic disorder in adolescent and adult psychiatric inpatients. *Journal of Clinical Psychiatry, 62,* 517–522.

Grant, J. E., Kim, S. W., & Eckert, E. D. (2002). Body dysmorphic disorder in patients with anorexia nervosa: Prevalence, clinical features, and delusionality of body image. *International Journal of Eating Disorders, 32,* 291–300.

Grant, J. E., Menard, W., Pagano, M. E., Fay, C., & Phillips, K. A. (2005). Substance use disorders in individuals with body dysmorphic disorder. *Journal of Clinical Psychiatry, 66,* 309–316.

Greenberg, J. L., Mothi, S. S., & Wilhelm, S. (2016). Cognitive-behavioral therapy for adolescent body dysmorphic disorder: A pilot study. *Behavior Therapy, 47,* 213–224.

Heron, K. E., Mason, T. B., Sutton, T. G., & Myers, T. A. (2015). Evaluating the real-world predictive validity of the Body Image Quality of Life Inventory using ecological momentary assessment. *Body Image, 15,* 105–108.

Jacobson, N. S., & Truax, P. (1991). Clinical significance: a statistical approach to defining meaningful change in psychotherapy research. *Journal of Consulting and Clinical Psychology, 59,* 12–19.

Jolanta, J. R. J., & Tomasz, M. S. (2000). The links between body dysmorphic disorder and eating disorders. *European Psychiatry, 15,* 302–305.

Jorge, R. T. B., Sabino Neto, M., Natour, J., Veiga, D. F., Jones, A., & Ferreirea, L. M. (2008). Brazilian version of the Body Dysmorphic Disorder Examination. *São Paulo Medical Journal, 126,* 87–95.

Joseph, A. W., Ishii, L., Joseph, S. S., Smith, J. I., Su, P., Bater, K., . . . Ishii, M. (2017). Prevalence of body dysmorphic disorder and surgeon diagnostic accuracy in facial plastic and oculoplastic surgery clinics. *JAMA Facial Plastic Surgery, 19,* 269–274.

Kaufman, J., Birmaher, B., Brent, D., Rao, U., Flynn, C., Moreci, P., . . . Ryan, N. (1997). Schedule for Affective Disorders and Schizophrenia for School-Age Children—Present and Lifetime Version (K-SADS-PL): Initial reliability and validity data. *Journal of the American Academy of Child and Adolescent Psychiatry, 36,* 980–988.

Kroenke, K., & Spitzer, R. L. (2002). The PHQ-9: A new depression diagnostic and severity measure. *Psychiatric Annals, 32,* 509–515.

Leone, J. E., Sedory, E. J., & Gray, K. A. (2005). Recognition and treatment of muscle dysmorphia and related body image disorders. *Journal of Athletic Training, 40,* 352–359.

Mancuso, S. G., Knoesen, N. P., & Castle, D. J. (2010). The Dysmorphic Concern Questionnaire: A screening measure for body dysmorphic disorder. *Australian and New Zealand Journal of Psychiatry, 44,* 535–542.

Marques, L., Weingarden, H. M., LeBlanc, N. J., & Wilhelm, S. (2011). Treatment utilization and barriers to treatment engagement among people with body dysmorphic symptoms. *Journal of Psychosomatic Research, 70,* 286–293.

Mataix-Cols, D., Fernández de La Cruz, L., Isomura, K., Anson, M., Turner, C., Monzani, B., . . . Krebs, G. (2015). A pilot randomized controlled trial of cognitive-behavioral therapy for adolescents with body dysmorphic disorder. *Journal of the American Academy of Child and Adolescent Psychiatry, 54,* 895–904.

Mayville, S., Katz, R. C., Gipson, M. T., & Cabral, K. (1999). Assessing the prevalence of body dysmorphic disorder in an ethnically diverse group of adolescents. *Journal of Child and Family Studies, 8,* 357–362.

Mosley, P. E. (2009). Bigorexia: Bodybuilding and muscle dysmorphia. *European Eating Disorders Review, 17,* 191–198.

Oosthuizen, P., Lambert, T., & Castle, D. (1998). Dysmorphic concern: Prevalence and associations with clinical variables. *Australian and New Zealand Journal of Psychiatry, 32,* 129–132.

Osman, S., Cooper, M., Hackmann, A., & Veale, D. (2004). Spontaneously occurring images and early memories in people with body dysmorphic disorder. *Memory, 12,* 428–436.

Phillips, K. A. (1996). *The broken mirror: Understanding and treating body dysmorphic disorder.* New York: Oxford University Press.

Phillips, K. A. (2006). An open-label study of escitalopram in body dysmorphic disorder. *International Clinical Psychopharmacology, 21,* 177–179.

Phillips, K. A. (Ed.). (2017). *Body dysmorphic disorder:*

Advances in research and clinical practice. New York: Oxford University Press.

Phillips, K. A., Atala, K. D., & Pope, H. G. (1995). Diagnostic instruments for body dysmorphic disorder. *Journal of Consulting and Clinical Psychology, 63,* 263–269.

Phillips, K. A., & Diaz, S. F. (1997). Gender differences in body dysmorphic disorder. *Journal of Nervous and Mental Disease, 185,* 570–577.

Phillips, K. A., Didie, E. R., Menard, W., Pagano, M. E., Fay, C., & Weisberg, R. B. (2006). Clinical features of body dysmorphic disorder in adolescents and adults. *Psychiatry Research, 141,* 305–314.

Phillips, K. A., Grant, J., Siniscalchi, J., & Albertini, R. S. (2001). Surgical and nonpsychiatric medical treatment of patients with body dysmorphic disorder. *Psychosomatics, 42,* 504–510.

Phillips, K. A., Hart, A. S., & Menard, W. (2014). Psychometric evaluation of the Yale–Brown Obsessive Compulsive Scale Modified for Body Dysmorphic Disorder (BDD-YBOCS). *Journal of Obsessive-Compulsive and Related Disorders, 3,* 205–208.

Phillips, K. A., Hart, A. S., Menard, L. W., & Eisen, L. J. (2013). Psychometric evaluation of the Brown Assessment of Beliefs Scale in body dysmorphic disorder. *Journal of Nervous and Mental Disease, 201,* 640–643.

Phillips, K. A., Hollander, E., Rasmussen, S. A., Aronowitz, B. R., Decaria, C., & Goodman, W. K. (1997). A severity rating scale for body dysmorphic disorder: Development, reliability, and validity of a modified version of the Yale–Brown Obsessive Compulsive Scale. *Psychopharmacology Bulletin, 33,* 17–22.

Phillips, K. A., & Menard, W. (2006). Suicidality in body dysmorphic disorder: A prospective study. *American Journal of Psychiatry, 163,* 1280–1282.

Phillips, K. A., Menard, W., Pagano, M. E., Fay, C., & Stout, R. L. (2006). Delusional versus nondelusional body dysmorphic disorder: Clinical features and course of illness. *Journal of Psychiatric Research, 40,* 95–104.

Phillips, K. A., Pinto, A., Hart, A. S., Coles, M. E., Eisen, J. L., Menard, W., & Rasmussen, S. A. (2012). A comparison of insight in body dysmorphic disorder and obsessive–compulsive disorder. *Journal of Psychiatric Research, 46,* 1293–1299.

Phillips, K. A., & Taub, S. L. (1995). Skin picking as a symptom of body dysmorphic disorder. *Psychopharmacology Bulletin, 31,* 279–288.

Pope, C. G., Pope, H. G., Menard, W., Fay, C., Olivardia, R., & Phillips, K. A. (2005). Clinical features of muscle dysmorphia among males with body dysmorphic disorder. *Body Image, 2,* 395–400.

Pope, H. G., Jr., Gruber, A. J., Choi, P., Olivardia, R., & Phillips, K. A. (1997). Muscle dysmorphia: An underrecognized form of body dysmorphic disorder. *Psychosomatics, 38,* 548–557.

Pope, H., Katz, D. L., & Hudson, J. (1993). Anorexia nervosa and reverse anorexia among 108 male bodybuilders. *Comprehensive Psychiatry, 34,* 406–409.

Ribeiro, R. V. E. (2017). Prevalence of body dysmorphic disorder in plastic surgery and dermatology patients: A systematic review with meta-analysis. *Aesthetic Plastic Surgery, 41,* 964–970.

Rief, W., Buhlmann, U., Wilhelm, S., Borkenhagen, A., & Brahler, E. (2006). The prevalence of body dysmorphic disorder: A population-based survey. *Psychological Medicine, 36,* 877–885.

Rosen, J. C., & Reiter, J. (1996). Development of the body dysmorphic disorder examination. *Behaviour Research and Therapy, 34,* 755–766.

Scahill, L., Riddle, M. A., McSwiggin-Hardin, M., Ort, S. I., King, R. A., Goodman, W. K., . . . Leckman, J. F. (1997). Children's Yale–Brown Obsessive Compulsive Scale: Reliability and validity. *Journal of the American Academy of Child and Adolescent Psychiatry, 36,* 844–852.

Schneider, S. C., Turner, C. M., Mond, J., & Hudson, J. L. (2017). Prevalence and correlates of body dysmorphic disorder in a community sample of adolescents. *Australian and New Zealand Journal of Psychiatry, 51,* 595–603.

Sheehan, D., Harnett-Sheehan, K., & Raj, B. (1996). The measurement of disability. *International Clinical Psychopharmacology, 11*(Suppl. 3), 89–95.

Sheehan, D. V., Sheehan, K. H., Shytle, R. D., Janavs, J., Bannon, Y., Rogers, J. E., . . . Wilkinson, B. (2010). Reliability and validity of the Mini International Neuropsychiatric Interview for Children and Adolescents (MINI-KID). *Journal of Clinical Psychiatry, 71,* 313–326.

Silverman, A. B., Reinherz, H. Z., & Giaconia, R. M. (1996). The long-term sequelae of child and adolescent abuse: A longitudinal community study. *Child Abuse and Neglect, 20,* 709–723.

Storch, E. A., Bussing, R., Jacob, M. L., Nadeau, J. M., Crawford, E., Mutch, P. J., . . . Murphy, T. K. (2015). Frequency and correlates of suicidal ideation in pediatric obsessive–compulsive disorder. *Child Psychiatry and Human Development, 46,* 75–83.

Summers, B. J., & Cougle, J. R. (2018). An experimental test of the role of appearance-related safety behaviors in body dysmorphic disorder, social anxiety, and body dissatisfaction. *Journal of Abnormal Psychology, 127,* 770–780.

Toh, W. L., Castle, D. J., Mountjoy, R. L., Buchanan, B., Farhall, J., & Rossell, S. L. (2017). Insight in body dysmorphic disorder (BDD) relative to obsessive–compulsive disorder (OCD) and psychotic disorders: Revisiting this issue in light of DSM-5. *Comprehensive Psychiatry, 77,* 100–108.

Tolin, D. F., Gilliam, C., Wootton, B. M., Bowe, W., Bragdon, L. B., Davis, E., . . . Hallion, L. S. (2018). Psychometric properties of a structured diagnostic interview for DSM-5 anxiety, mood, and obsessive–

compulsive and related disorders. *Assessment, 25,* 3–13.

Veale, D. (2009). Body Image Questionnaire—Child and Adolescent version. Retrieved from *www.kcl.ac.uk/ioppn/depts/psychology/research/ResearchGroupings/CADAT/Research/Body-Image-Questionnaires.aspx.*

Veale, D., De Haro, L., & Lambrou, C. (2003). Cosmetic rhinoplasty in body dysmorphic disorder. *British Journal of Plastic Surgery, 56,* 546–551.

Veale, D., Gournay, K., Dryden, W., Boocock, A., Shah, F., Willson, R., & Walburn., J. (1996). Body dysmorphic disorder: A cognitive behavioural model and pilot randomised controlled trial. *Behaviour Research and Therapy, 34,* 717–729.

Veale, D., Miles, S., Re ad, J., Troglia, A., Carmona, L., Fiorito, C., . . . Muir, G. (2015). Environmental and physical risk factors for men to develop body dysmorphic disorder concerning penis size compared to men anxious about their penis size and men with no concerns: A cohort study. *Journal of Obsessive-Compulsive and Related Disorders, 6,* 49–58.

Weingarden, H., Curley, E. E., Renshaw, K. D., & Wilhelm, S. (2017). Patient-identified events implicated in the development of body dysmorphic disorder. *Body Image, 21,* 19–25.

Weingarden, H., & Renshaw, K. D. (2015). Shame in the obsessive compulsive related disorders: A conceptual review. *Journal of Affective Disorders, 171,* 74–84.

Wilhelm, S. (2006). *Feeling good about the way you look: A program for overcoming body image problems.* New York: Guilford Press.

Wilhelm, S., Greenberg, J. L., Rosenfield, E., Kasarskis, I., & Blashill, A. J. (2016). The Body Dysmorphic Disorder Symptom Scale: Development and preliminary validation of a self-report scale of symptom specific dysfunction. *Body Image, 17,* 82–87.

Wilhelm, S., Phillips, K. A., & Steketee, G. (2013). *Cognitive-behavioral therapy for body dysmorphic disorder: A treatment manual.* New York: Guilford Press.

Wilhelm, S., Phillips, K. A., Didie, E., Buhlmann, U., Greenberg, J. L., Fama, J. M., . . . Steketee, G. (2014). Modular cognitive-behavioral therapy for body dysmorphic disorder: A randomized controlled trial. *Behavior Therapy, 45,* 314–327.

Woods, D. W., & Houghton, D. C. (2014). Diagnosis, evaluation, and management of trichotillomania. *Psychiatric Clinics of North America, 37,* 301–317.

PART VIII

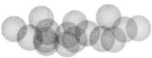

Health-Related Issues

CHAPTER 23

Pediatric Sleep

Lisa J. Meltzer

Sleep is ubiquitous, which means that every patient or research participant will engage in sleep for at least part of every day. Similar to breathing and eating, sleep is a critical health asset. However, 25–40% of youth without chronic illnesses or developmental disorders experience sleep problems at some point during childhood or adolescence (Mindell & Owens, 2015; Owens, 2005), with up to 80% of youth with chronic illnesses or developmental disorders experiencing sleep issues (Lewandowski, Ward, & Palermo, 2011; Robinson-Shelton & Malow, 2016). When children or adolescents do not obtain sufficient, high-quality sleep, every aspect of functioning is impacted, including their physical, mental, and social health. Thus, it is important to gain a basic foundational understanding of how sleep works, how to screen for sleep disorders and sleep problems, and how to integrate sleep assessment into clinical practice or research studies.

The Basics of Sleep

Sleep Stages

Sleep is not a passive, meaningless function, but rather a complex process in which our bodies and brains recover from the day and prepare for the next day. At bedtime, it takes most people between 10 and 20 minutes to fall asleep. When a child falls asleep immediately, that is a sign of insufficient or poor-quality sleep. When a child regularly takes more than 30–45 minutes to fall asleep every night, this can result in insomnia.

There are two primary stages of sleep: rapid eye movement (REM) and non–rapid eye movement (NREM) (Carskadon & Dement, 2010). Within NREM sleep there are three substages: N1 (light sleep), N2 (midstage sleep or "true" sleep), and N3 (deep sleep) (Mindell & Owens, 2015). Each stage of sleep serves a unique purpose. For example, during N3 sleep (which should occur primarily after sleep onset), growth hormone is released and executive functioning develops, while during REM sleep (which predominantly occurs in the last part of the night) memories and learning consolidate (Sheldon, 2014). Understanding the different types of sleep stages, and when they occur, is important when assessing for disorders of arousal (reviewed in the next section), including sleep terrors, sleepwalking, and nightmares.

Throughout the night, we cycle between each NREM and REM stage of sleep, with sleep cycles typically lasting about 50–60 minutes for infants and young children and 90–110 minutes in children and adolescents (Mindell & Owens, 2015). At the end of most sleep cycles, the brain has a brief arousal before returning to sleep. This is important to understand because frequent night wakings is one of the most common sleep complaints in younger children. However, night wakings are normal; the true issue is that the child is unable to return to sleep without assistance following a normal arousal.

Two-Process Model of Sleep and Wake

There are two major processes that facilitate sleep and wakefulness: Process S, which is dependent on duration of sleep and wake, and Process C, which is regulated by the circadian rhythm. These two processes work together to provide wakefulness during the day and promote consolidated sleep during the night.

Process S

Sleep pressure (or the need for sleep) builds every hour that a person is awake (Achermann & Borbely, 2010; Borbely, 1982). Once a certain threshold is reached, the sleep pressure is sufficient to help a person fall asleep. In the first part of the night, the high level of sleep pressure pushes a person into the deepest stage of sleep (N3). In addition, because of the high level of sleep pressure, if awakened during the first few hours of sleep, it is relatively easy to return to sleep. However, as the night passes, sleep pressure is alleviated; thus, it is often harder to return to sleep if awakened in the early morning hours.

However, Process S is also dependent on hours of wakefulness. In other words, a person has to be awake a certain number of hours before he or she has built enough sleep pressure to facilitate sleep onset. The amount of wakefulness needed changes with development (Jenni & Carskadon, 2005). Specifically, because sleep pressure builds more rapidly in young children, naps are developmentally appropriate for most children until the age of 3 years, with at least 25% of children still napping at age 5 years (National Sleep Foundation, 2004).

For most school-age children, after 12–14 hours of wakefulness, sleep pressure should be sufficient to facilitate sleep onset; thus, naps should not be observed in school-age children. Adolescents should be able to maintain wakefulness for 14–16 hours, although there is a biological need for many adolescents to have a short, 45-minute nap in the afternoon (Carskadon & Acebo, 2002).

Process C

The circadian pacemaker is located in the suprachiasmatic nuclei (SCN) and is regulated by external cues (called zeitgeibers, or "time givers"), in particular, the light–dark cycle. Darkness signals the brain to produce melatonin, which helps prepare the body for sleeping, while light suppresses melatonin production, which contributes to the promotion of wakefulness. During puberty, the onset of melatonin is delayed by 1–2 hours for most youth, resulting in significant challenges falling asleep early and waking in time for early school start times. This is one of the strongest factors behind the movement to delay middle and high school start times to 8:30 A.M. (American Academy of Pediatrics, 2014).

Research Domain Criteria

Sleep falls under the Research Domain Criteria (RDoC) of Arousal/Regulatory Systems, which are defined as "responsible for generating activation of neural systems as appropriate for various contexts and providing appropriate homeostatic regulation of such systems as energy balance and sleep" (NIMH Definitions of the RDoc Domains and Constructs, section 6). The three constructs are arousal, circadian rhythms, and sleep and wakefulness.

Each of these constructs highlight the different aspects of sleep and daytime functioning that are critical to health and well-being. The construct of arousal is "regulated by homeostatic drives," which is supported by Process S. The circadian rhythms construct focuses on the regulation of circadian systems by external stimuli (e.g., light), which is supported by Process C. Finally, the construct of sleep and wakefulness focuses on how these two processes interact to ensure a continuous pattern of alternating sleep and wakefulness, and how what happens during sleep affects neurobehavioral and other functions during wakefulness, as well as how homeostatic drive and experiences during wakefulness impact the quality and quantity of sleep.

Sleep and Mental Health

An entire volume could be dedicated to the dynamic interaction between sleep and mental health; thus, it is not possible to comprehensively review the literature that has considered different mental health disorders and sleep. This section highlights some of the most common associations found between sleep and mental health disorders to increase awareness among clinical child psychologists. Readers are referred to an excellent, detailed review article by Gregory and Sadeh (2016) for more information on this topic. In terms of assessment, questions and measures described later in this chapter can easily be woven into the daily clinical practice of psychologists who focus on mental health disorders.

Neurodevelopmental Disorders

Children with neurodevelopmental disorders including autism, ADHD, global developmental delays, and numerous syndromes (e.g., Williams, Down, Angelman) have been shown to have significantly more issues with sleep than typically developing children, including prolonged sleep-onset latency, frequent night wakings, and/or early sleep termination (Gregory & Sadeh, 2016). Although the mechanisms for the increased frequency of sleep disorders are still being explored, theories related to the inability to self-soothe and regulate at bedtime, anatomical differences that may dysregulate sleep, and issues with either reduced melatonin production or mistiming of melatonin release have been considered (Mazzone, Postorino, Siracusano, Riccioni, & Curatolo, 2018).

Mood Disorders

There is a strong relationship between sleep and depression, with studies consistently showing sleep issues (in particular insomnia and hypersomnia) among children and adolescents with depression, with reports that sleep disturbances (in particular insomnia) often precede the onset of depression (Alvaro, Roberts, & Harris, 2013; Lovato & Gradisar, 2014; Roberts & Duong, 2014). Clinically, children and adolescents with depression may also experience dysfunctional beliefs about sleep that make sleep initiation and maintenance more difficult (Clarke & Harvey, 2012). Alternatively, hyperinsomnia may be seen in youth with depression who do not want to engage with others or in activities. Instead, these youth will often sleep at least 12–16 hours, especially on weekends.

Anxiety Disorders

In addition to difficulties falling and staying asleep, youth with anxiety may experience a broader range of sleep issues, including bedtime resistance and nightmares (Alfano, 2018). At bedtime, anxiety may increase a child's fears, resulting in increased irrational thoughts that make sleep onset difficult. Similarly, children with separation anxiety may find bedtime particularly stressful, with co-sleeping often required in order to help the child fall asleep. Cognitive and physiological arousal can also delay sleep onset for youth with anxiety.

Clinical Assessment and Research Outcomes: Patterns, Habits, and Disorders of Sleep

"Do you (or your child) have problems sleeping?" This simple question is one of the easiest ways to quickly assess for sleep issues in clinical settings. A positive response would suggest the need for additional screening or measurement. Difficulties sleeping and daytime sleepiness are the most common symptoms that may indicate a sleep problem or sleep disorder. However, a negative response does not mean that sleep should be crossed off the list of symptoms or factors to be considered, as patients and parents may be unaware of underlying sleep disorders that may impact both sleep and wakefulness (Meltzer & Crabtree, 2015).

Sleep can easily be viewed through a biopsychosocial lens, with biological factors such as the two-process model of sleep contributing to sleep and wakefulness, along with different behavioral and environmental factors that can promote or interfere with sufficient sleep duration and good sleep quality. Not only is it important to identify these different factors to guide diagnoses and clinical treatment, but when determining research outcomes it is also essential to have a clear definition of what is being measured.

One way to conceptualize these factors is the "PHD of sleep:" sleep *Patterns*, sleep *Habits*, and sleep *Disorders*. This section provides an overview of each PHD construct to better assist readers with clinical questions that can be used for screening and/or treatment planning, as well as assist with the selection of measures to use in research studies. This is followed by a discussion of one of the most important sleep assessment tools, the sleep diary. The section concludes with case examples that highlight how different clinical questions and sleep diary data can be utilized. For a more detailed discussion of how to conduct a comprehensive sleep assessment, readers are referred to Meltzer and Crabtree (2015).

Sleep Patterns

Sleep Quantity

The most common cause of daytime sleepiness is not getting enough sleep; thus, it is important to ask how much sleep a child is obtaining. Although sleep need can vary significantly between children, there are recommended ranges of sleep duration, with most children falling within these ranges (Paruthi et al., 2016). One clear sign of insufficient sleep during the week is a difference of 2 or more hours of sleep between weekdays and weekends. In this case, the child is attempting to make up his or her sleep debt on the weekends. If a child is obtaining sufficient sleep for his or her age but is still excessively sleepy during the day, it is important to consider underlying sleep disorders that may be contributing to poor quality sleep.

Clinical Questions

"How many hours of sleep do you get on weekdays?"; "How many hours of sleep do you get on weekends?"

Common Research Outcomes

Total sleep time (TST; hours of sleep between bedtime and wake time), separating weekdays and weekends for older children and adolescents to measure for weekend oversleep (number of hours of extra sleep obtained on weekends vs. weekdays).

Sleep Schedule

Sleep schedules include bedtimes, wake times, and nap times. Having a consistent sleep schedule is important for keeping the circadian rhythm on track and to ensure that sufficient sleep pressure accumulates prior to bedtime. Inconsistent bedtimes and wake times, shifting sleep schedules by more than 1 hour on weekends, or improperly timed naps (i.e., too close to bedtime) can all interfere with a child's ability to fall asleep or wake in the morning, and may contribute to excessive daytime sleepiness. Sleep schedule questions can be used to calculate sleep opportunity (which is often used as a proxy for sleep duration).

Clinical Questions

"What time do you try to fall asleep at bedtime (weekdays and weekends)?"; "What time do you wake up in the morning to start your day (weekdays and weekends)?"; "Do you nap (and if yes, what time)?"

Common Research Outcomes

Bedtime (clock time the child attempted to fall asleep), wake time (clock time the child awakens in the morning to start the day), sleep opportunity or time in bed (TIB; hours between bedtime and wake time).

Sleep-Onset Latency

Sleep-onset latency is how long it takes a person to fall asleep. It is important to note that sleep-onset latency starts when the child attempted to fall asleep rather than what time the child got into bed, especially if the child reads or engages in other activities (e.g., phone, tablet use) before attempting to fall asleep. As previously described, a rapid sleep onset (e.g., "immediately" or "in just a couple of minutes") can be a sign of insufficient or poor-quality sleep. Similarly, a very prolonged sleep-onset latency may be a sign of insomnia or a delayed circadian rhythm.

Clinical Question

"Once you are in bed, turn off the lights, and try to fall asleep, how long does it take you to fall asleep?"

Common Research Outcome

Sleep-onset latency (SOL; duration in minutes or hours from reported bedtime to time child fell asleep).

Night Wakings

Although nighttime arousals are normal, prolonged night wakings can contribute to insufficient sleep duration and poor sleep quality. It is important to assess the timing and frequency of night wakings to help identify potential sleep disorders (described later). As a child gets older, parents may become less aware of when he or she wakes during the night (Meltzer et al., 2013; Paavonen et al., 2000). Thus, starting around the age of 8 years, children should directly be asked about night wakings.

Clinical Questions

"Once you fall asleep, do you wake up during the night?"; "If yes, how often?"; "How long are you awake?"

Common Research Outcomes

Night-waking frequency (NWF; number of times the child awakens between bedtime and wake time), night-waking duration (NWD; minutes/hours child is awake during night wakings), wake after sleep onset (WASO; cumulative time of night-waking durations representing amount of time child is awake between sleep onset and morning waking).

Naps

As previously mentioned, naps are age appropriate for younger children, and some adolescents may have a biological need for a short afternoon nap. However, if naps last too long, or occur too close to bedtime, it will be difficult to fall asleep, which in turn may result in insufficient sleep and daytime sleepiness. If a school-age child is reportedly getting sufficient nighttime sleep but still naps regularly, then this could be a sign of poor-quality sleep, and further screening for sleep disorders may be needed.

Clinical Questions

"Do you nap?"; "If yes, how often, at what time, and for how long?"

Common Research Outcomes

Nap frequency (number of naps per day or week), nap duration (length of naps).

Sleep Habits

Bedtime/Evening Routine

The activities that precede bedtime can greatly impact sleep quantity and quality. An inconsistent or exceptionally long bedtime routine can be quite stressful for both children and their parents. Bed-

time routines are critical for children of all ages and may contribute to many different aspects of development (Mindell & Williamson, 2018).

Clinical Questions

"Do you have a bedtime routine?"; "If yes, please describe what happens on a typical night between dinner and the time your child falls asleep."

Common Research Outcome

Bedtime routine (yes–no).

Sleep Location and Parental Presence

Where a child falls asleep and wakes up is important to assess, as many children fall asleep in one location and wake up in another. This may be a result of a child who does not have a consistent bedtime routine (e.g., falls asleep on the couch watching television and parents moves child to his or her room). However, changes in sleep location is more commonly a sign of a child who needs parental presence to fall asleep at bedtime, then following normal nighttime arousal, needs the parental presence to return to sleep. This most commonly presents as a child who falls asleep in his or her own bed with the parent present, but then moves to the parents' bed sometime during the night.

Clinical Questions

"Where does your child fall asleep"; "Does he or she fall asleep alone, or is someone in the room with him or her?"; "Where does your child wake up?"

Common Research Outcomes

Location where child falls asleep, wakes in the morning, and whether parent is present at bedtime (yes–no).

Caffeine Use

According to the American Academy of Pediatrics, children under age 12 years should not consume any caffeine, while adolescents should limit caffeine to 85–100 mg per day (Committee on Nutrition and the Council on Sports Medicine and Fitness, 2011). Caffeine is a wake-promoting drug that blocks adenosine, a chemical that makes us feel sleepy as it builds up over the day. Because caffeine has a half-life of approximately 4–6 hours, too much caffeine or improperly timed caffeine can interfere with SOL, which in turn may result in insufficient sleep and daytime sleepiness.

Clinical Questions

"How often do you drink beverages with caffeine?"; "What time do you drink your last caffeinated beverage of the day?"

Common Research Outcomes

Caffeine amount (per day), caffeine frequency (per day/week).

Sleep Environment

To ensure high-quality sleep, it is recommended that bedrooms be cool, dark, comfortable, and technology free. While few studies have examined the relationship between sleep duration/sleep quality and "cool, dark, and comfortable," several reports have clearly demonstrated an association between the presence of technology and shortened sleep duration or poor-quality sleep (Buxton et al., 2015; Gradisar et al., 2013; Mindell, Meltzer, Carskadon, & Chervin, 2009), even if the technology is not used in the hour prior to bedtime.

Clinical Questions

"Is there a nightlight or other light on at bedtime?"; "Is there technology in the bedroom (e.g., television, laptop, tablet, phone)?"

Common Research Outcomes

Presence of technology in the bedroom, use of technology in the hour prior to sleep onset.

Sleep Disorders

It is beyond the scope of this chapter to provide a comprehensive review of all pediatric sleep disorders. Thus, the following is a brief overview of common sleep disorders seen in children and adolescents.

Poor Sleep Quality

While not a diagnosable disorder per se, poor sleep quality is one of the most common clinical complaints. Using the questions outlined in this section, a clinician can better clarify *why* a child or adolescent has poor sleep quality (e.g., insufficient sleep, obstructive sleep apnea [OSA], poor sleep habits). However, overall sleep quality remains one

of the most common outcomes in research. It is important to remember that sleep quality is a subjective experience, and whenever possible, questions about sleep quality should be asked directly of children ages 8 years and older.

Excessive Daytime Sleepiness

Excessive daytime sleepiness (EDS, or hypersomnia) can be a result of both biological and behavioral factors described throughout the PHD of Sleep. However, it is important to recognize the most common signs of EDS, including (1) significant difficulties waking in the morning (e.g., multiple alarm clocks, parent throwing water on a child to wake him or her), (2) falling asleep in school (school-age children and adolescents), (3) regularly falling asleep on brief car rides (i.e., less than 10–20 minutes) regardless of time of day, (4) falling asleep during events or activities (e.g., birthday party, sporting events), and (5) changes in mood (e.g., irritable) or behavior (e.g., hyperactive) following a night of poor-quality/insufficient sleep.

Clinical Questions

"Following a night of poor-quality or not enough sleep, what do you notice different about yourself (your child) the next day?"; "Do you (your child) regularly fall asleep in school or on short car rides?"; "Is it difficult to wake up and get going in the morning?"

Insufficient Sleep

The most common cause of difficulties waking in the morning or daytime sleepiness is insufficient sleep. Before other diagnoses can be made, it is essential that children and adolescents have an age-appropriate sleep opportunity every night. Sleep opportunity can be determined using the sleep schedule questions. If a sufficient sleep opportunity is present, and the child still has difficulties falling asleep, frequent night wakings, difficulty waking in the morning, or daytime sleepiness, the following sleep disorders should be considered.

Insomnia

The hallmark features of insomnia are difficulties initiating sleep, difficulties maintaining sleep, or waking early and being unable to return to sleep

(American Academy of Sleep Medicine, 2014). Notably, in the third edition of the *International Classification of Sleep Disorders* (ICSD-3), these symptoms must occur within an age-appropriate sleep opportunity and be accompanied by daytime dysfunction, which can include sleepiness, academic impairments, or behavior problems. Insomnia can be screened with previously described sleep schedule, SOL, and night wakings questions.

Circadian Rhythm Sleep–Wake Disorders

Circadian rhythm sleep–wake disorders (CRSWDs) are a group of disorders in which the circadian rhythm is not in alignment with a person's typical day (American Academy of Sleep Medicine, 2014). Delayed sleep–wake phase disorder (DSWPD) is most commonly seen in adolescents who are unable to fall asleep at a "normal bedtime." Most youth with DSWPD are unable to fall asleep until between 1:00 and 4:00 A.M.; however, once asleep, their sleep quality is good. The problem is that early school start times prevent these youth from obtaining sufficient sleep duration, resulting in difficulties waking in the morning and excessive daytime sleepiness. One of the key features that differentiates insomnia from DSWPD is that when youth with the latter attempt to fall asleep at a later bedtime, they can fall asleep quickly and not wake during the night, whereas a youth with insomnia will likely have difficulties initiating or maintaining sleep regardless of the bedtime.

Clinical Questions

"If you go to bed later, do you fall asleep faster?"; "When are you most alert/awake, or when would you want to take your most important exams: morning, midday, or evening?" (Those who respond evening are likely to have a delayed circadian phase preference.)

Parasomnias

Sleepwalking, sleep talking, and sleep terrors are all disorders of arousal that fall under the term "parasomnias" (American Academy of Sleep Medicine, 2014). These disorders occur during the transition from sleep to wake or sleep to dreaming, with the child appearing awake, yet having no memory of the event. Sleepwalking children may engage in purposeful behaviors, and children with

sleep terrors may be distressed or appear fearful, while children with sleep talking may engage in nonsensical conversations. These events typically occur in the first part of the night, when children are coming out of slow wave sleep (NREM, Stage 3). Up to 40% of children experience at least one parasomnia episode in their lifetime, with approximately 1–7% of children having frequent events (American Academy of Sleep Medicine, 2014). Parasomnias are most often triggered by insufficient or poor-quality sleep (Mason & Pack, 2007); thus, it is important to screen for sufficient sleep duration, as well as underlying sleep disorders such as OSA, restless legs syndrome, or periodic limb movements in sleep.

Clinical Questions

"What time of night do these events occur?" Sleep terrors: "When your child wakes, is he or she responsive to your efforts to comfort him or herher?" All parasomnias: "Does your child recall these behaviors or events the next day?"

Recurrent Nightmares

While most people experience nightmares or frightening dreams, recurrent nightmares are found in approximately 1–5% of children (Li et al., 2011), with prevalence rates higher in children with generalized anxiety, a history trauma, and/or severe stress. Unlike parasomnias, nightmares typically occur in the last third of the night (when REM sleep occurs), with children recalling that they have had a nightmare (although they may not always recall the exact content).

Clinical Question

"How often do you [your child] have nightmares?"

Obstructive Sleep Apnea

Obstructions of the upper airway, including enlarged tonsils and/or adenoids, or obesity, can result in prolonged pauses in breathing (apneas). When these pauses are accompanied by drops in oxygen levels and are followed by arousals, this may be OSA (American Academy of Sleep Medicine, 2014). The resulting poor oxygenation and disrupted sleep most typically presents as daytime sleepiness, despite an adequate sleep opportunity. Approximately 1–4% of children have documented OSA (Lumeng & Chervin, 2008).

Frequent, loud snoring is also a primary symptom of OSA, with the American Academy of Pediatrics recommending that all children and adolescents who have regular snoring be further evaluated for OSA (Marcus et al., 2012). Other symptoms of OSA include breathing pauses, gasping for air, sleeping in upright positions or with the neck hyperextended, excessive sweating during sleep, and morning headaches. Secondary enuresis and comorbid daytime behavior problems may also be OSA signs. OSA is diagnosed by overnight polysomnography (PSG; a sleep study is described later in this chapter).

Clinical Questions

"Does your child snore; if yes, how often and how loud?"; "Does your child have pauses in breathing or gasp during sleep?" If a positive response is given for either question, additional questions may be used to assess for other symptoms (e.g., secondary enuresis, excessive sweating during sleep, morning headaches, etc.).

Restless Legs Syndrome/Periodic Limb Movement Disorder

Restless legs syndrome (RLS, also known as Willis–Ekbom disease) and periodic limb movement disorder (PLMD) are disorders that often occur together and may be very disruptive to either a child's ability to fall asleep or obtain good-quality sleep. RLS is a clinically diagnosed disorder, with symptoms of (1) uncomfortable feelings in the legs and/or the urge to move the legs; (2) these feelings occurring primarily at night, making it difficult to fall asleep or return to sleep; and (3) with discomfort is alleviated with rubbing or movement (American Academy of Sleep Medicine, 2014). Approximately 2–6% of children and adolescents are reported to have RLS (Picchietti et al., 2007, 2013), with 18–26% of children with attention-deficit/hyperactivity disorder (ADHD) experiencing RLS (Cortese et al., 2005). The prevalence of RLS may be an underestimate, however, as the "growing pains" many children experience may also be due to RLS. PLMD is characterized by bursts of repetitive movements during sleep that result in frequent arousals. Unlike RLS, PLMD can only be diagnosed by PSG, although parents often remark about how restless the child appears during sleep, with repetitive kicking or twitching that coincides with daytime sleepiness.

Clinical Questions

"At bedtime or during the night, do your arms or legs bother you?"; "Do you feel as if you need to move or rub your arms or legs at bedtime or during the night?"

Narcolepsy

The primary feature of narcolepsy is significant daytime sleepiness, even with a sufficient, age-appropriate amount of sleep at night. Youth with narcolepsy may also experience cataplexy, which is a sudden loss of muscle tone that occurs following a strong emotion such as laughter or anger. The other common symptoms for narcolepsy are sleep paralysis (the inability to move even though one is awake) and hypnogogic/hypnopompic hallucinations, which typically occur together at either sleep onset or sleep offset (American Academy of Sleep Medicine, 2014). Following symptom reports, narcolepsy is diagnosed by overnight PSG and a daytime napping study (called a multiple sleep latency test and described later in this chapter). There is often a significant delay between the onset of symptoms and the diagnosis of narcolepsy (Maski et al., 2017), so the prevalence in children and adolescents is not known. However, prevalence in the population is approximately 25–50 per 100,000 people (Longstreth, Koepsell, Ton, Hendrickson, & van Belle, 2007).

Clinical Questions

"How often do you [your child] fall asleep during school, on short car rides [<10 minutes], or during activities [e.g., birthday parties, family outings]?" (Other symptoms of narcolepsy need to be screened only if sleepiness and sufficient sleep duration are present together.)

Sleep Diary

A daily sleep diary is a subjective, prospective record of sleep. The most common variables measured by a sleep diary are bedtime, wake time, SOL, night waking frequency and duration, and daytime napping. Diaries can also include other questions of interest (e.g., caffeine use, sleepwalking episodes) depending on the clinical or research question. There are two primary formats for sleep diaries, a graphical version (Figure 23.1) or tabular version.

In the graphical version, patients/parents make notations to indicate bedtimes, wake times, night wakings, and naps, as well as shade boxes to indi-

Sleep Log

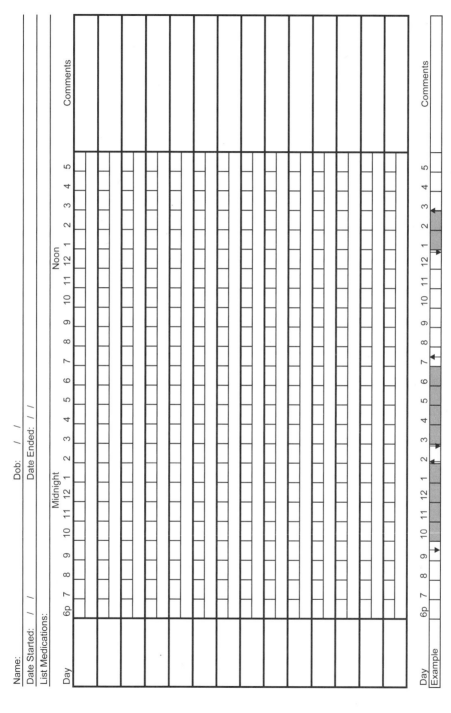

Name: _____ Dob: /   /

Date Started: /   / Date Ended: /   /

List Medications: _____

Key: down arrow = in bed   up arrow = out of bed   shaded = asleep (can have unshaded space between arrows, in bed not asleep)

FIGURE 23.1. Sleep log. From Meltzer and Crabtree (2015). Copyright © 2015 by American Psychological Association Books. Reproduced with permission.

cate when the child is actually asleep. The graphical version is most useful for clinical settings, as it provides a 1- to 2-week "snapshot" on a single page. This includes an examination of consistency of sleep patterns, as well as an identification of other potential issues (e.g., the contribution of late-afternoon napping to delayed sleep onset). However, this type of diary lacks precision, which makes it less useful for research studies in which sleep patterns are the outcome of interest.

In the tabular version (e.g., Consensus Sleep Diary; Carney et al., 2012), more details can be provided about each sleep variable (e.g., separating the time the child got into bed from the time the child attempted to fall asleep). These data can be used to provide average values, as well as values for variability in sleep patterns. Additional questions can be used depending on the presenting concern (e.g., sleep impacting daytime behavior; a question could be used to subjectively rate the child's daytime behavior, or the association between sleep and pain could include a pain rating scale for each day). In addition to the tabular diary's usefulness in research studies, it is also a better selection when using cognitive-behavioral therapy for insomnia (CBT-I), especially when monitoring treatment progress (e.g., calculating sleep efficiency).

One of the most significant limitations of sleep diaries is the potential for nonadherence. Just as in any daily measure, it is essential to establish ways to ensure diaries are completed each day rather than all at once at the end of the week. Some strategies that can be used for research studies is electronic sleep diaries that are sent each day (e.g., through REDCap), allowing the research team to monitor whether the diary has been completed by a certain time. Despite this limitation, sleep diaries are the most commonly used measure in pediatric sleep research, with multiple studies demonstrating their validity and reliability.

Sleep apps, which have grown in popularity with increased smartphone use, are currently limited by the lack of validation studies and ability for clinicians and researchers to easily extract data (Lee-Tobin, Ogeil, Savic, & Lubman, 2017). Even more problematic, most of these apps purport to provide outcomes (e.g., sleep stages) that are not possible to capture with current technology, and they often provide recommendations and information that are not based on empirical evidence or national guidelines (Khosla et al., 2018). That said, when patients present with sleep app data, it can provide information about sleep patterns (bedtime and wake time).

Clinical Case Examples

Preschool Bedtime Tantrums

Liam, a 4-year-old boy, is being treated for behavior problems. Although the parents have successfully implemented a number of behavior management techniques during the day, they still complain about difficulties with sleep, both at bedtime and through the night. Sleep patterns questions focus on bedtime, SOL, night wakings, and nap times, while sleep habits questions focus on sleep location and parental presence. In response to these questions, parents tell the clinician that Liam has a consistent bedtime of 7:00 P.M. but can take up to 2 hours to fall asleep. To avoid bedtime tantrums, they finally "give in" and one parent lies down with Liam around 8:30 P.M. to help him fall asleep. However, Liam will then wake the parents multiple times during the night. If it is before 2:00 A.M. one parent will walk Liam back to his bed and stay with him until he returns to sleep. During the week, Liam continues to nap at preschool, with naps ending as late as 3:30 P.M. With just a few questions, it becomes clear to the clinician that either Liam needs to give up his late-ending nap or his parents need to set a more realistic bedtime. In addition, his parents need to work on teaching Liam to fall asleep independently at bedtime; otherwise, he will continue to wake during the night following normal nighttime arousals and require parental assistance to return to sleep. Because his parents both get home from work late, they decide to allow Liam to continue to nap and push bedtime later, instead focusing on teaching him to fall asleep independently at bedtime.

Anxiety and Night Wakings

Emma, an 11-year-old girl, presents for treatment of anxiety. In the course of her clinical evaluation, her mother raises concerns about Emma's difficulties falling asleep and night wakings. A 2-week sleep diary confirms difficulties: a prolonged SOL and marked night wakings in which Emma appears quite distressed. Her mother worries these are anxiety related, although Emma denies these events. Clinical questions begin with bedtime, wake time, and SOL, but rather than simply asking about the frequency and duration of night wakings, questions related to the timing of Emma's night wakings and whether Emma is responsive to her mother's attempts to comfort her are added. Although Emma has a consistent bedtime every night, she reports feeling anxious and fearful at bedtime, which makes it difficult to fall asleep. On school mornings Emma is difficult to awaken, although on weekends she wakes spontaneously about 2 hours later than her school day wake time. As for her night wakings, Emma's mother reports that she can "almost time" when Emma will wake up, as it is typically 90 minutes after she falls asleep, and that Emma does not respond to her mother's attempt to comfort or wake her, but after a few minutes simply returns to sleep. Emma continues to deny these events. Together, this information suggests Emma is having sleep terrors, which are likely triggered by her anxiety and prolonged SOL during the week, resulting in insufficient sleep. As Emma makes progress with her generalized anxiety treatment and learns some coping strategies at bedtime, she begins falling asleep faster, waking easier in the morning, and has fewer sleep terror events.

Daytime Sleepiness and Inattention

Noah, a 9-year-old boy being evaluated for ADHD, is reportedly having significant difficulties with inattention at school and has recently started wetting the bed again, which his father feels may be related to bullying. His father reports that it is extremely difficult to wake Noah in the morning for school. A 2-week sleep diary shows a consistent bedtime and wake time, with few night wakings. Thus, in addition to standard sleep pattern questions, the clinician focuses on Noah's sleep quality, asking questions about whether he snores or is a restless sleeper. The father reports that Noah snores "louder than a Mack truck." The combination of snoring, secondary enuresis, and daytime sleepiness (including classroom inattention) leads to a referral for further evaluation for OSA. Following surgery to remove his enlarged tonsils and adenoids, a significant improvement is noted in Noah's ability to wake in the morning, as well as his ability to focus during school. His secondary enuresis also resolved without additional treatment.

Depression

Abby, a 16-year-old girl, presents for treatment of depression. During the initial evaluation, Abby reports significant difficulties falling asleep, and her parents report that during the school year, she is extremely difficult to wake. Over the first few weeks of the summer holiday, Abby has reportedly had her "days and nights mixed up," with a variable bedtime between 10:00 P.M. and 3:00 A.M.,

and a wake time typically around 11:00 A.M. or 12:00 P.M. A 2-week sleep diary shows that regardless of her bedtime, Abby rarely falls asleep before 3:00 A.M. In response to clinical questions to differentiate between insomnia and a delayed circadian phase, Abby reports that if she goes to bed later, she falls asleep much faster, and that once she is asleep, she rarely has night wakings. Abby also stated that she would much prefer to take her SATs at 7:00 P.M. than 7:00 A.M., as she is much more alert and awake in the evenings than the rest of the day. Together, this information suggests a delayed circadian rhythm.

Objective Measures of Sleep

Although a significant amount of information about the PHD of Sleep can be obtained through clinical questions and a sleep diary, there are times when more objective measures of sleep are required for clinical patients or research participants. This section reviews the three objective measures of sleep—overnight PSG, the daytime Multiple Sleep Latency Test (MSLT), and actigraphy—with both clinical and research examples provided to highlight situations when these measures might be selected.

Overnight Polysomnography

Overnight or nocturnal PSG includes multiple sources of data (*poly*) that capture sleep (*somno*) through a recording (*graphy*). PSG is conducted in a sleep laboratory, which typically is found in a hospital. The different channels of measurement include electroencephalography (EEG, electrical activity of the brain), electro-oculography (EOG, movements of the eyes), and electromyography (EMG, muscle activity). The information collected is used to determine stages of sleep (NREM, REM). Additional channels measure respiration and cardiac functioning. PSG is the "gold standard" for the diagnosis of OSA, central sleep apnea, and PLMD (Marcus et al., 2012).

In order to capture the multiple channels of data, multiple leads are affixed to the child's head, face, and body. This can be uncomfortable for many children, in particular those with sensory issues. Along with sleeping in a strange environment, these leads can result in an atypical night of sleep, with a "first-night effect" described as a limitation of PSG (Scholle et al., 2003). In addition, due to the significant cost, the need to travel to a specialized sleep laboratory, and limited number of beds available for PSG, it is rare for a child or adolescent to have more than one night of PSG. Finally, because of the unfamiliar environment and single night of data capture, PSG is less useful when insomnia or a circadian rhythm sleep disorder is suspected in the absence of OSA or PLMD.

Clinical Examples of When to Refer for PSG

- A child who is being evaluated for ADHD is reported to have symptoms of prominent snoring, witnessed apneas, and excessive daytime sleepiness. Thus, the clinician refers him for an overnight PSG to rule out OSA.
- Despite following a consistent sleep schedule and obtaining 9 hours of sleep every night, an adolescent with social anxiety complains of excessive daytime sleepiness. The parents report that no one in the family wants to share a bed with the teen on family vacations because she kicks so frequently throughout the night. In addition to treatment for her anxiety (that may be contributing to her excessive sleepiness) she is referred for an overnight PSG to rule out PLMD.

Research Examples Utilizing PSG

- To better understand the relationship between sleep architecture and measures of affective symptoms in children with generalized anxiety disorder (GAD), PSG is used to compare sleep in children with and without GAD (Palmer & Alfano, 2016).
- In children with and without eczema, PSG is used to objectively capture group differences in sleep quality and sleep disturbances, as well as compare sleep with neurocognitive outcomes (Camfferman, Kennedy, Gold, Simpson, & Lushington, 2013).

Multiple Sleep Latency Test

The MSLT is an objective measure of daytime sleepiness (Carskadon et al., 1986). Like PSG, the MSLT is performed in a sleep laboratory, using multiple leads to capture different types of data (EEG, EOG, EMG, etc.). However, the MSLT is conducted during the daytime, allowing the child or adolescent four to five opportunities to take a 20-minute nap, with naps spaced 2 hours apart. During MSLT, youth with excessive daytime sleepiness fall asleep faster and more often than youth who are not sleepy. An MSLT is necessary for the diagnosis of narcolepsy (American Academy of Sleep Medicine, 2014).

Although MSLT provides a clear, objective measure of daytime sleepiness, it is important to note that the limitations are similar to those of PSG, including cost, the need to travel to a dedicated sleep laboratory, child discomfort from multiple leads, and anxiety about sleeping in an unusual environment. In addition, it is essential to ensure that a youth does not have an underlying sleep disorder (e.g., OSA, PLMD) and is not sleep deprived coming into the MSLT. Thus, there is a need to include a sleep diary and when possible actigraphy (described in next section) to ensure sufficient sleep duration prior to this daytime napping test (American Academy of Sleep Medicine, 2014).

Clinical Example of When to Refer for MSLT

- An adolescent who is referred for truancy reports that even after taking one or two daily naps (each lasting more than 1 hour), he still sleeps 9–10 hours every night, is difficult to wake in the morning, and frequently falls asleep during class. The patient denies symptoms of OSA, PLMD, or any mental health disorders. A PSG plus MSLT (with 2 weeks of actigraphy prior to the study) is recommended to evaluate for narcolepsy.

Research Example Utilizing MSLT

- To examine the impact of early school start times on high school students, MSLT is used to compare objective daytime sleepiness of students from schools with a later (8:25 A.M.) and earlier (7:20 A.M.) start time (Carskadon, Wolfson, Acebo, Tzischinsky, & Seifer, 1998).

Actigraphy

Actigraphy is an ambulatory study that estimates sleep–wake patterns through movement. An *actigraph* is a wrist-watch-size device that uses accelerometry to measure movements, with the idea that when we are awake, movements are large and frequent, and while we sleep, movements are small and infrequent (Ancoli-Israel et al., 2015). Algorithms have been developed comparing actigraphy to overnight PSG to validate the estimation of sleep–wake patterns. Due to the nonintrusive nature of the devices, the ability to capture sleep–wake patterns over an extended period of time (e.g., 2 weeks) in the child's natural sleep environment, and the lower cost (relative to PSG), actigraphy provides useful information for clinicians who are seeking information beyond that captured by a clinical interview or sleep diary (especially when the patient/parent is a poor historian) (Meltzer, 2018). In addition, actigraphy is commonly used in pediatric sleep research to provide objective sleep outcomes (Meltzer, Montgomery-Downs, Insana, & Walsh, 2012). Common outcomes captured by actigraphy include *bedtime* (can only be scored with diary or event marker), *wake time* (can only be scored with diary or event marker), *sleep-onset time* (time actigraphy determines the child is asleep), *sleep-offset time* (time actigraphy determines the child is awake for the day), *sleep-onset latency* (time from reported bedtime to sleep onset time), *sleep opportunity* (duration from bedtime to wake time), *wake after sleep onset* (minutes of wake after sleep-onset time), *total sleep time* (total amount of time asleep between bedtime and wake time), and *sleep efficiency* (total sleep time divided by sleep opportunity, expressed as a percent).

Despite the many advantages of actigraphy over PSG, there remain a number of important considerations. First, although less expensive than PSG, there is a significant up-front cost for purchasing actigraphs and required support materials (e.g., interface, software, batteries), with each new device costing approximately $600–1,000. Second, because actigraphy relies solely on movement, a daily sleep diary is required to provide information about the different aspects of the child's sleep and day, including times the child attempted to fall asleep, times the device was removed, and whether it was a typical day. These supporting data are used for the most accurate scoring of data, and without a diary, certain variables (i.e., SOL, sleep opportunity, sleep efficiency) cannot be calculated. Third, artifacts may be present in actigraphy recordings (e.g., child sleeping in moving vehicle, adolescent awake but sitting still at a 2-hour movie). Finally, a minimum of 5 days of recording is required to ensure validity of data collection (Acebo et al., 1999), with additional data required if a comparison of weekday and weekend sleep patterns is desired.

The market for consumer wearable technology has exploded in recent years, providing the promise of an inexpensive way to measure sleep patterns and sleep quality. However, a number of studies in pediatric specific populations have demonstrated that these devices are currently inferior to validated actigraphs and polysomnography (Meltzer, Hiruma, Avis, Montgomery-Downs, & Valentin, 2015; Pesonen & Kuula, 2018; Toon et al., 2016), limiting their utility in empirical research studies.

Clinically, the current position of the American Academy of Sleep Medicine is that while these devices are not substitutes for medical evaluation, they may "enhance the patient–clinician interaction" (Khosla et al., 2018). For example, an adolescent who complains of difficulties waking for school may provide data from a device showing an inconsistent and late bedtime. This provides useful clinical information, in that (1) parents are often unaware of how late adolescents are going to bed, (2) it provides an explanation for daytime sleepiness, and (3) it provides a point to begin intervention.

Clinical Examples of When to Use Actigraphy

- Following successful treatment for difficulties falling asleep independently and frequent night wakings, parents report that a nonverbal, developmentally delayed 4-year-old child is now sleeping through the night, yet she remains difficult to awaken and continues to have behavior problems during the day. Actigraphy is used to examine the child's sleep–wake patterns and identifies that the child is in fact awake for 2–3 hours during the night but is no longer signaling for the parents' attention.
- An adolescent with autism complains of difficulties waking for school and daytime sleepiness, but both the patient and his mother are unable to provide a consistent report of his sleep patterns. Actigraphy is used to determine whether the teen is maintaining a consistent sleep schedule, allowing for a sufficient sleep opportunity. Two weeks of data also examine differences in his sleep patterns on weekdays versus weekends.

Research Examples Utilizing Actigraphy

- To evaluate the efficacy of different approaches to CBT-I (Internet, group, wait list), as well as whether the intervention also benefits psychopathology in adolescents, actigraphy is used to objectively assess total sleep time, SOL, and sleep efficiency (de Bruin, Bogels, Oort, & Meijer, 2018).
- Actigraphy is used to objectively measure sleep patterns for up to 12 nights in youth with acute musculoskeletal pain to examine the temporal relationship between sleep and pain, with outcomes including total sleep time, sleep efficiency, and wake after sleep onset (Lewandowski Holley, Rabbitts, Zhou, Durkin, & Palermo, 2017).

Subjective Measures of Sleep

There are over 300 subjective measures of sleep in children and adolescents. In order to identify which measures may be useful in a clinical setting or research study, it is important to clearly identify outcomes of interest based on the PHD of Sleep. Although not a comprehensive review of all measures available, this section provides information about many of the most commonly used measures in pediatric sleep, as well as some newer measures that hold significant potential for both clinical and research use. For quick reference, these measures are presented alphabetically, with Table 23.1 providing a comparison of validated ages, number of items, respondent, and outcomes captured.

Adolescent Sleep Hygiene Scale

The Adolescent Sleep Hygiene Scale (ASHS) is a self-report measure that captures sleep patterns and sleep habits, with four qualitative items to assess bedtimes and wake times, and 28 items to calculate nine subscales (Physiological, Cognitive, Emotional, Sleep Environment, Daytime Sleep, Substances, Sleep Stability, Bedtime Routine, and Bed Sharing) (LeBourgeois, Giannotti, Cortesi, Wolfson, & Harsh, 2005). The original version reported internal reliability, but validity was not examined. A revised version (ASHSr) reduced the ASHS to 24 items with five subscales (Physiological, Behavioral Arousal, Cognitive–Emotional, Sleep Stability, Sleep Environment, and Daytime Sleep). The ASHSr demonstrated satisfactory internal consistency, concurrent validity, and convergent validity (Storfer-Isser, LeBourgeois, Harsh, Tompsett, & Redline, 2013). The clinical utility of this measure is not clear due to the length and the grouping of individual items that might be targets of treatment. However, recent studies focusing on sleep in children with mental health issues and ADHD have included the ASHSr (Martin et al., 2018; Zhang et al., 2018).

Adolescent Sleep–Wake Scale

The Adolescent Sleep–Wake Scale (ASWS) is a 28-item self-report measure of sleep quality for adolescents, with original factors including going to bed, falling asleep, maintaining sleep, reinitiating sleep, and returning to wakefulness (LeBourgeois et al., 2005). The original version reported internal reliability, but validity was not examined. A more recent study found that a 10-item version

of the ASHS produced a three-factor model that included falling asleep and reinitiating sleep (revised), returning to wakefulness (revised), and going to bed (revised), with acceptable internal consistency and preliminary construct validity (Essner, Noel, Myrvik, & Palermo, 2015). In addition to the length, the clinical utility of this measure is unclear, as it groups symptoms of multiple disorders (e.g., RLS, insomnia) in the same scale. However, recent studies have included the ASWS in populations of adolescents with type 1 diabetes (Adler, Gavan, Tauman, Phillip, & Shalitin, 2017) or autism (Goldman et al., 2017).

Brief Infant Sleep Questionnaire

The Brief Infant Sleep Questionnaire (BISQ) was designed as a standardized screening tool for both research and clinical settings, and includes eight items focused on sleep patterns and habits, including total sleep time, sleep opportunity, sleep location, and methods of falling asleep (Sadeh, 2004). The BISQ showed good validity and reliability in the original study. An expanded version that included questions for toddlers was used in large international studies of sleep in young children (Mindell, Sadeh, Kohyama, & How, 2010; Sadeh, Mindell, Luedtke, & Wiegand, 2009). With only eight items, the BISQ is a good measure to provide standardized data within a clinical setting and has demonstrated research utility, including large population-based studies (Hysing, Sivertsen, Garthus-Niegel, & Eberhard-Gran, 2016) and treatment studies (Mindell et al., 2011a, 2011b).

Children's Report of Sleep Patterns

The Children's Report of Sleep Patterns (CRSP) is a self-report measure of sleep patterns, sleep habits, and sleep disorders for school-age children (Meltzer, Biggs, et al., 2012; Meltzer et al., 2013) and adolescents (Meltzer et al., 2014), with demonstrated reliability and validity. The CRSP includes 60 items, making it a lengthy measure for clinical or research use. However, the measure was designed and validated to allow for the selection of individual subscales (e.g., Bedtime Fears/Worries, Insomnia) or indices (e.g., caffeine use, sleep location) rather than requiring all items to calculate a total score. A new exploratory factor analysis was conducted on 155 school-age children, suggesting an alternative three-scale version. However, validity was not examined for this alternative version (Cordts & Steele, 2016). Parts of the CRSP have been used in studies of pediatric survivors of brain tumors (Brimeyer et al., 2016) and to examine the relationship between bullying and sleep in adolescents (Donoghue & Meltzer, 2018).

Children's Sleep Habits Questionnaire

The 45-item, parent reported Children's Sleep Habits Questionnaire (CSHQ) is one of the most widely used measures of pediatric sleep. Designed to be a clinical screener of major medical and behavioral sleep disorders in children ages 4–10 years, the CSHQ demonstrated reliability and validity, with a clinical cutoff score provided (Owens, Spirito, & McGuinn, 2000). The CSHQ has since undergone additional validation in toddlers and preschoolers (Goodlin-Jones, Sitnick, Tang, Liu, & Anders, 2008; Sneddon, Peacock, & Crowley, 2013), as well as in comparison to actigraphy and PSG (Markovich, Gendron, & Corkum, 2014). The CSHQ has also been translated into multiple languages. While 33 items is long for a clinical screener, the subscales focus on a number of symptoms that may aid in the diagnosis and monitoring of treatment for behavioral sleep problems, night wakings, parasomnias, sleep-disordered breathing, and daytime sleepiness.

Children's Sleep–Wake Scale

The Children's Sleep–Wake Scale (CSWS) is a 25-item, parent-report measure of behavioral sleep quality in children ages 2–8 years, and includes five factors (going to bed, falling asleep, maintaining sleep, reinitiating sleep, returning to wakefulness). The CSWS has been shown to be reliable and valid (LeBourgeois & Harsh, 2016). Similar to the ASWS, as a clinical and research tool, the CSWS is limited by the length and the grouping of symptoms of multiple disorders (e.g., RLS, insomnia) in the same scale.

Modified Epworth Sleepiness Scale

The original Epworth Sleepiness Scale (ESS) was an eight-item, self-report measure of daytime sleepiness for adults (Johns, 1991). Because some of the questions were not relevant for children, the measure was adapted for use in a study of youth with suspected sleep-disordered breathing (Melendres, Lutz, Rubin, & Marcus, 2004), and has been used in multiple studies, including a large randomized clinical trial for the treatment of OSA (Garetz et al., 2015). Notably, the modified version (mESS)

was not authorized by the copyright holder. Thus Dr. Johns developed and validated a new ESS for children and adolescents, the ESS-CHAD (Janssen, Phillipson, O'Connor, & Johns, 2017). The brief nature of this measure makes it a useful tool for screening daytime sleepiness in both clinical settings and research studies.

Morningness–Eveningness Scale for Children

The Morningness–Eveningness Scale for Children (M/E) is a reliable and valid measure of circadian preference in children and adolescents (Carskadon & Acebo, 1992; Carskadon, Vieira, & Acebo, 1993). With 10 items, the M/E includes questions about whether youth are most alert and awake in the morning, middle of the day, or evening. As a clinical tool, the M/E is brief and useful when a circadian phase delay is suspected, or when trying to differentiate between insomnia and circadian phase delay. The M/E is also useful in research studies when circadian preference is believed to be associated with different outcomes, such as substance use (Hasler et al., 2017) or behavioral/emotional problems in adolescents (Gau et al., 2007).

Obstructive Sleep Apnea–18

The Obstructive Sleep Apnea–18 (OSA-18) is an 18-item, caregiver-reported quality-of-life survey for patients with OSA. The original validation study demonstrated that the OSA-18 was associated with PSG parameters, as well as adenoid and tonsil size (Franco, Rosenfeld, & Rao, 2000), with a large randomized clinical trial also finding an association between the OSA-18 and OSA severity (Mitchell et al., 2015). However, two large studies have raised concerns about the validity of the OSA-18 as a diagnostic screener (Borgstrom, Nerfeldt, & Friberg, 2013; Walter et al., 2016). That said, the OSA-18 still has a place in clinical practice as a measure of subjective quality of life before and after treatment for OSA, as well as in research studies in which OSA patients' quality of life is of interest.

Pediatric Daytime Sleepiness Scale

The Pediatric Daytime Sleepiness Scale (PDSS) is an eight-item self-report measure of sleepiness in adolescents. This measure has been found to have good internal consistency, as well as construct and divergent validity (Drake et al., 2003; Perez-Chada et al., 2007). With eight items, this

TABLE 23.1. Summary Table of Subjective Sleep Measures

Measure	ASHS	ASWS	BISQ	CRSP	CSHQ	CSWS	mESS[c]
Validated ages (yr)	12–18	12–18	0–3	8–18	2–10	2–8	2–18
Items	32/24[a]	28/10[a]	13/25[b]	60	45	25	8
Respondent	Self	Self	Parent	Self	Parent	Parent	Self/Parent
Sleep patterns							
Total sleep time			✓		✓		
Sleep opportunity	✓			✓	✓		
Schedule/consistent	✓		✓	✓	✓		
Sleep-onset latency		✓	✓	✓	✓	✓	
Night wakings		✓	✓	✓	✓	✓	
Naps	✓		✓	✓	✓		
Daytime sleepiness				✓	✓		✓
Sleep habits							
Bedtime routine	✓		✓	✓			
Sleep location			✓	✓	✓		
Parent present		✓	✓	✓	✓	✓	
Caffeine	✓			✓			
Technology	✓			✓			
Sleep disorders							
Insomnia		✓		✓	✓	✓	
Parasomnia				✓	✓		
Nightmares				✓	✓		
OSA				✓	✓		
RLS				✓			
Circadian preference							
Quality/problem		✓	✓	✓	✓	✓	

Note. ASHS, Adolescent Sleep Hygiene Scale; ASWS, Adolescent Sleep–Wake Scale; BISQ, Brief Infant Sleep Questionnaire; CRSP, Children's Report of Sleep Patterns; CSHQ, Children's Sleep Habits Questionnaire; CSWS, Children's Sleep–Wake Scale; ESS, Epworth Sleepiness Scale; M/E, Morningness–Eveningness Questionnaire for Children; OSA, obstructive sleep apnea; PDSS, Pediatric Daytime Sleepiness Scale; PSQ, Pediatric Sleep Questionnaire; PROMIS: SD, PROMIS Sleep Disturbance; PROMIS: SRI, PROMIS Sleep-Related Impairment; RLS, restless legs syndrome; SDSC, Sleep Disturbance Scale for Children; SHS, Sleep Habits Survey.
[a]Number of items in revised version.
[b]Number of items in extended version.
[c]Number of items in new validated version is the Epworth Sleepiness Scale for Children and Adolescents (ESS-CHAD).
[d]PROMIS: SD and PROMIS: SRI both include validated eight-item and four-item short forms.

Measure	M/E	OSA-18	PDSS	PSQ	PROMIS: SD	PROMIS: SRI	SDSC	SHS
Validated ages (yr)	11–12	6 mo–12	11–15	2–18	8–18	8–18	6–15	13–19
Items	10	18	8	22	15/8/4[d]	13/8/4[d]	27	45
Respondent	Self	Parent	Self	Parent	Self	Self	Parent	Self
Sleep patterns								
Total sleep time							✓	✓
Sleep opportunity								✓
Schedule/consistent								✓
Sleep-onset latency							✓	✓
Night wakings								✓
Naps								✓
Daytime sleepiness		✓	✓	✓		✓	✓	✓
Sleep habits								
Bedtime routine								
Sleep location								✓
Parent present								
Caffeine								✓
Technology								
Sleep disorders								
Insomnia					✓		✓	
Parasomnia							✓	
Nightmares								
OSA		✓		✓			✓	
RLS								
Circadian preference	✓							✓
Quality/problem		✓		✓	✓			✓

measure can be useful to screen for sleepiness, as well as monitor sleepiness following interventions (Tan, Healey, Gray, & Galland, 2012). In addition, the PDSS can be used as an outcome measure in research studies or to help identify the impact of EDS on outcomes, as has been done in studies of youth with ADHD (Langberg, Dvorsky, Marshall, & Evans, 2013) or cystic fibrosis (Vandeleur et al., 2017). The PDSS has been translated into multiple languages.

Pediatric Sleep Questionnaire

The Pediatric Sleep Questionnaire (PSQ) is a 22-item caregiver-report measure that has been shown to be a valid screener for sleep-disordered breathing (Chervin et al., 2007; Chervin, Hedger, Dillon, & Pituch, 2000). There are four PSQ subscales—Sleep-Related Breathing Disorder, Snoring, EDS, and Inattentive/Hyperactive Behavior—and the measure has been translated into multiple languages. In both clinical settings and research studies, the PSQ can be used to identify those who are at highest risk for sleep-disordered breathing (Rosen et al., 2015), as well as to monitor symptoms of OSA before and after treatment (Wei, Mayo, Smith, Reese, & Weatherly, 2007).

PROMIS Sleep Disturbance and Sleep-Related Impairment Item Banks

With the recent focus on patient-centered approaches to health care, it is essential to have valid patient-reported outcome measures of sleep for children and adolescents. Two new measures were recently developed and validated for use in clinical settings or research studies, including large epidemiological studies (Bevans et al., 2018). The Patient-Reported Outcomes Measurement Information System (PROMIS) Pediatric Sleep Disturbance (SD) item bank includes 15 items that measure sleep disturbances and sleep quality. There are both eight-item and four-item SD short forms that can be administered. The PROMIS Pediatric Sleep-Related Impairment (SRI) item bank includes 13 items that measure daytime sleepiness and functioning related to sleep. The SRI also has both eight-item and four-item short forms that can be administered, with higher scores indicating poorer daytime functioning. Both item banks were validated and normed on a large national sample of children and adolescents, and have been shown to be reliable and valid, distinguishing between

clinical patients in a sleep center and the general population (Forrest et al., 2018). Both item banks are in the process of being translated into Spanish and other languages.

Sleep Disturbance Scale for Children

The Sleep Disturbance Scale for Children (SDSC) was developed to provide a standardized clinical measure of sleep disturbances across pediatric patients, providing an index score that is easy for clinicians to calculate (Bruni et al., 1996). The SDSC includes 27 parent-reported items and factors that focus on sleep patterns and sleep disorders. More recent studies have demonstrated slightly different factor structures in a clinical sample of children and adolescents (Marriner, Pestell, Bayliss, McCann, & Bucks, 2017) and preschoolers (Romeo et al., 2013). The SDSC has been translated into multiple languages.

Sleep Habits Survey

The Sleep Habits Survey (SHS) was developed to capture sleep–wake patterns and problems in large populations of high school students (Acebo & Carskadon, 2002; Wolfson & Carskadon, 1998). Six questions ask about sleep patterns (i.e., bedtime, sleep onset latency, wake time) for both weekdays and weekends. Additional individual items ($n = 7$) query sleep location, naps, caffeine, and perceived sleep quality/problems. The SHS also includes two sleepiness scales (10 items and four items), sleep quality (two items), circadian phase delay (six items), and circadian preference (10 items). The SHS has been shown to have good reliability (Acebo & Carskadon, 2002) and validity compared to both actigraphy and sleep diary (Wolfson et al., 2003).

Conclusions

As an important health asset, sleep is a variable that is essential to include in both clinical work and research studies. In clinical settings, insufficient or poor-quality sleep has a significant impact on presenting issues (e.g., depression, anxiety). In addition, sleep problems may interfere with treatment progress if a patient is unwilling or unable to engage in therapy or work on assignments between sessions. While research studies have highlighted the relationship between sleep and mental health disorders in children and adolescents, many questions remain unanswered about the bidirectional relationship between sleep and mental health. This chapter has provided an overview of how to integrate sleep into general clinical practice, as well as both objective and subjective measures of sleep that can be used in clinical settings and research studies.

REFERENCES

Acebo, C., & Carskadon, M. A. (2002). Influence of irregular sleep patterns on waking behavior. In M. A. Carskadon (Ed.), *Adolescent sleep patterns: Biological, social, and psychologyogical influences* (pp. 220–235). Cambridge, UK: Cambridge University Press.

Acebo, C., Sadeh, A., Seifer, R., Tzischinsky, O., Wolfson, A. R., Hafer, A., & Carskadon, M. A. (1999). Estimating sleep patterns with activity monitoring in children and adolescents: How many nights are necessary for reliable measures? *Sleep, 22,* 95–103.

Achermann, P., & Borbely, A. A. (2010). Sleep homeostasis and models of sleep regulation. In M. Kryger, T. Roth, & W. Dement (Eds.), *Principles and practices of sleep medicine* (5th ed., pp. 431–444). Philadelphia: Elsevier.

Adler, A., Gavan, M. Y., Tauman, R., Phillip, M., & Shalitin, S. (2017). Do children, adolescents, and young adults with type 1 diabetes have increased prevalence of sleep disorders? *Pediatric Diabetes, 18,* 450–458.

Alfano, C. A. (2018). (Re)Conceptualizing sleep among children with anxiety disorders: Where to next? *Clinical Child Family Psychology Review, 21*(4), 482–499.

Alvaro, P. K., Roberts, R. M., & Harris, J. K. (2013). A systematic review assessing bidirectionality between sleep disturbances, anxiety, and depression. *Sleep, 36,* 1059–1068.

American Academy of Pediatrics. (2014). School start times for adolescents. *Pediatrics, 134,* 642–649.

American Academy of Sleep Medicine. (2014). *International classification of sleep disorders: Diagnostic and coding manual* (3rd ed.). Westchester, IL: American Academy of Sleep Medicine.

Ancoli-Israel, S., Martin, J. L., Blackwell, T., Buenaver, L., Liu, L., Meltzer, L. J., . . . Taylor, D. J. (2015). The SBSM Guide to Actigraphy Monitoring: Clinical and research applications. *Behavioral Sleep Medicine, 13*(Suppl. 1), S4–S38.

Bevans, K. B., Meltzer, L. J., De La Motte, A., Kratchman, A., Viel, D., & Forrest, C. B. (2019). Qualitative development and content validation of the PROMIS Pediatric Sleep Health items. *Behavioral Sleep Medicine, 17,* 657–671.

Borbely, A. A. (1982). A two process model of sleep regulation. *Human Neurobiology, 1,* 195–204.

Borgstrom, A., Nerfeldt, P., & Friberg, D. (2013). Questionnaire OSA-18 has poor validity compared to polysomnography in pediatric obstructive sleep apnea. *International Journal of Pediatric Otorhinolaryngology, 77,* 1864–1868.

Brimeyer, C., Adams, L., Zhu, L., Srivastava, D. K., Wise, M., Hudson, M. M., & Crabtree, V. M. (2016). Sleep complaints in survivors of pediatric brain tumors. *Supportive Care in Cancer, 24,* 23–31.

Bruni, O., Ottaviano, S., Guidetti, V., Romoli, M., Innocenzi, M., Cortesi, F., & Giannotti, F. (1996). The Sleep Disturbance Scale for Children (SDSC) Construction and validation of an instrument to evaluate sleep disturbances in childhood and adolescence. *Journal of Sleep Research, 5,* 251–261.

Buxton, O. M., Chang, A. M., Spilsbury, J. C., Bos, T., Emsellem, H., & Knutson, K. L. (2015). Sleep in the modern family: Protective family routines for child and adolescent sleep. *Sleep Health, 1,* 15–27.

Camfferman, D., Kennedy, J. D., Gold, M., Simpson, C., & Lushington, K. (2013). Sleep and neurocognitive functioning in children with eczema. *International Journal Of Psychophysiology, 89,* 265–272.

Carney, C. E., Buysse, D. J., Ancoli-Israel, S., Edinger, J. D., Krystal, A. D., Lichstein, K. L., & Morin, C. M. (2012). The Consensus Sleep Diary: Standardizing prospective sleep self-monitoring. *Sleep, 35*(2), 287–302.

Carskadon, M. A., & Acebo, C. (1992). Relationship of a morningess/eveningness scale to sleep patterns in children. *Sleep Research, 21,* 367.

Carskadon, M. A., & Acebo, C. (2002). Regulation of sleepiness in adolescents: Update, insights, and speculation. *Sleep, 25,* 606–614.

Carskadon, M. A., & Dement, W. C. (2010). Normal human sleep: An overview. In M. Kryger, T. Roth, & W. C. Dement (Eds.), *Principles and practices of sleep medicine* (5th ed., pp. 16–26). Philadelphia: Elsevier.

Carskadon, M. A., Dement, W. C., Mitler, M. M., Roth, T., Westbrook, P. R., & Keenan, S. (1986). Guidelines for the multiple sleep latency test (MSLT): A standard measure of sleepiness. *Sleep, 9,* 519–524.

Carskadon, M. A., Vieira, C., & Acebo, C. (1993). Association between puberty and delayed phase preference. *Sleep, 16,* 258–262.

Carskadon, M. A., Wolfson, A. R., Acebo, C., Tzischinsky, O., & Seifer, R. (1998). Adolescent sleep patterns, circadian timing, and sleepiness at a transition to early school days. *Sleep, 21,* 871–881.

Chervin, R. D., Hedger, K., Dillon, J. E., & Pituch, K. J. (2000). Pediatric sleep questionnaire (PSQ): Validity and reliability of scales for sleep-disordered breathing, snoring, sleepiness, and behavioral problems. *Sleep Medicine, 1,* 21–32.

Chervin, R. D., Weatherly, R. A., Garetz, S. L., Ruzicka, D. L., Giordani, B. J., Hodges, E. K., . . . Guire, K. E. (2007). Pediatric sleep questionnaire: Prediction of sleep apnea and outcomes. *Archives of Otolaryngology–Head and Neck Surgery, 133,* 216–222.

Clarke, G., & Harvey, A. G. (2012). The complex role of sleep in adolescent depression. *Child and Adolescent Psychiatric Clinics of North America, 21,* 385–400.

Committee on Nutrition and the Council on Sports Medicine and Fitness. (2011). Sports drinks and energy drinks for children and adolescents: Are they appropriate? *Pediatrics, 127,* 1182–1189.

Cordts, K. P., & Steele, R. G. (2016). An evaluation of the Children's Report of Sleep Patterns using confirmatory and exploratory factor analytic approaches. *Journal of Pediatric Psychology, 41,* 993–1001.

Cortese, S., Konofal, E., Lecendreux, M., Arnulf, I., Mouren, M. C., Darra, F., & Dalla Bernardina, B. (2005). Restless legs syndrome and attention-deficit/hyperactivity disorder: A review of the literature. *Sleep, 28,* 1007–1013.

de Bruin, E. J., Bogels, S. M., Oort, F. J., & Meijer, A. M. (2018). Improvements of adolescent psychopathology after insomnia treatment: Results from a randomized controlled trial over 1 year. *Journal of Child Psychology and Psychiatry, 59,* 509–522.

Donoghue, C., & Meltzer, L. J. (2018). Sleep it off: Bullying and sleep disturbances in adolescents. *Journal of Adolescence, 68,* 87–93.

Drake, C., Nickel, C., Burduvali, E., Roth, T., Jefferson, C., & Pietro, B. (2003). The pediatric daytime sleepiness scale (PDSS): Sleep habits and school outcomes in middle-school children. *Sleep, 26,* 455–458.

Essner, B., Noel, M., Myrvik, M., & Palermo, T. (2015). Examination of the factor structure of the Adolescent Sleep–Wake Scale (ASWS). *Behavioral Sleep Medicine, 13,* 296–307.

Forrest, C. B., Meltzer, L. J., Marcus, C. L., De La Motte, A., Kratchman, A., Buysse, D. J., . . . Bevans, K. B. (2018). Development and validation of the PROMIS Pediatric Sleep Disturbance and Sleep-Related Impairment item banks. *Sleep, 41.* [Epub ahead of print]

Franco, R. A., Rosenfeld, R. M., & Rao, M. (2000). First place—resident clinical science award 1999: Quality of life for children with obstructive sleep apnea. *Otolaryngology–Head and Neck Surgery, 123,* 9–16.

Garetz, S. L., Mitchell, R. B., Parker, P. D., Moore, R. H., Rosen, C. L., Giordani, B., . . . Redline, S. (2015). Quality of life and obstructive sleep apnea symptoms after pediatric adenotonsillectomy. *Pediatrics, 135,* e477–e486.

Gau, S. S., Shang, C. Y., Merikangas, K. R., Chiu, Y. N., Soong, W. T., & Cheng, A. T. (2007). Association between morningness–eveningness and behavioral/emotional problems among adolescents. *Journal of Biological Rhythms, 22,* 268–274.

Goldman, S. E., Alder, M. L., Burgess, H. J., Corbett, B. A., Hundley, R., Wofford, D., . . . Malow, B. A. (2017). Characterizing sleep in adolescents and adults with autism spectrum disorders. *Journal of Autism and Developmental Disorders, 47,* 1682–1695.

Goodlin-Jones, B. L., Sitnick, S. L., Tang, K., Liu, J., & Anders, T. F. (2008). The Children's Sleep Habits Questionnaire in toddlers and preschool children. *Journal of Developmental and Behavioral Pediatrics, 29,* 82–88.

Gradisar, M., Wolfson, A. R., Harvey, A. G., Hale, L., Rosenberg, R., & Czeisler, C. A. (2013). The sleep and technology use of Americans: Findings from the National Sleep Foundation's 2011 Sleep in America poll. *Journal of Clinical Sleep Medicine, 9,* 1291–1299.

Gregory, A. M., & Sadeh, A. (2016). Annual Research Review: Sleep problems in childhood psychiatric disorders—a review of the latest science. *Journal of Child Psychology and Psychiatry and Allied Disciplines, 57,* 296–317.

Hasler, B. P., Franzen, P. L., de Zambotti, M., Prouty, D., Brown, S. A., Tapert, S. F., . . . Clark, D. B. (2017). Eveningness and later sleep timing are associated with greater risk for alcohol and marijuana use in adolescence: Initial findings from the National Consortium on Alcohol and Neurodevelopment in Adolescence study. *Alcoholism: Clinical and Experimental Research, 41,* 1154–1165.

Hysing, M., Sivertsen, B., Garthus-Niegel, S., & Eberhard-Gran, M. (2016). Pediatric sleep problems and social–emotional problems: A population-based study. *Infant Behavior and Development, 42,* 111–118.

Janssen, K. C., Phillipson, S., O'Connor, J., & Johns, M. W. (2017). Validation of the Epworth Sleepiness Scale for children and adolescents using Rasch analysis. *Sleep Medicine, 33,* 30–35.

Jenni, O. G., & Carskadon, M. A. (2005). Normal human sleep at different ages: Infants to adolescents. In *SRS basics of sleep guide* (pp. 11–19). Westchester, IL: Sleep Researcher Society.

Johns, M. W. (1991). A new method for measuring daytime sleepiness: The Epworth sleepiness scale. *Sleep, 14,* 540–545.

Khosla, S., Deak, M. C., Gault, D., Goldstein, C. A., Hwang, D., Kwon, Y., . . . Rowley, J. A. (2018). Consumer sleep technology: An American Academy of Sleep Medicine Position Statement. *Journal of Clinical Sleep Medicine, 14,* 877–880.

Langberg, J. M., Dvorsky, M. R., Marshall, S., & Evans, S. W. (2013). Clinical implications of daytime sleepiness for the academic performance of middle school-aged adolescents with attention deficit hyperactivity disorder. *Journal of Sleep Research, 22,* 542–548.

LeBourgeois, M. K., Giannotti, F., Cortesi, F., Wolfson, A. R., & Harsh, J. (2005). The relationship between reported sleep quality and sleep hygiene in Italian and American adolescents. *Pediatrics, 115,* 257–265.

LeBourgeois, M. K., & Harsh, J. R. (2016). Development and psychometric evaluation of the Children's Sleep–Wake Scale. *Sleep Health, 2,* 198–204.

Lee-Tobin, P. A., Ogeil, R. P., Savic, M., & Lubman, D. I. (2017). Rate my sleep: Examining the information, function, and basis in empirical evidence within sleep applications for mobile devices. *Journal of Clinical Sleep Medicine, 13,* 1349–1354.

Lewandowski, A. S., Ward, T. M., & Palermo, T. M. (2011). Sleep problems in children and adolescents with common medical conditions. *Pediatric Clinics of North America, 58,* 699–713.

Lewandowski Holley, A., Rabbitts, J., Zhou, C., Durkin, L., & Palermo, T. M. (2017). Temporal daily associations among sleep and pain in treatment-seeking youth with acute musculoskeletal pain. *Journal of Behavioral Medicine, 40,* 675–681.

Li, S. X., Yu, M. W., Lam, S. P., Zhang, J., Li, A. M., Lai, K. Y., & Wing, Y. K. (2011). Frequent nightmares in children: Familial aggregation and associations with parent-reported behavioral and mood problems. *Sleep, 34,* 487–493.

Longstreth, W. T., Koepsell, T. D., Ton, T. G., Hendrickson, A. F., & van Belle, G. (2007). The epidemiology of narcolepsy. *Sleep, 30,* 13–26.

Lovato, N., & Gradisar, M. (2014). A meta-analysis and model of the relationship between sleep and depression in adolescents: Recommendations for future research and clinical practice. *Sleep Medicine Reviews, 18,* 521–529.

Lumeng, J. C., & Chervin, R. D. (2008). Epidemiology of pediatric obstructive sleep apnea. *Procedures of the American Thoracic Society, 5,* 242–252.

Marcus, C. L., Brooks, L. J., Draper, K. A., Gozal, D., Halbower, A. C., Jones, J., . . . Spruyt, K. (2012). Diagnosis and management of childhood obstructive sleep apnea syndrome. *Pediatrics, 130,* 576–584.

Markovich, A. N., Gendron, M. A., & Corkum, P. V. (2014). Validating the Children's Sleep Habits Questionnaire against polysomnography and actigraphy in school-aged children. *Frontiers in Psychiatry, 5,* 188.

Marriner, A. M., Pestell, C., Bayliss, D. M., McCann, M., & Bucks, R. S. (2017). Confirmatory factor analysis of the Sleep Disturbance Scale for Children (SDSC) in a clinical sample of children and adolescents. *Journal of Sleep Research, 26,* 587–594.

Martin, C. A., Hiscock, H., Rinehart, N., Heussler, H. S., Hyde, C., Fuller-Tyszkiewicz, M., . . . Sciberras, A. (2020). Associations between sleep hygiene and sleep problems in adolescents with ADHD: A cross-sectional study. *Journal of Attention Disorders, 24,* 545–554.

Maski, K., Steinhart, E., Williams, D., Scammell, T., Flygare, J., McCleary, K., & Gow, M. (2017). Listening to the patient voice in narcolepsy: Diagnostic delay, disease burden, and treatment efficacy. *Journal of Clinical Sleep Medicine, 13,* 419–425.

Mason, T. B. A., & Pack, A. I. (2007). Pediatric parasomnias. *Sleep, 30,* 141–151.

Mazzone, L., Postorino, V., Siracusano, M., Riccioni, A., & Curatolo, P. (2018). The relationship between sleep problems, neurobiological alterations, core symptoms of autism spectrum disorder, and psychiatric comorbidities. *Journal of Clinical Medicine, 7.* [Epub ahead of print]

Melendres, M. C., Lutz, J. M., Rubin, E. D., & Marcus, C. L. (2004). Daytime sleepiness and hyperactivity in children with suspected sleep-disordered breathing. *Pediatrics, 114,* 768–775.

Meltzer, L. J. (2018). Sleep FAQs: When is actigraphy useful for the diagnosis and treatment of pediatric sleep problems? *Paediatric Respiratory Reviews, 28,* 41–46.

Meltzer, L. J., Avis, K. T., Biggs, S., Reynolds, A. C., Crabtree, V. M., & Bevans, K. B. (2013). The Children's Report of Sleep Patterns (CRSP): A self-report measure of sleep for school-aged children. *Journal of Clinical Sleep Medicine, 9,* 235–245.

Meltzer, L. J., Biggs, S., Reynolds, A., Avis, K. T., Crabtree, V. M., & Bevans, K. B. (2012). The Children's Report of Sleep Patterns—Sleepiness Scale: A self-report measure for school-aged children. *Sleep Medicine, 13,* 385–389.

Meltzer, L. J., Brimeyer, C., Russell, K., Avis, K. T., Biggs, S., Reynolds, A. C., & Crabtree, V. M. (2014). The Children's Report of Sleep Patterns: Validity and reliability of the Sleep Hygiene Index and Sleep Disturbance Scale in adolescents. *Sleep Medicine, 15,* 1500–1507.

Meltzer, L. J., & Crabtree, V. M. (2015). *Pediatric sleep problems: A clinician's guide to behavioral interventions.* Washington, DC: American Psychologyogical Association.

Meltzer, L. J., Hiruma, L. S., Avis, K., Montgomery-Downs, H., & Valentin, J. (2015). Comparison of a commercial accelerometer with polysomnography and actigraphy in children and adolescents. *Sleep, 38,* 1323–1330.

Meltzer, L. J., Montgomery-Downs, H. E., Insana, S. P., & Walsh, C. M. (2012). Use of actigraphy for assessment in pediatric sleep research. *Sleep Medicine Reviews, 16,* 463–475.

Mindell, J. A., Du Mond, C. E., Sadeh, A., Telofski, L. S., Kulkarni, N., & Gunn, E. (2011a). Efficacy of an internet-based intervention for infant and toddler sleep disturbances. *Sleep, 34,* 451–458.

Mindell, J. A., Du Mond, C. E., Sadeh, A., Telofski, L. S., Kulkarni, N., & Gunn, E. (2011b). Long-term efficacy of an internet-based intervention for infant and toddler sleep disturbances: One year follow-up. *Journal of Clinical Sleep Medicine, 7,* 507–511.

Mindell, J. A., Meltzer, L. J., Carskadon, M. A., & Chervin, R. D. (2009). Developmental aspects of sleep hygiene: Findings from the 2004 National Sleep Foundation Sleep in America Poll. *Sleep Medicine, 10,* 771–779.

Mindell, J. A., & Owens, J. A. (2015). *A clinical guide to pediatric sleep: Diagnosis and management of sleep problems* (3rd ed.). Philadelphia: Wolters Kluwer.

Mindell, J. A., Sadeh, A., Kohyama, J., & How, T. H. (2010). Parental behaviors and sleep outcomes in infants and toddlers: A cross-cultural comparison. *Sleep Medicine, 11*, 393–399.

Mindell, J. A., & Williamson, A. A. (2018). Benefits of a bedtime routine in young children: Sleep, development, and beyond. *Sleep Medicine Reviews, 40*, 93–108.

Mitchell, R. B., Garetz, S., Moore, R. H., Rosen, C. L., Marcus, C. L., Katz, E. S., . . . Redline, S. (2015). The use of clinical parameters to predict obstructive sleep apnea syndrome severity in children: The Childhood Adenotonsillectomy (CHAT) study randomized clinical trial. *JAMA Otolaryngology–Head and Neck Surgery, 141*, 130–136.

National Sleep Foundation. (2004). 2004 Sleep in America Poll. Retrieved May 11, 2007, from *www.sleepfoundation.org*.

Owens, J. A. (2005). Epidemiology of sleep disorders during childhood. In S. H. Sheldon, R. Ferber, & M. H. Kryger (Eds.), *Principles and practices of pediatric sleep medicine* (pp. 27–33). Philadelphia: Elsevier Saunders.

Owens, J. A., Spirito, A., & McGuinn, M. (2000). The Children's Sleep Habits Questionnaire (CSHQ): Psychometric properties of a survey instrument for school-aged children. *Sleep, 23*, 1043–1051.

Paavonen, E. J., Aronen, E. T., Moilanen, I., Piha, J., Rasanen, E., Tamminen, T., & Almqvist, F. (2000). Sleep problems of school-aged children: A complementary view. *Acta Paediatrica, 89*, 223–228.

Palmer, C., & Alfano, C. A. (2017). Sleep architecture relates to daytime affect and somatic complaints in clinically-anxious but not healthy children. *Journal of Clinical Child and Adolescent Psychology, 46*(2), 175–187.

Paruthi, S., Brooks, L. J., D'Ambrosio, C., Hall, W., Kotagal, S., Lloyd, R. M., . . . Wise, M. S. (2016). Recommended amount of sleep for pediatric populations: A statement of the American Academy of Sleep Medicine. *Journal of Clinical Sleep Medicine, 12*(6), 785–786.

Perez-Chada, D., Perez-Lloret, S., Videla, A. J., Cardinali, D., Bergna, M. A., Fernandez-Acquier, M., . . . Drake, C. (2007). Sleep disordered breathing and daytime sleepiness are associated with poor academic performance in teenagers: A study using the Pediatric Daytime Sleepiness Scale (PDSS). *Sleep, 30*, 1698–1703.

Pesonen, A. K., & Kuula, L. (2018). The validity of a new consumer-targeted wrist device in sleep measurement: An overnight comparison against polysomnography in children and adolescents. *Journal of Clinical Sleep Medicine, 14*, 585–591.

Picchietti, D., Allen, R. P., Walters, A. S., Davidson, J. E., Myers, A., & Ferini-Strambi, L. (2007). Restless legs syndrome: Prevalence and impact in children and adolescents—the Peds REST study. *Pediatrics, 120*, 253–266.

Picchietti, D. L., Bruni, O., de Weerd, A., Durmer, J.

S., Kotagal, S., Owens, J. A., & Simakajornboon, N. (2013). Pediatric restless legs syndrome diagnostic criteria: An update by the International Restless Legs Syndrome Study Group. *Sleep Medicine, 14*, 1253–1259.

Roberts, R. E., & Duong, H. T. (2014). The prospective association between sleep deprivation and depression among adolescents. *Sleep, 37*, 239–244.

Robinson-Shelton, A., & Malow, B. A. (2016). Sleep disturbances in neurodevelopmental disorders. *Current Psychiatry Reports, 18*(1), 6.

Romeo, D. M., Bruni, O., Brogna, C., Ferri, R., Galluccio, C., De Clemente, V, . . . Mercuri E. (2013). Application of the sleep disturbance scale for children (SDSC) in preschool age. *European Journal of Paediatric Neurology, 17*, 374–382.

Rosen, C. L., Wang, R., Taylor, H. G., Marcus, C. L., Katz, E. S., Paruthi, S., . . . Chervin, R. D. (2015). Utility of symptoms to predict treatment outcomes in obstructive sleep apnea syndrome. *Pediatrics, 135*, e662–e671.

Sadeh, A. (2004). A brief screening questionnaire for infant sleep problems: Validation and findings for an Internet sample. *Pediatrics, 113*, e570–e577.

Sadeh, A., Mindell, J. A., Luedtke, K., & Wiegand, B. (2009). Sleep and sleep ecology in the first 3 years: A web-based study. *Journal of Sleep Research, 18*, 60–73.

Scholle, S., Scholle, H. C., Kemper, A., Glaser, S., Rieger, B., Kemper, G., & Awacka, G. (2003). First night effect in children and adolescents undergoing polysomnography for sleep-disordered breathing. *Clinical Neurophysiology, 114*, 2138–2145.

Sheldon, S. H. (2014). The function, phylogeny and ontogeny of sleep. In S. H. Sheldon, R. Ferber, M. H. Kryger, & D. Gozal (Eds.), *Principles and practice of pediatric sleep medicine* (2nd ed., pp. 3–11). Philadelphia: Elsevier.

Sneddon, P., Peacock, G. G., & Crowley, S. L. (2013). Assessment of sleep problems in preschool aged children: An adaptation of the children's sleep habits questionnaire. *Behavioral Sleep Medicine, 11*, 283–296.

Storfer-Isser, A., LeBourgeois, M. K., Harsh, J., Tompsett, C. J., & Redline, S. (2013). Psychometric properties of the Adolescent Sleep Hygiene Scale. *Journal of Sleep Research, 22*, 707–716.

Tan, E., Healey, D., Gray, A. R., & Galland, B. C. (2012). Sleep hygiene intervention for youth aged 10 to 18 years with problematic sleep: A before–after pilot study. *BMC Pediatrics, 12*, 189.

Toon, E., Davey, M. J., Hollis, S. L., Nixon, G. M., Horne, R. S., & Biggs, S. N. (2016). Comparison of commercial wrist-based and smartphone accelerometers, actigraphy, and psg in a clinical cohort of children and adolescents. *Journal of Clinical Sleep Medicine, 12*, 343–350.

Vandeleur, M., Walter, L. M., Armstrong, D. S., Robinson, P., Nixon, G. M., & Horne, R. S. C. (2017).

How well do children with cystic fibrosis sleep?: An actigraphic and questionnaire-based study. *Journal of Pediatrics, 182,* 170–176.

Walter, L. M., Biggs, S. N., Cikor, N., Rowe, K., Davey, M. J., Horne, R. S., & Nixon, G. M. (2016). The efficacy of the OSA-18 as a waiting list triage tool for OSA in children. *Sleep and Breathing, 20,* 837–844.

Wei, J. L., Mayo, M. S., Smith, H. J., Reese, M., & Weatherly, R. A. (2007). Improved behavior and sleep after adenotonsillectomy in children with sleep-disordered breathing. *Archives of Otolaryngology–Head and Neck Surgery, 133,* 974–979.

Wolfson, A. R., & Carskadon, M. A. (1998). Sleep schedules and daytime functioning in adolescents. *Child Development, 69,* 875–887.

Wolfson, A. R., Carskadon, M. A., Acebo, C., Seifer, R., Fallone, G., Labyak, S. E., & Martin, J. L. (2003). Evidence for the validity of a sleep habits survey for adolescents. *Sleep, 26,* 213–216.

Zhang, J., Xu, Z., Zhao, K., Chen, T., Ye, X., Shen, Z., . . . Li, S. (2018). Sleep habits, sleep problems, sleep hygiene, and their associations with mental health problems among adolescents. *Journal of the American Psychiatric Nurses Association, 24,* 223–234.

CHAPTER 24

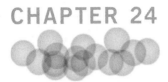

Risky and Impulsive Behaviors

Kevin M. King, Madison C. Feil, Katherine Seldin, Michele R. Smith,
Max A. Halvorson, and Kevin S. Kuehn

Adolescence is a developmental period characterized by increases in risky behaviors, and the personality, cognitive, and neural processes that seem to underlie them. Mortality rates overall are 200% higher in adolescence than in childhood, and many of the top causes of adolescent deaths are related to modifiable behaviors, such as motor vehicle accidents and accidents involving firearms (Dahl, 2004; Xu, Kochanek, & Murphy, 2018). The rates of nonfatal injuries reported to emergency rooms—such as those from falls, being unintentionally struck, or being in motor vehicle accidents—increase significantly in adolescence before declining into middle adulthood (Centers for Disease Control and Prevention [CDC], 2001;

Willoughby, Good, Adachi, Hamza, & Tavernier, 2013). Beyond direct risk of bodily harm, risky and impulsive behaviors in adolescence can have a long-term impact on individuals and society. In the United States in 2010, an estimated 6% of girls ages 15–19 became pregnant, with about 3% giving birth (Kost & Henshaw, 2014). By age 18, 12.4% and of adolescents will meet criteria for alcohol abuse, 12.7% for drug abuse (Swendsen et al., 2012), and the average high-risk adolescent can impose an estimated cost on society between $314,000 and $553,000 by the time he or she reaches the age of 18 (Cohen & Piquero, 2009). Risk taking and impulsive behavior are also core symptoms of various mental health disorders including attention-deficit/hyperactivity disorder (ADHD), borderline personality disorder, alcohol and substance use disorders, eating disorders, and bipolar disorder (Beauchaine & Neuhaus, 2008; Berg et al., 2015; Whiteside & Lynam, 2001). Many of these disorders first onset during adolescence (Kessler et al., 2005; Nagl et al., 2016), and risky and impulsive behaviors also seem to peak during this developmental period (Steinberg, 2007).

In this chapter, we focus on the assessment of risky behaviors, as well as their personality, motivational and cognitive underpinnings. Understanding the bases of risky behavior provides a lens for the clinical assessor to differentiate fleeting, contextually driven instances of risky behaviors from those that represent a larger pattern of risk behaviors that are more likely to lead to negative outcomes. We also outline normative developmental changes in these processes that occur during adolescence, as well as differences observed in adolescents with pathological levels of risk-taking behaviors, when able. We hope this will aid clinicians in understanding the larger developmental context of risky and impulsive behaviors in adolescents.

One theme of this chapter is that risky and impulsive behaviors are difficult to summarize with a single definition or measurement. In some cases, different measures capture similar constructs, yet call them by different names (i.e., the "jangle" fallacy). In other cases, measures with similar names can capture very different constructs (i.e., the "jingle" fallacy; Block, 1995; Kelley, 1927). Furthermore, many well-accepted and widely used measures have poor evidence of reliability or validity. In this chapter, we try to delineate distinct risk-related constructs, while describing the types of approaches commonly used to measure them.

The term "risky behavior" generally refers to specific behaviors (e.g., unprotected sex, binge drinking, or delinquent acts) that have the potential for immediate or long-term negative mental, physical, and social outcomes. The term "impulsive behaviors," or impulsivity, is used variously to describe behaving on a whim or impulse, acting without forethought, giving up easily, or seeking thrilling or exciting experiences. Impulsive behaviors are most typically discussed in the context of trait-like tendencies (e.g., "impulsivity" or "inhibition") and are believed to be the core cognitive and behavioral tendencies underlying, but not fully explaining, engagement in risky behaviors. Therefore, risky behaviors and impulsive behaviors are related but not fully overlapping constructs. Many impulsive behaviors may be considered risky, but others (e.g., an impulsive purchase or a spontaneous decision to get coffee with a friend) would not, and some risky behaviors may occur without much impulsiveness (e.g., skydiving, which requires a great deal of planning to engage in more than once).

Risky and impulsive behaviors can manifest as part of a larger psychological disorder (e.g., delinquent behaviors in the context of conduct disorder) (Moffitt, 1993) or may be present in an otherwise healthy individual (Casey, Getz, & Galván, 2008). Although many adolescents engage in some kinds of risky behaviors, a relatively smaller percentage of adolescents engage heavily in a wide variety of risk behaviors (Brener & Collins, 1998; Lindberg, Boggess, Williams, & Jones, 2000; Zweig, Lindberg, & McGinley, 2001). Because of the great diversity in how risky behaviors manifest in real life, and how their meaning can change depending on the presence of personality or contextual risk factors, it is particularly important to take care when assessing these behaviors in a clinical or research setting.

We first discuss the conceptualization and measurement of risky and impulsive behaviors, with an emphasis on the evidence (or lack thereof) for reliability, validity, and psychometrics of measures. We then provide some information on the developmental context of adolescence, and how normative neurobiological, cognitive, and personality changes parallel developmental changes in the prevalence of risky behaviors. We end with recommendations for nuanced assessment of risky behaviors in clinical settings.

Finally, we must caution readers of this chapter about the research we summarize in this chapter. There is increasing evidence that much research in the psychological sciences may not be replicable (Aarts et al., 2015; Ioannidis, 2005; Munafò et al., 2017; Tackett et al., 2017; Vazire, 2018), due to a reliance on underpowered samples, statistical significance rather than effect size, researcher practices that increase false-positive rates, a lack of transparency in research practices, and an academic culture that emphasizes positive and/or novel findings over credible and/or negative ones (Asendorpf et al., 2013; Button et al., 2013; Miguel et al., 2014; Silberzahn et al., 2018; Vazire, 2018). Although some fields (like personality psychology or population estimates of health-risk behaviors) are characterized by large samples and a culture of replication (Funder, 2016), less attention has been paid to replicability issues in developmental, neuroscience, and clinical research, in spite of the relatively complicated methodological issues that characterize these fields (King, Pullmann, Lyon, Dorsey, & Lewis, 2019; Tackett et al., 2017; Tackett, Brandes, King, & Markon, 2019). Skepticism is particularly important in light of the psychometric problems with many laboratory task measures of risky and impulsive behaviors, as unreliable measurements can still produce false-positive findings, particularly in small samples, which are especially prone to producing large and false effects (Kraemer, Mintz, Noda, Tinklenberg, & Yesavage, 2006). Unreliable measures, when combined with underpowered samples and publication bias for positive findings, may produce a literature that comprises *entirely* false positives.

Even meta-analyses, which are used to synthesize the published literature, are not free of bias. Meta-analyses are the scientific benchmark for calculating effect sizes across a body of studies; however, the replication crisis has raised some concerns about the reliability of these estimates. Stanley, Carter, and Doucouliagos (2018) conducted a meta-analysis of 12,065 different surveys and 200 meta-analyses, and found that only 8% of studies were adequately powered to detect effects, while the average psychological study has only 36% power. Heterogeneity, differences between studies, accounted for 74% of the median proportion of the observed variation within the published effect sizes, which means that the typical psychological research study is unlikely to replicate (Stanley et al., 2018). This meta-analysis suggests that pooling underpowered samples with large heterogeneity is unlikely to produce reliable effect sizes. Additionally, meta-analyses focus on published studies, of which there is likely to be systematic bias in the magnitude, direction, and level of significance in the published literature as compared to unpublished studies (Dickersin, 2005). Researchers have developed some selection methods (Hedges & Vevea, 2006) to minimize this form of bias; however, the assumptions of the researcher conducting the meta-analysis may still affect the reliability of effect sizes (McShane, Böckenholt, & Hansen, 2016).

In general, we believe that a healthy dose of skepticism is warranted in interpreting many of the findings we present in the current chapter.

Definitions and Distinctions of Risky and Impulsive Behaviors

Risky and impulsive behaviors are often operationalized differently depending on the setting in which they are assessed. In large-scale epidemiological studies, the term "health-risk behaviors" refers to engagement in specific behaviors that increase risk for negative health outcomes (e.g., risky driving, substance use, or unprotected sexual activity). In laboratory studies, the term "risky decision making" is used to describe choices made in the face of uncertainty (e.g., in a gambling task). "Impulsive traits" are typically measured with self-report of behavioral tendencies that may contribute to impulsive and risky behavior (e.g., lack of planning, sensation seeking, or a tendency toward acting on impulses). Finally, many behavioral

tasks aim to measure the cognitive processes that underlie impulsive behaviors, such as the ability to wait for a delayed reward or inhibit an automatic response. In this section, we describe in greater detail these different approaches for understanding and measuring risky and impulsive behaviors.

Health-Risk Behaviors

Health-risk behaviors are those that can lead, either directly or indirectly, to negative health outcomes, and were originally studied in an attempt to track precursors of disease (Kolbe, Kann, & Collins, 1993; Thompson, Nelson, Caldwell, & Harris, 1998). Underlying many top causes of death in the United States are seven modifiable risk behaviors: tobacco use, poor diet and inactivity, alcohol consumption, motor vehicle injuries, firearms, sexual behavior, and illicit drug use (Mokdad, Marks, Stroup, & Gerberding, 2004). For adolescents, the conceptualization of health-risk behaviors has expanded to include behaviors that can have a long-term impact on mental health, well-being, and economic opportunity (Kolbe et al., 1993). For example, the CDC has tracked adolescent health-risk behaviors since 1991 using the biennial Youth Risk Behaviors Surveillance System, which measures seatbelt usage, driving while intoxicated, or riding in a car with an intoxicated driver, or distracted driving; carrying a weapon, fighting, tobacco use, alcohol use, and illicit drug use; sexual behaviors and contraceptive use, poor diet, physical inactivity; excessive use of video games, computer, or television; sports injuries, poor sleep, use of indoor tanning equipment, and inadequate sun protection (Brener et al., 2013). Other national and international monitoring surveys additionally track a range of delinquent and criminal behavior in their assessment of youth health-risk behaviors (Arthur, Hawkins, Pollard, Catalano, & Baglioni, 2002; Enzmann et al., 2010; Esbensen & Huizinga, 1993). There is also an increasingly wide range of instruments designed to assess an individual's level of involvement in specific health-risk behaviors. For example, one review of available assessments for substance use in adolescents listed 23 unique instruments that measure the extent of involvement with alcohol and other drugs (Winters, 2003). Similarly, there are measures aimed at assessing involvement in risky sexual behaviors (Turchik & Garske, 2009), risky driving (Taubman-Ben-Ari, Mikulincer, & Gillath, 2004), delinquency (Krohn, Thornberry,

Gibson, & Baldwin, 2010), and other health-risk behaviors of adolescence. The vast majority of these measures are self-report, though in clinical settings, it is not uncommon for adolescent report to be verified by parent report, school or legal records, or potentially even objective measures such as in the case of drug testing. Table 24.1 provides prevalence estimates for a variety of risky behaviors across age.

Risky Decision Making

Risky decision making is most commonly assessed using laboratory tasks that allow researchers to observe decisions in scenarios in which the riskiness and/or the expected value of outcomes can be manipulated. Risky decisions are those whose outcome is uncertain and can be influenced by individuals' sensitivity to rewards and preference for risk (Defoe, Dubas, Figner, & Van Aken, 2015). Laboratory models of risky decision making allow researchers to carefully manipulate aspects of the risky decision (e.g., the relative influence of reward, punishment, and uncertainty) thought to influence risky decision-making preferences.

One widely used risky decision task using this model is the Iowa Gambling Task (IGT; Buelow & Suhr, 2009), in which participants are presented with four decks of cards—two of which are riskier (bigger gains and bigger losses) and have negative expected values (i.e., average losses over time), and two of which are safer and have positive expected values (i.e., average gains over time). Participants have no knowledge of the deck contents before the task begins and are instructed to try to win as much money as possible (Hooper, Luciana, Conklin, & Yarger, 2004; Schonberg, Fox, & Poldrack, 2011). Other tasks, such as the Columbia Card Task (CCT; Figner, Mackinlay, Wilkening, & Weber, 2009), provide explicit information about the amount and probability of gains and losses, and can measure risk taking in the presence of feedback about wins and losses ("hot") or the absence of feedback ("cold"). Other tasks attempt to measure decisions in the face of dynamic, intuitive, and unknown risk probabilities, such as the Balloon Analogue Risk Task (BART; Lejuez, Aklin, Zvolensky, & Pedulla, 2003), in which participants are simply instructed to click as many times as they like to inflate a virtual balloon and earn rewards, knowing that after a randomly selected number of clicks, the balloon will burst, and all rewards will be lost.

Impulsive Traits

Impulsive behaviors are generally those that occur due to an impulse or spur-of-the-moment decision, a lack of forethought or persistence, or thrill or excitement seeking (Smith et al., 2007). Impulsive traits are the stable patterns of behaviors, including consistent behavioral responses to situations (Baumert et al., 2017) that give rise to impulsive behaviors. Impulsive traits have long been conceptualized as personality traits and are commonly measured with retrospective self-report measures (Smith et al., 2007; Whiteside & Lynam, 2001), although more recent approaches have attempted to use behavioral and cognitive tasks (e.g., the Stroop task) to measure impulsive traits as well (King, Patock-Peckham, Dager, Thimm, & Gates, 2014; Sharma, Markon, & Clark, 2014). It is important to note that how researchers define and organize impulsive traits is heavily conflated with how traits are measured (King et al., 2014). Thus, it is impossible to define impulsive traits independent from how they are measured.

A second persistent challenge in this field is a lack of consistency among researchers in defining, labeling, and structuring impulsive traits. Both *jingle* and *jangle* fallacies are prevalent. For example, the tendency to plan ahead before acting has been variously labeled "impulse control," "planning," "premeditation," "good self-control," and "self-control" (King et al., 2014), in spite of these measures using similar or even identical items. The very same task may even be said to measure different constructs at different times. For example, the Stroop task has been described by different researchers as a measure of inattention, inhibition, and resistance to interference (Macleod, 1991). Another issue is the simple lack of specificity of some measures. For example, in the self-report domain, many measures aggregate distinct impulsive traits (e.g., sensation seeking and planning) (Smith et al., 2007). Below we attempt to summarize research that has attempted to bring some consilience to the organization of and relations between impulsive traits.

Self-Report Measures of Impulsive Traits

Self-report measures assess individuals' perceptions of the causes of their impulsive behaviors, in that they are asking people to look back over aggregations of their behaviors and rate the degree to which they acted "on the spur of the moment,"

TABLE 24.1. Prevalence Estimates of Risky Behaviors by Age

	Childhood	6th grade	9th grade	12th grade	Young adults (general population)	Young adults (college sample)	Adult
Driving while distracted (*read or sent texts or e-mails*)	—	—	12.9[a] (11.1–14.9) (*past 30 days*)	59.3[a] (55.8–62.6) (*past 30 days*)	Ages: 20–24 26.4[b]	—	Ages: 25–34 21.1[b]
Seatbelt use (*rarely or never*)	—	3.3[a]* (2.4–4.6)	6.2[a] (5.0–7.7)	5.9[a] (4.4–7.9)	Ages: 20–24 7.9[c] (7.3–8.4)	3.2[d]	Ages: 25–44 6.3[c] (6.0–6.6)
Carried a weapon	—	25.6[a]* (22.6–28.0) (*ever*)	15.3[a] (12.3–19.0) (*past 30 days*)	14.6[a] (12.2–17.5) (*past 30 days*)	—	—	. . . hard to find research on this for adult age ranges—thanks, gun lobby!
Fighting	6.9[e] (6.1–7.7) Ages: 6–11 (*bullies others*)	45.0[a]* (42.0–48.0) (*ever been in a physical fight*)	28.3[a] (25.3–31.5) (*past year*)	17.8[a] (14.9–21.1) (*past year*)	—	3.7[d] (*past year*)	—
Cigarette use	—	1.4[a]* (.92–2.6)	5.2[a] (3.8–7.0)	13.4[a] (10.9–16.2)	Ages: 20–24 13.2[c] (12.3–14.1)	7.7[d] (*past 30 days*)	Ages: 25–44 19.9[c] (19.3–20.6)
Alcohol use	—	14.3[a]* (12.3–16.8) (*ever drank*)	18.8[a] (16.4–21.4) (*past 30 days*)	40.8[a] (37.0–44.8) (*past 30 days*)	Ages: 20–24 52.0[c] (50.9–53.0) (*past 30 days*)	60.4[d] (*past 30 days*)	Ages: 25–44 60.6[c] (60.1–61.2) (*past 30 days*)
Binge drinking	—	—	7.3[a] (5.7–9.2) (*past 30 days*)	20.9[a] (18.1–24.1) (*past 30 days*)	Ages: 20–24 25.2[c] (24.4–26.1)	—	Ages: 25–44 23.9[c] (23.4–24.4)
Marijuana use	—	3.4[a]* (2.3–5.2) (*ever used*)	13.1[a] (11.1–15.4) (*past 30 days*)	25.7[a] (22.9–28.7) (*past 30 days*)	Ages: 18–25 22.1[d] (*past 30 days*)	22.4[d] (*past 30 days*)	Ages: 25–34 14.8[f] (*past 30 days*)

Sexually active	—	3.5[a]* (2.5–5.2) (ever had intercourse)	12.9[a] (11.3–14.7) (past 3 months)	44.3[a] (40.6–48.0) (past 3 months)	—	66.3[d] (past year)	—
Risky sexual behavior (no condom use)	—	Grades 6–8 40.8[a]* (35.7–46.2) (last intercourse)	45.5[a] (38.1–53.1) (last intercourse)	50.1[a] (46.4–53.9) (last intercourse)	—	54.1[d] (past 30 days)	—
Excessive computer time	Age: 6–11 42.2[e] (40.9–43.5) (2+ hours/day; includes phone)	35.6[a]* (32.9–38.5) (3+ hours/day; includes video games)	45.0[a] (41.7–48.2) 3+ hours/day; includes video games	39.2[a] (36.7–41.8) (3+ hours/day; includes video games)	—	—	—
Excessive TV use	Age: 6–11 48.3[e] (45.9–50.8) (2+ hours/day; includes video games)	23.8[a]* (21.3–26.6) (3+ hours/day)	20.9[a] (18.3–23.8) (3+ hours/day)	19.5[a] (17.7–21.5) (3+ hours/day)	—	—	—
Nonfatal injury hospitalizations (rate per 100,000)	Ages: 5–9 7.5[g] (6.0–9.0)	Ages: 10–14 8.6[g] (7.0–10.1)	Ages: 15–19 10.4[g] (8.7–12.2)	Ages: 20–25 10.7[g] (9.0–12.5)	—	Ages: 25–44 9.4[g] (8.0–10.9)	—
Injury deaths (rate per 100,000)	Ages: 5–9 3.85[g]	Ages: 10–14 4.11[g]	Ages: 15–19 19.65[g]	Ages: 20–25 43.5[g]	—	Ages: 25–44 52.7[g]	—
Arrests (rates per 100,000)	Ages: 10–12 507.3[h]	Ages: 13–14 2,579.90[h]	Age: 15 4,633.80[h]	Ages: 17–18 8,206.80[h]	Ages: 19–25 9,611.07[h]	—	Ages: 25–44 6,120.25[h]

Note. *Weighted average from states providing data.
[a]Center of Disease Control and Prevention (2017a)
[b]Schroeder, Peña, & Wilbur (2018)
[c]Centers for Disease Control and Prevention (2017b)
[d]American College Health Association (2018)
[e]Child and Adolescent Health Measurement Initiative, Data Resource Center for Child and Adolescent Health (2016)
[f]Substance Abuse and Mental Health Services Administration (2017)
[g]Centers for Disease Control and Prevention, National Center for Injury Prevention and Control (2016)
[h]Snyder, Cooper, & Mulako-Wangota (2014)

"without thinking," or "on impulse." Many theorists have suggested that self-regulated behavior emerges from a balance between automatic, appetitive, and fearful reactions to internal or external stimuli and the controlled, cognitive processes that direct those reactions toward appropriate behaviors (Carver, 2005; Posner & Rothbart, 2000). Current evidence suggests that when measured through self-report, there are three overarching impulsive traits (Carver, Johnson, & Joormann, 2008; Smith et al., 2007; Smith & Cyders, 2016; Whiteside & Lynam, 2001), two that reflect automatic and one that reflects controlled processes. Moreover, two of these facets comprise two moderately to highly correlated facets (King et al., 2014; Sharma et al., 2014). Some authors assert that this model of impulsive traits differentiates *too much*, in a way that may not be supported by biological evidence (Gullo, Loxton, & Dawe, 2014), arguing for a two-factor model of traits of "approach impulse" and "inhibitory control," but it does not appear that the evidence, reviewed below, supports this assertion.

Automatic Processes

Negative and Positive Urgency

Urgency reflects the tendency to experience strong impulses or urges, and to act rashly in response to strong negative (*negative urgency*) or positive (*positive urgency*) emotions. This trait is described by items such as "I have trouble controlling my impulses," "It is hard for me to resist acting on my feelings," and "When I am upset, I often do things I later regret." Urgency items were originally derived from the impulsivity facet of neuroticism (Whiteside & Lynam, 2001). Both negative and positive urgency have been studied extensively (Cyders et al., 2007), but most reports suggest that they are highly correlated ($r = .60–.80$), suggesting the majority of variance in each is overlapping. Moreover, they share variance with items tapping impulsivity regardless of the presence of emotion (i.e., "I often act on impulse"), as well as negative emotionality (Sharma et al., 2014). Taken together, this suggests that urgency reflects a tendency toward acting on impulses and emotions. A more recent theory suggests that urgency, sometimes also described as "emotional impulsivity," underlies shared variation across most psychological disorders (the "P factor") and reflects high reflexive impulsivity in the face of emotions (Carver, Johnson, & Timpano, 2017).

Sensation Seeking

Sensation seeking is the propensity to pursue novel, thrilling, and potentially dangerous activities. This factor is described by items such as "I'll try anything once," and "I sometimes like doing things that are a bit frightening." Sensation seeking has long been studied as an independent trait (Zuckerman, 1985), and consistently has been shown to be independent of both urgency and planning and persistence (Cross, Cyrenne, & Brown, 2013; Duckworth & Kern, 2011). Sensation seeking is related to the broad personality trait of extraversion—a trait defined by pursuit of social and environmental reward.

Controlled Processes: Planning and Persistence

Controlled processes are reflected in two traits derived from conscientiousness that are moderately associated across studies ($r = ~.40–.50$; e.g., Smith et al., 2007; Whiteside, Lynam, Miller, & Reynolds, 2005). The first facet, *planning*, describes the tendency to plan ahead and think carefully through decisions. People low in planning are thought to act without careful consideration of the consequences. The second facet, *persistence*, describes the ability to persist with difficult or boring tasks, particularly to serve a larger end goal. People low in persistence lose focus quickly and give up easily. The construct "grit," defined as perseverance and passion for long-term goals, is closely related to persistence, such that one integrative meta-analysis suggested that it had near-perfect overlap with measures of persistence and perseverance (Credé, Tynan, & Harms, 2017). Planning and persistence are moderately associated and can be viewed as either moderately related impulsive traits or as facets of one higher-order trait (Sharma et al., 2014).

Laboratory Measures of Risky and Impulsive Traits

Another approach to measuring impulsive traits has arisen from the neuropsychological tradition, using laboratory behavioral tasks to assess the processes that might lead to impulsive behaviors. Because researchers tend to measure only a few tasks (or a single task) in most empirical studies, as well as other psychometric issues (described below), there is less clarity on how these tasks should be organized (Eisenberg, Bissett, Canning, et al., 2018; Sharma, Kohl, Morgan, & Clark, 2013). Below we discuss two general types of laboratory measures: measures of delay ability that tap preference for shorter versus longer reward delays (e.g., the Delay Discounting Task [DDT]), and measures of response inhibition that tap the ability to stop an initiated response and to engage in an alternative response (Hamilton, Littlefield, et al., 2015; Hamilton, Mitchell, et al., 2015). We then discuss the conflicting psychometric evidence on the organization, reliability, and validity of such tasks.

Delay Ability

Delay ability reflects a preference for larger, later rewards over smaller, sooner rewards, and is measured with intertemporal choice tasks, such as the paper-and-pencil Monetary Choice Questionnaire (MCQ; Kirby, Petry, & Bickel, 1999), or the two-choice impulsivity task (Dougherty, Mathias, Marsh, & Jagar, 2005). All tasks require participants to make a choice between pairs of rewards with different magnitudes and different delay periods, such as an immediate $0.50 reward or a $1,000 reward in 5 years. Tasks can vary in terms of whether they provide real or hypothetical rewards, but most evidence suggests that there are few differences in validity across task type (Duckworth & Kern, 2011; Hamilton, Mitchell, et al., 2015). Discounting of future over immediate rewards is known to follow a hyperbolic trajectory, where the value of a given reward declines quickly for short delays, but this decline slows as the delay becomes longer. Multiple outcomes of interest can be computed from task data, including the slope of the hyperbolic curve (the *discounting rate k*), the area under the curve (AUC), and the percent of large rewards chosen (Hamilton, Mitchell, et al., 2015).

Inhibition

Inhibition, the ability to resist or inhibit an appealing or prepotent response in favor of a more advantageous one, is most frequently used as a behavioral measure of impulsive behaviors. Measures of inhibition are often (but not always) derived from a larger body of measures of executive function (Miyake & Friedman, 2012). Some researchers have made further distinctions between the ability to inhibit an automatic response, as in the go/no-go task, and the ability to inhibit an already initiated response, as in a stop-signal task (Hamilton, Littlefield, et al., 2015). In the go/no-go task, for example, participants are frequently given a "go" signal, and rarely are given a "no-go" signal. The frequency of successful "no-go" trials is used as an indicator of inhibition. On the other hand,

a stop-signal task also prompts frequent responses but occasionally provides a delayed cue to inhibit responding. Again, the frequency of successful inhibition (sometimes paired with the delay time) is an indicator of inhibition. However, it is important to note that inhibition tasks have been classified in many different ways in the literature, and it is subsequently difficult to provide a definitive, empirically based classification scheme. For example, the Stroop task has been categorized as both a measure of inhibition, because participants must inhibit the automatic reading response in favor of naming the color of the word, and a measure of resistance to interference, because of the presentation of conflicting information (King et al., 2014).

Methodological Considerations in Assessment Tools

Self-Report Measures

Psychometric Properties

Self-report measures of risky behaviors and impulsive traits generally have good-to-excellent psychometric properties. The test–retest reliability and internal consistency of self-reported behavior and traits is generally excellent, with average estimates above the threshold of acceptability ($r > .75$, alpha $> .70$). Although researchers sometimes come to different conclusions about the number of factors underlying impulsive traits, most common self-report measures are supported by exploratory or confirmatory factor analysis, which suggest that items have generally reported high factor loadings and low-to-moderate correlations across factors (with the exception of negative and positive urgency, described earlier). For example, in one study, Sharma and colleagues (2013) conducted a meta-analysis of 125 studies reporting on 58 different self-report subscales used to measure impulsive traits. Using exploratory principle components analysis, results supported the presence of three relatively distinct traits across all measures that correspond to planning/persistence, urgency, and sensation seeking. Eisenberg, Bissett, Enkavi, and colleagues (2018) used 56 subscales from 23 self-report measures of impulsive traits given to 522 adult participants via Amazon's Mechanical Turk (MTurk). Exploratory factor analyses again differentiated sensation seeking from other impulsive traits, but (contrary to many prior studies) urgency loaded weakly on a facet with planning, while persistence was noted as a separate facet. The difference between these studies is that Sharma and colleagues (2014) relied more heavily on personality-derived measures, sampling more heavily from measures derived from the Big Five (Costa & McCrae, 1995), whereas Eisenberg, Bissett, Enkavi, and colleagues used a broad array of measures intended to measure self-regulation specifically.

Improving the Validity of Self-Report Measures

There is some concern about bias in self-report measures. Self-reports require people to retrospectively recall their behavior, which may be biased because it involves active reconstruction processes that are influenced by factors related to the encoding and recall of a memory, the emotional salience of a memory, and heuristics involved in judging a response to an item (Shiffman et al., 2008). Some biases have been associated with facets of personality, raising the possibility that certain impulsive traits are associated with particularly biased recall. For example, urgency was derived from a facet of neuroticism, and neuroticism is related to a propensity to store and retrieve negative memories from long-term memory (Eysenck & Mogg, 1992; Ruiz-Caballero & Bermúdez, 1995). Thus, between-person differences in impulsive traits themselves may influence the accuracy of retrospective recall.

Accuracy of recall may be improved with Timeline Followback (TLFB) or experience sampling. TLFB helps the individual to retrospectively recall daily behaviors with the aid of specific prompting of an interviewer (Sobell, 2003). These measures are routinely used in research studies of alcohol and drug use (Dawson, 2003) but can be generalized to measure instances of any discrete behavior, and increase the accuracy and reliability of retrospective recall of concrete behaviors (Hjorthøj, Hjorthøj, & Nordentoft, 2012; Pedersen, Grow, Duncan, Neighbors, & Larimer, 2012). Another example of methodological improvement on the self-report measure is the use of daily diary, experience sampling, and ecological momentary assessment (EMA) methods to reduce recall bias in self-report (Shiffman et al., 2008). These measures ask participants to report on behaviors that have happened in the very recent past (the previous day, or shorter), eliminating the need for participants to recall distant behaviors or to generalize about "typical" behavior (Tomko et al., 2014).

Several other factors can influence the accuracy of self-reports of health-risk or impulsive behaviors, including response styles (e.g., a tendency to avoid extreme responses), social desirability, or self-presentation biases (Brener, Billy, & Grady, 2003; Paulhus & Vazire, 2005). For example, in one study, 17% of participants with a confirmed sexually transmitted infection (STI) endorsed lifetime or recent abstinence from vaginal intercourse (Brown et al., 2012), and the belief that fewer peers engaging in sex was associated with inaccurate reporting of recent sexual behavior, suggesting that perceived norms and social undesirability of behaviors can lead to inaccurate reporting.

Administration mode also influences the accuracy of self-reporting. In general, adolescents reported lower levels of health-risk behaviors in home-administered surveys compared to school-administered surveys (Brener et al., 2003, 2006), and during in-person compared to self-administered interviews (Brener et al., 2003). This effect varies according to the sensitivity of the behaviors. For example, in home-administered surveys, adolescents underreported drug and alcohol use, violence, and sexual behavior but not physical activity or tobacco use, compared to adolescents in a school-based survey (Brener et al., 2006). Some research has suggested that most adolescents prefer (and are most honest) answering health-risk behavior screening items using electronic devices compared to clinician interview, in clinical settings (Jasik, Berna, Martin, & Ozer, 2016). The literature about validity of adolescent self-report of health-risk behavior supports the notion that confidentiality has an impact on adolescent willingness to self-report many health-risk behaviors (Brener et al., 2003), and the ability of clinicians to keep adolescents' report of these behaviors confidential will vary based on the behavior, the treatment setting, and the discretion of the clinician.

Inattentive, careless, and mischievous responses are a concern when estimating the prevalence of risk behaviors (Meade & Craig, 2012). A small subset of adolescents has been found to respond to surveys in "mischievous" patterns—typically overendorsing more severe health-risk behaviors (Meade & Craig, 2012; Pape & Storvoll, 2006; Robinson-Cimpian, 2014), while other surveys have provided estimates of careless or inattentive responding that range from 5 to 40% (Curran, 2016; Kim, McCabe, Yamasaki, Louie, & King, 2018). Beyond biasing population estimates of these behaviors, the low prevalence of health-risk behaviors means that inattentive, careless or mischievous respondents can have a significant impact on correlations between risk behaviors and their predictors or outcomes. For example, King,

Kim, and McCabe (2018) show that the true correlation between two variables can be inflated by as much as .20 depending on the proportion of bad respondents and the degree of skew in the data. Many surveys of health-risk behaviors include efforts to screen out these types of responses, for example, by including items assessing the use of fictitious drugs or excluding responses with highly unlikely combinations of responses (Credé, 2010; Kim et al., 2018; Pape & Storvoll, 2006).

In spite of potential biases in self-report data, there is substantial evidence that self-reports exhibit reasonable convergent validity across methods. For example, Brener and colleagues (2003) reported relatively good validity of self-reported risky behaviors, such that they generally converged with other measures (e.g., alcohol and drug use, dietary behaviors, injury and violence). Multiple studies have used more objective measures (e.g., urinalysis, court records, STI test results) to demonstrate that self-reported health-risk behaviors are generally accurate. For example, self-report of alcohol and drug use has been shown to be largely concordant with biological markers (Dawson, 2003; Dillon, Turner, Robbins, & Szapocznik, 2005; Simons, Wills, Emery, & Marks, 2015). Other studies have shown that self-report of personality (including impulsive traits) has at least moderate convergence with interview methods (Smith et al., 2007), informant report (Connolly, Kavanagh, & Viswesvaran, 2007; McCrae & Costa, 1987; Paulhus & Vazire, 2005), and EMA of behavior (Sharma et al., 2014).

Predictive Validity of Trait Models

In general, self-reported traits have excellent predictive validity, predicting a wide range of psychopathology using retrospective, longitudinal, and EMA data (Berg et al., 2015; Eisenberg, Bissett, Enkavi, et al., 2018; Sharma et al., 2014). Parent report of children's impulsive traits at age 3 predicted objective measures (e.g., court, tax, and medical records) of health and well-being up to 30 years later (Moffitt et al., 2011). Several meta-analyses have shown robust associations between self-reported impulsive traits and psychopathology (Berg et al., 2015; Coskunpinar, Dir, & Cyders, 2013; Stautz & Cooper, 2013), and real-world impulsive behavior (Sharma et al., 2014). It is also important to note that there is variability in the degree to which specific impulsive traits are associated with psychopathology. For example, borderline personality disorder is most strongly associated

with urgency and low planning, while aggression is associated with urgency and sensation seeking (Berg et al., 2015). In a meta-analysis of alcohol use and impulsivity factors, drinking quantity was most strongly associated with low planning, binge drinking was most strongly associated with sensation seeking, and alcohol problems were associated with urgency (Coskunpinar et al., 2013). Differentiating between different facets of impulsivity can help us understand how different types of impulsive behaviors vary from one another, and who is likely to be at risk for involvement in specific risk-taking behaviors.

Behavioral Task Measures

Psychometric Properties

Construct operationalization across studies is even more problematic for behavioral task measures. There is a wide variety of behavioral tasks, and each task may be scored differently across studies, with little empirical evidence to guide standardization of administration or scoring. For example, for inhibition tasks, scoring options include reaction time, overall task time, error count, correct responses, proportion of correct to incorrect responses, and difference scores, among others (Scarpina & Tagini, 2017). Authors have noted similar variability for risk-taking and delay tasks (Eisenberg, Bissett, Canning, et al., 2018; Hamilton, Littlefield, et al., 2015; Hamilton, Mitchell, et al., 2015). This methodological variance vastly complicates the ability to compare tasks across studies of reliability and validity for these tasks.

Extant evidence for behavioral tasks suggests that, at best, they have modest psychometric properties. The one exception is delay ability, which has shown moderate to high test–retest reliability up to 1 year later, and good convergence across multiple measures (Hamilton, Mitchell, et al., 2015; Odum, 2011; Weafer, Baggott, & de Wit, 2013). On the other hand, laboratory measures of risky decision making and inhibition have much less psychometric support. First, it has frequently been noted that few studies have reported on the reliability of these tasks (Buelow & Suhr, 2009; Sharma et al., 2014). Those that have report low-to-moderate test–retest reliabilities for risky decision-making and inhibition measures (median r = .54) (Enkavi et al., 2019; Weafer et al., 2013). Enkavi and colleagues (2019) compared multiple task outcomes from multiple risky decision-making, delay, and inhibition tasks, and showed that difference measures, which are commonly used as an indicator of inhibition (e.g., the difference in reaction times between inhibition and noninhibition conditions), had almost no reliability across tasks (mean = .25, SD = .24). Although latent factors formed from those tasks did have adequate reliability, they failed to predict meaningful variance in real-world outcomes, or conform to a priori groupings of tasks (Enkavi et al., 2019).

Behavioral tasks may do a poor job of capturing reliable individual differences because many of them aim to maximize an experimental effect, such as reaction times to a go versus no-go condition or differentiating choices in the face of varying risks and rewards. By maximizing within-individual differences, between-individual differences become harder to detect (Hedge, Powell, & Sumner, 2018), limiting their utility as an indicator of individual differences. In other words, if a task is designed so that *everyone* shows the effect, individual differences might be inadvertently obscured. The poor evidence of reliability for these tasks is further confounded by evidence that many tasks have very strong practice effects. Several studies indicating that stability in some working memory and inhibition tasks may be *almost entirely* accounted for by practice effects (Salthouse, 2014; Sullivan et al., 2017), suggesting that the modest estimates of test–retest reliability may actually *overestimate* the amount of between-person variance in these tasks. There is also evidence to suggest that strategies in gambling tasks may be learned, inflating reliability estimates (Buelow & Suhr, 2009; Toplak, Sorge, Benoit, West, & Stanovich, 2010). Finally, recent evidence suggests that aggregating information across multiple trials of a task contaminates between-person variation with trial-by-trial variation and can dramatically attenuate between-person associations (Rouder & Haaf, 2018). Until psychometric issues with behavioral tasks are resolved, we recommend against their use for measuring between-person differences in the cognitive and motivational processes underlying impulsive and risky behaviors.

Within-Method Convergence

As noted earlier, prior studies have reported good-to-excellent cross-task convergence for measures of delay ability (Hamilton, Mitchell, et al., 2015; MacKillop et al., 2016). However, the evidence for convergence within measures of risky decision making and inhibition is weaker, with some reviews suggesting there is no consistent latent structure for tasks (Sharma et al., 2014). Multiple factor-analytic studies have reported factors that fit the data well, although the specific configurations of inhibition, delay, and risky decision-making tasks vary with each analysis (Eisenberg, Bissett, Enkavi, et al., 2018; Miyake et al., 2000; Miyake & Friedman, 2012; Rey-Mermet, Gade, & Oberauer, 2018; Reynolds, Ortengren, Richards, & de Wit, 2006; Stahl et al., 2014; Venables et al., 2018). In spite of the "well-fitting" nature of these models, there are several indications that these factor-analytic studies are not discovering strong latent structure among these tasks. First, studies routinely report low to modest, r = .00–.30, correlations among measures of inhibition, and factor loadings that are often weak to modest, lambda < .30–.50 (MacKillop et al., 2016; Miyake et al., 2000; Rey-Mermet et al., 2017; Reynolds et al., 2006; Stahl et al., 2014; Venables et al., 2018). Indeed, one reanalysis of six datasets with large samples and multiple measures of executive function suggested that inhibition could not be differentiated from the broader factor of cognitive speed (Jewsbury, Bowden, & Strauss, 2016). In a meta-analysis of 98 studies reporting correlations between at least two inhibition, delay, and risky decision-making tasks, performance on the BART was uncorrelated with all other tasks (including the IGT), while the IGT was associated with both delay and inhibition tasks (Sharma et al., 2014), Given the poor evidence of reliability or convergent validity for behavioral tasks, it is impossible to discern whether predictive validity for these tasks has any meaning. Thus, we strongly recommend against their use in research or clinical settings without further development of psychometric models of individual differences in task performance (Rouder & Haaf, 2018).

Predictive Validity of Task Measures

As may be expected given the poor psychometric properties of behavioral task measures, the extant evidence suggests they have weak predictive validity. In one meta-analytic study, commission errors on measures such as the go/no-go task or the continuous performance task were at best weakly associated with most forms of psychopathology (e.g., ADHD and addiction; Hedges's g = .31–.49), and exhibited substantial heterogeneity in effects (Wright, Lipszyc, Dupuis, Thayapararajah, & Schachar, 2014). Another meta-analysis suggested that some studies have found inhibition deficits among those with alcohol dependence (g = .40–.53), but associations with other addictive behaviors depended on the specific task, which suggests that effects may be unreliable (Smith, Mattick,

Jamadar, & Iredale, 2014). Moreover, both of these meta-analyses had relatively few (n < 10) samples for each specific meta-analytic association, undermining confidence in the stability of the reported effect sizes. In contrast, delay discounting was shown to be weakly (r = .14) associated with a broad range of alcohol-related outcomes in a large (n = 64) meta-analysis (Amlung, Vedelago, Acker, Balodis, & MacKillop, 2017), and strongly associated with ADHD diagnosis (n = 25; Cohen's d = 0.43) (Jackson & MacKillop, 2016).

Convergence of Self-Report and Behavioral Measures

As might be expected, there is little evidence that behavioral tasks used to measure delay, risky decision making, or inhibition converge with self-report measures of impulsive traits. This is in part because behavioral task and self-report measures have low overlap in construct representation (Cyders & Coskunpinar, 2011) or the theoretical mechanisms that lead to item or task responses (Whitely, 1983). Most studies report task–trait correlations that are very small or close to zero (Cyders & Coskunpinar, 2012; de Ridder, Lensvelt-Mulders, Finkenauer, Stok, & Baumeister, 2012; Duckworth & Kern, 2011; Eisenberg, Bissett, Enkavi, et al., 2018; MacKillop et al., 2016; Sharma et al., 2014). For example, in a large (n = 989) sample of early adolescents (ages 9–16), indicators of inhibition (go/no-go), risky decision making (IGT), and working memory (digit span and trail making tests) shared almost no common variance with one another, with parent report of temperament (effortful control), or with internalizing and externalizing symptoms (r < .20). Tasks may not always reflect the complex interplay between learning histories and situations that people face in the real world, while self-report measures filter impulsive behaviors through a retrospective lens that may bias individuals' explanations of their own behavior (Cyders & Coskunpinar, 2011).

Developmental Changes in Risky Behaviors and Impulsive Traits

Adolescence, the transitional period between childhood and adulthood, is marked by substantial changes in neurobiological, cognitive, behavioral, and social systems. The timing of these changes suggests that they may underlie the occurrence of health-risk behaviors during adolescence (Casey, 2015; Casey et al., 2008; Shulman et al., 2016;

Steinberg, 2008), yet attempts to demonstrate that these changes relate to real-life risk taking have garnered mixed results (for reviews, see Crone & Dahl, 2012; Romer, Reyna, & Satterthwaite, 2017). In this section, we begin by outlining typical trajectories for health-risk behaviors in adolescence, then describe key developmental changes that occur during adolescence, and how those changes relate to adolescent risk taking. Last, we address common misconceptions about the origins of risk taking during this developmental period.

Developmental Changes in Health-Risk Behaviors

The prevalence of health- risk behaviors varies across age. Evidence from large-scale population-based surveys suggests that most risk behaviors increase in prevalence during early-to-middle adolescence and peak in late adolescence and young adulthood, before decreasing into adulthood (Brener & Collins, 1998; Dahl, 2004; Defoe et al., 2015; Gardner & Steinberg, 2005; Mata, Josef, & Hertwig, 2016; Steinberg, 2007; Willoughby et al., 2013). For example, risky driving behaviors are higher among 20- to 25-year-olds than in 15- to 19-year-olds (Jonah, 1990), binge drinking peaks between ages of 21 and 23 (Chassin, Colder, Hussong, & Sher, 2016), and risky sexual behaviors are highest in the 4 years following high school (Fergus, Zimmerman, & Caldwell, 2007). Though prevalence of criminal behavior varies greatly based on individual factors and the nature of the crime, population age–crime curves typically indicate that delinquency peaks in late adolescence and early adulthood (Loeber & Farrington, 2014).

Within any given age, there is heterogeneity in risk behavior involvement. Most health-risk behaviors are positively skewed, with many adolescents abstaining altogether and a smaller proportion of adolescents engaging in a wide variety of health-risk behaviors (though engaging in multiple health-risk behaviors becomes more common with age, peaking in young adulthood) (Bjork & Pardini, 2015; Brener & Collins, 1998; Lindberg et al., 2000; Vaughn, Salas-Wright, Delisi, & Maynard, 2014; Zweig et al., 2001). For example, in a study looking at the health-risk behaviors of 12- to 17-year-olds from a nationally representative sample of over 18,000 youth, Vaughn and colleagues (2014) found that 73% of adolescents fell into a "normative" group with uniformly low levels of all risk behaviors measured, whereas only 5% of adolescents had both the highest average of health-risk behaviors and most wide-ranging. Thus, typical adolescent development is marked by a modest increase in health-risk behaviors, which peaks between midadolescence and young adulthood, while a small subset of adolescents who exhibit early, broad, severe, and persistent involvement in health-risk behaviors. In the following sections we outline developmental changes in biological, psychological, and social factors as they relate to adolescent risk taking.

Neurobiological Changes during Adolescence Related to Risk Taking

That neurobiological systems associated with processes thought to underlie health-risk behaviors (e.g., risky decision making, impulsive traits, delay ability and inhibition) exhibit different rates of development in adolescence compared to childhood has led some authors to attribute changes in health-risk behaviors observed during adolescence to the neurobiological changes that characterize adolescence (Casey et al., 2008; Shulman et al., 2016; Steinberg, 2010).

Pubertal and Hormonal Changes

Biological changes associated with puberty, by most considered the biological onset of adolescence, are triggered by increases in pubertal hormones (estrogen and testosterone), typically around ages 9–10 for girls and 10–11 for boys (Peper & Dahl, 2013). These hormonal changes have cascading effects on the development of many body systems, including the brain (Peper & Dahl, 2013). Pubertal status has long been associated with increases in risky behavior in terms of self-reports of health-risk behaviors and performance on risky decision-making tasks (Braams, van Duijvenvoorde, Peper, & Crone, 2015; Collado, MacPherson, Kurdziel, Rosenberg, & Lejuez, 2014). Some research has suggested that increases in testosterone and estrogen may be linked to reduced delay ability and increases in risky choices and health-risk behaviors (Apicella, Carré, & Dreber, 2015; Boyer, 2006; Forbes et al., 2010; Vermeersch, T'Sjoen, Kaufman, & Vincke, 2008), and individual differences in sensation seeking have long been attributed to testosterone (Roberti, 2004).

Neural Development

Adolescence is marked by substantial reorganization and development of many neural systems that may underlie risky and impulsive behaviors, such as the limbic system and the prefrontal cortex. In general, development of the limbic system is characterized by curvilinear development, with accelerated development around the pubertal transition and a peak during midadolescence, while the prefrontal cortex appears to develop in a relatively linear fashion into adulthood. Activity in the limbic system has been associated with sensitivity to reward, thought to be related to delay ability and risky decision making (Galván, Hare, Voss, Glover, & Casey, 2007; Telzer, Fuligni, Lieberman, & Galván, 2013). During adolescence, there is heighted response to reward in the limbic system and dampened response to punishment (Humphreys et al., 2016; Luna, Paulsen, Padmanabhan, & Geier, 2013; McCormick & Telzer, 2017; van der Schaaf, Warmerdam, Crone, & Cools, 2011). On the other hand, functioning of the prefrontal cortex has been associated with inhibition and other executive functions (Luna et al., 2013; Ordaz, Foran, Velanova, & Luna, 2013), and the prefrontal cortex continues its development in a relatively slow, linear process through early adulthood (Luna et al., 2013).

The "dual systems" model of adolescent risk taking posits that the difference in the development of the limbic system and the prefrontal cortex creates an "imbalance" during adolescence that is skewed toward more impulsive, reward-driven, and risky behavior (Steinberg, 2010). This model is supported by parallel trajectories of adolescent development in performance on laboratory behavioral tasks (Defoe et al., 2015; Huizinga, Dolan, & van der Molen, 2006; Steinberg et al., 2008), self-reports of impulsive traits (Harden & Tucker-Drob, 2011; Steinberg et al., 2008), and risky behaviors (Duell et al., 2018), many of which exhibit steep increases that peak during adolescence, followed by later declines (e.g., performance on risky decision tasks, delay ability, sensation seeking, and health-risk behaviors) or linear increases (inhibition, planning, and persistence). Many variations on this model that have been proposed to integrate new findings differ in the proposed timing of development of the two systems (Casey, 2015; Luna et al., 2013; Steinberg, 2008), but most theorize that asymmetrical changes in neurobiological systems explain age differences in risk taking.

However, some authors have argued that the dual systems model does not accurately describe the more nuanced changes in both brain function and behavior that occur during adolescence (Defoe et al., 2015; Pfeifer & Allen, 2012; Romer et al., 2017; Willoughby et al., 2013). For example, there is evidence that limbic system activity may be related to positive adaptation and reduced risk taking (Telzer, 2016; Telzer et al., 2013). Some longitudinal research indicates that psychometrically sound measures of planning/persistence and/or sensation seeking do not follow the trajectory of development proposed by the dual systems model (King, Fleming, Monahan, & Catalano, 2011; King, Lengua, & Monahan, 2013; Littlefield, Stevens, Ellingson, King, & Jackson, 2016; Monahan, King, Shulman, Cauffman, & Chassin, 2015), and that the development of the two are highly correlated (Littlefield et al., 2016), even in data for which authors conclude otherwise (King, Littlefield, et al., 2018; Shulman, Harden, Chein, & Steinberg, 2014). No research has connected individual differences in the development of neurobiological, behavioral task, or self-report measures, further undermining the credibility of this research. Moreover, some authors have pointed out that the predicted period of time during which adolescent risk taking should be highest based on the dual systems model—early adolescence—does not line up well with the consistent findings that real-world risk behaviors peak in late adolescence and early adulthood (Willoughby et al., 2013). As we noted earlier, research suggests that most adolescents do not engage in a wide variety of risk behaviors (Bjork & Pardini, 2015), in spite of the evidence for broad neurobiological changes during adolescence, and no research has connected individual differences in neurobiological development to age-related increases in risky health behaviors. Finally, the noted unreliability and poor psychometric properties of many laboratory behavioral tasks measuring risky decision making and inhibition means that research relying on these tasks may have unusually high false-positive rates, making a true integration of this literature difficult, if not impossible.

Changes in Peer Affiliation

Adolescence is a time of shifting social opportunities and expectations, which may increase the potential for risk behaviors. Adolescents spend more time with their peers than in any other social context (Myers, Doran, & Brown, 2007). Susceptibility to peer influence peaks during mid-adolescence (Monahan, Steinberg, & Cauffman, 2009; Steinberg & Monahan, 2007), and adolescence is marked by both heightened desire for affiliation and sensitivity to social evaluation (Somerville, 2013). Adolescents remain connected to peer groups and media messaging even when at home:

In a 2015 study in the United States, an estimated 67% of teens ages 13–18 had smartphones of their own with unrestricted Internet access, compared to only 24% of 8- to 12-year-olds, and spent an average of 160 minutes engaged with their phones each day (Common Sense Media). Peers have long been identified as a central influence on delinquent and risk behavior (Dishion & Tipsord, 2011), and adolescents make more risky decisions, display preferences for immediate versus delayed rewards, and exhibit heightened activity in neural systems associated with reward when exposed to peers as compared to being alone (Albert, Chein, & Steinberg, 2013; Chein, Albert, O'Brien, Uckert, & Steinberg, 2011; Geier, Terwilliger, Teslovich, Velanova, & Luna, 2010; O'Brien, Albert, Chein, & Steinberg, 2011). Again, however, we urge cautious interpretation of these findings, as they often have relied on unreliable measures of individual differences in risk preference.

Changes in Risk Evaluation

By mid-adolescence, youth are able to evaluate the risks of many behaviors as well as adults can (Reyna & Farley, 2006; Reyna & Rivers, 2008; Romer et al., 2017). Indeed, Romer and colleagues (2017) suggest that adolescents could be considered "hyperrational," inasmuch as they rely on assessments of the risks and benefits of their behavior to guide their actions *even more* than adults do. This "hyperrationality" may in fact promote risk taking in situations where negative consequences are perceived to be unlikely (Reyna & Farley, 2006). In fact, adolescents perceive themselves as *more* vulnerable to certain negative outcomes than adults do, often overestimating the likelihood of negative outcomes in the face of risk (Reyna & Farley, 2006). However, there seems to be a marked difference in how risk is evaluated in different situations. For example, Tymula and colleagues (2012) found that adolescents are more likely to take risks in ambiguous situations when compared to adults. This may be because adolescents are prone to reward seeking despite ambiguity, while adults may be primed to be risk-averse in the face of ambiguity. This finding may also reflect the bias toward novel action that often is seen in adolescence (Romer, 2010; Romer & Hennessy, 2007). These findings emphasize the point that adolescents' approach to risk is not necessarily one of broad-band disinhibition but may at times represent a different pattern of processing risk and reward information than what is normative in adulthood.

Sociodemographic Correlates of Risky Behavior

Involvement in risky behaviors is associated with many demographic factors beyond the individual differences we discussed earlier. In an assessment setting, it is important to consider the base rates of different behaviors in contextualizing any risky behavior. First, males generally tend to engage in more risky behavior than females. For example, males exhibit larger increases, higher peak rates, and slower declines in criminal behavior across adolescence (Salas-Wright, Nelson, Vaughn, Gonzalez, & Córdova, 2017). There are myriad social and contextual factors at play as well. For instance, Chung, Hill, Hawkins, Gilchrist, and Nagin (2002) found that among early adolescents who had committed minor offenses by age 13, those with more antisocial peers, poorer engagement at school, and living in neighborhoods with more drugs were more likely to escalate their offending throughout adolescence.

Many of the prevalence rates listed earlier are primarily in the context of westernized cultures, although some recent research suggests that the general trend of age differences in risk taking is found in multiple cultures across the world (Duell et al., 2018; Steinberg et al., 2018). However, there are indications that the absolute rate of risk behavior varies across cultures. One cross-national study suggested that adolescents in China engage in risky behaviors such as delinquency, cigarette smoking, and alcohol use at overall lower rates than American adolescents (Jessor et al., 2003). Similarly, first-generation immigrants in the United States are less likely to engage in risky sexual behavior, substance use, and delinquent behavior than second- and third-generation immigrants across several different countries of origin (Hussey et al., 2007; Trejos-Castillo & Vazsonyi, 2009; Willgerodt & Thompson, 2006).

Considerations in the Assessment of Risky Behaviors

We have discussed the operationalization, measurement, and developmental context of risky and impulsive behaviors in adolescence. It is important to note that not every occurrence of a health-risk behavior necessarily results in harm and, in fact, most do not. Understanding health-risk behaviors when they are observed in clinical practice requires consideration of contextual and individual-difference factors that provide more information about whether an occurrence of the behavior was part of a larger pattern of behavior, or with full knowledge of the risk involved.

In a typical clinical setting, presented with an adolescent engaging in some or many risky behaviors, it is necessary to integrate many of these factors into a holistic assessment in order to understand these risky behaviors in the context of the adolescent's developmental and social context. First, it is important to understand the degree to which any risky behavior is normative for an adolescent, relative to other same-age peers. Many resources (such as the Youth Risk Behaviors Survey, the CDC, and the Monitoring the Future survey) provide normative data for a wide variety of risky behaviors. Interventions that provide normative feedback about risky behavior (e.g., alcohol use) have been shown to be broadly effective (e.g., Lewis et al., 2014). Moreover, given that only some adolescents engage in a broad array of risky behaviors, it is important to screen for engagement in other risky behaviors to understand whether any one risky behavior represents a general pattern of risk, or a more focused behavior. This may also extend to assessing impulsive traits, which may help a clinician differentiate whether an adolescent is likely to engage in further risky behaviors. However, given the lack of clinical evidence for the utility of any of these assessments, we would caution clinicians against relying exclusively on single assessments. One limitation of the literature is that research largely focuses on how to predict involvement in risky behaviors, but not how to predict *how* risky they are for a given person. One exception is alcohol use, with its long line of research differentiating between involvement and problems with alcohol (Chassin et al., 2016). In understanding the potential impact of a given risky behavior, it may be important for a clinician to assess many features of risky behavior involvement to better understand the potential for immediate or long-term harm.

A Research Agenda

Given the problems we identified with many of the measures of the underlying propensity toward risky behaviors, we provide some suggestions to guide future developmental work. Given the paucity of strong psychometric research on laboratory behavioral tasks, it is critical for research to focus on understanding and improving the psychometric performance of such tasks, including the consideration of novel psychometric models (Rouder & Haaf, 2018). Although multitrait-multimethod (MTMM) studies are ideal (Strauss & Smith, 2009), few successful MTMM studies have been completed for impulsive traits due to the psychometric challenges across self-report and laboratory tasks discussed earlier. This is in part because most MTMM studies have attempted to connect disparate measures of impulsive and risky behaviors (e.g., tasks and self-report) that may reflect entirely different levels of psychological processes (Cyders & Coskunpinar, 2011). It may be more profitable to consider methods of assessment that are closer variants of the measure at hand (e.g., peer ratings or narrative interviews compared with self-report), as a few prior studies have done (Smith et al., 2007). Finally, researchers should also attend to the state–trait distinction (Hertzog & Nesselroade, 1987), and work to develop psychometrically sound measures of impulsive states as well as traits (e.g., Tomko et al., 2014). This type of research may lead to tools that allow clinicians to better understand not only *who* is at risk for risky and impulsive behaviors but also *when* those risks manifest.

Future research in this area must include improvements in measurement and greater clarity in conceptualization. Understanding the role of bias and improving measures to maximize between person differences and more cogent operationalization of risk are critical next steps in measurement. Both context and individual personality characteristics must also be considered when estimating risk involvement.

REFERENCES

Aarts, A. A., Anderson, J. E., Anderson, C. J., Attridge, P. R., Attwood, A., Axt, J., . . . Zuni, K. (2015). Estimating the reproducibility of psychological science. *Science, 349*(6251).

Albert, D., Chein, J. M., & Steinberg, L. (2013). The teenage brain: Peer influences on adolescent decision making. *Current Directions in Psychological Science, 22*(2), 114–120.

American College Health Association. (2018). *American College Health Association-National College Health Assessment: II. Reference Group Executive Summary Spring 2018.* Silver Spring, MD: Author.

Amlung, M., Vedelago, L., Acker, J., Balodis, I., & MacKillop, J. (2017). Steep delay discounting and addictive behavior: A meta-analysis of continuous associations. *Addiction, 112*(1), 51–62.

Apicella, C. L., Carré, J. M., & Dreber, A. (2015). Testosterone and economic risk taking: A review. *Adaptive Human Behavior and Physiology, 1*(3), 358–385.

Arthur, M. W., Hawkins, J. D., Pollard, J. A., Catalano, R. F., & Baglioni, A. J. (2002). Measuring risk and protective factors for substance use, delinquency, and other adolescent problem behaviors: The communities that care youth survey. *Evaluation Review, 26*(6), 575–601.

Asendorpf, J. B., Conner, M., De Fruyt, F., De Houwer, J., Denissen, J. J. A., Fiedler, K., . . . Wicherts, J. M. (2013). Recommendations for increasing replicability in psychology. *European Journal of Personality, 27*(2), 108–119.

Baumert, A., Schmitt, M., Perugini, M., Johnson, W., Blum, G., Borkenau, P., . . . Wrzus, C. (2017). Integrating personality structure, personality process, and personality development. *European Journal of Personality, 31*(5), 503–528.

Beauchaine, T. P., & Neuhaus, E. (2008). Impulsivity and vulnerability to psychopathology. In T. P. Beauchaine & S. P. Hinshaw (Eds.), *Child and adolescent psychopathology* (pp. 129–156). Hoboken, NJ: Wiley.

Berg, J. M., Latzman, R. D., Bliwise, N. G., Lilienfeld, S. O. (2015). Parsing the heterogeneity of impulsivity: A meta-analytic review of the behavioral implications of the UPPS for psychopathology. *Psychological Assessment, 27*(4), 1129–1146.

Bjork, J. M., & Pardini, D. A. (2015). Who are those "risk-taking adolescents"?: Individual differences in developmental neuroimaging research. *Developmental Cognitive Neuroscience, 11*, 56–64.

Block, J. (1995). A contrarian view of the five-factor approach to personality description. *Psychological Bulletin, 117*(2), 187–215.

Boyer, T. W. (2006). The development of risk-taking: A multi-perspective review. *Developmental Review, 26*(3), 291–345.

Braams, B. R., van Duijvenvoorde, A. C., Peper, J. S., & Crone, E. A. (2015). Longitudinal changes in adolescent risk-taking: A comprehensive study of neural responses to rewards, pubertal development, and risk-taking behavior. *Journal of Neuroscience, 35*(18), 7226–7238.

Brener, N. D., Billy, J. O., & Grady, W. R. (2003). Assessment of factors affecting the validity of self-reported health-risk behavior among adolescents: Evidence from the scientific literature. *Journal of Adolescent Health, 33*(6), 436–457.

Brener, N. D., & Collins, J. L. (1998). Co-occurrence of health-risk behaviors among adolescents in the United States. *Journal of Adolescent Health, 22*(3), 209–213.

Brener, N. D., Eaton, D. K., Kann, L., Akinbami, L., Brown, B., Chandler, K., . . . Turner, C. (2006). The association of survey setting and mode with self-reported health risk behaviors among high school students. *Public Opinion Quarterly, 70*(3), 354–374.

Brener, N. D., Kann, L., Shanklin, S., Kinchen, S., Eaton, D. K., Hawkins, J., & Flint, K. H. (2013). Methodology of the youth risk behavior surveillance system—2013. *Morbidity and Mortality Weekly Report: Recommendation and Reports, 62,* 1–20.

Brown, J. L., Sales, J. M., Diclemente, R. J., Salazar, L. F., Vanable, P. A., Carey, M. P., . . . Stanton, B. (2012). Predicting discordance between self-reports of sexual behavior and incident sexually transmitted infections with african american female adolescents: Results from a 4-city study. *AIDS and Behavior, 16*(6), 1491–1500.

Buelow, M. T., & Suhr, J. A. (2009). Construct validity of the Iowa gambling task. *Neuropsychology Review, 19*(1), 102–114.

Button, K. S., Ioannidis, J. P. A., Mokrysz, C., Nosek, B. A., Flint, J., Robinson, E. S. J., & Munafò, M. R. (2013). Power failure: Why small sample size undermines the reliability of neuroscience. *Nature Reviews Neuroscience, 14*(5), 365–376.

Carver, C. S. (2005). Impulse and constraint: Perspectives from personality psychology, convergence with theory in other areas, and potential for integration. *Personality and Social Psychology Review, 9*(4), 312–333.

Carver, C. S., Johnson, S. L., & Joormann, J. (2008). Serotonergic function, two-mode models of self-regulation, and vulnerability to depression: What depression has in common with impulsive aggression. *Psychological Bulletin, 134*(6), 912–943.

Carver, C. S., Johnson, S. L., & Timpano, K. R. (2017). Toward a functional view of the p factor in psychopathology. *Clinical Psychological Science, 5*(5), 880–889.

Casey, B. J. (2015). Beyond simple models of self-control to circuit-based accounts of adolescent behavior. *Annual Review of Psychology, 66*(1), 295–319.

Casey, B. J., Getz, S., & Galván, A. (2008). The adolescent brain. *Developmental Review, 28*(1), 62–77.

Centers for Disease Control and Prevention. (2001). National estimates of nonfatal injuries treated in hospital emergency departments—United States, 2000. *Morbidity and Mortality Weekly Report, 50*(17), 340–346.

Chassin, L., Colder, C. R., Hussong, A. M., & Sher, K. J. (2016). Substance use and substance use disorders. In D. Cicchetti (Ed.), *Developmental psychopathology* (3rd ed., Vol. 3, pp. 833–897). Hoboken, NJ: Wiley.

Chein, J. M., Albert, D., O'Brien, L., Uckert, K., & Steinberg, L. (2011). Peers increase adolescent risk taking by enhancing activity in the brain's reward circuitry. *Developmental Science, 14*(2), F1–F10.

Child and Adolescent Health Measurement Initiative, Data Resource Center for Child and Adolescent Health. (2016). Washington, DC: Health Resources and Services Administration, Maternal and Child Health Bureau in collaboration with the U.S. Census Bureau.

Chung, I. J., Hill, K. G., Hawkins, J. D., Gilchrist, L. D., & Nagin, D. S. (2002). Childhood predictors of offense trajectories. *Journal of Research in Crime and Delinquency, 39*(1), 60–90.

Cohen, M. A., & Piquero, A. R. (2009). New evidence on the monetary value of saving a high risk youth. *Journal of Quantitative Criminology, 25*(1), 25–49.

Collado, A., MacPherson, L., Kurdziel, G., Rosenberg, L. A., & Lejuez, C. W. (2014). The relationship between puberty and risk taking in the real world and in the laboratory. *Personality and Individual Differences, 68,* 143–148.

Connolly, J. J., Kavanagh, E. J., & Viswesvaran, C. (2007). The convergent validity between self and observer ratings of personality: A meta-analytic review. *International Journal of Selection and Assessment, 15*(1), 110–117.

Coskunpinar, A., Dir, A. L., & Cyders, M. A. (2013). Multidimensionality in impulsivity and alcohol use: A meta-analysis using the UPPS model of impulsivity. *Alcoholism: Clinical and Experimental Research, 37*(9), 1441–1450.

Costa, P. T., & McCrae, R. R. (1995). Domains and facets: Hierarchical personality assessment using the revised NEO Personality Inventory. *Journal of Personality Assessment, 64*(1), 21–50.

Credé, M. (2010). Random responding as a threat to the validity of effect size estimates in correlational research. *Educational and Psychological Measurement, 70*(4), 596–612.

Credé, M., Tynan, M. C., & Harms, P. D. (2017). Much ado about grit: A meta-analytic synthesis of the grit literature. *Journal of Personality and Social Psychology, 113*(3), 492–511.

Crone, E. A., & Dahl, R. E. (2012). Understanding adolescence as a period of social–affective engagement and goal flexibility. *Nature Reviews Neuroscience, 13*(9), 636–650.

Cross, C. P., Cyrenne, D.-L. M., & Brown, G. R. (2013). Sex differences in sensation-seeking: A meta-analysis. *Scientific Reports, 3,* 2486.

Curran, P. G. (2016). Methods for the detection of carelessly invalid responses in survey data. *Journal of Experimental Social Psychology, 66,* 4–19.

Cyders, M. A., & Coskunpinar, A. (2011). Measurement of constructs using self-report and behavioral lab tasks: Is there overlap in nomothetic span and construct representation for impulsivity? *Clinical Psychology Review, 31*(6), 965–982.

Cyders, M. A., & Coskunpinar, A. (2012). The relationship between self-report and lab task conceptualizations of impulsivity. *Journal of Research in Personality, 46*(1), 121–124.

Cyders, M. A., Smith, G. T., Spillane, N. S., Fischer, S., Annus, A. M., & Peterson, C. (2007). Integration of impulsivity and positive mood to predict risky behavior: Development and validation of a measure of positive urgency. *Psychological Assessment, 19*(1), 107–118.

Dahl, R. E. (2004). Adolescent brain development: A period of vulnerability and opportunities. *Annals of the New York Academy of Sciences, 102*(1), 1–22.

Dawson, D. A. (2003). Methodological issues in measuring alcohol use. *Alcohol Research and Health, 27*(1), 18–29.

de Ridder, D. T. D., Lensvelt-Mulders, G., Finkenauer, C., Stok, F. M., & Baumeister, R. F. (2012). Taking stock of self-control: A meta-analysis of how trait self-control relates to a wide range of behaviors. *Personality and Social Psychology Review, 16*(1), 76–99.

Defoe, I. N., Dubas, J. S., Figner, B., & Van Aken, M. A. G. (2015). A meta-analysis on age differences in risky decision making: Adolescents versus children and adults. *Psychological Bulletin, 141*(1), 48–84.

Dickersin, K. (2005). Publication bias: Recognizing the problem, understanding its origins and scope, and preventing harm. In H. R. Rothstein, A. J. Sutton, & M. Borenstein (Eds.), *Publication bias in meta-analysis: Prevention, assessment and adjustments* (pp. 9–33). Chichester, UK: Wiley.

Dillon, F. R., Turner, C. W., Robbins, M. S., & Szapocznik, J. (2005). Concordance among biological, interview, and self-report measures of drug use among African American and Hispanic adolescents referred for drug abuse treatment. *Psychology of Addictive Behaviors, 19*, 404–413.

Dishion, T. J., & Tipsord, J. M. (2011). Peer contagion in child and adolescent social and emotional development. *Annual Review of Psychology, 62*, 189–214.

Dougherty, D. M., Mathias, C. W., Marsh, D. M., & Jagar, A. A. (2005). Laboratory behavioral measures of impulsivity. *Behavior Research Methods, 37*(1), 82–90.

Duckworth, A. L., & Kern, M. L. (2011). A meta-analysis of the convergent validity of self-control measures. *Journal of Research in Personality, 45*(3), 259–268.

Duell, N., Steinberg, L., Icenogle, G., Chein, J., Chaudhary, N., Di Giunta, L., . . . Chang, L. (2018). Age patterns in risk taking across the world. *Journal of Youth and Adolescence, 47*(5), 1052–1072.

Eisenberg, I. W., Bissett, P. G., Canning, J. R., Dallery, J., Enkavi, A. Z., Whitfield-Gabrieli, S., . . . Poldrack, R. A. (2018). Applying novel technologies and methods to inform the ontology of self-regulation. *Behaviour Research and Therapy, 101*, 46–57.

Eisenberg, I. W., Bissett, P., Enkavi, A. Z., Li, J., MacKinnon, D., Marsch, L., & Poldrack, R. (2018). Uncovering mental structure through data-driven ontology discovery. *Nature Communications, 19*, Article 2319.

Enkavi, A. Z., Eisenberg, I. W., Bissett, P. G., Mazza, G. L., Mackinnon, D. P., & Marsch, L. A. (2019). A large-scale analysis of test-retest reliabilities of self-regulation measures. *Proceedings of the National Academies of Science in the USA, 116*, 5472–5477.

Enzmann, D., Marshall, I. H., Killias, M., Junger-Tas, J., Steketee, M., & Gruszczynska, B. (2010). Self-reported youth delinquency in Europe and beyond: First results of the second international self-report delinquency study in the context of police and victimization data. *European Journal of Criminology, 7*(2), 159–183.

Esbensen, F.-A., & Huizinga, D. (1993). Gangs, drugs, and delinquency in a survey of urban youth. *Criminology, 31*, 565–589.

Eysenck, M. W., & Mogg, K. (1992). Clinical anxiety, trait anxiety, and memory bias. In S.-Å. Christianson (Ed.), *The handbook of emotion and memory: Research and theory* (pp. 429–450). Hillsdale, NJ: Erlbaum.

Fergus, S., Zimmerman, M. A., & Caldwell, C. H. (2007). Growth trajectories of sexual risk behavior in adolescence and young adulthood. *American Journal of Public Health, 97*(6), 1096–1101.

Figner, B., Mackinlay, R. J., Wilkening, F., & Weber, E. U. (2009). Affective and deliberative processes in risky choice: Age differences in risk taking in the Columbia Card Task. *Journal of Experimental Psychology: Learning, Memory, and Cognition, 35*, 709–730.

Forbes, E. E., Ryan, N. D., Phillips, M. L., Manuck, S. B., Worthman, C. M., Moyles, D. L., . . . Dahl, R. E. (2010). Healthy adolescents' neural response to reward: Associations with puberty, positive affect, and depressive symptoms. *Journal of the American Academy of Child and Adolescent Psychiatry, 49*(2), 162–172.

Funder, D. C. (2016). Why doesn't personality psychology have a replication crisis? Retrieved from *https://funderstorms.wordpress.com/2016/05/12/why-doesnt-personality-psychology-have-a-replication-crisis.*

Galván, A., Hare, T., Voss, H., Glover, G., & Casey, B. J. (2007). Risk-taking and the adolescent brain: Who is at risk? *Developmental Science, 10*(2), 8–14.

Gardner, M., & Steinberg, L. (2005). Peer influence on risk taking, risk preference, and risky decision making in adolescence and adulthood: An experimental study. *Developmental Psychology, 41*(4), 625–635.

Geier, C. F., Terwilliger, R., Teslovich, T., Velanova, K., & Luna, B. (2010). Immaturities in reward processing and its influence on inhibitory control in adolescence. *Cerebral Cortex, 20*(7), 1613–1629.

Gullo, M. J., Loxton, N. J., & Dawe, S. (2014). Addictive behaviors impulsivity?: Four ways five factors are not basic to addiction. *Addictive Behaviors, 39*(11), 1547–1556.

Hamilton, K. R., Littlefield, A. K., Anastasio, N. C., Cunningham, K. A., Fink, L. H. L., Wing, V. C., . . . Potenza, M. N. (2015). Rapid-response impulsivity: Definitions, measurement issues, and clinical implications. *Personality Disorders: Theory, Research, and Treatment, 6*(2), 168–181.

Hamilton, K. R., Mitchell, M. R., Wing, V. C., Balodis, I. M., Bickel, W. K., Fillmore, M., . . . Moeller, F. G. (2015). Choice impulsivity: Definitions, measurement issues, and clinical implications. *Personality Disorders: Theory, Research, and Treatment, 6*(2), 182–198.

Harden, K. P., & Tucker-Drob, E. M. (2011). Individual differences in the development of sensation seeking and impulsivity during adolescence: Further evidence for a dual systems model. *Developmental Psychology, 47*(3), 739–746.

Hedge, C., Powell, G., & Sumner, P. (2018). The reliability paradox: Why robust cognitive tasks do not produce reliable individual differences. *Behavior Research Methods, 50*(3), 1166–1186.

Hedges, L. V., & Vevea, J. (2006). Selection method approaches. In H. R. Rothstein, A. J. Sutton, & M. Borenstein (Eds.), *Publication bias in meta-analysis: Prevention, assessment and adjustments* (pp. 145–174). Hoboken, NJ: Wiley.

Hertzog, C., & Nesselroade, J. R. (1987). Beyond autoregressive models: Some implications of the trait–state distinction for the structural modeling of developmental change. *Child Development, 58*(1), 93–109.

Hjorthøj, C. R., Hjorthøj, A. R., & Nordentoft, M. (2012). Validity of Timeline Follow-Back for self-reported use of cannabis and other illicit substances—systematic review and meta-analysis. *Addictive Behaviors, 37*(3), 225–233.

Hooper, C. J., Luciana, M., Conklin, H. M., & Yarger, R. S. (2004). Adolescents' performance on the Iowa Gambling Task: Implications for the development of decision making and ventromedial prefrontal cortex. *Developmental Psychology, 40*(6), 1148–1158.

Huizinga, M., Dolan, C. V, & van der Molen, M. W. (2006). Age-related change in executive function: Developmental trends and a latent variable analysis. *Neuropsychologia, 44*(11), 2017–2036.

Humphreys, K. L., Telzer, E. H., Flannery, J., Goff, B., Gabard-Durnam, L., Gee, D. G., . . . Tottenham, N. (2016). Risky decision making from childhood through adulthood: Contributions of learning and sensitivity to negative feedback. *Emotion, 16*(1), 101–109.

Hussey, J. M., Hallfors, D. D., Waller, M. W., Iritani, B. J., Halpern, C. T., & Bauer, D. J. (2007). Sexual behavior and drug use among Asian and Latino adolescents: Association with immigrant status. *Journal of Immigrant and Minority Health, 9*(2), 85–94.

Ioannidis, J. P. A. (2005). Why most published research findings are false. *PLOS Medicine, 2*(8), 0696–0701.

Jackson, J. N. S., & MacKillop, J. (2016). Attention-deficit/hyperactivity disorder and monetary delay discounting: A meta-analysis of case–control studies. *Biological Psychiatry: Cognitive Neuroscience and Neuroimaging, 1*(4), 316–325.

Jasik, C. B., Berna, M., Martin, M., & Ozer, E. M. (2016). Teen preferences for clinic-based behavior screens: Who, where, when, and how? *Journal of Adolescent Health, 59*(6), 722–724.

Jessor, R., Turbin, M. S., Costa, F. M., Dong, Q., Zhang, H., & Wang, C. (2003). Adolescent problem behavior in China and the United States: A cross-national study of psychosocial protective factors. *Journal of Research on Adolescence, 13*(3), 329–360.

Jewsbury, P. A., Bowden, S. C., & Strauss, M. E. (2016). Integrating the switching, inhibition, and updating model of executive function with the Cattell–Horn–Carroll model. *Journal of Experimental Psychology: General, 145*(2), 220–245.

Jonah, B. A. (1990). Age differences in risky driving. *Health Education Research, 5*(2), 139–149.

Kelley, T. L. (1927). *Interpretation of educational measurements.* Yonkers-on-Hudson, NY: World Book.

Kessler, R. C., Berglund, P., Demler, O., Jin, R., Merikangas, K. R., & Walters, E. E. (2005). Lifetime prevalence and age-of-onset distributions of DSM-IV disorders in the National Comorbidity Survey Replication. *Archives of General Psychiatry, 62*(6), 593–602.

Kim, D. S., McCabe, C. J., Yamasaki, B. L., Louie, K. A., & King, K. M. (2018). Detecting random responders with infrequency scales using an error balancing threshold. *Behavior Research Methods, 50*, 1960–1970.

King, K. M., Fleming, C. B., Monahan, K. C., & Catalano, R. F. (2011). Changes in self-control problems and attention problems during middle school predict alcohol, tobacco, and marijuana use during high school. *Psychology of Addictive Behaviors, 25*(1), 69–79.

King, K. M., Kim, D. S., & McCabe, C. J. (2018). Random responses inflate statistical estimates in heavily skewed addictions data. *Drug and Alcohol Dependence, 183*, 102–110.

King, K. M., Lengua, L. J., & Monahan, K. C. (2013). Individual differences in the development of self-regulation during pre-adolescence: Connections to context and adjustment. *Journal of Abnormal Child Psychology, 41*(1), 57–69.

King, K. M., Littlefield, A. K., McCabe, C. J., Mills, K. L., Flournoy, J., & Chassin, L. (2018). Longitudinal modeling in developmental neuroimaging research: Common challenges, and solutions from developmental psychology. *Developmental Cognitive Neuroscience, 33*, 54–72.

King, K. M., Patock-Peckham, J. A., Dager, A. D., Thimm, K., & Gates, J. R. (2014). On the mismeasurement of impulsivity: Trait, behavioral, and neural models in alcohol research among adolescents and young adults. *Current Addiction Reports, 1*(1), 19–32.

King, K. M., Pullmann, M. D., Lyon, A. R., Dorsey, S., & Lewis, C. C. (2019). Using implementation science to close the gap between the optimal and typical practice of quantitative methods in clinical science. *Journal of Abnormal Psychology, 128*, 547–562.

Kirby, K. N., Petry, N. M., & Bickel, W. K. (1999). Heroin addicts have higher discount rates for delayed rewards than non-drug-using controls. *Journal of Experimental Psychology: General, 128*(1), 78–87.

Kolbe, L. J., Kann, L., & Collins, J. L. (1993). Overview of the Youth Risk Behavior Surveillance System. *Public Health Reports, 108*(Suppl. 2), 2–10.

Kost, K., & Henshaw, S. (2014). *U.S. Teenage pregnancies, births and abortions, 2010: National and state trends by age, race and ethnicity.* New York: Guttmacher Institute.

Kraemer, H. C., Mintz, J., Noda, A., Tinklenberg, J., & Yesavage, J. A. (2006). Caution regarding the use of pilot studies to guide power calculations for study proposals. *Archives of General Psychiatry, 63*(5), 484–489.

Krohn, M. D., Thornberry, T. P., Gibson, C. L., & Baldwin, J. M. (2010). The development and impact of self-report measures of crime and delinquency. *Journal of Quantitative Criminology, 26*(4), 509–525.

Lejuez, C. W., Aklin, W. M., Zvolensky, M. J., & Pedulla, C. M. (2003). Evaluation of the Balloon Analogue Risk Task (BART) as a predictor of adolescent real-world risk-taking behaviours. *Journal of Adolescence, 26*(4), 475–479.

Lewis, M. A., Patrick, M. E., Litt, D. M., Atkins, D. C., Kim, T., Blayney, J. A., . . . Larimer, M. E. (2014). Randomized controlled trial of a web-delivered personalized normative feedback intervention to reduce alcohol-related risky sexual behavior among college students. *Journal of Consulting and Clinical Psychology, 82*(3), 429–440.

Lindberg, L. D., Boggess, S., Williams, S., & Jones, J. (2000). *Multiple threats: The co-occurrence of teen health risk behaviors.* Washington, DC: Office of the Assistant Secretary for Planning and Evaluation, U.S. Department of Health and Human Services.

Littlefield, A. K., Stevens, A. K., Ellingson, J. M., King, K. M., & Jackson, K. M. (2016). Changes in negative urgency, positive urgency, and sensation seeking across adolescence. *Personality and Individual Differences, 90,* 332–337.

Loeber, R., & Farrington, D. P. (2014). Age–crime curve. In G. Bruinsma & D. Weisburd (Eds.), *Encyclopedia of criminology and criminal justice* (pp. 12–18). New York: Springer-Verlag.

Luna, B., Paulsen, D. J., Padmanabhan, A., & Geier, C. (2013). The teenage brain: Cognitive control and motivation. *Current Directions in Psychological Science, 22*(2), 94–100.

MacKillop, J., Weafer, J., C. Gray, J., Oshri, A., Palmer, A., & de Wit, H. (2016). The latent structure of impulsivity: Impulsive choice, impulsive action, and impulsive personality traits. *Psychopharmacology, 233*(18), 3361–3370.

Macleod, C. M. (1991). Half a century of research on the Stroop effect: An integrative review. *Psychological Bulletin, 109*(2), 163–203.

Mata, R., Josef, A. K., & Hertwig, R. (2016). Propensity for risk taking across the life span and around the globe. *Psychological Science, 27*(2), 231–243.

McCormick, E. M., & Telzer, E. H. (2017). Failure to retreat: Blunted sensitivity to negative feedback supports risky behavior in adolescents. *NeuroImage, 147,* 381–389.

McCrae, R. R., & Costa, P. T. (1987). Validation of the five-factor model of personality across instruments and observers. *Journal of Personality and Social Psychology, 52*(1), 81–90.

McShane, B. B., Böckenholt, U., & Hansen, K. T. (2016). Adjusting for publication bias in meta-analysis: An evaluation of selection methods and some cautionary notes. *Perspectives on Psychological Science, 11*(5), 730–749.

Meade, A. W., & Craig, S. B. (2012). Identifying care-less responses in survey data. *Psychological Methods, 17*(3), 437–455.

Miguel, E., Camerer, C., Casey, K., Cohen, J., Esterling, K. M., Gerber, A., . . . Neumark, D. (2014). Social science: Promoting transparency in social science research. *Science, 343*(6166), 30–31.

Miyake, A., & Friedman, N. N. P. (2012). The nature and organisation of individual differences in executive functions: Four general conclusions. *Current Directions in Psychological Science, 21*(1), 8–14.

Miyake, A., Friedman, N. P., Emerson, M. J., Witzki, A. H., Howerter, A., & Wager, T. D. (2000). The unity and diversity of executive functions and their contributions to complex "frontal lobe" tasks: A latent variable analysis. *Cognitive Psychology, 41*(1), 49–100.

Moffitt, T. E. (1993). Adolescence-limited and life-course-persistent antisocial behavior: A developmental taxonomy. *Psychological Review, 100*(4), 674–701.

Moffitt, T. E., Arseneault, L., Belsky, D., Dickson, N., Hancox, R. J., Harrington, H., . . . Caspi, A. (2011). A gradient of childhood self-control predicts health, wealth, and public safety. *Proceedings of the National Academy of Sciences of the USA, 108*(7), 2693–2698.

Mokdad, A. H., Marks, J. S., Stroup, D. F., & Gerberding, J. L. (2004). Actual causes of death in the United States, 2000. *Journal of the American Medical Association, 291*(10), 1238–1245.

Monahan, K. C., King, K. M., Shulman, E. P., Cauffman, E., & Chassin, L. (2015). The effects of violence exposure on the development of impulse control and future orientation across adolescence and early adulthood: Time-specific and generalized effects in a sample of juvenile offenders. *Development and Psychopathology, 27*(2015), 1–18.

Monahan, K. C., Steinberg, L., & Cauffman, E. (2009). Affiliation with antisocial peers, susceptibility to peer influence, and antisocial behavior during the transition to adulthood. *Developmental Psychology, 45*(6), 1520–1530.

Munafò, M. R., Nosek, B. A., Bishop, D. V. M., Button, K. S., Chambers, C. D., Percie Du Sert, N., . . . Ioannidis, J. P. A. (2017). A manifesto for reproducible science. *Nature Human Behaviour, 1*(1), 1–9.

Myers, M. G., Doran, N. M., & Brown, S. A. (2007). Is cigarette smoking related to alcohol use during the 8 years following treatment for adolescent alcohol and other drug abuse? *Alcohol and Alcoholism, 42*(3), 226–233.

Nagl, M., Jacobi, C., Paul, M., Beesdo-Baum, K., Höfler, M., Lieb, R., & Wittchen, H.-U. (2016). Prevalence, incidence, and natural course of anorexia and bulimia nervosa among adolescents and young adults. *European Child and Adolescent Psychiatry, 25*(8), 903–918.

O'Brien, L., Albert, D., Chein, J. M., & Steinberg, L. (2011). Adolescents prefer more immediate rewards when in the presence of their peers. *Journal of Research on Adolescence, 21*(4), 747–753.

Odum, A. L. (2011). Delay discounting: Trait variable? *Behavioural Processes, 87*(1), 1–9.

Ordaz, S. J., Foran, W., Velanova, K., & Luna, B. (2013). Longitudinal growth curves of brain function underlying inhibitory control through adolescence. *Journal of Neuroscience, 33*(46), 18109–18124.

Pape, H., & Storvoll, E. E. (2006). Teenagers' "use" of non-existent drugs: A study of false positives. *Nordic Studies on Alcohol and Drugs, 23*, 43–58.

Paulhus, D. L., & Vazire, S. (2005). The self-report method. In R. W. Robins, R. C. Fraley, & R. F. Krueger (Eds.), *Handbook of research methods in personality psychology* (pp. 224–239). New York: Guilford Press.

Pedersen, E. R., Grow, J., Duncan, S., Neighbors, C., & Larimer, M. E. (2012). Concurrent validity of an online version of the timeline followback assessment. *Psychology of Addictive Behaviors, 26*(3), 672–677.

Peper, J. S., & Dahl, R. E. (2013). The teenage brain: Surging hormones—brain–behavior interactions during puberty. *Current Directions in Psychological Science, 22*(2), 134–139.

Pfeifer, J. H., & Allen, N. B. (2012). Arrested development?: Reconsidering dual-systems models of brain function in adolescence and disorders. *Trends in Cognitive Sciences, 16*(6), 322–329.

Posner, M. I., & Rothbart, M. K. (2000). Developing mechanisms of self-regulation. *Development and Psychopathology, 12*(3), 427–441.

Rey-Mermet, A., Gade, M., & Oberauer, K. (2017). Should we stop thinking about inhibition?: Searching for individual and age differences in inhibition ability. *Journal of Experimental Psychology: Learning, Memory, and Cognition, 44*(4), 501–526.

Reyna, V. F., & Farley, F. (2006). Risk and rationality in adolescent decision making: Implications for theory, practice, and public policy. *Psychological Science in the Public Interest, 7*(1, Suppl.), 1–44.

Reyna, V. F., & Rivers, S. E. (2008). Current theories of risk and rational decision making. *Developmental Review, 28*(1), 1–11.

Reynolds, B., Ortengren, A., Richards, J. B., & de Wit, H. (2006). Dimensions of impulsive behavior: Personality and behavioral measures. *Personality and Individual Differences, 40*(2), 305–315.

Roberti, J. W. (2004). A review of behavioral and biological correlates of sensation seeking. *Journal of Research in Personality, 38*(3), 256–279.

Robinson-Cimpian, J. P. (2014). Inaccurate estimation of disparities due to mischievous responders: Several suggestions to assess conclusions. *Educational Researcher, 43*(4), 171–185.

Romer, D. (2010). Adolescent risk taking, impulsivity, and brain development: Implications for prevention. *Developmental Psychobiology, 52*(3), 263–276.

Romer, D., & Hennessy, M. (2007). A biosocial-affect model of adolescent sensation seeking: The role of affect evaluation and peer-group influence in adolescent drug use. *Prevention Science, 8*(2), 89–101.

Romer, D., Reyna, V. F., & Satterthwaite, T. D. (2017). Beyond stereotypes of adolescent risk taking: Placing the adolescent brain in developmental context. *Developmental Cognitive Neuroscience, 27*, 19–34.

Rouder, J. N., & Haaf, J. M. (2019). A psychometrics of individual differences in experimental tasks. *Psychonomic Bulletin and Review, 26*, 452–467.

Ruiz-Caballero, J. A., & Bermúdez, J. (1995). Neuroticism, mood, and retrieval of negative personal memories. *Journal of General Psychology, 122*(1), 29–35.

Salas-Wright, C. P., Nelson, E. J., Vaughn, M. G., Gonzalez, J. M. R., & Córdova, D. (2017). Trends in fighting and violence among adolescents in the United States, 2002–2014. *American Journal of Public Health, 107*(6), 977–982.

Salthouse, T. A. (2014). Why are there different age relations in cross-sectional and longitudinal comparisons of cognitive functioning? *Current Directions in Psychological Science, 23*(4), 252–256.

Scarpina, F., & Tagini, S. (2017). The Stroop Color and Word Test. *Frontiers in Psychology, 8*, 557.

Schonberg, T., Fox, C. R., & Poldrack, R. A. (2011). Mind the gap: Bridging economic and naturalistic risk-taking with cognitive neuroscience. *Trends in Cognitive Sciences, 15*, 11–19.

Schroeder, P., Peña, R., & Wilbur, M. (2018). *National survey on distracted driving attitudes and behaviors–2015.* Washington, DC: National Highway Traffic Safety Administration.

Sharma, L., Kohl, K., Morgan, T. A., & Clark, L. A. (2013). "Impulsivity": Relations between self-report and behavior. *Journal of Personality and Social Psychology, 104*(3), 559–575.

Sharma, L., Markon, K. E., & Clark, L. A. (2014). Toward a theory of distinct types of "impulsive" behaviors: A meta-analysis of self-report and behavioral measures. *Psychological Bulletin, 140*(2), 374–408.

Shiffman, S., Stone, A. A., Hufford, M. R., Rev, A., Psychol, C., Shiffman, S., . . . Hufford, M. R. (2008). Ecological momentary assessment. *Annual Review of Clinical Psychology, 4*(5), 1–32.

Shulman, E. P., Harden, K. P., Chein, J. M., & Steinberg, L. (2014). The development of impulse control and sensation-seeking in adolescence: Independent or interdependent processes? *Journal of Research on Adolescence, 26*(1), 1–8.

Shulman, E. P., Smith, A. R., Silva, K., Icenogle, G., Duell, N., Chein, J. M., & Steinberg, L. (2016). The dual systems model: Review, reappraisal, and reaffirmation. *Developmental Cognitive Neuroscience, 17*, 103–117.

Silberzahn, R., Uhlmann, E. L., Martin, D. P., Anselmi, P., Aust, F., Awtrey, E., . . . Nosek, B. A. (2018). Many analysts, one data set: Making transparent how variations in analytic choices affect results. *Advances in Methods and Practices in Psychological Science, 1*(3), 337–356.

Simons, J. S., Wills, T. A., Emery, N. N., & Marks, R. M. (2015). Quantifying alcohol consumption: Self-report, transdermal assessment, and prediction of dependence symptoms. *Addictive Behaviors, 50*(2015), 205–212.

Smith, G. T., & Cyders, M. A. (2016). Integrating affect and impulsivity: The role of positive and negative urgency in substance use risk. *Drug and Alcohol Dependence, 163*(Suppl. 1), S3–S12.

Smith, G. T., Fischer, S., Cyders, M. A., Annus, A. M., Spillane, N. S., & McCarthy, D. M. (2007). On the validity and utility of discriminating among impulsivity-like traits. *Assessment, 14*(2), 155–170.

Smith, J. L., Mattick, R. P., Jamadar, S. D., & Iredale, J. M. (2014). Deficits in behavioural inhibition in substance abuse and addiction: A meta-analysis. *Drug and Alcohol Dependence, 145*, 1–33.

Snyder, H. N., Cooper, A. D., & Mulako-Wangota, J. (2014). *Bureau of Justice Statistics: Arrest rates by age for all offenses.* Washington, DC: Bureau of Justice Statistics.

Sobell, L. C. (2003). Alcohol Timeline Followback (TLFB). In *Assessing alcohol problems: A guide for clinicians and researchers* (pp. 301–305). Bethesda, MD: National Institute on Alcohol Abuse and Alcoholism.

Somerville, L. H. (2013). Special issue on the teenage brain: Sensitivity to social evaluation. *Current Directions in Psychological Science, 22*(2), 121–127.

Stahl, C., Voss, A., Schmitz, F., Nuszbaum, M., Tüscher, O., Lieb, K., & Klauer, K. C. (2014). Behavioral components of impulsivity. *Journal of Experimental Psychology: General, 143*(2), 850–886.

Stanley, T. D., Carter, E. C., & Doucouliagos, H. (2018). What meta-analyses reveal about the replicability of psychological research. *Psychological Bulletin, 144*(12), 1325–1346.

Stautz, K., & Cooper, A. (2013). Impulsivity-related personality traits and adolescent alcohol use: A meta-analytic review. *Clinical Psychology Review, 33*(4), 574–592.

Steinberg, L. (2007). Risk taking in adolescence: New perspectives from brain and behavioral science. *Current Directions in Psychological Science, 16*(2), 55–59.

Steinberg, L. (2008). A social neuroscience perspective on adolescent risk-taking. *Developmental Review, 28*(1), 78–106.

Steinberg, L. (2010). A dual systems model of adolescent risk-taking. *Developmental Psychobiology, 52*(3), 216–224.

Steinberg, L., Albert, D., Cauffman, E., Banich, M., Graham, S., & Woolard, J. (2008). Age differences in sensation seeking and impulsivity as indexed by behavior and self-report: Evidence for a dual systems model. *Developmental Psychology, 44*(6), 1764–1778.

Steinberg, L., Icenogle, G., Shulman, E. P., Breiner, K., Chein, J., Bacchini, D., . . . Takash, H. M. S. (2018). Around the world, adolescence is a time of heightened sensation seeking and immature self-regulation. *Developmental Science, 21*(2), 1–13.

Steinberg, L., & Monahan, K. C. (2007). Age differ-

ences in resistance to peer influence. *Developmental Psychology, 43*(6), 1531–1541.

Strauss, M. E., & Smith, G. T. (2009). Construct validity: Advances in theory and methodology. *Annual Review of Clinical Psychology, 5*, 1–25.

Substance Abuse and Mental Health Services Administration. (2017). *Key substance use and mental health indicators in the United States: Results from the 2016 National Survey on Drug Use and Health.* Washington, DC: Author.

Sullivan, E. V., Brumback, T., Tapert, S. F., Prouty, D., Fama, R., Thompson, W. K., . . . Pfefferbaum, A. (2017). Effects of prior testing lasting a full year in NCANDA adolescents: Contributions from age, sex, socioeconomic status, ethnicity, site, family history of alcohol or drug abuse, and baseline performance. *Developmental Cognitive Neuroscience, 24*, 72–83.

Swendsen, J., Burstein, M., Case, B., Conway, K. P., Dierker, L., He, J., & Merikangas, K. R. (2012). Use and abuse of alcohol and illicit drugs in US adolescents: Results of results of the National Comorbidity Survey-Adolescent Supplement. *Archives of General Psychiatry, 69*(4), 390–398.

Tackett, J. L., Brandes, C. M., King, K. M., & Markon, K. E. (2019). Psychology's replication crisis and clinical psychological science. *Annual Review of Clinical Psychology, 15*, 579–604.

Tackett, J. L., Lilienfeld, S. O., Patrick, C. J., Johnson, S. L., Krueger, R. F., Miller, J. D., . . . Shrout, P. E. (2017). It's time to broaden the replicability conversation: Thoughts for and from clinical psychological science. *Perspectives on Psychological Science, 12*(5), 742–756.

Taubman-Ben-Ari, O., Mikulincer, M., & Gillath, O. (2004). The multidimensional driving style inventory—scale construct and validation. *Accident Analysis and Prevention, 36*(3), 323–332.

Telzer, E. H. (2016). Dopaminergic reward sensitivity can promote adolescent health: A new perspective on the mechanism of ventral striatum activation. *Developmental Cognitive Neuroscience, 17*, 57–67.

Telzer, E. H., Fuligni, A. J., Lieberman, M. D., & Galván, A. (2013). Ventral striatum activation to prosocial rewards predicts longitudinal declines in adolescent risk taking. *Developmental Cognitive Neuroscience, 3*(1), 45–52.

Thompson, B. L., Nelson, D. E., Caldwell, B., & Harris, J. R. (1998). Assessment of health risk behaviors. *American Journal of Preventive Medicine, 16*(2), 48–59.

Tomko, R. L., Solhan, M. B., Carpenter, R. W., Brown, W. C., Jahng, S., Wood, P. K., & Trull, T. J. (2014). Measuring impulsivity in daily life: The momentary impulsivity scale. *Psychological Assessment, 26*(2), 339–349.

Toplak, M. E., Sorge, G. B., Benoit, A., West, R. F., & Stanovich, K. E. (2010). Decision-making and cognitive abilities: A review of associations between Iowa Gambling Task performance, executive functions, and intelligence. *Clinical Psychology Review, 30*(5), 562–581.

Trejos-Castillo, E., & Vazsonyi, A. T. (2009). Risky sexual behaviors in first and second generation Hispanic immigrant youth. *Journal of Youth and Adolescence, 38*(5), 719–731.

Turchik, J. A., & Garske, J. P. (2009). Measurement of sexual risk taking among college students. *Archives of Sexual Behavior, 38*(6), 936–948.

Tymula, A., Belmaker, L. A. R., Roy, A. K., Ruderman, L., Manson, K., Glimcher, P. W., & Levy, I. (2012). Adolescents' risk-taking behavior is driven by tolerance to ambiguity. *Proceedings of the National Academy of Sciences of the USA, 109*(42), 17135–17140.

van der Schaaf, M. E., Warmerdam, E., Crone, E. A., & Cools, R. (2011). Distinct linear and non-linear trajectories of reward and punishment reversal learning during development: Relevance for dopamine's role in adolescent decision making. *Developmental Cognitive Neuroscience, 1*(4), 578–590.

Vaughn, M. G., Salas-Wright, C. P., Delisi, M., & Maynard, B. R. (2014). Violence and externalizing behavior among youth in the United States: Is there a severe 5%? *Youth Violence and Juvenile Justice, 12*(1), 3–21.

Vazire, S. (2018). Implications of the credibility revolution for productivity, creativity, and progress. *Perspectives on Psychological Science, 13*(4), 411–417.

Venables, N. C., Foell, J., Yancey, J. R., Kane, M. J., Engle, R. W., & Patrick, C. J. (2018). Quantifying inhibitory control as externalizing proneness: A cross-domain model. *Clinical Psychological Science, 6*(4), 561–580.

Vermeersch, H., T'Sjoen, G., Kaufman, J. M., & Vincke, J. (2008). Estradiol, testosterone, differential association and aggressive and non-aggressive risk-taking in adolescent girls. *Psychoneuroendocrinology, 33*(7), 897–908.

Weafer, J., Baggott, M. J., & de Wit, H. (2013). Test–retest reliability of behavioral measures of impulsive choice, impulsive action, and inattention. *Experimental and Clinical Psychopharmacology, 21*(6), 475–481.

Whitely, S. E. (1983). Construct validity: Construct representation versus nomothetic span. *Psychological Bulletin, 93*(1), 179–197.

Whiteside, S. P., & Lynam, D. R. (2001). The Five Factor Model and impulsivity: Using a structural model of personality to understand impulsivity. *Personality and Individual Differences, 30*(4), 669–689.

Whiteside, S. P., Lynam, D. R., Miller, J. D., & Reynolds, S. K. (2005). Validation of the UPPS Impulsive Behaviour Scale: A four-factor model of impulsivity. *European Journal of Personality, 19*(7), 559–574.

Willgerodt, M. A., & Thompson, E. A. (2006). Ethnic and generational influences on emotional distress and risk behaviors among Chinese and Filipino American adolescents. *Research in Nursing and Health, 29*(4), 311–324.

Willoughby, T., Good, M., Adachi, P. J. C., Hamza, C., & Tavernier, R. (2013). Examining the link between adolescent brain development and risk taking from a social–developmental perspective. *Brain and Cognition, 83*(3), 315–323.

Winters, K. C. (2003). Assessment of alcohol and other drug use behaviors among adolescents. In J. P. Allen & V. P. Wilson (Eds.), *Assessing alcohol problems: A guide for clinicians and researchers* (2nd ed., pp. 101–123). Bethesda, MD: National Institutes of Health.

Wright, L., Lipszyc, J., Dupuis, A., Thayapararajah, S. W., & Schachar, R. (2014). Response inhibition and psychopathology: A meta-analysis of Go/No-Go task performance. *Journal of Abnormal Psychology, 123*(2), 429–439.

Xu, J., Kochanek, K. D., & Murphy, S. L. (2018). Deaths: Final data for 2016. *National Vital Statistics Reports, 67*(5), 76.

Zuckerman, M. (1985). Biological foundations of the sensation-seeking temperament. In J. Strelau, F. A. Farley, & A. Gale (Eds.), *The biological bases of personality and behavior: Vol. 1. Theories, measurement techniques, and development* (pp. 97–113). Washington, DC: Hemisphere.

Zweig, J. M., Lindberg, L. D., & McGinley, K. A. (2001). Adolescent health risk profiles: The co-occurrence of health risks among females and males. *Journal of Youth and Adolescence, 30*(6), 707–728.

Author Index

Subject Index